HUMAN PHARMACOLOGY

MOLECULAR TO CLINICAL

HUMAN PHARMACOLOGY

MOLECULAR TO CLINICAL

THEODORE M. BRODY, Ph.D.
Professor Emeritus, Department of Pharmacology and Toxicology
College of Human Medicine
Michigan State University
East Lansing, Michigan

JOSEPH LARNER, M.D., Ph.D.
Alumni Professor, Department of Pharmacology
University of Virginia School of Medicine
Charlottesville, Virginia

KENNETH P. MINNEMAN, Ph.D.
Professor, Department of Pharmacology
Emory University Medical School
Atlanta, Georgia

HAROLD C. NEU, M.D.
Professor and Chief, Division of Infectious Diseases
Departments of Medicine and Pharmacology
Columbia University College of Physicians and Surgeons
Chief, Division of Infectious Diseases Columbia-Presbyterian Hospital
New York, New York

SECOND EDITION

with **436** *illustrations*

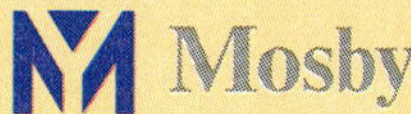

St. Louis Baltimore Berlin Boston Carlsbad Chicago
London Madrid Naples New York Philadelphia
Sydney Tokyo Toronto

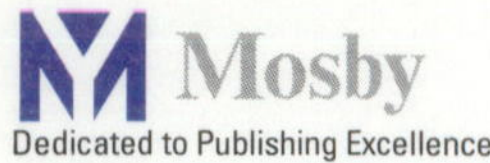

Managing Editor: Emma D. Underdown
Project Manager: Mark Spann
Production Editor: Elizabeth Fathman
Designer: David Zielinski
Manufacturing Supervisor: Betty Richmond
Cover Photograph: © Dennis Kunkel

SECOND EDITION

Printed in the United States of America
Composition by Clarinda
Printing/binding by Von Hoffman

Mosby-Year Book, Inc.
11830 Westline Industrial Drive
St. Louis, Missouri 63146

Library of Congress Cataloging in Publication Data

Human pharmacology : molecular to clinical / Theodore M. Brody ... [et al.].-- 2nd ed.
p. cm.
Includes bibliographical references and index.
ISBN 0-8016-7928-1
1. Pharmacology. 2. Chemotherapy. I. Brody, Theodore M.
[DNLM: 1. Pharmacology. 2. Drug Therapy. QV 4 H918 1995]
RM300.H86 1995
615.5′8--dc20
DNLM/DLC
for Library of Congress 94-21774
CIP

95 96 97 98 / 9 8 7 6 5 4 3 2

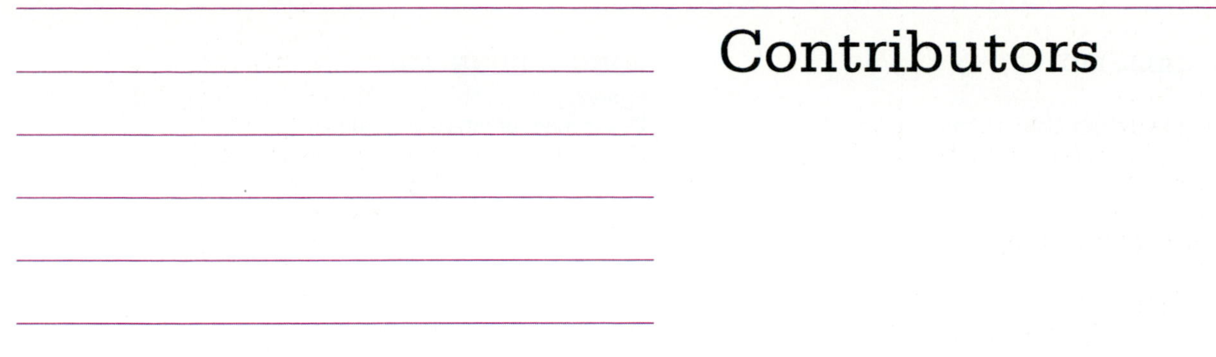

Contributors

TAI AKERA, MD, PhD
Vice President
MSD Research Laboratories—Japan
Minato-Ku, Tokyo
Japan

BARRIE ASHBY, PhD
Associate Professor
Department of Pharmacology
Temple University School of Medicine
Philadelphia, Pennsylvania

WILLIAM D. ATCHISON, PhD
Director of Neuroscience Program
Professor of Pharmacology and Toxicology
Department of Pharmacology and Toxicology and Neuroscience
Michigan State University
East Lansing, Michigan

RICHARD L. ATKINSON, MD
Professor
Department of Nutritional Sciences
University of Wisconsin
Madison, Wisconsin

ROBERT L. BALSTER, PhD
Professor
Department of Pharmacology and Toxicology
Medical College of Virginia
Virginia Commonwealth University
Richmond, Virginia

LOUIS A. BARKER, PhD
Professor
Department of Pharmacology
Louisiana State University Medical Center
New Orleans, Louisiana

JAMES L. BENNETT, PhD
Professor
Department of Pharmacology and Toxicology
Michigan State University College of Osteopathic Medicine
East Lansing, Michigan

JAMES P. BENNETT, JR., MD, PhD
Associate Professor
Departments of Neurology Behavioral Medicine & Pharmacology
University of Virginia School of Medicine;
Clinical Neurologist
Department of Neurology
University of Virginia Health Sciences Center
Charlottesville, Virginia

DAVID A. BRASE, PhD
Clinical Pharmacology Fellow
Department of Pharmacology
Meharry Medical College
Nashville, Tennessee

THEODORE M. BRODY, PhD
Professor Emeritus
Department of Pharmacology and Toxicology
College of Human Medicine
Michigan State University
East Lansing, Michigan

THOMAS F. BURKS, PhD
Professor
Department of Pharmacology
Executive Vice President
Office of Research and Academic Affairs
The University of Texas Houston Health Science Center
Houston, Texas

EDWARD J. CAFRUNY, MD, PhD
Distinguished Professor Emeritus
Graduate School of Biomedical Sciences
University of Medicine and Dentistry of New Jersey
Newark, New Jersey

ROBERT S. CALL, MD
Instructor
Department of Allergy and Clinical Immunology
University of Virginia School of Medicine
Charlottesville, Virginia

GEORGE P. CHROUSOS, MD
Chief
Department of Pediatric Endocrinology
National Institute of Child Health and Development
National Institute of Health
Bethesda, Maryland

RICHARD C. DART, MD, PhD
Director
Rocky Mountain Posion Center;
Director of Section Medical Toxicology
Department of Internal Medicine
Denver General Hospital
Denver, Colorado

RICHARD A. DEITRICH, PhD
Professor
Department of Pharmacology
University of Colorado School of Medicine
Denver, Colorado

WILLIAM L. DEWEY, PhD
Vice President for Research and Graduate Studies
Department of Pharmacology and Toxicology
Virginia Commonwealth University
Richmond, Virginia

EDWARD F. DOMINO, MD
Professor
Department of Pharmacology
University of Michigan School of Medicine
Clinical Pharmacologist
Department of Psychiatry
Ann Arbor Veterans Administration Medical Center
Ann Arbor, Michigan

PETER H. DOUKAS, PhD
Professor
Department of Pharmaceutical Sciences
Temple University School of Pharmacy
Philadelphia, Pennsylvania

ANN D. DUNN, PhD
Research Associate Professor
Department of Internal Medicine
University of Virginia School of Medicine
Charlottesville, Virginia

JOHN T. DUNN, MD
Professor
Department of Internal Medicine
University of Virginia School of Medicine;
Staff
Department of Internal Medicine
University of Virginia Health Sciences Center
Charlottesville, Virginia

PAUL D. ELLNER, PhD
Professor Emeritus
Departments of Microbiology and Pathology
Columbia University College of Physicians and Surgeons
New York, New York

WILLIAM S. EVANS, MD
Professor
Department of Internal Medicine
University of Virginia School of Medicine;
Attending Physician
Department of Internal Medicine
University of Virginia Hospital
Charlottesville, Virginia

GREGORY D. FINK, PhD
Professor
Department of Pharmacology and Toxicology
Michigan State University
College of Human Medicine
East Lansing, Michigan

HAROLD E. FOX, MD, MSc
Acting Chairman
Department of Obstetrics and Gynecology
Columbia University College of Physicians and Surgeons;
Acting Director
Sloane Hospital for Women
Presbyterian Hospital in the City of New York
New York, New York

MICHAEL K. FRITSCH, MD, PhD
Post-doctoral Fellow
Laboratory of Biochemistry
National Institutes of Health
Bethesda, Maryland

WILLIAM T. GERTHOFFER, PhD
Associate Professor
Department of Pharmacology
University of Nevada School of Medicine
Reno, Nevada

ACHILLE GRAVANIS, PhD
Associate Professor
Department of Pharmacology
University of Crete Medical School
Iraklion, Greece

BRENDA J. GROSSMAN, MD
Medical Officer, Blood Services
American Red Cross
St. Louis, Missouri

DANIEL H. HAVLICHEK, Jr., MD
Associate Professor
Department of Medicine
Michigan State University
College of Human Medicine
East Lansing, Michigan

STEPHEN G. HOLTZMAN, PhD
Professor
Department of Pharmacology
Emory University School of Medicine
Atlanta, Georgia

JOSEPH R. HUME, PhD
Professor
Department of Physiology
University of Nevada School of Medicine
Reno, Nevada

STEVEN J. JACOBS, MD
Adjunct Associate Professor
Department of Medicine
University of North Carolina School of Medicine
Chapel Hill, NC

THOMAS T. KAWABATA, PhD
Research Scientist
Human and Environmental Safety Division
The Procter and Gamble Company
Cincinnati, Ohio

JAMES M. LARNER, MD
Assistant Professor
Departments of Internal Medicine and Radiology
University of Virginia;
Attending Physician
Department of Radiology
University of Virginia Health Sciences Center
Charlottesville, Virginia

JOSEPH LARNER, MD, PhD
Alumni Professor
Department of Pharmacology
University of Virginia School of Medicine
Charlottesville, Virginia

THOMAS J. LAUTERIO, PhD
Associate Professor
Department of Internal Medicine and Physiology
Eastern Virginia Medical School
Norfolk, Virginia

JOHN C. LAWRENCE, Jr., PhD
Associate Professor
Department of Molecular Biology and Pharmacology
Washington University School of Medicine
Saint Louis, Missouri

JOHN S. LAZO, PhD
Professor and Chairman
Department of Pharmacology
University of Pittsburgh School of Medicine
Pittsburgh, Pennsylvania

ANDREW N. MARGIORIS, MD
Associate Professor
Department of Clinical Chemistry
Medical School of Crete
Iraklion, Greece

ROBERT H. MCDONALD, Jr., MD
Professor
Department of Medicine
University of Pittsburgh School of Medicine;
Staff
Presbyterian-University Hospital
Pittsburgh, Pennsylvania

DAVID C. B. MILLS, PhD
Associate Professor
Department of Pharmacology
Sol Sherry Thrombosis Research Center
Temple University Hospital
Philadelphia, Pennsylvania

KENNETH P. MINNEMAN, PhD
Professor
Department of Pharmacology
Emory University Medical School
Atlanta, Georgia

BERNARD L. MIRKIN, MD, PhD
Professor
Department of Pediatrics and Pharmacology
Northwestern University Medical School;
Head and Director
Children's Memorial Institute for Education and Research
Children's Memorial Hospital
Chicago, Illinois

KENNETH E. MOORE, PhD
Professor and Chairman
Department of Pharmacology and Toxicology
Michigan State University College of Human Medicine
East Lansing, Michigan

ALBERT E. MUNSON, PhD
Professor
Department of Pharmacology and Toxicology
Medical College of Virginia/Virginia Commonwealth University
Richmond, Virginia

FERN E. MURDOCH, PhD
Assistant Professor
Department of Biochemistry
Uniformed Services University of the Health Sciences
Bethesda, Maryland

HAROLD C. NEU, MD
Professor and Chief
Division of Infectious Diseases
Departments of Medicine and Pharmacology
Columbia University College of Physicians and Surgeons
Chief, Division of Infectious Diseases
Columbia-Presbyterian Hospital
New York, New York

JOHN J. O'NEILL, PhD
Professor Emeritus
Department of Pharmacology
Temple University School of Medicine
Philadelphia, Pennsylvania

JOHN D. PALMER, MD, PhD
Professor and Acting Head
Department of Pharmacology
Assistant Professor
Department of Internal Medicine
University of Arizona College of Medicine;
Attending Physician and Consultant
Department of Internal Medicine
Veterans Administration Medical Center
Tucson, Arizona

THOMAS A.E. PLATTS-MILLS, MD, PhD
Professor and Head
Division of Allergy and Clinical Immunology
University of Virginia School of Medicine
Charlottesville, Virginia

RICHARD H. RECH, PhD
Professor
Department of Pharmacology and Toxicology
Michigan State University College of Human Medicine
East Lansing, Michigan

ROBERT R. RUFFOLO, JR., PhD
Vice President and Director
Pharmacological Sciences, U.S., U.K., Europe, and Australia
SmithKline Beecham Pharmaceuticals
King of Prussia, Pennsylvania

I. GLENN SIPES, PhD
Professor and Head
Department of Pharmacology and Toxicology
University of Arizona College of Pharmacy
Tucson, Arizona

J. BRYAN SMITH, PhD
Professor and Chairman
Department of Pharmacology
Temple University Medical School
Philadelphia, Pennsylvania

MICHAEL J. SOLLENBERGER, MD
Assistant Professor
Bowman Gray School of Medicine
Winston-Salem, North Carolina

GARY E. STEIN, PharmD
Associate Professor
Department of Medicine
Michigan State University College of Human Medicine
East Lansing, Michigan

PAULA H. STERN, PhD
Professor
Department of Pharmacology
Northwestern University Medical School
Chicago, Illinois

JANET L. STRINGER, MD, PhD
Assistant Professor
Department of Pharmacology
Baylor College of Medicine
Houston, Texas

YUNG-FONG SUNG, MD
Associate Professor
Department of Anesthesiology
Emory University School of Medicine;
Chief
Department of Anesthesiology
Ambulatory Surgery Center/Emory Clinic and Wesley Woods Geriatric Hospital
Atlanta, Georgia

JOHN E. THORNBURG, DO, PhD
Professor
Department of Pharmacology
Michigan State University College of Osteopathic Medicine
East Lansing, Michigan

PAL L. VAGHY, MD
Associate Professor
Department of Medical Biochemistry
Ohio State University College of Medicine
Columbus, Ohio

ELIZABETH A. VANDEWAA, PhD
Research Scientist
Department of Comparative Biosciences
University of Wisconsin Medical School
Madison, Wisconsin

ROBERT M. WARD, MD
Associate Professor
Department of Pediatrics
University of Utah Medical Center;
Medical Director
Newborn Critical Care Services
Primary Children's Medical Center
Salt Lake City, Utah

SANDRA P. WELCH, PhD
Assistant Professor
Department of Pharmacology and Toxicology
Medical College of Virginia
Richmond, Virginia

DAVID P. WESTFALL, PhD
Professor and Chairman
Department of Pharmacology
University of Nevada School of Medicine
Reno, Nevada

STEPHEN J. WINTERS, MD
Professor
Department of Medicine
University of Pittsburgh School of Medicine
Pittsburgh, Pennsylvania

Preface

The unique aspects of this edition, as well as the earlier edition, continue to be the relation of the mechanism of action of a drug at a molecular or cellular level to its action in the intact human, with its full component of biochemical, physiological, and pathological influences. Pharmacology, a discipline bridging basic and clinical science, is increasingly directed toward developing new drugs and therapeutic agents based on sound mechanistic principles. For example, coincident with the explosion of information in the molecular biology, biochemistry, and physiology of receptors and signaling mechanisms; the neurobiology of transmitters; and the immunochemistry of monoclonal antibodies and lymphokines, an aim of pharmacology is to develop new drugs and therapeutic agents of greater selectivity than previously thought possible. Classical physiological responses to drugs and fundamental studies of disease processes in clinical medicine also continue to contribute important insights for drug development. Accordingly, in this book appropriate, balanced emphasis is placed on both basic and clinical mechanistic aspects with the goal of providing the student with a sound fundamental understanding of the discipline, in a text of reasonable size, to better prepare for future self-learning in pharmacology.

The text is unique in its overall organization and ease of use, including a focus on drug classes and prototypical drugs to treat disease, the use of boxes and tables to summarize factual data related to basic principles, and the emphasis on relevant fundamental clinical information. Illustrations stress current models of mechanisms. Chapter sections, boxes, tables, and figures can be used conveniently, either separately or in any order desired by the instructor or student. Chapters were invited from authoritative experts who are well-versed in both basic and clinical aspects of the subject. Content has been carefully selected to meet the immediate needs of medical and related professional students within the framework of either a standard or an innovative professional curriculum. This book was also designed to provide residents and practicing physicians with easy access to clinical information related to drug use.

A number of important modifications and additions have been made in the second edition. Two new Editors have been added, together with a significant number of new chapter contributors. Based on comments from both faculty and student reviewers, significant chapter updating and revisions have been instituted. Importantly, at the end of each chapter a *New Directions* section outlines approaches to future drug development or use. Representative questions are also provided for student self-assessment, with the answers listed in the back of the book. New chapters include pharmacological gene therapy and novel drugs produced by recombinant biotechnology. The book may be particularly suitable for those programs currently using, or those contemplating, a problem-based learning mode.

A strength of the first edition on which we have built is the consistent chapter format. Such a presentation allows the student to navigate easily through the chapter to find the specific information he or she seeks. To this end, each section of the book is introduced by an appropriate summary to focus and highlight the content of that section. Each chapter is subdivided into the following headings:

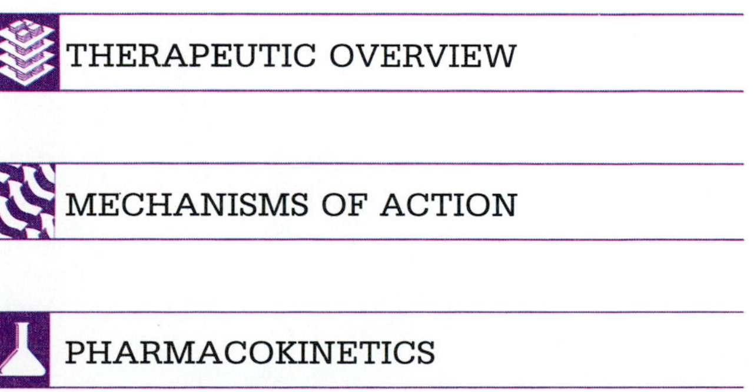

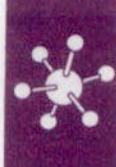

RELATION OF MECHANISMS OF ACTION TO CLINICAL RESPONSE

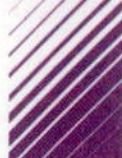

SIDE EFFECTS, CLINICAL PROBLEMS, AND TOXICITY

NEW DIRECTIONS

Numerous color-coded tables and boxes help emphasize important information for quick access. Each chapter now has an overview box summarizing the specific drug classes covered in that chapter. Other standardized boxes and tables throughout the chapters list the pharmacokinetics, clinical problems, and trade names. The full-color illustrations have been refined and increased in number to reinforce pharmacological and therapeutic concepts; these were generated by the authors and editors to enable the student to visualize important mechanisms described in the text.

This edition continues to offer currently important special topics not ordinarily emphasized in standard pharmacology texts. These include full chapters on the nutritional aspects of pharmacology, perinatal/neonatal pharmacology, and gerontological pharmacology.

We trust that the revisions in content, together with an increase in the number of color-coded tables, boxes, and figures, make this second edition even more user friendly and valuable to the student of pharmacology.

Theodore M. Brody
Joseph Larner
Kenneth P. Minneman
Harold C. Neu

Reviewers

EDITORIAL CONSULTANTS

GREGORY D. FINK, PhD
Professor
Department of Pharmacology and Toxicology
Michigan State University College of Human Medicine
East Lansing, Michigan

JAMES C. GARRISON, PhD
Professor and Chairman
Department of Pharmacology
University of Virginia Health Sciences Center
Charlottesville, Virginia

REVIEWERS

LELAND A. BABITCH
Wayne State University School of Medicine

ELIZABETH BIANCHI
University of Florida College of Medicine

STEVEN L. BRODY, MD
Department of Medicine
Washington University School of Medicine

WILLIAM CACINI, PhD
Department of Pharmacology
University of Cincinnati College of Pharmacy

DAVE CHASEN
Jefferson Medical College

MARGARITA L. CONTRERAS, PhD
Department of Pharmacology and Toxicology
Michigan State University College of Human Medicine

JOHN A. EDWARDS
University of Wisconsin Medical School

ERIC GUNTHER
Robert Wood Johnson Medical School

WALEED HASSEN
Eastern Virginia Medical School

SHAWN K. HASSLER
University of Miami School of Medicine

WARREN HEIDEMAN, PhD
Department of Pharmacology
University of Wisconsin Medical School

DAVID W. HENRY, MS, FASHP
University of Kansas Medical Center

MAHESH KRISHNAN
Jefferson Medical College

ROGER P. MAICKEL, PhD
Department of Pharmacology and Toxicology
Purdue University College of Pharmacy

ROBERT L. MAROIS, PhD
Albany College of Pharmacy

MARK S. MESKIN, PhD, RD
Department of Pharmacology and Nutrition
University of Southern California College of Medicine

LEONARD L. NAEGER, PhD
Department of Pharmacology
St. Louis University College of Pharmacy

ROBERT B. NELSON, PhD
Department of Pharmacology
University of Wyoming School of Pharmacy

WILLIAM J. O'CONNOR
New York University School of Medicine

S. MICHAEL OWENS, PhD
Department of Pharmacology and Toxicology
University of Arkansas for Medical Sciences

PAUL POLISHUK
University of Wisconsin Hospital and Clinics

DAVID E. POTTER, PhD
Department of Pharmacology and Toxicology
Morehouse School of Medicine

LAWRENCE RICE, MD
Department of Medicine, Hematology Section
Baylor College of Medicine and Methodist Hospital

CHANLAND ROONPRAPUNT
New York University School of Medicine

ROBERT J. ROBERTS, MD, PhD
Department of Pediatrics and Pharmacology
University of Virginia School of Medicine

ALAN ROGOL, MD, PhD
Department of Pediatrics and Pharmacology
University of Virginia School of Medicine

ALBERT I. SORIANO
Eastern Virginia Medical School

CARY STEWART
Loma Linda University School of Medicine

JOSEPH R. STIMERS, PhD
Department of Pharmacology
University of Arkansas for Medical Sciences

STEPHEN A. SWISHER
Saint Louis University School of Medicine

NATHAN M. THIELMAN, MD
Department of Internal Medicine
University of Virginia School of Medicine

MARK J. WINN, PhD*
Department of Pharmacology
University of Alabama

LYNN R. WILLIS, PhD
Department of Pharmacology and Toxicology
Indiana University School of Medicine

LYNN C. YEOMAN, PhD
Department of Pharmacology
Baylor College of Medicine

*deceased

Contents

PART I

GENERAL PRINCIPLES

Part I describes principles that apply to essentially all drugs. These principles pertain to administration, distribution to different body sites, general mechanisms by which drugs produce beneficial effects, and mechanisms for drug disappearance from the body. Because of differences in chemical structure, not all drugs undergo the same specific processes. Examples of drug groups in some of the key processes are given. Examples in Chapter 4 explain how to determine specific pharmacokinetic parameter values based on realistic data, but actual drug names are omitted to emphasize principles rather than values for specific drugs.

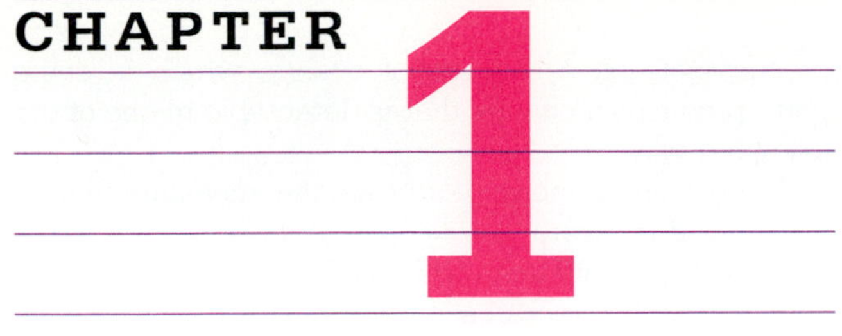

CHAPTER 1 Introduction and Definitions

THEODORE M. BRODY

THERAPEUTIC IMPORTANCE OF DRUGS

Both physicians and patients acknowledge the major role played by drugs in modern therapy. Many millions of prescriptions are written each year in the United States, containing more than 700 active ingredients available in several thousand different pharmaceutical preparations or delivery forms. Additionally, approximately 100,000 over-the-counter nonprescription preparations are available. These nonprescription items vary from a single high-purity active ingredient, such as aspirin mixed with tableting materials, to mixtures of several ingredients, many of which have questionable efficacy.

Despite the proliferation of active chemical compounds for the treatment of diseases, new and better drugs are still needed. The search is intensive and provokes nationwide interest when a new chemical compound is discovered that provides symptomatic relief or cures a previously untreatable disease. A similar response arises when a new drug is reported that provides as good or better relief compared with existing compounds but with fewer undesirable side effects. The enthusiasm of discovery, however, should be tempered by a healthy skepticism. Is the new drug effective when exposed to a larger patient population? Do potential side effects and toxicity limit its usefulness? Problems frequently arise because the mechanism of action and therefore the safety of the drug may be poorly understood and an early decision to allow clinical use of the agent may profoundly affect the well-being of patients.

THE SCOPE OF PHARMACOLOGY

For hundreds of years most drugs were highly impure mixtures of only vaguely known composition and primarily of plant or animal origin. A physician was required to know only what effects to expect from a preparation. How the mixture produced such effects was beyond the knowledge of that day. Over the past 60 years the situation has changed greatly. Today a physician is required to know the overt expected effects, and the precise mechanism by which the beneficial effect is brought about.

This broader knowledge of how drugs interact with body constituents to produce therapeutic effects is termed **pharmacology.** This term covers the spectrum from the molecular level to the whole body and relies heavily on knowledge of biochemistry, physiology, molecular biology, and organic chemistry. The elucidation of molecular mechanisms of drug response, the development of new drugs, and the formulation of clinical guidelines for safe and effective use of drugs in therapy or prevention of disease states and in relief of symptoms are all part of pharmacology.

UNDERSTANDING DRUG ACTIONS AT THE MOLECULAR LEVEL

As recently as the 1920s, relatively few therapeutically beneficial active ingredients (by today's standards) existed. Most active ingredients were used in only partially purified forms. Since then, vastly improved tools and methods for the purification of chemical compounds have been developed and chemical structures have been elucidated. It is possible to identify which compounds in the earlier crude mixtures produced the beneficial effects and which the undesirable responses. Techniques of synthetic organic chemistry are applied not only to define the structure of each parent drug, but also to synthesize thousands of structural analogs and to test these analogs for pharmacological activity. These efforts resulted in the current research thrust to develop structure–activity relationships for different classes of drugs.

Another breakthrough which occurred in the 1940s, resulted from the realization that microorganisms could produce compounds (antibiotics) capable of killing other microorganisms. This led to the discovery and subsequent fermentative production of thousands of potentially useful antibiotics. Chemical structures of these antibiotics were more complex than those of previous drugs. Therefore, deciphering structures required additional time and delayed synthesis of analogs. Thus, during the 1940s and 1950s, pharmacology depended heavily on organic chemistry to provide the information to synthesize new drugs and develop an understanding of relationships between chemical structures and pharmacological activity.

Developments in biochemistry during the 1960s and continuing today also have had a major influence in establishing the current molecular emphasis in pharmacology. Sophisticated purification techniques provide greatly improved insights into qualitative and quantitative molecular mechanisms of cellular processes. It is now possible to identify, isolate, and characterize body fluid or tissue constituents when drugs initiate their beneficial effects. Therefore, processes of how drugs act can be approached from two directions: (1) drugs can be studied as chemical compounds of known structure and (2) tissue or body fluid sites where the drugs act can also be chemically characterized. The pace of defining the nature of drug sites of action accelerated greatly in the 1980s as a result of advances in molecular biology and genetic engineering. Cellular or body fluid constituents that are present in concentrations too small to be isolated and characterized can now be produced in milligram and even gram quantities through gene cloning and expression in foreign cell lines. Therefore, understanding of how drugs or other compounds act on body constituents at the molecular level is expected to increase greatly over the coming years. This knowledge will provide a sound basis for rational drug use in successful medical therapy, as well as provide a foundation for development of improved drugs with minimal unwanted side effects.

CLINICAL USE OF DRUGS

Important Factors in Rational Drug Therapy

Information on the molecular mechanism of action of drugs provides a valuable link between basic medical science and clinical medicine. As mentioned earlier, information available through pharmacology depends on principles of biochemistry and physiology. Clinically, the initial molecular action of a drug in an individual patient cannot be detected. Instead, the initial molecular process sets off a cascade of events, which at some point produces a change that is detectable in one of the following ways:

1. With instruments, such as the measurement of blood pressure
2. By laboratory tests on body fluid or tissue samples
3. Through direct observation of the patient by the physician

This cascade concept is illustrated in Figure 1-1 for digitalis and its action on the heart and how this leads to reduced edema. In this example a digitalis glycoside is administered to a patient with congestive heart failure. After it reaches the blood, the drug interacts with and binds to a specific site on the cardiac muscle membrane. This site is Na^+, K^+-ATPase, an enzyme that controls the intracellular concentrations of both Na^+ and K^+. The glycoside inhibits a normal function of this enzyme, which is to extrude intracellular Na^+ during the cardiac cycle, resulting in an increase in the intracellular concentration of this ion in the cardiac muscle cell. This leads to a series of biochemical events culminating in an increase in the force of cardiac contraction, an increase in renal perfusion, and a subsequent reduction in the edema; the latter is obvious to both physician and patient. One of the more difficult aspects of pharmacology is providing rational explanations that link the initial drug-induced molecular events to clinical observations.

In a given clinical situation the choice of drug to obtain a desired therapeutic effect may be simple or complicated. In either case, numerous factors should be considered:

1. Each patient is different. Many, but not all, will respond adequately to the selected drugs. This is largely because of patient-to-patient or biological variability. Some patients may require very large doses of drugs before a response is observed. Others may be exquisitely sensitive to normal doses. With several drug classes, differences in drug responses may be hereditary.
2. Therapy may have been initiated without all the data. In life-threatening situations or in disease states that prove difficult to diagnose, drug therapy often must be started before all of the laboratory results or physician reports are received.
3. Patient status changes. The drug and the size and frequency of the dose may need to be modified as the patient's condition improves or worsens.
4. Multiple drugs may have been used. Many hospitalized patients receive five to 10 different drugs concurrently, outpatients may be taking two to four drugs, and some elderly patients may be taking up to 12 drugs. The opportunity for drug in-

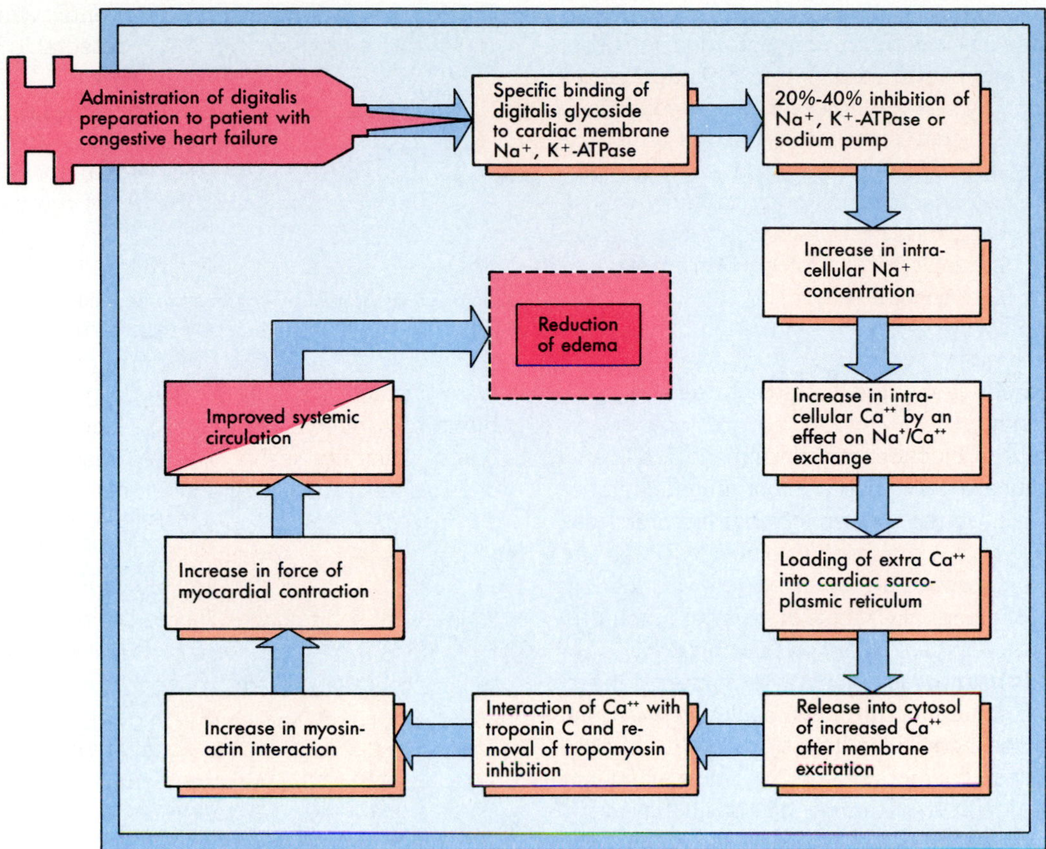

FIGURE 1-1 Initial molecular interaction of digitalis with a body constituent and the subsequent cascade of events that results in an observable pharmacological response. In 1785 the Scottish physician William Withering published his famous treatise on the effect of the foxglove, or digitalis, on the treatment of dropsy (edema). After 200 years of research, it is recognized that a series of events is initiated by the interaction of a digitalis glycoside with a protein embedded in the cardiac cell membrane. The red boxes indicate events that are readily detectable or observable.

teractions increases exponentially as the number of drugs being taken increases.

These factors and others make the selection of a specific drug and the dosage schedule for an individual patient difficult, and therefore selection involves an element of experimentation.

Individual patients may respond differently to the same drug therapy regimen. The drug may bring about the desired therapeutic result or various unwanted results, including toxicity, lack of effectiveness, or a change in the course of the disease. Such occurrences may result from rapid or slow disposition of the drug by the patient, an inappropriate dosing schedule, a drug–drug interaction, incorrect diagnosis, or a change in disease state. In dealing with these uncertainties, the physician trained to understand the mechanisms of action, principal routes of disposition, and pharmacological and toxic effects of drugs has an advantage. This physician assesses the patient's pharmacological response as well as the validity of the diagnosis, with each drug used. This aids in choosing a subsequent course of therapy. The course of the disease and therapeutic intervention with drugs should be viewed as dynamic rather than static processes.

Therapeutic Index

Drugs must produce beneficial effects to qualify for government approval for clinical use (see Chapter 65). In addition, all drugs in high doses produce toxic responses. The range between the concentration of drug needed to produce the therapeutic response and that which produces a toxic response is a key factor in classifying a drug as easy or difficult to use. The ratio of these concentrations is called the **therapeutic index** (also called the **margin of safety**) and is expressed as the minimum concentration (or dose) that produces toxicity divided by the minimum concentration (or dose) that gives the therapeutic response in a patient population. When this ratio is 2.0 or less, the compound can be difficult to use in patients without encountering significant toxicity. Such is the case with the cardiac drug digoxin, where the therapeutic index is close to 2.0. When the therapeutic index is considerably larger, there is less chance that toxicity will be encountered when the recommended dosage is used.

TERMINOLOGY

Basic Terms

General terms of the pharmacology literature are listed in Table 1-1 with their definitions. The terms **action, effect,** and **response** are used interchangeably in this book. All refer to the result of an interaction of a drug with some biological entity within the body.

Pharmacodynamics is a general term often defined as the study of fundamental or molecular interactions between drug and body constituents, which through a subsequent series of events results in a pharmacological response. In many instances the basic molecular mechanism may be unknown; then the pharmacological response must be described at a higher level of biochemical or physiological complexity. Pharmacodynamics is used by some investigators to relate response to drug concentration.

Table 1-1 Definitions

Term	Definition
Pharmacology	The study of drugs. Observable interaction between drug and body constituent. May be at any level of organization. Also includes how the drug is transformed by body tissues.
Pharmacodynamics	Broad term defined in several ways, but generally a more precise description of the fundamental action of a drug on a physiological or biochemical level.
Pharmacokinetics	Drug concentrations in body fluids and tissues that influence how those concentrations vary with time. Fate of the drug during its sojourn through the body.
Drug receptor	Specific macromolecule, peptide, protein, organ, cell type, enzyme, membrane component, nucleic acid, etc., where the initial molecular event occurs with the drug, leading to the therapeutic response. "Site of action" of drug.
Pharmacogenetics	Field of pharmacology that examines relationship of genetic factors to variations in drug response.
Toxicology	Study of effects, antidotes, and detection of poisons and description of effects of drug overdose.

Pharmacological Response

Pharmacological response is initiated by a drug at its site of action on its so-called receptor (see Chapter 2). For most drugs, the magnitude of pharmacological response increases as the concentration of drug increases at the site. When the drug's action is reversible, the pharmacological response decreases as the concentration of drug decreases. But not all drugs act reversibly. The clinical use of drugs would be more precise if procedures existed to (1) measure the magnitude of the response and (2) monitor the magnitude in a specific patient. Unfortunately, these methods exist for only a few drugs. One of these drugs is the neuromuscular blocking agent succinylcholine. Figure 1-2 shows an example of the pharmacological response and how it varies with time in a patient.

Figure 1-2 also offers a description of **magnitude of effect.** Specifically the magnitude of pharmacological effect is defined as the percentage of neuromuscular blockade achieved. Thus, 0% blockade corresponds to the predrug condition, whereas 100% blockade represents complete paralysis. The blockade is calculated as

$$\%\ \text{blockade} = \left(1.0 - \frac{F}{F_0}\right)100 \qquad \textbf{(1)}$$

In this expression, F_0 and F are measured in millimeters. The results for various times and for an F_0 of 53 mm are illustrated in Figure 1-2. Succinylcholine is a reversibly acting drug; thus, the system returns to the predrug state after disappearance of the drug. The initial increased magnitude of effects results from a gradual buildup of drug at the neuromuscular junction (site of action) after a single-bolus intravenous injection. Succinylcholine is rapidly hydrolyzed in plasma to essentially inactive compounds, thus accounting for the rapid disappearance of the drug at the site of action.

Pharmacokinetic Variables

As previously stated, for most drugs the magnitude of pharmacological effect depends on the concentration of drug at the site of action. The factors that influence the rates of delivery, distribution, and disappearance of drug to or from the site of action must be understood from a clinical standpoint. Factors involved in how the concentration of drug varies with time in body fluids or tissues are the substance of pharmacokinetics. These

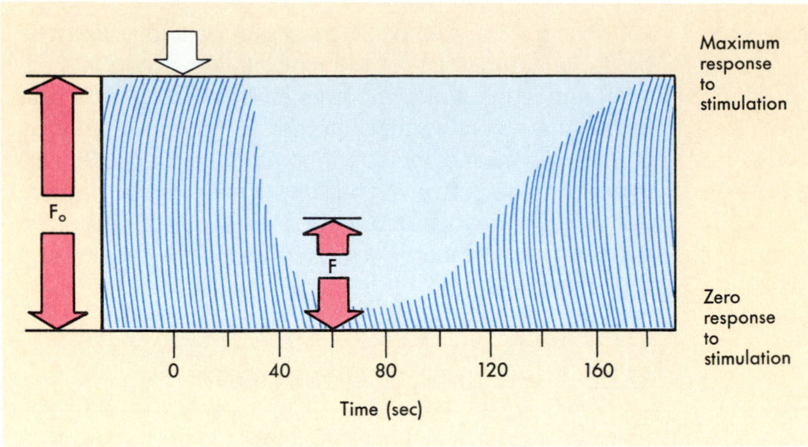

FIGURE 1-2 Pharmacological response of neuromuscular blocking agent succinylcholine in a 6-year-old patient undergoing surgery. Plot shows force exerted by thumb (attached to strip chart recorder pen) after repeated electrical stimulation of ulnar nerve. F_0 is force before drug and F after drug. Succinylcholine administered intravenously (4 mg/m ^{2}) at arrow. Magnitude of effect is defined in text. Blockade calculated from illustration and Equation 1.

Time (sec)	Blockade (%)	Time (sec)	Blockade (%)
0	0	55	84
30	12	72.5	90
35	38	135	38
45	72	175	2

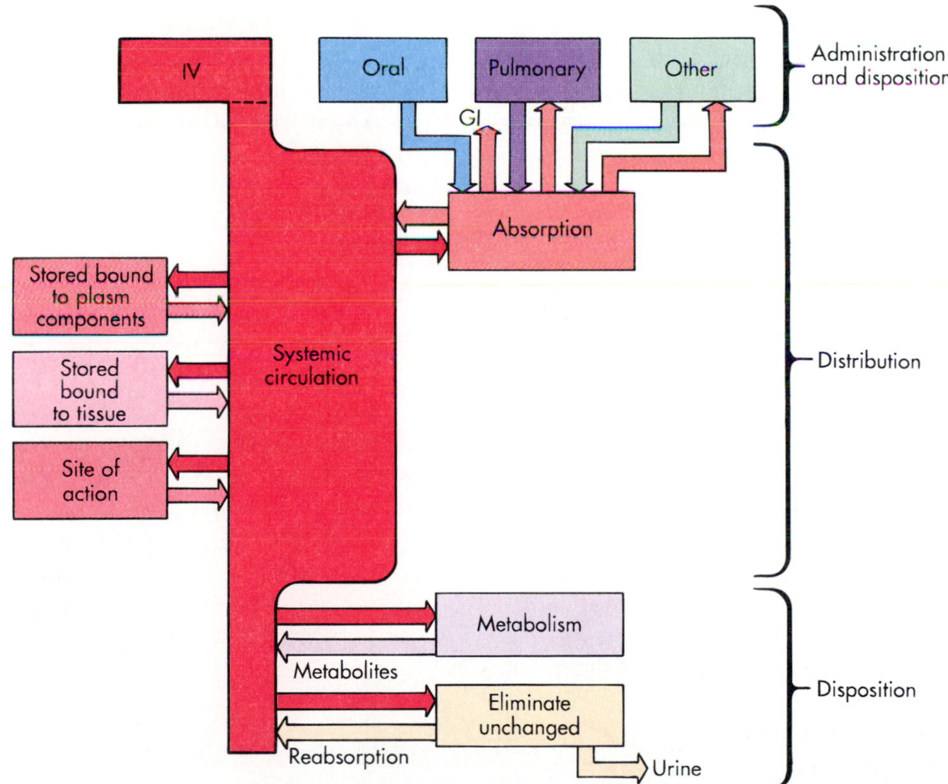

FIGURE 1-3 Factors influencing concentration of drug at site of action and at different times after administration. Free drug molecules are those that are not bound to blood constituents or to other body components. The circulatory system is shown as the major pathway for drug delivery to the site of action.

factors, outlined in Figure 1-3 and discussed extensively in Chapter 4, include:

Input site, input rate, dosage form, and dosage schedule
Rate of absorption, bioavailability
Location of site of action, ease of crossing membranes
Binding to plasma and tissue constituents
Pathways and rates of elimination or metabolism
Influence of disease states, other drugs, genetic factors

PHARMACOGENETICS

Pharmacogenetics is that area of pharmacology concerned with unanticipated or unusual responses to drugs that may have a hereditary basis for their action. These effects should be distinguished from toxic or side effects of drugs that can generally be anticipated, or from allergic manifestations. Generally, pharmacogenetic differences in responses to drugs indicate an inherited defect that results in variability of the metabolic machinery of the body to convert the drug or chemical to an inert metabolite. Thus, pharmacogenetic factors may produce either a diminished or an enhanced response to a drug. A discussion of pharmacogenetic problems relating to drug use, with some relevant examples, is presented in Chapter 7.

TOXICOLOGY

Toxicology is the science of poisons. Drugs, which are primarily foreign substances to the body, can be considered to be poisons because they can produce undesirable or "toxic" effects if administered in large enough doses. Thus, any beneficial effects of therapeutic agents must be balanced against their potential to do harm. An agent that produces significant toxic effects may be prescribed when that drug is used in a lifesaving situation. The use of such a drug for treating a trivial clinical problem should not be condoned, however. Wherever the specific pharmacological effects of a drug or chemical are described in this book, these are generally followed by a characterization of the side effects, potential hazards, and signs and symptoms associated with its use. **Signs** are objective measurements made primarily by the physician and include laboratory findings. **Symptoms** are subjective events described by the patient. Chapter 62 provides information on chemicals found in the environment that present significant health hazards to humans.

SELF-ASSESSMENT QUESTIONS

1. The knowledge of how drugs interact with body constituents to produce therapeutic effects is termed:
   a. Pharmacy
   b. Pharmacokinetics
   c. Pharmacology
   d. Biochemistry
   e. Pharmacognosy
2. The ratio between the drug concentration required to produce a toxic response and that which elicits the therapeutic action in a patient population is called:
   a. The minimal effective dose
   b. The therapeutic index
   c. The margin of safety
   d. The ED_{50}
   e. b and c are correct
3. Factors involved in how the concentration of drug in the body varies with time is called:
   a. Pharmacodynamics
   b. Pharmacogenetics
   c. Clinical chemistry
   d. Pharmacokinetics
   e. None of the above
4. Difficulty in drug selection and dosing schedule for an individual patient is attributable to:
   a. Patient-to-patient variability in drug response
   b. Change in the disease status of the patient
   c. Variability in drug disposition
   d. a and c only are correct
   e. a, b, and c are correct

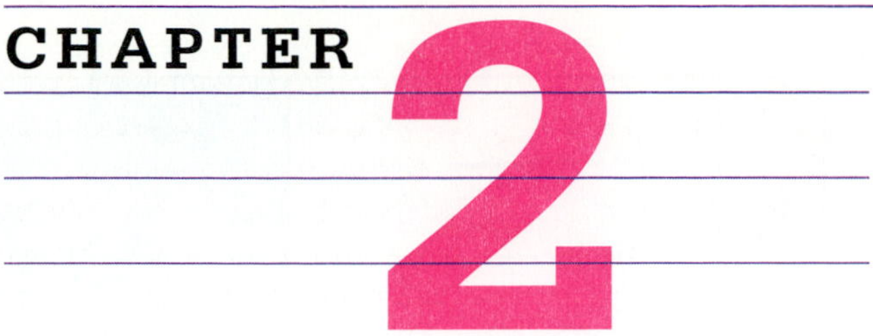

Sites of Action: Receptors

THEODORE M. BRODY

PHARMACOLOGICAL RESPONSE

In the previous chapter the point is made that pharmacological responses are initiated by molecular interactions of drugs with cells, tissues, or other body constituents. The key word is "molecular." What specific biological molecules must be present? How do drugs and biological molecules interact to produce changes? How are these changes converted into observable responses? In this chapter these questions are addressed, especially for the large group of drugs that act through receptors.

AXIOMS OF SITES OF ACTION

For most drugs the site of action is at a specific biological molecule, generally termed a **receptor,** which may be, for example, a membrane or a membrane protein, or a cytoplasmic or extracellular enzyme. In some cases a drug shows organ or tissue selectivity for the biological molecule; for example, selectivity may be more pronounced in cardiac compared with pulmonary tissue. Although the actions of a few drug types such as osmotic diuretics (Chapter 19) and general anesthetic agents (Chapter 30) may not involve receptors, the concept of receptors as sites of drug action is so important to understanding pharmacology that the remainder of this chapter is devoted to the description of receptors and how they interact with drugs at the molecular level.

The first axiom of a molecular drug-initiated response is that the drug molecule and the biological target must come together; they do not act at a distance. But if mere interaction is all that is required, then there is no way to build selectivity into the scheme. Therefore the second axiom is that the interaction must result in selective binding of the drug to the biological target before the response can take place. This brings into focus the concept of **molecular level recognition.** The biological molecules to which drugs bind must have molecular locales that are both spatially and energetically favorable for binding of specific drug molecules. These locales are termed "receptors" in a general sense, though, as is pointed out in the next section, a more restricted definition of receptors is usually applied in classical pharmacology.

Essentially all drug binding sites discovered so far are on proteins, glycoproteins, or proteolipids. This is not surprising because proteins undergo folding to form unique three-dimensional structures. Thus it is logical to conclude that proteins contain special binding sites of the correct three-dimensional shape to accommodate drug molecules. Receptors, enzyme active sites, enzyme allosteric regulatory or binding sites, and antibody and antigen binding sites all possess molecular recognition capabilities. Actually, enzymes constitute the site of action of many drugs, with selective binding of the drug usually resulting in inhibition of catalytic activity. From

ABBREVIATIONS

cAMP	Cyclic adenosine monophosphate
cDNA	Complementary deoxyribonucleic acid
CNS	Central nervous system
DAG	1,2-diacylglycerol
GABA	Gamma-aminobutyric acid
GDP	Guanosine diphosphate
GTP	Guanosine triphosphate
IP_3	Inositol 1,4,5-trisphosphate
MAPK	Mitogen-activated protein kinase
Na^+, K^+-ATPase	Sodium-potassium-adenosine triphosphatase
NMDA	*N*-methyl-D-aspartate
PIP_2	Phosphatidylinositol 4,5-bisphosphate

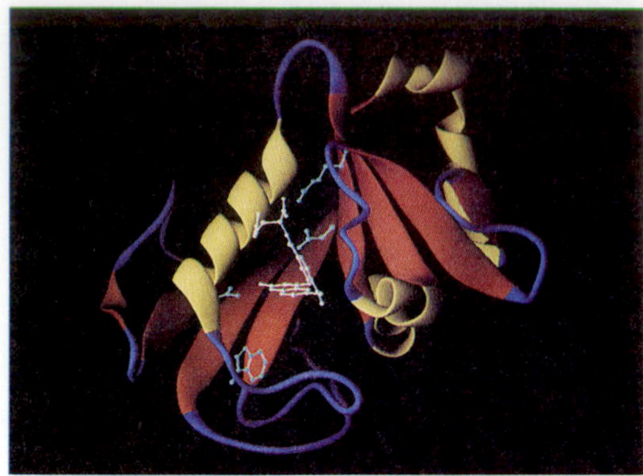

FIGURE 2-1 Ribbon representation of human dihydrofolate reductase with methotrexate (in white) modeled into the left substrate cleft. α Helices, yellow; β strands, orange; connecting loops, blue. Also shown (in pale blue) are side chains of some key binding residues (Trp-24, Glu-30, Asn-64, Arg-70). (Courtesy Jay F. Davies II and Joseph Kraut.)

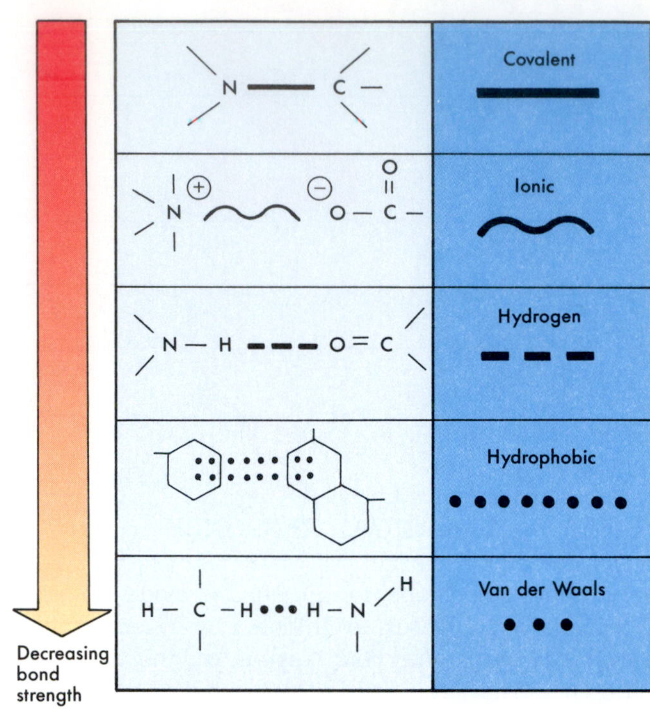

FIGURE 2-2 Types of chemical bonds and attractive forces between molecules that are pertinent to drugs binding to sites of action.

the standpoint of classical pharmacology, however, drug binding sites on enzymes are *not* called receptors. Because drug binding sites are found predominantly on proteins, a discussion of protein folding as it relates to the three-dimensional structure and the formation of binding sites is included here before going on to describe receptors of the classical type.

PROTEIN FOLDING

The three-dimensional shape that a particular protein assumes is the net result of its primary, secondary, and tertiary structures. The primary structure is the sequence of amino acids, connected through amide bonds; the secondary structure consists of the spatial restrictions caused by sulfur bridges and ionic interactions; and tertiary features result from steric factors and weak attraction and repulsion forces between atoms, including hydrogen bond formation. The denaturing process results in unfolded or random chains devoid of tertiary structure. Four features contribute to the tertiary structure of native proteins: (1) α helix, (2) β sheets, (3) β folds, and (4) random sections. Sequences of roughly 8 to 30 amino acids can form a spiral in the shape of an α helix, with 3.6 amino acid residues required per 360-degree angle turn and 0.54 nm in length per turn.

The enzyme dihydrofolate reductase (Figure 2-1) is the site of action for the antitumor drug methotrexate (see Chapter 43). When the drug binds to the enzyme, the latter is inactivated. The tertiary structure of this enzyme and how it binds to methotrexate have been established using enzyme from *Escherichia coli* and was recently estimated for enzyme from humans (see Figure 2-1). With the *E. coli* enzyme, the amino acid residues involved in binding of the drug appear too far apart in the drug-free enzyme to accommodate multipoint drug binding. Yet, despite this spatial misalignment, the interaction of enzyme and drug does occur at multiple sites. This problem can be resolved by introducing the concept of **induced fit,** which assumes that binding to one or more of the residues causes a conformational change in the enzyme that modifies the tertiary structure to bring the other amino acid residues involved in binding closer to the drug. Induced fit is believed to apply to the binding of methotrexate to the human enzyme and also the functioning of classical receptors and other enzymes.

A short discussion of the principal types of chemical bonds is included here. These bond types apply to the interactions between drugs and classical receptors and to those between drugs and enzymes. The major types of chemical bonds are summarized in Figure 2-2. Covalent bonds require considerable energy to break and are classified as irreversible when formed in drug–receptor interactions. Ionic bonds also are strong but under some circumstances can be reversed by a change in pH. Other bond types are weak but can exert considerable influence when several bonds interact with the same drug molecule.

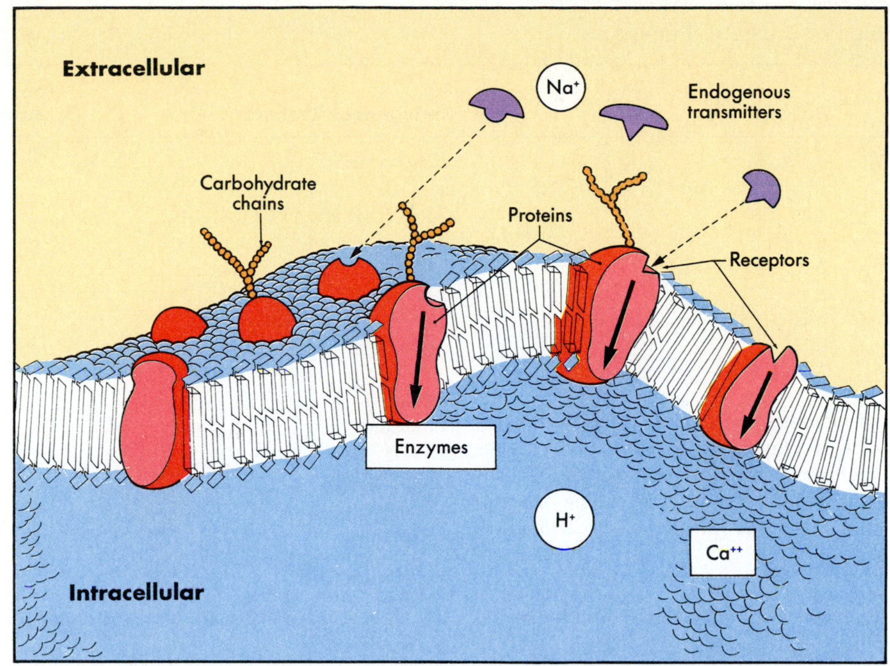

FIGURE 2-3 Proteins embedded in cell membranes generally extend further on both extracellular and intracellular sides. Attached to the proteins on the extracellular side are carbohydrate (glycosylation) chains. Also shown on the extracellular side of some of the proteins are receptor sites to which endogenous transmitter compounds bind. Arrows indicate the direction of communication to the other side of the membrane.

CLASSICAL RECEPTORS AND LIGAND BINDING

In the classical sense the term **receptor** is reserved for proteins, which usually are imbedded in a cellular or subcellular membrane and facilitate communication between the two sides of the membrane. This concept is shown schematically in Figure 2-3 for several proteins.

Membranes of cells consist of phospholipid bilayers. The bilayer forms because of the physicochemical properties of the phospholipid constituents and their interaction with water. Phospholipid molecules have two distinct regions and are thus termed **amphipathic.** One region is nonpolar, consisting of tails of the fatty acyl chains. The other region is very polar, consisting of charged phosphate, choline, and ethanolamine headgroups. It is the potential interaction of these distinct regions with hydrogen bonds of water that determines the structural organization of a membrane. Disruption of hydrogen bonds of water by the nonpolar lipid region is energetically very unfavorable. Therefore, these nonpolar regions tend to avoid contact with water by facing inward and self-associating. Disruption of the hydrogen bonds of water by polar headgroups is energetically more than compensated for by the formation of new polar interactions between water molecules and the headgroups. Therefore, contact of the polar groups with water is favored. These types of interactions are optimized by the bilayer structure.

Protein constituents of the membrane are either peripheral proteins, associated with the external or internal surfaces of the membrane, or integral proteins, deeply imbedded in the bilayer and sometimes spanning the membrane. As might be anticipated by their function of recognizing ligands at the external surface of the cell and transmitting information to inside the cell, membrane receptors span the membrane. Like phospholipids, membrane receptors are amphipathic. They contain distinct domains that have polar hydrophilic surfaces and that are exposed to the aqueous solvent on either side of the membrane. These polar domains are separated by transmembrane regions of hydrophobic nonpolar components.

Characteristically, transmembrane regions of receptors are formed by α helices that are composed of 19 to 24 sequential amino acids having nonpolar side groups. Several basic amino acids constitute the cytoplasmic end of the transmembrane sequence. These are believed to interact with phosphate headgroups of the bilayer and to anchor the receptor so that it cannot slip

Table 2-1 Examples of Classical Receptors

Type	Subtype*	Endogenous Transmitter	Ion Channel	Secondary Messenger
acetylcholine	nicotinic	acetylcholine	×	—
	muscarinic: M_1, M_2, M_3, M_4, M_5	acetylcholine		×
adrenergic	α_1, α_2	epinephrine and norepinephrine		×
	β_1, β_2, β_3	epinephrine and norepinephrine	—	×
GABA	A	GABA	×	—
	B	GABA	?	×
acidic amino acids	NMDA, kainate, quisqualate	glutamate or aspartate	×	?
opiate	μ, μ_1, κ, δ, ϵ	enkephalins	×†	×
serotonin	5-HT_1, 5-HT_2, 5-HT_3	5-HT	—	×
dopamine	D_1, D_2, D_3, D_4, D_5	dopamine	—	×
adenosine	A_1, A_2	adenosine	—	×
glycine	—	glycine	×	—
histamine	H_1, H_2, H_3	histamine	—	×
insulin	—	insulin	—	×
glucagon	—	glucagon	—	×
ACTH	—	ACTH	—	×
steroids	—	several	—	special

ACTH, Adrenocorticotrophic hormone.

*Other subtypes in various stages of documentation have been proposed, especially where no endogenous transmitter is defined yet.

†Results not clear.

into or out of the bilayer. This characteristic sequence of 19 to 24 nonpolar amino acids, flanked by several basic amino acids, is used to identify presumptive membrane-spanning domains within the amino acid sequences of membrane receptors.

Although movement of membrane receptors into and out of the bilayer is restricted by the amphipathic nature of the receptor, lateral diffusion of the receptor within the plane of the membrane can occur, unless specifically restrained by interaction with the intracellular cytoskeletal elements. This lateral diffusion has been demonstrated experimentally by labeling receptors with fluorescent-tagged ligands and measuring the rates of diffusion of the fluorescent tags into membrane areas rendered nonfluorescent by photobleaching. Lateral diffusion of receptors is an important concept because it means that membrane receptors can interact freely with other membrane proteins. Indeed, many receptors depend on such interactions to trigger a response to receptor–ligand binding.

In the classical case, an endogenous compound is present on one side of the membrane only by binding to the proper "receptor," the endogenous compound transmits a molecular change to the other side of the membrane. Neurotransmitters, hormones, growth factors, odorants, and a host of other compounds are part of the growing list of endogenous materials for which classical receptors have been discovered. For the remainder of this chapter the term **receptor** is limited to this classical definition.

The idea that drugs might act by first binding to a receptive substance in the cell is attributed to Langley's work in the late 1800s and early 1900s and to Ehrlich's studies of a few years later. It was not until the 1920s and the 1930s that drug–receptor interactions were approached from a quantitative standpoint by both Clark and Gaddum. During the 1960s, receptor proteins were isolated and purified by highly selective chromatography techniques; in the 1970s, the amino acid sequence of receptor subunits was determined. During the 1980s, the primary amino acid sequence of many receptors was determined from the nucleic acid sequence of their complementary DNA (cDNA). This structural information predicts that most receptors are members of families of related proteins, leading to significant insight to the function of these proteins. As the 1990s unfold, evidence is accumulating on the three-dimensional structure of several of the key receptors, with the result that our molecular understanding of receptors will increase greatly and introduce possibilities for improved drug design.

Table 2-1 contains a list of certain receptors relevant to the action of therapeutically useful drugs. Additional receptors are known to exist in human tissues and may become pertinent to drug actions in the future. For many receptors, subtypes have been identified. These subtypes may represent variants of the receptor coding sequence (e.g., β-adrenergic receptors), though certain subtypes couple to different signal-generating molecules and activate separate signaling pathways (e.g., histamine H_1 and H_2 receptors).

Receptor identification and classification is based in

large part on ligand-binding specificity. The experimental procedures to perform ligand–receptor binding measurements are important and are briefly described here. Using radiolabeled ligands, it is possible to obtain accurate measurements of the concentrations of bound, as well as free, drugs. Receptor preparations, with the receptor solubilized or still intact in the membrane, are mixed with radiolabeled ligand.

After equilibrium binding is established, the bound and free ligand must be separated rapidly (often in 1 second or less) to maintain the binding equilibrium. Then the concentration of bound ligand can be determined by measuring the amount of radioactivity associated with the high-molecular-weight receptor after separation. For the reversible binding of ligand and receptor, the equilibrium expression can be written

$$L + R \underset{k_{-1}}{\overset{k_1}{\rightleftharpoons}} LR \quad (1)$$

In this expression

L = free ligand

R = unoccupied receptor

LR = ligand–receptor complex

The association and dissociation rate constants are k_1 and k_{-1}, respectively. At equilibrium, the rates of association and dissociation are equal. Therefore the law of mass action can be employed to give

$$k_1[L][R] = k_{-1}[LR] \quad (2)$$

In equation 2 the use of [] denotes concentration. Rearrangement gives

$$\frac{[L][R]}{[LR]} = \frac{k_{-1}}{k_1} = K_d \quad (3)$$

Here K_d is the equilibrium binding constant, or just the binding constant. Now, only *[L]* and *[LR]* can be determined experimentally for most systems. Therefore, *[R]* is defined in terms of the total receptor concentration $[R_T]$ and that part which is bound *[LR]*, as

$$[R] = [R_T] - [LR] \quad (4)$$

Substituting in equation 3 and rearranging gives

$$\frac{[LR]}{[L]} = \frac{[R_T]}{K_d} - \frac{[LR]}{K_d} \quad (5)$$

This can also be expressed as

$$\frac{[B]}{[F]} = \frac{[B_m]}{K_d} - \frac{[B]}{K_d} \quad (6)$$

In equation 6

[B] = concentration of bound ligand

[F] = concentration of free ligand

$[B_m]$ = maximum possible concentration of bound ligand, which is assumed to be the same as the concentration of total receptor.

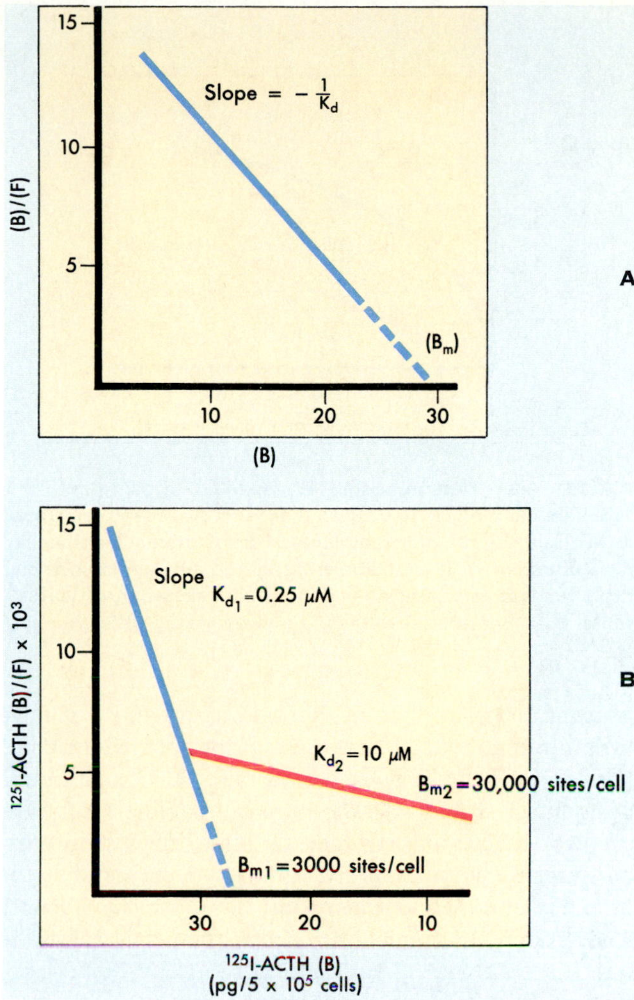

FIGURE 2-4 Scatchard plot of ligand–receptor binding to obtain values for K_d and B_m. **A,** The simple case of one binding site with one K_d. **B,** A case in which the ligand (shown here as ACTH) binds to sites with two different K_d values. The lines in the figure represent straight lines that would be drawn from the experimental data points. *ACTH,* Adrenocorticotrophic hormone.

The formulation B_m was developed by Scatchard to describe the association of one ligand with one binding site. A plot of *[B]/[F]* versus *[B]* should be linear when a single subtype of binding site is involved. If ligand binding occurs at more than one subtype of binding site, the plot is curved and the interpretation becomes more difficult. Scatchard plots (equation 6) are shown for the simple case of one subtype of binding site and for the more complex case of two subtypes (Figure 2-4). Typically, Scatchard plots are used to obtain values for K_d and $[B_m]$.

When performing ligand–receptor binding measurements, care must be taken to differentiate between specific binding of ligand to receptor sites and nonspecific binding of ligand to adsorption sites that likely are

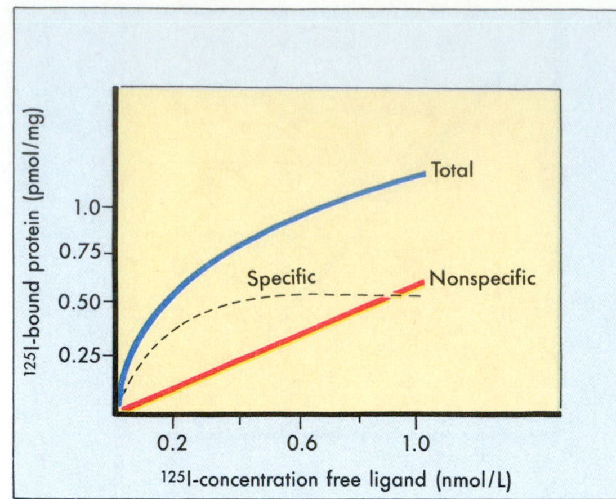

FIGURE 2-5 Determination of specific binding of ^{125}I-radiolabeled β-blocking drug to β-adrenergic receptors. "Total" data obtained with only radiolabeled drug added. "Nonspecific" data obtained with radiolabeled drug and also nonradiolabeled drug present (nonradiolabeled drug concentration at least 10 times K_d). "Specific" results obtained by taking difference.

present on the protein or the membrane and that have nothing to do with the receptor of interest. Nonspecific ligand binding increases linearly with the concentration of ligand, whereas specific binding reaches saturation, as evidenced by the plateau (Figure 2-5). Separate experimental determinations are used to obtain the amounts of total and nonspecific ligand that are bound. The amount or concentration of specifically bound ligand is obtained by subtracting the nonspecific component from the total. The nonspecific values are obtained by the addition of a large excess of nonradiolabeled ligand (that saturates the specific sites) to the radiolabeled ligand in the binding assay. Thus all the specific sites are occupied by the nonradioactive ligand.

RECEPTOR MECHANISTIC CONCEPTS

The major features of receptors are summarized schematically in Figure 2-6 and are also described in the box . The details of how these features are used, particularly to carry out transmembrane signal transmission, is a complex process with many of the details still not clear at the molecular level. Several key points are emphasized here before describing the mechanistic processes of specific ligand–receptor signal transmission systems and their modulation by drugs. The key points are as follows:

1. Receptors are membrane proteins having one or more subtypes of binding sites with glycosylated pendant chains on the extracellular side. Special lipids also may be associated with the protein.

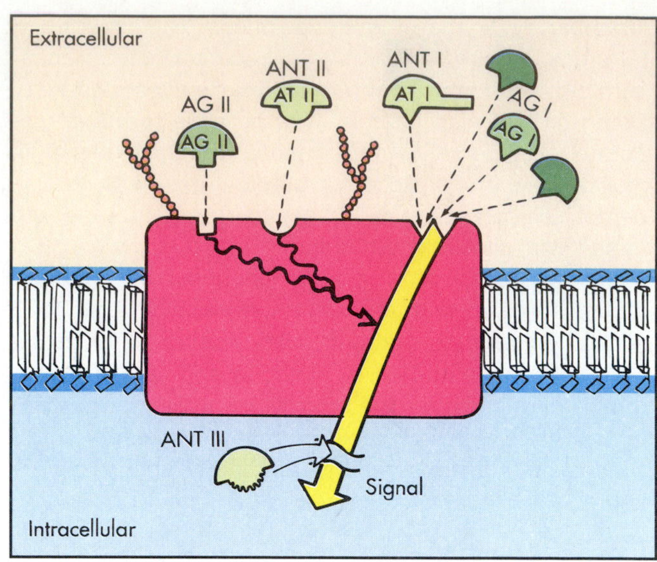

FIGURE 2-6 Major features of classical receptors. These include embedding in a membrane, glycosylated chains on the extracellular side, binding sites on the extracellular side for an endogenous transmitter *(dark green symbol)* with two molecules needing to be bound (as shown here) to activate transmembrane signal. Drugs can use many targets (*AG,* Agonist; *ANT,* antagonist): (1) AG I and ANT I compete with endogenous transmitter for activation sites, AG I to enhanced and ANT I to block signal; (2) AG II and ANT II enhances or block signal, respectively, by binding to allosteric sites that influence *(wavy line)* signal transmission; (3) ANT III blocks signal within the membrane or at intracellular signal reception points.

2. Binding of the endogenous compound specific for that receptor results in activation of the receptor (probably by inducing a conformational change) and transmission of a signal through the membrane to the intracellular side. Sometimes two or more molecules of endogenous compound must bind per receptor to generate a signal. The binding is usually reversible. Sometimes two molecules of ligand-bound receptor associate to form a dimer and initiate signalling (Chapter 34).
3. The magnitude of the transmembrane signal may depend on the percentage of the available receptors that are occupied by the endogenous compound or on the rate of occupancy. This topic is discussed in Chapter 3.
4. Drugs can enhance, diminish, or block the generation, transmission, or receipt of the signal by several approaches. These approaches are classified according to whether the drug produces a signal (or enhances the signal produced by an endogenous ligand) or diminishes the signal.

The terms **agonist** and **antagonist,** as introduced here, represent drugs that enhance or diminish a response. These terms are described in greater detail in Chapter 3. The approaches are as follows:

1. Agonist I: the drug binds to the same site as the endogenous compound and produces the same type of

FEATURES OF RECEPTORS

Protein; lipoprotein, glycoprotein
Molecular weight, 45–200 kilodaltons
Subunits, subtypes depending on tissue
Frequently glycosylated; glycolipid anchoring groups
K_d of drug binding to receptor (1–100 nM), binding reversible, stereoselective
Specifity of binding not absolute, leading to drug binding to several receptor types
Receptors saturable because of finite number of receptors
Specific binding of receptor results in signal transduction via second messenger to intracellular site
May require more than one drug molecule to bind to receptor to generate signal
Magnitude of signal depends on number of receptors occupied or on receptor occupancy rate. Signal is amplified by intracellular mechanisms
By acting on receptor, drugs can enhance, diminish, or block generation or transmission of signal
Drugs are receptor modulators and do not confer new properties on cells or tissues
Receptors must have properties of recognition and transduction
Receptors can be upregulated or downregulated

signal, usually of magnitude equal to to greater than that of the endogenous agent.

2. Agonist II: the drug binds to a different site on the extracellular side than does agonist I, producing no signal by itself; however, an enhanced signal is generated when the endogenous agent also binds to its site. This is an **allosteric action.**
3. Antagonist I: the drug binds to the site used by the endogenous agent and diminishes or blocks the signal generated by the endogenous agent.
4. Antagonist II: the drug binds to an allosteric site on the extracellular side, similar to agonist II, but produces a diminished signal generated by the endogenous agent.
5. Antagonist III: the drug dissolves in the membrane or crosses the membrane and intercepts the signal generated by the endogenous agent within the membrane or on the intracellular side.

The approaches by which drugs interact with classical membrane receptor complexes are discussed in general terms later in this chapter and in Chapter 3. However, the discussions that relate these approaches to specific drugs are found in chapters that deal with those drugs.

An important topic of ligand–receptor binding is that of transmembrane signal transmission. As the mechanisms for transmission of the ligand–receptor-activated signal through the membrane and for activation of metabolic or other processes on the intracellular side become better understood at the molecular level, the opportunities for modulation by drugs become more apparent. So far, four mechanisms for signal transmission are known. Three specific examples are given later in this chapter. The mechanisms are listed as follows:

1. Direct receptor control of ion channels (ligand gated or voltage gated)
2. Receptor-controlled generation of second messengers (G-protein/cAMP or G-protein/phosphoinositide systems)
3. Receptor internalization and recycling-polypeptide redistribution
4. Receptor-initiated phosphorylation involving tyrosine kinase activity (discussed in Chapter 34)

The remainder of this chapter contains descriptions of several key receptor systems that function to open or close channels to allow certain ions to pass through the cell membrane, as well as a discussion of receptor-based second messenger systems. The chapter ends with an overview of some of the common features that are beginning to emerge for many of the key receptor systems.

SPECIFIC RECEPTOR EXAMPLES

Nicotinic Acetylcholine Receptors

The nicotinic acetylcholine receptor is a well-characterized, ligand-gated ion channel. This receptor is found on the muscle cell end plate in the neuromuscular junction at all autonomic ganglia and in the central nervous system (CNS). The role of the acetylcholine receptor is to convert the binding of the neurotransmitter, acetylcholine, into an electrical signal in the cells of the organ containing the receptor. It does this, for example, by opening a pore for the Na^+ or K^+ ions to pass through the cell membrane, leading to depolarization of the cell's membrane potential.

The acetylcholine receptor consists of five subunits of four different types. The subunits are all glycosylated. The protein subunit molecular weights are as follows:

alpha (α)	50,200 daltons
beta (β)	53,700 daltons
delta (δ)	57,600 daltons
gamma (γ)	56,300 daltons

Because the α subunit appears twice and the carbohydrate adds another 20,000 daltons, the receptor total molecular weight is approximately 288,000 daltons. The data presented here are for acetylcholine receptors from the electroplaque membrane of the *Torpedo californica* electric eel. The quantities of this receptor in human tissues are minute; the availability of receptor from the electric fish organ is much greater, and the differences in structure of the receptor from fish versus humans appear to be small.

A view of the receptor from the extracellular side shows a nearly pentameric symmetrical arrangement of the subunits in α, γ, δ, α, and β order (clockwise) (Figure 2-7). Different subunit arrangements occur in other tissues. Approximately 10% of the acetylcholine-gated change activity is obtained with only an α, β, and γ combination. All the subunits appear necessary for holding the acetylcholine and other binding sites in the proper conformation for normal binding and for full channel-opening activity. Approximate dimensions of the receptor and the water-filled central channel also are included.

Normally the channel is closed. Channel opening occurs when two molecules of acetylcholine bind to the receptor. Because the binding sites for acetylcholine, agonists, competitive antagonists, and bungarotoxin (a channel-blocking compound) all are on the α subunit, and both α subunit acetylcholine binding sites must be occupied for channel opening to occur. Binding of acetylcholine opens the pore to at least 0.65 nm, enough to allow the passage of partially hydrated cations, particularly sodium or potassium. Anions are blocked from passage through the channel. Protons appear to block the channel. The mechanism of channel opening is not known, though binding of acetylcholine causes the release of four to six calcium ions per receptor molecule. It is postulated that the calcium ions help stabilize the membrane-spanning portions. The calcium release may augment the conformational change brought about by acetylcholine binding, thus causing the channel to open. With acetylcholine binding, the mean channel open time is 1 to 2 ms. A subsequent influx of calcium ions may be the mechanism that causes the channel to close.

The amino acid sequence of the α subunit in relation to the cell membrane is shown in Figure 2-8. It is

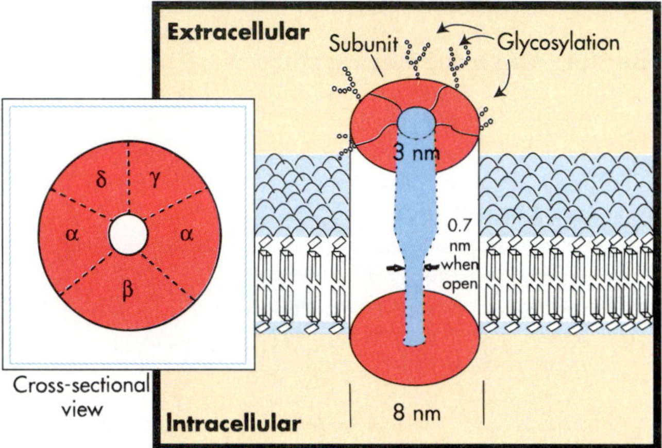

FIGURE 2-7 Schema of acetylcholine receptor shows the pentameric arranagement of α, β, γ, and δ subunits, glycosylation, ion channel, and approximate dimensions.

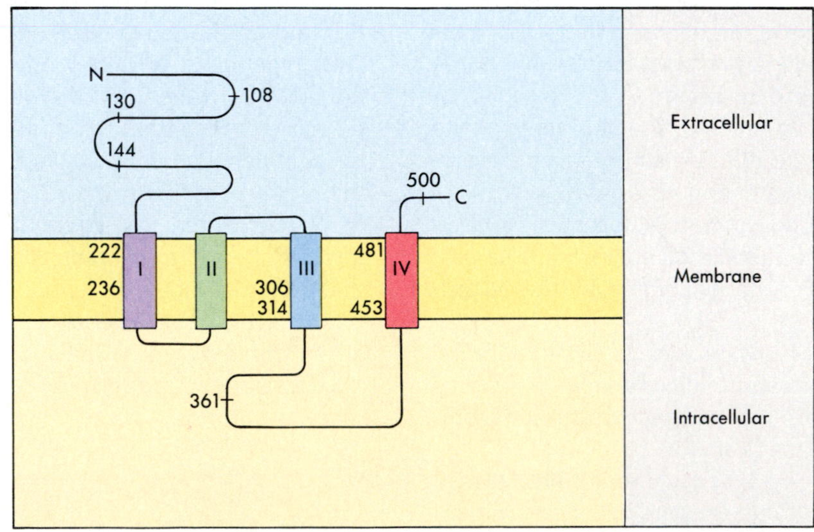

FIGURE 2-8 Proposed model for topology of amino acid chain in subunit of acetylcholine receptor, showing four (I, II, III, IV) helical, hydrophobic, transmembrane regions each 20 to 30 residues long. Numbers indicate approximate positions of amino acid residues starting from amino *(N)* end. Experimental data indicate that *N* and *C* (carboxyl) ends are on extracellular side of membrane. (Developed from Claudio T: Molecular genetics of acetylcholine receptor-channels. In Glover DM, Hames BD, editors: *Molecular neurobiology,* Oxford, 1989, IRL Press.)

controversial whether four or five helical, hydrophobic transmembrane regions are present in the single, roughly 500–amino acid chain that constitutes each subunit.

Prolonged contact of the acetylcholine receptor with elevated concentrations of agonist results in inactivation (desensitization) of the receptor. The mechanism for this is only postulated and includes the concept of two conformational states (Figure 2-9). In a low-affinity conformation, the channel can be opened when two molecules of agonist bind; in a high-affinity conformation, the channel cannot be opened.

Sodium-Channel Receptors

Voltage-dependent sodium channels are present in the membranes of excitable nerve, cardiac, and skeletal muscle cells. The sodium ion–channel receptor system is subject to voltage-controlled channel opening, also termed **gating,** whereas the nicotinic acetylcholine ion–channel system is controlled by ligand binding. In their resting state, these cells maintain the intracellular sodium-ion concentration at a much lower level (more negative voltage) than that in the extracellular environment. This is accomplished by means of the Na^+, K^+-ATPase pump. The sodium channels can be opened by voltage gating, brought about by membrane depolarization. Channel opening allows a transient influx of Na^+ ions to take place before inactivation and return to the resting state can occur. Local anesthetic agents bind to sodium channels and block the transient increase in membrane sodium ion permeability, thereby blocking nerve conduction.

The structure of the sodium channel is shown schematically in Figure 2-10. The α subunit (molecular weight approximately 260,000) is heavily glycosylated and has four similar domains, each containing six hydrophobic α-helix transmembrane regions. The β_1 and β_2 subunits (molecular weight 36,000 and 33,000 daltons respectively) also are glycosylated.

Depolarization of the membrane causes a voltage-driven conformational change in the sodium channel that moves approximately 6 positive charges into the extracellular space and an equivalent number of negative charges into the intracellular region. One can explain this by considering the transmembrane helical domains to have a sequence of positive charges paired with negative charges on nonhelix parts of the subunit. Sliding of each helix, to move 1 or 2 positive charges into the extracellular space, could be accomplished by a rotation of approximately 60 degrees and a linear displacement of approximately 0.5 nm.

Acidic Amino Acid Receptors

It is now recognized that L-glutamate, L-aspartate, and possibly other acidic amino acids and peptides play a major role as excitatory neurotransmitters in the mammalian central nervous system. An ion channel is associated with their receptor, and both ligand gating and

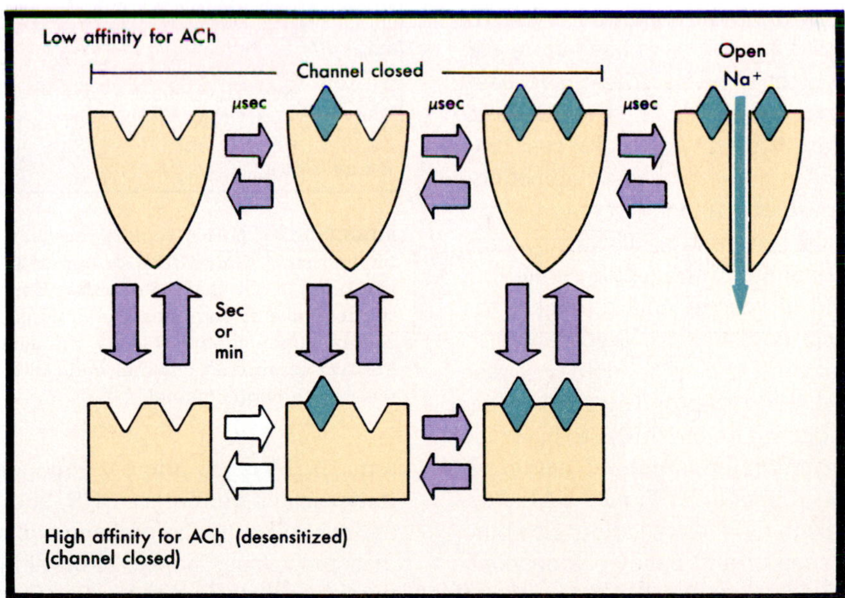

FIGURE 2-9 Acetylcholine receptor becomes desensitized in the presence of prolonged elevated concentrations of acetylcholine. The concept of two receptor conformational states has been suggested, but this still leaves some of the experimental observations only partially explained.

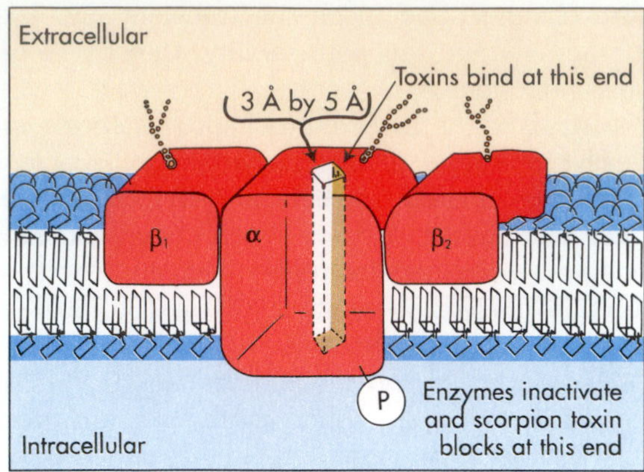

FIGURE 2-10 How the voltage-gated sodium channel from the human brain may be assembled in the membrane. The α subunit is believed to have six helix transmembrane domains, with the channel roughly a 0.3 by 0.5 nm rectangular hole formed by four of the transmembrane helices within this subunit. The α subunit also is phosphorylated *(P)*. At least one of the binding sites for inactivation of the increased sodium-ion permeability is located on the intracellular side of the α subunit. The location of the binding site for local anesthetics is presumed to be inside the channel.

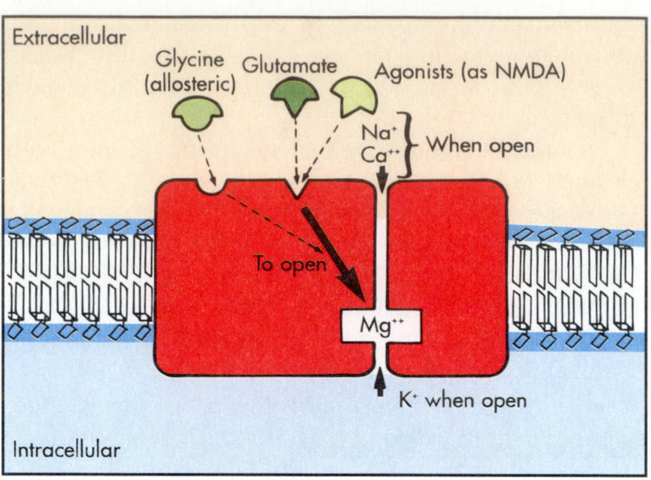

FIGURE 2-11 Suggested components of acidic amino acid receptors in CNS. Channel shown in resting stage. Depolarization by agonist binding or voltage gating releases blockade by magnesium ions and lets potassium ions pass outward and Na^+ and Ca^{++} pass into the nerve cell. Glycine acts to augment agonist effect.

voltage gating appear to be involved in control of channel opening. The evidence indicates that this receptor system may be a target for development of new drugs for use as anticonvulsants or analgesics and possibly for treating epilepsy and some neurodegenerative disorders.

The glutamate receptor system is often characterized using three agonists: *N*-methyl-D-aspartate (NMDA), kainate, and quisqualate. Glutamate and aspartate can open the channel, but most of the studies have been done with the more potent test compounds. NMDA usually produces larger ion-channel conductances than kainate or quisqualate. Amino acid or test compound–induced depolarization results in an ion current in which Na^+ and Ca^{++} flow into the cell and K^+ flows out. Magnesium ions block the channel in the resting state, but depolarization, by ligand or voltage gating, causes the magnesium ions to become dislodged. Glycine, which is an inhibitory transmitter in the spinal cord, can also bind to the acidic amino acid receptor. Glycine binding enhances the ability of glutamate or NMDA to open the channel, presumably through an allosteric action. A schema of the receptor is shown in Figure 2-11. Psychoactive compounds, such as phencyclidine, also bind to the channel of this receptor and behave as noncompetitive antagonists.

GABA Type A Receptors

Another important ligand-gated ion-channel receptor is the type A γ-aminobutyric acid (GABA) receptor system. GABA is the primary endogenous inhibitory transmitter in the vertebrate CNS, and its inhibitory actions are enhanced by the presence of barbiturates or benzodiazepines (see Chapter 25 and Figure 2-12). The GABA type A receptor consists of α and β subunits and possibly γ or δ subunits, with four or five total subunits constituting a functional receptor assembly. The types and number of subunits in a receptor assembly may vary with the species and possibly with anatomical location. Binding of GABA results in opening of a chloride-ion

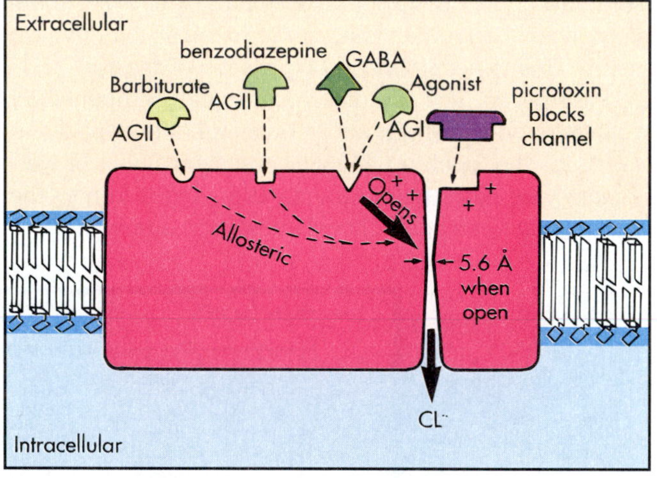

FIGURE 2-12 GABA type A receptor, showing four different binding sites. Only GABA or agonists that bind to the GABA site bring about channel opening. Benzodiazepines and barbiturates have strong allosteric actions. Picrotoxin binds to the channel opening and blocks the channel noncompetitively. Positive charges at channel ends filter out positive ions from passing through channel.

channel. Benzodiazepines and barbiturates bind at other site in allosteric fashion to augment the GABA-channel opening. Sequence analysis shows that each subunit probably has four helix regions that are believed to span the membrane, with a long extracellular section on the amino end of each subunit that serves as the proposed site for the binding domains.

G-PROTEIN–BASED SECOND MESSENGER RECEPTORS

A large group of receptors use second messenger systems for their transmembrane signaling mechanism. In these systems, ligand–receptor binding results in a sequence of reactions, usually within the membrane, that includes activation or inhibition of an enzyme that controls the formation of second messenger compounds. These messengers can move within the membrane or within the intracellular space and modify the activity of intracellular signaling pathways. Cyclic adenosine monophosphate (cAMP) and inositol trisphosphate (IP_3) are the principal second messenger and are described further.

In systems using cAMP as a second messenger, binding of the ligand to the receptor results in activation or inhibition of adenylate cyclase, the enzyme that catalyzes the formation of cAMP from ATP. The mechanism involves intermediary G-proteins as part of the signaling complex. Examples of receptors that activate adenylate cyclase include the β-adrenergic, histamine H_2, and dopamine D_1 subtypes. Adenylate cyclase inhibition occurs with the muscarinic M_2, α_2-adrenergic, dopamine D_2, opiate μ and δ, adenosine A_1, and GABA type B receptors.

G-proteins form a family of membrane-associated proteins that serve a key role in receptor modification of adenylate cyclase activity. The guanosine groups are the source of the "G" terminology. G-proteins provide the link between the ligand-activated receptor protein and the effector enzyme adenylate cyclase. G-proteins exist in two states: an inactive state, in which GDP is bound to the protein, and an active form, in which GTP is bound to protein. Activation of the receptor by a ligand causes the receptor to interact with the α subunit of the G-protein, yielding release of bound GDP and binding of GTP. The active, GTP-bound form of the protein then interacts with adenylate cyclase.

G-proteins have intrinsic GTPase activity, which spontaneously hydrolyzes bound GTP to bound GDP and thereby converts the G-protein from an active to an inactive form. The resulting GDP remains tightly bound to the protein and facilitates binding of the inhibitory βγ subunits to the α subunit (see discussion following). As the number of cycles of GTP binding and hydrolysis increases, the ligand–receptor complex promotes a greater number of α subunits into the active state and thus stimulates adenylate cyclase activity.

Based on their functional and biochemical properties, the G-proteins that couple receptors to effects (especially to adenylate cyclase) can be divided into the following four functional groups:

1. G_s, which couples stimulatory receptors to adenylate cyclase
2. G_i, which couples inhibitory receptors to adenylate cyclase
3. G_o (and perhaps G_i), which are believed to couple to ion channels
4. G_q, which couples receptors to activation of phospholipase C

The G-proteins consist of the following three subunits:

1. 6,000- to 8,000-dalton molecular weight γ unit
2. 35,000- to 36,000-dalton molecular weight β unit
3. 39,000- to 52,000-dalton molecular weight α unit

The α subunits provide the major structural and functional differences between the various G-proteins. The α subunit interacts with the receptor and the effector enzyme (i.e., adenylate cyclase) and accounts for activation/deactivation of the G-protein through binding and hydrolysis of GTP. The α subunit from each type of G-protein has a unique region, which imparts the specificity. The interaction with the β and γ subunits and the hydrolysis of GTP are attributed to regions of the α subunit that are common for numerous types of G-proteins. The genes for the α subunits from 17 different G-proteins have been cloned and sequenced, and it is clear from the structural point of view that the α subunits can be grouped into five families of proteins with similar functional properties. There is particularly strong homology (i.e., commonality) among the GTP-binding regions of these subunits with respect to amino acid sequence and to location within the protein. Four noncontiguous regions of the α subunit are involved, with protein folding accounting for the positioning of the four regions in proximity to one another. Several lines of evidence demonstrate that the C-terminal region of the α subunit interacts with receptors. This region thus has displayed considerable variation among α subunits from different G-proteins. Less is known about the regions involved in interaction with the β and γ subunits and with the effector enzyme.

One result emerging from the information revealed by the cDNA clones of the α subunits is that there appear to be more types of α subunits than are needed to account for the known biochemical and functional classes of α subunits. It is likely that regulation of new effector systems by G-proteins will be discovered. These systems will be possible targets for development of new drugs.

The β and γ subunits of G-proteins form a tightly as-

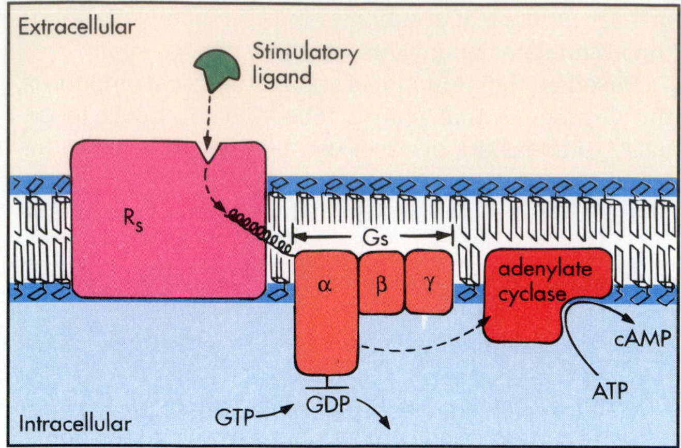

FIGURE 2-13 Components for ligand–receptor binding induced activation of adenylate cyclase. Binding of ligand to stimulatory receptor, R_s, produces conformation change that is coupled to carboxy terminus of α-helix domain of α subunit of G_s. This activates G_s by displacing bound GDP with GTP to give active α_s. G_s dissociates, with active α_s moving to adenylate cyclase location and activating this enzyme. The β γ subunits are released and freed for other signaling functions. Similar scheme can be shown for inhibition of adenylate cyclase using R_i and G_i.

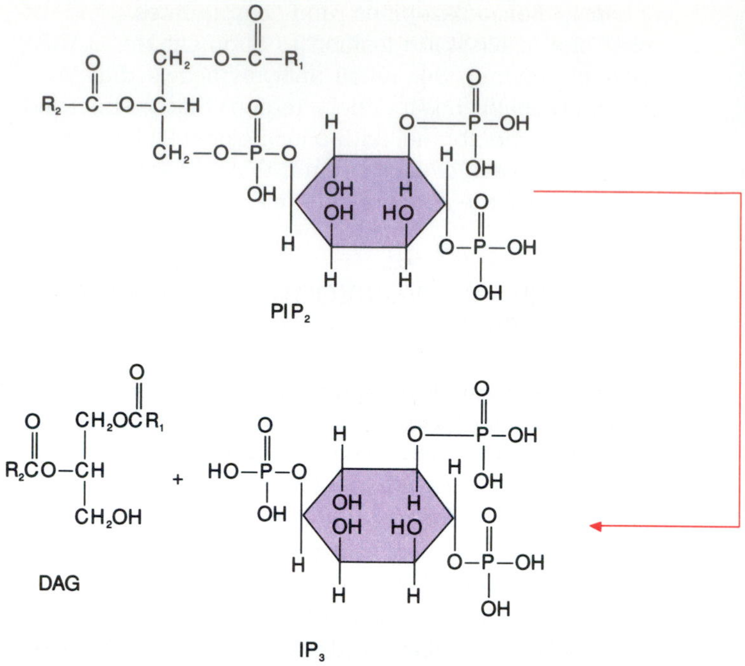

FIGURE 2-14 Chemistry of phosphoinositides. R_1 and R_2 represent lipids. R_1 is often a stearate derivative and R_2 a multiple double-bond long-chain lipid. PIP_2 is phosphatidylinositol 4,5-bisphosphate; IP_3 is inositol 1,4,5-trisphosphate; and DAG is 1,2-diacylglycerol.

sociated functional unit. As with the α subunits, multiple genes for the β and γ subunits have been discovered. There are currently four different β and seven different γ subunits known. The role that these different proteins play in the G-protein signaling pathway is just beginning to emerge.

On activation of G_s or G_i, the α subunit dissociates from the βγ subunits. In the common situation, the GTP-α_s or GTP-α_i forms interact with adenylate cyclase to produce enzyme activation or inhibition respectively. Enzyme activation by the βγ complex occurs, but its role in the transmembrane signaling system is not well understood. On GTP hydrolysis by the α subunit previously described, the α and β γ subunits recombine and reestablish the basal state of the system. The G-protein adenylate cyclase system is shown schematically in Figure 2-13 for G_s. Activated G_i can inhibit the enzyme directly or it can work indirectly by inhibiting activated G_s.

The other system for ligand–receptor generation of a second messenger system involves the enzyme phospholipase C. This phosphodiesterase type of enzyme catalyzes the hydrolysis of membrane phospholipids known as **phosphoinositides.** The hydrolysis releases two compounds, IP_3 and DAG, both of which appear to function as second messengers. Examples of receptors that use this signaling system include the α-adrenergic, muscarinic M_1 or M_2, serotonin 5-HT_2, and thyrotropin-releasing hormone (TRH) receptors.

Activation of phospholipase C by receptors occurs by a mechanism analogous to that used to activate adenylate cyclase. The major pathway is for the receptor to activate the α subunit of the G_q, which interacts directly with phospholipase C. The activated G-protein increases phospholipase C activity and dramatically increases the rate of hydrolysis of phosphatidylinositol 4,5-bisphosphate (PIP_2). The two second messengers generated are inositol 1,4,5-trisphosphate (IP_3) and 1,2-diacylglycerol (DAG). IP_3 is very water soluble and can migrate into the intracellular fluid, where it binds to the IP_3 receptor in the endoplasmic reticulum and causes the release of stored calcium ions. Hydrolysis of IP_3 terminates the signal by removing its activity. The degradation products undergo rephosphorylation to regenerate PIP_2. The chemical structures of the messengers generated from PIP_2 (IP_3 and DAG) are shown in Figure 2-14. The other second messenger, DAG, is highly lipid soluble and migrates within the membrane. DAG activates the enzyme protein kinase C, which in turn modulates many intracellular processes by causing covalent phosphorylation of proteins.

All three second messengers discussed above—cAMP, IP_3, and DAG—eventually lead to the activation of protein kinases that produce the cellular response by initiating the phosphorylation of important regulatory proteins. cAMP activates the cAMP-dependent protein kinase, IP_3 (through its release of Ca^{++} ion) activates a host of Ca^{++}- and calmodulin-dependent protein kinases, and DAG activates the family of enzymes known as protein kinase C. The phosphorylation of the key intracellular enzymes by these kinases leads to modification (both activation and inactivation) of cellular enzymes, leading to the characteristic response caused by activation of the receptor.

As noted, modulation of localized intracellular Ca^{++} concentrations is one of the regulatory features attributed to second messengers, such as IP_3. Several types of transmembrane calcium-ion channels also play key roles in the modulation of localized intracellular Ca^{++} concentrations. These calcium channels function primarily by voltage gating and possibly by ligand gating. The three types of voltage-gated calcium channels (L, N, and T) differ in the voltage needed for activation and in binding specificities. Whether these Ca^{++} channels operate by similar mechanisms as the ion channels described earlier in this chapter or whether second messengers are involved is not yet clear. Chapter 16 describes the processes of calcium-channel drugs in further detail.

RECEPTORS WITH INTRINSIC TYROSINE KINASE ACTIVITY

A large group of receptors for growth factors including insulin, epidermal growth factor, platelet-derived growth factor, hepatocyte growth factor, etc., are large proteins (molecular weight, MW, of 150,000 to 200,000 daltons) that pass through the plasma membrane of the cell once. Their extracellular domain contains regions that bind the growth factor, and their intracellular domain contains a kinase activity capable of phosphorylating proteins on tyrosine residues. Both the receptor itself and other intracellular proteins become phosphorylated on tyrosine after binding of the growth factor. Occupation of these receptors leads to multiple intracellular events with both immediate (e.g., activation of phospholipase C) and long-term (e.g., cell growth) consequences. A common feature of the this class of receptors is that the autophosphorylation of the receptor on tyrosine residues leads to formation of a domain in the receptor that promotes binding of other signaling molecules. Thus, one consequence of activation of this class of receptors is that complexes of signaling molecules are organized within the cell. These complexes activate a separate signaling pathway (the MAP kinase pathway), eventually leading to cell division. Another common feature of this class of receptors is that activation of the receptor leads to receptor internalization and downregulation of the receptor (described further). A detailed description of these receptors is provided in Chapter 34.

RECEPTOR DESENSITIZATION AND TURNOVER

The loss of response in an organ (e.g., smooth muscle) on exposure to an agonist is commonly called **tachyphylaxis.** When applied to a receptor, however, this phenomenon is termed **desensitization.** It is a general property of receptor systems. Several schemes have been devised to explain the mechanism by which receptor are desensitized on continuous exposure to agonists. One such proposal visualizes the receptor existing in two functional states, one of which is resting and activatable; the other is the desensitized state. In the absence of ligand, the receptor is present in the activatable state, and on ligand addition a greater fraction of ligand is bound to the desensitized state of the receptor because it is the one of higher affinity for the ligand. As the ligand dissociates from the higher-affinity state, desensitization dissipates. When the desensitization involves receptors occupied by a specific class of agonists, such as those activating the nicotinic acetylcholine receptor, it is termed **homologous desensitization.** Under conditions in which the response of the target receptor can be diminished by several different classes of agents, the term **heterologous desensitization** is used. An example of the latter would be where agonists share a similar pathway for activation, such as the G_s-stimulation of adenylyl cyclase, common to many receptors. Many mechanisms leading to the desensitization of receptors have been established. These include decreases in receptor number (see below), a decrease in affinity of binding of agonist to receptor, phosphorylation of the receptor by specific kinases, and a decrease of coupling of the receptor to its second messenger system.

As receptors are processed within the cell after transcription of the receptor gene, they are ultimately fused into the cell or plasma membrane. Here either they tend to be randomly dispersed on the membrane surface or they may be concentrated in a specialized area of the membrane, called the *coated-pit region.* When receptors are exposed to agonists, the receptors move in the plane of the membrane and appear to concentrate in the coated pits. It is this region of the cell membrane that is internalized into the cell by endocytosis, where they may be degraded by lysosomes or ultimately recycled back into the cell membrane. Thus, this hypothesis is proposed for the mechanism of **downregulating** of receptors, resulting in a smaller receptor number and perhaps in desensitization. It should be emphasized that the basis for this proposition is derived from studies of only a limited number of receptor systems and does not include G-protein–linked receptors, which are targets of many major drug classes. Thus, receptor downregulation may occur after continuous agonist exposure, or from blockade of degradation or uptake of a neurotransmitter or hormone normally activating that receptor. On the other hand, exposure of the receptor to an antagonist, or inhibition of synthesis or release of the cognate neurotransmitter or hormone, can increase receptor processing and number. This phenomenon is called **upregulation** and can result in receptor supersensitivity. Receptor desensitization and supersensitivity, as they relate to the central nervous system, are considered in Chapter 22 and, as they relate to hormones, in Chapter 34.

FAMILIES (HOMOLOGY) AND HETEROGENEITY OF RECEPTORS

Classification of receptors of relevance to pharmacology traditionally is based on ligand-binding specificity. However, the application of the techniques of molecular biology and structural chemistry to the study of receptors is suggestive that alternative classification schemes based on the structure or composition of receptors may emerge. The amino acid sequences of a large number of receptors are available and indicate the existence of commonality among many receptors. For example, the nicotinic acetylcholine, glycine, GABA type A, and acidic amino acid (glutamate) receptors all show extensive homology in sequences, an indication that these receptors belong to the same genetic family. Significant homology in sequences also is found between the large family of G-protein–coupled receptors, including those for important drugs such as β-adrenergic agonists and antagonists.

Some of the apparent heterogeneity of receptor or channel subtypes, wherein a given receptor subtype appears to function differently depending on the type of tissue or anatomical location where it is found, may be attributable to genetic variations. For example, different genes are known to produce functional acetylcholine muscarinic receptors of the same subtype, and many ligands activate more than one G-protein through several receptor subtypes. One example is norepinephrine, which activates adenylate cyclase through the β-adrenergic receptor, inhibits this same enzyme through the α_2-adrenergic receptor, and activates phospholipase C through the α_1-adrenergic receptor, all through different members of the G-protein family.

It is clear that the existence of multiple receptor types in different tissues linked to multiple signalling systems provides fertile ground for new advances in the development of therapeutically useful drugs.

REFERENCES

Catterall WA: Excitation-contraction coupling in vertebrate skeletal muscle: a tale of two calcium channels, *Cell* 64:871, 1991.

Dohlman HG, Thorner J, Caron MC, Lefkowitz RJ: Model systems for the study of seven-transmembrane segment receptors, *Annu Rev Biochem* 60:349-400, 1991.

Galzi JL, Revah F, Bessis A, and Changeux JP: Functional architecture of the nicotinic acetylcholine receptor from electric organ to brain. *Annu Rev Pharmacol* 31:37-72, 1991.

Kaziro Y, Itoh H, Kozasa T, et al: Structure and function of signal-transducing GTP-binding proteins, *Annu Rev Biochem* 60:349-400, 1991.

Taylor P, Insel PA: Molecular basis of drug action: In Pratt WE, Taylor P, editors: *Principles of drug action,* vol 2, New York, 1990, Churchill Livingstone.

SELF-ASSESSMENT QUESTIONS

1. A drug acting by a receptor-based mechanism may have several side effects in addition to its primary therapeutic action because:
   a. The receptor for the drug may be located in multiple tissues, some of which are not involved in the therapeutic response.
   b. The drug may be bound to more than one receptor with different K_d values.
   c. The receptors for the drug may be linked to different second messenger systems to produce several cellular responses.
   d. a and c are correct.
   e. All of the above are correct.
2. Binding of a drug to a receptor generally:
   a. Involves covalent binding between receptor and drug.
   b. Involves more than one type of weak bond between drug and receptor.
   c. Requires long-lasting stable bonds between drug and receptor.
   d. Has a similar affinity for the several stereoisomers of the drug.
   e. Is characterized by high K_d values.
3. The graph below shows Scatchard plots for the binding of drugs A and B to their respective receptors. Based on the graph, which of the following statements is true?

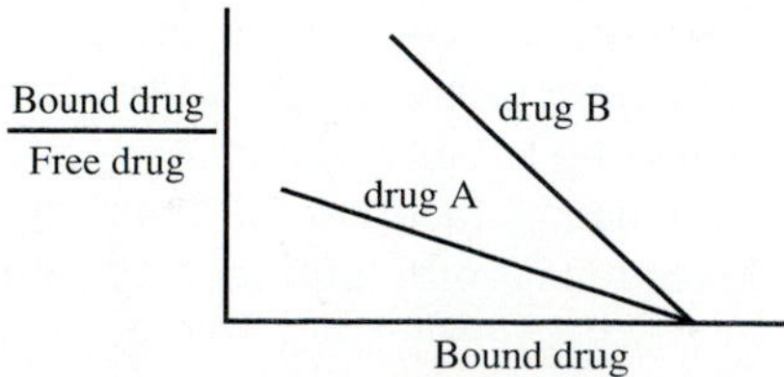

a. Drugs A and B have the same affinity and the same number of binding sites.
b. The binding of drug A is characterized by a higher affinity of binding and a greater number of receptors than that observed in the binding of drug B.
c. The binding of drug A is characterized by a lower affinity of binding and fewer receptors than that observed for drug B.
d. The binding of drug A is characterized by a higher affinity of binding than that observed for drug B. However, the number of receptors is equal.
e. The binding of drug A is characterized by a lower affinity for binding than that observed for the binding of drug B, but there are equal numbers of receptors.

4. Long or continuous exposure of a receptor to an agent that is an antagonist can:
   a. Result in a phenomenon called upregulation.
   b. Desensitize the receptor.
   c. Produce tachyphylaxis
   d. Cause downregulation of the receptor.
   e. b and c are correct.
5. Which of the following statements is true regarding responses mediated by drug receptors that are linked either to ion channels or G-proteins to produce a cellular response?
   a. The onset of responses produced by drugs that affect ion-channel systems is more rapid than that of responses mediated by G-protein systems.
   b. Amplification of the signal occurs when the receptor is linked to a G-protein system to produce a second messenger.
   c. Production of a second messenger can result in second messenger modification of the drug receptor interaction.
   d. a and b are correct.
   e. All of the above are correct.
6. Which of the following is NOT a feature of receptors:
   a. By acting on receptors, drugs can enhance diminish or block generation or transmission of signals.
   b. K_d of drug binding to receptors is generally in the range of 1 to 100 micromolar (μM).
   c. Specificity of drug binding to receptors is not absolute.
   d. It may require more than one drug molecule to bind to a receptor to elicit a response.
   e. Receptors are frequently glycosylated.

CHAPTER 3

Concentration–Response Relationships

THEODORE M. BRODY

HOW MUCH DRUG IS NEEDED

The binding of drug molecules to receptors leads to enhancement, inhibition, or blockade of molecular signals. This applies to "classical" receptors, as well as to enzyme inhibitors. The change in molecular signal is amplified through a sequence of biochemical and physiological processes to produce an "observable" pharmacological response. The question is how much drug is needed to obtain a desired magnitude and duration of response. This chapter defines the types of relationships between response and concentration. Chapter 4 is a discussion of the relationships between concentration and time.

Because the binding between drug and receptor molecules occurs according to the law of mass action, the concentrations of drug and receptor are key variables. Therefore it is appropriate to address the question of how much drug is needed to produce a given response in terms of "concentration–response" relationships. When concentration data are not available, "dose–response" relationships are used.

ABBREVIATIONS	
cAMP	Cyclic adenosine monophosphate
E	Magnitude of effect
ED_{50}	Effective dose in 50% of subjects
E_m	Maximum effect
I_{50}	Concentration that elicits 50% inhibition of enzyme activity
K_d	Dissociation constant

GRADED AND QUANTAL RESPONSES

Quantification of Responses

There can be more than one measure of the pharmacological response produced by a drug. Figure 3-1 illustrates the neuromuscular blocking agent succinylcholine, using data replotted from Figure 1-2. The response is defined as the **percentage blockade of neuromuscular transmission** and is found by determination of the force of contraction of the thumb muscle on repeated electrical stimulation of the ulnar nerve. This is an example of a "graded" response. It is characterized by the magnitude of the response increasing continuously with greater concentration of unbound drug at the receptor site. Succinylcholine acts by binding to the acetylcholine receptor on the muscle cell surface and causing membrane depolarization, described in greater detail in Chapter 11. Succinylcholine undergoes such rapid hydrolysis that concentration data are not available, but the ease of quantifying the magnitude of pharmacological response makes this a good example for demonstrating the concept of a graded response. Actually, the outer membrane of each muscle cell contains several thousand nicotinic acetylcholine receptor sites. Each molecule of succinylcholine is assumed to elicit the same degree of membrane depolarization when a molecule of drug binds to an unoccupied receptor site. In other words, each receptor molecule can be occupied or unoccupied; there are no intermediate degrees of occupancy for individual receptor molecules. Thus the increasing magnitude of neuromuscular blockade and the corresponding decreasing contraction of muscle fiber is the net result of many receptor sites on individual cells being occupied by drug and also of many muscle cells attempting to respond to the electrical stimulation.

A large number of drugs produce a graded pharmacological response; however, there are other drugs in

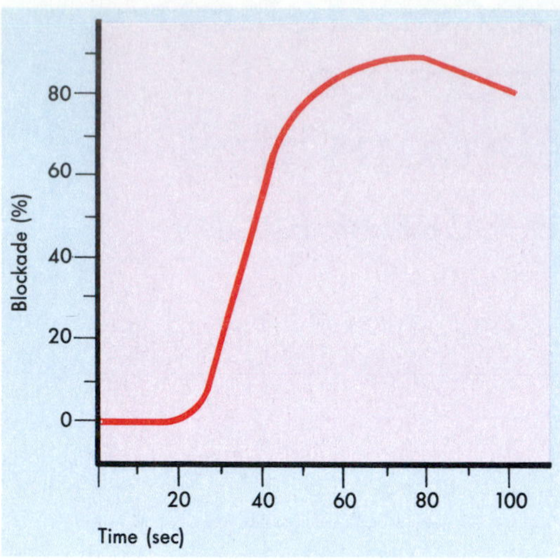

FIGURE 3-1 Magnitude of the pharmacological response for neuromuscular blockade by succinylcholine administered as a single intravenous injection and monitored by recording the force of thumb jerk on repeated electrical stimulation of the ulnar nerve. Results shown only for the first 100 seconds after injection.

which the observable response can be described only in terms of an all-or-none event. This is called a **quantal** response. (It should be emphasized however, that although the overt response may be *quantal* the underlying molecular mechanism may still depend on the interaction of the drug with a specific number of receptors in a *graded* fashion.) For example, the subject either does or does not respond to a pinprick pain stimulus in the presence of a particular concentration of pain suppressant. If the subject feels no pain, the response to the drug is positive. Because of intersubject variations, not all persons show a positive quantal response at the same concentration of drug. Thus the frequency of response to a given concentration of drug becomes the important variable in reporting quantal effects, whereas the magnitude of response is the comparable variable for a graded effect. This distinction will become more evident after the two types of responses are described further. It is possible to convert a graded response to a quantal basis by defining some criterion, such as a 25 mm Hg decrease in systolic blood pressure with a specific dose of an antihypertensive drug, and noting which subjects meet the criterion. However, it is not possible to convert many quantal responses to a graded basis.

Graded Responses

Similar to the ligand–receptor binding equilibrium expression developed in the previous chapter, an expression for the fraction of receptors occupied, Y, at equilibrium is developed here (see equation 3). The symbols are

D = concentration of free (i.e., unbound) drug
R = concentration of unoccupied receptor
DR = concentration of drug-bound receptor
R_T = concentration of total receptor

The law of mass action is applied as

$$\mathrm{D + R \underset{k-1}{\overset{k_1}{\rightleftharpoons}} DR} \quad \textbf{(1)}$$

$$\mathrm{k-1\,[D]\,[R] = k_{-1}\,[DR] = k_1\,[D]\,([R_T] - [DR])} \quad \textbf{(2)}$$

$$\mathrm{Y = \frac{[DR]}{[R_T]} = \frac{[D]}{K_d + [D]}} \quad \textbf{(3)}$$

$$\mathrm{K_d = \frac{k_{-1}}{k_1}}$$

In the classical theory for a graded response, the **magnitude of effect** *(E)* is assumed to be directly proportional to the fraction of the receptors occupied (receptor-occupancy theory), and the **maximum effect** (E_m) is supposed to occur when all of a given subtype is occupied by drug. Because some of the experimental results are not compatible with this theory, however, a modified theory has been introduced (1) to enable the maximum effect to occur without all the receptors of a given subtype being occupied and (2) to relate the effect to the concentration of occupied receptors through a stimulus *(S)*, which in turn is governed by the fraction of receptor sites that are occupied. Modification number one uses the concept of "spare" receptors, discussed later in this chapter, to explain some of the experimental observations. Modification number two (see equation 4) adapts the theory to allow several different groups of compounds to act at the same receptor subtype without the need for spare receptors.

The modified theory can be expressed quantitatively as

$$\mathbf{E} = \mathrm{hS \text{ and } S = \epsilon Y}$$

$$\mathbf{E} = \mathrm{\frac{h\epsilon[D]}{K_d + [D]}} \quad \textbf{(4)}$$

In these expressions, h is an undefined function that relates E to the stimulus, S, and ϵ is the proportionality factor between S and the fraction of occupied receptors, Y. In Figure 3-2, equation 4 is plotted with h and ϵ both constant and with the product $h\epsilon$ equal to E_m. In Figure 3-2, *A*, the plot of equation 4 is shown with an arithmetic scale for concentration. The resulting curved line is difficult to fit to experimental data, particularly when appreciable scatter is present. Therefore, several alter-

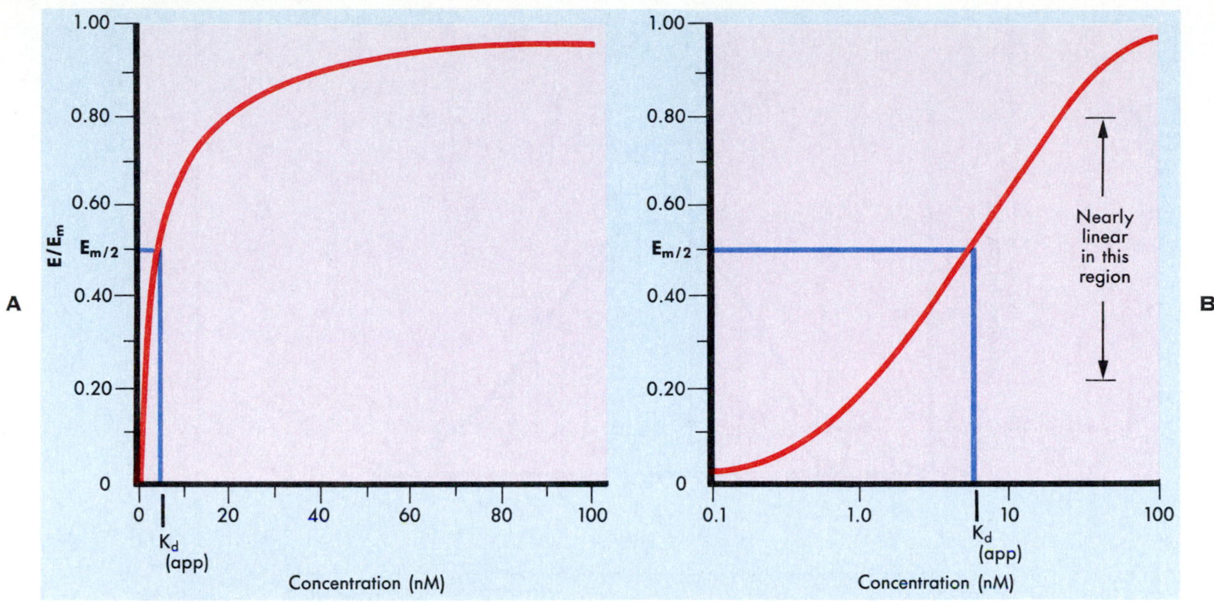

FIGURE 3-2 Concentration–response curve for graded response. **A,** Arithmetic scales. **B,** Log concentration scale. K_d *(app)* is arbitrarily taken to be 4.5 nM.

native approaches have been developed in which the data are replotted and thus transform at least part of the curve into a nearly straight line. This is desirable because it is easier to fit the data to a linear expression, especially with the natural variations often found in clinical studies. One of these transformations is used in Figure 3-2, *B,* where the concentration is plotted on a logarithmic, instead of an arithmetic, scale. This is an empirically based transformation, but it results in essentially a straight line between approximately 20% and 80% of the maximum response. More complex transformation techniques that linearize the curve from Figure 3-2, *A,* over the entire range of concentrations are available, but such techniques are beyond the scope of this book. The log concentration–response curve in Figure 3-2, *B,* is used later in this chapter to describe characteristics of agonist and antagonist drugs.

Graded log concentration–response curves (see Figure 3-2, *B*) are obtained after different amounts of drug are administered to a single subject. If a group of 50 subjects were given just enough drug to achieve a plasma concentration (e.g., 10 nM), a variety of magnitudes of effect could be expected. In other words, interpatient variation results in a different magnitude of effect in individual patients, and mean values for E_m and for the concentration that produces $E_m/2$ can be obtained for the general patient population. However, the logarithmic concentration-graded response curve shown in Figure 3-2, *B,* is for a single subject.

In defining the term *Y* in equation 3, the approach sometimes is called the **receptor occupancy theory,** which postulates that the net response from a cell, or more realistically from a mass of cells in a tissue bed, depends on the fraction of receptor molecules of a given subtype that are occupied by the drug. An alternative concept to the occupancy theory for explaining receptor concentration–response data is the rate theory. The rate theory postulates that the rate of drug–receptor binding, rather than the fraction of the sites occupied, is the controlling factor. So far no experiments have been devised to determine which theory is closer to the physical situation. The quantitative expressions have the same form for the occupancy and rate theories. The occupancy theory provides a more useful working concept, however, and is thus the more widely cited of the two approaches.

Quantal Responses

Mentioned earlier, the frequency of the response (that is, the number of subjects that respond to a given concentration or dose of drug) is the key factor in describing quantal responses. For a large group of subjects, one can organize the results by noting the minimum concentration of drug needed to obtain a response in each of the subjects. By plotting the number of subjects that respond versus the minimum concentration or dose required for the response, one obtains a distribution curve

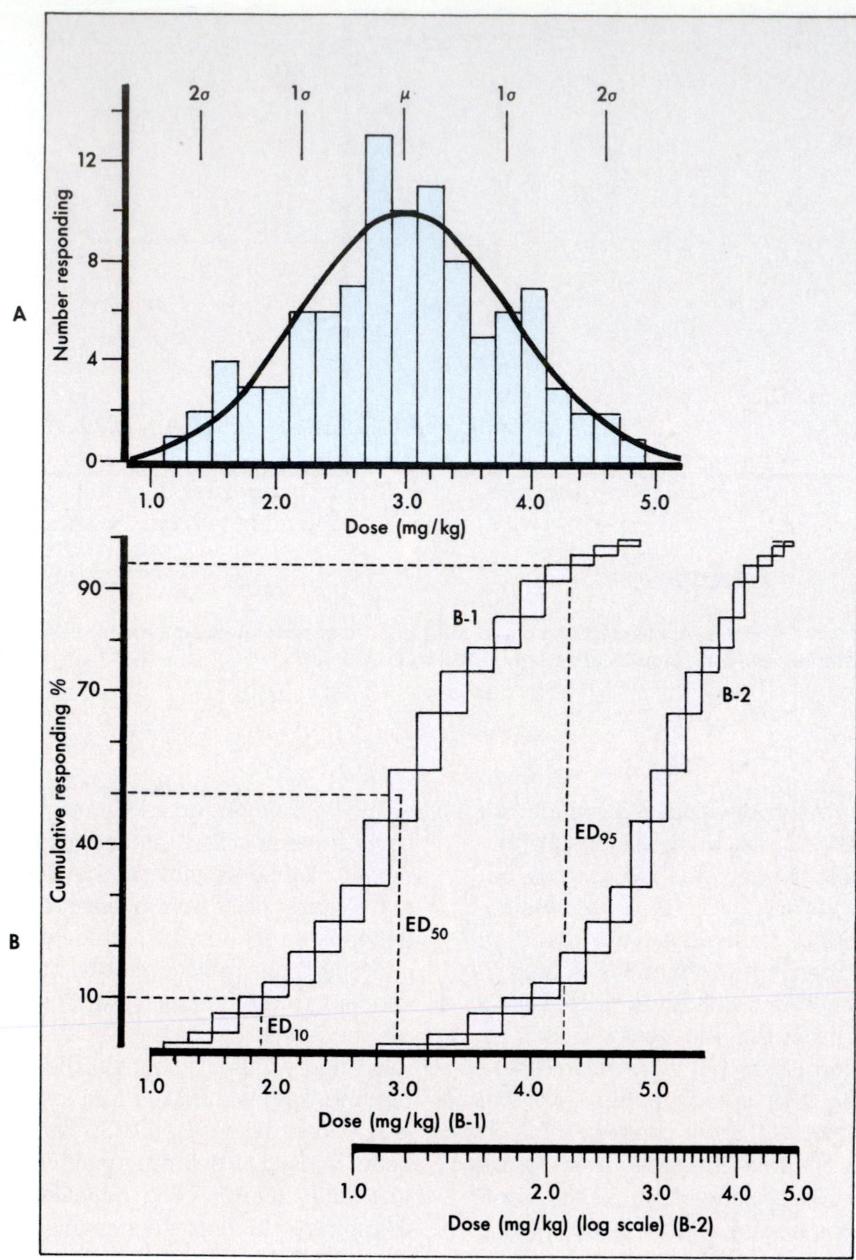

FIGURE 3-3 Quantal effects. Typical set of data after administration of increasing doses of drug to a group of subjects and observation of minimum dose at which each subject responds. Data shown are for 100 subjects; dose increased in 0.2 mg/kg of body weight increments. Mean (μ) (and median) dose is 3.0 mg/kg; standard deviation ($\bar{v}$) is 0.8 mg/kg. **A,** Results plotted as histogram *(bar graph)* showing number responding at each dose; smooth curve is normal distribution function calculated for μ of 3.0 and $\bar{v}$ of 0.8. **B,** Data of **A** replotted as cumulative percentage responding versus dose with dose shown in B-1 on arithmetic scale (as in **A**) and in B-2 on logarithmic scale. The reason for showing two dose scales is discussed in the text. ED (effective dose) values are shown for doses at which 10%, 50%, or 95% of subjects respond.

with most of the subjects clustered about the median value (half of the subjects on either side).

It is usually not possible to know what type of statistical distribution the experimental data are likely to follow. The normal or gaussian distribution often is encountered, however, and is used here to explain several features of concentration–response or dose–response curves as applied to quantal effects. A set of typical quantal dose–response data is shown in Figure 3-3, *A*. One hundred subjects received increasing doses of a drug until all the subjects responded. The number responding is plotted against the minimum dose needed to obtain the response, resulting in the histogram.

One of the first steps with a set of data such as this is to decide what statistical distribution can be used to represent the spread in the data. Because the results in the example have a mean of 3.0 mg of drug per kilogram of body weight and a standard deviation of 0.8 mg drug/kg body weight, one approach is to calculate the normal distribution function for such a mean and standard deviation and compare the shape of the normal function with that of the histogram. The smooth curve is the calculated normal function, with the shape giving reasonably good agreement with the shape of the histogram. Thus the statistical parameters of the normal distribution can be used with reasonably good reliability to predict the range of variability expected with this drug for use with the general population.

The histogram or normal distribution function is not a practical form in which to use dose–response data. A more linearized presentation of the data is desirous. Linearization can be accomplished in several ways, one of which is to replot the data as the *cumulative* percentage responding versus the dose, as shown in Figure 3-3, *B-1*. This converts the bell-shaped curve of Figure 3-3, *A*, into an S-shaped plot, with the region between, approximately 20% and 80%, forming essentially a straight line. This transformation from a histogram to an S-shaped cumulative response arithmetic plot has a firm theoretical basis.

Quantal response data often are presented in the literature as S-shaped dose-cumulative response curves with the dose plotted on a logarithmic, rather than an arithmetic, scale (see Figure 3-3, *B-2*). Notice that the arithmetic *(B-1)* and logarithmic *(B-2)* dose scales give S-shaped cumulative plots that are essentially linear over the 20% to 80% region. The log transformation again has an empirical basis. The key factor in deciding whether the dose or the log dose gives the more accurate representation is based on the distribution function. The histogram, with the dose plotted on an arithmetic scale, agrees well with the shape of the normal distribution function, and so the cumulative curve in *B-1* is the more accurate representation. If the histogram had been plotted with the dose on a logarithmic scale and the shape had agreed more closely with that for the normal distribution function, the cumulative curve in *B-2* would be the more accurate.

There are numerous situations in which the response to a drug is skewed in one direction. For example, a drug that changes heart rate has a much larger range over which the rate can be increased than decreased without lethal consequences. Such a skewed response pattern is sometimes fitted better to a skewed distribution function, as is obtained by use of the logarithmic scale for the concentration or dose. The choice of the distribution function and whether to use an arithmetic or logarithmic scale must be determined empirically for each drug or type of drug.

The values labeled ED (see Figure 3-3) denote the **effective dose** (or effective concentration) at which 50% (ED_{50}), 95% (ED_{95}), or 10% (ED_{10}) of the subjects respond. With animal studies, a value for the lethal dose (LD_{50}) also may be obtained; this is the dose (or concentration) that causes death in 50% of the animals.

AGONISTS AND ANTAGONISTS

The term **agonist** is defined in the previous chapter as a compound that activates receptor-based processes. It is assumed that agonists bind reversibly to the receptor (see Chapter 2). The concentration–response curves for a series of agonist drugs, which bind to the same receptor subtype and produce the same maximum effect, are shown schematically in Figure 3-4. The term **potency** is used to differentiate between a series of such compounds. Drug *A* is the most potent of the four because it can produce 50% of the maximum effect with the smallest concentration of drug. Drug *D* is the least potent of the four. The most potent agent has the smallest apparent K_d and the least potent has the largest ap-

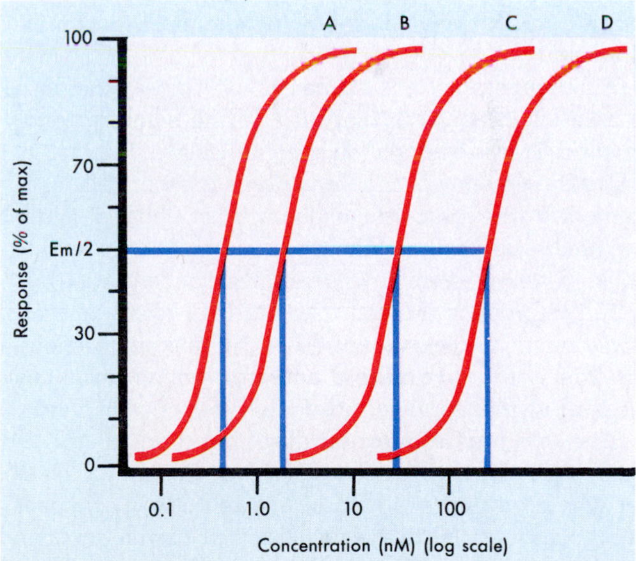

FIGURE 3-4 Schema of log concentration–response curves for a series of agonists *(A, B, C, and D)*. Note that all the drugs are shown having the same maximum response. The most potent drug produces $E_m/2$ at the lowest concentration; thus drug A is the most potent. Concentration of each drug needed to produce 50% of maximum response (ED_{50}) also shown. Concentration values are arbitrary.

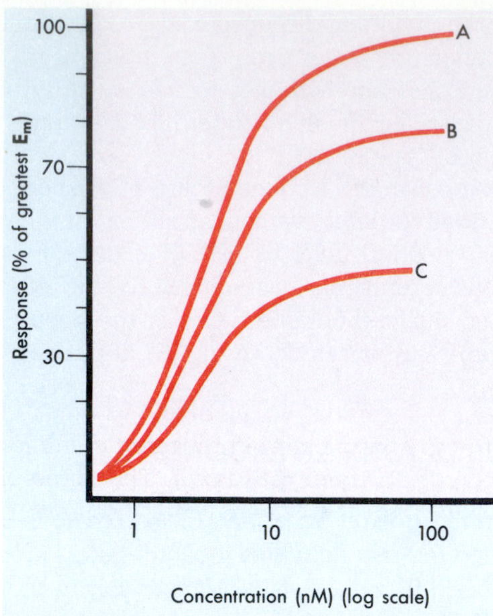

FIGURE 3-5 Series of agonists that vary in efficacy (E_m) at essentially constant potency. Drug *A* is the most efficacious and drug *C* the least. Concentrations are arbitrary but in therapeutic plasma concentration range for many drugs.

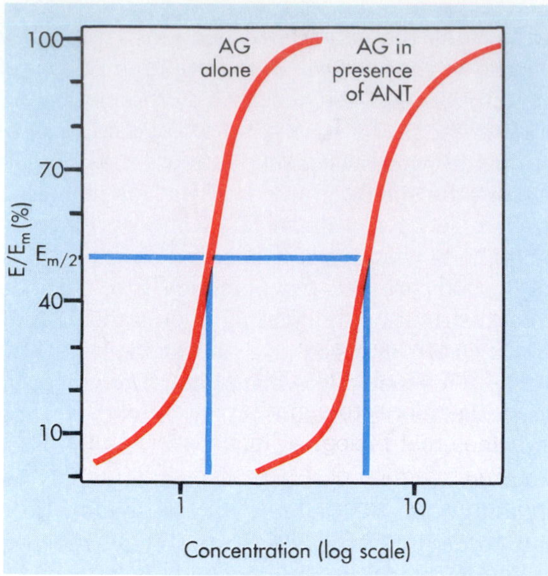

FIGURE 3-6 Competitive antagonism, where both the agonist *(AG)* and the antagonist *(ANT)* compete to bind reversibly to the same subtype of receptor sites.

parent K_d. Another term often associated with potency is that of **affinity**—the reciprocal of the apparent K_d. It should be recognized that the term "apparent K_d" is used for convenience to convey relative affinity. The term K_d should be used strictly for a ligand–receptor interaction.

Another parameter is **efficacy.** This term applies also to a series of agonists that bind to the same receptor subtype. This is exemplified schematically in Figure 3-5, where the potency of the three drugs is essentially constant, with the most efficacious agonist defined as the one that can produce the greatest maximum effect. Thus, *potency* refers to the relative concentration required to produce a given magnitude of effect, and *efficacy* refers to the magnitude of the maximum effect. An older term is **intrinsic activity,** which describes the relative maximum effects for a series of compounds.

The term **partial agonist** describes drugs of low efficacy that do not produce a very large maximum effect yet where all the receptors of a given subtype appear to be occupied. Further explanation of partial agonists depends on the development of a better molecular level understanding of the relationship between receptor occupancy and stimulus for such drugs. These drugs are also weak antagonists.

Agonist drugs may compete with endogenous ligands, transmitters, or substrates for receptor binding sites. However, the concentrations of the endogenous compounds usually are not known or else they vary considerably at the receptor site, and so this type of competitive binding is addressed only qualitatively.

Antagonists are defined in the previous chapter as compounds that inhibit or block receptor activity. The main classifications of antagonists are competitive/noncompetitive and reversible/irreversible. Other terminology is proposed to describe certain antagonist drugs, but only the main types are given here. In competitive antagonism, the antagonist and an agonist compete for reversible binding to the same receptor sites. The log concentration–effect curve for the agonist is displaced to higher concentrations by the presence of the antagonist (Figure 3-6). The action of a competitive antagonist can be overcome by use of an excess of agonist, essentially to displace the antagonist molecules from the vicinity of the receptor site.

Other forms of antagonism by drugs can be characterized as not capable of being reversed by excess agonist. With noncompetitive antagonists, the result is typically a decrease in the maximum effect obtainable by the agonist, though some shift to slightly higher agonist concentrations also may be needed to obtain a given magnitude of effect in the presence of the antagonist. Noncompetitive or other forms of antagonism take place by the antagonist binding to other sites on the receptor from where the agonist binds. For example, certain toxins and drugs are believed to bind to the ion channel of the γ-aminobutyric acid (GABA) receptor and to block the channel much as a cork plugs the opening of a bottle. The antagonist binding in such cases may be very strong but may eventually show reversibility. Other antagonists may bind irreversibly, especially those that produce irreversible inhibition of enzymes.

The potency of some antagonists, particularly those that act by inhibiting the activity of an enzyme, are often expressed as the **I_{50} value.** This is simply the concentration of antagonist needed to elicit 50% inhibition of enzyme activity.

SPARE RECEPTORS

Frequently, the measured biological response elicited by a compound binding to receptors is proportional to the fraction of receptors that are occupied. Usually, however, a maximal biological response is achieved when only a small fraction of the receptors are occupied. This phenomenon is referred to as a situation involving "spare" receptors. It usually occurs when the measured biological response is separated from the initial receptor-triggering event by several intervening amplification steps, one of which becomes fully activated before all the receptor molecules are occupied. For example, a receptor type produces a biological response by stimulating the production of cyclic adenosine monophosphate (cAMP). The cAMP in turn activates a protein kinase, which initiates a cascade of events ultimately leading to the measured response. In this example, submaximal concentrations of cAMP maximally activate the kinase. Thus further receptor occupancy leading to higher cAMP concentrations will not result in further kinase activity or in an increase in the measured response.

There are interesting consequences of spare receptors. The concentration–response curve is shifted to smaller ligand concentrations, as compared with the curve location for saturation of the receptor sites. Small changes in the number of receptors have no effect on the maximal response but change the sensitivity to the ligand. In addition, partial agonists may still produce a maximal biological response but probably at a higher receptor occupancy than is required for a full agonist. This is exemplified when one observes that a full agonist can produce 100% response with only 50% of the receptors occupied, if half of the total receptors are assumed to be present as spare receptors. For the partial agonist, 100% response (reduced in magnitude as compared with the maximum full agonist response) occurs when all the receptors appear to be occupied; this can easily occur at a higher fractional occupancy than is needed for the full agonist–50% spare receptor case.

SPECIAL EFFECTS

The development of tolerance and the placebo effect are two experimentally observed conditions that do not fit into the receptor-occupancy scheme of drug response.

Narcotic analgesics, opioids, and some other drugs that act primarily on the central nervous system may after one or more doses bring about a dampened response in which the magnitude of effect is decreased for subsequent doses of the same size as the initial dose. The dampened response is called **tolerance.** Some types of tolerance may be the result of changes in the concentration of drug at the receptor site and evolve from pharmacokinetic considerations discussed in Chapter 4. Other types of tolerance may be caused by changes that are receptor mediated. A name for tolerance that is manifest by rapid repeated administration of certain drugs is **tachyphylaxis.** The forms of drug tolerance and their management are discussed further in the relevant drug chapters.

The **placebo effect** is a usually beneficial therapeutic result that apparently arises from psychological factors. If a patient is told that this new compound will bring considerable beneficial changes—but unknown to the patient is an inert material instead of the new compound—beneficial effects are often observed in as many as 35% of subjects. This placebo effect is not predictable but can be a contributing factor to benefit the clinical condition of a patient.

SUMMARY

Although an exact quantitative expression that relates drug response to drug concentration remains to be developed, the receptor occupancy theory provides a useful working model. For the types of response that vary continuously with the concentration of drug (graded response), the key variable is the magnitude of effect. For the all-or-none case frequency becomes the key variable. Classification of drugs as to whether they act as agonists, partial agonists, antagonists, or some other category and concepts of potency, efficacy, competitive/noncompetitive antagonists, tolerance, and the placebo effect all help to provide some organizational framework applicable to many classes of drugs.

REFERENCES

Ariens EJ, Simonis AM, van Rossum JM: Drug-receptor interaction and relation between stimulus and effect. In Ariens EJ, editor: *Molecular pharmacology,* vol 1, 1964, Academic Press.

Goldstein A: *Biostatistics,* New York, 1971, Macmillan Co.

Paton WDM: A theory of drug action based on the rate of drug-receptor combination, *Proc R Soc* 154B:21, 1961.

Stephenson RP: A modification of receptor theory, *Br J Pharmacol* 11:379, 1956.

SELF-ASSESSMENT QUESTIONS

1. This is a typical histogram obtained by administering various doses of a drug to patients and noting responders. Which statement(s) is/are correct?

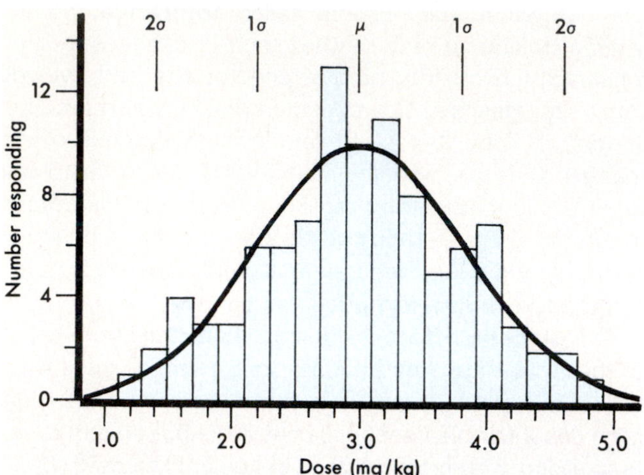

   a. A curve similar to that above can be obtained when increasing doses of a narcotic drug are administered to a group of patients and the minimum dose at which each patient responds or fails to respond to a painful stimulus is noted.
   b. The above curve is called a quantal dose–response curve.
   c. The above curve is an example of a graded dose–response curve.
   d. It is an example of a cumulative dose–response curve.
   e. a and b are correct.
2. The above graph indicates that:
   a. Approximately half of the patient population will respond to a dose of 3 mg/kg or less.
   b. Those patients on the right hand side of the graph are more sensitive to the drug than those of the left hand side of the graph.
   c. The therapeutic index or margin of safety is low.
   d. a and c are correct.
   e. All of the above are correct.
3. The curves below represent responses to several agonists that bind to the same receptor subtype and indicate that:

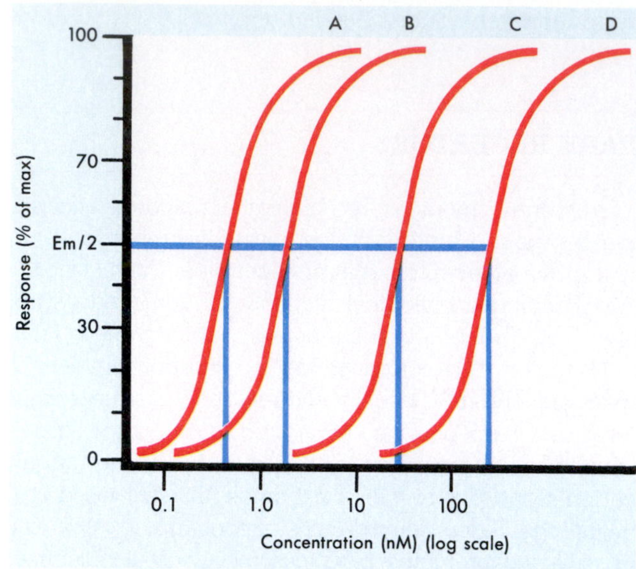

   a. Drug A is more potent than drug D.
   b. Drug A has greater efficacy than drug B has.
   c. Drug A has many spare receptors.
   d. a, b, and c are correct.
   e. b and c are correct.
4. From the above curves:
   a. Curve D could be considered to be a partial antagonist of the receptor.
   b. A curve almost identical to curve D could be obtained if a receptor subtype antagonist were mixed with agonist A.
   c. Agonist A has the largest apparent K_d.
   d. All of the above are correct.
   e. All of the above are incorrect.

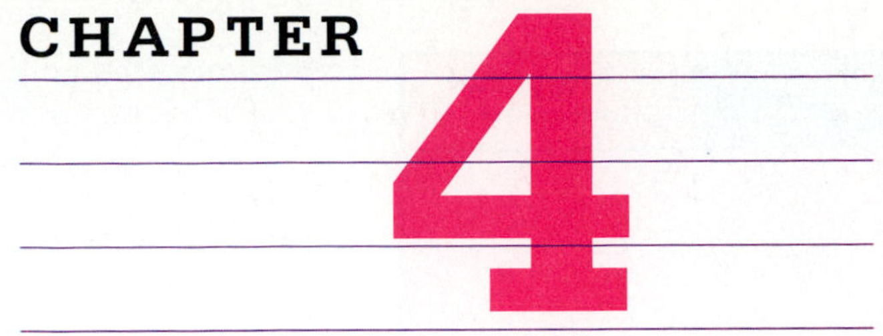

Clinical Pharmacokinetics and Dosing Schedules

THEODORE M. BRODY

DRUG CONCENTRATIONS

Before using drugs for therapeutic intervention in individual patients, the choice of drug must be made. An observable pharmacological effect or end point may be selected and the rate of drug input manipulated until this end point is achieved. With some drugs this approach works well. For example, blood pressure can be monitored in a hypertensive patient (Figure 4-1, drug *A*) and the rate of input for a drug modified until blood pressure is reduced to the desired level.

For other drugs, this approach for selecting the rate of drug input does not work. This failure is usually caused by one or more of the following factors:

1. Observable effect or end point is not possible.
2. Therapeutic index of drug is small.
3. Changes in condition of the patient require modification in rate of drug input.

For example, an antibiotic with a narrow therapeutic index is being used to treat a severe infection (Figure 4-1, drug *B*). It is often difficult to quantify the progress of antibiotic therapy because an observable effect is not available. In addition, drug *B* is assumed to have a narrow therapeutic index, which affects the patient if the antibiotic concentration becomes excessive. Another example in which the site of inflammation may be in a major organ and thus not accessible even for visual observation is shown (Figure 4-1, drug *C*). Thus, for drug *C* an observable effect again is not possible.

ABBREVIATIONS	
C_{ss}	steady state clearance
IM	intramuscular, intramuscularly
IV	intravenous, intravenously
SC	subcutaneous, subcutaneously
$t_{1/2}$	half-life
T	dosing interval

Another factor that could necessitate adjustments in the rates of input of drugs *A, B,* or *C* is a change in the condition of the patient. If each drug is eliminated from the body through the kidneys and the patient's kidney function changes, the rate of input of drugs *A, B,* or *C* will need modification. Reasons for this are discussed later in this chapter. The point here is that the lack of an observable effect for drugs *B* and *C* could cause the adjustments in drug input rates to be implemented and without knowing whether such changes will benefit the patient.

An alternative approach, also listed in Figure 4-1, is to define a target concentration of drug rather than an observable effect as the end point. The **plasma concentration** of drug is usually selected because patient tissue samples cannot be obtained (see Figure 4-1, drug *C*) or the location of the specific site to be sampled may be uncertain (see Figure 4-1, drug *B*). Thus, for drugs in which an observable effect is not available or where the **therapeutic index** (toxic : therapeutic concentration ratio) is less than about 2.5, a target plasma concentration of drug can be a useful guideline for achieving the therapeutic response without incurring toxic side effects. Similarly, a target level drug concentration in plasma can be used to guide modifications in drug input rates needed to compensate for changes in patient conditions that bring about slower or faster rates of drug disappearance.

The major goals of this chapter are listed as follows:

1. Description of factors that control the plasma concentration of drug
2. Showing how plasma concentration of drug changes with time for different routes and schedules of drug administration.
3. Demonstration of how drug input rates and dosing schedules can be developed or modified on a

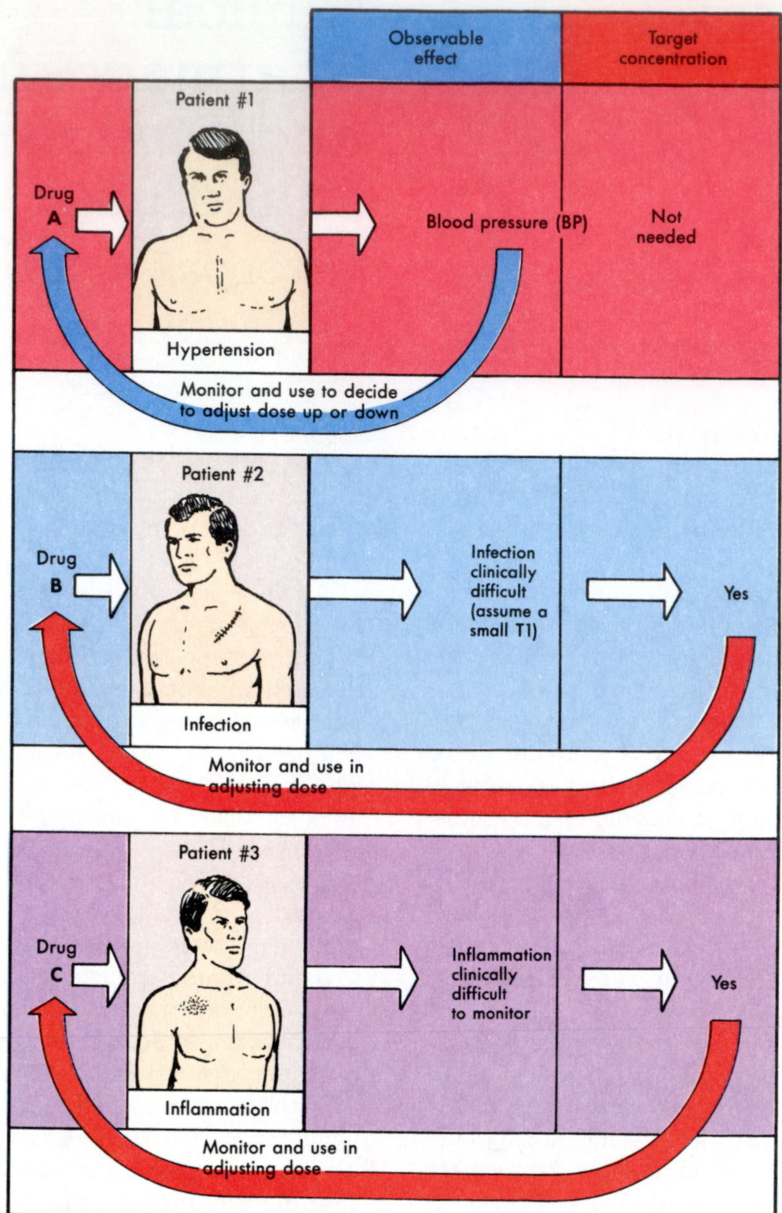

FIGURE 4-1 Concept of target plasma concentration of drug as an alternative approach to use of observable effect for determining if drug input rate is sufficient or needs to be modified. *TI,* Therapeutic index.

rational basis to achieve the plasma target concentration of drug

In most clinical situations, it is desirable to maintain the magnitude of pharmacological response at the target level for prolonged periods. To accomplish this, the plasma concentration of drug must also be maintained near a target level over the same period. Multiple doses or continuous administration of drug is required, with dose size and frequency of administration constituting the **dosing schedule** or **dosing regimen.** In providing instructions for the treatment of a patient, the dosing schedule, the choice of drug, and the mode and route of administration must be specified. Pharmacokinetic considerations have a major role in establishing the dosing schedule, or in adjusting an existing schedule, to increase effectiveness of the drug or to reduce symptoms of toxicity.

Before addressing how to design or adjust a dosing schedule, several key pharmacokinetic parameters and principles must be described. For clarity, a single acute dose of drug is presented here and used in a later part of this chapter for the design or modification of multiple dosing regimens. The relevant pharmacokinetic concepts and parameters can be developed and used in the rational design of dosing schedules from several perspectives. The emphasis in this chapter is to stress the physical meaning of the principles and parameters and also to provide sufficient mathematical background for those readers who desire a somewhat greater in-depth coverage. The key equations are enclosed in boxes to highlight their importance.

ROUTES OF ADMINISTRATION

Major routes of drug administration are divided into (1) **enteral,** those drugs entering the body via the gastrointestinal (GI) tract and (2) **parenteral,** those entering the body by a route other than the GI tract. The main routes are given in Table 4-1. The oral route is the most widely prescribed because it can be conveniently used by the patient. However, poor absorption in the GI tract, first-pass destruction in the liver, delays in stomach emptying, degradation by stomach acidity, and complexation with food may preclude oral administration. Intramuscular (IM) and subcutaneous (SC) routes bypass these problems. In many cases absorption into the circulatory system is rapid for drugs given by the intramuscular (IM) route and only slightly slower for subcutaneously (SC) administered compounds. The intravenous (IV) route advantage is a rapid onset of action as well as a controlled rate of administration; however, this is countered by the disadvantages of possible infection, coagulation problems, and a greater incidence of anaphylactoid reactions. Most drugs given by injection, especially by the IV route, require administration by a trained person.

The major routes are reviewed in terms of the relevant pharmacokinetic concepts and the time course of plasma concentration of drug. Chapter 6 describes approaches to drug delivery and targeting of drugs to specific organs or tissues.

DOSE ADJUSTMENT FOR SIZE OF PATIENT

The average male adult weighs approximately 70 kg and has a body surface area of 1.7 square meters. The dosage of drug often is scaled to give a constant mg/kg of body weight for adults of different size. For some drugs, and especially with children, the scaling works better when based on mg/m^2 of body surface area. Body surface area correlates with cardiac output and glomerular filtration rate better than body weight does. Body weight is still favored by many clinicians, however. Because the therapeutic plasma concentration can cover a considerable range without evidence of toxicity or ineffectiveness, many drugs require only gross scaling.

Table 4-1 Main Routes of Drug Administration

PER OS, BY MOUTH	
Oral	(Swallowed)
Sublingual	(Under the tongue)
Buccal	(In the cheek pouch)
INJECTION	
IV	(Intravenous)
IM	(Intramuscular)
SC	(Subcutaneous)
IA	(Intraarterial)
Intrathecal	(Into subarachnoid space)
PULMONARY	
RECTAL	
TOPICAL	

SINGLE DOSES

Single-Dose IV Injection and Plasma Concentration of Drug

If a drug is injected as a single bolus over 5 to 30 seconds into a vein and blood samples are taken periodically and analyzed for unchanged drug, the results appear as in Figure 4-2, *A.* The concentration will be greatest a few minutes after injection, when the distribution of drug throughout the circulatory system has equilibrated. This initial mixing of drug and blood is essentially completed after several passes through the heart. Drug leaves the plasma by a variety of processes, as follows:

1. Slow distribution across membranes to tissue or other body fluids
2. Elimination of unchanged drug by renal or biliary routes
3. Exhalation through the pulmonary pathway if the drug is volatile
4. Metabolism to other active or inactive compounds

Some of the drug in the plasma is bound to plasma proteins or other plasma constituents; this binding equilibrium is reached very rapidly. Similarly, a considerable fraction of the injected dose may pass through capillary walls and bind to extravascular tissue. Tissue binding also reaches equilibrium in a short time. The values of drug concentration plotted on the vertical scale in Figure 4-2, *A,* represent the sum of free drug and bound drug.

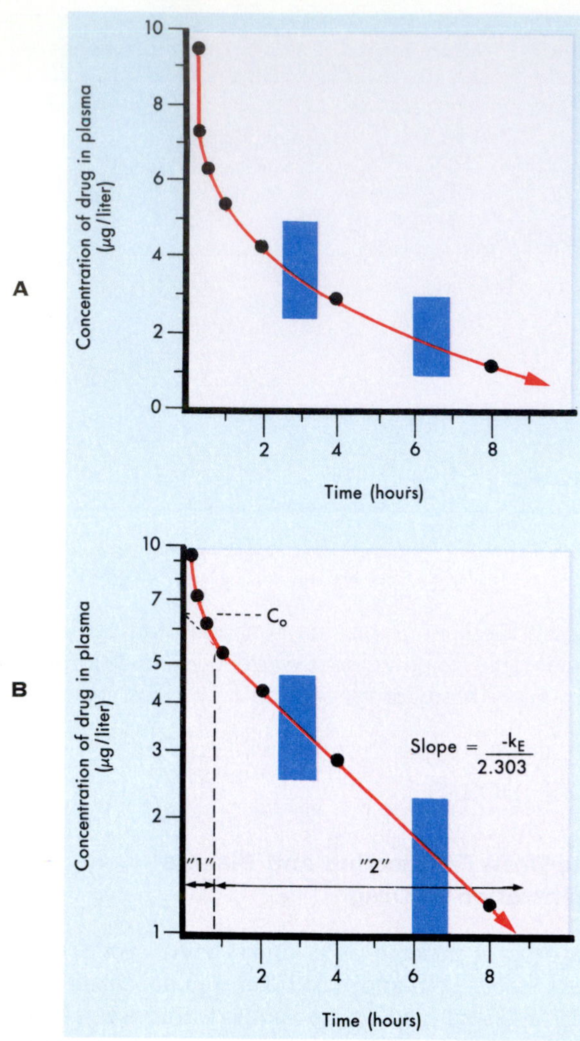

FIGURE 4-2 Plasma or serum concentration of drug as a function of time after IV injection of a single bolus over 5 to 30 seconds. **A,** Arithmetic plot. **B,** Same data with concentrations plotted on a logarithmic scale. The *1* represents the distribution (or alpha) phase and *2* the elimination-metabolism (or beta) phase. Fractional decrease in concentration is constant for a fixed time interval during the straight-line portion of **B,** shown here as an 18.6% decrease for any 1-hour period *(shaded areas).*

The data in Figure 4-2, *A,* can be presented in a more useful format if the concentrations are plotted on a logarithmic scale (Figure 4-2, *B*), resulting in data points on a straight line. The portion marked *"1"* represents the **distribution phase** (also called **alpha phase**), wherein the main process is redistribution of drug across membranes and into body regions that are *not* well perfused by capillary beds. In phase 2 **(beta phase** or **elimination/metabolism phase),** distribution is supplanted by elimination and metabolism as the principal influences governing the gradual decrease in the plasma concentration of drug. In many clinical situations the duration of time of the distribution phase is very short compared with that of the elimination and metabolism phase. Thus the distribution phase can be minimized in many clinical situations.

If the distribution phase in Figure 4-2, *A* or *B,* is neglected, the equation of the line becomes

$$C(t) = C_0\, e^{-k_E t} \qquad (1)$$

where

$C(t)$ = Concentration of drug in the plasma as a function of time

C_0 = Concentration at time zero

e = Base for natural logarithms

k_E = First-order rate constant for the elimination/metabolism phase

t = Time

Equation 1 is a curve when plotted on an arithmetic scale (Figure 4-2, *A*); however, equation 1 becomes a straight line when plotted on a semilogarithmic scale (Figure 4-2, *B*). This is evident by taking the natural logarithm (ln, base *e*) of each side of equation 1 to give equation 2 and then converting from natural (ln, base *e*) to common (log, base 10) logarithms in equation 3, using the relationship that ln × equals (2.303)(log *x*) and noting that ln *e* is 1.0.

$$\ln C(t) = \ln C_0 + (-k_E\, t) \ln\ e \qquad (2)$$

$$\log C(t) = \log C_0 - \frac{k_E t}{2.303} \qquad (3)$$

Thus, from equation 3, a plot of log C(t) versus t (Figure 4-2, *B*) should be a straight line of slope $-k_E/2.303$ and concentration axis intercept log C_0. Both k_E and C_0 can be obtained from such a plot, provided that the data can be represented by a linear relationship. A characteristic of an equation 1 type of curve is that *for a given duration the fractional change in concentration is fixed and independent of the time at which the interval is begun.* Thus, for an interval of 4 hours, the fractional change in concentration is the same whether the interval is started at 1, 3, 5, 8, or some other number of hours after injection.

In situations where the elimination-metabolism is rapid, the error in describing C(t) becomes appreciable when the distribution phase is omitted. Therefore, the expression for C(t) with both the distribution and the elimination/metabolism phases included is given as

$$C(t) = C_0^d\, e^{-k_d t} + C_0\, e^{-k_E t} \qquad (4)$$

where k_d is the first-order rate constant for the distribution processes and $C_0^{\,d}$ is the extrapolated time zero-concentration component for the distribution phase.

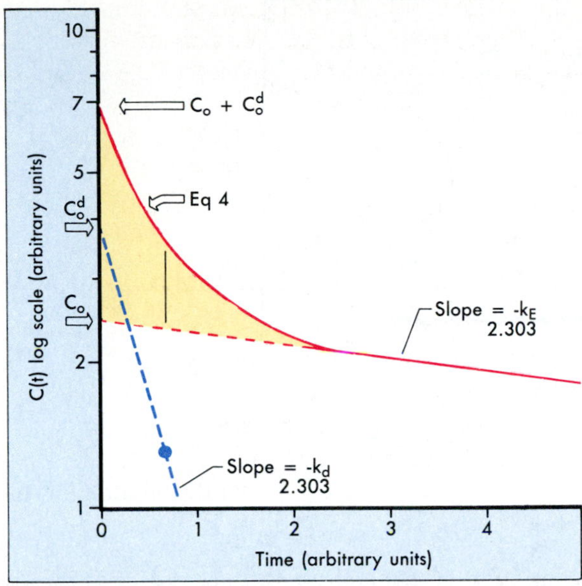

FIGURE 4-3 Semilogarithmic plot of plasma concentration of drug versus time where the distribution phase is included. Solid line represents equation 4 with terms for distribution and elimination-metabolism. The solid line can be obtained by nonlinear curve fitting of the data points (not shown) to equation 4 using one of the many available computer programs. Equation 4 can also be obtained by graphical means in which extrapolation of the linear portion of the data (elimination-metabolism phase) is used to obtain C_0 and k_E. The differences between the data points and the extrapolated line in the distribution phase (*double arrow vertical line at 0.65 time units* and plotted as 1.3 concentration units) *(shaded area)* are plotted and extrapolated linearly to obtain $C_0{}^d$ and k_d.

The actual concentration of drug at time zero is the sum of $C_0{}^d$ and C_0. Equation 4 and each of the component terms are plotted in Figure 4-3. The meaning of each of the parameters can be understood more clearly (see Figure 4-3). It is an inherent assumption that the distribution occurs much more rapidly than the elimination-metabolism, and so k_d is much greater than k_E. Therefore the distribution term becomes zero after only a small portion of the dose is eliminated or metabolized, and equation 4 reduces to equation 1 at these longer times. By back extrapolation of the linear postdistribution data, the value of C_0 can be obtained, whereas k_E can be determined from the slope. The concentration component responsible for the distribution phase (shaded area in Figure 4-3) is obtained as the difference between the actual concentration and the extrapolated elimination-metabolism line, and this difference is plotted to give the line of slope $(-)k_d/2.303$ and intercept $C_0{}^d$. Because C(t) for many drugs can be described adequately in terms of the monoexponential of equation 1, the remainder of this chapter deals only with the post-distribution phase and equation 1.

Rate Constants and Half-Lives

The monoexponential equation 1 for C(t) was given earlier but without any explanation of how such an expression is developed and what functional meaning is inherent in the derivation. Experimental data for many drugs show that the rates of drug elimination, metabolism, absorption, and distribution generally are directly proportional to concentration. Such a process follows **first-order kinetics** because the rate varies with the first power of the concentration. This is shown quantitatively as:

$$\frac{dC(t)}{dt} = -k_E\, C(t) \tag{5}$$

where dC(t)/dt is the rate of change of concentration, and k_E is the proportionality constant, also called **rate constant.** The negative sign denotes that the concentration is being decreased by elimination-metabolism.

Rate processes also can occur through **zero-order kinetics** where the rate is independent of the concentration. Two prominent examples are the metabolism of ethanol and the metabolism of aspirin at high doses. Under such conditions that process becomes saturated and the rate of metabolism becomes independent of the concentration of drug.

For those who desire an in-depth explanation of the derivation of equation 1, notice that equation 5 can be rearranged and integrated to obtain equation 1 as:

$$\frac{dC(t)}{C(t)} = -k_E\, dt \tag{6}$$

$$\int_{C_o}^{C(t)} \frac{dC(t)}{C(t)} = -k_E \int_o^t dt \tag{7}$$

$$\ln C(t) - \ln C_0 = -k_E t \tag{8}$$

$$C(t) = C_0\, e^{-k_E t} \tag{1}$$

In the above expression, k_E has the units of time^{-1}. Now any first-order rate constant is related to the half-life of the process by the following expression:

$$k = \frac{0.70^*}{t_{1/2}} \tag{9}$$

That equation 9 is correct is shown by expressing the time in equation 1 in terms of the number of half-lives ($n\ t_{1/2}$) to give:

$$\frac{C(t)}{C_0} = e^{-k_E n t_{1/2}} \tag{10}$$

*Rounded off from 0.693.

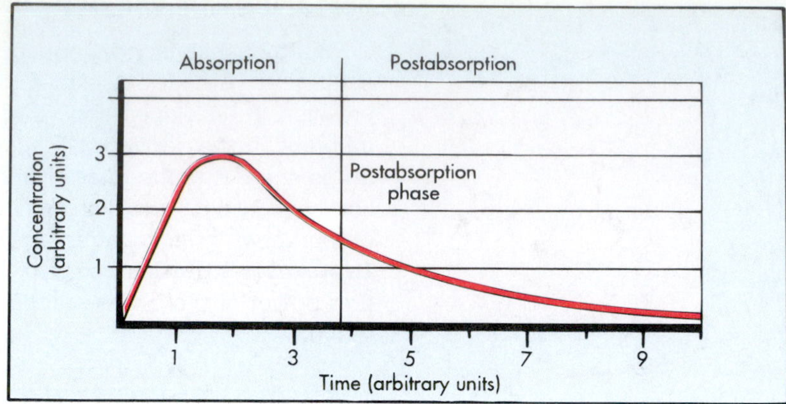

FIGURE 4-4 Typical profile for plasma concentration of drug versus time after oral administration and with the usual condition that the rate constant for drug absorption is at least 10 times larger than that for drug elimination-metabolism.

Half-life is defined as the time it takes for the concentration to decrease to half the value it had at the start of the time interval. Thus, by definition $C(t)/C_0$ is 0.5 and n is 1.0 in equation 10. Taking the ln of each side gives $0.7 = -k_E\ t_{1/2}$, which can be rearranged to equation 9 for k_E. Notice that the ln of 2 is 0.693 but is rounded off here to 0.70 and that the half-life and k_E are constants that do not change with concentration as long as the plot of log C(t) versus t is a straight line. The value of $t_{1/2}$ can be read directly from a graph of log C(t) versus t as shown in the example with Figure 4-8. Values of $t_{1/2}$ for the elimination-metabolism phase range in practice from several minutes to days or longer for different drugs. In addition, the $t_{1/2}$ may vary widely between patients receiving the same dose or in some cases can vary with dose in a given patient.

Single Oral Dose and Plasma Concentration of Drug

The plot of C(t) versus time after oral administration is different from that after IV injection only during the drug absorption phase. The two plots become identical for the postabsorption or elimination-metabolism phase. A typical plot of the plasma concentration of drug versus time after oral administration is shown in Figure 4-4. Initially there is no drug in the plasma because the preparation must be swallowed, undergo dissolution if administered as a tablet, be absorbed in the stomach or small intestine, and await stomach emptying if absorption is mainly in the small intestine. As the plasma concentration of drug increases because of rapid absorption, the rate of elimination-metabolism also increases because elimination and metabolism usually are **first-order processes** where the rates increase directly with increasing concentration of drug. The peak concentration is reached when the rates of absorption and disappearance are equal. The expression for the plasma concentration of drug and how the concentration changes with time is given in equation 11.

$$C(t) = \frac{C_0\ k_a\ F}{(k_a - k_E)}\ (e^{-k_E t} - e^{-k_a t}) \qquad \textbf{(11)}$$

In this expression, k_a is the first-order rate constant for absorption of drug in the stomach or intestine and F is the fraction of the dose that is absorbed and enters the systemic circulation. For a drug to be useful, k_a must be at least 10 times larger than k_E; otherwise the drug will disappear as soon as it enters the systemic circulation and the concentration will not increase to therapeutically useful levels. The definition of F, the **bioavailability,** is discussed later in this chapter. The experimental determination of k_a is difficult, and a knowledge of the absorption rate constant is usually of little value clinically. However, one can still obtain the half-life corresponding to k_E from data in the postabsorptive phase by plotting log C(t) versus t and obtaining the slope of the linear portion.

Binding of Drug to Plasma Constituents

The rates of drug disappearance and the concentration of free unbound drug available to the site of action are influenced greatly if a significant portion of the dose is bound to plasma constituents. In general, clinical laboratory assays for plasma drug concentrations are based on the total (bound plus unbound) concentration of drug. A knowledge of the concentration of free drug would be most useful clinically for those drugs that are highly bound to plasma components because it is only the free drug that is available to interact at the receptor. However, the range of therapeutic concentrations of

DRUGS THAT BIND APPRECIABLY TO SERUM OR PLASMA CONSTITUENTS

BIND PRIMARILY TO ALBUMIN	BIND PRIMARILY TO α_1-ACID GLYCOPROTEIN	BIND PRIMARILY TO LIPOPROTEINS
barbiturates	alprenolol	amitriptyline
benzodiazepines	bupivacaine	nortriptyline
bilirubin*	desmethylperazine	
digotoxin	dipyridamole	
fatty acids*	disopyramide	
penicillins	etidocaine	
phenytoin	imipramine	
phenylbutazone	lidocaine	
probenecid	methadone	
streptomycin		
sulfonamides	prazosin	
tetracycline	propranolol	
tolbutamide	quinidine	
valproic acid	verapamil	
warfarin		

*May displace drugs in some disease states.

free drug for highly bound compounds is extremely narrow and often beyond the sensitivity limits of available assays.

The binding of drugs to plasma or serum constituents involves primarily albumin, α_1-acid glycoprotein, or lipoprotein (see box). Serum albumin is the most abundant protein in human plasma, with a normal concentration of approximately 4.0 g/100 ml. This material is synthesized in the liver at roughly 140 mg/kg of body weight/day under normal conditions but often at greatly decreased rates in certain disease states. Albumin has a molecular weight of 68,000 daltons, no appreciable carbohydrate component, and a net electrical charge of 19 negative groups of pH 7.4. Many acidic drugs bind strongly to albumin, but because of the normally high concentration of plasma albumin, the binding does not saturate the sites. Basic drugs bind primarily to α_1-acid glycoprotein, which has a molecular weight of 40,000 with 41% carbohydrate including sialic acid, and is present in plasma at a concentration of 0.08 g/100 ml. Less is known about drug binding to lipoproteins. Disease states often cause major changes in plasma albumin, α_1-acid glycoprotein concentrations, or in the binding affinities of these materials for specific drugs. Drugs that are highly bound to plasma proteins present a scenario for drug interactions that are discussed in Chapter 7. The influence of protein binding on drug disposition is covered in Chapter 5.

Volume of Distribution

The actual volume in which drug molecules are distributed within a patient's body cannot be measured. However, an **apparent volume of distribution** (V_d) can be obtained, which may be of some clinical usefulness. A method for obtaining a value for V_d is to determine the time zero concentration, C_0, after IV injection and, by using equation 12 and knowing the dose (D), to calculate V_d.

$$C_0 = \frac{D}{V_d} \tag{12}$$

If C_0 has the units of milligrams per liter and D of milligrams, then V_d would be in liters. Another method for obtaining V_d is described later in this chapter (see equation 16). In some cases it is meaningful to compare the apparent volume of distribution with typical body-water volumes. The following volumes in liters and percentage of body weight apply to adult humans:

BODY WATER	BODY WEIGHT (%)	VOLUME (APPROX. LITERS)
Plasma	4	3
Extracellular	20	14
Total body	60	45

Experimental values of the volume of distribution vary from 5 to 10 liters for drugs such as warfarin and tolbutamide to 15,000 to 40,000 liters for chloroquine and quinacrine in a 70 kg adult. How can one calculate apparent volumes of distribution grossly in excess of the total body volume? This can occur as a result of protein binding of drug and of using plasma as the sole source of samples for determination of V_d (Figure 4-5). For a drug such as warfarin that is 97% bound to plasma albumin at therapeutic concentrations, nearly all the dose initially is in the plasma, and so a plot of log plasma C(t) versus time, when extrapolated back to time zero, gives a large value for C_0 (for bound plus unbound drug). Using equation 12, $V_d = D/C_0$, we find that the resulting value of V_d is small and usually in the range of 2 to 10 liters. At the other extreme is a drug such as chloroquine, which is strongly bound to tissue sites but weakly bound to plasma proteins. Most of the dose initially is at tissue sites, thereby resulting in quite small concentrations in plasma samples. Thus a plot of log-plasma C(t) versus time and will give a small value to C_0 (for bound plus unbound drug), which can result in apparent V_d values greatly in excess of the total body volume.

The volume of distribution can serve as a guide in determining whether a drug is bound primarily to plasma or tissue sites and possibly whether the drug is distributed primarily into plasma or into extracellular spaces.

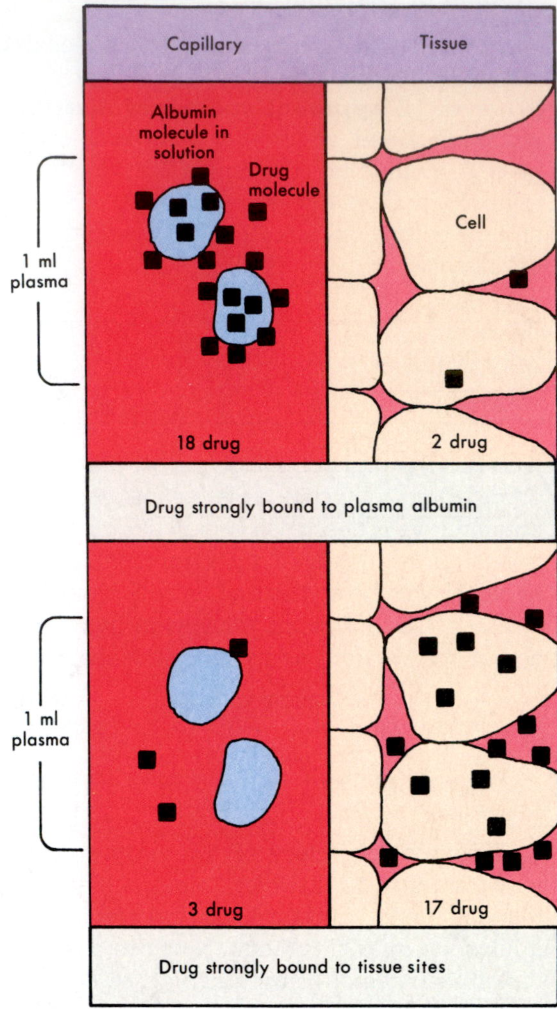

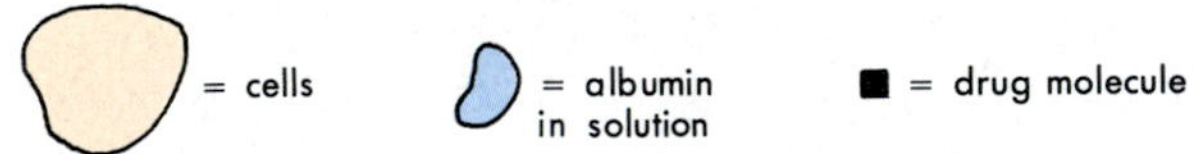

FIGURE 4-5 Influence of drug binding to plasma protein versus tissue sites on apparent volume of distribution. Numbers represent relative quantity of drug in 1 ml of plasma as compared with adjacent tissue. Only the plasma is sampled to determine V_d and the albumin-bound drug is included in the sample.

Drug Clearance

Clearance is a pharmacokinetic parameter that is useful clinically for describing the capability of the patient to dispose of a particular drug. The discussion in this chapter is limited to **total body clearance.** Chapter 5 includes descriptions of renal clearance, hepatic clearance, and other specific organ or specific mechanisms of clearance that constitute total body clearance.

The plot of plasma C(t) versus time (see Figure 4-2) shows the concentration of drug decreasing with time. The corresponding rate (such as milligrams per minute) at which drug is being removed from the plasma can be indicated as $dX(t)/dt$, where $X(t)$ represents the quantity (mg) of drug. The rate of drug removal by various processes is assumed to follow first-order kinetics with respect to the plasma concentration of drug, and the total body clearance can be perceived as the proportionality constant between the rate and the concentration. Thus,

$$\frac{dX(t)}{dt} = (\text{clearance})_p\, C(t) = (Cl)_p\, C(t) \qquad \textbf{(13)}$$

where p indicates "total body" removal from the **plasma.** Total body clearance thus has the units of volume/time, such as milliliters per minute, and can be considered as the volume of plasma from which all drug molecules need to be removed each minute to achieve the rate of removal (Figure 4-6). It is sometimes easier to rearrange equation 13 to obtain equation 14 for the definition of total body clearance.

$$(Cl)_p = \frac{dX(t)/dt}{C(t)} = \frac{\text{rate of removal of drug (in mg/min)}}{\text{plasma concentration of drug (in mg/ml)}} \qquad \textbf{(14)}$$

Two methods are available for obtaining values for $(Cl)_p$ for a given drug in an individual patient. The first method requires that the half-life and the apparent volume of distribution be known and used as:

$$(Cl)_p = \frac{0.7\, V_d}{t_{1/2}} = k_E\, V_d \qquad \textbf{(15)}$$

The second method is based on obtaining an empirical solution to equation 13, as follows:

$$\int_0^{X_0} dX = X_0 = (Cl)_p \int_0^{\infty} C(t)\, dt \qquad \textbf{(16)}$$

where X_0 is the dose, or that part of the dose that enters the systemic circulation. The integral of C(t) dt is the same as the area under the curve of concentration versus time. Thus one obtains the clearance by dividing the dose that enters the systemic circulation by the area under the curve.

The area under the curve, the dose, and the value of k_E also can be used with equation 16 to obtain a value for the apparent volume of distribution.

Bioavailability and First-Pass Effect

When a drug is administered by IV injection, all the dose enters the systemic circulation, but this may not

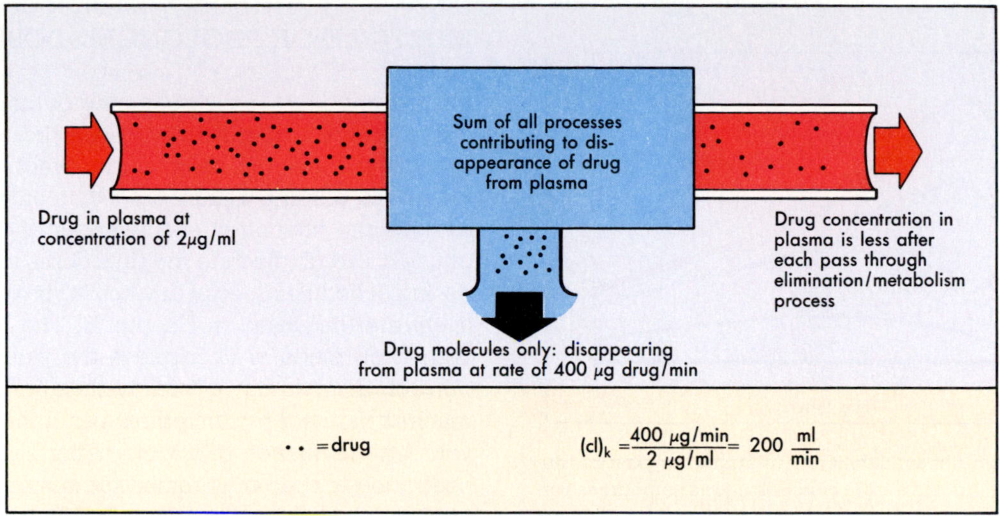

FIGURE 4-6 Concept of total body clearance of drug from plasma. Only *some* of the drug molecules disappear from the plasma on each pass of blood through kidneys, liver, or other sites that contribute to drug disappearance (elimination-metabolism). In this example, it required 200 ml of plasma to account for the amount of drug that disappears each minute (400 μg/min) at the concentration of 2 μg/ml. The total body clearance is thus 200 ml/min.

be true for drugs administered by other routes, especially for drugs given orally. Dissolution of tablets can vary greatly between manufacturers of the same drug and is a major source of differences in drug bioavailability. The fraction of the dose that enters the systemic circulation when given orally, for example, compared with that which enters when given by IV injection, is called the **bioavailability** or the **bioequivalence** (F). Physical or chemical processes that account for reduced bioavailability ($F < 1$) include poor solubility of drug or incomplete absorption of drug in the gastrointestinal tract and rapid metabolism of drug during its first pass through the liver (discussed later). Differences in bioavailability in oral preparations result from the inert ingredients present and the tableting process itself. Values of F are obtained by use of equation 17, as follows:

$$F = \frac{X_{O(oral)}}{X_{O(IV)}} = \frac{(Cl)_{P(oral)} \int_0^\infty C(t)\, dt_{(oral)}}{(Cl)_{P(IV)} \int_0^\infty C(t)\, dt_{(IV)}} \quad (17)$$

$$\text{or } F = \frac{(AUC)_{(oral)}}{(AUC)_{(IV)}}$$

AUC is the area under the curve, and the clearance is assumed to be independent of the route of administration. This assumption is valid for most drugs but is not followed in a few unexplained cases. The problem of bioavailability was first recognized in the 1970s when unexplained low plasma concentrations of digoxin, a digitalis glycoside, in several patients were traced to variable absorption from the GI tract. The digoxin was administered in tablet form as different lots from the same manufacturer or from different suppliers. Typical plots in Figure 4-7 show that the area under the curve can be considerably different. Thus, for drugs in which absorption from the GI tract is not always 100%, the drug formulations must now pass a bioavailability test that verifies that bioavailability is constant, within certain limits, among lots.

The potential problem of changes in bioavailability is a major consideration in choosing between substitution of generic compounds and specifying a brand name. If substitution of a different brand or a generic product is made and neither the physician nor the patient is aware of the substitution, the bioavailability may be changed greatly without any compensating modification made in the dose. This can in some instances have life-threatening consequences.

Low bioavailability can also result when the drug is well absorbed from the GI tract, but subsequent metabolism of the drug is high during its transit from the splanchnic capillary beds through the liver and into the systemic circulation. The drug concentration in the plasma is at its highest level during this "first pass" through the liver. Therefore, drugs that are subject to liver metabolism may encounter a very significant reduction in the concentration of active compound during this first pass. For example, the first-pass effect of lido-

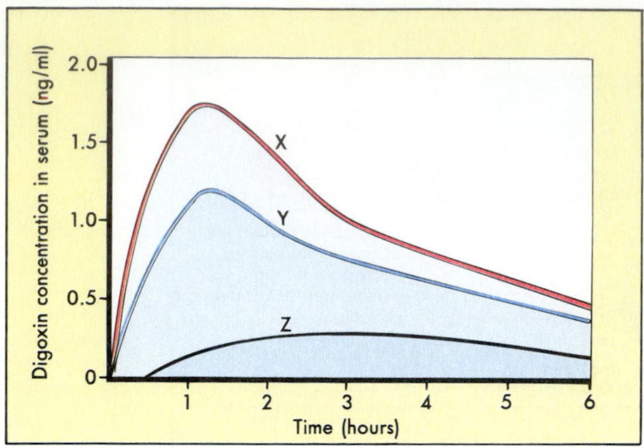

FIGURE 4-7 Before bioavailability regulations for pharmaceutical preparations, digoxin serum concentrations sometimes varied appreciably between brands and even between lot numbers of the same brand. The curves shown here are for a group of subjects receiving single 0.5 mg oral doses of each of the following digoxin tablets: *X* from company no. 1; *Y* and *Z*, two different lots, from company no. 2. The area under the curve differs greatly, thus showing that the bioavailabilities varied greatly, roughly from 0.8 to 0.4. For drugs in which the therapeutic index is less than about 2.5 and the bioavailability is less than about 0.95, arbitrary switching of brands or poor control of tableting operations by drug suppliers can result in serious situations in patients.

caine is so large that this drug is not administered orally. Some drugs that show strong first-pass effects include:

- acetylsalicylic acid (aspirin): an analgesic, anti-arthritis agent
- desipramine: an antidepressant
- hydralazine: an antihypertensive
- isoproterenol: a bronchodilator
- lidocaine: an antiarrhythmic
- methylphenidate: a central nervous system stimulant
- morphine: an analgesic
- pentazocine: an analgesic
- propoxyphene: an analgesic
- propranolol: an antihypertensive

Sample Calculations of Pharmacokinetic Parameters

Figure 4-8 is a semilogarithmic plot of a highly plasma protein–bound drug at two different doses. The slopes are parallel within the experimental error of the assays, demonstrating that the pharmacokinetics are the same at the two doses. The calculations of $t_{1/2}$, k_E, C_0, V_d, Cl_p (see equations 13 to 15), and the area under the curve is given for one of the sets of data in the figure legend.

MULTIPLE OR PROLONGED DOSING

As mentioned at the beginning of this chapter, most drugs require administration over a prolonged period to achieve the desired therapeutic effect. Two principal modes of administration are commonly employed to achieve the prolonged effectiveness: (1) continuous IV infusion and (2) discrete multiple doses on a designated dosing schedule. Special devices for prolonged drug delivery are discussed in Chapter 6. The basic objective with each mode is to increase the plasma concentration of drug until a steady-state concentration is reached that will produce the desired therapeutic effect with little evidence of toxicity. This steady-state concentration is then maintained for minutes, hours, days, or even longer as required by the clinical situation. The steady-state concentration must be maintained at greater than the minimum concentration needed to produce a pharmacological response yet below the concentration that produces toxicity. Pharmacokinetic considerations for designing or adjusting a continuous infusion or a discrete multiple dosing schedule are described in the next two sections.

Continuous Intravenous Infusion

The continuous intravenous infusion mode of administration is used when it is necessary to obtain a rapid onset of drug action and to maintain the action for an extended period under controlled conditions. Continuous infusions normally are administered in a hospital or emergency setting.

In continuous infusion, the drug is administered at a fixed rate. The plasma concentration of drug gradually increases and then plateaus at a concentration where the rate of infusion equals the total rate of elimination/metabolism. A typical plasma concentration profile is shown in Figure 4-9. The plateau (C_{ss}) is also called the **steady-state concentration** (see equation 19).

The concentration curve in Figure 4-9 is described by equation 18 for simple cases in which the distribution phase is omitted and where k_0 is the rate of infusion of drug in amount/time (that is, mg/min, mg/min/kg of body weight, or mg/min/m^2 of body surface area).

$$C(t) = \frac{k_0}{k_E V_d}(1 - e^{-k_E t}) \qquad \textbf{(18)}$$

From equation 18, C_{ss} can be described by equation 19:

$$C_{ss} = \frac{k_0}{k_E V_d} = \frac{\text{infusion rate}}{\text{total body clearance}} \qquad \textbf{(19)}$$

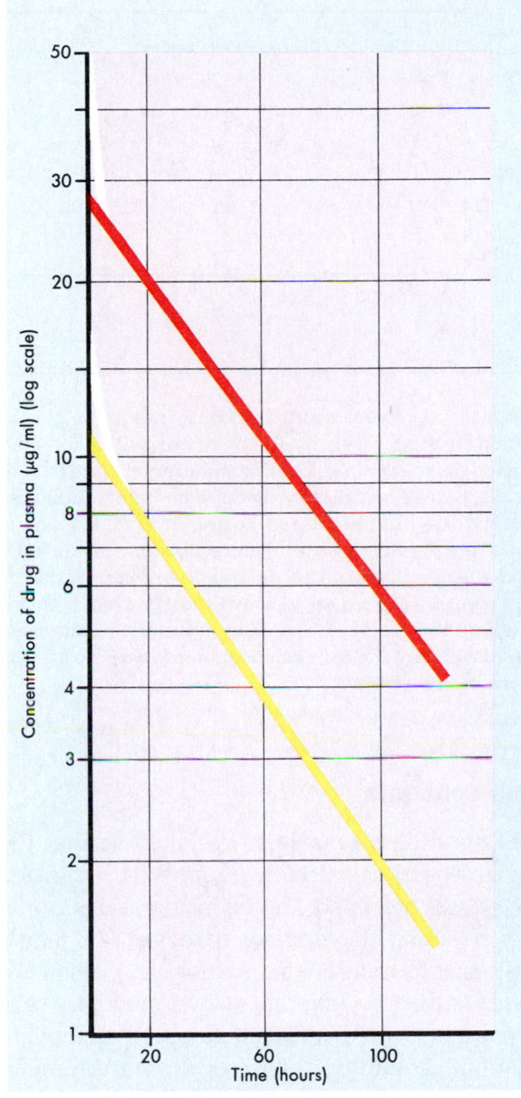

$$V_d = D/C_o = \frac{(100 \text{ mg})(1000\ \mu g/mg)}{(10.7\ \mu g/ml)} = 9{,}300 \text{ ml}$$

To get the slope read two points from the line and solve text equation 3.

At $t = 20$ hr, $C = 7.6\ \mu g/ml$

At $t = 100$ hr, $C = 1.92\ \mu g/ml$

$$\text{Thus: } \log 7.6 = \log C_o - \frac{k_E}{2.303}(20) = 0.8808$$

$$\log 1.92 = \log C_o - \frac{k_E}{2.303}(100) = 0.2833$$

$$+\frac{k_E}{2.303}(80) = 0.5975$$

$$-\text{slope} = \frac{k_E}{2.303} = 0.00746$$

$$k_E = 0.017 \text{ hr}^{-1}$$

$$t_{1/2} = \frac{0.7}{k_E} = 0.7/0.017 = 41 \text{ hr}$$

To check $t_{1/2}$ note from the plot that C is 10 μg/ml at 4 hr and 5 μg/ml at about 44 hr giving an estimate of 40 hr for $t_{1/2}$. This agrees well with the above value from the slope.

$$(Cl)_p = k_E V_d = (0.017 \text{ hr}^{-1})(9{,}300 \text{ ml}) = 158 \text{ ml/hr}$$

Area Under Curve (AUC):

$$AUC = \int C(t)\,dt = C_o\int_o^{120} e^{-k_E t}\,dt = C_o\left.\frac{e^{-k_E t}}{-k_E}\right|_0^{120} =$$

$$-\frac{10.7}{0.017}(0.13 - 1.00) = 547 \frac{\mu g,\ hr}{ml} = AUC$$

Need to add an additional 15% to correct for the drug that disappears between 120 hours and infinite hours.

FIGURE 4-8 Use of plasma concentration versus time data to determine values for key pharmacokinetic parameters. Concentrations are plotted for drug administered by IV injection as single doses of 200 mg *(red line)* and 100 mg *(yellow line)* on two separate occasions. The yellow line was fitted by the linear least-squares method on the semilogarithmic plot and extrapolated to time zero to get a C_0 of 10.7 μg/ml. White line indicates distributive phase.

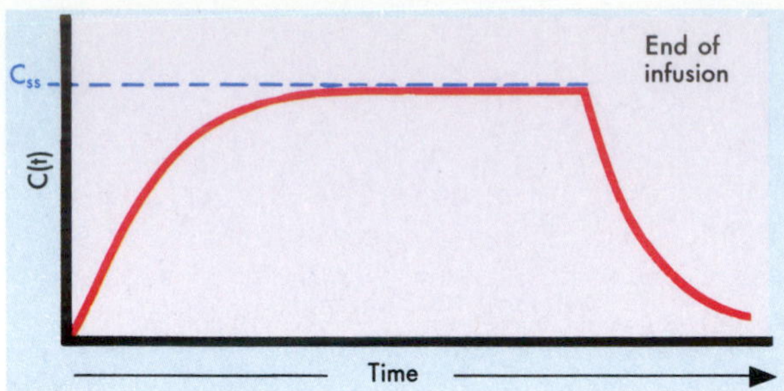

FIGURE 4-9 Typical profile showing how plasma concentration of drug varies with time for continuous IV injection at a constant rate and without a loading dose. C_{ss} is the concentration at the plateau, or steady state, where the rate of drug input equals the rate of drug disappearance. At the end of the infusion, the decay in the concentration will react as it would for any acute IV injection with C_0 being equal to C_{ss}.

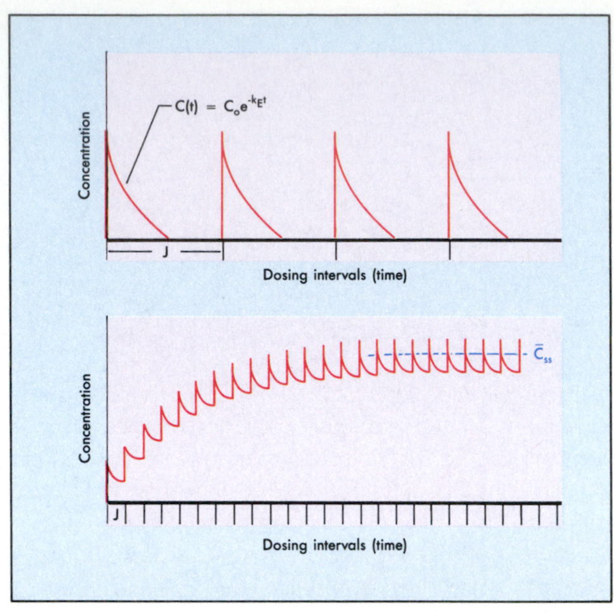

FIGURE 4-10 Discrete multiple-dosing profile of plasma concentration of drug given by IV injections with the same dose given each time. In part *A*, the dosing interval (T) is long enough so that each dose completely disappears before administration of the next dose. In part *B*, the dosing interval is much shorter so that drug from previous injection is still present when the next dose is administered. Accumulation results in part *B*, with $\overline{C}_{ss}$ representing the mean concentration of drug at the plateau level, where the mean rate of drug input equals the mean rate of drug disappearance for each dosing interval. No loading dose is shown in this profile.

There is little point in memorizing equation 19 because a functional understanding of steady state and a knowledge of the units of each term enable equation 19 to be developed as needed. Key points are as follows:

1. At steady state the rate of drug input must equal the rate of drug disappearance.
2. The input rate is the infusion rate (mg/min).
3. What is needed to convert C_{ss} in milligrams per liter to the disappearance rate in milligrams per minute?
4. The answer is a term with units of liters per minute. Clearance has those units.
5. Thus, at steady state:

$$k_0 = C_{ss}\,(Cl)_p = C_{ss}\,\frac{V_d 0.7}{t_{1/2}} \tag{20}$$

This approach of determining operational conditions and ascertaining that the units are consistent is a much more useful approach to learning and applying pharmacokinetics than simply memorizing the pharmacokinetic equations.

The plateau level concentration is influenced by the infusion rate, the drug disappearance half-life, the apparent volume of distribution, and the total body clearance. Of these factors, only the infusion rate can be modified as needed. For example, if the plateau level concentration is at 2.0 ng/ml with an infusion rate of 16 μg/hr and it is determined that the concentration is too high and that it is determined approximately 1.5 ng/ml would be better, you can achieve the lower value by decreasing the infusion rate to 12 μg/hr. A 25% reduction in infusion rate should give a 25% decrease in the plateau concentration. The length of time necessary to achieve a new plateau concentration is discussed later.

Dosing Schedule

Multiple dosing usually is specified so that the size of the dose and the dosing interval (i.e., the time between doses) are fixed. Two considerations are important in selecting the **dosing interval** (T). Smaller intervals result in minimal fluctuations in plasma concentration of drug; however, the interval must be a relatively standard number of hours to help ensure compliance by the patient. In addition, for oral dosing the milligrams per dose must be compatible with the size of the available tablets or other pharmaceutical preparations. Thus, an oral dosing schedule of 28 mg every 2.8 hours is impractical because the drug probably is unavailable as a 28 mg tablet. Clearly, a schedule of taking a tablet at 2.8-hour intervals is also impractical. More practical dosing intervals, particularly for patient compliance, are every 6, 8, 12, or 24 hours.

The plasma concentration of drug versus time is shown in Figure 4-10 for multiple dosing by repeated IV injections. T is selected so that all the drug from the previous dose disappears before the next dose is injected (see Figure 4-10, *A*). There is no accumulation of drug; therefore, no plateau or steady state is reached.

If a plateau concentration is desired, the dosing interval must be short enough so that drug from the previous dose is still present when the next dose is administered. In this way the plasma concentration gradually increases until the drug lost by elimination-metabolism during a dosing interval is equal to the dose of drug added at the start of the dosing interval. When this equality is achieved, the mean concentration for a dosing interval, $\overline{C}_{ss}$ (with the bar indicating 'mean'), has plateaued. The stepwise accumulation is exemplified by the plot of plasma concentration of drug versus time for multiple IV injections with the dosing interval roughly equivalent to the half-life of drug disappearance (see Figure 4-10, *B*). The average rate (over a dose interval) of drug input is constant at D/T. The rate of drug disappearance is very small during the first dosing interval but increases with drug concentration during subsequent intervals until the average rate of disappearance and the average rate of input are equal. For significant accumulation, the dosing interval must be at least as short as the half-life and preferably shorter.

At the plateau, the mean concentration of drug, $\overline{C}_{ss}$ again is equal to the input rate divided by the clearance, just as for continuous infusion.

$$\overline{C}_{ss} = \frac{D/T}{(Cl)_p} \quad \textbf{(21)}$$

From equation 21 it is evident that the size of the dose or the duration of the dosing interval can be changed to modify the mean plateau concentration of drug. The quantitative description of the entire curve (see Figure 4-10, *B*) for repetitive IV injections or for a modified curve for repetitive oral doses has been determined but these equations are complex and of use primarily in pharmacokinetic research studies.

Loading Dose

If all of the multiple doses are the same size, the term **maintenance dose** can be used. In certain clinical situations, however, a more rapid onset of action is required. One can achieve this by giving a much larger, or **loading, dose** just before the start of the smaller maintenance dose regimen. A single IV loading dose (bolus) is often used before starting a continuous IV infusion is started, or a parenteral or oral loading dose may be used at the start of discrete multiple dosing. Ideally, the loading dose is calculated to raise the plasma drug concentration immediately to the plateau concentration and the maintenance doses are designed to maintain the same plateau concentration. Multiplying the plateau concentration by the apparent volume of distribution results in a value for the loading dose. However, the uncertainty in the V_d in individual patients usually leads to a more conservative loading dose to prevent overshooting the plateau and encountering toxic concentrations. This is particularly important to avoid with drugs that have a small therapeutic index.

Duration of Time to Steady State

For a continuous IV infusion or a series of discrete multiple doses, the time to reach the plateau concentration or to move from one plateau concentration to another depends only on the half-life of the drug. This principle can be shown using equation 18, which describes the time course of plasma concentration of drug for a continuous infusion. After replacement of k_E with $0.7/t_{1/2}$ from equation 9 and designation of the time as *n* number of half-lives ($n\ t_{1/2}$), the exponent becomes $-0.7n$, and equation 18 reduces to

$$\frac{C(t)}{C_{ss}} = 1 - e^{-0.7n} \quad \textbf{(22)}$$

This is solved for several values for *n*, to give:

n	$C(t)/C_{ss}$
0	0
1	0.50
2	0.75
3	0.88
3.3	0.90
4	0.94
5	0.97

During each half-life, 50% of the change in concentration is achieved from the starting point to the new plateau. From a practical standpoint, 90% of the change to get to the plateau is considered as having reached the new plateau, and so the duration is simply 3 to 4 half-lives.

PRACTICAL PHARMACOKINETIC PRINCIPLES

Example 1 Figure 4-11 is a plot of plasma concentration of a drug at different times during a continuous infusion at 3 mg/min for 70 minutes. Calculate k_E, $t_{1/2}$, $(Cl)_p$, V_d, the concentration 20 minutes after the infusion is stopped; and the infusion rate and loading dose to achieve a plateau of 7 mg/L.

From the plateau concentration of 5.0 mg/L and the infusion rate of 3 mg/min and knowing that input rate must equal disappearance rate, one can find that the $(Cl)_p$ must be (3 mg/min)/(5 mg/1000 ml), or 600 ml/min. Note that the concentration reaches 50% of its plateau

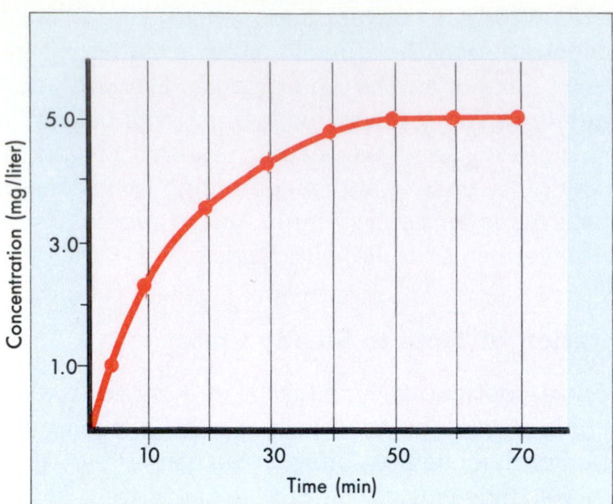

FIGURE 4-11 Data on plasma concentration of a drug at different times for an IV infusion at 3 mg/min for 70 minutes for use in example 1, for obtaining pharmacokinetic parameter values and for estimating the conditions to be used to accomplish other dosing goals.

during the first half-life, the value of 0.50 C_{ss} is 2.50 mg/L. From the graph this is achieved at 11.5 minutes after the start of the infusion. Thus $t_{1/2}$ is 11.5 minutes (relatively fast) and k_E becomes 0.061 min^{-1} from the equality of k_E and $0.7/t_{1/2}$. Because $(Cl)_p$ is k_E V_d, the value for V_d is 9.8 liters (or 10 liters). After the infusion is stopped, the concentration is described by 5.0 exp(−0.061(20)), which solves to give 1.5 mg/L. For a plateau concentration of 7 mg/L, the infusion rate should be 40% greater or 4.2 mg/min. A loading dose of 68 mg will place the concentration at 7 mg/L; a practical loading dose might be 50 mg.

Example 2 A patient has received a cardiac drug, digoxin, orally at 0.25 mg (one tablet/day) for several weeks, and symptoms of appreciable toxicity appeared recently. A blood sample was taken and assayed to give a plasma concentration of 3.2 ng/ml. This is in the toxic range. You do not want to drop the plasma concentration too low but decide to try reducing it to 1.5 ng/ml. What new dosing schedule should be used and how long will it take to reach the new plateau?

The once-a-day dosing interval is convenient; so you now specify 0.125 mg/day (one-half tablet/day); a 50% reduction in the plateau level requires a 50% decrease in dose. There are two options for reaching the lower plateau: (1) immediately switch to the 0.125 mg/day dosing rate and achieve the 1.6 ng/ml concentration in approximately four half-lives (you do not know what the half-life for digoxin is in your patient) or (2) terminate all digoxin dosing for an unknown number of days until the concentration reaches 1.6 ng/ml and then begin again at a dosing schedule of 0.125 mg/day. The second procedure undoubtedly will be more rapid, but you must determine how many days to wait. You decide to stop all digoxin dosing, wait 24 hours from the previous 3.2 ng/ml sample, and get another blood sample. The concentration now has decreased to 2.7 ng/ml or by about one sixth in a day. From equation 1, the fractional decrease each day should remain constant. Therefore a decrease of one sixth of the remaining concentration each day gives 2.25 ng/ml after day 2, 1.85 ng/ml after day 3, and 1.55 ng/ml after day 4. Therefore, by withholding drug for a total of 4 days, you can reduce the plasma concentration to 1.6 ng/ml. Because the half-life is calculated to be 3.8 days in this patient, switching to the 0.125 mg/day dosing rate without withholding drug would have required 12 to 15 days to reach the 1.6 ng/ml concentration.

An additional example is given in Chapter 5 under the section on modified renal function and drug elimination to illustrate how changing the dosing schedule compensates for a decreased drug-elimination capability by the patient.

SUMMARY

Pharmacokinetics provides a firm basis for the design of dosing regimens and for the characterization of the kinetics of drug disposition. The topic is approached here from a functional rather than a rigorous mathematical standpoint to show that pharmacokinetic considerations can be used readily in everyday clinical medicine without resorting to a large number of equations. The major points include the following:

1. Half-life
2. Clearance
3. Bioavailability and first pass
4. Results of plasma protein–binding of drugs
5. Concept of the apparent volume of distribution
6. Exponential disposition of drug (first-order decline) in which the same fraction of drug is disposed of per unit time
7. Concept that the rates of drug input and disappearance are equal at the steady-state or plateau concentrations.
8. How to modify a dosing regimen to achieve a desired change in plateau concentration
9. Concept that the time to reach the plateau depends only on the disappearance half-life of the drug
10. The use of a loading dose to accelerate the onset of the desired therapeutic effect

REFERENCES

Notari RE: *Biopharmaceutics and clinical pharmacokinetics,* ed 4 (practical aspects, worked examples), New York, 1987, Marcel Dekker.

Roland M, Tozer TN: *Clinical pharmacokinetics,* Philadelphia, 1980, Lea & Febiger.

Shargel L, Yu ABC: *Applied biopharmaceutics and pharmacokinetics,* ed2, Norwalk, Conn., 1985, Appleton-Century-Cofts.

Wilkinson GR: Clearance approaches in pharmacology, *Pharmacol Rev* 39:1, 1987.

SELF ASSESSMENT QUESTIONS

1. A drug was present in the plasma shortly after intravenous administration at a concentration of 300 μg/ml. Eight hours later, the plasma concentration was determined at 75 μg/ml. Assuming first-order kinetics, the half-life ($t_{1/2}$) of the drug is approximately:
   a. 30 minutes
   b. 60 minutes
   c. 2 hours
   d. 4 hours
   e. 6 hours
2. Under the same conditions as above, now assume that the drug disappears from plasma through zero-order kinetics. It takes approximately how long for the original blood concentrations to be reduced by 50%?
   a. 1 hour
   b. 3 hours
   c. 4 hours
   d. 5 hours
   e. 7 hours
3. A drug is administered intravenously in a dose of 200 mg to an 80 kg male patient. After 4 hours the plasma concentration was 1.5 mg/ml. Assume that the apparent V_d is 10% of body weight. The total amount of drug in body fluids at 4 hours is approximately:
   a. 15 mg
   b. 30 mg
   c. 60 mg
   d. 90 mg
   e. 120 mg
4. A single dose of a drug is given to an 85 kg female patient. The drug is known to have an apparent volume of distribution of 20% of body weight and elimination half-life of 2 hours. The total body clearance of this drug is:
   a. 20 mg/min
   b. 50 mg/min
   c. 100 mg/min
   d. 170 mg/min
   e. 340 mg/min
5. If 50 mg of a drug is given orally every 6 hours to a 70 kg male patient. The $t_{1/2}$ of the drug is 6 hours, and it disappears according to first-order kinetics. Ninety percent of a steady-state concentration of the drug will be achieved in:
   a. 4 to 6 hours
   b. 6 to 12 hours
   c. 18 to 24 hours
   d. 36 to 48 hours
   e. No finite time
6. If under the same conditions it is desirable to achieve approximately the same steady-state plasma concentration and therapeutic effect immediately, without accumulation of the drug and the potential toxicity, the appropriate dosing regimen should be:
   a. 25 mg every 3 hours
   b. 50 mg every 3 hours
   c. 100 mg every 12 hours
   d. 100 mg for the first dose and then 50 mg every 6 hours
   e. 100 mg for the first dose and then 50 mg every 3 hours

CHAPTER 5

Absorption, Distribution, Metabolism, and Elimination

THEODORE M. BRODY

WHAT HAPPENS TO DRUGS

In nearly all cases drugs must traverse membranes to reach their site of action. Therefore the ease by which a compound crosses membranes is the key to assessment of the rates and extent of absorption and distribution of the drug throughout the several body compartments. An objective of this chapter is to provide guidelines for assessing how specific drugs cross membranes and what variables are most important.

Drugs are transported by blood flow throughout the circulatory system and, except for a few targeting techniques discussed in Chapter 6, end up at tissues and organs where their presence is beneficial and also in some areas where their presence may be detrimental. Because of the potential importance of this problem, special mention is made in this chapter about drug distribution to the brain. Drug distribution to the fetus is considered in Chapter 63.

The principal routes by which drugs disappear from the body are by elimination of unchanged drug or by metabolism to other pharmacologically active or inactive compounds that may be subject to further elimination or metabolism. The mechanisms of the elimination processes and the principal chemical pathways involved in drug metabolism also are described. Some additional metabolic pathways that are of primary application in the detoxification of nontherapeutic compounds that may enter the body are discussed in Chapter 62 on toxicology.

ABBREVIATIONS	
$(Cl)_r$	Renal clearance
CNS	Central nervous system
CSF	Cerebrospinal fluid
GI	Gastrointestinal
NAD	Nicotinamine adenine dinucleotide
NADP	Nicotinamine adenine dinucleotide phosphate
pH	Logarithm of the reciprocal of the hydrogen-ion concentration
pK_a	Logarithm of the reciprocal of the dissociation constant
UDP	Uridine diphosphate
V_{max}	Maximum rate of reaction

ABSORPTION AND DISTRIBUTION

Transport of Drugs Across Membranes

Drugs that are administered orally (PO), intramuscularly (IM), or subcutaneously (SC) must cross membranes to be absorbed and to enter the systemic circulation. Not all agents need to enter the systemic circulation, but even those drugs given orally to treat gastrointestinal (GI) tract infections, stomach acidity, and other diseases within the GI tract often cross membranes and are absorbed into the general circulation. Drugs administered by intravenous (IV) injection also must cross capillary membranes to leave the systemic circulation and reach extracellular and intracellular sites of action. Even materials directed against platelets or other blood-borne elements must cross membranes. The renal elimination of drugs also requires the traversing of membranes.

Membranes are highly lipidic in chemical composition and thus strongly hydrophobic within the lipid bilayer. Most drugs, on the other hand, must have some affinity for water (i.e., hydrophilic) or they cannot dissolve and be transported by blood and other body fluids to their sites of action.

Several factors that favor the ability of a drug to cross membranes are listed in the box. Compounds that con-

CHARACTERISTICS OF DRUG MOLECULES THAT FAVOR DRUG TRANSPORT ACROSS MEMBRANES

Uncharged	Low molecular weight
Nonpolar	High lipid solubility

tain electrical charges or in which the electronic distribution is distorted toward one end of the molecule because of the nature of the atoms involved (imparts polarity to the compound) are not compatible with the uncharged nonpolar lipid environment. In addition the ordered structure of a lipid membrane does not allow many pores to exist; thus only small molecules in molecular weight normally can pass through the membrane. Large molecular weight proteins, for example, cannot pass through many membranes by simply dissolving in the membrane and diffusing to the other side. With proteins, active transport is often required, sometimes using carrier molecules to accomplish transmembrane transport. Most high molecular weight polypeptides and proteins cannot be administered orally because there are no mechanisms for their absorption from the GI tract, even if they could survive the high acidity of the stomach or the proteolytic enzymes of the GI tract.

As a general rule, drugs that have high lipid solubility cross membranes better than those with low lipid solubility. This is exemplified in Figure 5-1 for three different barbiturates. The oil/water equilibrium partition coefficient is a measure of the degree of lipid solubility. The drug is added to a mixture of equal volumes of oil and water and the mixture is agitated to promote solubilization of the compound in each phase. When equilibrium is attained, the phases are separated and assayed for drug. The ratio of the two concentrations becomes the partition coefficient. Therefore, larger numbers for the partition coefficient represent greater lipid solubility. Absorption across the stomach wall is greater for the barbiturate that has the largest lipid solubility (see Figure 5-1).

Many drugs, because of their chemical structure, behave as acids or bases in that they can take up or release a hydrogen ion. Within some ranges of pH, these drugs will carry an electrical charge, whereas in other pH ranges the compounds will be uncharged. It is the uncharged form of a drug that is lipid-soluble and therefore crosses biological membranes readily. In the barbiturate example, the compounds were selected so that the pK_a (the logarithm of the reciprocal of the dissociation constant) of each material was very similar. Otherwise, the differences in absorption could have been caused by variation in the degree of electrical charges on the three compounds. Further study of the pH influence will help predict the distribution of a drug between body compartments that differ in pH.

Influence of pH on Drug Distribution

The pH values of the major body fluids are shown in Table 5-1. The range is wide, from pH 1 to about pH 8. To predict how a drug will be distributed with gastric juice at pH 1.0 on one side of the membrane and blood at pH 7.4 on the other side, one determines the degree of dissociation of the drug at each of these pH values.

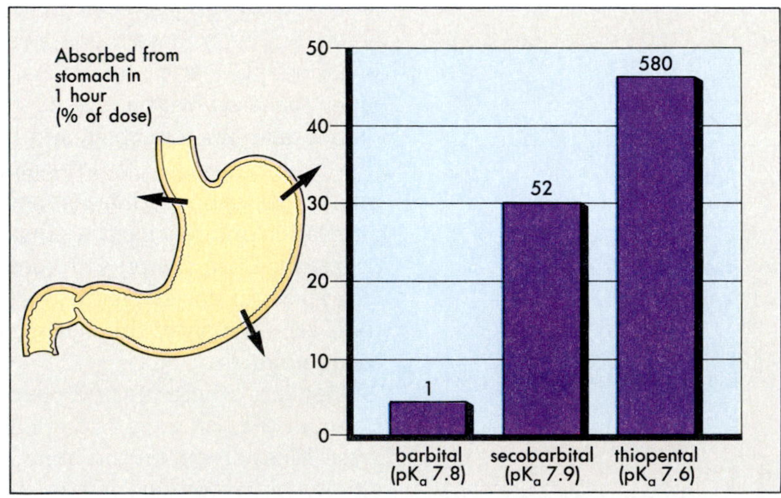

FIGURE 5-1 Increased lipid solubility influences the amount of drug absorbed from the stomach for three barbiturate compounds. The number above each column is the oil/water equilibrium partition coefficient. The compounds have roughly equivalent pK_a values, and so the degree of ionization is similar for all three drugs.

Table 5-1 pH of Selected Body Fluids

Fluids	pH
Gastric juice	1.0 to 3.0
Small intestine: duodenum	5.0 to 6.0
Small intestine: ileum	8
Large intestine	8
Plasma	7.4
Cerebrospinal fluid (CSF)	7.3
Urine	4.0 to 8.0

An acid is defined as a compound that can dissociate and release a hydrogen ion; whereas a base can take up a hydrogen ion. By this definition, RCOOH and RNH_3^+ are both acids and $RCOO^-$ and RNH_2 are bases. The equilibrium dissociation expression and the equilibrium dissociation constant (K_a) can be described for an acid HA or BH^+ and a base A^- or B as shown below. The convention for K_a requires that the acid appear on the left and the base on the right of the dissociation equation:

$$HA \leftrightharpoons A^- + H^+ \quad K_a = \frac{[A^-]\,[H^+]}{(HA)} \tag{1}$$

$$BH^+ \leftrightharpoons B + H^+ \quad K_a = \frac{(B)\,[H^+]}{[BH^+]} \tag{2}$$

The negative log of both sides gives

$$-\log K_a = -\log\,[H^+] - \log \frac{[A^-]}{(HA)} \tag{3}$$

$$-\log K_a = -\log\,[H^+] - \log \frac{(B)}{[BH^+]} \tag{4}$$

By definition the negative log of $[H^+]$ is expressed as pH and the negative log of K_a is pK_a. Therefore equations 3 and 4 can be simplified and rearranged to give

$$pH = pK_a + \log \frac{[A^-]}{(HA)} \tag{5}$$

$$pH = pK_a + \log \frac{(B)}{[BH^+]} \tag{6}$$

Equations 5 and 6 are the acid and base forms, respectively, of the Henderson-Hasselbalch equation and can be used to calculate the pH of the solution when the pK_a and the ratios of $[A^-]/(HA)$ or $(B)/[BH^+]$ are known. In pharmacology it is often of interest to calculate the ratios of $[A^-]/(HA)$ or $(B)/[BH^+]$ when the pH and the pK_a are known. For this calculation equations 5 and 6 are rearranged to equations 7 and 8:

$$pH - pK_a = \log \frac{[A^-]}{(HA)} \tag{7}$$

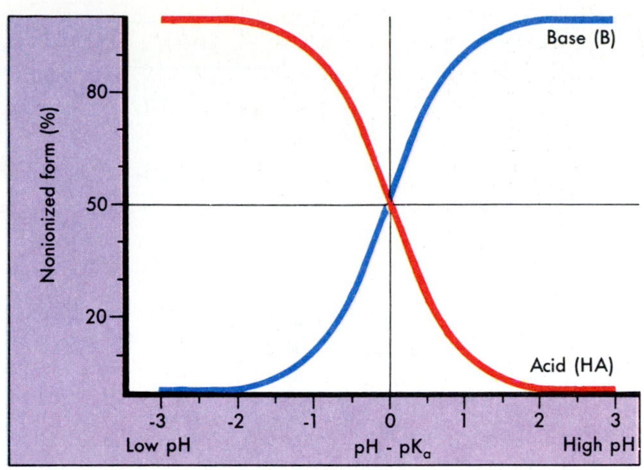

FIGURE 5-2 Degree of acidic or basic drug in nonionized (uncharged) form (*HA*, acid; *B*, base) at different pH values, with pH expressed relative to the drug pK_a.

$$pH - pK_a = \log \frac{(B)}{[BH^+]} \tag{8}$$

The results are plotted in Figure 5-2 to show the fraction of the nonionized (HA or B) forms. The pK_a is the pH when the drug is 50% dissociated. Applying equations 7 and 8 to an acidic drug with a pK_a of 6.0 enables one to calculate the degree of ionization for this drug in the stomach or blood (assume the blood pH is 7.0 for ease of calculation) as follows:

Stomach: $1.0 - 6.0 = \log Y$; $\log Y = -5$, or $Y = 10^{-5}$; $Y = [A^-] / (HA) = 0.00001$; if (HA) is 1.0, then $[A^-]$ is 0.00001 and the compound is ionized very little.

Blood: $7.0 - 6.0 = \log Y$; $\log Y = +1$, or $Y = 10^{+1}$; $Y = [A^-] / (HA) = 10.0$; if (HA) is 1.0, then $[A^-]$ is 10.0 and the compound is ionized considerably.

The drug is ionized very little in the stomach but appreciably in blood, and so the compound should cross readily in the stomach-to-plasma direction but hardly at all in the reverse direction.

Another example is shown in Figure 5-3 for a basic drug. This approach is particularly useful for predicting whether drugs can be absorbed in the stomach, upper intestine, or not at all. Figure 5-4 provides a summary of the pH effect on drug absorption in the GI tract for several acidic and several basic drugs. Another area of application is in predicting which drugs will undergo tubular reabsorption, which will be discussed later in this chapter.

Most drugs that cross membranes do so by simple passive diffusion. The concentration gradient across the membrane becomes the driving force that establishes the rate of diffusion, with the direction from the high toward the low drug concentration. Other mechanisms of transmembrane drug transport such as active transport, facilitated diffusion, or pinocytosis also exist.

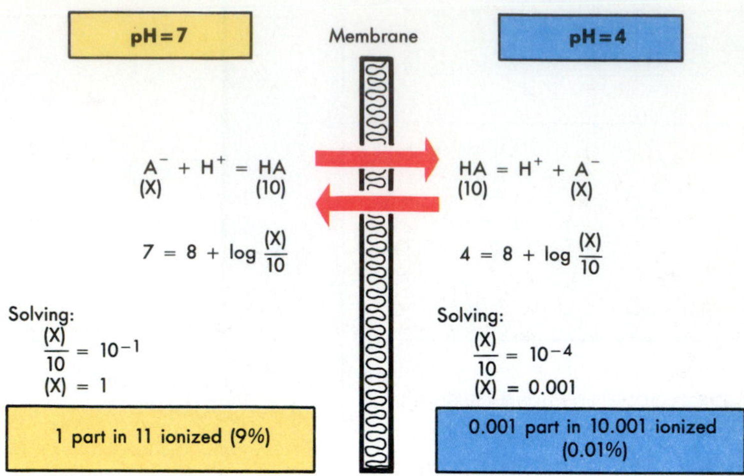

FIGURE 5-3 Equilibrium distribution of drug when pH is 4 on one side and 7 on the other side of membrane for an acid drug with a pK_a of 8.0. Nonionized form, HA, of the drug can readily cross the membrane. Thus HA has the same concentration on both sides of the membrane. The concentration of nonionized drug is arbitrarily set at 10 μg/ml, and the expressions are solved to determine the concentration of ionized species at equilibrium.

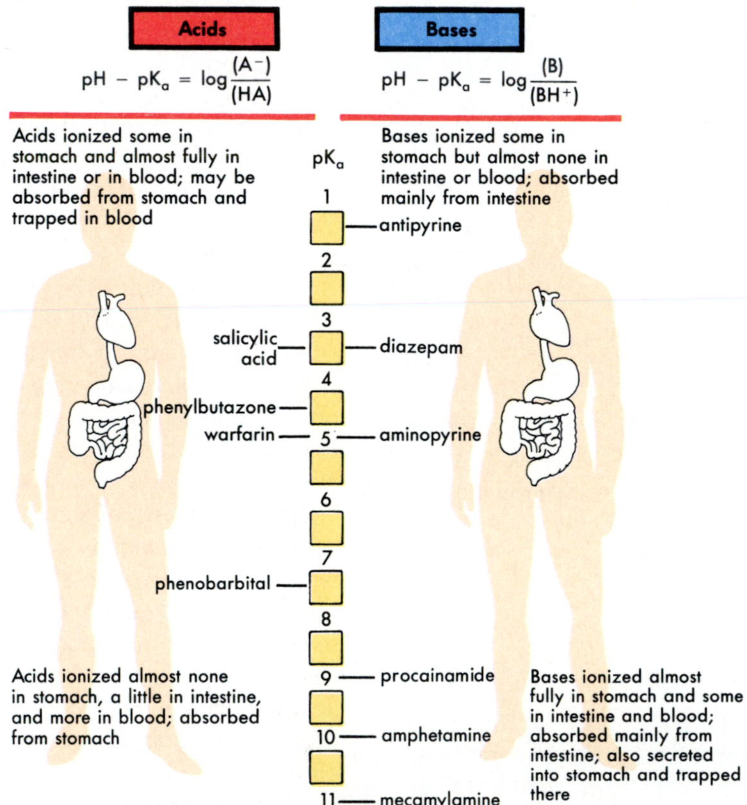

FIGURE 5-4 Summary of pH effect on degree of ionization of several acidic and basic drugs. Statements in corners refer to compounds with extremes of pK_a values and allow prediction of where drugs with various pK_as will be absorbed.

Distribution to Special Organs and Tissues

Blood flow rates determine the maximum amount of drug per minute that can be delivered to specific organs and tissues at a given plasma concentration of drug. Tissues that are well perfused can receive a large quantity of drug, provided that the drug can cross the membranes or other barriers present between the plasma and tissue. Similarly, tissues, such as fat, that are poorly perfused receive drug at a slow rate, and so the concentration of drug in fat may still be increasing long after the concentration in plasma has started to decrease.

Two areas of special importance are the brain and the fetus. Many drugs do not readily enter the brain. Capillaries in the brain differ structurally from those in other tissues, with the result that a barrier exists between blood within the brain capillaries and extracellular fluid in brain tissue. This **blood-brain barrier** hinders the transport of drugs and other materials from blood into brain tissue. The blood-brain barrier is found throughout the brain and spinal cord at all regions central to the arachnoid membrane, except for the floor of the hypothalamus and the area postrema. The structural differences between brain and nonbrain capillaries and how these differences influence blood-brain transport of solutes are shown schematically in Figure 5-5. Nonbrain capillaries have fenestrations (openings) between the endothelial cells through which solutes move readily by passive diffusion, with compounds having molecular weights greater than about 25,000 daltons undergoing transport by pinocytosis. In brain capillaries tight junctions are present because there are no fenestrations, and pinocytosis appears to be greatly reduced. Special transport systems are available at brain capillaries for glucose, amino acids, amines, purines, nucleosides, and organic acids; all other materials apparently must cross the two endothelial membranes plus the endothelial cytoplasm to move from capillary blood to tissue extracellular fluid. Thus the main route of drug entry into central nervous system (CNS) tissue appears to be by passive diffusion across membranes. This restricts the available compounds as potential drugs for treating brain disorders. At the same time, the potential effects of many compounds on the CNS are not known; for these compounds the blood-brain barrier acts as a safety buffer. The only other generalization that can be made now is that most highly lipid-soluble drugs cross the blood-brain barrier. In infants and the elderly, the blood-brain barrier may not be completely intact and drugs may diffuse into the brain.

An alternative approach for drug delivery to brain tissue is by intrathecal injection into the subarachnoid space and the cerebrospinal fluid (CSF). However, injection into the subarachnoid space can be difficult to perform safely because of the small volume of this region and the proximity to easily damaged nerves. In addition, drug distribution within the CSF and across the CSF-brain barrier can be slow and show large interpatient variations; however, for some drugs there may not be another route.

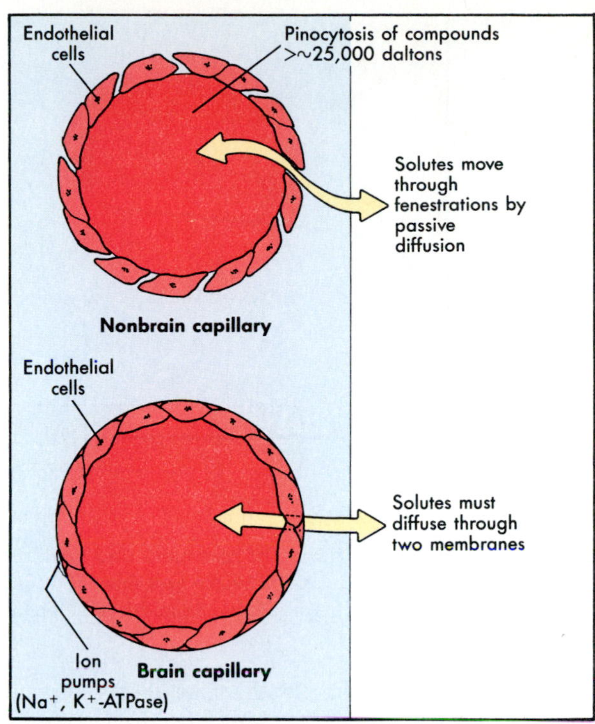

FIGURE 5-5 Structural differences between nonbrain and brain capillaries. In brain capillaries, lack of openings between endothelial cells in capillary wall requires drugs and other solutes to pass through two membranes to move from blood to tissue or the reverse. Ion pumps are mainly on the outer membrane of the brain endothelial cells and maintain a concentration difference between the two fluid regions.

METABOLISM AND ELIMINATION OF DRUGS

The term **elimination** refers to the removal of drug without any chemical changes being involved. For some drugs this is the only route of disappearance; for most drugs only some of the dose is removed unchanged. Elimination of drugs occurs primarily by renal mechanisms into the urine and to some extent by mixing with bile salts for solubilization followed by transport into the intestinal tract. The terms **metabolism** and **biotransformation** refer to the disappearance of a drug when it changes chemically into another compound, termed a **metabolite.** Some drugs are administered as inactive **"prodrugs,"** which must be metabolized into the pharmacologically active form. Although drug metabolism

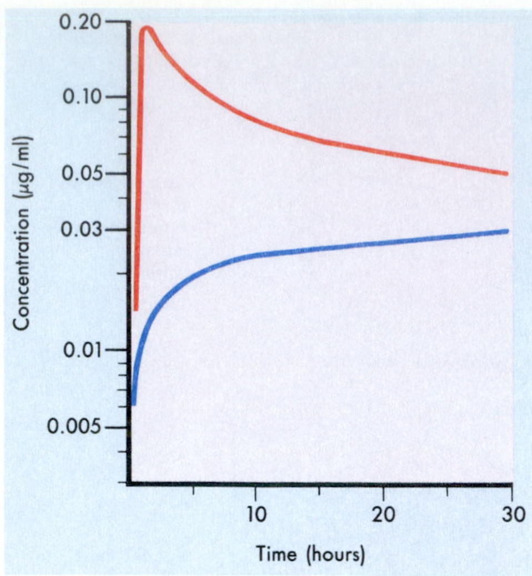

FIGURE 5-6 Plasma concentration of diazepam *(red line)* and its main metabolite *(blue line)* after a single oral dose of 10 mg of diazepam in humans. The metabolite is desmethyldiazepam.

occurs largely in the liver, most other tissues and organs, especially the lung, carry out varying degrees of drug metabolism. A few drugs become essentially irreversibly bound to tissues and are metabolized or otherwise removed over long periods of time. Finally, drugs also may be excreted in feces, exhaled through lungs, or secreted through sweat or salivary glands.

Metabolism of Drugs

When drugs are metabolized, the change is usually an increase in water solubility often accompanied by a decrease in lipid solubility or an increase in the polarity of the products. The result is the production of compounds that can be excreted in the urine more readily. Some drugs are administered as prodrugs in an inactive or less active form to promote absorption, to overcome potential destruction by stomach acidity, or to minimize exposure to highly reactive chemical species. Thus drug-metabolizing systems convert the prodrug into a more active species on entry into the systemic circulation. In other situations, drugs that are administered as the active species are metabolized to form products, which may be "active" and produce pharmacological effects similar to or different from those generated by the parent drug. An example is diazepam (Figure 5-6), an antianxiety compound that is demethylated to an active metabolite. The half-life of the parent drug is about 30 hours, whereas that of the metabolite averages about 70 hours. Thus the effect of the metabolite is present long after the parent drug has disappeared. In this case the magnitude of the pharmacological effect is much less for the metabolite than for the parent drug, but in general the lingering presence of active metabolites makes the precise control of the magnitude of pharmacological effect more difficult to achieve. In the case of diazepam the therapeutic index is large enough so that precise control is not required.

Drug metabolism takes place primarily in the liver, through microsomal and in some cases nonmicrosomal enzyme systems. However, considerable drug-metabolizing capability often is found in other body sites, including the placenta, GI tract bacteria and intestinal tissue.

Although a myriad of different types of chemical reactions are observed in drug metabolism, most of the reactions can be categorized into the following four groups:

Oxidation
Conjugation
Reduction
Hydrolysis

Oxidation and conjugation are most important and are discussed further. Simple examples are given for reduction and hydrolysis.

Oxidation can take place at many different sites on a drug molecule and can appear as one of many chemical reactions. Typically, an oxygen atom may be inserted to convert $—CH_2—$ to —CHOH— or $—CH(NH_2)—$ to —CH(O)—. By definition, an oxidation reaction requires the transfer of one or more electrons and includes a final electron acceptor. A large fraction of drug-oxidation reactions operate under the control of the cytochrome P-450 mixed-function oxidase system. The overall net reaction can be summarized as

$$R + NAD(P)H + H^+ + O_2 = RO + NAD(P)^+ + H_2O$$

where *R* = the drug, *NADH* or *NADPH* = reduced nicotinamide adeninedinucleotide cofactors, and *NAD* or *NADP* = oxidized cofactors.

In this reaction molecular oxygen serves as the final electron acceptor. **Cytochrome P-450s** are a family of iron-containing proteins that include flavin and NADP and NAD cofactor electron and proton transfer components. The iron undergoes a cycle that starts in the ferric oxidation state, when the drug binds to cytochrome P-450, and includes reduction to the ferrous state, activation of oxygen, and eventual regeneration of the ferric state. Free radical or ion-radical groups are formed at one or more parts of the cycle. The subcellular site of this enzyme system is the endoplasmic reticulum. The reaction cycle is summarized in Figure 5-7. Cytochrome P-450s are very complex systems of enzymes in which the detailed molecular chemistry is still ongoing. If drug metabolism by the cytochrome P-450 route leads to the generation of highly reactive free radical groups, this must be considered in drug design to minimize the for-

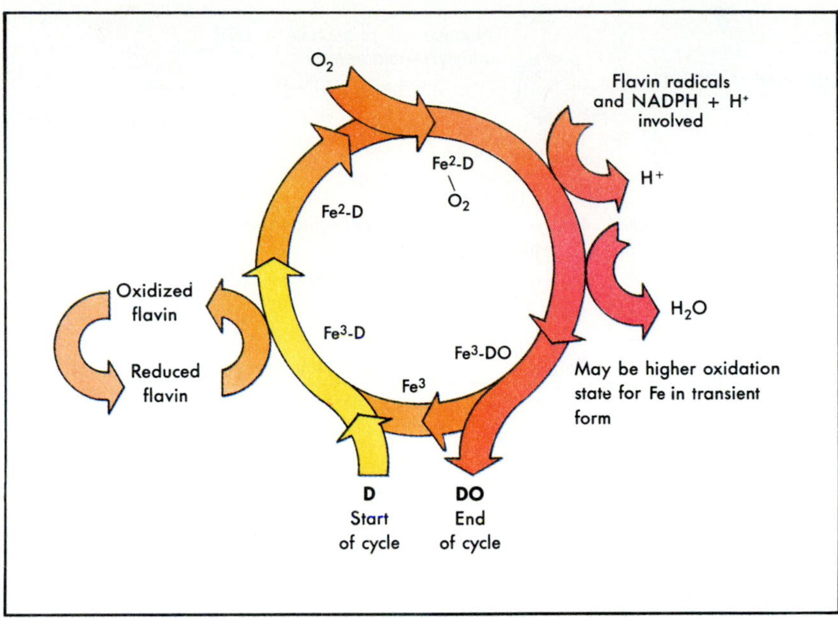

FIGURE 5-7 Simplified model of cytochrome P-450 mixed-function oxidase reaction sequence. *D* is the drug undergoing oxidation to product *DO*. Molecular oxygen serves as the final electron acceptor. Flavin cofactor systems are involved at several sites. The iron of the cytochrome P-450 is involved in binding and electron transfer with changes in valence state.

mation of reactive and potentially toxic drug metabolites.

Conjugation, the second major type of drug metabolism, involves coupling another group to the drug molecule so that the resulting product will have greater water solubility or other features for enhanced renal or biliary elimination. Conjugation, like other metabolism processes, requires the presence of drug-metabolizing enzymes. In addition, groups that are being coupled need to be "activated" through participation of high-energy phosphate compounds. For example, glucuronic acid can be conjugated, in the presence of the enzyme uridine diphosphate (UDP)–glucuronosyl transferase, to compounds of the general types ROH, RCOOH, RNH_2, or RSH, where *R* represents the remainder of the drug molecule. However, glucuronic acid must first be activated. This occurs by the reaction of glucose-1-phosphate with uridine triphosphate followed by oxidation of the resulting product to activated glucuronic acid. The reaction sequence is shown in Figure 5-8 for the formation of the ROH glucuronide of salicylic acid. Another glucuronide could be formed through conjugation with the RCOOH group. Several endogenous materials, including bilirubin, thyroxine, and steroids also undergo conjugation with activated glucuronic acid in the presence of UDP-glucuronosyl transferase. Conjugation occurs with activated glycine, acetate, sulfate, and other groups besides glucuronate.

Typical drug metabolism reduction and hydrolysis reactions are shown in Figure 5-9.

Drug Metabolizing Enzyme Kinetic Factors Numerous chemical reactions that participate in the metabolism of drugs are governed by enzyme catalysts. Therefore the kinetics of drug metabolism can be approximated by the single substrate relationship

$$v = \frac{V_{max}(S)}{K + (S)} \qquad (9)$$

In this expression

v = rate of reaction

V_{max} = maximum rate of reaction

(S) = concentration of drug

K = Michaelis constant

$\mathbf{V_{max}}$ is directly proportional to the concentration of enzyme. If a change occurs in the concentration of enzyme, there should be a proportional change in the rate of drug metabolism.

A wide variety of drugs, environmental chemicals, air pollutants, and components of cigarette smoke stimulate the synthesis of higher concentrations of drug-metabolizing enzymes. This process, termed **enzyme induction,** can be used clinically to elevate the level of hepatic drug-metabolizing enzymes. In the treatment of drug overdoses it is sometimes useful to stimulate enzyme induction to increase the rate of drug metabolism. Enzyme induction can be achieved clinically by the ad-glucose–1–phosphate + [uridine triphosphate: OH, N, O, N, R–P–P–P] $\xrightarrow{\text{glucose—1—phosphate + UTP uridylyltransferase}}$ UDP–glucose + P–P (pyrophosphate)

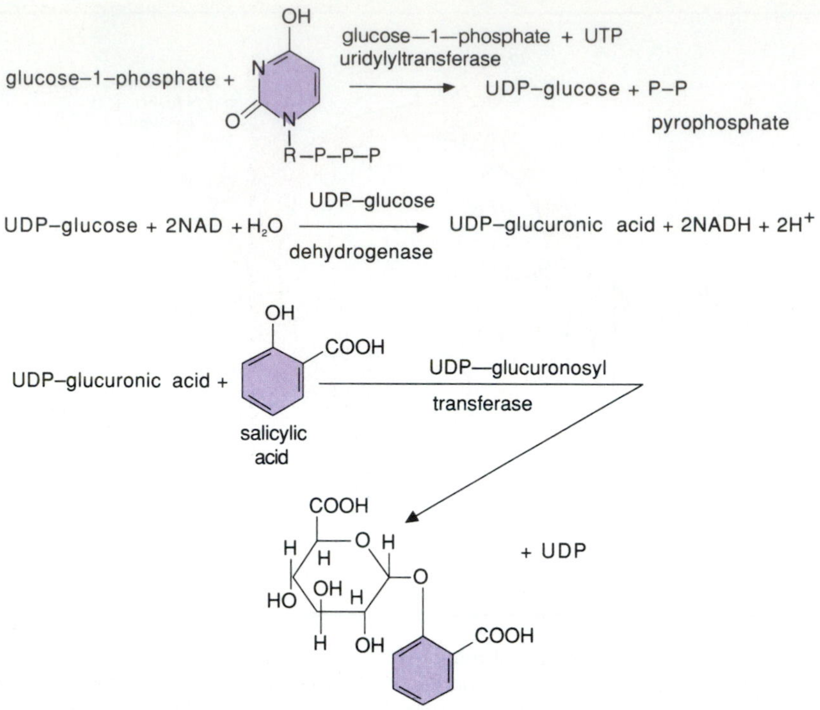

UDP–glucose + 2NAD + H_2O $\xrightarrow[\text{dehydrogenase}]{\text{UDP–glucose}}$ UDP–glucuronic acid + 2NADH + $2H^+$

UDP–glucuronic acid + salicylic acid $\xrightarrow[\text{transferase}]{\text{UDP—glucuronosyl}}$ [salicyl phenolic glucuronide] + UDP

FIGURE 5-8 Sequence of reactions for conjugation of salicylic acid to form salicyl phenolic glucuronide. *P* is phosphate. Enzyme names are from International Union of Biochemistry nomenclature listing. The glucuronic acid must first be activated, with glucose-1-phosphate coupling with high-energy UTP to UDP-glucose, by oxidation to UDP-glucuronic acid before conjugation can occur.

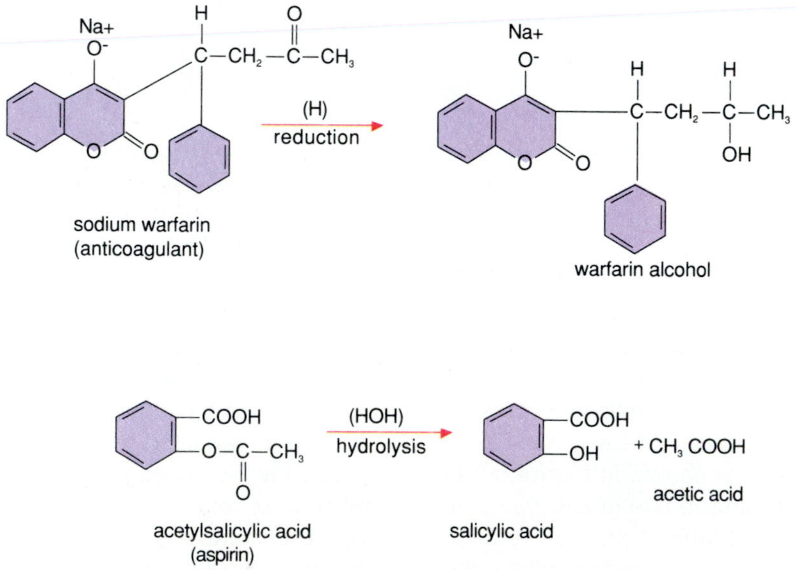

sodium warfarin (anticoagulant) $\xrightarrow[\text{reduction}]{\text{(H)}}$ warfarin alcohol

acetylsalicylic acid (aspirin) $\xrightarrow[\text{hydrolysis}]{\text{(HOH)}}$ salicylic acid + CH_3COOH (acetic acid)

FIGURE 5-9 Representative reduction and hydrolysis reactions for metabolism of drugs.

ministration of barbiturates; the induction can be observed after about 24 hours in humans. For example, phenobarbital and the highly reactive air pollutant 3,4-benzo*[a]*pyrene can increase the rate of oxidation of the CNS muscle relaxant zoxazolamine in animals (Figure 5-10). Because cigarette smoke contains compounds that can promote induction, chronic cigarette smokers have considerably higher levels of hepatic and lung drug-metabolizing enzymes, especially aryl hydroxylase.

Drug metabolism reactions typically follow first order kinetics in humans receiving therapeutic concentrations of drugs. Equation 9 reduces to a first-order expression when the concentration of drug is much smaller than the Michaelis constant. Thus, for nearly all drugs within their normal therapeutic range of concentrations, the hepatic or other drug metabolizing systems operate far below saturation. An exception is the metabolism of salicylic acid in humans, in which saturation of the available enzymes can occur at elevated drug concentrations. Aspirin is used extensively for the treatment of inflammatory diseases, with the optimum therapeutic concentration only slightly below the concentration where signs of toxicity appear. Aspirin is hydrolyzed to salicylic acid, which in turn has several routes for elimination (Figure 5-11). Two salicylic acid metabo-

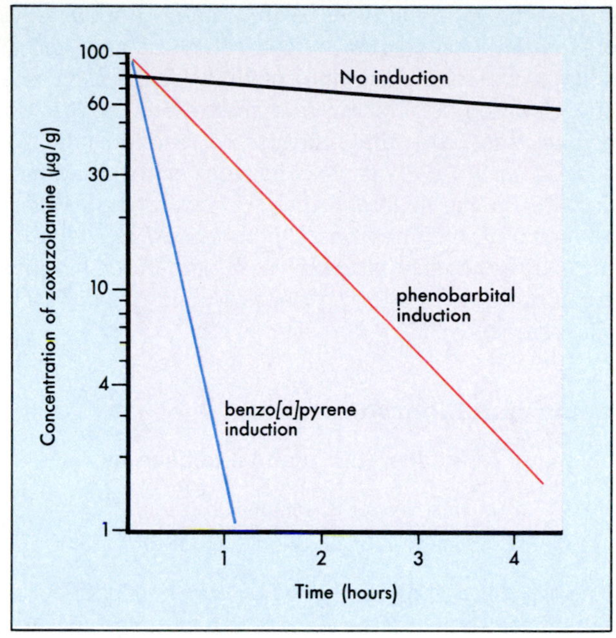

FIGURE 5-10 Example of enzyme induction. Zoxazolamine administered by intraperitoneal injection to rats. For induction studies phenobarbital or 3,4-benzo*[a]*pyrene was injected twice daily for 4 days before injection of the zoxazolamine. Drug concentration is expressed as microgram of drug/gram of tissue.

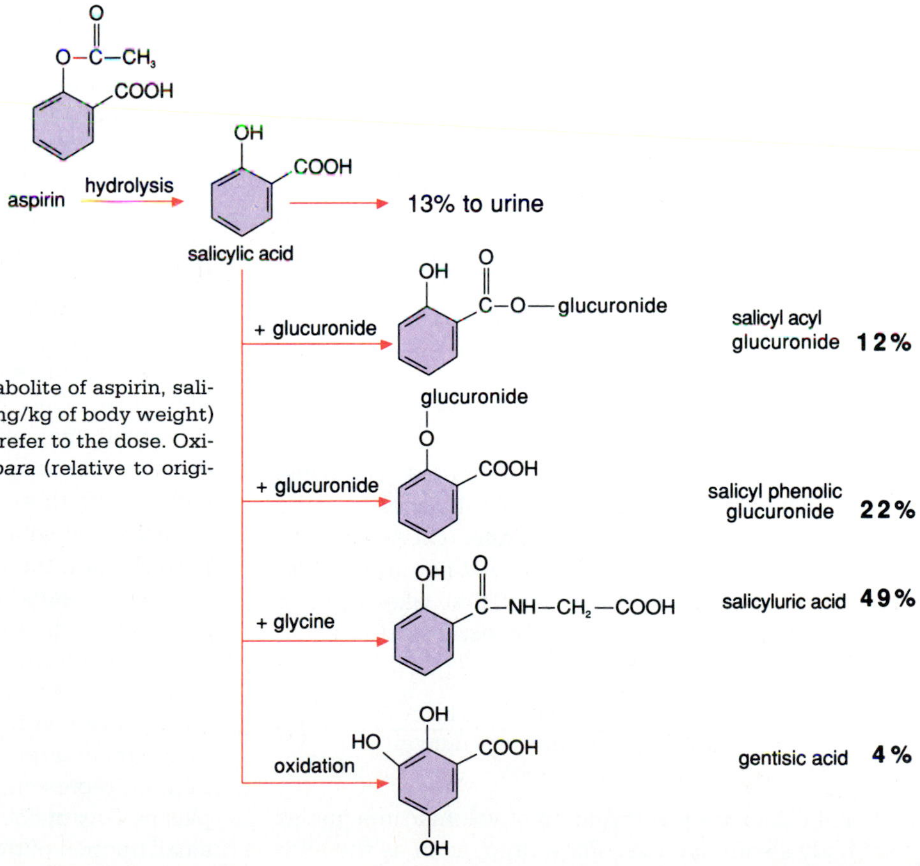

aspirin — hydrolysis → salicylic acid → 13% to urine

+ glucuronide → salicyl acyl glucuronide **12%**

+ glucuronide → salicyl phenolic glucuronide **22%**

+ glycine → salicyluric acid **49%**

oxidation → gentisic acid **4%**

FIGURE 5-11 Disposition of primary metabolite of aspirin, salicylic acid, at a single dose of 4 grams (54 mg/kg of body weight) in a healthy adult. The percentage values refer to the dose. Oxidation produces a mixture of *ortho* and *para* (relative to original OH group) isomers.

lism pathways are subject to saturation in humans: (1) conjugation with glycine to form salicyuric acid and (2) conjugation with glucuronic acid to form salicyl phenolic glucuronide. For enzyme saturation, the kinetics become zero order and the rate of reaction becomes constant at V_{max}. This is consistent with equation 9 when (S) is much larger than K. Saturation of drug-metabolizing enzymes has a pronounced influence on drug-plateau concentrations. With zero-order kinetics, elimination rates no longer depend upon dose or blood concentration.

Hepatic and Biliary Clearance

Hepatic clearance, $(Cl)_h$, can be defined as

$$\frac{\text{rate of hepatic removal of drug}}{\text{concentration of drug in portal vein}} \qquad \textbf{(10)}$$

Likewise, biliary clearance, $(Cl)_b$, can be defined in a similar manner with the bile flow rate times the drug concentration in the bile a measure of the rate of biliary removal of drug. Direct measurement of hepatic or biliary clearance in humans is not practical because of the high risk in obtaining appropriate blood samples. The concept of hepatic and biliary clearance is included here to emphasize that the concept of clearance can be applied to any body region or organ system, as long as sample points can be designated.

A complicating result of biliary elimination of a drug sometimes occurs when the drug is reabsorbed from the GI tract and returned to the systemic circulation. This is termed **enterohepatic cycling** and can result in a measurable increase in the plasma concentration of drug several half-lives after the drug originally was administered and will delay the eventual disposition of the drug.

Renal Elimination of Drugs

The removal of unchanged drug by the renal route is one of the processes that is included in "total body clearance," or the sum of removal by all routes. The same general definition of clearance can also be applied to the renal route to define **renal clearance,** $(Cl)_r$, as the volume of plasma that needs to be cleared per unit time to account for the rate of drug removal that takes place in the kidneys. This definition can be expressed in equation form as

$$(Cl)_r = \frac{\text{rate of drug removal by the kidneys}}{\text{plasma concentration of drug in renal artery}} \qquad \textbf{(11)}$$

Renal clearance has the units of volume/time just as total body clearance does. For a drug, such as the antibiotic cephalexin, that is removed entirely by renal elimination, the renal clearance and the total body clearance are equal. In this example renal clearance can be determined from plasma data if one plots the log plasma concentration of cephalexin versus time after an IV injection. For other drugs, where only part of the dose is removed by renal elimination, data must be obtained for the appearance of unchanged drug in the urine to calculate renal clearance. For example, the rate of drug removal by the renal route can be estimated if one collects urine volumes over known time intervals and assays each urine volume for the concentration of unchanged drug. If the rates of drug removal are plotted against mean plasma concentration of drug for each urine volume interval, the slope will be an estimate of the renal clearance of that drug. Other techniques are available for determination of renal clearance, but their use is limited.

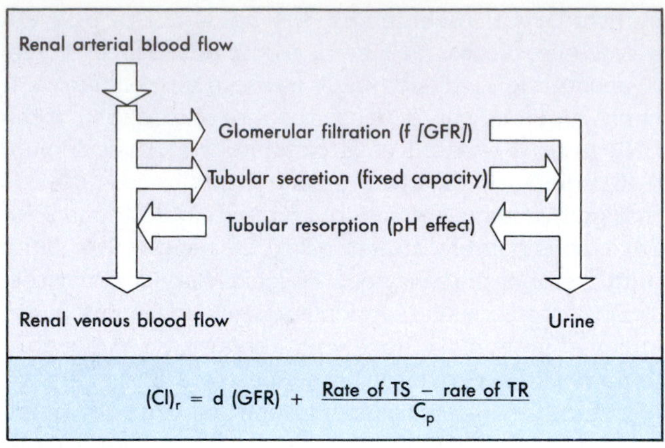

FIGURE 5-12 Summary of renal clearance $(Cl)_r$ mechanisms. C_p, Renal arterial blood concentration of drug; *f*, fraction of drug in plasma not bound; *GFR*, glomerular filtration rate of drug; *TR*, tubular resorption of drug; *TS*, tubular secretion of drug.

The mechanisms by which the renal clearance of drugs takes place are the same as those responsible for the renal elimination of endogenous substances. Glomerular filtration, tubular secretion, and tubular reabsorption are those mechanisms (Figure 5-12).

Molecules smaller than those of about 15A° readily pass through the glomeruli, with approximately 125 ml of plasma cleared each minute in a healthy adult. This figure of 125 ml/min is independent of the plasma concentration of drug, and so removal by glomerular filtration, expressed in milligrams per minute, shows a linear increase with higher plasma concentration of drug in the renal artery. The glomerular filtration rate of 125 ml/min represents less than 10% of the total renal plasma flow of 650 to 750 ml/min, indicating that only a small fraction of the total renal plasma flow is cleared of drug by this mechanism on each pass through the kidneys. Because albumin and other plasma protein molecules do not pass through the glomeruli, drug molecules that are bound to these plasma proteins are retained. Inulin and creatinine can be used to assess the glomerular filtration capability of renal function in individual patients because these materials show very little binding to plasma proteins and do not undergo appreciable tubular secretion or reabsorption. These materials are discussed later in regard to dosing schedules for patients who have impaired renal function.

Tubular secretion is a second mechanism for renal clearance of drugs. This is an active process that occurs in the proximal tubule, with different details pertinent to the secretion of acids and bases. Compounds that are secreted usually also undergo glomerular filtration, and so renal clearance is the sum of both routes. Because tubular secretion involves active transport by carrier groups and since there are a limited number of carrier groups, the process can become saturated. The volume of plasma that can be cleared per unit time by tubular secretion varies with the concentration of drug in plasma. This is in contrast to glomerular filtration, where the *volume filtered per unit time* is independent of the plasma concentration of drug. At very low plasma concentrations of drug, tubular secretion can operate at its maximum rate of clearing approximately 650 ml/min. If the concentration of drug in the arterial plasma is 4 ng/ml, clearing 650 ml/min removes 2600 ng each minute. If the concentration of the same drug increases to 200 ng/ml and tubular secretion is saturated, the tubules will still remove only 2600 ng/min by secretion, and so the clearance by tubular secretion falls to 13 ml/min. If drug disappearance studies show that the renal clearance is considerably greater than 125 ml/min, tubular secretion must be involved because there is no other explanation for such a high clearance. In tubular secretion, both bound drug and free drug are removed. Tubular transit time is long enough so that binding dissociation can take place for those compounds in which the concentration change along the tubule is sufficient to shift the binding equilibrium and release additional drug.

The third mechanism affecting the renal clearance of drugs is reabsorption of filtered or secreted drug from the tubules back into the venous blood of the nephrons. Although this process may be active or passive, for most drugs it occurs by simple passive diffusion. Drugs that are readily reabsorbed are characterized by high lipid solubility or by a significant fraction of the drug in a nonionized form at urine pH and in the ionized form at plasma pH. For example, salicylic acid with a pK_a of 3.0 is about 99.99% in the ionized form at pH 7.4 (per equation 5) but only about 90% ionized at pH 4.0. Thus, some reabsorption of salicylic acid could be expected from acidic urine. In drug overdose, the manipulation of urine pH is sometimes used to prevent reabsorption. Ammonium chloride administration leads to acidification of the urine and sodium bicarbonate administration to alkalinization. Some additional examples are given in the box below.

EFFECT OF URINE PH ON RENAL CLEARANCE FOR DRUGS THAT UNDERGO TUBULAR RESORPTION

Bases	Acids
CLEARED RAPIDLY BY MAKING URINE MORE ACIDIC	CLEARED RAPIDLY BY MAKING URINE MORE ALKALINE
amphetamine	acetazolamide
chloroquine	nitrofurantoin
imipramine	phenobarbital
levophanol	probenecid
mecamylamine	salicylates
quinine	sulfathiazole

Modified Renal Function and Drug Elimination The renal clearance of drugs may be less in neonates, geriatric patients, and those with improperly functioning kidneys. The effects of patient age on renal clearance of drugs are discussed in Chapters 7, 63, and 64. The modification of dosing regimens to compensate for changing renal function is discussed here.

The following situation is typical:

1. It is desired to use a particular drug in a patient.
2. This drug usually is disposed of primarily through renal elimination.
3. The patient's renal function is inadequate.

The problem is whether a safe dosing schedule can be worked out for the desired drug in this patient. In many cases the problem can be solved. However, some measure of the degree of renal function is necessary. Creatinine clearance is a standard clinical determination that can be used to obtain an approximate measure of renal function. Creatinine is selected instead of inulin clearance because the assay and methodology with inulin are more difficult. To determine the rate of urinary excretion of creatinine, urine is collected over a known period (often 24 hours) and pooled, its volume is measured, and the urine assayed for creatinine. At the midpoint of the urine collection period, a serum sample is obtained and assayed for creatinine. The creatinine clearance is calculated from equation 12 as follows:

$$(Cl)_{Cr} = \frac{\text{rate of urinary excretion of creatinine (mg/min)}}{\text{serum concentration of creatinine (mg/ml)}} = \text{ml/ml} \quad \textbf{(12)}$$

Determination of the creatinine clearance for the patient gives a measure of glomerular filtration function. In addition the relationship between the rate constant for renal elimination of unchanged drug and creatinine clearance must be demonstrated. For the usual case of first-order renal elimination the relationship is linear, and so a creatinine clearance of 50% of normal means that renal elimination of this drug would be expected to operate at 50% and the rate of drug input should be reduced accordingly. For example, a drug that is administered 100 mg every 6 hours (400 mg in 24 hours) to a patient with normal creatinine clearance could be given 40 mg every 12 hours (80 mg in 24 hours) if the creatinine clearance decreased to only 20% of normal. Other pathways for disappearance of this drug retain their normal functionality.

Extraction Ratio

An alternative approach to the calculation of renal clearance or hepatic clearance is to multiply the blood flow rate to the organ by the **extraction ratio.** This ratio is that fraction of drug removed from each unit volume of blood per pass through the kidneys or liver respectively. For drugs with a high extraction ratio, the limiting step in drug removal is the rate of delivery to the organ (i.e., the blood flow rate). At the other extreme (i.e., a low extraction ratio) the rate of removal of drugs is little influenced by blood-flow rate but is strongly influenced by changes in the degree of plasma protein binding of the drug. The extraction ratio is a valid alternative approach for clearance concepts; however, few experimental results are available to apply this approach to humans other than as a research tool.

SUMMARY

Understanding the major routes of disposition of a drug and the factors that influence the functionality and capacity of each route can aid profoundly in the safe and effective use of drugs, especially in patients in whom the state of the disease has compromised one or more of the main drug disposition routes. The multiple routes for the disposition of aspirin and its hydrolysis product, salicylic acid (see Figure 5-11), represent the complexity of drug disappearance.

REFERENCES

Guengerich FP, Macdonald TL: Chemical mechanisms of catalysis by cytochromes P-450: a unified view, *Acc Chem Res* 17:9, 1984.

LaDu, BN, Mandel HG, Way EL, editors: *Fundamentals of drug metabolism and drug disposition,* Baltimore, 1971, Williams & Wilkins.

Lewis DVF: Physical methods in the study of the active site geometry of cytochromes P-450, *Drug Metab Rev* 17:1, 1986.

SELF-ASSESSMENT QUESTIONS

1. Cell membranes are composed of:
   a. Phospholipids.
   b. Receptor proteins.
   c. DNA.
   d. a and b are correct.
   e. All of the above are correct.
2. All of the following tend to lower the plasma concentration of a drug *except*
   a. Metabolic biotransformation.
   b. Renal tubular reabsorption.
   c. Binding to plasma proteins.
   d. Renal secretion.
   e. Biliary excretion.
3. What is the approximate percentage of a weak acid ($pK_a = 5.4$) in the nonionized form in plasma having a pH of 7.4?
   a. 99%
   b. 90%
   c. 10%
   d. 1%
   e. 0.1%
4. To facilitate excretion of sodium pentobarbital by the kidney:
   a. Sodium bicarbonate is effective because of its "common ion" effect.
   b. Ammonium chloride, an acidic compound, is used because it promotes the elimination of another weak acid, sodium pentobarbital.
   c. Sodium bicarbonate promotes alkalinization of the urine, retarding reabsorption of the weak acid.
   d. Ammonium chloride acidifies the urine enhancing renal excretion of sodium pentobarbital.
   e. None of the above is correct.
5. Passive diffusion of a drug across a lipid membrane is enhanced if:
   a. It is highly polar.
   b. It contains a quaternary nitrogen.
   c. A substantial gradient exists between extracellular and intracellular concentrations.
   d. The drug is water soluble as well as very lipid soluble.
   e. c and d are correct.
6. Drug oxidations frequently involve all of the following *except*
   a. Cytochrome P-450 proteins.
   b. NADH or NADPH cofactors.
   c. Liver endoplasmic reticulum.
   d. Esterases.
   e. Molecular oxygen.
7. Conjugation reactions
   a. Occur with weak acids but not weak bases.
   b. Do not require the presence of drug-metabolizing enzymes.
   c. Need activation by high-energy phosphate compounds.
   d. Can involve amino acids.
   e. c and d are correct.

CHAPTER 6

Drug Delivery Strategies and Gene Therapy

THEODORE M. BRODY

DELIVERY GOALS

Direct placement of drugs into the oral or gastrointestinal (GI) cavities in the form of discrete multiple doses for absorption is the major mode of drug administration for hospitalized and nonhospitalized patients. With this mode of administration, the plasma concentration of drug increases and decreases during a dosing interval, even if the mean concentration has reached a plateau. Depending on the length of the dosing interval in relation to the disappearance half-life of the drug, the concentration may decrease to below the minimum effective concentration for a significant portion of the dosing interval. In addition, the drug is distributed throughout the entire circulatory system and into many different tissue beds, even though the site of therapeutic action may be localized to a single organ or tissue type.

Clinically, it is therapeutically advantageous with some drug types (1) to minimize fluctuations in plasma drug concentration, (2) to be able to target drugs to the site of therapeutic action with minimal exposure of other body compartments to unwanted effects of the drug, and (3) for the rate of drug delivery to vary depending on the measured concentration of some constituent in blood or other body fluid. Some clinical progress has been made in achieving each of these delivery goals for certain drugs.

Recent advances in molecular medicine have led to a new approach to the treatment of certain disease states. Instead of delivery of a drug to the circulation with the objective that it will affect a specific condition, the concept of **gene therapy** envisions the treatment of disease by the delivery of a human gene to a target organ with the subsequent production of a "gene product," or protein, which acts as the "drug." There are two routes that research in this field have followed. The most obvious is **gene-replacement therapy,** in correction of hereditary conditions in which there is defective production of an essential enzyme or protein, attributable to the gene. Here, the goal is to insert the normal gene into a cell so that a sufficient amount of product is now available to ameliorate the problem. The second approach is in attempts to treat acquired diseases. This has been called **gene-addition therapy.** An example is the use of cytokine gene transfer into tumor cells, in an attempt to stimulate the immune response against these cells. An extended discussion of these new strategies in pharmacotherapy is also presented in this chapter.

ABBREVIATIONS	
CNS	central nervous system
DNA	deoxyribonucleic acid
RNA	ribonucleic acid
mRNA	messenger RNA

PROLONGED-RELEASE PREPARATIONS

With drug administration by discrete multiple doses, there is an increase and a decrease in drug concentration during the span of a dosing interval. Often such fluctuation is not desirable. Intravenous therapy can be used to minimize fluctuation, but this is generally a hospital-based procedure. Another approach is to administer a larger dose of the drug but to extend the duration of drug absorption over a longer interval. Thus a wide variety of clinically available dosage forms with extended drug release-absorption have become available as "sustained-release" pharmaceutical preparations.

One such method involves coating drug tablets with materials that dissolve slowly in the GI tract or at IM or SC injection sites. Others include administration of the

CATEGORIES OF DRUG-POLYMER RELEASE MECHANISMS
Diffusional migration of drug
Chemical reaction of polymer or drug linkages with body constituents
Magnetic control of release rates
Solvent action on polymer release of drug

drug as a drug-salt or drug–ion exchange resin complex, which undergo slow dissociation before absorption. Some sustained-release preparations prolong absorption for up to 15 to 20 hours. However, release rates may vary as a result of local fluctuations in pH.

Relatively constant drug-release rates, not influenced by pH or other factors, can be obtained by the use of drug-polymer systems. These are designed to release drug at a relatively constant rate by slow diffusion. Polymer systems can be divided into the four categories listed in the box. Only the first category is widely used clinically.

Diffusional release of drug from an implanted polymer system is shown schematically in Figure 6-1. Two types of arrangements for storing the drug for release are available. In Figure 6-1, *A,* the drug is stored in a hollow reservoir within the polymer container, and the rate of drug release is dependent on the steepness of the concentration gradient between the reservoir and the fluid surrounding the delivery device. The steeper the gradient, the more rapid the rate of release for a given polymer system. The rate of release also is dependent on the diffusion coefficient for the random migration of drug molecules through the tangled polymer chains. In an alternative drug storage arrangement (see Figure 6-1, *B*), the drug is distributed uniformly throughout the polymer matrix, but the rate of release is dependent on the concentration gradient and the drug diffusion coefficient within the matrix.

The reservoir devices are expensive and have the inherent disadvantage of releasing a large quantity of drug if the device has a mechanical rupture or defects. However, mechanical damage to a matrix storage device would not cause the sudden release of drug. For very small molecular weight drugs (i.e., 100 to 200 daltons), diffusional control of the release rate is more difficult to maintain than with larger molecular weight compounds without resorting to thicker membranes of very tightly cross-linked polymers and thus larger devices. With either storage arrangement the stability of the drug for prolonged holding at 37° C without significant degradation is a factor that must be proved for each drug-polymer system.

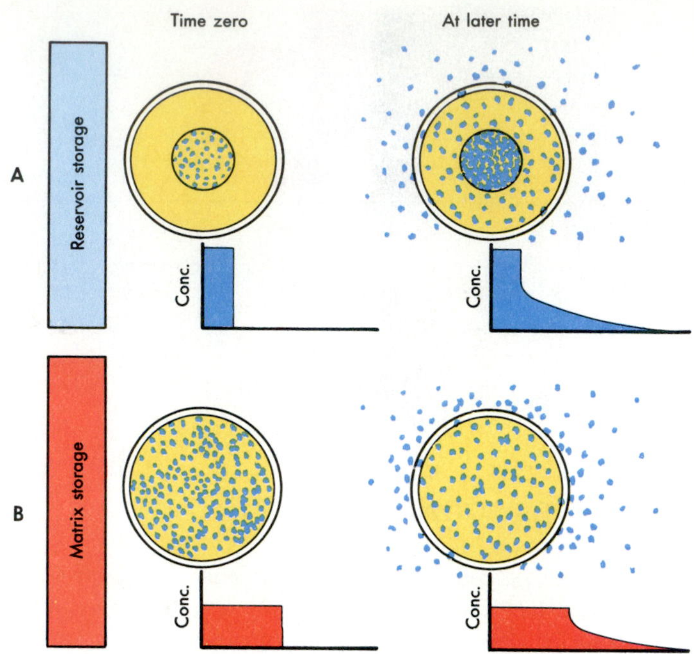

FIGURE 6-1 Diffusional release of drug from drug-polymer system in which drug is stored in a reservoir surrounded by the polymer or stored dispersed within the polymer matrix. See text for further discussion.

A wide variety of alternatives exist for the anatomical placement of diffusional drug-release devices. The controlled delivery of drugs to the eye and to the systemic circulation are two of the examples that are currently in clinical use. Pilocarpine is normally administered several times a day as eyedrops for the treatment of glaucoma. However, the reservoir type of diffusional-release devices (Figure 6-2) are available for insertion under the lower eyelid. These deliver pilocarpine at a constant rate for up to a week and thus give continuous, instead of intermittent, exposure of the eye to pilocarpine. In addition, transdermal matrix-storage diffusional-delivery devices are in clinical use, for example, for placement on the skin to deliver scopolamine for the prevention of motion sickness, nitroglycerin for the treatment of cardiac angina (Figure 6-3), estradiol for the treatment of menopausal problems, and clonidine for the systemic treatment of hypertension.

Transdermal diffusional drug-delivery devices operate on the principle that diffusion through the polymer membrane is slower than that through the skin or other membranes and therefore controls the rate of absorption of the drug. The device must not be placed on a hard epidermal layer; otherwise, diffusion through the skin is greatly reduced. Transdermal delivery of drugs may be advantageous for certain compounds in that the hepatic first-pass effect, transit through the gastric acid, and ex-

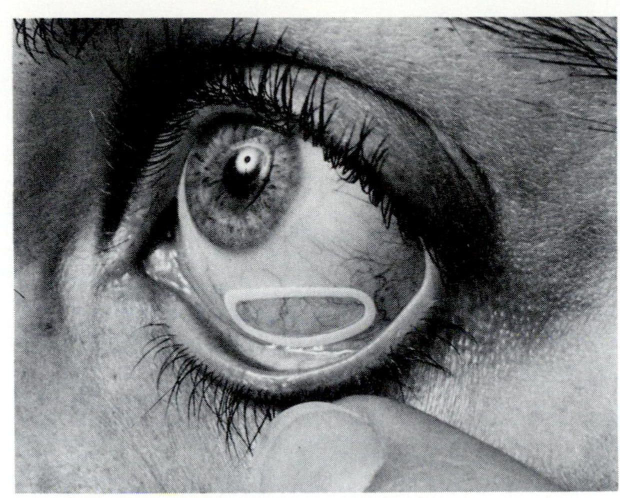

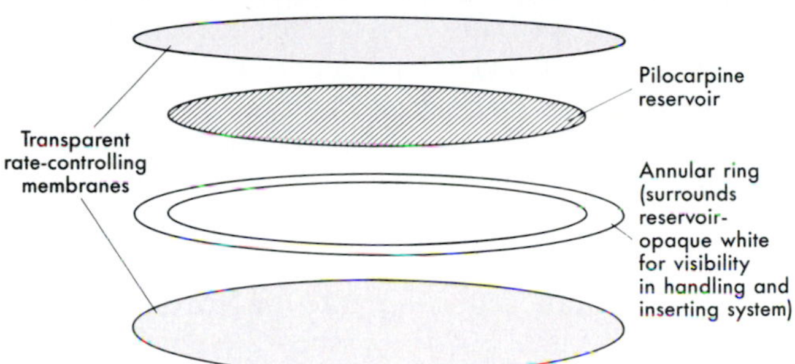

FIGURE 6-2 Ocusert ocular therapeutic system for delivery of pilocarpine (see Chapter 9) for treatment of glaucoma. Flexible wafer is placed under the eyelid and provides drug for a week. Eyelid is shown displaced to expose device. The expanded view denotes the purpose of each of the components. (Courtesy ALZA Corporation, Palo Alto, Calif.)

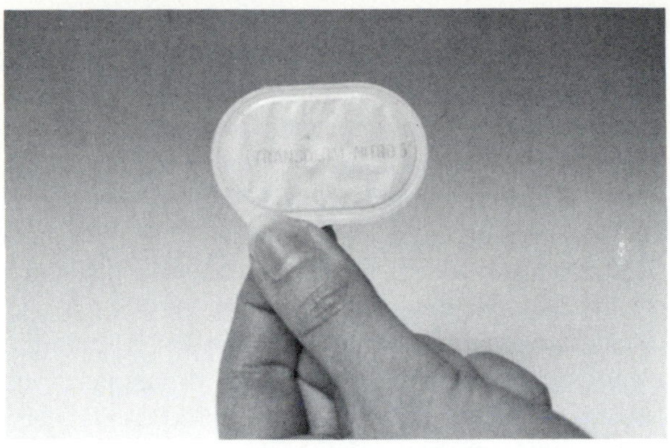

FIGURE 6-3 Transderm-Nitro delivery system for controlled release of nitroglycerin for prevention of angina (see Chapter 17). Patches are applied by means of an adhesive surface usually on the chest. Nitroglycerin diffuses from the matrix at a controlled rate of about 0.02 mg/cm^2/hr and is absorbed through the skin into the systemic circulation. A typical intermittent dosage schedule of 12 to 14 hours with the patch on, followed by 10 to 12 hours off, provides drug delivery at 0.4 mg/hr. The intermittent schedule reduces development of tolerance. A new patch is used every day. (Courtesy Summit Pharmaceuticals, Division of CIBA-Geigy Corporation, Summit, NJ.)

posure to digestive enzymes are bypassed. In addition, the duration of drug administration can be stopped or extended as needed, and the problem of poor patient compliance usually is less than that with repeated oral dosing. However, a drug must have enough lipid solubility to diffuse through the skin at an appreciable rate to be suitable for transdermal delivery.

The second category of drug-polymer release is release by chemical reaction. Two approaches appear promising: chemical erosion of the polymer matrix and chemical release of pendant drug molecules covalently attached to polymer chains (Figure 6-4). For the chemical erosion approach, the polymers undergoing clinical trials are selected such that endogenous hydrolytic enzymes catalyze polymer cleavage. As the polymer matrix disintegrates, drug is uniformly distributed throughout the matrix and is released into the surrounding body fluid. Likewise, hydrolytic enzymes present in body fluids catalyze the cleavage of pendant drug molecules

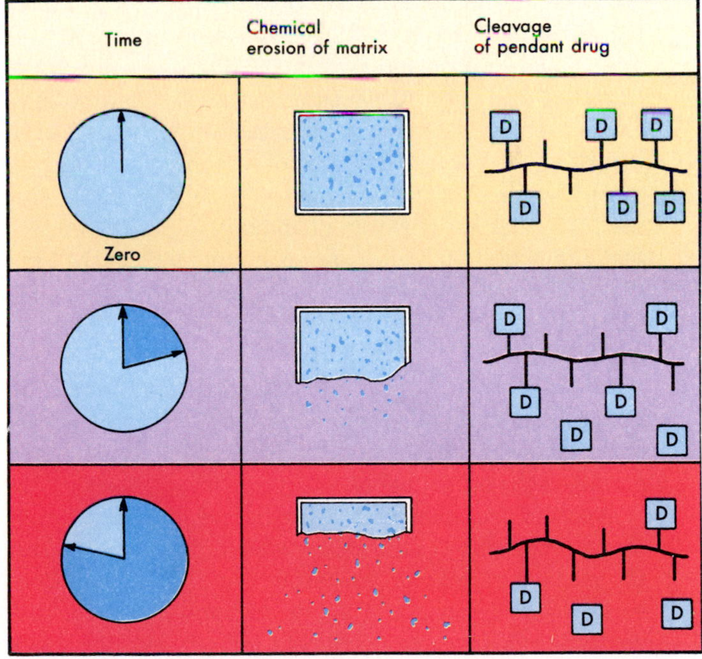

FIGURE 6-4 Drug release by chemical reaction. One approach involves chemical erosion of the polymer matrix and corelease of drug distributed throughout the matrix. The other involves chemical cleavage of drug attached covalently to polymer chains.

from polymer chains in the second approach. Both approaches require the careful selection of polymers to ensure that the products of the polymer erosion are nontoxic. In addition, disposition of the polymer remaining after release of the pendant drug may require surgical removal, if the preparation initially was inserted by surgical implantation.

The third and fourth categories of drug-polymer release mechanisms have only research use (see box). One category uses magnetic materials dispersed throughout the drug-polymer matrix, with the diffusionally controlled rate of release of drug augmented by imposition of an oscillating magnetic field. The other category uses solvent action to raise the osmotic pressure in the space surrounding an implanted drug-filled container, with the increased pressure forcing drug solution out a small opening in the device. Routine clinical use of the latter two categories remain under investigation.

TARGETING OF DRUGS

Drugs that are administered for eradication of tumor cells will be most effective if delivered primarily to the tumor and minimally to other parts of the body. Likewise, a disorder within the central nervous system (CNS) or a severe infection within the pulmonary cavity may be more aggressively treated with drugs if the delivery can be targeted to the CNS or pulmonary spaces respectively. Current extensive research examines cellular, physiological, and anatomical differences between diseased and normal tissues or between different body tissues for leads that may be exploited for purposes of targeting drugs to those cells or tissues. For example, drug-filled albumin microspheres, 15 to 30 μm in diameter, deposit nearly 99% in pulmonary capillary beds after IV injection but lodge approximately 90% in the liver if the microsphere diameter is reduced to 1 to 3 μm. The IV injection of drug-filled microspheres may become a clinically useful means of targeting drugs to these two organs, if the safety considerations caused by plugged capillary beds and scavenging of partially disintegrated albumin spheres from the circulatory system can be resolved favorably.

Another example is the use of carrier molecules, such as glycoproteins or antibodies with recognition sites on the surface of cells of the target organ or tissue. Cell-surface glycoproteins, attached to liposomes, viral envelopes, and erythrocyte ghosts (empty red blood cell membranes) are under study as carriers. In particular, antibodies against tumor cell-surface antigens are under clinical study as carriers for targeting drugs to specific types of tumors.

CONTROLLED VARIABLE RATE DRUG DELIVERY

The delivery of insulin for control of blood glucose concentrations in type I insulin-dependent diabetes mellitus patients is the prime example in which a controlled yet variable rate of drug delivery is needed. Ideally, closed-loop control with an in vivo glucose sensor continuously monitoring the concentration of blood glucose and directing the operation of an implanted, rechargeable insulin-delivery pump is viewed as the needed device. Actually, all the components for such a device are available and workable except the glucose sensor. As a result of the lack of a suitable sensor for in vivo measurement of glucose concentrations, insulin-delivery pumps have been used in patients on an open-loop basis, with blood sampling and in vitro assay for glucose concentrations followed by manual correction of the pumping rate. Patient trials show therapeutic benefits with improved control of blood glucose concentrations; however, costs are high and some problems have developed, particularly with patient compliance.

A variety of implantable pumps are available for infusion of drug by IV, SC, or IM modes. Pumps are powered by batteries or by vapor pressure of a fluorocarbon sealed within the pump unit. Pump reservoirs hold 25 to 35 ml of drug solution. Problems such as thermal stability of the drug for prolonged storage at body temperature, clogging of the outlet orifice, and refilling of the pump reservoir remain to be solved. A significant number of clinical applications are evident for open-loop, as well as closed-loop, delivery of drugs in the endocrine, CNS, anticancer, and immunosuppressant areas.

GENE THERAPY

Advances in the ability to manipulate mammalian genetic material have provided new strategies for research and treatment of human disease through gene transfer and gene therapy. **Gene transfer** is the delivery of exogenous deoxyribonucleic acid (DNA) that encodes for a therapeutic protein to a mammalian cell that can then direct the production of the protein. Gene therapy is the application of this concept for the treatment of hereditary or acquired diseases and employs a wide variety of technologies for DNA delivery to cells. The phases of gene delivery, expression, and action of the gene product are analogous to conventional drug therapy, and each gene therapy system has its own specific pharmacological characteristics that must be appreciated.

GENE THERAPY VECTORS
Plasmid-based vectors plasmid plasmid with liposome plasmid linked to ligand Virus-based vectors retrovirus adenovirus adeno-associated virus herpes simplex virus

Genes that are transferred to cells must contain all components necessary to direct the production of ribonucleic acid (RNA) that will result in functional protein production. The transferred DNA must therefore contain promoter elements necessary for transcription and the entire protein coding region of the gene. Other elements to enhance RNA stability, such as a polyadenylation sequence, are often included.

To introduce this DNA into mammalian cells, several methods can be used. One can introduce in vitro, DNA into cells by microinjection, by coprecipitation with calcium phosphate, or by increasing cell permeability by electrical shock (electroporation). By these techniques one can insert DNA into only a small number of cells, and therefore these techniques have limited use for therapeutic application. Instead, more efficient vehicles have been developed for gene transfer that make possible in vivo gene delivery. Vehicles for DNA delivery include a variety of plasmid- and virus-based vectors (see box). Examples include recombinant plasmids, plasmid mixed with lipid micelles called *liposomes,* and genetically engineered, recombinant DNA or RNA viruses that can carry exogenous genes, infect mammalian cells, and transfer the functional genetic material to that cell. For gene therapy, the most widely investigated vehicles for gene transfer are genetically engineered retrovirus vectors derived from the Moloney murine leukemia retrovirus. Additionally, gene-transfer vectors have been developed from adenovirus and herpes simplex virus. Virus-based vectors are engineered to maximize the safety of gene transfer by modification of the viral genome so that normal virus replication does not occur.

The concept of gene transfer is similar, regardless of vector used (Figure 6-5). The introduction of foreign genes into cells begins with the identification and cloning of a gene. That gene then can be inserted into a plasmid or grown in bacteria; then alone, or combined with one of the many vehicles for gene transfer, it can be delivered to target cells. After administration, the vehicle carrying the DNA enters the cell by passing through the host cell membrane or by active transfer through a specific receptor site. The DNA then is taken up into the nucleus where it can function. If a retrovirus vector is used, DNA can be permanently, though randomly, integrated into the host cell genome. In most systems, the host cell machinery supplies enzymes necessary for the transcription of the DNA into messenger RNA (mRNA), which then can be translated by the host cell into protein. This protein can function intracellularly or extracellularly either to replace a hereditary deficient or defective protein or to provide an additional therapeutic function. The protein may be one that (1) functions intracellularly, such as the enzyme adenosine deaminase, used to correct the mutation in lymphocytes responsible for the severe combined immunodeficiency syndrome; (2) a cell membrane protein, such as the chloride-channel cystic fibrosis transmembrane conductance regulator, that is mutant in cystic fibrosis; or (3) a secreted protein, such as the cytokine interleukin-2, used for anticancer therapy.

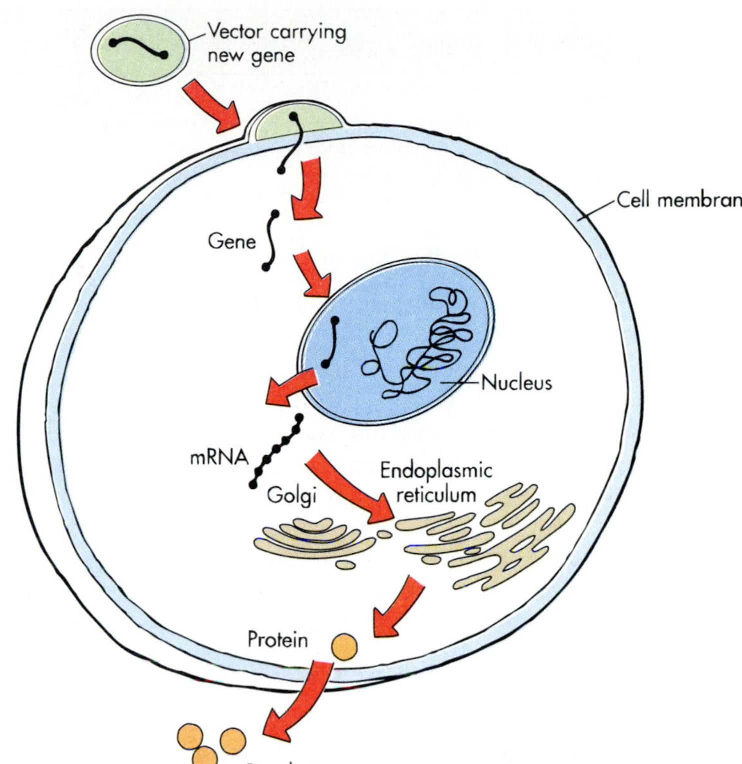

FIGURE 6-5 Generalized schema of gene transfer of a gene encoding for a secreted protein. The vector carrying an exogenous gene is taken up by the target cell and transferred to the nucleus, where the DNA is transcribed to mRNA. The mRNA travels to the Golgi and endoplasmic reticulum, where it is translated to protein. The therapeutic protein is then secreted into the circulation.

Table 6-1 Some Current Human Gene Therapy Studies*

Disease	Gene	Target cell
Severe combined immunodeficiency	adenosine deaminase	Lymphocyte
Cystic fibrosis	cystic fibrosis transmembrane regulator	Lung epithelium
Hemophilia	factors VIII, IX	Skin fibroblast Vascular endothelium
Duchenne's muscular dystrophy	dystrophin	Muscle
Gaucher's disease	glucocerebrosidase	Liver
Acquired immunodeficiency syndrome	cell toxin, antisense	Lymphocytes
Thrombosis	tissue plasminogen activating factor	Vascular endothelium
Solid tumors	interleukin-2, tumor necrosis factor, HLA	Tumor cells

*Only some protocols have been approved for clinical trial.

Two basic experimental approaches have been used for gene therapy. The first is to remove the target cells from the affected individual, add the normal gene to the cells in vitro, and return these modified cells to the donor. If a target cell expressing a mutation can be removed from an organ, modified in vitro, and then returned to that organ where they now function correctly, then the disease may be ameliorated. This strategy has been widely used in animal models for the transfer of new genes to bone marrow cells and was also used in the first approved human gene therapy protocol for the correction of adenosine deaminase deficiency. In these studies, T lymphocytes, which are known to be the critical functional site of the deficient enzyme, were removed from the blood and infected in vitro with a retrovirus vector containing the normal adenosine deaminase gene. The genetically modified lymphocytes were reinfused, where they functioned normally and improved the clinical status of the treated individuals.

This strategy cannot be applied to all diseases because it is virtually impossible to remove and then replant a large number of cells from organs such as the heart, lung, or brain. Therefore, a second approach must be used. In this case, genes must be delivered to the target organ or organs in vivo in a highly efficient manner. This method, called **in vivo gene transfer,** has been successful in several experimental models, such as the transfer of the chloride channel transmembrane regulator gene to lung cells by aerosolization into the airway to treat cystic fibrosis, and the injection of a "healthy" dystrophin gene, for the treatment of muscular dystrophy, into skeletal muscle.

Although gene therapy is in its infancy, several clinical trials involving a variety of creative approaches for the treatment of hereditary and acquired diseases are underway (Table 6-1). For example, gene therapy is being used for the treatment of hereditary hypercholesterolemia caused by low-density lipoprotein receptor deficiency, by addition of the normal gene for the low-density lipoprotein receptor into resected defective hepatocytes, which are then injected into the liver. In addition, cancer therapies that are an attempt to enhance the immune response to tumors are in progress. These involve the use of a retrovirus for the transfer of genes for interleukin-2 and tumor necrosis factor to tumor cells, or the use of liposomes for the transfer of human leukocyte–associated antigens by direct injection into tumors. Using analyses identical to that employed in the assessment of other kinds of pharmacotherapy, a major research effort is underway to determine the utility of gene therapy for the treatment of many other diseases, including acquired immunodeficiency syndrome, leukemia, and hemophilia.

REFERENCES

Anderson WF: Human gene therapy, *Science* 256:808, 1992.

Juliano RL, editor: Biological approaches to the controlled delivery of drugs, *Ann NY Acad Sci* 507:1, 1987.

Langer R: Implantable controlled release systems. In Ihler GM, editor: *Methods of drug delivery,* New York, 1986, Pergamon Press.

Mecklenburg RS, Benson EA, Benson JW Jr, et al: Long-term metabolic control with insulin pump therapy, *N Engl J Med* 313:465, 1985.

Miller AD: Human gene therapy comes of age, *Nature* 357:455, 1992.

Poste G: Drug targeting in cancer therapy. In Gregoriadis G, Poste G, Senior J, et al, editors: Receptor mediated targeting of drugs, New York, 1985, Plenum Publishing Co.

Verma IM: Gene therapy, *Sci Am,* pp 68-72, 81, 82, 84, Nov 1990.

SELF-ASSESSMENT QUESTIONS

1. Drug-polymer sustained-release preparations:
   a. Are the most commonly used preparations to extend the duration of drug absorption.
   b. Vary in release rates, depending on tissue pH.
   c. Release drugs at a relatively constant rate by slow diffusion.
   d. a and c are correct.
   e. All of the above are correct.
2. Transdermal drug delivery devices:
   a. Generally increase patient compliance.
   b. Can be used effectively only with lipid-soluble drugs.
   c. Avoid the effects of gastric acid.
   d. a and c are correct.
   e. All of the above are correct.
3. Vectors for gene transfer include the following *except:*
   a. Recombinant plasmids.
   b. Plasmids mixed with microsomes.
   c. Genetically engineered leukemia retrovirus.
   d. Genetically engineered herpes simplex virus.
   e. All of the above are correct.
4. Gene therapy:
   a. Can be used where there is defective production of an enzyme or protein attributable to a gene.
   b. Can be used in hereditary conditions.
   c. Can be used in the treatment of certain acquired diseases.
   d. a and b are correct.
   e. All of the above are correct.

CHAPTER 7

Issues in Therapeutics

THEODORE M. BRODY

CLINICAL PROBLEM AREAS

Several problem areas arise in the clinical use of drugs. These include drug interactions, genetic factors, dosage modifications required for the extremes of patient age (pediatric and geriatric), and drug reactions. The first three topics are discussed in this chapter, with more extensive coverage of the pharmacological considerations specific for pediatric or geriatric patients included in Chapters 63 and 64 respectively. This chapter also contains a list of drugs for which the therapeutic index is small and where the plasma concentration of drug is often monitored to assist in achieving the target concentration with minimal toxic side effects. Allergic responses to drug are also considered.

DRUG INTERACTIONS

One of the four factors mentioned (Chapter 1) for the individual clinical use of drugs is that patients often receive more than one drug. Hospitalized patients, for example, receive an average of five to ten drugs, and outpatients may take two to four preparations. Some geriatric patients receive as many as 12 drugs concurrently. With so many drugs administered, especially in hospitalized patients, there are numerous opportunities for drug interactions to occur.

In this context, a **drug interaction** refers to a change in the magnitude or duration of the pharmacological response of one drug because of the presence of another drug. A classical example is the patient receiving chronic warfarin anticoagulant therapy, to which a 14-day regimen of the antiinflammatory agent, phenylbutazone, is added. Warfarin and phenylbutazone are each approximately 97% bound to plasma albumin at therapeutic concentrations, with both drugs competing for the same albumin binding sites. Introduction of phenylbutazone displaces some of the albumin-bound warfarin, thereby increasing the concentration of unbound warfarin by as much as 50% to 100%. The magnitude of the anticoagulant effect of warfarin can become dangerously high. The dose of warfarin must therefore be reduced before the start of phenylbutazone administration.

The physician should be aware of which drugs a patient is receiving and recognize the possibilities for drug interactions when adding new drug or discontinuing a currently used drug. Most pharmacies maintain records of drugs currently used by individual patients and can provide this information to other members of the health care team. Compendia are also available that list drug interactions.

In anticipation of changes in the pharmacological direction of therapy, steps sometimes need to be taken to modify existing dosing schedules to compensate for an anticipated interaction, or, where possible, to select another drug that does not participate in this interaction. Drug interactions can result in elevated concentrations of drug by displacement of protein-bound drug or reduced rates of drug disposition, including elevation to toxic concentrations. Drug interactions also can result in more rapid disappearance of drug, with the plasma concentration decreasing to below the minimum effective value. Both of these situations are undesirable. Being able to predict the direction and extent of the expected change in concentration or in magnitude of effect arises primarily from an understanding of the mechanisms by which the interaction occurs.

Drug interactions occur by several principal mechanisms. These include acceleration or inhibition of drug metabolism; displacement of plasma protein-bound drug; impaired uptake of drug from the gastrointestinal (GI) tract; altered renal clearance of drug; modifications in receptors or blockade of receptor channels; and changes in electrolyte balance, body fluid pH, or rates of protein synthesis. The more frequently encountered mechanisms are illustrated schematically in Figure 7-1. A partial listing of specific drug interactions is contained in Table 7-1. Some appreciation of the drug types that are most often associated with drug interactions can be obtained from Table 7-2. This empirical approach singles out the drug types in which the major interaction problems arise. A discussion of specific interactions with the oral anticoagulants is included in Chapter 21.

Detailed descriptions of specific drug interactions are available in the pharmacology literature.*

PHARMACOGENETICS

Variation in drug responses can result from genetic differences in drug disposition. The study of these disorders is called **pharmacogenetics.** Differences in drug disposition are inherited similarly to inborn errors of metabolism but with two major differences. Patients with pharmacogenetic disorders may lead normal lives and never encounter difficulties unless challenged with the drug capable of producing the aberrant response. Also, a nutrient or its metabolite is not involved; rather, the problem substrate is obviously a drug. Pharmacogenetic differences result in either enhancement or reduction in intensity of response to a drug, with the drug duration of action lengthened or shortened. Infrequently the effects of a drug in a patient may differ qualitatively from normal.

Usually a plot of the plasma drug concentration curve in a population of patients receiving the same dosage of that drug results in a normal bell-shaped curve. However, if a genetic factor or factors are involved, the population distribution curve becomes bimodal (or sometimes multimodal), an indication of separate populations, one sensitive and one less sensitive to the drug (Fig. 7-2). Some of the more widely encountered pharmacogenetic variations and the mechanisms by which these genetic differences occur are now discussed.

Genetic modification of enzyme activity associated with the biotransformation of specific drugs is a major mechanism encountered in pharmacogenetics. One such example is **acetylation polymorphism.** *N*-Acetylation is one of several metabolic reactions by which drugs and other chemicals are detoxified, acetylating aromatic amines and hydrazines. Primary sites for acetylation in humans are liver and gastrointestinal mucosa. Differences in *N*-acetylation were originally recognized in tuberculosis patients treated with isoniazid, a drug metabolized principally by this mechanism. By determining the plasma concentration at a specific time

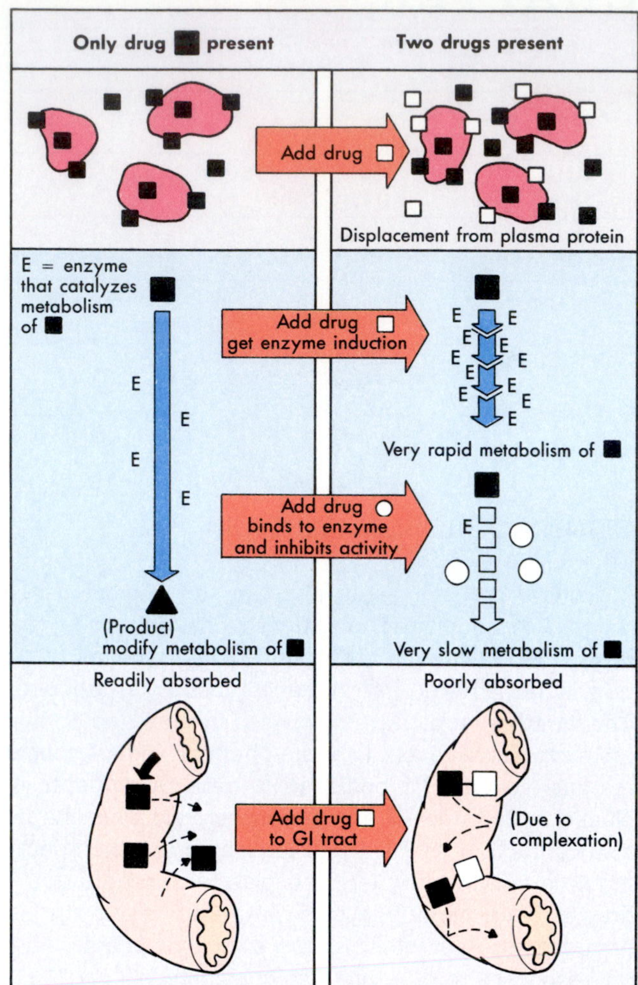

FIGURE 7-1 Frequently encountered mechanisms by which drug interactions occur.

after a fixed dose of isoniazid, patients were classified as either slow or rapid acetylators, an indication that *N*-acetylating activity is distributed bimodally in humans. Acetylation polymorphism has now been found to influence the metabolizing of many drugs and chemicals (see box) in addition to isoniazid. This phenomenon varies widely with race and geographic distribution; 45% of the United States population (white and African-American) are slow acetylators and 55% are rapid, whereas 90% of Orientals are slow acetylators.

Thus, acetylation polymorphism has important clinical and toxicological significance. Acetylation phenotype modulates metabolism of drugs with free amino groups such as sulfonamides, hydralazine, procainamide, dapsone, and aminoglutethamide, as well as isoniazid. Metabolism of carcinogenic aromatic amines such as benzidine and β-naphthylamine are also influenced. Affected too are drugs such as sulfasalazine,

*One journal that is particularly useful is *Clinical Pharmacology and Therapeutics.*

Table 7-1 Drug Interactions

Site	Substance	Circumstances of Interaction
GI tract	tetracyclines	Complex with Al^{+3}, Ca^{++}, or Mg^{++} antacids or with aluminum hydroxide gels or milk; decrease absorption
	cholestyramine	Acts as ion-exchange resin to complex with acidic compounds such as warfarin and prevents warfarin absorption
	metoclopramide	Speeds up gastric emptying; increases absorption of acetaminophen
Protein binding in blood	salicylates nonsteroidal antiinflammatory agents oral hypoglycemic agents long-lasting sulfonamides	In each case, other drugs are present that bind to the same region on the protein and therefore displace some of the substance
Renal clearance	probenecid	Inhibits renal secretion of indomethacin; decreases clearance
	salicylates	Inhibit renal secretion of phenylbutazone, sulfinpyrazone, indomethacin, and probenecid; decrease clearance
	sulfinpyrazone	Inhibits renal secretion of salicylates; decreases clearance
	phenylbutazone	Inhibits renal secretion of acetoheximide; decreases clearance
	thiazide diuretics	Decrease lithium clearance
	tricyclic antidepressants	Interact with methylphenidate or guanethidine
Drug metabolism	ethanol	Speeds up metabolism of phenytoin, tolbutamide, and warfarin
	antihistamines	Speed up metabolism of phenobarbital or progesterone
	phenytoin	Speeds up metabolism of corticosteroids or warfarin
	barbiturates	Speed up metabolism of digitoxin, phenytoin, griseofulvin, phenylbutazone, warfarin, or testosterone
	glutethimide	Speeds up metabolism of warfarin
	phenylbutazone	Inhibits metabolism of tolbutamide or warfarin
	chloramphenicol	Inhibits metabolism of hexobarbital or tolbutamide
	allopurinol	Inhibits metabolism of 6-mercaptopurine or azathioprine
	cimetidine	Inhibits metabolism of benzodiazepines or propranolol
	desipramine	Inhibits metabolism of amphetamine
	methylphenidate	Inhibits metabolism of warfarin, some anticonvulsants, and tricyclic antidepressants

Table 7-2 Estimated Tendency of Drug Classes to Participate in Drug-Drug Interactions

Drug Class	Interactions/Drug*
Anticoagulants, oral	43
Antidiabetics	16
Monoamine oxidase inhibitors	16
Phenothiazines	10
Anticonvulsants	10
Tricyclic antidepressants	6
Digitalis glycosides	6
Antiarrhythmics	5.9
Salicylates	4
Hormones	3
Diuretics	2.9
Antihypertensives	2.9
Antiinfective agents	2.2
Antineoplastic agents	1.7
Others	0.7

*Results obtained by counting the number of interactions of major clinical significance as listed in Hanston PD and Horn JR: *Drug interactions,* ed. 6, Philadelphia, 1989, Lea & Feibiger. For example, 26 combinations of antihypertensives and other drugs were reported to produce significant interactions. Twenty-six divided by the nine different antihypertensive agents listed produces a frequency of 2.9 interactions for each type of antihypertensive drug.

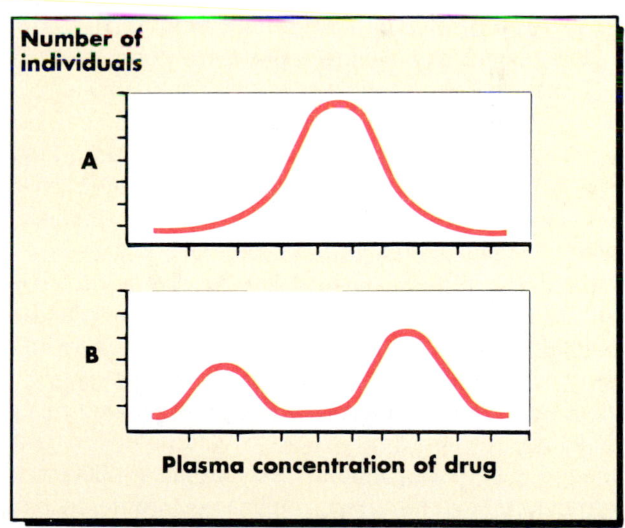

FIGURE 7-2 **A,** Frequency distribution curve shows the normal variability in plasma concentrations when a fixed dose of drug *X* is administered to a large population of patients. **B,** Frequency distribution curve under the same conditions with drug *Y,* indicating a bimodal curve typical of a pharmacogenetic alteration.

SOME DRUGS AND CHEMICALS THAT UNDERGO *N*-ACETYLATION

isoniazid
hydralazine
procainamide
dapsone
sulfonamides
clonazepam
nitrazepam
aminoglutethimide
β-naphthylamine
benzidine
phenelzine

clonazepam, and nitrazepam; compounds without a free amino group, but with one introduced during their metabolic biotransformation. Slow acetylation is responsible for such toxic effects as peripheral neuropathy in patients treated with isoniazid, for lupus erythematosus during procainamide and hydralazine treatment, for hemolytic anemia during sulfasalazine treatment, and for urinary bladder cancer after environmental exposure to benzidine.

Another drug-metabolizing enzyme found in a genetically altered form is cholinesterase in plasma and liver, also termed pseudocholinesterase or butyrylcholinesterase. This enzyme catalyzes the hydrolysis of succinylcholine, used as a muscle relaxant during surgery (see Chapter 11.) Some patients do not hydrolyze a standard dose of succinylcholine rapidly, resulting in prolonged muscle relaxation and an ensuing apnea. In these patients, atypical plasma cholinesterase is present, with the abnormally long duration of drug action resulting from a reduced affinity of the aberrant enzyme for succinylcholine. The atypical enzyme gene has a worldwide distribution, with an allele frequency of approximately 2% in many populations, but it is rare to undetectable in blacks, Filipinos, Eskimos, and the Japanese population. Another enzyme variant has been found; it is several times more active than the normal enzyme, thus producing resistance to administered succinylcholine.

Genetic differences among cytochrome P-450 monooxygenases have also been implicated in differences in metabolic clearances of several drug classes. An example is the variability of responses seen in patients treated with the antihypertensive debrisoquine. Introduced in the United Kingdom in the 1960s, debrisoquine is normally hydroxylated to an inactive product in liver. Liver biopsy studies established that those patients who were poor metabolizers of debrisoquine had a deficiency

DRUGS CAPABLE OF INDUCING HEMOLYTIC ANEMIA IN G6PD-DEFICIENT PATIENTS

acetophenetidin	*p*-aminosalicylic acid
chloramphenicol	primaquine
chloroquine	sulfonamides
nitrofuran derivatives	Vitamin K analogs

in cytochrome P-450 monooxygenase activity resulting from ineffective binding of substrate to the enzyme. The impaired metabolism of other drugs in some patients is now also considered to result from an aberrant or deficient cytochrome P-450 monooxygenase protein. These include drugs such as metiamide, dextromethorphan, phenytoin, nortriptyline, phenformin, and metoprolol. Although some of these drugs are hydroxylated, others are demethylated or deethylated, an indication that several different cytochrome P-450 proteins may be involved.

Many drugs can induce hemolytic anemia in patients genetically deficient in red blood cell glucose-6-phosphate dehydrogenase (see box). This enzyme, part of the hexose monophosphate shunt in red blood cells, is a primary source of the reduced form of nicotinamide adenine dinucleotide phosphate (NADPH), a cofactor for glutathione reductase, which normally reduced oxidized glutathione. Hemolysis of red blood cells can result from the cells' inability to maintain sufficient reduced glutathione. Glutathione is critical for maintaining protein sulfhydryl groups in the reduced state, thus preventing enzyme denaturation and promoting erythrocyte membrane integrity. Many glucose-6-phosphate dehydrogenase variants have been identified, and it has been estimated that a variant is present in approximately 200 million people worldwide.

These specific examples emphasize the importance of considering genetic variation in evaluating abnormal responses to drugs in patients.

DRUG ALLERGY

Another clinical problem is that of undesirable immunological responses to drugs. These are frequently called "drug allergies," a broad term encompassing genetic variations already discussed, and toxic effects of drugs resulting from idiosyncratic reactions. Drug allergy, or **hypersensitization,** is discussed here in the context of drug-induced activations of immunological reactions with drugs acting as antigens. Although normally we consider the immune system as beneficial and protective, adverse reactions occur when the system is challenged by certain antigens. The nature and intensity vary with antigen type and site of contact. A common feature of hypersensitivity is that a response occurs only after a previous exposure. Exposure may be either to the parent drug or to a metabolite. Subsequent exposure to the same drug, or a closely related species, then induces the allergic or hypersensitive reaction. Because the presence of considerable interindividual differences is a common feature, genetic factors are at least in part responsible for many allergic responses.

Drug hypersensitivities can be classified into four types, depending on the nature of the immune response.

Type I, or **immediate,** or **anaphylactoid reaction,** involves IgE antibodies produced by drugs that bind to the surface of mast cells and basophils. The interaction of the allergen with several IgE antibodies results in cross-linking of antibodies, with subsequent degranulation of mast cells and basophils, releasing histamine, leukotrienes, serotonin, and prostaglandins. These released mediators trigger a rapid immune reaction, leading to bronchiolar constriction, capillary dilatation, or urticaria. If severe, the reaction can result in anaphylactic shock.

Type II, or **cytotoxic** or **autoimmune responses,** involve IgG and IgM antibodies and complement. The allergen binds to a protein on the surface of a vascular cell, red or white blood cell, or platelet, evoking an antibody response. The drug-protein complex bound to the antibody activates the complement system, resulting in cytolysis and cell death. Methyldopa, for example, may cause hemolytic anemia by this mechanism, and thrombocytopenia purpura may occur with quinidine use.

In the type III, or **immune complex—mediated reaction,** antigen-antibody complexes interact and are deposited in tissues such as the vascular endothelium or cell basement membrane, activating the complement system and promoting an acute inflammatory reaction. If deposited in the vascular endothelium, serum sickness may occur. Other type III reactions include arteritis, urticaria, and granulocytopenia. Stevens-Johnson syndrome is an example of a severe skin and mucous membrane manifestation resulting from sulfonamide administration.

Type IV, the **cell-mediated response,** is a delayed type of hypersensitivity involving T lymphocytes, macrophages, and neutrophils occurring primarily in skin. In this reaction, the allergen combines with skin proteins, evoking the immune response. Sensitized T lymphocytes release lymphokines activating macrophages and neutrophils. The infiltration of these cells produces a local inflammatory response. Halothane-induced hepatitis is an example that may result from a type IV reaction.

Many factors may predispose individuals to allergic responses to drugs and chemicals. A physician should be familiar with a patient's drug history. This may be difficult because many patients are unaware of prior exposure to a particular drug or drug class. Allergens frequently may be present in over-the-counter drugs, in foods, or in the environment. A patient also may not be aware that an allergic reaction has occurred with earlier drug use because mild reactions to many drugs are not uncommon and are often overlooked. Recent studies indicate that documented allergic reactions account for as few as 10% of all adverse effects to drugs. Although allergies generally can occur with any route of drug administration, the oral route is less likely to result in sensitization, whereas topical drug application presents the greatest risk. Continuous exposure of workers to industrial chemicals is a frequent cause of allergic dermatitis. Some drug classes are more likely to cause hypersensitivity reactions than others, and although there is no method to estimate the allergic potential of any drug, as with most untoward responses to drug therapy, the physician is well advised to limit the number of drugs prescribed.

DOSING MODIFICATIONS FOR PEDIATRIC AND GERIATRIC PATIENTS

Pharmacokinetic as well as pharmacological response differences exist between young adults and infants and between young adults and the elderly. The differences must be appreciated for safe and beneficial use of drugs in patients at the extremes of age. Some pharmacokinetic considerations are mentioned here, but an in-depth discussion is available in Chapters 63 and 64.

Numerous physiological changes take place during the life-span, from infant, through young adult, to the geriatric years. These changes are important to drug pharmacokinetics and are discussed here; they include liver metabolic function, renal elimination capabilities, and body composition.

Liver metabolism and renal elimination of drugs are usually diminished at the extremes of age. The ability of the newborn infant to dispose of drugs is often limited. Liver drug metabolizing enzyme systems may be present at birth only in extremely low activities; renal elimination capabilities also may be depressed. Both hepatic and renal drug disposition is reduced in infants, as shown in Table 7-3. In infants, renal tubular secretion may not be well developed, and renal blood flow may be less than expected. After 40 years of age, liver mass decreases at a rate of approximately 1% per year, resulting in a diminished ability to metabolize drugs. What is not clearly defined is whether the intrinsic drug

Table 7-3 Comparative Body Size and Renal Clearance Capacity Between Infants and Adults

Parameter	Infants	Adults
Body weight, kg	3.5	70
Body water, %	77	58
Inulin clearance		
ml/min/kg	0.85	1.85
ml/min	3	130
$t_{1/2}$ min	630	220
p-Aminohippuric acid clearance		
ml/min/kg	3.4	9.2
ml/min	12	650
$t_{1/2}$ min	160	43

metabolizing activity of each molecule of enzyme also diminishes with increased age. Renal elimination in the elderly also shows diminished glomerular filtration and tubular secretion clearance mechanisms. Thus it may be desirable to assess filtration capability in individual patients by determining creatinine clearance.

Changes in body composition also occur on aging. Infants contain the highest proportion of total body water in relation to body weight. The proportion of total body water decreases with aging and is accompanied by an increased proportion of body fat. Such changes in body composition can profoundly influence the distribution of a drug into the various body compartments, tissues, and fluids. The target plasma concentration of a drug thus may be different for the three age groups as a result of the modified distribution pattern. These changes are shown schematically in Figure 7-3.

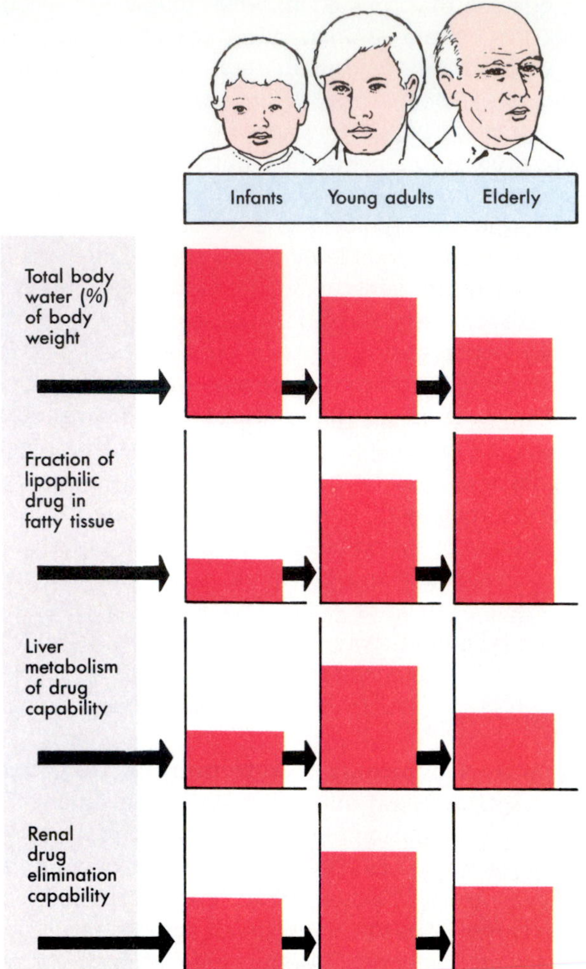

FIGURE 7-3 Areas of boxes indicate relative size or capability of function at each age.

MONITORING PLASMA DRUG CONCENTRATIONS

Development of suitably sensitive assays for the quantitative determination of drug concentrations in small samples of patient blood and at therapeutic concentrations of drug has made it possible to monitor blood drug concentrations as a guide to the rapid achievement and maintenance of the desired target concentrations. Table 7-4 lists target concentration ranges for drugs that are most difficult to use without encountering toxic symptoms. A range of concentrations is given for each drug to compensate for differences in distribution and in the rates of drug absorption and disposition in individual patients because values for pharmacokinetic and pharmacological response parameters are not known for individual patients. Monitoring of blood drug concentrations for the compounds

Table 7-4 Serum Concentrations of Drugs at Target Therapeutic and Estimated Toxic Concentrations

	Concentrations (μg/ml)	
Drugs	**Therapeutic**	**Toxic**
carbamazepine	5-12	
digitoxin	0.013-0.025	>0.035
digoxin	0.0010-0.0022	>0.0025
diphenylhydantoin	10-20	>25
ethosuximide	50-100	
gentamicin	8-12	
lidocaine	1.5-5	>9
lithium	0.6-1.2*	
nortriptyline	0.050-0.080	
phenobarbital	15-30	>40
procainamide	4-8	>10
propranolol	0.030-0.120	
quinidine	2-4	>6
salicylate	150-300	>300
theophylline	10-20	>20

*Milliequivalents/liter.

in Table 7-4 may help in nonstandard situations to provide guidance in adjusting dosing schedules or obtaining a therapeutic drug concentration with a minimum of toxicity. However, the routine monitoring of drug blood concentrations is usually not warranted after the plateau concentration is reached and maintained for several dosing intervals.

SUMMARY

An unexpected response to the therapeutic dosing regimen of a drug occasionally occurs. The practitioner must quickly define the cause of the unexpected response and adjust the administration of the drug to the situation if necessary. Possible causes include drug interaction, genetic variation, histamine release, immunological reaction, and incorrect adjustment of dose for patient age. Other unknown causes may also be responsible. In many cases dosing adjustment can be made so that the originally planned drug type can be used.

REFERENCES

Hansten PD, Horn JR: *Drug interactions,* ed 6, Philadelphia, 1989, Lea & Febiger.

Pratt WB, Tayler P, editors: *Principles of drug action,* ed 3, New York, 1990, Churchill Livingstone.

Schmucker DL: Aging and drug disposition: an update, *Pharmacol Rev* 37:133, 1985.

Weber WW, Hein DW: *N*-Acetylation pharmacogenetics, *Pharmacol Rev* 37:25, 1985.

SELF-ASSESSMENT QUESTIONS

1. All statements about drug interactions are true *except:*
   a. Can result in a change in magnitude of a pharmmacological response
   b. Can result in a change in duration of a pharmacological response
   c. Can result in a more rapid disappearance of drug
   d. Can result in inhibition of biotransformation of drug
   e. All of the above are true
2. Which of the following generally occur significantly in a normal elderly population compared with young adults:
   a. An increase in total body water, thus decreasing free drug concentrations in body fluids
   b. An increase in drug metabolizing activity, reducing pharmacological intensity and duration of many drugs
   c. A decrease in plasma proteins, increasing free drug concentrations in the elderly
   d. A decrease in vascular permeability, which decreases the transport of drugs across the blood-brain barrier in the elderly patient
   e. a, c, and d are correct
3. Pharmacogenetic differences in drug response:
   a. May result from the drug or any of its metabolites.
   b. Cannot be identified from population studies.
   c. Most frequently involve a single genetic factor and a specific substrate (drug).
   d. Are present in approximately 10% of the United States population.
   e. All of the above are correct.
4. Acetylation polymorphism occurs with:
   a. Catecholamines.
   b. Isoniazid, procainamide, and hydralazine.
   c. Compounds that originally do not possess a free amino group but with one introduced after biotransformation of these compounds.
   d. b and c are correct.
   e. All of the above are correct.
5. A genetic variant of pseudocholinesterase has been implicated in an abnormal response to average doses of:
   a. Acetylcholine.
   b. Carbachol.
   c. Succinylcholine.
   d. Acetaminophen.
   e. Aspirin.
6. Drug allergy is a term for a reaction:
   a. That does not include genetic factors.
   b. That is a form of hypersensitization.
   c. That does not necessarily occur after a prior exposure to the drug but is observed on initial exposure.
   d. In which drugs act as antibodies.
   e. All of the above are correct.
7. Cell-mediated hypersensitivity:
   a. Exhibits a delayed response.
   b. Is characterized by T lymphocytes and neutrophil involvement.
   c. Occurs when the drug (or allergen) combines with skin proteins, evoking a local response.
   d. Is the cause of halothane-induced hepatitis.
   e. All of the above are correct.

PART II

PERIPHERAL AUTONOMIC NERVOUS SYSTEM: DRUGS AFFECTING TRANSMISSION AND FUNCTION

The autonomic nervous system controls key visceral processes, including cardiac output, blood flow to specific organs, glandular secretions, waste elimination, sexual function, and other processes necessary for life. Many of the autonomic actions take place outside of the central nervous system (CNS), either at junctions along the nerve fibers that innervate specific organs or at the junction of the nerve with the organ innervated. Drugs developed to treat disease states that require modification of autonomically controlled functions can be divided into agents that act in the peripheral nervous system and those that act in the CNS. Part II pertains to drug actions that occur in the peripheral nervous system and specifically in the peripheral portion of the autonomic nervous system. Drug actions that occur in the CNS are described in Part III.

Chapter 8 describes the peripheral autonomic nervous system, with special emphasis on sites and biochemical or physiological processes in which clinically used drugs act. The approach is to treat the two main neurotransmitter systems of the peripheral autonomic nervous system separately. Thus Chapter 9 covers the parasympathetic nervous system in which acetylcholine is the endogenous transmitter, and Chapter 10 covers the sympathetic nervous system with norepinephrine as the endogenous transmitter. Because of the wide scope of actions of peripheral autonomic innervation, many of the drugs presented in Part II are mentioned in subsequent parts as having therapeutic actions in other disease states not mentioned in this part. Other therapeutic actions and the drugs involved are discussed in other appropriate chapters, with reference to Chapters 9 or 10.

Because the neuromuscular blocking agents act at peripheral sites, they also are included in this part (Chapter 11).

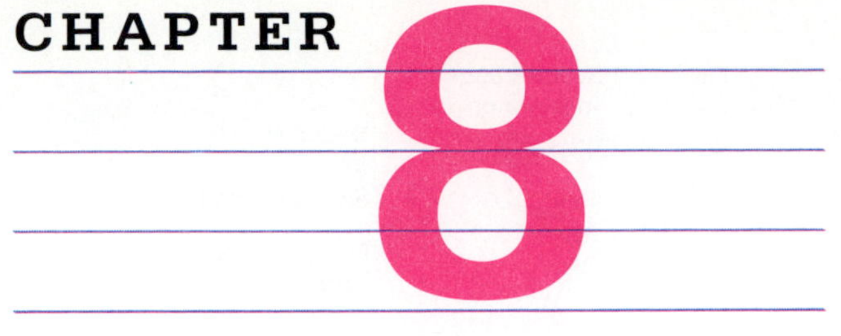

Physiology and Biochemistry of the Peripheral Nervous System

ROBERT R. RUFFOLO, JR.

The autonomic nervous system represents a peripheral efferent nervous system that provides innervation to the heart, blood vessels, visceral organs, glands, and virtually all other organs that are composed in part of smooth muscle. The autonomic nervous system is widely distributed throughout the body and serves to regulate the functions of these organs in a manner that is generally beyond conscious control. Hence, the autonomic nervous system is often referred to as the involuntary nervous system. Although the efferent outflow of the autonomic nervous system provides innervation to most structures in the body, one notable exception is skeletal muscle, which is under conscious, voluntary control originating from higher centers in the central nervous system (CNS). Nerves having cell bodies within the CNS that innervate the skeletal muscles are termed **somatic nerves** and are functionally and anatomically different from autonomic nerves.

Autonomic nerves are actually composed of two neuron systems, termed *preganglionic* and *postganglionic,* based on anatomical location relative to the **ganglia,** or relay centers. A **preganglionic neuron** has its cell body in the spinal cord or brain and is modulated by higher centers in the brain and by spinal reflexes. The axon originating from the cell body of a preganglionic neuron leaves the spinal cord from the cranial, thoracic, lumbar, or sacral regions and forms a synaptic connection in the autonomic ganglia with the cell body of the postganglionic autonomic nerve fiber. The **postganglionic neurons** send their axons directly to the effector organs to complete the pathway of autonomic innervation of the peripheral involuntary visceral organs.

ABBREVIATIONS	
ATP	adenosine triphosphate
cAMP	cyclic adenosine monophosphate
CNS	central nervous system
DOPA	3,4-dihydroxyphenylalanine
G protein	guanine nucleotide regulatory protein

The function of the peripheral autonomic nerves is to modulate the ongoing activity of the involuntary visceral organs by eliciting excitatory or inhibitory responses. Although neuronal connections for the somatic nervous system are located entirely within the CNS, virtually all autonomic nerves have ganglia located outside the CNS. Furthermore, most somatic nerves that control motor function are myelinated and transmit impulses rapidly, whereas most postganglionic autonomic nerves are nonmyelinated and conduct impulses at relatively slower rates. Most preganglionic neurons, however, are also myelinated and conduct impulses rapidly.

DIVISIONS OF THE PERIPHERAL AUTONOMIC NERVOUS SYSTEM

There are two major divisions of the peripheral autonomic nervous system: **sympathetic** and **parasympathetic.** Many anatomical and functional differences distinguish these two separate entities. An anatomical depiction of divisions is presented in Figure 8-1.

Sympathetic Nervous System

Cell bodies for preganglionic neurons of the sympathetic division of the autonomic nervous system originate in the intermediolateral cell column of the spinal cord at the thoracic and lumbar levels. Relatively short preganglionic neurons leave the spinal cord at the thoracic and lumbar levels (called **thoracolumbar outflow**). These short preganglionic axons send projections to the sympathetic ganglia outside of the spinal vertebrae. These 22 segmentally arranged ganglia consist of two chains located bilaterally with respect to the spinal cord. Postganglionic neurons with their cell bodies located in the paravertebral sympathetic chain gan-

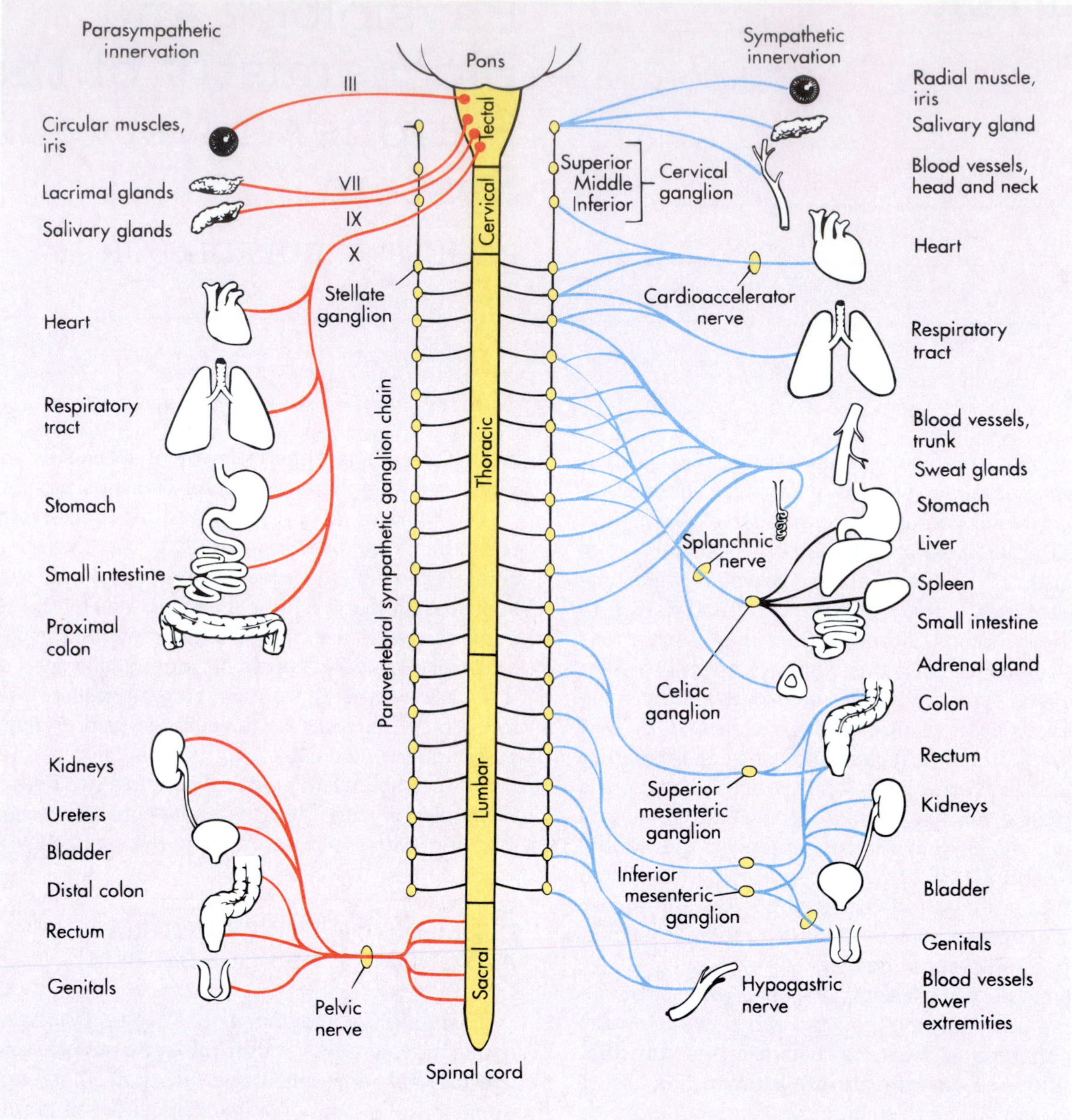

FIGURE 8-1 Schema of the autonomic nervous system depicting the functional innervation of peripheral effector organs and the anatomical origin of peripheral autonomic nerves from the spinal cord. Although both paravertebral sympathetic ganglia chains are presented, the sympathetic innervation to the peripheral effector organs is shown only on the right part of the figure, whereas parasympathetic innervation of peripheral effector organs is depicted on the left. The roman numerals on nerves originating in the tectal region of the brainstem refer to the cranial nerves that provide parasympathetic outflow to the effector organs of the head, neck, and trunk.

glia send relatively long postganglionic fibers to their effector organs.

Most preganglionic sympathetic neurons synapse in the paravertebral sympathetic ganglia. However, a few preganglionic sympathetic fibers pass through these vertebral ganglia without making synaptic connections and travel by way of the splanchnic nerves to the prevertebral ganglia located in front of the vertebral column. These ganglia are situated in the pelvis and abdomen and are named the **celiac, superior mesenteric,** and **inferior mesenteric (hypogastric) ganglia** (see Figure 8-1). Terminal ganglia lie close to the organs they innervate, namely, the urinary bladder and rectum.

The neurotransmitter that mediates synaptic transmission between preganglionic and postganglionic nerve fibers in the sympathetic pathway is **acetylcholine.** In contrast, the neurotransmitter liberated by the long postganglionic sympathetic nerves and mediating the end-organ responses at the neuroeffector junctions is **norepinephrine.** Sites that use acetylcholine as the neurotransmitter are termed **cholinergic,** whereas those that use norepinephrine are called **adrenergic.** (See Chapter 10 for additional comments on terminology.)

The adrenal medulla contains chromaffin cells, embryologically and anatomically homologous to the sympathetic ganglia in that they are derived from the neural crest. The adrenal medulla, unlike the postganglionic sympathetic nerve terminals, releases epinephrine as the primary catecholamine. The chromaffin cells of the adrenal medulla are innervated by typical preganglionic sympathetic nerve terminals, whose neurotransmitter is acetylcholine.

Parasympathetic Nervous System

The parasympathetic division of the autonomic nervous system differs greatly from the sympathetic division. Cell bodies giving rise to preganglionic **parasympathetic nerves** have their origins in the brain and spinal cord. They leave the brain and spinal cord at the cranial and sacral levels, giving rise to the term **craniosacral outflow.** The cranial (tectobulbar) portion of the parasympathetic outflow innervates structures in the head, neck, thorax, and abdomen. These fibers travel in the oculomotor (III), facial (VII), glossopharyngeal (IX), and vagal (X) cranial nerves. The sacral division of the parasympathetic nervous system forms the pelvic nerve and innervates the remainder of the intestines and the pelvic viscera, including the bladder and reproductive organs.

The preganglionic neurons of the parasympathetic division of the autonomic nervous system are extremely long, such that the parasympathetic ganglia are located in, or near, the effector organs. As such, the postganglionic parasympathetic neurons are short. The neurotransmitter mediating synaptic transmission in the parasympathetic ganglia is acetylcholine. Acetylcholine is also the neurotransmitter liberated by postganglionic parasympathetic nerves innervating the effector organs.

Autonomic Regulation of Peripheral Involuntary Organs

Most organs of the body receive dual innervation consisting of sympathetic and parasympathetic components of the autonomic nervous system. In general, the parasympathetic and sympathetic neurons mediate opposing responses in the effector organ, although some exceptions to this generalization exist. Because balance exists in most organs between the sympathetic and parasympathetic divisions of the autonomic nervous system, blockade or inhibition of one system leads to exaggeration in the response mediated by the other. Some organs of the body, such as the vasculature and the spleen, receive only one type of innervation, which in these specific cases is sympathetic.

Regarding thoracolumbar sympathetic outflow, one preganglionic neuron may ramify and ultimately synapse with many postganglionic sympathetic neurons, leading to diffusion of sympathetic responses. In contrast, the craniosacral parasympathetic preganglionic neurons form, in general, only single synaptic connections with postganglionic parasympathetic neurons, resulting in a more discrete and localized response (Auerbach's plexus in the small intestine is a notable exception). This anatomical distinction between the sympathetic and parasympathetic divisions of the autonomic nervous system has profound physiological significance. *Activation of sympathetic outflow,* resulting from anger, fear, or stress, prepares the body for a ready state of activation characteristic of the "fight or flight" response. Thus, heart rate is accelerated, blood pressure is increased, perfusion to skeletal muscle is augmented as a result of the redirection of blood flow away from the skin and splanchnic region, blood glucose is elevated, bronchioles and pupils are dilated, and piloerection occurs. In contrast, because the parasympathetic system is organized in a more discrete and localized manner, *activation of parasympathetic outflow* is associated with conservation of energy and maintenance of organ function during periods of minimal activity. Activation of parasympathetic outflow produces a reduction in heart rate and blood pressure, activation of gastrointestinal movements, and emptying of the urinary bladder and rectum. Furthermore, glandular cells such as lacrimal, salivary, and mucous cells are activated, and smooth muscle of the bronchial tree is contracted, with the result that bronchi are constricted. Based on responses involved, it is clear that widespread activation of the parasympathetic nervous system is not beneficial.

Although the parasympathetic nervous system is essential for life, the sympathetic nervous system is not, and animals completely deprived of the sympathetic nervous system will survive, albeit with a lower level of efficiency. A decrease in sympathetic tone to visceral organs occurs during times of stress, when activation of sympathetic outflow to other organs (e.g., heart, vasculature) is essential.

NEUROTRANSMITTERS IN THE PERIPHERAL AUTONOMIC NERVOUS SYSTEM

Transmission Process

The concept of neurochemical transmission is firmly established as the mechanism by which nerves interact with effector organs of the body. The basic premise is that a nerve releases a chemical mediator, termed a **neurotransmitter,** that diffuses across a small but defined area, the **neuroeffector junction,** to interact with a receptor on the effector organ, thereby evoking a response in the effector organ. The nerve terminal contains all the necessary apparatus for the synthesis, storage, release, and subsequent inactivation of the neurotransmitter. The effector organ contains, on its cell surface membrane, the receptor with which the neurotransmitter interacts, the enzymes necessary for its degradation, and intracellularly the "signal transduction" mechanisms for information transfer from the receptor to the "cellular machinery," producing the end-organ response.

Transmission of information from preganglionic neurons to postganglionic neurons, or from postganglionic neurons to the effector organs, involves the chemical transmission of nerve impulses for the sympathetic and parasympathetic divisions of the autonomic nervous system. The sequence of events is illustrated for the sympathetic and parasympathetic ganglia, as well as for the postganglionic sympathetic and parasympathetic neurons, in Figure 8-2. Electrical impulses, originating from within the CNS, result in local depolarization of the neuronal membrane as a result of the selective increase in the permeability of sodium ions that flow inwardly in the direction of their electrochemical gradient. Repolarization of the membrane follows immediately and results from the selective increase in permeability to potassium ions. These ionic flows are mediated by separate and distinct ion channels. The transmembrane ion fluxes, which are ion currents, result in the generation of an action potential that is propagated throughout the length of the axon. The arrival of the action potential at the preganglionic or postganglionic nerve terminal triggers the quantal release of neurotransmitter stored in intracellular vesicles. The synthesis of the neurotransmitter occurs in the nerve terminal, where it is maintained in the storage vesicles until an action potential stimulus is received. The adrenergic storage vesicles in sympathetic nerve terminals and in adrenal chromaffin cells range in diameter from 40 to 130 nm whereas cholinergic storage vesicles in parasympathetic and ganglia terminals range in diameter from 20 to 40 nm.

The release of neurotransmitter after the arrival of an action potential occurs through a calcium-dependent process known as **exocytosis.** In this process the storage vesicle migrates to the nerve terminal membrane, fuses with the neuronal plasma membrane, opens to the extracellular space, and allows the contents of the storage vesicle, including the neurotransmitter, to be discharged into the synaptic cleft. The neurotransmitter diffuses across the synaptic cleft or the neuroeffector junction and interacts with a specific receptor located on the cell body of the postganglionic neuron or on the effector organ. In both sympathetic and parasympathetic ganglia, the neurotransmitter released by preganglionic neurons is acetylcholine. Activation of the postjunctional membrane receptors on the cell body of postganglionic neurons leads to an increase in ion permeability, and therefore to ionic conductance, in the postganglionic neuron (see Chapters 2 and 22). This increase in permeability of ions ultimately results in the generation of an action potential, which is propagated along the length of the postganglionic nerve. As at preganglionic nerve terminals, neurotransmitter is released when the action potential reaches the postganglionic sympathetic and parasympathetic nerve terminals. As indicated previously, the neurotransmitter liberated by postganglionic sympathetic nerve terminals is norepinephrine, whereas the neurotransmitter in the postganglionic parasympathetic neuron is acetylcholine. The response mediated in the effector organ subsequent to the release of the neurotransmitter is dependent on the neurotransmitter and the nature of the postjunctional receptor subtype present in the effector organ. These autonomic receptors are discussed in greater detail later in this chapter and in Chapters 2, 9, 10, and 12.

After release of the neurotransmitter, the effect of the neurotransmitter must be rapidly terminated to avoid excessive activation of the postjunctional elements. Most cholinergic synapses and neuroeffector junctions contain the highly selective enzyme acetylcholinesterase, which rapidly hydrolyzes acetylcholine into the two inactive products acetic acid and choline, thereby terminating the effect of the neurotransmitter. Choline is then rapidly taken up into the cholinergic nerve by an active neuronal membrane pump for use again in the synthesis of acetylcholine by the enzyme, choline acetyltransferase, present in the cytoplasm of the cholinergic nerves. Acetylcholine then accumulates in the storage vessels of the cholinergic nerve terminal until required for release, thereby conserving the neurotransmitter.

At adrenergic neuroeffector junctions, the response to norepinephrine is not terminated by enzymatic deactivation. Instead, termination occurs by a combina-

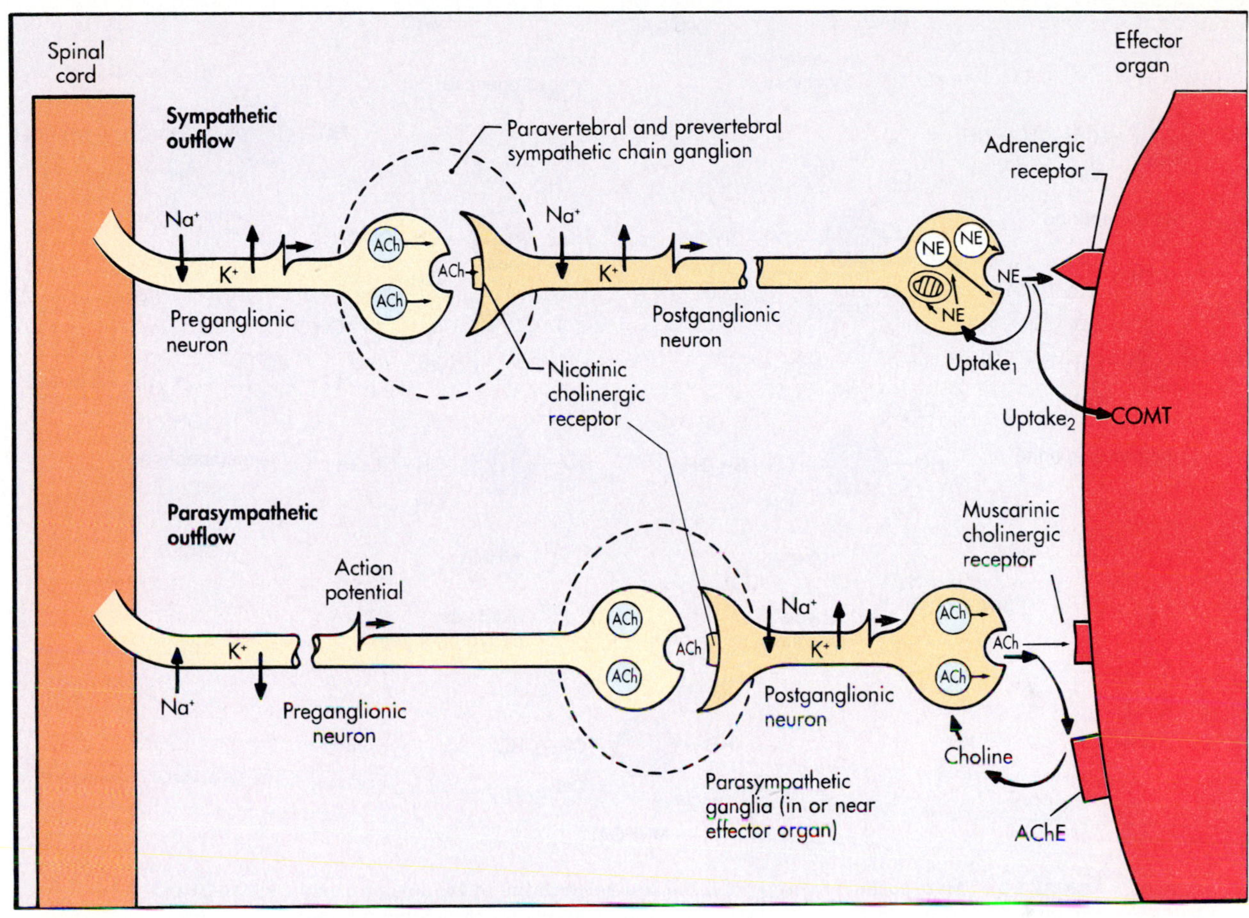

FIGURE 8-2 Schema of neurochemical transmission in the sympathetic and parasympathetic divisions of the peripheral autonomic nervous system. The neurotransmitter liberated in both sympathetic and parasympathetic ganglia is acetylcholine *(ACh)*, which is released on the arrival of an action potential to the preganglionic nerve terminal. ACh liberated from preganglionic neurons in the sympathetic and parasympathetic ganglia diffuses across the synaptic cleft to interact with nicotinic cholinergic receptors on cell bodies of the postganglionic neurons. The interaction of ACh with ganglionic cholinergic receptors results in the generation and propagation of action potentials that elicit the release of neurotransmitter at the postganglionic nerve terminal (neuroeffector junction). The neurotransmitter liberated from postganglionic sympathetic nerves is norepinephrine *(NE)*, which diffuses across the neuroeffector junction to stimulate the adrenergic receptors and elicit the end-organ response. Most of the liberated NE is taken back up into the sympathetic nerve terminal *(uptake$_1$)* and is either stored in the adrenergic storage vesicles or is metabolized by monoamine oxidase *(MAO)* located in the mitochondria. A smaller amount of the liberated NE may diffuse away from the adrenergic receptors and be accumulated by extraneuronal cells *(uptake$_2$)* after which it may be metabolized by the enzyme catechol-*O*-methyltransferase *(COMT)*. A similar process occurs at the postganglionic parasympathetic neuroeffector junction except that the neurotransmitter released is ACh, which diffuses across the synaptic cleft and activates muscarinic cholinergic receptors on the effector organ. The liberated ACh is rapidly metabolized by acetylcholinesterase *(AChE)* into choline. Choline is taken up into the parasympathetic nerve terminal and used to synthesize additional ACh, which is subsequently stored.

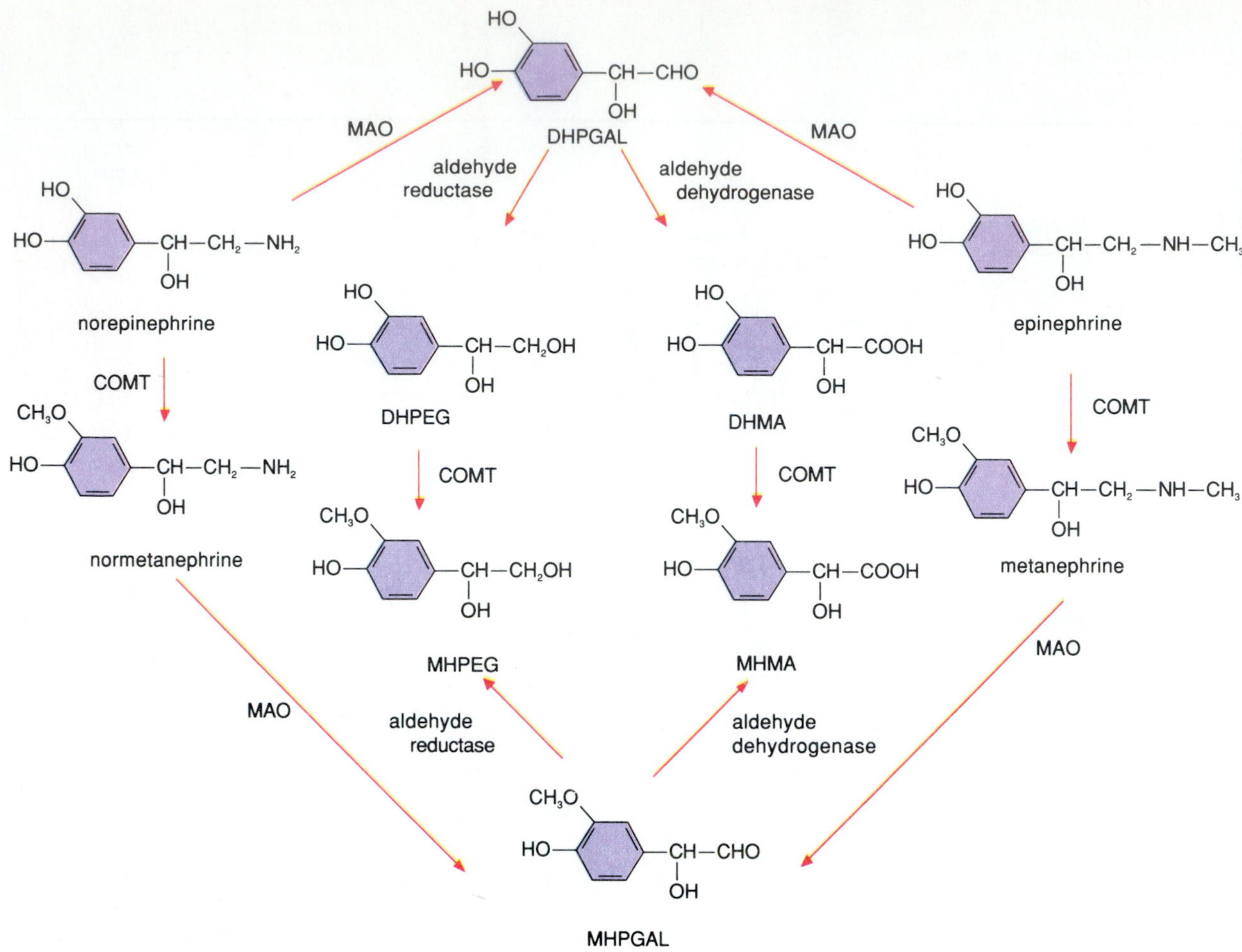

FIGURE 8-3 Metabolism of norepinephrine and epinephrine by monoamine oxidase (MAO) and catechol-O-methyltransferase *(COMT)*. The abbreviations for the individual metabolites are as follows: *DHPGAL*, 3,4-dihydroxyphenylglycol aldehyde; *DHPEG*, 3,4-dihydroxyphenylethylene glycol; *DHMA*, 3,4-dihydroxymandelic acid; *MHPEG*, 3-methoxy-4-hydroxyphenylethylene glycol; *MHMA*, 3-methoxy-4-hydroxymandelic acid; *MHPGAL*, 3-methoxy-4-hydroxyphenylglycol aldehyde.

tion of neuronal reuptake of the neurotransmitter into the sympathetic nerve by an energy-dependent amine uptake pump, called **uptake$_1$** and by simple diffusion away from the region of the receptors and subsequent uptake by an extraneuronal process referred to as **uptake$_2$**. Norepinephrine, accumulated in sympathetic nerves by uptake$_1$, has two fates (Figure 8-3). It may be oxidatively deaminated by the enzyme monoamine oxidase in the mitochondria of the sympathetic nerve terminal or sequestered in storage vessels for subsequent release. Norepinephrine diffusing away from the receptors to the extraneuronal site of uptake$_2$ may be inactivated by *O*-methylation through the enzyme catechol-*O*-methyltransferase. The metabolism of the catecholamines norepinephrine and epinephrine by the catabolic enzymes monoamine oxidase and catechol-*O*-methyltransferase results in inactive degradation products that have been identified and quantitated in tissues, blood, and urine. The scheme for the metabolic breakdown of the catecholamines is well established (see Figure 8-3).

Biosynthesis of Neurotransmitters

Catecholamines The pathway for the biosynthesis of the catecholamines epinephrine and norepinephrine is well understood (Figure 8-4). The precursor for the synthesis of all catecholamines is the amino acid tyrosine. Tyrosine is first hydroxylated in the *meta* position by the enzyme tyrosine hydroxylase to form the catechol derivative 3,4-dihydroxyphenylalanine. Tyrosine hydroxylase is the rate-limiting enzyme in the biosyn-

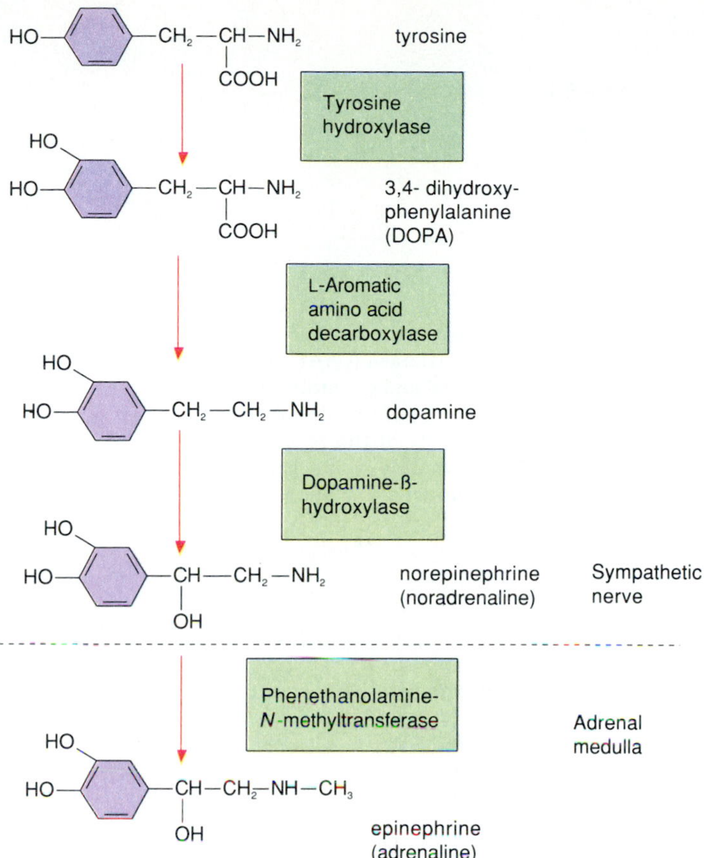

FIGURE 8-4 Steps in the enzymatic biosynthesis of the catecholamines dopamine, norepinephrine (noradrenaline), and epinephrine (adrenaline). The enzymes involved in each catalytic step are enclosed in boxes. The first three enzymatic steps occur in postganglionic sympathetic nerve terminals leading to the synthesis of norepinephrine, and all four enzymatic steps occur in the adrenal medulla, resulting in the synthesis of epinephrine.

thesis of all catecholamines, and this step takes place in the cytoplasm of the postganglionic sympathetic nerve terminal. 3,4-Dihydroxyphenylalanine (dopa) is subsequently decarboxylated by the enzyme L-aromatic amino acid decarboxylase to form dopamine, and this step also occurs in the cytoplasm. Dopamine is then actively accumulated by the storage vesicles in the sympathetic nerve terminals, and during this transport process, dopamine is β-hydroxylated by the enzyme dopamine-β-hydroxylase, which is associated with the adrenergic storage vesicle. The product, norepinephrine, is retained within the storage vesicle in association with adenosine triphosphate (ATP) until released on the arrival of an action potential at the sympathetic nerve terminal. Dopamine-β-hydroxylase represents the terminal enzyme in the biosynthesis of catecholamines in the postganglionic sympathetic neuron. As such, adrenergic nerves release only norepinephrine as the neurotransmitter.

In contrast, in the adrenal medulla, norepinephrine and epinephrine coexist. The synthesis of epinephrine in the adrenal gland occurs because of the presence of the enzyme phenethanolamine-*N*-methyltransferase, which *N*-methylates norepinephrine to form epinephrine in the cytoplasm. Cytoplasmic epinephrine is then accumulated in storage granules in the chromaffin cell and stored until released. In the adult human, epinephrine accounts for approximately 80% of the catecholamines in the adrenal medulla, with norepinephrine making up the remainder.

Acetylcholine The biosynthesis of acetylcholine in cholinergic neurons occurs by the acetylation of choline, catalyzed by the enzyme choline acetyltransferase, with acetyl coenzyme A serving as the acetyl donor (Figure 8-5). Choline is actively accumulated into the axoplasm of the neuron from extraneuronal sites by a high-affinity choline uptake process. The synthesis of acetylcholine from choline occurs in the axoplasm with acetylcholine actively accumulated in storage vesicles in the cholinergic nerve terminal, releasing neurotransmitter on the arrival of sufficient action potential stimuli.

NEUROTRANSMITTER RECEPTORS IN THE PERIPHERAL AUTONOMIC NERVOUS SYSTEM

Acetylcholine and norepinephrine use different pharmacological receptors to mediate their end-organ responses, and each neurotransmitter may interact with many receptor subtypes (see Chapter 2). The classification of the numerous receptor subtypes is primarily based on pharmacological studies, but it is evident that the end-organ response is as much a function of the receptor mediating that response as it is of the neurotransmitter that elicits the response. A listing of the adrenergic and cholinergic receptor subtypes is presented in Figure 8-6, with examples of agents that stimulate (agonists) or block (antagonists) these receptor subtypes.

Adrenergic Receptors

In the classic study of Ahlquist, the graded actions of a series of sympathomimetic amines provided the first evidence that the neurotransmitter norepinephrine and the adrenal catecholamine epinephrine could activate more than one type of adrenergic receptor. For stimulation of smooth muscle in the vasculature, uterus, ureter, and dilator pupillae, and for the inhibition of intestinal smooth muscle, the following rank order of potency was obtained: epinephrine > norepinephrine > α-methylnorepinephrine > α-methylepinephrine > iso-

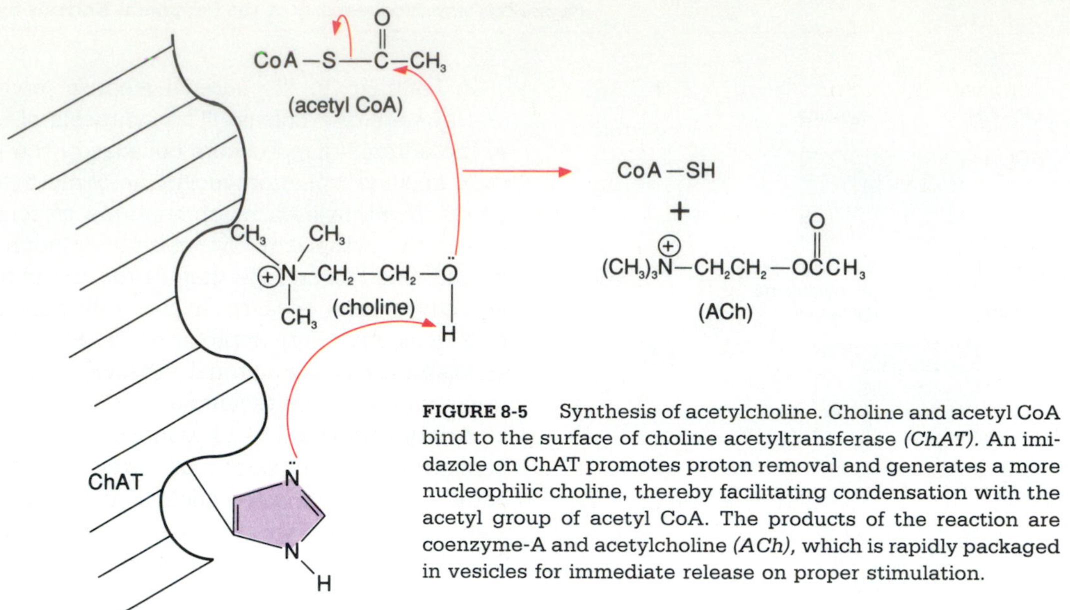

FIGURE 8-5 Synthesis of acetylcholine. Choline and acetyl CoA bind to the surface of choline acetyltransferase *(ChAT)*. An imidazole on ChAT promotes proton removal and generates a more nucleophilic choline, thereby facilitating condensation with the acetyl group of acetyl CoA. The products of the reaction are coenzyme-A and acetylcholine *(ACh)*, which is rapidly packaged in vesicles for immediate release on proper stimulation.

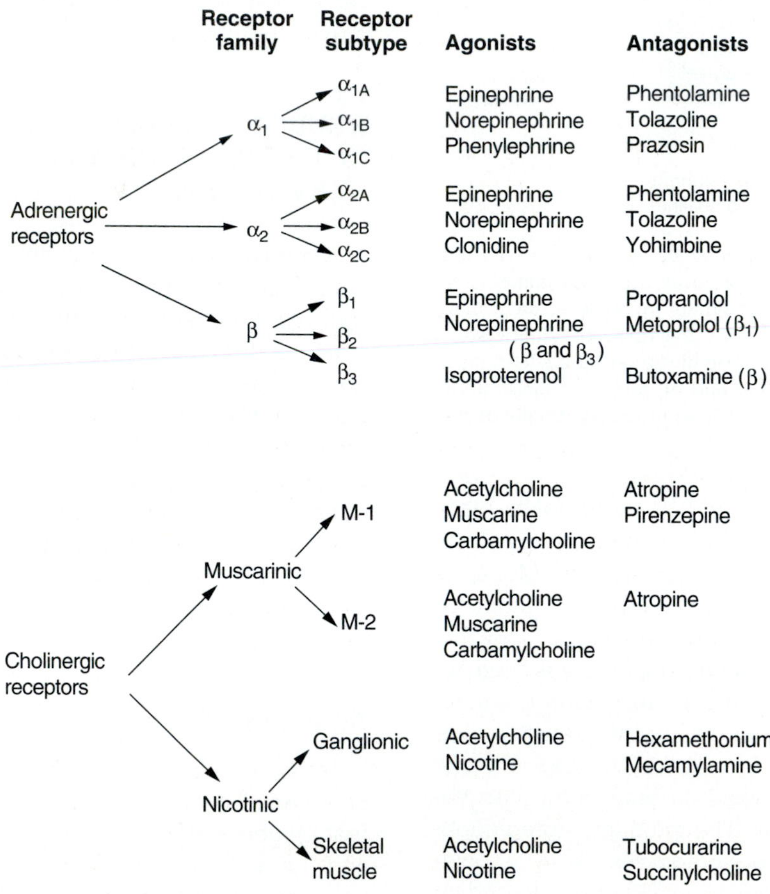

FIGURE 8-6 Division of the adrenergic receptors and cholinergic receptors into individual receptor subtypes. Some of the drugs that stimulate (agonists) or block (antagonists) each of the individual adrenergic and cholinergic receptor subtypes are listed.

proterenol. In contrast, the rank order of potency for these same agonists for inhibition of vascular and uterine smooth muscle and for stimulation of the myocardium was isoproterenol > epinephrine > α-methylepinephrine > α-methylnorepinephrine > norepinephrine. Based on these distinct potency orders, it was proposed that two types of adrenergic receptors existed, those being termed α when the first potency order described above was obtained, and the other β, when the second order of potency was obtained. The existence of distinct α- and β-adrenergic receptors was subsequently confirmed by the development of selective α- and β-adrenergic receptor antagonists.

For many years, only two adrenergic receptors were known to exist, the α and β types as defined. Subsequent studies indicated that β-adrenergic receptors could be subdivided into β_1, β_2, and β_3 subtypes. Thus the β_1 subtypes are characterized by the following rank order of potency: isoproterenol > epinephrine = norepinephrine. In contrast, β_2 subtypes are characterized by the following order of potency: isoproterenol > epinephrine >> norepinephrine. β_3 receptors show an order of potency of isoproterenol > norepinephrine > epinephrine. The development of β-adrenergic receptor antagonists with high selectivities for either the β_1 or β_2 subtypes has confirmed this subclassification (although none of the typical β-adrenergic antagonists can potently inhibit β_3 receptors).

In an analogous manner, studies have confirmed that α-adrenergic receptors do not represent one homogeneous population but may be further subdivided into at least two types, termed α_1 and α_2, each of which are now known to comprise additional subtypes (see Figure 8-6 and Chapter 22). α_1-Adrenergic receptors are defined as those showing high potency to selective agonists, such as methoxamine and phenylephrine, and specific blockade by prazosin. α_2-Adrenergic receptors are characterized by high potency to specific agonists such as clonidine and α-methylnorepinephrine, and selective antagonism by yohimbine. Recent studies in which the genes for adrenergic receptors were cloned using molecular biology techniques have confirmed the existence of three major families of adrenergic receptors: α_1, α_2, and β. Each of these may be further subdivided into three or more subtypes (Figure 8-6), which represent separate and distinct molecular entities (see Chapters 2 and 22). Amino acid sequences of the adrenergic receptors show a high degree of homology for subtypes within a given adrenergic receptor family. All the adrenergic receptors possess seven hydrophobic regions, an indication that the amino acid chain may traverse the membrane seven times. Additional research will determine what classification systems may be appropriate for the adrenergic receptors and other membrane receptors.

Cholinergic Receptors

As expected, differences in responses mediated by acetylcholine result from actual differences in cholinergic receptors (see Figure 8-6). The actions of acetylcholine can be mimicked in certain organs by the alkaloid muscarine, whereas in other organs the response to acetylcholine is more closely mimicked by the alkaloid nicotine. Thus, responses evoked by acetylcholine or by activation of the parasympathetic nervous system are described as being **nicotinic** or **muscarinic** and have led to the subclassification of cholinergic receptors as nicotinic cholinergic receptors or muscarinic cholinergic receptors. The response of most autonomic effector cells in peripheral visceral organs is typically muscarinic, whereas the responses in parasympathetic and sympathetic ganglia, as well as responses of skeletal muscle, are nicotinic. The nicotinic receptors of autonomic ganglia and skeletal muscle are not homogeneous because they can be blocked by different antagonists. Thus tubocurarine effectively blocks nicotinic responses in skeletal muscle, whereas hexamethonium is more effective in blocking nicotinic responses in autonomic ganglia, thereby confirming heterogeneity in nicotinic cholinergic receptors.

Muscarinic receptors also may be divided into at least two subtypes, M_1 and M_2, based on the pharmacologic specificities of certain agonists and antagonists. Atropine blocks both M_1 and M_2 muscarinic cholinergic receptors to nearly equivalent extents. However, the drug pirenzepine has proved to be a selective antagonist of the M_1 subtype. In general, muscarinic cholinergic receptors with the pharmacological profile characteristic of the M_1 subtype are found in autonomic ganglia and in the CNS, whereas M_2-receptors exist at neuroeffector junctions of organs innervated by the parasympathetic system.

Molecular biology is currently used to explore the heterogeneity of cholinergic receptors and where they fit into the genetic classification scheme being developed for receptors. The cholinergic receptor population, similar to the adrenergic receptor population is complex. For example, five different human genes that produce functional acetylcholine muscarinic receptors of the same family but with subtle structural and mechanistic differences have been identified.

Prejunctional Autoreceptors

In recent years, the functional significance of prejunctional autoreceptors has been established. Their distribution and function are illustrated schematically in Figure 8-7. On most adrenergic and cholinergic nerve terminals, the existence of prejunctional α-adrenergic receptors, belonging to the α_2 subtype, have been identified. Activation of these receptors by the released neu-

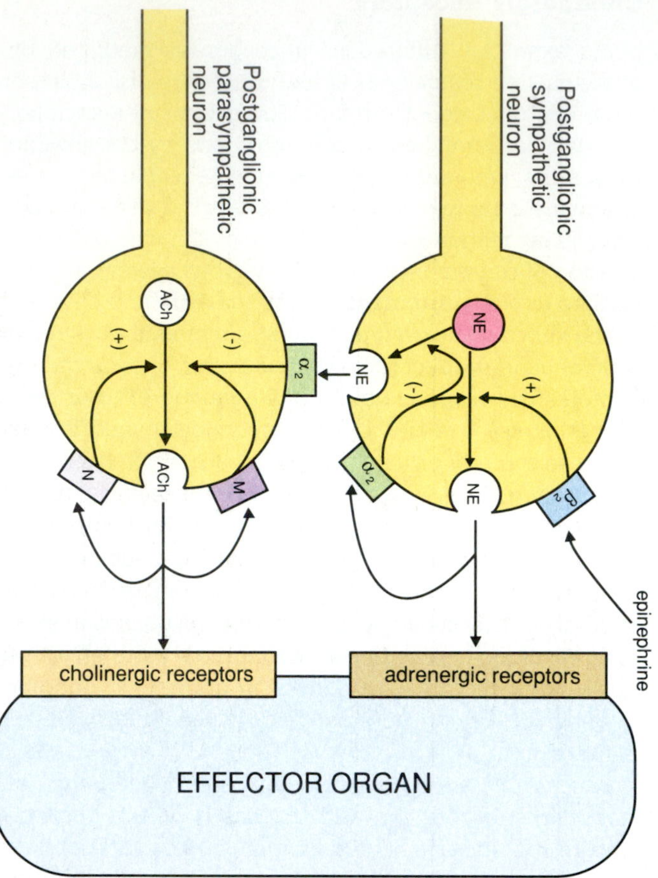

FIGURE 8-7 Schema of the presynaptic autoreceptors that regulate neurotransmitter release in adrenergic and cholinergic neurons. Presynaptic α_2- and β_2-adrenergic receptors exist on sympathetic nerve terminals and inhibit and facilitate, respectively, the release of the neurotransmitter, norepinephrine *(NE)*. Presynaptic muscarinic *(M)* and nicotinic *(N)* cholinergic receptors exist on cholinergic neurons and inhibit and facilitate, respectively, the release of the neurotransmitter acetylcholine *(ACh)*. Presynaptic α_2-adrenergic receptors also exist on cholinergic neurons and inhibit acetylcholine release.

rotransmitter norepinephrine or by exogenously administered α_2-adrenergic receptor agonists, decreases the release of norepinephrine. This presynaptic inhibitory autoreceptor mechanism may be involved in the normal regulation of neurotransmitter release as evidenced by the fact that blockade of this prejunctional α_2-receptor leads to an enhanced overflow of the neurotransmitter norepinephrine. Presynaptic α_2-receptors also exist on most cholinergic nerve terminals; and when these presynaptic α_2 subtype receptors are activated, the release of acetylcholine is inhibited. These prejunctional α_2-receptors on cholinergic nerves may be activated by exogenously administered α_2-receptor agonists and may also play a physiological role in regulating the release of acetylcholine when activated by norepinephrine liberated from postganglionic sympathetic neurons that impinge on postganglionic cholinergic nerve terminals.

Presynaptic β-adrenergic receptors, belonging to the β_2 subtype, have also been identified on adrenergic nerve terminals. Activation of these receptors by β_2-receptor agonists, such as epinephrine, leads to facilitation of norepinephrine release, an effect that is opposite to that observed with presynaptic α_2-adrenergic receptor activation. The physiological role of the presynaptic β_2-subtype receptor is not known.

Presynaptic muscarinic cholinergic receptors have also been proposed to exist on postganglionic parasympathetic neurons, and when activated, these receptors mediate a decrease in the release of acetylcholine. Prejunctional nicotinic cholinergic receptors may also exist on cholinergic nerve terminals and facilitate the release of acetylcholine.

MECHANISMS OF SIGNAL TRANSDUCTION USED BY AUTONOMIC RECEPTORS

Detailed intracellular molecular events that are set into motion when a cell-surface receptor is stimulated by a neurotransmitter are beginning to be understood for the peripheral autonomic receptors. These mechanisms of signal transduction use ion channels or enzyme activation-inhibition with secondary messengers. A brief summary of signal transduction as used by autonomic receptors follows.

β-Adrenergic Receptors

Stimulation of β_1-, β_2-, and β_3-receptors leads to the activation of the membrane-bound enzyme adenylate cyclase, which catalyzes conversion of ATP to cyclic adenosine monophosphate (cAMP). The activation of adenylate cyclase by β_1-, β_2-, and β_3-receptors involves G proteins (see Chapter 2), which couple the β-receptor subtypes to the catalytic enzyme. These coupling proteins, or guanine nucleotide regulatory proteins (G proteins) are essential for receptor-mediated activation of adenylate cyclase. The sequence of events is believed to be as follows:

1. β-Adrenergic receptor agonists bind to β_1-, β_2-, or β_3-receptors.
2. Resulting receptor-agonist complex binds to the stimulatory G protein, termed G_s (the role of the α, β, and γ subunits of the G proteins is discussed in Chapter 2).
3. Formation of the receptor-agonist-stimulatory G protein complex facilitates displacement of guanine diphosphate by guanine triphosphate on the stimulatory G protein.

4. Complex between stimulatory G protein and guanosine triphosphate dissociates from the receptor-agonist complex and interacts with the catalytic subunit of adenylate cyclase, thereby promoting the conversion of ATP to cAMP.
5. cAMP then activates an intracellular enzyme, cAMP-dependent protein kinase, which phosphorylates phosphorylase b kinase and a number of intracellular proteins, leading to a pharmacological response.

α_2-Adrenergic Receptors

In many systems, α_2-receptors are coupled to the inhibition of adenylate cyclase and result in the opposite effect of that observed for activation of the β-adrenoceptors. Thus, α_2-receptors are coupled to adenylate cyclase in an inhibitory manner through an inhibitory G protein termed G_i (see Chapter 2 for details). When α_2-receptors are activated, the inhibitory G protein ultimately inhibits the catalytic activity of adenylate cyclase, thereby leading to a reduction in intracellular concentrations of cAMP that decreases the activation of cAMP-dependent protein kinase.

Although the inhibition of adenylate cyclase by α_2-receptor activation occurs in many systems, α_2-receptors also may use other mechanisms of signal transduction. For example, in the human platelet, activation of α_2-receptors leads to stimulation of a sodium-hydrogen exchange system that produces an influx of sodium and an efflux of hydrogen ions. The net effect is intracellular alkalinization leading to elevated intracellular calcium, activation of membrane-bound phospholipase A_2, release of arachidonic acid, and enzymatic conversion to thromboxane A_2 to produce platelet aggregation (see Chapters 18 and 21).

In blood vessels, a different mechanism for signal transduction is used by α_2-adrenergic receptors. Although details have not been fully elucidated, it appears that the effects of α_2-receptor activation are mediated by a G protein that leads to activation of a membrane calcium channel, resulting in the influx of calcium from extracellular sites.

α_1-Adrenergic Receptors

α_1-Receptors produce their effects through increases in intracellular phosphatidylinositol turnover. That is, activation of the α_1-adrenergic receptor leads to stimulation of membrane-bound phospholipase C, the latter being coupled to the α_1-receptor by a G protein. The activation of phospholipase C results in the hydrolysis of phosphatidylinositol bisphosphate to produce diacylglycerol and inositol-1,4,5-trisphosphate. Diacylglycerol activates protein kinase C, in part by sensitizing it to Ca^{++}, which leads to phosphorylation of a set of intracellular proteins. Inositol-1,4,5-trisphosphate acts to mobilize calcium from the endoplasmic reticulum into the cytosol. Thus, diacylglycerol and inositol-1,4,5-trisphosphate are intracellular messengers that lead to pharmacological responses mediated by α_1-receptor activation.

Muscarinic Cholinergic Receptors

Muscarinic cholinergic receptors may use a signal transduction process that is similar to that of α_1-adrenergic receptors, in that they produce effects through increases in intracellular phosphatidylinositol turnover. Thus, activation of the muscarinic cholinergic receptor leads to association with a G protein and activation of phospholipase C. The subsequent generation of diacylglycerol and inositol-1, 4, 5-trisphosphate from phosphatidylinositol bisphosphate after hydrolysis by phospholipase C ultimately mediates the muscarinic cholinergic effects.

In some cells, activation of muscarinic receptors can lead to the inhibition of adenylate cyclase and a decrease in intracellular cAMP concentrations, in a manner similar to that described previously for α_2-adrenergic receptors.

Nicotinic Cholinergic Receptor

Details of signal transduction for nicotinic cholinergic responses have not been fully elucidated. Activation of the nicotinic cholinergic receptor does not require interaction with a G protein. Rather, the nicotinic cholinergic receptor itself can form an ion channel (selective for cations), which, when activated by acetylcholine, undergoes a conformational change that results in opening of the ion channel.

FUNCTIONAL RESPONSES MEDIATED BY PERIPHERAL AUTONOMIC NERVOUS SYSTEM

Many organs of the body receive adrenergic and cholinergic innervation, and responses in these organs represent a complex interplay between these two divisions of the autonomic nervous system. It is usual for one type of innervation to predominate over the other, and so an organ may be predominantly under the control of only one division of the autonomic nervous system, although both components are usually present and can modulate any given response. Organs receiving dual innervation from the sympathetic and parasympathetic divisions of

Table 8-1 Responses Elicited in Effector Organs by Stimulation of Sympathetic and Parasympathetic Nerves

Effector Organ	Adrenergic Response	Primary Receptor Involved	Cholinergic Response	Dominant Response*
Heart				
Rate of contraction	Increase	β_1	Decrease	C
Force of contraction	Increase	β_1	Decrease	C
Blood vessels				
Arteries (most)	Vasoconstriction	α_1 (α_2)	—	A
Skeletal muscle	Vasodilatation	β_2	—	A
Veins	Vasoconstriction	α_2 (α_1)	—	A
Bronchial tree	Bronchodilation	β_2	Bronchoconstriction	C
Splenic capsule	Contraction	α_1	—	A
Uterus	Contraction	α_1	Variable	A
Vas deferens	Contraction	α_1	—	A
Prostatic capsule	Contraction	α_1	—	A
GI tract	Relaxation	α_2 (β_3)	Contraction	C
Eye				
Radial muscle, iris	Contraction (mydriasis)	α_1	—	A
Circular muscle, iris	—		Contraction (miosis)	C
Ciliary muscle	Relaxation	β	Contraction (accommodation)	C
Kidney	Renin secretion	β_1	—	A
Urinary bladder				
Detrusor	Relaxation	β	Contraction	C
Trigone and sphincter	Contraction	α_1	Relaxation	A, C
Ureter	Contraction	α_1	Relaxation	A
Insulin release from pancreas	Decrease	α_2	—	A
Fat cells	Lipolysis	β_1 (β_3)	—	A
Liver glycogenolysis	Increase	α_1 (β_2)	—	A
Hair follicles, smooth muscle	Contraction (piloerection)	α_1	—	A
Nasal secretion	Decrease	α_1 (α_2)	Increase	C
Salivary glands	Increase secretion	α_1	Increase secretion	C
Sweat glands	Increase secretion	α_1	Increase secretion	C

**A*, Adrenergic, *C*, cholinergic

the autonomic nervous system include the heart, eye, bronchial tree, gastrointestinal tract, urinary bladder, and reproductive organs. Some organs receive only a single type of innervation, generally that of the sympathetic nervous system. Thus, blood vessels, spleen, and piloerector muscles receive predominantly an adrenergic innervation. As indicated earlier, the predominant cholinergic receptor located postjunctionally on the visceral effector organs and mediating the response to acetylcholine is the muscarinic cholinergic receptor of the M_2 subtype. In contrast, the α- or β-adrenergic receptor subtypes can mediate the adrenergic responses to nerve stimulation in the various visceral effector organs receiving adrenergic innervation.

A detailed account of the adrenergic and cholinergic responses that occur in many important organs of the body is presented in Table 8-1. In most instances sympathetic and parasympathetic nerves mediate physiologically opposing effects. That is, if one system inhibits a certain function, the other system usually enhances that function. The responses presented in Table 8-1 represent only those mediated by stimulation of sympathetic or parasympathetic nerves, and therefore they represent responses mediated by the neurotransmitter interacting only with autonomic receptors located directly in the neuroeffector junction. However, autonomic receptors are also found at sites away from the neuroeffector junction. These receptors may be different from the receptors or receptor subtypes located directly in the neuroeffector junction. For example, although vascular smooth muscle generally has no cholinergic innervation, it has a full complement of cholinergic receptors. Although these "extrajunctional" receptors are functional and may mediate responses to exogenously administered drugs, they probably play little or no physiological role in the normal autonomic response mediated by sympathetic or parasympathetic nerves. They are therefore not listed in Table 8-1.

Table 8-2 Mechanisms of Pharmacologic Agents in the Peripheral Nervous System

Action	Mechanism(s) of Action	Example
Ganglion blockade	Interferes with transmission of nerve impulses between preganglionic and postganglionic neurons	Hexamethonium Mecamylamine
Inhibition of neurotransmitter synthesis	Inhibition of enzymes in biosynthesis	α-Methyltyrosine (inhibits tyrosine hydroxylase) Fusaric acid (inhibits dopamine-β-hydroxylase)
Inhibition of neurotransmitter release	Interference with adrenergic neurotransmission	Bretylium Guanethidine
Promotion of neurotransmitter release	Activation of nicotinic ganglionic cholinergic receptors	Nicotine
	Release of cytoplasmic stores of norepinephrine	Tyramine Ephedrine Amphetamine
Inhibition of neurotransmitter storage	Blockade of norepinephrine accumulation by cytoplasmic granules	Reserpine
Inhibition of neuronal uptake	Blockade of amine uptake$_1$ pump, thereby increasing synaptic concentrations of norepinephrine	Cocaine Imipramine
Inhibition of neurotransmitter metabolism	Inhibition of enzymes in metabolic pathway	Pargyline (inhibits monoamine oxidase) Physostigmine (inhibits acetylcholinesterase)
Stimulation of autonomic receptors	Stimulation of α- and β-receptors	Phenylephrine (activates α_1-receptors) Isoproterenol (activates β-receptors)
Blockade of autonomic receptors	Blockade of α- and β-receptors	Prazosin Phentolamine (blocks α-receptors) Propranolol (blocks β-receptors)

Effect of Pharmacological Agents

Pharmacological agents that alter the adrenergic and cholinergic divisions of the autonomic nervous system are discussed in detail in Chapters 9 to 11. The purpose of this discussion is to present a brief overview of the points of pharmacological intervention (Table 8-2) that are possible in the peripheral autonomic nervous system and a few examples of the drugs that interfere at these points.

Ganglionic Blockers Drugs that block autonomic ganglia interfere with the transmission of nerve impulses from preganglionic nerve terminals to the cell bodies of postganglionic neurons. Because the neurotransmitters (acetylcholine) and receptors (nicotinic) are identical in autonomic ganglia of both sympathetic and parasympathetic nerves, ganglionic blockers appear to impede both divisions of the autonomic nervous system equally. However, the end-organ response may show a predominant adrenergic or cholinergic effect. The reason for this is that the degree of innervation by the adrenergic and cholinergic nervous system, and the extent of the adrenergic and cholinergic dominance in a given organ, may not be equivalent (see Table 8-1). Therefore, interruption of ganglionic transmission will have the overall effect of selectively eliminating that component of the autonomic nervous system that generally dominates, leading to a response that is characteristic of the less dominant component. For example, in the heart the cholinergic system generally dominates over the adrenergic component at the level of the sinoatrial node. The administration of a ganglionic blocker therefore has the greatest effect on the cholinergic component, resulting in an apparent adrenergic end-organ effect (i.e., tachycardia). The classic ganglionic blockers are hexamethonium and mecamylamine, although they now have limited clinical use.

Drugs That Inhibit Synthesis of Neurotransmitter Several enzymes are necessary for the biosynthesis of norepinephrine and epinephrine from tyrosine (see Figure 8-4). Tyrosine hydroxylase, the rate-limiting enzyme, is inhibited by α-methyltyrosine. The next enzyme, L-aromatic amino acid decarboxylase, is inhibited by carbidopa and α-methyldopa. The latter also is a substrate for the decarboxylase, which converts it to α-methyl-norepinephrine, a potent and highly selective α_2-adrenergic receptor agonist.

Dopamine is synthesized in the cytoplasm and transported into storage vesicles. There the third enzyme associated with the storage vesicle membrane, dopamine-β-hydroxylase, hydroxylates dopamine to norepinephrine, which is stored in the adrenergic vesicles in association with ATP. Fusaric acid is a selective inhibitor of dopamine-β-hydroxylase and produces a significant reduction in norepinephrine concentrations and a concomitant increase in dopamine concentrations.

Dopamine-β-hydroxylase is the terminal enzyme in the biosynthesis of catecholamines in postganglionic sympathetic nerve terminals, and norepinephrine is found in high concentrations in these neurons. However, in the adrenal medulla, there is a fourth enzyme that catalyzes the formation of epinephrine, the major catecholamine in the adrenal gland. The fourth enzyme, phenethanolamine-*N*-methyltransferase, can be inhibited by agents such as 2,3-dichloro-α-methylbenzylamine.

As previously stated, synthesis of acetylcholine occurs by acetylation of choline through the enzyme choline acetyltransferase, using acetyl coenzyme A (see Figure 8-5). Although there are no potent and specific inhibitors of choline acetyltransferase, the biosynthesis of acetylcholine can be indirectly inhibited with the experimental drug hemicholinium, which blocks the high-affinity system that transports choline into the cholinergic nerve terminal. This results in considerable depletion of acetylcholine in cholinergic neurons.

Drugs That Inhibit Release of Neurotransmitter Release of norepinephrine from postganglionic sympathetic nerve terminals involves an exocytotic process in which the storage vesicle membrane fuses with the neuronal membrane, allowing the storage vesicle to release its contents into the neuroeffector junction. Bretylium and guanethidine are two drugs that inhibit this process and are classified as adrenergic neuronal blocking agents, which interfere with adrenergic neurotransmission.

The release of acetylcholine also occurs through exocytosis. Botulinus toxin prevents the release of acetylcholine from all types of cholinergic nerve fibers. Because the cholinergic nervous system is essential for survival, botulinus toxin is lethal.

Drugs That Promote Release of Neurotransmitter Two processes can promote the release of norepinephrine from postganglionic sympathetic nerve terminals. One is by activation of nicotinic ganglionic cholinergic receptors by nicotine, which generates action potentials in the cell body of the postganglionic neuron. The action potentials are propagated to the nerve terminal and activate the calcium-dependent exocytotic release of norepinephrine from storage vesicles into the synaptic cleft. The second process is through tyramine, ephedrine, or amphetamine, which are indirectly acting sympathomimetic amines evoking the release of cytoplasmic stores of norepinephrine. These drugs enter the sympathetic nerve terminal by the amine uptake$_1$ pump and displace cytoplasmic norepinephrine, which passively diffuses through the neuronal membrane into the synaptic cleft by a process that does not involve calcium or exocytosis.

The release of acetylcholine from postganglionic cholinergic nerve terminals can be evoked by activation of ganglionic nicotinic cholinergic receptors by nicotine. As is the case for the release of norepinephrine, nicotine elicits the generation of action potentials, which ultimately produce the exocytotic release of acetylcholine. There are no known drugs that displace acetylcholine from neuronal stores and thereby indirectly elicit release of this neurotransmitter. Because acetylcholine is a positively charged quaternary ammonium compound, it cannot readily penetrate the neuronal membrane. Therefore the ability of cholinergic agents to promote the release of acetylcholine is limited.

Drugs That Interfere with Storage of Neurotransmitter Norepinephrine is synthesized, accumulated, and stored in the cytoplasmic storage granules until subsequent release through exocytosis. An energy-dependent amine-uptake pump in the storage vesicle membrane accumulates catecholamines. Reserpine blocks uptake of catecholamines into the storage vesicles, thereby decreasing the amount of norepinephrine available for release on nerve stimulation. This leads to complete depletion of catecholamines from postganglionic sympathetic nerve terminals.

No known drugs interfere with the accumulation of acetylcholine by the cholinergic storage vesicles. However, the experimental drug hemicholinium leads to depletion of acetylcholine stores in cholinergic neurons by interfering with the accumulation of choline.

Drugs That Affect Neuronal Uptake After exocytotic release of norepinephrine from postganglionic sympathetic nerve terminals, most of the released catecholamine is actively reaccumulated in the sympathetic nerve terminal by uptake$_1$. Agents such as cocaine and imipramine block this amine uptake pump and thereby increase synaptic concentrations of norepinephrine, enhancing or facilitating adrenergic neurotransmission.

Acetylcholine is not taken up into cholinergic neurons after its release. As already discussed, high-affinity uptake for choline is present, which is inhibited by hemicholinium.

Drugs That Inhibit Metabolism of Neurotransmitter Two enzymes involved in the metabolism of the catecholamines are monoamine oxidase and catechol-*O*-methyltransferase. Monoamine oxidase is inhibited by the drugs pargyline or tranylcypramine, and catechol-*O*-methyltransferase is inhibited by other catechols, such as pyrogallol. Inhibition of monoamine oxi dase and catechol-*O*-methyltransferase results in higher concentrations of norepinephrine in peripheral tissues but does not enhance the responses of neuroeffector organs to sympathetic nerve stimulation (see Chapter 10).

Acetylcholinesterase is the major enzyme catalyzing the hydrolysis of acetylcholine and terminating the cholinergic effect. Acetylcholinesterase is inhibited by physostigmine and other drugs, which enhance the magnitude and duration of effects elicited by stimulation of cholinergic neurons.

Drugs That Block Autonomic Receptors Older prototypic α-adrenergic blockers are phenoxybenzamine, phentolamine, and tolazoline, which block both α_1- and α_2-adrenergic receptors. Developed more recently, prazosin blocks α_1-receptors and yohimbine blocks α_2-receptors with relatively high selectivity.

The prototypic β-receptor blockers such as propranolol block both β_1- and β_2-adrenergic receptors with little selectivity. Newer and more selective β-receptor blockers include metoprolol, a relatively selective β_1-receptor antagonist, and butoxamine, a selective β_2-receptor antagonist.

Most effector organs of the autonomic nervous system that contain muscarinic cholinergic receptors are blocked in a competitive manner by atropine. Nicotinic cholinergic receptors are of two types: those existing in skeletal muscle and those present in autonomic ganglia. Nicotinic cholinergic receptors in skeletal muscle are selectively antagonized by tubocurarine (Chapter 11) and ganglionic nicotinic receptors are selectively inhibited by hexamethonium or mecamylamine.

Drugs That Stimulate Autonomic Receptors The neurotransmitter norepinephrine activates α_1-, α_2-, and β_1-and β_3-adrenergic receptors with relatively weak activity at β_2-receptors. Epinephrine, however, activates all known adrenergic receptor subtypes with similar potency. Some drugs that selectively activate each of the receptor subtypes have been discovered. Phenylephrine is a potent and highly selective α_1-receptor agonist, and clonidine is a selective α_2-receptor agonist. Isoproterenol is equally effective at stimulating all β-adrenergic receptor subtypes. However, dobutamine has been proposed as a selective β_1-receptor agonist, whereas terbutaline is a selective agonist of β_2-receptors.

Acetylcholine activates both muscarinic and nicotinic cholinergic receptors, as well as each of the individual subtypes of these cholinergic receptors. Muscarinic cholinergic receptors may be selectively stimulated by the alkaloid muscarine or by synthetic agonists, such as carbamylcholine. Nicotinic cholinergic receptors may be selectively stimulated by the alkaloid nicotine, and selective stimulation of ganglionic nicotinic cholinergic receptors can be achieved with dimethylphenylpiperazinium.

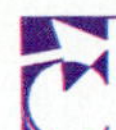

NEW DIRECTIONS

The major focus of research in the autonomic nervous system currently centers around the types and subtypes of adrenergic and cholinergic receptors. There are currently believed to exist three subtypes of the α_1-adrenergic receptor, three or four subtypes of the α_2-adrenergic receptor, three subtypes of the β-adrenergic receptor, and at least five subtypes of the muscarinic cholinergic receptor. Many of these receptors have now been cloned, and it is indeed possible that there are still additional adrenergic and cholinergic receptors that have yet to be identified.

The role of prejunctional adrenergic and cholinergic receptors in both physiological and pathophysiological states also continues to be explored, and the search continues for new drugs that will selectively activate or inhibit these receptors. Prejunctional autoreceptors may represent an important mechanism whereby chemical neurotransmission can be regulated both in the periphery and in the CNS. Because the autonomic nervous system plays a pathophysiological role in many diseases of peripheral organs, including the heart, kidney, gastrointestinal tract, and reproductive system, the ability to regulate selectively the autonomic function to these organs continues to be a major objective.

REFERENCES

Berthelsen S, Pettinger WA: A functional basis for classification of α-adrenergic receptors, *Life Sci* 21:595, 1977.

Gilman AG: Guanine nucleotide-binding regulatory proteins and dual control of the adenylate cyclase, *J Clin Invest* 73:1, 1984.

Langer SZ: Presynaptic regulation of the release of catecholamines, *Pharmacol Rev* 32:337, 1980.

Trendelenburg U: A kinetic analysis of the extraneuronal uptake and metabolism of catecholamines, *Rev Physiol Biochem Pharmacol* 87:33, 1980.

von Euler US: Synthesis, uptake and storage of catecholamines in adrenergic nerves: the effects of drugs. In Blaschko H, Muscholl E, editors: *Catecholamines: handbook of experimental pharmacology,* vol 33, Berlin, 1972, Springer-Verlag.

SELF-ASSESSMENT QUESTIONS

1. Which of the following is *not* a characteristic of the parasympathetic nervous system?
   a. Acetylcholine is the neurotransmitter at parasympathetic ganglia
   b. Acetylcholine is the neurotransmitter for postganglionic neurotransmission
   c. Long unmyelinated postganglionic neurons
   d. Cell bodies for preganglionic neurons originating in the brainstem and sacral region of the spinal cord
   e. Essential for life
2. The sympathetic nervous system is characterized by all of the following *except:*
   a. Cell bodies for preganglionic sympathetic neurons originate in the brain.
   b. The neurotransmitter for preganglionic sympathetic neurons is acetylcholine.
   c. Postganglionic sympathetic neurons are long.
   d. Postganglionic sympathetic nerve terminals have an active uptake process for norepinephrine termed *uptake*$_1$.
   e. Has nicotinic cholinergic receptors at the paravertebral ganglia.
3. Which of the following adrenergic receptors results in the activation of adenylate cyclase as the major component of its signal-transduction process?
   a. α_1-adrenergic receptor
   b. α_2-adrenergic receptor
   c. β_1-adrenergic receptor
   d. β_2-adrenergic receptor
   e. c and d
4. Stimulation of prejunctional or presynaptic α_2-adrenoceptors on postganglionic sympathetic neurons causes the following:
   a. Inhibition of acetylcholine release
   b. Stimulation of epinephrine release
   c. Stimulation of norepinephrine release
   d. Inhibition of norepinephrine release
   e. Has no effect on neurotransmitter release
5. Which of the following signal transduction processes can be used by muscarinic cholinergic receptors?
   a. Inhibition of adenylate cyclase
   b. Stimulation of adenylate cyclase
   c. Activation of phospholipase C
   d. Stimulation of a sodium-hydrogen exchange system
   e. a and c
6. Activation of the parasympathetic nervous system results in which of the following responses?
   a. An increase in heart rate
   b. Vasoconstriction
   c. Bronchoconstriction
   d. Renin secretion
   e. Relaxation of the gastrointestinal tract

CHAPTER 9

Drugs Affecting the Parasympathetic Nervous System and Autonomic Ganglia

JOHN J. O'NEILL
PETER H. DOUKAS

MAJOR DRUGS

- cholinomimetic agonists (e.g., pilocarpine, bethanechol)
- muscarinic blocking drugs (e.g., atropine sulfate, scopolamine)
- ganglionic blocking drugs (e.g., trimethaphan camsylate)
- cholinesterase inhibitors (e.g., physostigmine, neostigmine)

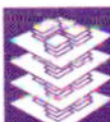

THERAPEUTIC OVERVIEW

The parasympathetic branch of the autonomic nervous system consists of neural pathways that use acetylcholine as the neurochemical transmitter. The parasympathetic division innervates primarily the gastrointestinal tract, eye, heart, respiratory tract, glands, and bladder (see Chapter 8). Although there are relatively few disease states with dysfunctions of cholinergic sites of the peripheral autonomic nervous system, cholinergic sites are still key points for pharmacological intervention for restoration of normal body functions. Because of the widespread accessibility and actions of the cholinergic system and the co-innervation of most organs and tissues by the parasympathetic and sympathetic divisions, two factors are of prime importance in pharmacological intervention: (1) the need for organ/tissue selectivity in the cholinergic-targeted drugs being used and (2) knowledge of the neuroeffector action of the sympathetic pathway when the input from the parasympathetic (cholinergic) division is blocked.

Knowing which cholinergic sites possess the muscarinic and which have the nicotinic subtype of acetylcholine receptors allows one to select a drug for the specific receptor subtype (see Chapter 8). Neuroeffector junctions of the parasympathetic division generally have muscarinic subtypes, whereas ganglionic synapses have nicotinic subtypes. Although the association of particular receptor subtypes with ganglia and with neuroeffector junctions provides a convenient operating classification, the relationship is actually more complex. Some junctions and some synapses have only postjunctional or postsynaptic cholinergic receptors and others contain both postjunctional and prejunctional or postsynaptic and presynaptic receptors. These may be the nicotinic or the muscarinic subtype of receptors, with the functions of the prejunctional or presynaptic control pathways not well understood.

In the previous chapter, sites and mechanisms of potential pharmacological intervention in the adrenergic or cholinergic portions of the peripheral autonomic nervous system are listed. The major mechanisms discussed in Chapter 8 by which drugs affect the cholinergic system are:

1. Stimulation of neuroeffector pathways by agonists
2. Blockade of neuroeffector receptors by antagonists
3. Inhibition of acetylcholine metabolism
4. Blockade (or stimulation) of ganglionic receptors

The effects and therapeutic uses of cholinergic-targeted drugs are summarized in Table 9-1.

A special type of neuroeffector junction, which uses acetylcholine as a neurochemical transmitter but is not part of the autonomic nervous system, exists between skeletal muscles and the somatic nerves that innervate these muscles. The actions of the receptors at these junctions are similar to the nicotinic receptors in the parasympathetic system. A group of drugs termed

ABBREVIATIONS

acetyl Co-A	acetyl coenzyme A

Table 9-1 Tissue/Organ Effects and Therapeutic Applications of Cholinergic-Targeted Drugs

Tissue/Organ	Effect	Condition Treated or Use
MUSCARINIC AGONISTS		
Eye	Contraction of ciliary muscle and sphincter muscle of iris	Glaucoma
Gastrointestinal tract	Increased peristaltic movement, sphincter relaxation	Adynamic ileus
Urinary bladder	Increased contraction of detrusor muscle, sphincter relaxation	Urinary retention
Vascular smooth muscle	Dilatation (minor effect)	—
Bronchial smooth muscle	Bronchoconstriction	—
Glands	Secretion	—
Heart	Negative inotropic, chronotropic, and dromotropic effect	—
ACETYLCHOLINESTERASE INHIBITORS		
Skeletal muscle	Increased muscle activity	Myasthenia gravis
Eye	Similar to agonists	Glaucoma
MUSCARINIC BLOCKING AGENTS		
Eye	Mydriasis	Refraction studies
Gastrointestinal tract	Decreased muscle actions and secretions	Spasm, hypermotility; preoperative medication
Urinary bladder	Relaxation, constriction of sphincter	Urinary incontinence
Bronchiolar smooth muscle	Decreased muscle action and secretions	Surgery, asthma
Brain	Blockade of central nervous system receptors	Parkinson's disease, motion sickness
Heart	Vagal blockade, tachycardia, increased atrioventricular nodal transmission	—
Glands	Salivary secretion, sweat glands blocked	—

neuromuscular blocking agents disrupt somatic nerve–skeletal muscle signal transmission by blocking these receptors. These drugs are described in Chapter 11.

Several central nervous system (CNS) problems associated with the cholinergic system, such as Alzheimer's and Parkinson's disease, are discussed in Chapter 27.

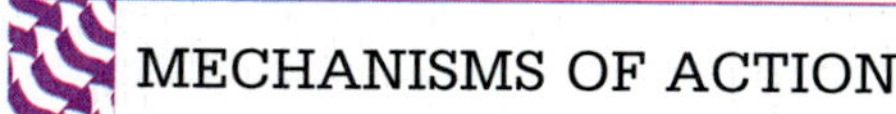

MECHANISMS OF ACTION

The structure and molecular mechanisms of the nicotinic acetylcholine receptor are described in Chapter 2, and the biochemistry and physiology of the peripheral autonomic nervous system, including cholinergic and adrenergic neurochemical transmission, are discussed in Chapter 8. Some additional topics that pertain specifically to cholinergic neurochemical transmission are described in this section.

Synthesis and Release of Acetylcholine

Acetylcholine is synthesized at neuroeffector and ganglionic junctions from the immediate precursors acetylcoenzyme A(acetyl CoA) and choline by action of choline acetyltransferase. This enzyme is present in the cytosol in soluble form, with a small amount bound to membranes. Its activity is strongly dependent on ionic strength.

Neuronal cells depend on exogenous choline because they are deficient in the transmethylating system required to convert precursors such as ethanolamine to choline. It is estimated that the transmethylating enzyme is present in these cells in less than 1% of the concentration found in liver. Choline-containing phospholipids, lecithins, or lysolecithins are the usual precursors. They may arise from dietary sources or by synthesis in the liver from phosphatidyl ethanolamine and *S*-adenosylmethionine. Choline is transported through the blood in phospholipid form from the liver to the nerve cells and is then released through the action of a phospholipase. The choline is then taken up into cholinergic nerve terminals by a sodium-dependent high-affinity choline uptake system. Although no therapeutically useful drugs act by blocking the uptake or the synthesis of acetylcholine at the nerve terminals, hemicholinium has been used experimentally to block choline uptake in animals.

Although the source of choline for acetylcholine formation is well understood, the origin of the acetyl moiety is yet unclear. Pyruvate is the immediate precursor but is converted to acetyl CoA exclusively in mitochondria and must be translocated to the cytosol, the site of acetylcholine synthesis. Intramitochondrial condensation of acetyl CoA and oxaloacetate to citrate may oc cur. Citrate is readily transported to the cytosol, where it is cleaved to acetyl CoA. It is clear that acetylcholine synthesis is tightly regulated, and the transmitter is packaged in small vesicles that protect acetylcholine from hydrolysis by intracellular and extracellular cholinesterases.

If we assume that acetylcholine containing vesicles from humans are similar in composition to synaptic vesicles of the electric eel, vesicles from cerebral tissue are estimated to contain 100 nmol of acetylcholine per mg of protein. In contrast, the phrenic nerve contains only 1 nmol of acetylcholine/mg protein, requiring a very rapid turnover and making this tissue especially vulnerable to various neurotoxins that inhibit acetylcholine release.

The arrival of a sufficient action potential at the nerve terminal triggers the Ca^{++}-dependent release of acetylcholine from vesicles. The release is quantal and transient. Without nerve stimulation, there is a small leakage of acetylcholine from nerve endings, which could come directly from the cytoplasm. However, this leakage contributes little to the total fraction of acetylcholine released after nerve stimulation. For example, botulinus toxin in an extremely low dose is known to block the release of acetylcholine from cholinergic nerve endings. It is administered locally into muscles of the orbit in the management of blepharospasm and strabismus. This treatment produces a long-lasting interruption of neuromuscular transmission and a reduction of spasmodic ocular movements.

Acetylcholine, after its release from nerve terminals, reacts with postsynaptic receptors or is hydrolyzed to terminate transmitter action. Unlike the catecholamines of the adrenergic system, the intact transmitter molecule is not taken back up into the prejunctional nerve cell; rather, only its hydrolysis product, choline, is taken up and reused.

Stimulation of Muscarinic or Nicotinic Receptors (Agonists)

Terminology for muscarinic and nicotinic receptors resulted from early use of the natural alkaloids muscarine and nicotine, and the physiological effects each produced in the autonomic nervous system. In keeping with this terminology, drugs that produce the same response as that obtained by stimulating the parasympathetic nervous system are termed **cholinomimetic,** and the effects produced are either **nicotinic** or **muscarinic,** depending on the subtype of the receptor. A similar distinction is used to classify antagonists at cholinergic receptors as antimuscarinic, or antinicotinic, although **blocking agents** is the descriptive term often used.

Muscarinic receptors are linked to G proteins and second messenger systems described in Chapters 2 and 8.

Some receptors exist postjunctionally and others exist on prejunctional nerve terminals (Figure 8-7). This has led to the additional terminology of autoreceptors or heteroreceptors. If a neurotransmitter is released from a nerve terminal and reacts with a receptor on its own prejunctional nerve ending, that receptor is termed an **autoreceptor.** Such a mechanism has been invoked to explain feedback regulation of release; elevated junctional concentrations of neurotransmitter would react with these prejunctional autoreceptors to slow further release.

A **heteroreceptor** is present on prejunctional structures but responds to substances other than the neurotransmitter released at the terminal. For example, the α_2-adrenergic agonist clonidine (Chapter 10) acts prejunctionally on cholinergic terminals to suppress acetylcholine outflow. Prejunctional α_2-adrenergic heteroreceptors are present on the splanchnic nerve and are stimulated by epinephrine and norepinephrine. This inhibits acetylcholine release from the nerve and decreases its interaction at adrenal nicotinic receptors, thus diminishing further release of catecholamines from the adrenal medulla.

Cholinergic agonists or cholinomimetic agents produce pharmacological effects by binding to muscarinic or nicotinic postjunctional receptors. The structures of pilocarpine, carbachol, bethanechol, methacholine (the latter compound used for diagnostic but not therapeutic purposes) and, as additional reference materials, acetylcholine, muscarine, and nicotine are shown in Figure 9-1.

Muscarinic Blocking Drugs

The naturally occurring alkaloid atropine and its related compounds are classified as **antimuscarinic** or muscarinic blocking drugs because they competitively block the actions of acetylcholine at both central and peripheral muscarinic receptors. Structurally related drugs include l-hyoscine, or scopolamine. Numerous derivatives and analogs have been synthesized to provide a large number of antimuscarinic agents.

The muscarinic blocking agents, such as atropine, compete with acetylcholine for both M_1 and M_2 muscarinic receptors. Other drugs discriminate between subtypes, with pirenzepine having high affinity for M_1-receptors and bethanecol for M_2. Muscarinic blocking agents may be more effective in blocking exogenous acetylcholine, or injected agonists, than in inhibiting responses to postganglionic nerve stimulation. Under the latter circumstances, a high local concentration of acetylcholine is achieved at or near the receptor, requiring

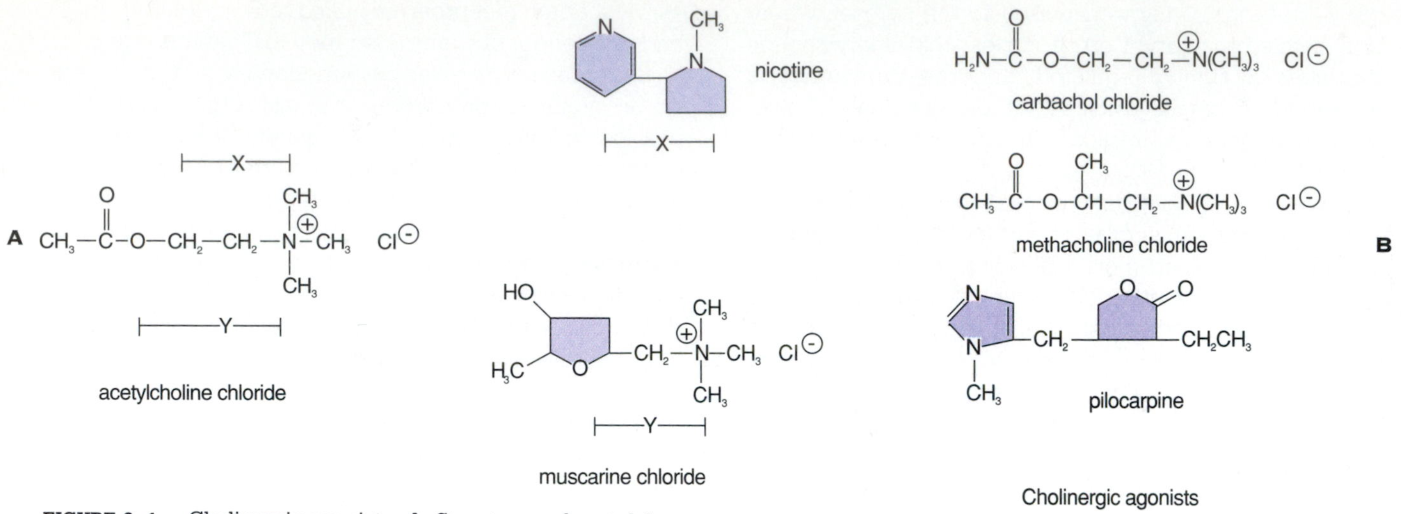

FIGURE 9-1 Cholinergic agonists. **A,** Structures of acetylcholine and naturally occurring prototypes. The distance and torsional angle between the ester and quaternary ammonium groups are critical for agonist activity. The distance between the two nitrogens of nicotine corresponds closely to *X* in acetylcholine, whereas that between the ether oxygen and the positive charge in muscarine corresponds to *Y*. **B,** Some cholinergic agonists that are used clinically and for diagnostics.

a greater concentration for competitive blockade.

Other drugs that block muscarinic receptors include antidepressants, neuroleptics, and antihistamines (Figure 9-2). At normal therapeutic doses they elicit atropinelike effects, including urinary retention, adynamic ileus, dry mouth, and blurring of vision, especially in the elderly patient.

Ganglionic Blocking and Stimulating Drugs

Ganglionic transmission is modulated by the effects of released acetylcholine acting directly on nicotinic receptors and indirectly on small cells that contain and release dopamine. Dopamine acts on receptors on the ganglion cell bodies to modulate ganglionic activity (Figure 9-3). In addition, there is evidence that peptides such as substance P further modulate electrical events associated with ganglionic transmission, though the mechanism is still not clear. Substance P is present mainly in the CNS and is discussed further in Chapter 22. In the autonomic nervous system, substance P is found at sympathetic ganglia and in the gastrointestinal wall. It appears to be selective for nicotinic receptors but not for those present at the skeletal muscle end plate. Substance P may provide another site for the future development of more selective cholinergic drugs.

Because it is difficult to limit ganglionic blockade to either parasympathetic or sympathetic division, or to specific organs, these agents are infrequently used clinically. Trimethaphan camsylate is available for injection for use in hypertensive crisis, and mecamylamine has been used orally. Nicotine is important toxicologically and produces ganglionic stimulation followed by depression. A dermal patch containing nicotine has been developed for use by individuals attempting to reduce their craving for cigarettes.

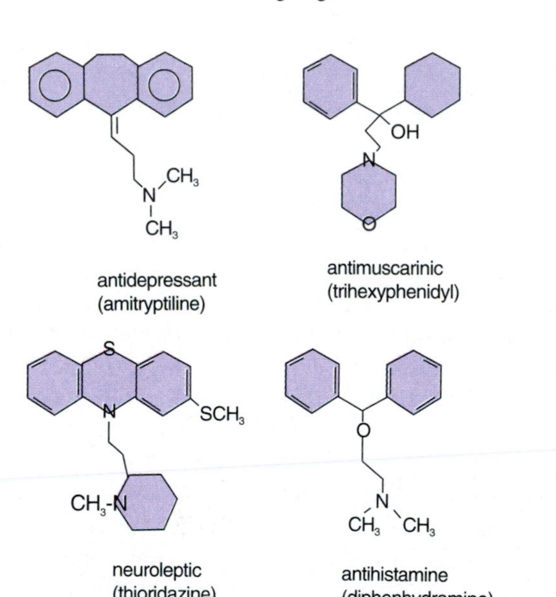

FIGURE 9-2 Structural similarities between antimuscarinic agents and other therapeutic categories that impart antimuscarinic side effects to the latter compounds.

Inhibition of Acetylcholine Metabolism

The indirect-acting cholinomimetics produce their pharmacological action by blocking the enzymatic hydrolysis of acetylcholine. Inhibitors of acetylcholinesterase and plasma pseudocholinesterase significantly increase local acetylcholine concentrations, which can be

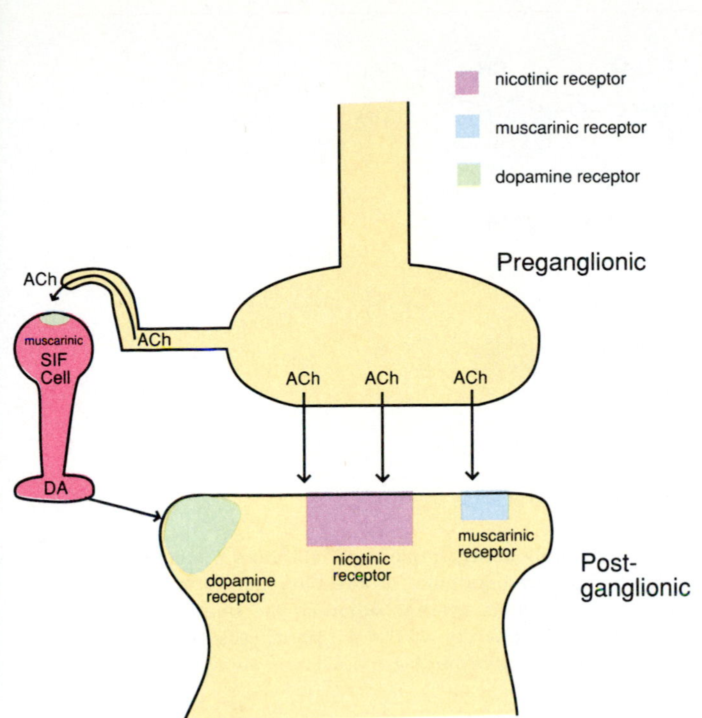

FIGURE 9-3 Ganglionic synapse. Acetylcholine *(ACh)* released from the preganglionic cell binds to nicotinic and muscarinic receptors postsynaptically on cell bodies. Also shown are small intensely fluorescent *(SIF)* cells, which possess muscarinic receptors on their outer membrane, and vesicles that contain dopamine. When released on appropriate stimulation, the dopamine interacts with dopamine receptors on the postsynaptic cell body and modulates the postsynaptic effect of ACh.

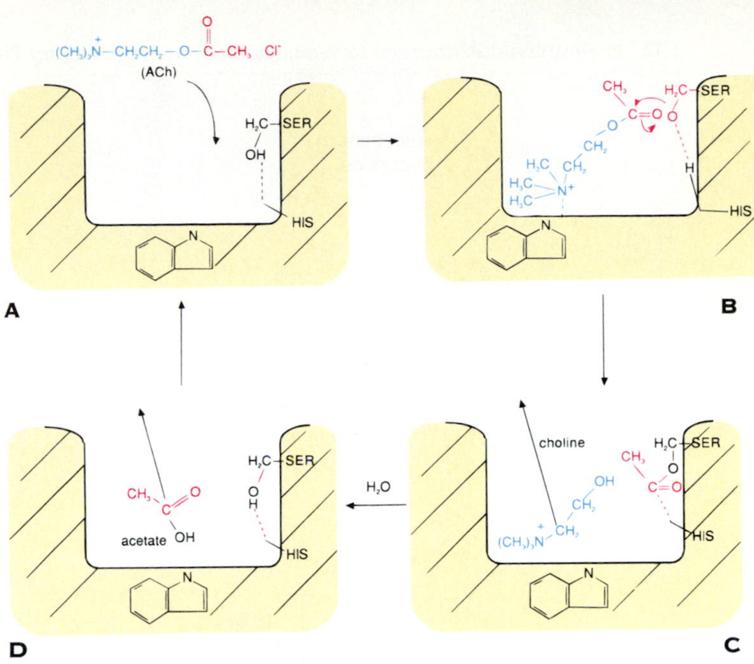

FIGURE 9-4 **A,** Hydrolysis of acetylcholine *(ACh)* by acetylcholinesterase. **B,** Activated serine OH attacks the carbonyl of ACh, **C,** becomes acetylated, and **D,** is eventually hydrolyzed to acetate and the free enzyme.

either therapeutic or life threatening, depending on the extent of enzyme inhibition.

As shown in Figure 9-4, the active region of acetylcholinesterase contains an esteratic site containing aromatic amino acids, which offer the possibility of pi-bonding and an esteratic site containing a serine hydroxyl. The enzymatic hydrolysis of acetylcholine involves initial electrostatic attraction of the positively charged quaternary nitrogen to the aromatic pocket and subsequent nucleophilic attack by the serine–OH (activated by an adjacent histidine), leading to acetylation of the serine. The acetylated enzyme is rapidly hydrolyzed to acetate and free enzyme, enabling reuse of the enzyme and rapid turnover of acetylcholine. The deacetylation step is rate limiting.

There are two types of cholinesterase inhibitors: *reversible* carbamates and related compounds (Figure 9-5) and *irreversible* organophosphates (Figure 9-6). Some of the latter are highly toxic and are not used clinically, but human exposure occurs through use of pesticides.

Simple quaternary amines (i.e., tetraethylammonium ion) can weakly inhibit acetylcholinesterase by hindering access of acetylcholine. More potent, though transient, inhibition is produced by the drug edrophonium, which in addition to associating with the aromatic pocket also forms a hydrogen bond with the neighboring histidine. Prolonged inhibition is mediated by carbamate-containing molecules such as physostigmine and pyridostigmine, which behave as substrates and carbamylate the serine–OH at the esteratic site in a manner analogous to the previously described acetylation. Decarbamylation occurs much more slowly than does deacetylation. It is estimated that the half-life of acetylcholine hydrolysis by deacetylation is 40 microseconds, whereas that for decarbamylation is approximately 30 minutes or longer. Thus, in the presence of carbamylating drugs, acetylcholine accumulates, producing prolonged effects.

The carbamates also have agonist, desensitizing, and channel-blocking properties at sensitive nicotinic sites. The implications of these activities await further study, especially at the low concentrations that produce cholinesterase inhibition. At higher concentrations physostigmine exerts a blocking action at sympathetic ganglia. The quaternary amine-containing carbamates have nicotinic blocking and anticholinesterase activity.

Irreversible cholinesterase inhibitors act by covalently phosphorylating the hydroxyl group of serine on the enzyme (see Figure 9-6). A few organophosphates, which show selective toxicity against insects but not against mammals, are used in agriculture mainly as pesticides. Some phosphorus compounds become active only after biotransformation. For example, parathion is converted to the very toxic analog paraoxon. The time

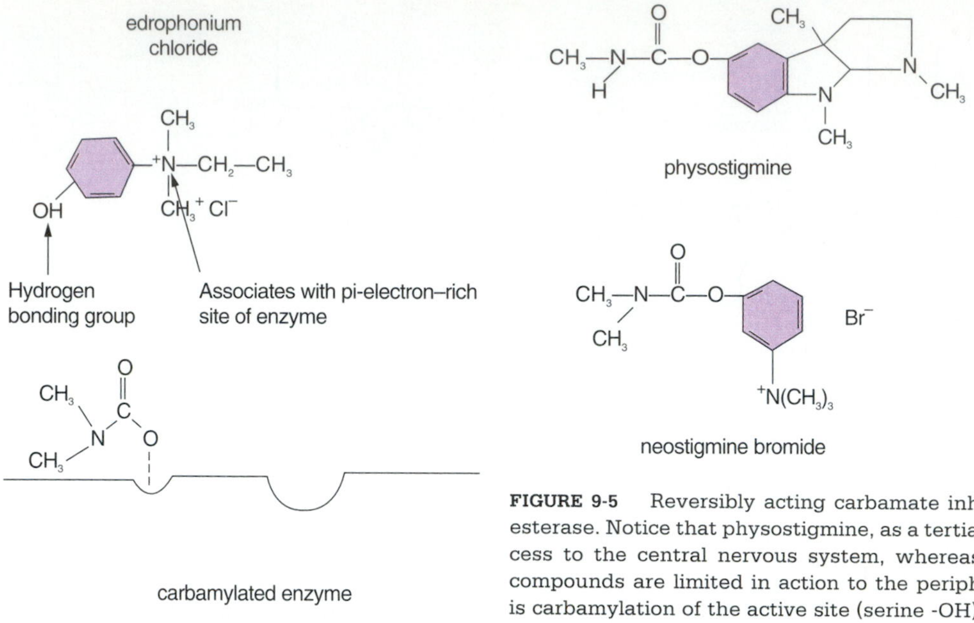

FIGURE 9-5 Reversibly acting carbamate inhibitors of cholinesterase. Notice that physostigmine, as a tertiary amine, has access to the central nervous system, whereas the quaternary compounds are limited in action to the periphery. Also shown is carbamylation of the active site (serine -OH) by neostigmine.

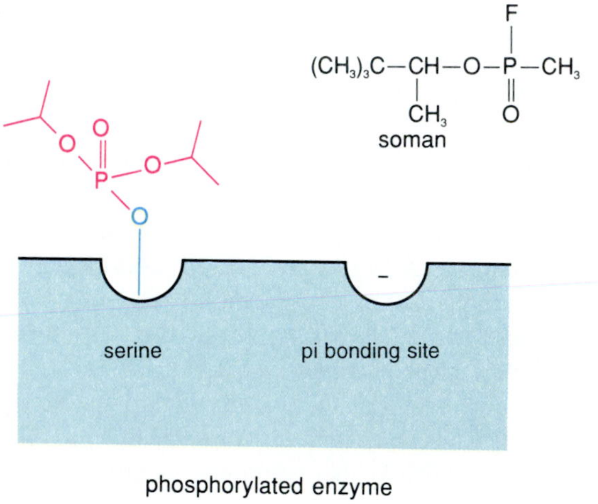

FIGURE 9-6 Organophosphate inhibitors of acetylcholinesterase. Also shown is phosphorylation of the active site (serine −OH) after reaction with isoflurophate. Soman is highly toxic and irreversible. Isoflurophate and echothiophate (not shown) are used clinically for topical ophthalmology applications.

required for transformations accounts for the delay before toxic signs appear. Malathion is a widely used pesticide that is much safer than others currently in use. It, too, must be bioactivated in vivo, but its oxidation product is rapidly metabolized by the plasma esterases.

The enzymes that hydrolyze acetylcholine are classified according to substrate specificity and distribution. The cholinesterase type found distributed throughout the nervous system and present in the red blood cell membrane is specific for acetylcholine with much lower affinity for other choline esters. It is termed "true," or **erythrocyte cholinesterase.** The neuronal enzyme is synthesized in cell bodies throughout the central and peripheral nervous systems, secreted by the Golgi apparatus, and transported along the axon by "fast" axoplasmic flow to the nerve terminals. Its presence at somatic nerve muscle junctions, ganglia, parasympathetic neuroeffector junctions, and throughout the brain and spinal cord has been demonstrated histochemically.

Cholinesterase is extensively distributed in brain and spinal cord, especially in dorsal root ganglia where acetylcholine is absent, and there is a high concentration of various peptides such as substance P. It has been suggested that cholinesterase in the dorsal horn may act as a peptidase, thus producing substance P from precursors. Tissues highest in true cholinesterase activity include preganglionic fibers to sympathetic and parasympathetic ganglia, postganglionic parasympathetic and somatic motor fibers, and sympathetic axons that innervate sweat glands. The enzyme may exist in monomeric, dimeric, and tetrameric forms and may contain a segment with a collagenlike structure for attachment to membranes.

Plasma cholinesterase or **pseudocholinesterase** is more widely distributed than true cholinesterase. Plasma contains several forms of pseudocholinesterase. Unlike the erythrocyte enzyme, pseudocholinesterase has a very broad substrate specificity, with the following order of preference: benzoyl > butyryl > propionyl > acetyl esters of choline. It is sometimes referred to as **butyrylcholinesterase** because it has greater activity against this substrate, with the possible exception of benzoylcholine. Because of its liver origin, plasma concentrations of the enzyme in combination with aspartate aminotransferase and alanine transaminase are useful as a measure of liver function. Its presence is important when the neuromuscular blocking agent succinylcholine is used, as discussed in Chapter 11. In addition to plasma, it is found in glial cells. Unlike true cholinesterase, the function of pseudocholinesterase in nerve tissue is unclear.

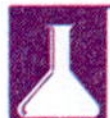

PHARMACOKINETICS

The pharmacokinetics of many of the cholinergic drugs have not been well studied in humans. This is partly because of a lack of analytical methods and partly because of the rapid and intense actions that ensue with small drug concentrations. Moreover, these drugs are given by many routes with variable onsets and durations, depending on their clinical use.

Cholinomimetic Agonists

The hydrolytic lability of *acetylcholine* limits its therapeutic application to a few topical applications, chiefly in ophthalmology. The available synthetic choline esters are charged and thus are poorly absorbed and distributed. The principal differences among these compounds are in their relative resistance to hydrolysis by acetylcholinesterase.

Pilocarpine is available for topical application as a solution or in an extended delivery device (see Chapter 6) placed into the conjunctival sac and providing continuous drug release for 7 days.

Muscarinic Blocking Drugs

Among the muscarinic blockers, the tertiary amines cross membranes readily and penetrate the CNS, whereas the quaternary ammonium compounds fail to traverse the membrane, or do so only poorly and thus are limited in their distribution (Table 9-2).

Atropine is rapidly absorbed after oral or parenteral administration. When applied topically to the eye, it is absorbed from the surrounding mucous membranes unless drainage from the conjunctiva is prevented by light pressure on the drainage canal. Atropine has a plasma half-life of approximately 2 hours and is well distributed throughout the body. Most of an administered dose is eliminated within 12 hours in the urine. Ten to fifty percent is unchanged and the remainder is excreted as unidentified metabolites. The half-life in children younger than 2 years of age and in the elderly is considerably longer. Quaternary nitrogen derivatives of atropine are poorly absorbed, quantitatively, between 10% and 25%

USES OF INDIVIDUAL CHOLINERGIC DRUGS

CHOLINOMIMETICS

1. Glaucoma
   - Pilocarpine
   - Carbachol
2. Urinary retention
   - Bethanechol

MUSCARINIC BLOCKING AGENTS

1. Antispasmodics:
   - atropine sulfate
   - scopolamine hydrobromide
   - methylscopolamine bromide
   - *l*-hyoscyamine sulfate
   - clinidium bromide
   - glycopyrrolate
   - isopropamide iodide
   - methantheline bromide
   - propantheline bromide
2. Antiparkinsonism:
   - biperiden lactate
   - procyclodin hydrochloride
   - trihexphenidyl hydrochloride
   - benztropine mesylate
3. Bronchial disorders:
   - atropine sulfate
   - ipratropium bromide
4. Mydriatic and cycloplegic
   - atropine sulfate
   - cyclopentolate hydrochloride
   - homatropine hydrobromide
   - scopolamine hydrobromide
   - tropicamide
   - eucatropine hydrochloride
5. Motion sickness
   - scopolamine hydrobromide
6. Anesthetic premedication
   - atropine sulfate
   - glycopyrrolate
   - scopolamine hydrobromide

CHOLINESTERASE INHIBITORS

1. Myasthenia gravis
   - pyridostigmine bromide
   - neostigmine bromide
   - edrophonium chloride
2. Glaucoma
   - physostigmine sulfate
   - demecarium bromide
   - echothiophate iodide
   - isoflurophate

Table 9-2 Muscarinic Blocking Drugs

Drug	Comments
TERTIARY AMINES	
atropine sulfate	Preoperative medication; treatment of anticholinesterase poisoning
scopolamine hydrobromide	Preoperative medication in childbirth
homatropine hydrobromide	Mydriatic and cycloplegic; used for mild anterior uveitis
adiphenine hydrobromide	To treat pyloric and biliary spasm, dysmenorrhea
dicyclomine	Alleviates gastrointestinal spasm, dysmenorrhea: pylorospasm and biliary distention
oxyphencyclimine	Antisecretory compound in peptic ulcer
cyclopentolate	Mydriatic, cycloplegic; may cause severe CNS effects
tropicamide	Mydriatic, cycloplegic
benztropine methanesulfonate	Antagonizes extrapyramidal symptoms of antiparkinson drugs and the phenothiazines
trihexyphenidyl	Similar uses as benztropine methanesulfonate
QUATERNARY AMINES	
atropine methylbromide (and methylnitrate)	Mydriatic, cycloplegic, antispasmodic in pyloric stenosis
methscopolamine bromide	Decreases gastric hyperacidity and hypermotility; fewer CNS effects than scopolamine
homatropine methylbromide	Restricted to gastrointestinal tract, diminish gastric acidity and spasm
ipratropium	Aerosol to diminish secretions in chronic emphysema
glycopyrrolate	Spasmolytic for ulcer therapy; preoperative drying of secretion
tridihexethyl chloride	Antispasmodic, preoperative to dry secretions
isopropamide iodine	May be used with cimetidine in Zollinger-Ellison syndrome
methantheline bromide	Spasmolytic to treat peptic ulcer: may precipitate exfoliative dermatitis
propantheline bromide	Spasmolytic in peptic ulcer; high doses may produce neuromuscular block
clidinium bromide	Spasmolytic in combination with chlordiazepoxide in management of "psychogenic" ulcer

of the oral dose. A small fraction is excreted unchanged.

Scopolamine, the epoxy analog of atropine, is available in a sustained delivery patch for topical skin application behind the ear, with a constant delivery rate over 3 days.

Other Drugs

Nicotine is available as a transdermal patch, or bound to an ion-exchange resin as a chewing gum. The nicotine is released slowly for buccal absorption and is used as a possible aid in the cessation of smoking.

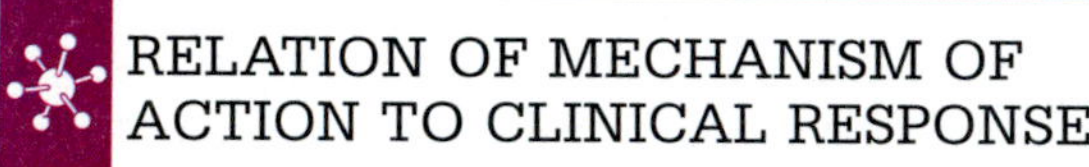

RELATION OF MECHANISM OF ACTION TO CLINICAL RESPONSE

The major uses of the important cholinergic drugs are listed in the box on page 103.

Cholinomimetic Agonists

Drugs can act by stimulating muscarinic receptors and thereby achieve organ or tissue selectivity because muscarinic sites are located predominantly at neuroeffector junctions and in the CNS. The route of administration also can be used to achieve organ selectivity (i.e., topical applications for the eye). Nicotinic receptors are present in autonomic ganglia, at skeletal muscle motor end plates (see Chapter 11), on adrenal medullary cells, and in the CNS.

In the eye, sustained increased intraocular pressure may result in glaucoma (described in anticholinesterase section). Some forms of this disease can be alleviated by administration of cholinomimetic drugs (e.g., pilocarpine) and anticholinesterases. But glaucoma can also be precipitated by the use of muscarinic receptor blocking drugs.

Pilocarpine Pilocarpine acts on smooth muscles of the eye to constrict the pupil (miosis), causing a spasm of accommodation, and a transient increase in intraocular pressure followed by a decrease that is longer lasting. Pilocarpine is a miotic of choice in initial maintenance therapy in primary open-angle glaucoma and in conjunction with other drugs in the emergency treatment of acute angle-closure glaucoma. It penetrates the eye after topical application, and miosis begins in 15 to 30 minutes, persisting for up to 8 hours. Reduction of intraocular pressure is maximal in 2 to 4 hours. Pilocarpine acts to increase aqueous outflow and possibly to reduce aqueous production. It is generally better tolerated than other miotics.

Carbachol Carbachol, a carbamyl ester of choline, shares similar properties with bethanechol. In contrast to acetylcholine, carbachol stimulates the urinary and gastrointestinal tracts fairly selectively. Its principal use, however, is in ophthalmology for cataract surgery or in other procedures in which rapid miosis is desired. For the chronic treatment of open-angle glaucoma, higher concentrations of carbachol are employed. Carbachol is often effective in reducing intraocular pressure when resistance to physostigmine or pilocarpine develops.

Bethanechol Chloride Bethanechol chloride is another choline ester that acts directly on effector cells. Its actions are like those of acetylcholine, but its effects are more persistent, again because of its resistance to hydrolysis by cholinesterases. It has no nicotinic effects and its actions on autonomic ganglia are minimal. However, its effects are much more pronounced on the urinary bladder and gastrointestinal tract. It is used to facilitate emptying of the neurogenic bladder and is frequently administered to patients after surgery or parturition. In patients with spinal cord injury, it is sometimes used to enhance weak detrusor muscle contractions for bladder evacuation. The drug is also used in children with "lazy bladder" syndrome.

Muscarinic Blocking Drugs

Atropine Atropine, the prototype muscarinic blocking agent will be discussed in detail. Table 9-2 lists other drugs in this class with brief comments regarding their use.

Atropine acts on muscarinic receptors to block parasympathetic effects on smooth muscle, cardiac muscle, and glandular cells. By blocking vagal activity there is an increased firing rate of the sinoatrial node and facilitation of conduction at the atrioventricular node. In gastrointestinal hypermotility and excessive gastric secretion, atropine is effective in blocking parasympathetic stimulation, diminishing these activities. A large number of atropinelike drugs with antimuscarinic actions have applicability in allaying symptoms associated with peptic ulcer (see Chapter 54). By blocking glandular secretions in the lung and mouth, atropine is useful as a preoperative medication and as palliative treatment to decrease pulmonary edema and bronchoconstriction in anticholinesterase poisoning.

The primary uses of muscarinic blocking agents are in ophthalmology and gastroenterology. Atropine and the tertiary and quaternary amines (see Table 9-2) are used to relax gastrointestinal smooth muscle and in various procedures involving the eye.

Atropine is applied topically for preoperative mydriasis (pupil dilatation) frequently in combination with phenylephrine. It is also widely used for treating anterior uveitis adjunctively with topical corticosteroids or for postoperative mydriasis. The use of phenylephrine enhances mydriasis, with less atropine needed for the desired effect. Where a mydriatic-cycloplegic (paralysis of accommodation) of lesser duration is desired (atropine effects may persist from days to weeks), the shorter-acting agents such as cyclopentolate, homatropine, and tropicamide may be used. Mydriatic-cycloplegics are also used to break down adhesions (posterior synechiae) and in ciliary block glaucoma.

Atropine as an antispasmodic produces variable undesirable clinical responses. Some of the synthetic tertiary amines have more uniform bioavailability than most of the naturally occurring alkaloids have, and their central effects are less prominent. Because quaternary compounds are permanently charged and unable to cross the blood-brain barrier, they remain in the periphery and seldom exhibit CNS effects. The quaternary amide *clidinium bromide* is characterized by the absence of any CNS actions and is widely prescribed as an antispasmodic. Despite the large number of synthetic agents available, preparations of the belladonna alkaloids are still used because few clear differences aid in the selection of an antispasmodic that may be used for gastrointestinal disturbances.

Atropine is often administered preoperatively to diminish salivary secretions. It is also used with cholinesterase inhibitors to reverse the action of neuromuscular blocking agents and to limit the effect of acetylcholine accumulation to the neuromuscular junction. In addition to its availability as a tertiary amine, atropine analogs are available as quaternary salts to limit access to the CNS.

Scopolamine Although there are few qualitative differences between atropine and scopolamine as muscarinic blocking drugs, quantitative differences limit the usefulness of the latter. Scopolamine is more potent centrally and, even at relatively low doses, can induce hallucinations and aberrant behavior in susceptible individuals. This is frequently observed in children premedicated with scopolamine before general anesthesia. Because of these actions, the drug is not widely used as an antisecretory or antispasmodic agent. Its action on the iris to produce mydriasis and on the ciliary muscle to produce cycloplegia is greater than the corresponding effects of atropine. It also produces xerostomia, or dry mouth, as atropine does. Atropine has less pronounced CNS effects. Atropine is more effective in promoting vagal slowing of the heart, in decreasing intestinal activity, in relaxing constricted bronchiolar smooth muscle, and in demonstrating a longer duration of action, particularly on the iris. Atropine is important as an antidote to treat poisoning by carbamate and organophosphate, agricultural insecticides that inhibit cholinesterases. Atropine also acts to reduce sphincter and bladder tone on the urinary tract and has a mild antispamodic action on the biliary tract.

Ganglionic Blocking Drugs

Historically, ganglionic blocking drugs were used for their ability to lower systemic blood pressure in hypertensive patients. However, these agents now have only limited use because of their broad actions resulting from inhibition of both sympathetic and parasympathetic systems. They have been supplanted by more selective and predictable antihypertensive drugs. Nevertheless, ganglionic blockers are important because they provide a basis for understanding the underlying principles of ganglionic function and reflex effects. Many of the prominent side effects of a wide variety of therapeutic agents result from actions on the autonomic system, though their major actions are elsewhere. Generalized ganglionic blockade leads to atony of the bladder and the gastrointestinal tract. Actions on ciliary ganglion cause cycloplegia, and actions on superior cervical ganglion produce dry mouth and anhidrosis.

The greatest problem from ganglionic blockade is that of orthostatic hypotension, resulting from the loss of postural reflexes. The cardiovascular system depends on sympathetic innervation to maintain blood pressure. The effects of ganglionic blockade on blood pressure in the recumbent position may be small, but a precipitous decrease in pressure can take place when the patient is sitting or standing. Thus orthostatic hypotension poses a major problem to the ambulatory patient. This effect may become less pronounced with continued use of the drug. The action of ganglion blocking agents on cardiac rate depends on the relative importance of vagal tone, which is greater in well-conditioned patients and much less in sedentary patients. Usually, mild tachycardia with hypotension indicates fairly complete ganglionic blockade. As a result of the hypotension, the decrease in venous return after blockade of sympathetic ganglia can result in diminished cardiac output. In contrast to the systemic circulation, cerebral blood flow is less affected because circulation to the brain is under tight autoregulation. Only when a substantial decrease in mean blood pressure occurs is there a significant decrease in cerebral blood flow. In elderly patients, in whom vessels may be sclerotic, a precipitous decrease in blood pressure can produce a rebound increase that can result in a cerebral vascular accident (a stroke).

Trimethaphan camsylate is administered intravenously in hypertensive crises. It is also used in surgical procedures involving highly vascularized tissues and has a short duration of action.

Inhibitors of Acetylcholine Metabolism

The primary target organs in which the anticholinesterase drugs act are the eye; the skeletal muscle neuromuscular junctions; the gastrointestinal, urinary, and respiratory tracts; and the heart and other tissues that receive parasympathetic innervation. In most respects the cholinesterase-inhibitor drugs produce effects similar to those of direct-acting cholinergic agonists.

The major clinical use for the anticholinesterases is in the treatment of glaucoma. There are two types of primary glaucoma, open-angle and angle-closure, depending on the configuration of the angle of the anterior chamber of the eye at the point where reabsorption of the aqueous humor takes place. Open-angle glaucoma can be successfully managed with cholinesterase inhibitors, particularly the irreversibly acting drugs, whereas angle-closure glaucoma may be treated initially with pilocarpine but generally requires surgery for correction. These agents relieve the elevated intraocular pressure of open-angle glaucoma by promoting outflow of the aqueous humor and perhaps also by diminishing secretion. This results from contraction of the ciliary muscle and the sphincter of the iris. When this occurs, the trabecular meshwork at the base of the ciliary muscle is opened and the iris is pulled away, widening the angle at the anterior chamber and facilitating flow of the aqueous humor into Schlemm's canal. The intraocular pressure in the anterior chamber of the eye is thus reduced. This action is shown schematically in Figure 9-7.

Physostigmine and Other Drugs to Treat Glaucoma Physostigmine is used to treat open-angle glaucoma and sometimes to treat accommodative esotropia, a strabismus resulting from excessive accommodation. Physostigmine is a tertiary amine, extremely lipid soluble, but not well tolerated. Among the long-acting miotics used to treat open-angle glaucoma are the organophosphates, *echothiophate* and *isoflurophate. Demecarium,* a synthetic bis-quaternary compound, is also used in open-angle glaucoma and esotropia. These latter compounds are generally instilled into the conjunctival sac at 12- to 48-hour intervals. They reduce intraocular pressure maximally in 1 day but tend to predispose to cataracts with prolonged use and are generally reserved for situations in which the shorter-acting cholinomimetics are not effective. The quaternary nitrogen in echothiophate essentially limits its distribution and does not allow ready systemic absorption after topical application. *Isoflurophate,* however, is lipophilic and can readily enter the systemic circulation after topical application to the eye.

Edrophonium Chloride, Neostigmine, and Pyridostigmine Another important use of the anticholinesterases is in the treatment of myasthenia gravis. This disease is characterized by a progressive weakness of skeletal muscle resulting from an impairment in neuromuscular transmission. The disorder stems at least in

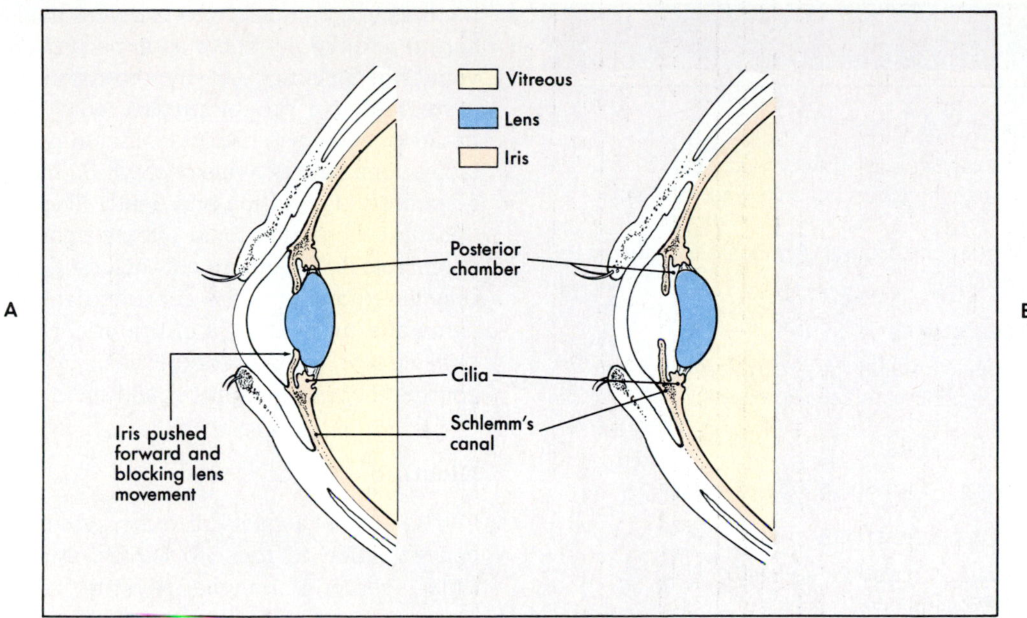

FIGURE 9-7 Treatment of glaucoma with cholinergic agonists or cholinesterase inhibitors. **A,** Before application of drug. **B,** After application of drug.

part from a reduction in the number of postsynaptic acetylcholine receptors. Because myasthenia gravis is an autoimmune disease, it is proposed that the loss of receptors is brought about by antigenic modulation, and so the acetylcholine receptors are degraded and are turned over at a more rapid rate than normal. Thus the rate of neurotransmitter-receptor binding is reduced and muscle fatigue results. Frequently used drugs to treat this disorder are the reversible carbamate ester anticholinesterases pyridostigmine and neostigmine.

The short-acting cholinesterase inhibitors, edrophonium chloride, neostigmine, and pyridostigmine, are used to reverse neuromuscular blockade (see Chapter 11), based on competitive antagonism between acetylcholine and the blocking drug. In this situation, the concentration of acetylcholine is permitted to increase by inhibiting acetylcholinesterase, thereby enhancing the ability of acetylcholine to compete for nicotinic receptors at the neuromuscular junction.

Edrophonium may also be used in the treatment of atrioventricular nodal reentrant tachycardia, particularly when carotid sinus massage is ineffective. The termination of the tachycardia is effected by the increase in acetylcholine released at the node, thereby reducing atrioventricular node conduction velocity. Edrophonium is the preferred anticholinesterase because of its rapid onset and short duration of action.

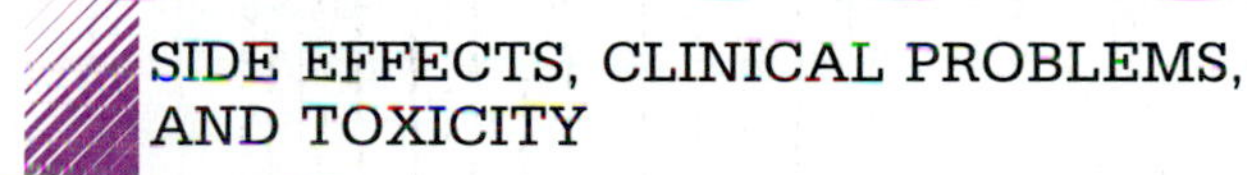

SIDE EFFECTS, CLINICAL PROBLEMS, AND TOXICITY

Clinical problems are summarized in the box on p. 108.

Cholinomimetic Agonists

With *pilocarpine* administration, stinging and local irritation may occur, and ciliary spasm and miosis may be troublesome initially. Allergic reactions are rare. In the patient with asthma, stimulation of bronchial smooth muscle by improperly administered pilocarpine may precipitate a full-blown asthmatic attack.

Bethanechol may cause symptoms associated with excessive parasympathetic activity, such as flushing of skin, sweating, nausea, cramps and diarrhea, asthmatic attacks, and a decrease in systemic blood pressure. These effects may be counteracted by atropine administered SC. Bethanechol should not be given IV or IM because acute circulatory failure and cardiac arrest can result. This drug also should not be used in the presence of anatomical or functional urinary tract obstruction. Its use should be avoided in patients who have problems associated with the detrusor muscle unless an effective external sphincter relaxant is given at the same time because of vesicoureteral reflux or other adverse

CLINICAL PROBLEMS

CHOLINOMIMETIC AGONISTS

Excessive parasympathetic activity: decreased blood pressure, bronchoconstriction, sweating, GI discomfort

At high concentrations, excess ganglionic activity

Mushroom toxicity

MUSCARINIC BLOCKERS

Blocks secretions, causes urinary retention, mydriasis, tachycardia, hypertension, constipation

GANGLIONIC BLOCKERS

Lack of selectivity makes drugs difficult to use

CHOLINESTERASE INHIBITORS

Side effects similar to those for agonists

Organophosphate compound toxicity

effects. Because it increases intestinal motility, bethanechol should not be given to patients with peptic ulcer or patients who have had intestinal resection or anastomosis.

The major toxicity from muscarinic agonists results not from therapeutic use but from eating certain varieties of mushrooms, most commonly *Amanita muscaria* and other species, particularly the *Inocybes,* in which the muscarine content is high. After ingestion of these fungi, toxic signs develop rapidly and are maximal within 2 hours. The toxic signs include salivation, sweating, tearing, nausea, vomiting, diarrhea, visual disturbances, bradycardia, hypotension, and shock. In *Amanita muscaria* poisoning, typical CNS symptoms consist of irritability, confusion, restlessness, hallucinations, and convulsions. These symptoms contrast with those produced by *Amanita phalloides,* which contain nonmuscarinic substances highly toxic to the liver, resulting in hepatotoxicity that is sometimes fatal. Treatment of mushroom poisoning requires parenteral administration of atropine, specifically to counteract the cholinergic symptoms. Mild sedatives are also given to treat the central effects of other substances present in mushrooms, which appear to be indole related in structure. In some situations, other supportive therapy may also be indicated.

Muscarinic Blocking Drugs

There are several undesirable effects associated with therapeutic doses of the muscarinic blocking agents. These include urinary retention, dry mouth, cycloplegia, mydriasis, anhidrosis, and tachycardia. Larger doses result in additional effects such as photophobia, nausea, vomiting, flushing, and hypertension. Central nervous system effects are prominent with overdoses of the naturally occurring alkaloids, including excitement, hallucinations, and convulsions, which may be followed by respiratory depression and death. The quaternary nitrogen drugs produce toxic effects characteristic of ganglionic blockade and do not include CNS effects. All anticholinergic agents are contraindicated in acute glaucoma and in conditions of the urinary and gastrointestinal tracts where decreases in smooth muscle contractility and motility would have adverse results.

Nicotine

The natural alkaloid *nicotine,* which is found in high concentration in tobacco leaves, stimulates the nicotinic receptor at ganglia. Nicotine has no therapeutic action but is medically important because of its potential toxicity.

Complex changes that occur after nicotine administration are both stimulant and depressant. The drug can cause an increased heart rate by stimulating sympathetic ganglia, or a decrease in heart rate by acting on parasympathetic ganglia. It stimulates adrenal release of epinephrine, accelerating heart rate and raising systemic blood pressure. Similar actions are produced by nicotine on the carotid and aortic bodies. Nicotine acts centrally to produce tremor and convulsions. Respiration is stimulated by nicotine at low doses by an indirect activation of reflex pathways and directly at high doses by stimulation of the medulla. It produces vomiting by stimulating the chemoreceptor trigger zone in the area postrema. Although this action may be lifesaving, large doses of nicotine ultimately depress the CNS, and death results from respiratory depression caused by skeletal muscle end plate depolarization blockade. Nicotine is rapidly absorbed percutaneously, orally through the buccal membranes, and through the respiratory tree. Treatment after oral ingestion includes gastric lavage and artificial respiration; oxygen should be used if respiratory function is greatly affected.

Inhibitors of Acetylcholine Metabolism

The acute toxicity of organophosphorus compounds is the result of inhibiting the actions of cholinesterase enzymes, leading to accumulation of acetylcholine. These compounds are absorbed through the respiratory tract, conjunctiva, or skin. Exposure to high concentrations causes CNS effects. The accumulation of acetylcholine at nerve endings produces typical muscarinic and nicotinic actions. The duration of symptoms, if un-

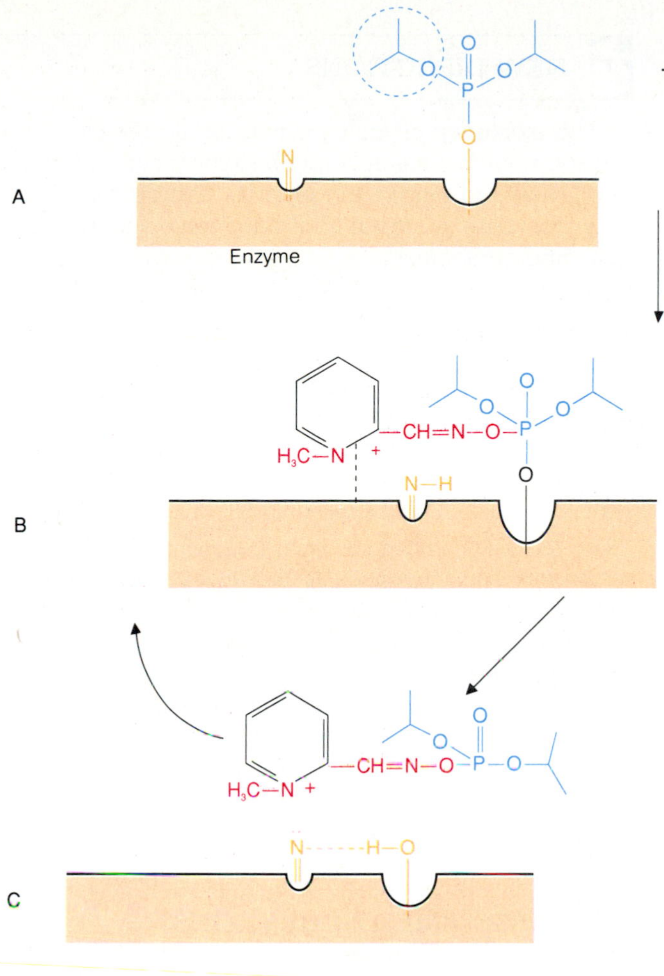

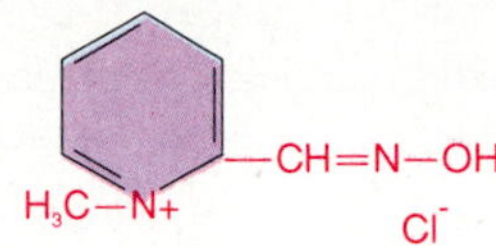

FIGURE 9-8 Reactivation of organphosphorus-inactivated cholinesterase by pralidoxime chloride. **A,** Inactive diisopropylphosphorylated enzyme, **B,** forming new covalent bond. **C,**Pralidoxime diisopropylphosphate is released, and enzyme is regenerated.

treated, depends on the reversibility of the inhibition of the cholinesterase. With *echothiophate* this may be less than 24 hours. With earlier agents such as soman or sarin, the irreversible effects may persist for several days to months.

Mild exposure leads to pupillary constriction, tightness of the chest, watery discharge from the nose, and wheezing. In *severe* exposure, the symptoms become intensified and, in addition to visual disturbances, muscle fasciculation becomes generalized. Excessive secretions lead to pulmonary edema after bronchoconstriction; there is subsequent pronounced muscle weakness and respiratory movements become shallow and intermittent. Central depression of respiratory control further intensifies the respiratory problems, which, if untreated, can lead to respiratory failure and death. These symptoms are accompanied by CNS effects, beginning with anxiety, restlessness, and emotional instability often leading to seizures. Profound long-term effects are manifested as headache, tremor, loss of short-term memory, confusion, apathy, and depression. The irreversibly acting organophosphates are a highly toxic group of compounds that collectively are capable of inhibiting more than a hundred different enzymes including the pancreatic enzymes chymotrypsin and trypsin, various kallikreins, thrombin and enzymes involved in clotting, and most importantly the cholinesterases.

Treatment of Toxicity In treating an individual exposed to an anticholinesterase, the first step is to remove the source to prevent further exposure. This may involve removal of clothing and possible lavage, or, if the environment is contaminated, evacuation to an uncontaminated area. The appearance of symptoms of poisoning requires prompt administration of atropine to block most sites of acetylcholine action except at neuromuscular junctions or other nicotinic sites. In mild cases, atropine can be administered over a 24-hour period. Eye symptoms, after local absorption of an anticholinesterase, are not relieved by systemic administration of atropine and require direct instillation of an ophthalmic solution of atropine or homatropine.

The use of *atropine* is palliative in nature; it relieves the symptoms of poisoning but does not reverse the inhibition of cholinesterases that results in neuromuscular activation and muscle paralysis. Reversal of mild organophosphate poisoning can be achieved by administration of pralidoxime (see Figure 9-8 for structure; the mechanism of reversal also is shown). With pralidoxime, regeneration of the enzyme occurs extremely rapidly compared with natural restoration. *Pralidoxime* acts as a site-directed nucleophile, which can regenerate the enzyme. When a cholinesterase is phosphorylated, it can undergo a process in which an alkyl or alkoxy group is lost. This results in a phosphorylated enzyme that is inherently more stable and also more resistant to a reactivator such as pralidoxime. It is therefore important that pralidoxime treatment be instituted early after organophosphate exposure. Pralidoxime does not antagonize the toxicity produced by the carbamates.

TRADE NAMES

In addition to generic and fixed-combination preparations, the following trade-named materials are available in the United States.

CHOLINOMIMETIC AGONISTS

Akarpine, Isopto Carpine, Pilocar, pilocarpine HCl
Miochol, acetylcholine chloride
Miostat, carbachol chloride
Myotonachol, Urecholine, bethanechol
Nicorette, nicotine
Ocusert, pilocarpine delivery device
Pilagan, pilocarpine nitrate

MUSCARINIC BLOCKING DRUGS

Akineton, biperiden HCl
Artane, trihexyphenidyl HCl
Atrovent, ipratropium bromide
Bentyl, dicyclomine HCl
Cogentin, benztropine mesylate
Isopto Atropine, atropine sulfate
Isopto Homatropine, homatropine HBr
Isopto Hyoscine, scopolamine HBr
Kemadrin, procyclidine
Pamine, methscopolamine bromide
Pathilon, tridihexethyl chloride
Pro-Banthine, propantheline bromide
Quarzan, clidinium bromide
Robinul, glycopyrrolate
Transdermscop, methscopolamine delivery device

GANGLIONIC BLOCKING DRUGS

Arfonad, trimethaphan camsylate
Inversine, mecamylamine HCl

ENZYME INHIBITORS

Antilirium, physostigmine salicylate
Floropryl, isoflurophate
Humorsol, demecarium bromide
Mestinon, Regonol, pyridostigmine bromide
Phospholine Iodide, echothiophate iodide
Prostigmin, neostigmine bromide

DIAGNOSTIC USE ONLY

Enlon, Reversol, Tensilon, edrophonium chloride
Provocholine, methacholine chloride

TREATMENT OF ANTICHOLINESTERASE INHIBITION

Protopam, pralidoxime chloride

NEW DIRECTIONS

The existence of multiple muscarinic receptor subtypes (m_1 to m_5) has recently become clear. Efforts are being made to exploit the pharmacological differences between these subtypes to develop more selective agonists and antagonists.

REFERENCES

Dolly JO, Barnard EA: Nicotinic acetylcholine receptors: an overview, *Biochem Pharm* 33:841, 1984.

Donati F, Lahoud J, McCready D, et al: Neostigmine, pyridostigmine and edrophonium as antagonists of deep pancuronium blockade, *Can J Anaesth* 34:589, 1987.

Elston JS, Lee JP, Powell CH, et al: Treatment of strabismus in adults with botulinum toxin A, *Br J Ophthalmol* 68:718-724, 1985.

Hartvig P, Wiklund L, Lindstrom B: Pharmacokinetics of physostigmine after intravenous, intramuscular and subcuous administration in surgical patients, *Acta Anaesth Scand* 26:297, 1982.

Kerlavage AR, Fraser CM, Venter JC: Muscarinic receptor structure: molecular biological support for subtypes. *Trends Pharmacol Sci* 8:426, 1987.

SELF-ASSESSMENT QUESTIONS

1. A 60-year-old male patient complains of difficulty reading in artificial light. After diagnosis of lens opacity, he is admitted to the surgical floor and undergoes cataract removal. After surgery, acetylcholine chloride (Miochol) is administered intraocularly to:
   a. relax the circular muscle of the iris.
   b. ensure complete miosis.
   c. decrease tearing from lacrimal secretion.
   d. decrease the flow of aqueous humor.
   e. all of the above
2. An elderly female patient is found to exhibit elevated intraocular pressure and is diagnosed as suffering from open-angle glaucoma. Her physician calls for 0.25% pilocarpine (Isopto Carpine), 2 gtt every 6 hours. The anticipated effect of administering pilocarpine eyedrops would be to:
   a. relax ciliary muscles.
   b. improve accommodation.

c. relax sphincter muscle of iris.
d. stimulate trabecular meshwork.
e. contract ciliary muscle and pull on trabecular network to relieve pressure.

3. A factory worker in a plant manufacturing chemical insecticides accidently ingests a residual white powder from a barrel labeled "Poisonous Material." He complains of a tightness in the chest and difficulty with vision. In the hospital emergency room he is found to have pinpoint pupils and profuse salivation. It is assumed he has been exposed to an anticholinesterase inhibitor. The most appropriate medication for his condition would be:
   a. atropine sulfate.
   b. physostigmine (Isopto-Eserine).
   c. edrophonium (Tensilon).
   d. propantheline (Pro-Banthine).
   e. atropine plus pralidoxime
4. Several hours after the factory worker's initial relief of symptoms, the symptoms return and are now more intense. At this time the toxic substance has been identified as Parathion, which is known to undergo biotransformation to the oxygen analog, Paraoxon, a highly toxic irreversible anticholinesterase. The most appropriate treatment combination would be:
   a. atropine in large doses given parenterally.
   b. parenteral pralidoxime and artificial respiration.
   c. Oral pralidoxime plus atropine.
   d. Parenteral pralidoxime, atropine, and artificial respiration.
   e. none of the above
5. If untreated, the cause of death from an anticholinesterase poisoning would be expected to be:
   a. hypertension.
   b. hypotension.
   c. congestive heart failure.
   d. respiratory failure.
   e. combination of b and c
6. The most toxic substance known that affects the cholinergic nervous system is an exotoxin secreted by the anaerobe *Clostridium botulinum*. There are several forms of botulinus toxin, all of which are highly toxic after ingestion of contaminated food. The toxin produces respiratory paralysis by:
   a. blocking nicotinic receptors.
   b. blocking release of acetylcholine from nerve endings.
   c. blocking peristalsis.
   d. causing circulatory collapse.
   e. stimulating the vagus nerve.

CHAPTER 10

Drugs Affecting the Sympathetic Nervous System

KENNETH E. MOORE

MAJOR DRUGS

albuterol
amphetamine
atenolol
clonidine
cocaine
epinephrine
isoproterenol
methyldopa
norepinephrine
phentolamine
phenylephrine
prazosin
propranolol

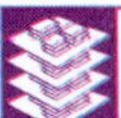

THERAPEUTIC OVERVIEW

The peripheral sympathetic nervous system modulates the activity of smooth muscle, cardiac muscle, and glandular cells. Transfer of information from terminals of most sympathetic neurons to the effector organs is mediated by norepinephrine. Exceptions are those few anatomically sympathetic neurons that project to sweat glands and to some blood vessels in the neck, face, and skeletal muscles that use acetylcholine as a transmitter. The actions resulting from activation of sympathetic neurons are reinforced by epinephrine and norepinephrine secreted into the circulation from the adrenal medulla (sympathoadrenal discharge). Outside of the United States, epinephrine and norepinephrine are known as adrenaline and noradrenaline, respectively, from which the adjectives "adrenergic" and "noradrenergic" are derived.

Drugs that facilitate or mimic the actions of the sympathoadrenal system are termed **sympathomimetics;** drugs that block or reduce these actions are termed **sympatholytics.** Because the sympathetic nervous system modulates the activity of many organ systems throughout the body, drugs that modify the actions of these neurons produce a variety of responses, and many of these drugs are important clinically. Because of their wide diversity of actions, however, these drugs also have a multiplicity of undesirable side effects.

By mimicking or facilitating the actions of norepinephrine on vascular smooth muscle, sympathomimetics constrict arterioles and veins and therefore can be administered locally to (1) reduce superficial bleeding, (2) slow diffusion of locally administered drugs (e.g., local anesthetics), (3) decongest mucous membranes, and (4) reduce formation of aqueous humor so as to lower intraocular pressure in glaucoma. Systemic administration of sympathomimetics causes generalized constriction of blood vessels leading to increases in peripheral vascular resistance and mean arterial blood pressure. These drugs are used to increase blood pressure in some hypotensive states (e.g., neurogenic shock resulting from spinal anesthesia or spinal cord injury). By increasing blood pressure, sympathomimetics cause a reflex slowing of the heart rate and for this reason can be used therapeutically to treat paroxysmal atrial tachycardia.

Epinephrine and other adrenergic drugs have strong stimulatory effects on cardiac muscle and are used to treat cardiogenic shock. These drugs also reduce the tone of various smooth muscles. By relaxing bronchial smooth muscle, adrenergic drugs are useful in treating

ABBREVIATIONS

cAMP	Cyclic adenosine monophosphate
COMT	catechol-*O*-methyl transferase
GI	gastrointestinal
L-dopa	dihydroxyphenylalanine
MAO	monoamine oxidase

bronchospasm resulting from allergies, and by reducing the tone of pregnant uterus smooth muscle cells, adrenergic drugs delay delivery in premature labor. Drugs that mimic epinephrine contract radial smooth muscle in the iris, causing dilatation of the pupil and thereby facilitate eye examinations.

Drugs that reduce the actions of the sympathetic nervous system on vascular smooth muscle are used to treat essential hypertension and hypertensive emergencies. Drugs that reduce the actions of norepinephrine and epinephrine on cardiac muscle are used to treat cardiac dysrhythmias, angina pectoris, and other cardiac disorders (e.g., postmyocardial infarction). These drugs also have utility in treating migraine headaches, glaucoma, essential tremor, and some symptoms of anxiety.

The major drugs in use are summarized in the box.

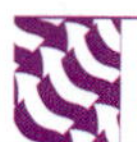

MECHANISMS OF ACTION

Noradrenergic Transmission Processes

The molecular structures of receptors and second-messenger signal systems are discussed in Chapter 2, and the anatomy, biochemistry, and physiology of the sympathetic nervous system are discussed in Chapter 8. Additional aspects of the dynamic processes that occur at a noradrenergic nerve terminal and the sites at which drugs act to modify these processes are described here.

Sympathetic noradrenergic neurons exhibit extensive branching. Fine preterminal axons at the end organs contain numerous beadlike enlargements, called **varicosities,** which may be the sites where norepinephrine is released into the neuroeffector junction. A schema of a varicosity and some of the chemical events that occur at the neuroeffector junction is depicted in Figure 10-1.

The chemical sequence in the synthesis of norepinephrine is also illustrated in Figure 8-4. L-Tyrosine is transported into the neuronal varicosity where it is converted to L-3,4-dihydroxyphenylalanine (dopa). This rate-limiting step in the synthesis of all catecholamines is catalyzed by tyrosine hydroxylase. The newly synthesized dopa is rapidly decarboxylated to dopamine by aromatic L-amino acid decarboxylase, also known as dopa decarboxylase. In dopaminergic neurons within the central nervous system (see Figure 23-4), this is the last step in the synthetic process, and dopamine is released as a neurotransmitter. Noradrenergic neurons in the central (see Figure 24-1) and the peripheral sympathetic nervous systems contain dopamine β-hydroxylase, which catalyzes the conversion of dopamine to norepinephrine. Because this enzyme is located within synaptic vesicles, dopamine must be actively transported into these vesicles before it can be converted to norepinephrine. When synthesized, norepinephrine is bound to adenosine triphosphate (ATP) and stored within the vesicle until released.

When the nerve action potential arrives at the varicosity, calcium channels open, allowing Ca^{++} to enter the neuron and cause the norepinephrine-containing vesicles to migrate and fuse with the neuronal membrane. Through exocytosis, the vesicles expel their contents into the neuroeffector junction. Thus the synaptic vesicles serve as the site for the final step in the synthesis of norepinephrine, store high concentrations of norepinephrine in a protective environment, and serve as a vehicle for the release process. In the neuroeffector junction, norepinephrine is free to bind to α_1-, α_2-, β_1, and β_3-adrenergic receptor sites on the presynaptic and postsynaptic membranes; the type of receptor depends on the organ innervated. Activation of α_2-"autoreceptors" on the presynaptic neuronal membrane inhibits the further release of norepinephrine. The biochemical events that occur in postjunctional cells subsequent to the binding of norepinephrine to the various receptors are presented in Chapter 8.

After norepinephrine has reacted with presynaptic or postsynaptic receptors, it is removed by the high-affinity uptake$_1$ system, which transports the amine back into the varicosity. Here norepinephrine can be transported into the protective environment of the synaptic vesicle for eventual re-release or can be oxidatively deaminated by monoamine oxidase (MAO) located on the external membrane of mitochondria. The biologically inactive deaminated metabolites (3,4-dihydroxyphenylethylene glycol; 3,4-dihydroxymandelic acid) are then lost from the neuron, circulate in the bloodstream, and eventually are excreted in the urine. Norepinephrine can also be transported into the postjunctional cell by the uptake$_2$ system, where it is *O*-methylated by catechol-*O*-methyltransferase (COMT) to normetanephrine. The transport of norepinephrine by the uptake$_1$ transporter is the major mechanism that terminates the actions of this amine at receptor sites. Preventing the metabolism of norepinephrine by the administration of inhibitors of COMT and MAO does not enhance the transmission process at sympathetic neuron terminals. Catechol-*O*-methyltransferase and MAO, however, play important roles in metabolizing circulating catecholamines (norepinephrine and epinephrine) and some exogenously administered sympathomimetic amines.

Norepinephrine is also synthesized in and released from chromaffin cells in the adrenal medulla. In addition, however, many cells in the adrenal medulla contain an additional synthetic enzyme, phenylethanolamine

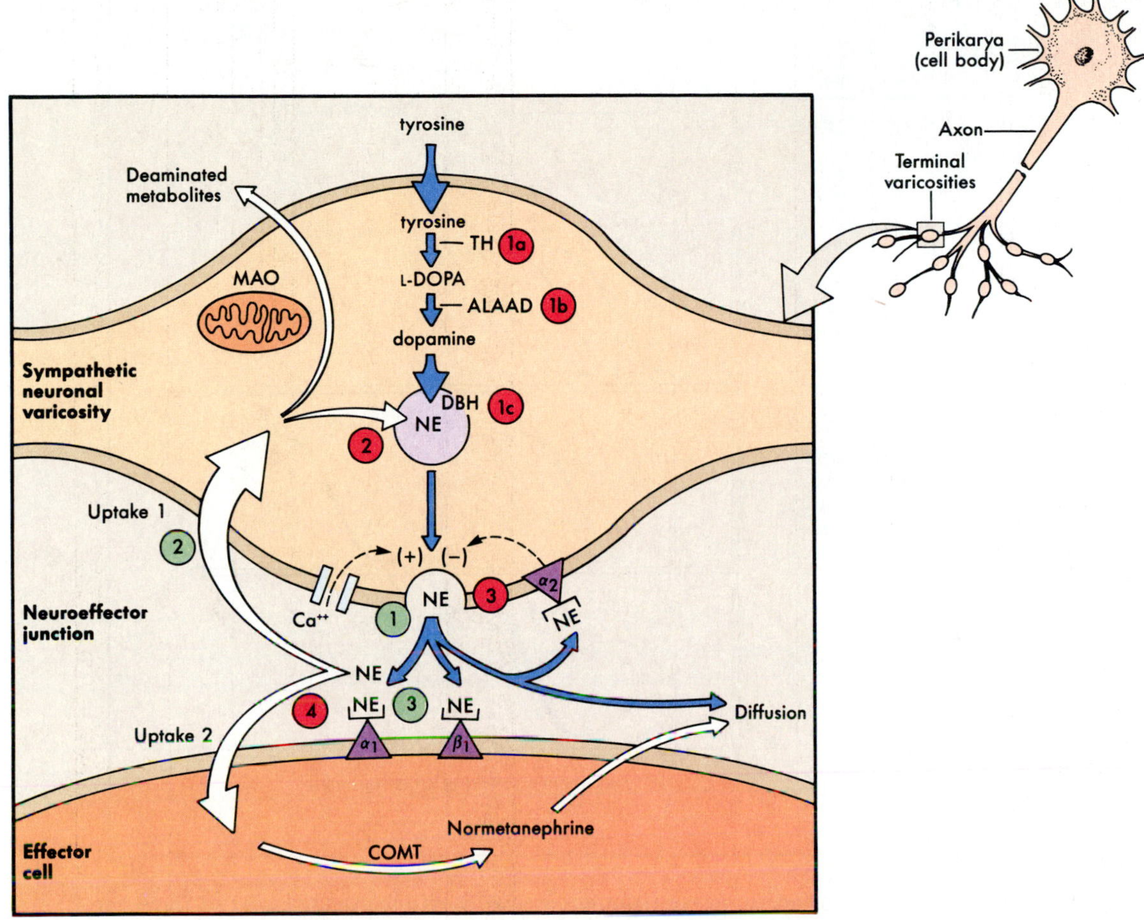

FIGURE 10-1 Prejunctional and postjunctional sites of action of drugs that modify noradrenergic transmission at a sympathetic neuroeffector junction. L-Tyrosine is actively transported into the axoplasm of the neuron, where it is converted first to L-dopa by tyrosine hydroxylase *(TH)* and then to dopamine by aromatic L-amino acid decarboxylase *(ALAAD)*. Dopamine is actively transported into synaptic vesicles, where it is converted by dopamine β-hydroxylase *(DBH)* to norepinephrine *(NE)*. The arrival of a nerve action potential at the varicosity causes the influx of calcium ions, which promotes the exocytotic release of NE into the neuroeffector junction where NE can activate receptors on postjunctional smooth muscle or glandular cells (α_1, or α_2) or cardiac cells (β_1) or on the prejunctional neuronal membrane (α_2). Activation of the latter receptor inhibits the further release of NE. The action of NE is terminated by transport back into the varicosity, uptake$_1$. In the varicosity, NE can be stored in the synaptic vesicle or metabolized by monoamine oxidase *(MAO)* to inactive deaminated products. NE is also lost from the neuroeffector junction by diffusion and by transport into the postjunctional cell, uptake$_2$, where it is metabolized to normetanephrine by catechol-*O*-methyltransferase *(COMT)*. Sites at which drugs enhance or mimic this noradrenergic transmission process are identified by *green numbers; red numbers* identify sites where drugs *block* or *reduce* this process.

Drugs that enhance or mimic noradrenergic transmission

1. Facilitate release (e.g., amphetamine)
2. Block reuptake (e.g., cocaine)
3. Receptor agonists (e.g., phenylephrine)

Drugs that reduce noradrenergic transmission

1. Inhibit synthesis (e.g., 1a, α-methyltyrosine; 1b, carbidopa; 1c, disulfiram)
2. Disrupt vesicular storage (e.g., reserpine)
3. Inhibit release (e.g., guanethidine)
4. Receptor antagonists (e.g., phentolamine)

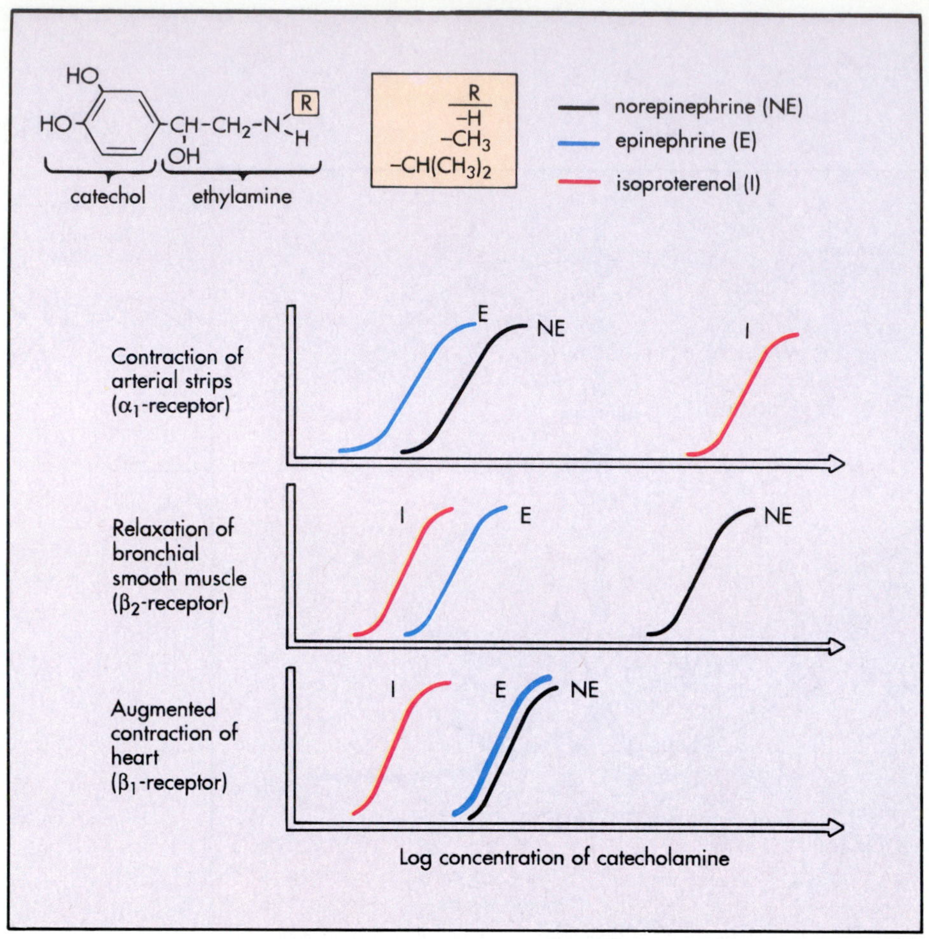

FIGURE 10-2 Dose-response curves (arbitrary scales) show relative potencies of three catecholamines on experimental muscle preparations. Changes in force of contraction or relaxation for each muscle tissue hung in separate tissue baths after addition of progressively increasing concentrations of each catecholamine.

N-methyltransferase, which catalyzes the conversion of norepinephrine to epinephrine. Chromaffin cells of the adrenal medulla are innervated by sympathetic preganglionic cholinergic neurons and release catecholamines into blood rather than into a neuroeffector junction. The released epinephrine is transported by blood to various organs where it activates α-and β-receptors on the surface of glandular, smooth muscle, and cardiac muscle cells. Like norepinephrine, epinephrine binds to α_1-, α_2- β_1, and β_3-receptors but also activates β_2-adrenergic receptors on smooth muscle. Circulating catecholamines, whether administered as drugs or released from the adrenal medulla, are taken up by the $uptake_1$ process in sympathetic nerves or are metabolized by enzymes in the liver.

Drugs modify the transmission processes at terminals of sympathetic neurons by increasing or decreasing the noradrenergic signal at the postsynaptic receptor sites (Figure 10-1). Sympathomimetics may mimic noradrenergic transmission by acting directly on postsynaptic receptors (e.g., phenylephrine), indirectly to facilitate norepinephrine release (e.g., amphetamine), or by blocking the neuronal reuptake ($uptake_1$) of this amine (e.g., cocaine). Sympatholytics reduce noradrenergic transmission by inhibiting synthesis (e.g., α-methyltyrosine), disrupting vesicular storage (e.g., reserpine), inhibiting release (e.g., guanethidine), or blocking receptors (e.g., phentolamine).

Summary of Catecholamine Activation of Adrenergic Receptors

In 1948, after comparing the actions of several sympathomimetic amines, Ahlquist proposed that these drugs acted on two different types of receptors, which he designated α and β (see Chapter 8). It was shown

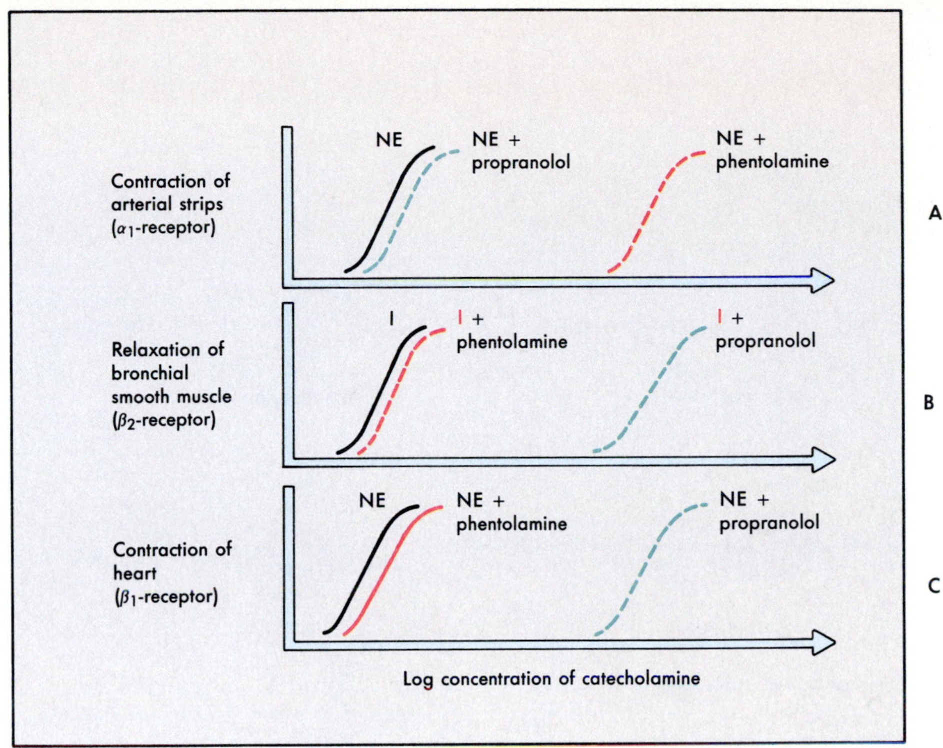

FIGURE 10-3 Change in force of contraction or relaxation (arbitrary scale) of different tissues hung in separate tissue baths after addition of increasing concentrations of catecholamine in absence and presence of a fixed concentration of an αadrenergic (phentolamine), or β-adrenergic (propranolol) receptor blocking drug. *NE,* Norepinephrine; *I,* isoproterenol.

subsequently, by examination of the actions of adrenergic agonists and antagonists, that there are three subtypes of β receptors, β_1, β_2, and β_3. The characteristics of β_1 and β_2 receptors are revealed when dose-response curves for three different catecholamines are examined on three separate tissues; these effects are schematically depicted in Figure 10-2. Norepinephrine and epinephrine are endogenous catecholamines released from the adrenal medulla, neurons in the brain, and peripheral postganglionic sympathetic neurons; isoproterenol is a synthetic catecholamine congener.

These amines augment the contraction of cardiac muscle and induce smooth muscle either to contract or to relax, depending on the receptor subtype located on the tissue cells. The three catecholamines have different potencies at these receptors. Contraction of arterial strips is mediated by α_1-receptors, and the relative potencies of the three catecholamines on this tissue is epinephrine > norepinephrine >>> isoproterenol. The relaxation of bronchial smooth muscle is mediated by β_2-receptors with the relative potencies of the three amines being isoproterenol > epinephrine >>> norepinephrine. The β_1-receptors located on cardiac muscle cells (cardiac β-receptors) are activated by the catecholamines with a potency relationship of isoproterenol > epinephrine = norepinephrine. The results of experiments such as those depicted in Figure 10-2 indicate that at reasonable pharmacological doses epinephrine activates α_1, β_1 and β_2-adrenergic receptors, norepinephrine activates α_1-and β_1-adrenergic receptors, and isoproterenol activates β_1- and β_2-receptors (see Chapter 8).

Confirming evidence is shown in Figure 10-3, using dose-response curves for the actions of norepinephrine or isoproterenol on different tissues in the presence of drugs that block α- or β-adrenergic receptors. Phentolamine, a competitive antagonist at α_1-receptors, causes a parallel shift to the right of the norepinephrine-induced contractions of arterial strips (Figure 10-3, *A*). Propranolol, a competitive antagonist at both β_1-and β_2-adrenergic receptors, causes a parallel shift to the right of responses mediated by β_2-receptors (Figure 10-3, *B*) and cardiac β_1-receptors (Figure 10-3, *C*).

α_2-Receptors are located on platelets and postsynaptically on a variety of target tissues (blood vessels, pancreas, enteric cholinergic neurons). Activation of α_2-receptors located on the terminals of sympathetic neurons reduces the release of norepinephrine (Figure 10-1).

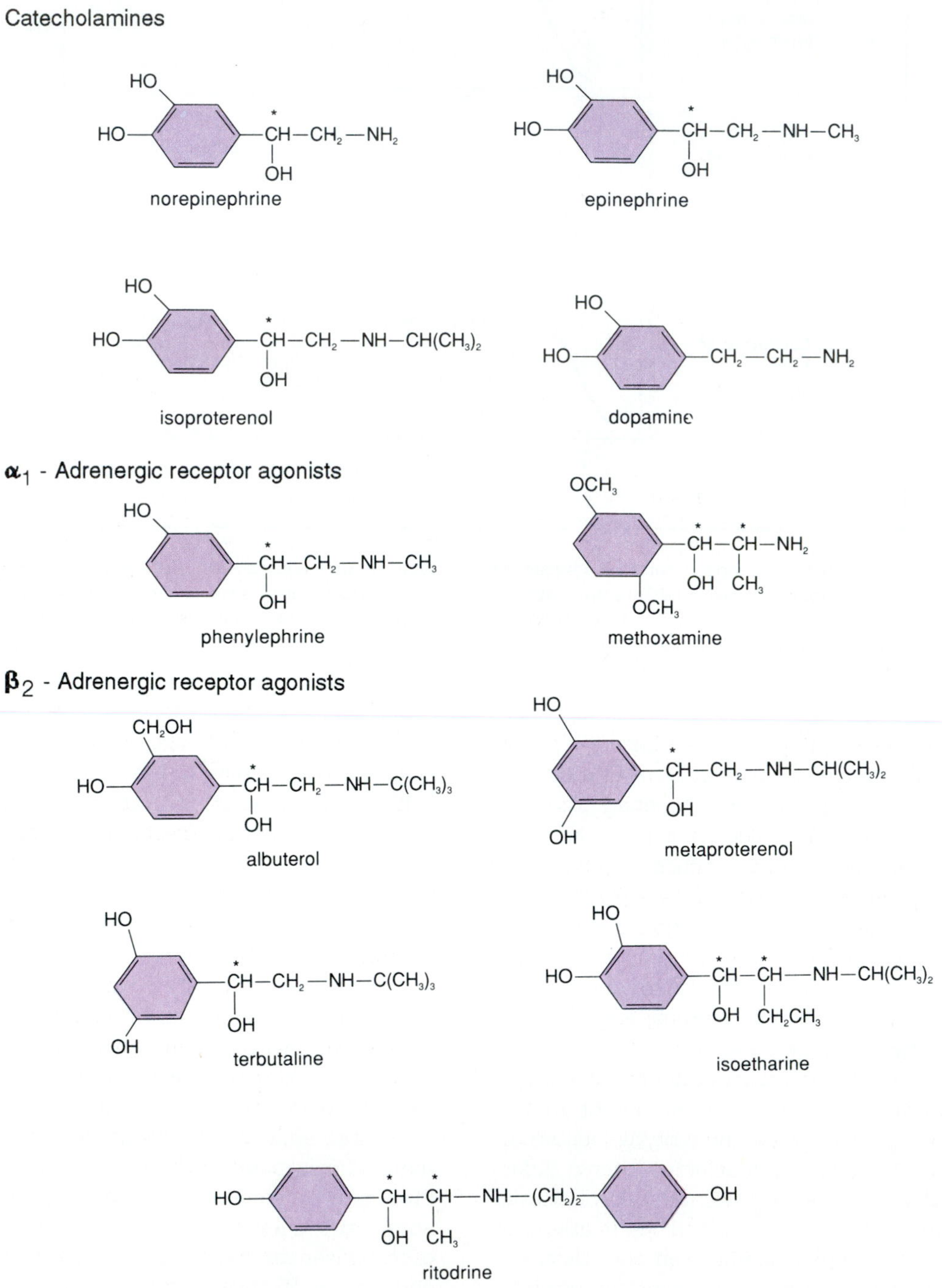

Catecholamines

norepinephrine

epinephrine

isoproterenol

dopamine

α_1 - Adrenergic receptor agonists

phenylephrine

methoxamine

β_2 - Adrenergic receptor agonists

albuterol

metaproterenol

terbutaline

isoetharine

ritodrine

FIGURE 10-4 Sympathomimetic agonists; direct-acting. Asterisk indicates asymmetric carbon. See text for further details.

β_1 - Adrenergic receptor agonists

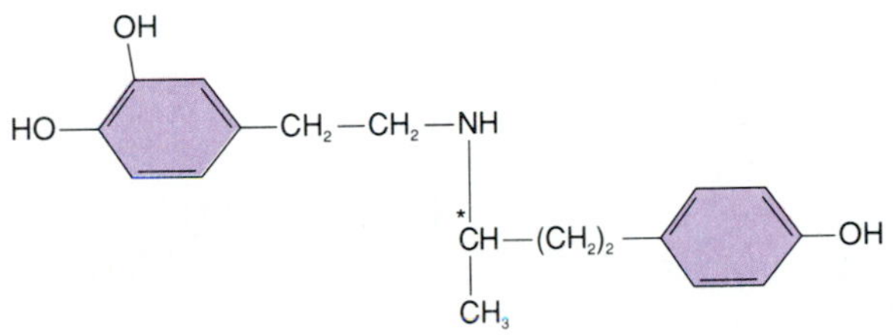

dobutamine

FIGURE 10-4, cont'd For legend see opposite page. See the text for further information.

α_2-Receptors are also located both presynaptically and postsynaptically on neurons in the brain; activation of these receptors reduces central sympathetic outflow (see Chapter 12).

Direct-acting Sympathomimetics

Receptor agonists mimic the effects of sympathoadrenal discharge by combining directly with postjunctional receptors (see site 3 [green] in Figure 10-1). Some drugs combine selectively with specific adrenergic receptors and mimic the effects of the endogenous ligands epinephrine and norepinephrine. Each endogenous catecholamine activates several different receptors (norepinephrine binds to α_1-, α_2-, β_1, and β_3-receptors, and epinephrine binds to α_1-, α_2-, and β_1-, and β_2-receptors), but some sympathomimetic amines selectively activate a single receptor type. For example, phenylephrine preferentially activates α_1-receptors, and clonidine activates α_2-receptors. Similarly, dobutamine and terbutaline are relatively specific agonists at β_1- and β_2-receptors respectively. The structures for some of the clinically important adrenergic agonists are shown in Figure 10-4.

Indirect-acting Sympathomimetics

Indirect-acting sympathomimetics do not activate receptors directly but facilitate the release of norepinephrine from sympathetic neuronal varicosities, or block the reuptake of norepinephrine by the uptake$_1$ transporter in the neuronal membrane. Amphetamine and chemically related drugs produce their sympathomimetic effects by facilitating the release of norepinephrine from the sympathetic nerve terminal (see site 1 [green] in Figure 10-1). The effects of these drugs in the central nervous system are described in Chapter 32.

Because norepinephrine is removed from the sympathetic neuroeffector junctional receptor sites by active transport back into the nerve terminals, sympathomimetic responses can be obtained by administration of drugs that block the uptake$_1$ amine transporter in the neuronal membrane (see site 2 [green] in Figure 10-1). Cocaine and tricyclic antidepressants, such as desimipramine, exert their sympathomimetic effects in this manner. The structure and discussion of cocaine is presented in Chapter 32, with similar information for tricyclic antidepressants in Chapter 24.

Because neuronal reuptake and not metabolism is the primary mechanism by which norepinephrine and epinephrine are removed from the neuroeffector junction, it is not surprising that drugs that inhibit the metabolism of these amines have little or no sympathomimetic actions. On the other hand, inhibitors of MAO (e.g., pargyline) or COMT (e.g., tropolone) can enhance the actions of exogenously administered sympathomimetic amines that are substrates for these enzymes (see Figure 10-1). This has some important toxicological implications. For example, the actions of tyramine, a sympathomimetic amine present in a variety of foods, are greatly enhanced in patients treated with an MAO inhibitor (Chapter 24).

Indirect-acting sympathomimetics can be recognized from the reduction in their actions if the effector organ is denervated (i.e., when there are no noradrenergic neurons innervating the cells) or if reserpine has been administered previously to deplete norepinephrine stores in sympathetic nerve terminals (Figure 10-5). An indirect sympathomimetic amine that releases norepinephrine must gain access to the noradrenergic neuron before effecting the release of the transmitter. Nonpolar, lipid-soluble drugs (e.g., amphetamine) can diffuse across the neuronal membrane, whereas polar, water-soluble compounds (e.g., tyramine) achieve access to the varicosity only by the uptake$_1$ transporter.

As noted in Figure 10-5, treatments that reduce or block the effects of the indirect-acting sympathomimetic amine tyramine enhance the effects of epinephrine, which acts directly on the adrenergic receptors. The enhanced effects of a direct-acting sympathomimetic in denervated tissues result from two temporally distinguishable effects. The early (2 to 3 days) increase in response to epinephrine results from the loss of uptake$_1$ sites in the neuronal membrane. As the neuron degenerates, the transporter sites primarily responsible for terminating the actions of epinephrine at the receptor sites are lost. Later augmentation of the actions of epinephrine occurs several days to weeks after denervation and is secondary to an increase (upregulation) in postjunctional receptors. Cocaine causes a prompt increase in the response to epinephrine by blocking the uptake$_1$ system. Reserpine, however, disrupts amine transport in the synaptic vesicle membrane but not in the neuronal membrane; it does not, therefore, alter the transport of the amine from the neuroeffector junction into the varicosity.

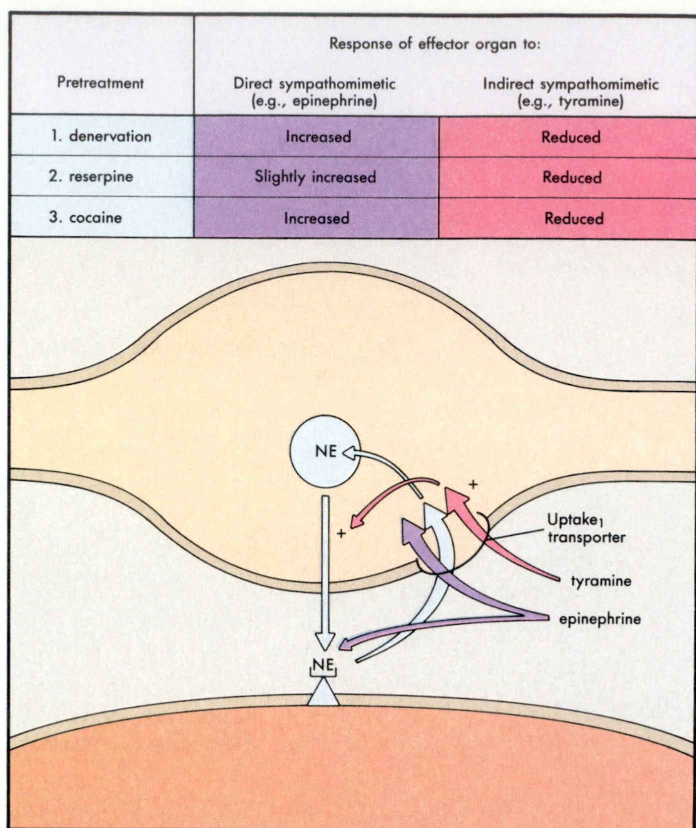

Pretreatment	Response of effector organ to: Direct sympathomimetic (e.g., epinephrine)	Indirect sympathomimetic (e.g., tyramine)
1. denervation	Increased	Reduced
2. reserpine	Slightly increased	Reduced
3. cocaine	Increased	Reduced

FIGURE 10-5 Comparison of direct- and indirect-acting sympathomimetics. *NE,* Norepinephrine.

Sympatholytics

Inhibition of Synthesis, Storage, or Release of Norepinephrine The synthesis of catecholamines can be disrupted at several steps, but effective in vivo blockade is obtained only when tyrosine hydroxylase, the enzyme catalyzing the first and rate-limiting step, is inhibited (see site 1a in Figure 10-1). This can be effected clinically with α-methyltyrosine (metyrosine). Several compounds can inhibit the other biosynthetic enzymes (e.g., aromatic L-amino acid decarboxylase is inhibited by carbidopa and dopamine β-hydroxylase is inhibited by disulfiram [see sites 1b and 1c in Figure 10-1]). These drugs have some experimental utility, but they do not effectively block endogenous catecholamine synthesis when administered clinically. On the other hand, carbidopa is clinically important because, by blocking peripheral decarboxylase activity, it reduces the side effects resulting from the formation of dopamine in the peripheral tissues of patients with Parkinson's disease treated with L-dopa.

Disruption of vesicular storage also modifies noradrenergic transmission (see site 2 [red] in Figure 10-1). Reserpine, for example, disrupts the ability of the synaptic vesicles to transport and store dopamine and norepinephrine, and so the intraneuronal amines are not protected from MAO. Inhibition of release is also a mechanism for modulation of the adrenergic response (see site 3 [red] in Figure 10-1). Drugs such as bretylium and guanethidine are transported into and become incorporated in the membranes of noradrenergic nerve terminals and prevent the release of norepinephrine in response to drugs and nerve action potentials.

Antagonists Antagonists have a high affinity for adrenergic receptors but lack intrinsic activity and thus effectively block the receptors (see site 4 [red] in Figure 10-1). The early antagonists blocked α-receptors (phenoxybenzamine) or β-receptors (propranolol). There are now available drugs that specifically block α_1-(prazosin), α_2-(idazoxan), or β_1-(metoprolol) receptors. These selective antagonists have valuable therapeutic advantages over the original, broad-spectrum adrenergic receptor blockers. Many of these antagonists are discussed further in Chapters 12 and 13.

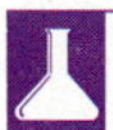

PHARMACOKINETICS

Detailed pharmacokinetics for many of these drugs have not been studied in humans because of the short duration of action, intense nature of the effects, or limited clinical use of the preparations. Available pharmacokinetic parameters are summarized in Table 10-1.

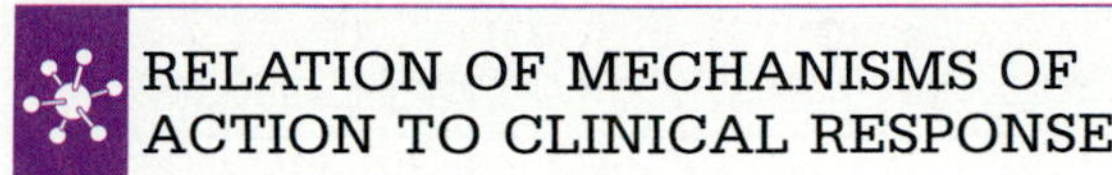

RELATION OF MECHANISMS OF ACTION TO CLINICAL RESPONSE

Direct and Reflex Cardiovascular Actions of Adrenergic Agents

The sympathetic nervous system plays an important role in regulating the cardiovascular system; thus, adrenergic drugs have pronounced effects on this system. These drugs alter the rate and force of contraction of the heart and the tone of blood vessels (and conse-

Table 10-1 Pharmacokinetic Parameters

Drug	Route of Administration	t½	Disposition	Remarks
DIRECT-ACTING SYMPATHOMIMETICS				
norepinephrine	IV	—	M	
epinephrine	IV, inhalation, topical	—	M	
isoproterenol	IV, inhalation	—	M	
dopamine	IV	~ 2 min	M	
phenylephrine	Oral, topical	—	M	primarily topical
methoxamine	IV, IM	—	—	
mephentermine	Slow IV, IM	—	M	
albuterol	Oral, inhalation	3.6 hr	R(30%) M(50%)	
metaproterenol	Oral, inhalation	~ 3 hr	M (main)	
terbutaline	IV, oral, inhalation	~ 6 hr	M (60%) first pass; crosses placenta	
isoetharine	Inhalation	—	—	
ritodrine	IV, oral	12 hr oral	R (90%)	bioavailability 30% (oral)
bitolterol	Inhalation	~ 4 hr	M (main)	
dobutamine	IV	2 min	M (main)	
INDIRECT-ACTING SYMPATHOMIMETICS				
amphetamine	Oral, exchange resin	—	R	
ephedrine	Oral, SC, IM, IV, topical	3-6 hr	R	
phenylpropanolamine	Oral	—	R	
pseudoephedrine	Oral	—	R	
SYMPATHOLYTICS: BLOCKERS				
phenoxybenzamine	IV, oral	24 hr oral	M, R, B	25% absorbed
phentolamine	IV, IM	19 min	R (13%) M	
tolazoline	IV	3-10 hr (neonates)		
prazosin	Oral	2.5 hr	M (main), B	>90% pb
propranolol	Oral	4 hr	M	
nadolol	Oral	22 hr	R (90%)	
timolol	Oral	4 hr	M 50% first pass, R	10% pb
pindolol	Oral	3.5 hr 7hr (elderly)	M (60%) no first pass R (40%)	40% pb
acebutolol	Oral	3.5 hr 10 hr(am)	M (main, active met (AM) R, B	
atenolol	Oral	6.5 hr	R (90%)	50% absorbed, 10% pb
metoprolol	IV, oral, inhalation	5 hr	M (90%), 50% first pass R (50%)	12% pb
esmolol	IV	9 min	M (98%), weak met R	
labetolol	IV, oral	5.5 hr	M (65%), first pass	50% pb

Continued.

Table 10-1 Pharmacokinetic Parameters—cont'd

Drug	Route of Administration	t½	Disposition	Remarks
OTHER SYMPATHOLYTICS				
α-methyl tyrosine (metyrosine)	Oral	3.5 hr	R (85%)	
reserpine	Oral	33 hr		96% pb, 50% bioavailability
bretylium	IV	7.8 hr	R (90%)	
guanethidine	Oral	1.5 da 4-8 da†	R M	
guanadrel	Oral	10 hr	R (85%)	
REDUCTION OF CENTRAL SYMPATHETIC OUTFLOW				
clonidine	Oral‡	12 hr	R (50%)	
methyldopa	Oral	105 min	M R	
guanabenz	Oral	6 hr	M (90%)	—
guanfacine	Oral	17 hr	M (50%) R (50%)	70% pb

B, Biliary; *first pass,* liver first-pass effect; *inhalation* inhalation as an aerosol; *M,* Metabolism; *pb,* plasma protein bound; *R,* renal, unchanged drug.
*Ester hydrolysis, gives weekly active metabolite.
†Terminal elimination phase.
‡Transdermal adhesive patch, 1 week.

quently blood pressure) by interacting directly with receptors located on cardiac and vascular smooth muscle cells. As a consequence of these direct actions, compensatory reflex adjustments take place. To understand the overall actions of adrenergic drugs on the heart and blood vessels, the cardiovascular reflexes must be considered.

Mean arterial blood pressure is maintained to deliver blood to all organs. It does not fluctuate widely because of feedback mechanisms that evoke compensatory secondary responses that maintain homeostasis. Homeostatic control of blood pressure is exerted primarily by baroreceptor reflexes (Figure 10-6). Baroreceptors are stretch receptors located in the walls of the heart and blood vessels, primarily in the carotid sinus and aortic arch, that are activated by distention of the blood vessels. Increased blood pressure increases the impulse traffic in the afferent neurons (baroreceptor neurons) that project to vasomotor centers in the medulla. Impulses generated in the baroreceptors inhibit the tonic discharge of sympathetic neurons projecting to the heart and blood vessels and activate vagal fibers projecting to the heart. When a drug such as phenylephrine, which contracts vascular smooth muscle, is administered, the peripheral resistance and consequently the blood pressure increase (Figure 10-7). The resulting increase in pressure within the carotid sinus and aortic arch increases impulse traffic in the afferent baroreceptor neurons and thereby reduces sympathetic nerve activity but increases vagal nerve activity. As a consequence, the heart rate decreases **(bradycardia).** If a drug such as histamine, which relaxes vascular smooth muscle, is administered, the blood pressure decreases, reducing impulse traffic in the afferent buffer neurons. Consequently, sympathetic nerve activity increases and vagal nerve activity decreases, resulting in an increase in heart rate **(tachycardia).**

In summary, drugs that cause vasoconstriction (e.g., α_1-adrenergic receptor agonists) secondarily cause reflex slowing of the heart. On the other hand, drugs that cause vasodilatation (e.g., α_1-adrenergic receptor blocking drugs) produce tachycardia through the baroreceptor reflex mechanism. Thus, when one is considering the actions of adrenergic drugs on the cardiovascular system, the direct actions of the drug on appropriate effector organs and compensatory reflex actions secondary to the direct actions must be considered.

Direct-acting Sympathomimetics

Epinephrine is a prototype of direct-acting sympathomimetic drugs because it activates all known subtypes of adrenergic receptors. The effects of direct-acting sympathomimetic drugs on selected tissues and organ systems are discussed here. Epinephrine is discussed first, and the properties of the more selective sympathomimetics are then compared with the prototype.

Cardiac Actions By activating cardiac β_1-adrenergic receptors, epinephrine alters the strength, rate, and rhythm of cardiac contractions; these actions

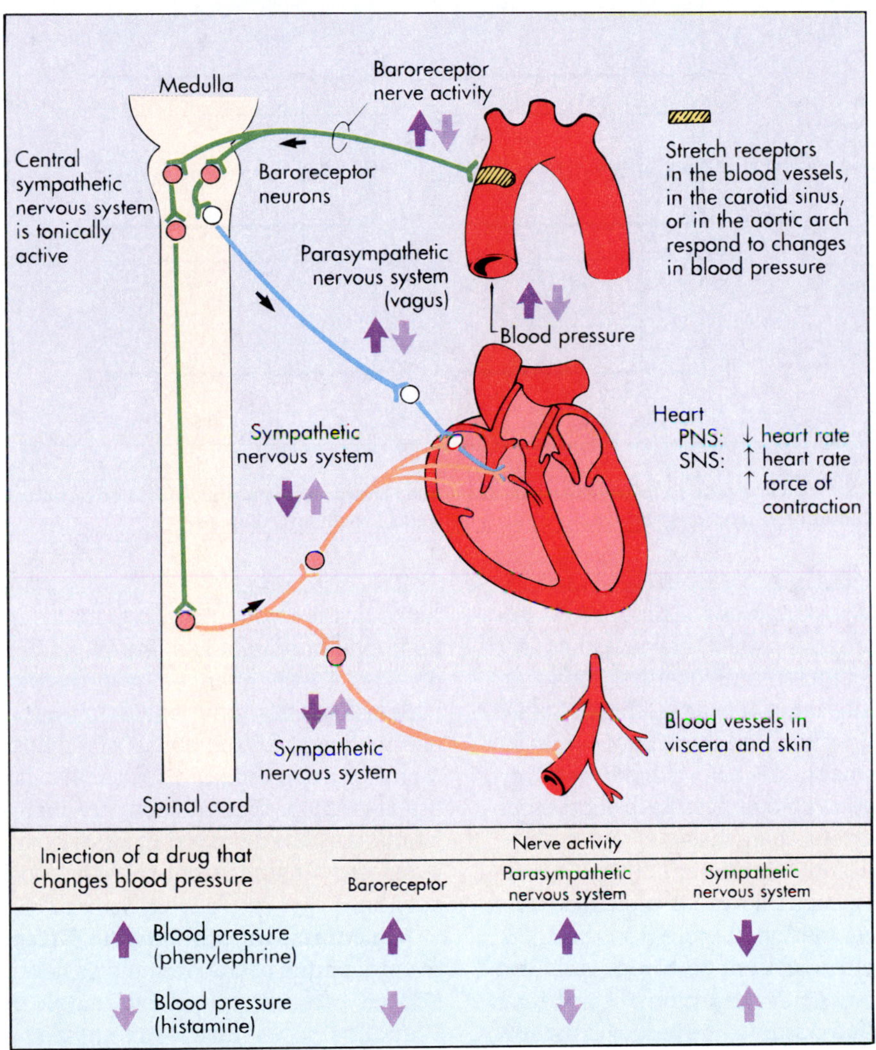

Injection of a drug that changes blood pressure	Nerve activity		
	Baroreceptor	Parasympathetic nervous system	Sympathetic nervous system
↑ Blood pressure (phenylephrine)	↑	↑	↓
↓ Blood pressure (histamine)	↓	↓	↑

FIGURE 10-6 Baroreceptor control of blood pressure and heart rate. *SNS,* Sympathetic nervous system; *PNS,* parasympathetic nervous system.

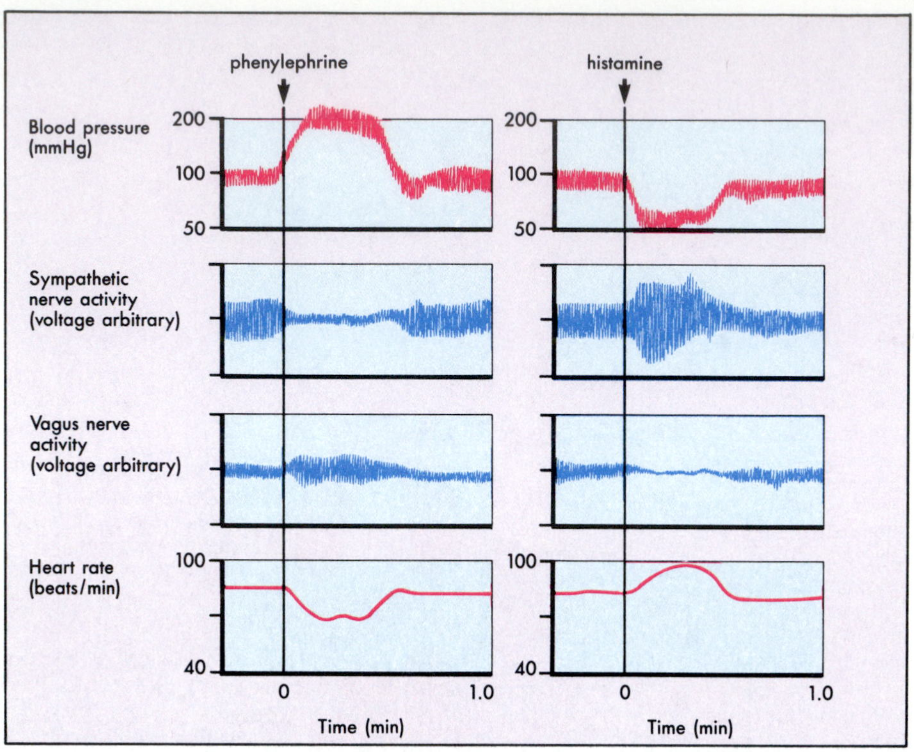

FIGURE 10-7 Responses to IV injections of drugs that cause vasoconstriction (phenylephrine) or vasodilatation (histamine) by acting directly on vascular smooth muscle.

may be either desirable or dangerous. Epinephrine increases the force of contraction (positive inotropic effect) by activating β_1-receptors on myocardial cells and increases the rate of contraction (positive chronotropic effect) by activating β_1-receptors on pacemaker cells in the sinoatrial node. Epinephrine also accelerates the rate of myocardial relaxation so that systole is shortened to a relatively greater extent than diastole. Thus, during the action of epinephrine, the fraction of time spent in diastole is increased, which allows for increased filling of the heart. The combination of increased diastolic filling time, more forceful ejection of blood, and increased rates of contraction and relaxation of the heart result in increased cardiac output. The initial increase in heart rate after the administration of epinephrine may be followed by slowing of the heart (bradycardia) as a result of reflex activation of the vagus nerve. The reflex bradycardia is blocked by muscarinic antagonists such as atropine. Reflex slowing of the heart is more pronounced after the administration of norepinephrine because, lacking β_2-adrenergic receptor agonist properties, it causes a greater increase in total peripheral resistance than epinephrine.

In addition to activating β_1-receptors on pacemaker cells in the sinoatrial node, epinephrine also activates conducting tissues, increasing conduction velocity and reducing the refractory period in the atrioventricular node, the bundle of His, Purkinje fibers, and ventricular muscle. These changes and the activation of latent pacemaker cells may lead to alterations in the rhythm of the heart. Large doses of epinephrine may cause tachycardia, premature ventricular systoles, and possibly fibrillation; these effects are more likely to occur in hearts that are diseased or have been sensitized by halogenated hydrocarbons (e.g., certain anesthetic agents).

Vascular Smooth Muscle Effects The responses to epinephrine of smooth muscle cells in different organs depend on the type of adrenergic receptors present. Vascular smooth muscle is regulated primarily by α_1- or β_2-receptor–containing cells, depending on the location of the vascular bed. Epinephrine is a powerful vasoconstrictor in some vascular beds; it activates α_1-receptors to contract smooth muscle cells in precapillary resistance vessels (arterioles) in skin, mucosa, and kidney, and in veins. At low doses, epinephrine relaxes vascular smooth muscle in skeletal muscle, liver, and gut as a result of activation of β_2-receptors. Thus, epinephrine increases blood flow in skeletal muscle and some splanchnic beds but reduces flow in the skin and kidney.

Systemic administration of epinephrine alters cerebral and coronary blood flow, but the changes are not attributable to the direct actions of the amine on α- or β_2-receptors on vascular smooth muscle in the brain and heart. Epinephrine-induced changes in cerebral blood flow primarily reflect changes in systemic blood pressure. Epinephrine increases coronary blood flow by inducing a relatively greater duration of diastole and metabolic changes (increased production of vasodilatory metabolites and the release of adenosine) secondary to increased work of the heart.

Other Smooth Muscle Effects Epinephrine is a potent bronchodilator. It relaxes bronchial smooth muscle by activating β_2-receptors. Epinephrine is a physiological antagonist to endogenous bronchoconstrictors (e.g., histamine, 5-hydroxytryptamine) and can be lifesaving in the treatment of acute asthmatic attacks (Chapter 58). This drug also relaxes smooth muscle in various organs by activating β_2-receptors. It reduces the frequency and amplitude of gastrointestinal (GI) contractions, decreases the tone and contractions of the pregnant uterus, and relaxes the detrusor muscle of the urinary bladder. Epinephrine, however, contracts smooth muscle of the splenic capsule and of GI and urinary sphincters by activating α_1-receptors. Epinephrine can contribute to urinary retention by relaxing the detrusor muscle and contracting the trigone and sphincter of the urinary bladder.

The radial pupillary dilator muscle of the iris contains α_1-receptors and contracts in response to activation of sympathetic neurons, causing mydriasis. Because epinephrine is a highly polar molecule, it does not readily penetrate the cornea when instilled into the conjunctival sac. Application of less polar, more lipid-soluble α-adrenergic agonists (e.g., phenylephrine) causes mydriasis. Instillation of epinephrine, however, lowers intraocular pressure, possibly by reducing formation of aqueous humor by the ciliary bodies, the latter involving a mechanism that is not well understood.

Because epinephrine and other catecholamines such as *norepinephrine, isoproterenol,* and *dopamine* are polar and cannot penetrate the blood-brain barrier, systemic administration of these amines has no direct cerebral action. Nevertheless, possibly through a secondary reflex action, systemic administration of epinephrine can cause anxiety, restlessness, and headache.

Metabolic Effects Epinephrine exerts many metabolic effects, some of which are secondary to an action of epinephrine on secretion of insulin and glucagon. The predominant action of epinephrine on islet cells of the pancreas is the inhibition of insulin secretion through activation of α_2-receptors and the stimulation of glucagon secretion through β_2-receptors.

The major metabolic effects of epinephrine are increased circulating concentrations of glucose, lactic acid, and free fatty acids. In humans, these effects are attributable to activation of β-receptors on the surface of liver, skeletal muscle, heart, and adipose cells (Figure 10-8). Subsequent to binding to β-receptors, G proteins and adenylate cyclase are activated by epinephrine. The increase in cyclic adenosine monophosphate (cAMP) activates cAMP-dependent protein kinase. This leads to phosphorylation and activation of other kinases, including phosphorylase *b* kinase, with subsequent additional phosphorylations of enzymes, including phosphorylase and lipase, both of which become activated. In fat, lipase catalyzes the breakdown of triglycerides to free fatty acids. The characteristic "calorigenic action" of epinephrine, which is reflected in a 20% to 30% increase in oxygen consumption, may be attributable in part to the breakdown of triglycerides in brown adipose tissue. In liver, phosphorylase catalyzes the breakdown of glycogen to glucose. In muscle, glycogenolysis and glycolysis produce lactic acid, which is released into the blood. The release of glucose from the liver is accompanied by the efflux of potassium, so that epinephrine induces hyperglycemia and a brief period of hyperkalemia. The hyperkalemia is followed by a more pronounced hypokalemia, as the potassium released from the liver is taken up by skeletal muscle.

Miscellaneous Actions Secretion of sweat from glands located on the palms of the hands and forehead is increased during psychological stress. The effect is mediated by α_1-receptors. Systemic administration of epinephrine does not activate these glands, but secretion of sweat in these areas can be induced by local injection of epinephrine. Epinephrine modulates the secretion of several hormones, though usually the physiological relevance and pharmacological effects are not pronounced. On the other hand, the secretion of insulin is inhibited by activation of α_2-receptors and slightly stimulated by activation of β_2-receptors. The secretion of glucagon is also stimulated by β_2-receptor activation. Epinephrine, by acting on β-receptors, also causes the release of renin from the juxtaglomerular apparatus in the kidney.

Other Direct-acting Sympathomimetics Several clinically useful, directly acting sympathomimetics differ from epinephrine in that they relatively selectively activate α- or β-receptors. The properties of some of these compounds are compared with those of epinephrine.

Norepinephrine has a low potency at β_2-receptors; thus the actions of clinically relevant doses of norepinephrine can be predicted because this amine stimulates only α- and cardiac β_1-adrenergic receptors. Norepinephrine produces only vasoconstriction in vascular beds and therefore increases diastolic blood pressure. Because total peripheral resistance increases, reflex

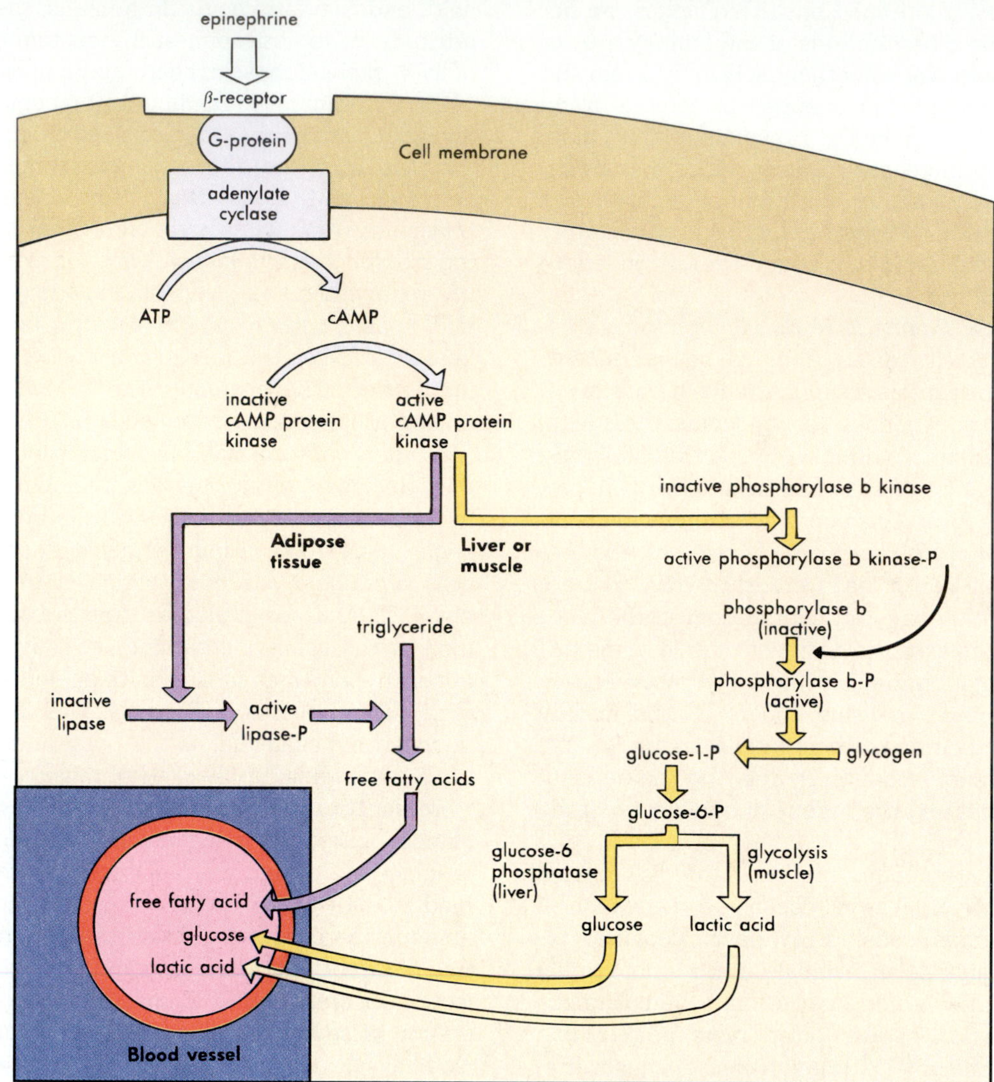

FIGURE 10-8 Mechanisms by which epinephrine (and other adrenergic agonists) exert metabolic effects in adipose, liver, heart, and skeletal muscle cells.

slowing of the heart rate is more pronounced with norepinephrine than with epinephrine. Unlike epinephrine, norepinephrine does not relax bronchial smooth muscle, and metabolic responses (e.g., hyperglycemia) are much less pronounced than they are with epinephrine.

Phenylephrine and *methoxamine* are synthetic selective α_1-receptor agonists. They differ from norepinephrine in that they do not activate β_1-receptors and therefore do not stimulate the heart. These drugs increase total peripheral resistance by causing vasoconstriction in most vascular beds. Consequently they produce a reflex slowing of the heart that can be blocked by atropine. These drugs are less potent but longer acting than norepinephrine.

Isoproterenol is a potent β-agonist; it differs from epinephrine in that it does not have α-adrenergic receptor agonist properties. It reduces total peripheral resistance, resulting in a considerable reduction in diastolic blood pressure. Further, it has a considerable stimulatory effect on the heart; tachycardia results from a combined direct action on β_1-receptors and a reflex action secondary to the hypotension. Like epinephrine, it relaxes bronchial smooth muscle and induces metabolic effects. Clinically, isoproterenol may be inhaled as an aerosol or injected subcutaneously to relieve bronchoconstriction resulting from allergies, drugs, or asthma. However, when used for this purpose, the side actions of isoproterenol on the heart, resulting from its β_1-agonist property, can be troublesome. Accordingly, efforts have been made to develop β-agonists that are relatively specific

Table 10-2 Actions of Selected Sympathomimetics on Heart Rate

Sympathomimetic Amine	Activated Receptors	Blood Pressure (Total Peripheral Resistance)	Heart Rate Effect		
			Reflex	Direct	Reflex and Direct
norepinephrine	α, β_1	↑	↓*	↑	↓ or ↑
phenylephrine	α_1	↑	↓*	0	↓
isoproterenol	β_1, β_2	↓	↑	↑	↑↑
dobutamine	β_1	0	0	↑	↑

*Blocked by atropine.

for the β_2-receptors and have less action on the β_1-cardiac receptors.

Metaproterenol, terbutaline, albuterol, bitolterol, and *ritodrine* are relatively specific agonists at β_2-adrenergic receptors. Because these drugs have little effect on β_1-receptors, they have less tendency to stimulate the heart. Nevertheless, selectivity for β_2-receptors is not absolute, and at higher doses these drugs stimulate the heart directly. These drugs also differ from isoproterenol in that they are effective orally and have a longer duration of action. The selective β_2-receptor agonists also relax vascular smooth muscle in skeletal muscle and relax smooth muscle in bronchi and uterus. Because of their relative selectivity for β_2-receptors, these drugs provide a therapeutic advantage over isoproterenol in that they are less likely to stimulate the heart. Although the pharmacological properties of all the β_2-agonists are similar, ritodrine is marketed as a tocolytic agent; that is, it relaxes uterine smooth muscle and thereby arrests premature labor. Ritodrine can be administered intravenously in emergency situations and orally for maintenance therapy, though there are recent reports that question the drug's utility for delaying labor. All other drugs are marketed as bronchodilators for the treatment of bronchospasm and bronchial asthma (Chapter 58). They can be administered by inhalation, parenterally, or orally. When used orally, the selective β_2-agonists have an advantage over ephedrine (see later discussion) because they do not penetrate the blood-brain barrier and thus lack central nervous system stimulant properties.

Dopamine and dobutamine are relatively specific for β_1-receptors and are used to stimulate the heart. *Dopamine* is an endogenous catecholamine with important actions as a neurotransmitter in the brain (see Chapter 23). In peripheral sympathetic neurons and in the adrenal medulla, dopamine serves as a precursor for the synthesis of norepinephrine and epinephrine; the endogenous amine, however, does not have noticeable sympathomimetic actions. The circulating concentrations of dopamine are low, and the compound has a very short half-life. When administered by IV infusion, the drug has a characteristic action on cardiac muscle and vascular smooth muscle in the kidney and gut. It produces a positive inotropic action on the heart directly by stimulating β_1-receptors and indirectly by releasing norepinephrine. Dopamine relaxes smooth muscle in some vascular beds, specifically in the kidney and mesenteric arteries, by activating dopamine receptors on smooth muscle cells (this effect is blocked by dopamine receptor antagonists such as haloperidol [Chapter 23], and not by β-adrenergic receptor antagonists such as propranolol). Because it can dilate the renal vascular bed, dopamine increases glomerular filtration rate, sodium excretion, and urinary output. Dopamine is administered by IV infusion for treatment of shock as a result of myocardial infarction, trauma, or renal failure. High doses of dopamine have α-agonist effects. For example, local ischemia results if during IV infusion dopamine leaks into the region surrounding the vein. If such an accident occurs, the ischemia can be treated by infiltration of the region with an α-receptor antagonist such as phentolamine.

Dobutamine is a relatively specific β_1-receptor agonist that, like dopamine, increases myocardial contractility without greatly altering total peripheral resistance. It has less effect on heart rate than isoproterenol does because it does not produce reflex tachycardia. Like dopamine, dobutamine is administered by IV infusion to treat acute cardiac failure. Dobutamine differs from dopamine in that it does not increase blood flow in the renal vascular bed.

Table 10-2 contains a comparison of the direct and reflex actions of selected sympathomimetics on heart rate.

Indirect-acting Sympathomimetics

Some drugs that do not interact directly with adrenergic receptors have sympathomimetic actions as a result of their ability to cause the release of norepinephrine from sympathetic neurons or block neuronal reuptake of released norepinephrine. Some of these drugs (e.g., amphetamine, ephedrine, cocaine) have noticeable stimulant actions in the brain; these central stimu-

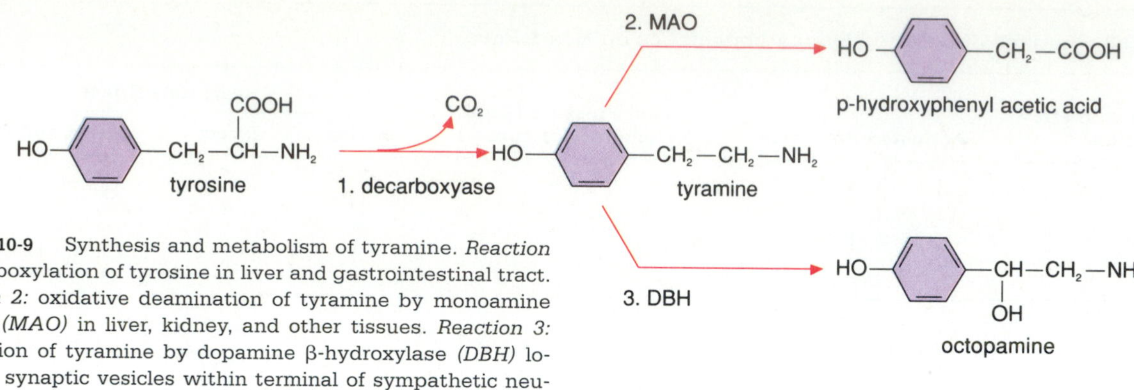

FIGURE 10-9 Synthesis and metabolism of tyramine. *Reaction 1:* decarboxylation of tyrosine in liver and gastrointestinal tract. *Reaction 2:* oxidative deamination of tyramine by monoamine oxidase *(MAO)* in liver, kidney, and other tissues. *Reaction 3:* β-oxidation of tyramine by dopamine β-hydroxylase *(DBH)* located in synaptic vesicles within terminal of sympathetic neurons.

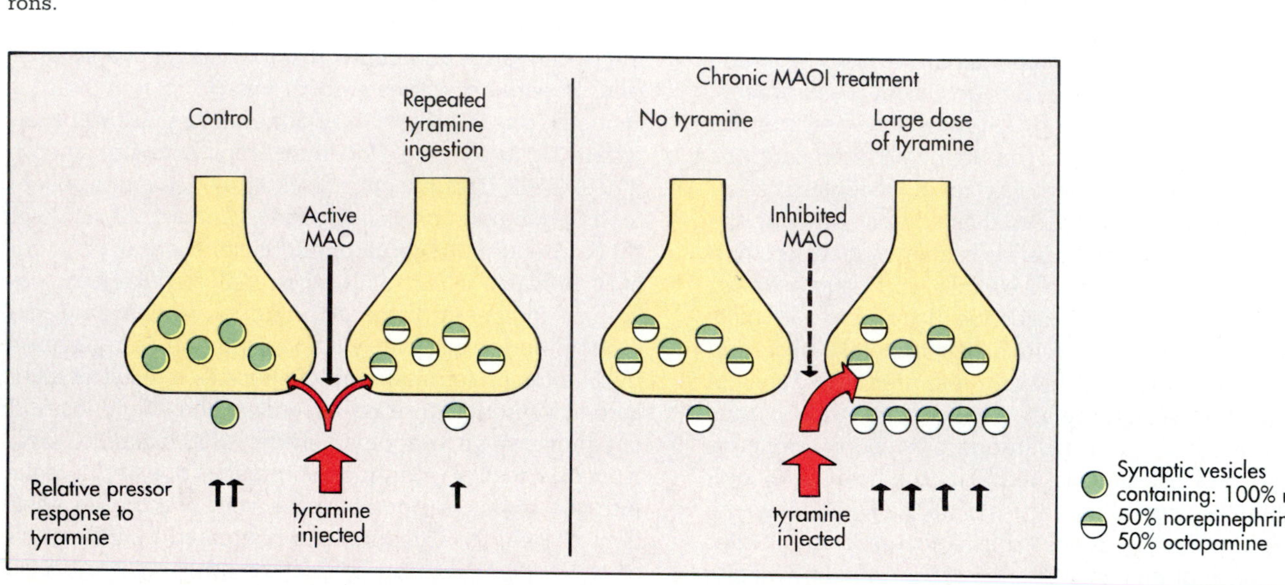

FIGURE 10-10 Schema of **A,** acute response to an ingestion of tyramine; **B,** tolerance to repeated ingestions of tyramine; **C,** chronic treatment with a monoamine oxidase inhibitor *(MAOI);* **D,** effects of tyramine after chronic MAOI pretreatment. The relative increase in blood pressure is denoted by the number of arrows.

lant actions are discussed in Chapter 32. The following sections focus on the sympathomimetic properties of these drugs.

Tyramine is not employed therapeutically, but it has pharmacological and toxicological importance because (1) it is widely used as an experimental tool to study mechanisms of norepinephrine release, (2) it is present in a variety of foods (e.g., ripened cheese, fermented sausage, wines), and (3) it is formed in the liver and GI tract as a result of the decarboxylation of tyrosine (see Figure 10-9).

Tyramine does not have an intrinsic action on adrenergic receptors (e.g., it does not affect denervated organs) but enters the norepinephrine nerve terminal by way of the amine transporter and causes release of norepinephrine (see Figure 10-5). The release of norepinephrine causes the sympathomimetic actions of tyramine. Tachyphylaxis, a form of rapid tolerance that manifests by repeated administration of the drug, develops to the sympathomimetic actions of injected tyramine. After tyramine enters the noradrenergic neuron, it is transported into the synaptic vesicle, where it is converted to octopamine by dopamine β-hydroxylase (Reaction 3, Figure 10-9). Octopamine then displaces norepinephrine, fills the synaptic vesicles, and is subsequently released as a "false transmitter." With repeated injections, tachyphylaxis develops as tyramine releases progressively more octopamine, which does not activate α- or β-adrenergic receptors, and less norepinephrine (compare *A* and *B* in Figure 10-10).

Even though tyramine is continually synthesized from dietary tyrosine, significant quantities of the amine are not found in blood or tissues because it is rapidly metabolized by MAO (reaction 2, Figure 10-9). In pa-

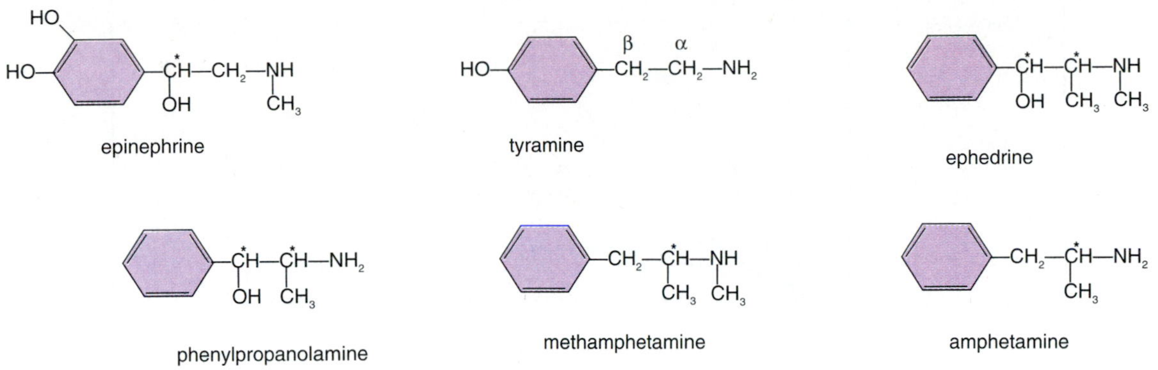

FIGURE 10-11 Comparison of structures of indirect-acting sympathomimetics with that of epinephrine. Asterisk indicates asymmetric carbon.

tients treated chronically with an MAO inhibitor, the circulating concentration of tyramine increases and is taken up by sympathetic nerve terminals (Figure 10-10, *C*). Here tyramine is converted to octopamine, which partially displaces norepinephrine. As a consequence, less norepinephrine is released when the sympathetic nervous system is activated; this leads to a reduction in blood pressure (Figure 10-10, *C*). Patients receiving repeated doses of MAO inhibitors experience orthostatic hypotension.

A more serious adverse effect that accompanies therapy with MAO inhibitors occurs if a patient consumes food containing tyramine. Normally there is no pharmacological response to tyramine-containing foods because the amine is rapidly destroyed by MAO. When this enzyme is inhibited, however, the consumed tyramine exerts a strong pharmacological action by releasing amine stores from terminals of sympathetic neurons (Figure 10-10, *D*). Enough norepinephrine is released to produce a severe hypertensive response. Patients treated with MAO inhibitors are cautioned to avoid foods containing tyramine, but if such foods are accidentally consumed, the hypertensive crisis can be treated by administration of an α-adrenergic receptor antagonist such as phentolamine.

Amphetamine and ephedrine are related chemically to epinephrine (Fig. 10-11) but exert their sympathomimetic effects primarily by facilitating the release or blocking the neuronal reuptake of norepinephrine. The chemical structure of *ephedrine* differs from epinephrine in two important respects: it lacks ring hydroxyl groups and has a methyl substitution on the α carbon. As a consequence, ephedrine is not a substrate for either COMT or MAO and thus has a longer duration of action than exogenously administered epinephrine. The lack of ring hydroxyl groups also makes ephedrine less polar and more lipid soluble than epinephrine, and so it readily traverses cell membranes and the blood-brain barrier. Consequently, in contrast to epinephrine, ephedrine is effective orally and has a stimulant action in the brain. Ephedrine has two asymmetric carbons, and thus there are four isomers of the compound: *d*- and *l*-ephedrine and *d*- and *l*-pseudoephedrine. *l*-Ephedrine is the most potent sympathomimetic isomer, but the racemic mixture of ephedrine is also available for clinical use, as is *d*-pseudoephedrine.

Ephedrine exerts sympathomimetic effects by acting directly on β_2-receptors and by releasing norepinephrine, which activates α-and β_1-receptors. Ephedrine has been used therapeutically to treat mild cases of asthma, but because of its central stimulant actions, it is no longer recommended for chronic treatment and has been largely replaced by newer, more selective β_2-agonists (Chapter 58).

Pseudoephedrine has little β_2-agonist activity and consequently is not effective in treating asthma. It has less central stimulant actions than ephedrine has and is therefore widely used in over-the-counter nasal decongestant oral preparations.

Phenylpropanolamine is administered topically and orally to relieve nasal congestion. It is widely available

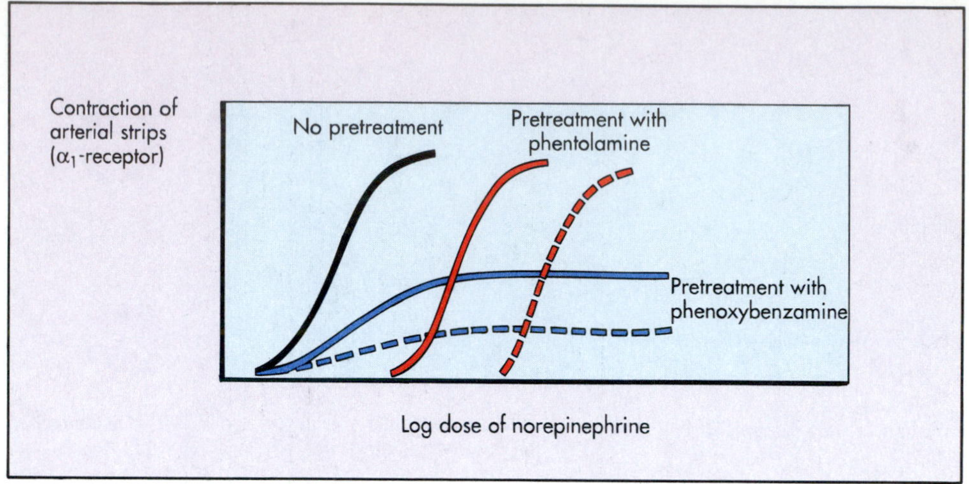

FIGURE 10-12 Comparison of effects of a reversible (phentolamine) and an irreversible (phenoxybenzamine) inhibitor of α-adrenergic receptors. Changes in the force of contraction of arterial strips were recorded after addition of increasing concentrations of norepinephrine in the absence and in the presence of low and high concentrations of phentolamine and low and high concentrations of phenoxybenzamine. The broken lines are larger doses of the antagonist.

as a component of over-the-counter drug preparations for relief of upper respiratory conditions that accompany the common cold and is often combined with analgesics, anticholinergics, antihistaminics, and caffeine. Phenylpropanolamine has fewer central stimulant actions than ephedrine, but it has been widely used with limited success as an anorectic in the treatment of obesity.

Methamphetamine and *amphetamine* exist as *d*- and *l*-optical isomers. Acting on peripheral sympathetic neurons, *d*- and *l*-amphetamine are equipotent, but in the CNS the *d*-isomer is three to four times more potent than the *l*-isomer. Amphetamine is used therapeutically only for its central stimulant action (see Chapter 32), and to minimize peripheral sympathomimetic actions only the *d*-isomer is employed. Unlike ephedrine, amphetamine does not directly activate β_2-receptors but exerts its sympathomimetic actions by facilitating release and blocking reuptake of norepinephrine. Amphetamine has relatively more central stimulant and less peripheral sympathomimetic effects than ephedrine has. The central stimulant actions of amphetamine appear to result from its ability to release and block reuptake of released dopamine in limbic regions of the brain.

Cocaine has central stimulant and peripheral sympathomimetic actions similar to those of amphetamine. It blocks the neuronal uptake of norepinephrine; unlike amphetamine it does not facilitate amine release.

Drugs that Block α-Adrenergic Receptors

Compounds that bind covalently to the α-receptor, such as phenoxybenzamine, produce an irreversible blockade; compounds such as phentolamine bind reversibly and produce a competitive blockade. The characteristics of the effects of reversible and irreversible α-adrenergic blocking drugs are schematically depicted in Figure 10-12. Blockade produced by the reversible antagonist phentolamine is surmountable; as more agonist (i.e., norepinephrine) is administered, it becomes a more effective competitor with phentolamine for the α-receptor. If more phentolamine is administered, the dose-response curve shifts in a parallel manner to the right. Blockade produced by the irreversible blocker phenoxybenzamine cannot be overcome by the addition of more norepinephrine. After administration of phenoxybenzamine, the response to norepinephrine depends on the number of receptors not covalently bound to phenoxybenzamine. If more phenoxybenzamine is administered, the dose-response curve for norepinephrine becomes more shallow.

Phenoxybenzamine and *phentolamine* block both α_1- and α_2-receptors; they differ primarily in their potency and duration of action. These drugs are very effective in blocking the actions of α-adrenergic agonists and the actions of the sympathetic nervous system on smooth muscle. By blocking sympathetic tone to blood vessels they cause vasodilatation, the effect being proportional to the degree of sympathetic tone. α-Receptor blocking drugs cause only a small decrease in recumbent blood pressure but produce a sharp decrease during compensatory vasoconstriction that occurs on standing because reflex sympathetic control of capacitance vessels (veins) is blocked. This results in **orthostatic** or **postural hypotension** accompanied by reflex tachycardia.

The effects of α-adrenergic receptor blockade on

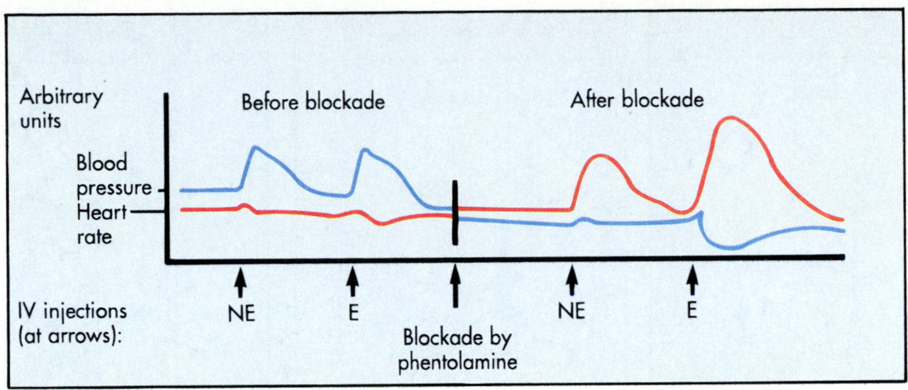

FIGURE 10-13 Schema of effects of the IV injections of norepinephrine *(NE)* and epinephrine *(E)* on mean blood pressure and heart rate before and after blockade of α-adrenergic receptors by phentolamine (see Figure 10-7).

mean blood pressure and heart rate to IV norepinephrine and epinephrine are illustrated in Figure 10-13. The IV injection of large doses of norepinephrine and epinephrine increase peripheral resistance and produce a brief increase in mean blood pressure by activating α-adrenergic receptors on vascular smooth muscle. In response to increased blood pressure, a reflex decrease in sympathetic tone and an increase in vagal tone to the heart occur; these are mediated by the baroreceptor reflex (see Figure 10-6). Although this should result in a slower heart rate, the reflex bradycardia is masked by the cardiac stimulatory actions of norepinephrine and epinephrine mediated by direct activation of β_1-receptors. Because of these opposing actions, it is difficult to predict the effects of these two catecholamines on heart rate (see Table 10-2). After the administration of phentolamine, the α-receptors are blocked, thereby reducing sympathetic tone on blood vessels and slightly lowering blood pressure. This is accompanied by a reflex increase in heart rate. With α-receptors now blocked, the administration of norepinephrine has little effect on blood pressure, whereas heart rate is increased because of the direct action of the drug on cardiac β_1-receptors. Because blood pressure does not greatly increase, no opposing reflex bradycardia occurs. When epinephrine is administered, the former pressor response is converted to a strong depressor response (epinephrine "reversal"). This results because, with α-receptors blocked, the activation of β_2-receptors by epinephrine is unmasked. Epinephrine now causes a pronounced tachycardia as a result of both the direct activation of cardiac β_1-receptors and the reflex tachycardia in response to the decrease in blood pressure. Thus, when α-adrenoceptors are blocked, epinephrine (an agonist at α- and β-receptors) resembles isoproterenol (an agonist at β-receptors).

Phenoxybenzamine and phentolamine block both α_1- and α_2-adrenergic receptors. The tachycardia that occurs after administration of these drugs is attributable in part to the blockade of α_2-receptors located on terminals of sympathetic noradrenergic neurons (Figure 10-14). Activation of these receptors inhibits release of norepinephrine (see Figure 10-14, *A*); this feedback inhibition is disrupted when α_2-receptors are blocked so that release of norepinephrine is increased. This has little consequence when postsynaptic receptors are α_1 because the α-receptor antagonists mentioned above block these receptors. In the heart, however, where the postsynaptic adrenergic receptors are β_1, the effects of sympathetic nerve activation are enhanced when the α_2-receptors are blocked. Thus, by blocking α_2-receptors, phenoxybenzamine and phentolamine increase norepinephrine release and thereby enhance reflex tachycardia (see Figure 10-14 *B*).

Prazosin is a relatively specific α_1-adrenoceptor antagonist. It causes less tachycardia than the nonselective α-receptor antagonists because the α_2-adrenoceptors, which when activated reduce norepinephrine release, are not blocked by this drug (see Figure 10-14 *C*).

The major side effects of α-adrenergic receptor antagonists are related to a reduced sympathetic tone at α-receptors. These effects include orthostatic hypotension, tachycardia (not pronounced with prazosin), inhibition of ejaculation, and nasal stuffiness. Some adverse effects of these drugs are not related to their α-blocking properties; for example, phenoxybenzamine acts centrally to cause nausea, vomiting, sedation, and weakness, whereas phentolamine stimulates the gastrointestinal tract, causing abdominal pain and diarrhea.

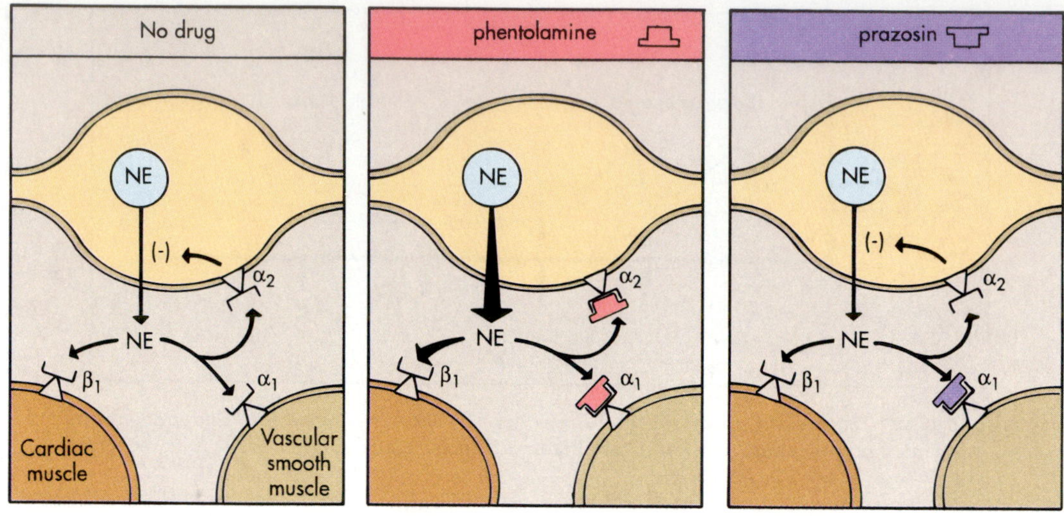

FIGURE 10-14 Comparison of actions of phentolamine (α_1- and α_2-antagonist) and prazosin (α_1-antagonist) at noradrenergic neuroeffector junctions in cardiac muscle (β_1-adrenergic receptors) and vascular smooth muscle (α_1-adrenergic receptors). (⎍ , antagonist).

Drugs That Block β-Adrenergic Receptors

The prototype of nonselective β-adrenergic blocking drugs is *propranolol.* Compounds introduced more recently differ from propranolol in duration of action and receptor subtype selectivity. Propranolol is a potent reversible antagonist at both β_1- and β_2-adrenergic receptors. As with all adrenergic receptor blocking drugs, the pharmacological effects depend on the activity of the sympathoadrenal system. When impulse traffic in the sympathetic neurons and circulating concentrations of norepinephrine and epinephrine are high (e.g., during exercise), the effects of the drugs are more pronounced, with the most profound effects of propranolol on the cardiovascular system. Propranolol blocks the positive chronotropic and inotropic effects resulting from administration of β-adrenergic agonists and from activation of the sympathetic nervous system. It reduces the rate and contractility of the heart at rest, but the effects are more dramatic during physical exercise. The drug may precipitate acute failure in an uncompensated heart. Propranolol, but not other β-blockers, has a direct membrane-stabilizing action (local anesthetic action) independent of its β-receptor blocking properties, which may contribute to its cardiac antiarrhythmic effect.

The acute administration of propranolol does not greatly affect blood flow because vascular smooth muscle is not tonically activated by circulating concentrations of epinephrine. As a result of compensatory reflexes, the drug does cause slightly increased peripheral resistance. Propranolol administered chronically is an effective antihypertensive agent. How it lowers blood pressure is not completely clear, but this effect probably results from several actions, including reduced cardiac output and reduced release of renin from the juxtaglomerular apparatus.

Propranolol blocks the metabolic actions of β-adrenergic drugs and the sympathoadrenal system. It inhibits the increase in plasma free fatty acids and glucose resulting from lipolysis in fat and glycogenolysis in liver, heart, and skeletal muscle, which can present a problem to patients with diabetes. Insulin-induced hypoglycemia is augmented by propranolol because the drug disrupts the compensatory glycogenolysis and glucose release resulting from increased sympathoadrenal activity. The β_1-selective blockers are less likely to delay recovery from hypoglycemia and to cause hypertension when the hypoglycemia releases epinephrine. β-Adrenergic receptor blocking drugs also reduce the premonitory tachycardia associated with insulin-induced hypoglycemia, and so patients must learn to recognize sweating (induced by activation of cholinergic sympathetic neurons) as a symptom of low blood glucose concentrations.

Propranolol has few serious side actions in healthy individuals but can produce adverse effects in patients suffering from various disease states; heart failure may develop. Propranolol is usually contraindicated in patients with sinus bradycardia, partial heart block, and compensated congestive heart failure. Sudden withdrawal of propranolol from long-term patients can cause "withdrawal symptoms" such as angina, tachycardia, and dysrhythmias. Rebound hypertension may occur in patients taking propranolol to control blood pressure when the drug is discontinued. These withdrawal symptoms probably result from the development of supersensitive β-receptors (disuse supersensitivity) and can be minimized by reducing dosage of the drug gradually.

The ability of propranolol to increase airway resistance is of little clinical importance in normal individuals but can be hazardous in patients with obstructive pulmonary disease or asthma, who may experience life-threatening increases in airway resistance. The newer cardioselective (β_1) receptor antagonists should be used in these patients, but even these drugs should be used with caution because they are not completely devoid of β_2-receptor blocking properties.

Nadolol is a nonselective β-receptor blocking drug that is less lipid soluble than propranolol and less likely to cause central effects. It has a significantly longer duration of action than most other β-blockers. *Timolol* is another nonselective β-adrenergic blocker administered orally for treatment of hypertension and angina pectoris or as an ophthalmic preparation for treatment of glaucoma.

Carteolol, pindolol, and *penbutolol* are nonselective β-adrenergic receptor blocking drugs that have partial agonist properties. As a result of their modest intrinsic sympathomimetic properties, these drugs cause less slowing of resting heart rate and fewer abnormalities of serum lipids than other blockers. Pindolol is relatively short acting; the other two drugs have longer durations of action. These drugs are used to treat hypertension.

Labetalol is a reversible antagonist of α_1-, β_1-, and β_2-adrenergic receptors. Consequently, it has hemodynamic effects similar to a combination of propranolol (β_1- and β_2-receptor blockade) and prazosin (α_1-receptor blockade). Unfortunately, it also has similar side effects to both drugs (e.g., orthostatic hypotension, nasal congestion, bronchospasm). It is a potent hypotensive agent and is used in the treatment of hypertension.

Nonselective β-adrenergic receptor antagonists, by blocking β_2-receptors, can precipitate bronchospasm in patients with obstructive pulmonary disease. At low doses, *acebutolol, atenolol, metoprolol,* and *esmolol* are more selective in blocking β_1-receptors on cardiac muscle than in blocking β_2-receptors on bronchiolar and vascular smooth muscle and are less likely to increase bronchoconstriction in patients with asthma than the nonselective β-blockers are. Presumably because they block cardiac stimulation and renin release induced by sympathoadrenal activation, these β_1-blockers are useful in treatment of hypertension and angina pectoris. Esmolol is a β_1-antagonist that is rapidly metabolized by esterases in red blood cells and has a very short half-life. It is used for emergency treatment of sinus tachycardia and atrial flutter or fibrillation.

Drugs That Interfere with Sympathetic Neuronal Function

Drugs that disrupt synthesis, storage, or release of norepinephrine or act in the brain to reduce sympathetic neuronal activity have been used primarily in the treatment of hypertension.

Guanethidine is the prototype of a class of drugs that impair the release of norepinephrine from postsynaptic sympathetic neurons. Guanethidine and related drugs (bretylium, guanadrel) are polar compounds that do not readily penetrate the blood-brain barrier but rather are selectively taken up by the norepinephrine transporter in terminals of sympathetic neurons and stored within synaptic vesicles. Guanethidine depletes norepinephrine stores within these neurons and the drug can be subsequently released as a "false transmitter." The pharmacological properties of guanethidine, however, relate to its ability to prevent the release of norepinephrine in response to nerve action potentials and indirect-acting sympathomimetics (e.g., tyramine, amphetamine).

The pharmacological consequences of the action of guanethidine are less specific than the receptor antagonists previously discussed because the drug depresses the response of α- and β_1-adrenergic receptors approximately equally. Chronic oral administration of guanethidine reduces sympathetic tone to all organs. In the cardiovascular system, guanethidine reduces blood pressure, heart rate, and cardiac output. In the gastrointestinal tract, it increases motility and causes diarrhea. Because of its side effects, guanethidine is reserved for the treatment of moderate to severe hypertension. Because the drug is highly ionized, it is poorly and irregularly absorbed from the GI tract and does not significantly traverse the blood-brain barrier. After it accumulates in sympathetic noradrenergic neurons, its effects persist, generally causing cumulative responses that last for several days after termination of the drug. The troublesome side effects of the drug are caused by disruption of sympathetic tone to various organs; these include orthostatic hypotension, nasal stuffiness, impaired ejaculation, and diarrhea (the parasympathetic neuronal influence on GI smooth muscle is unopposed by the sympathetic nervous system).

Guanadrel mimics the action of guanethidine, differing only in its pharmacokinetic profile. When compared with guanethidine, guanadrel has a more rapid onset and a shorter duration of action. *Bretylium* acts similarly

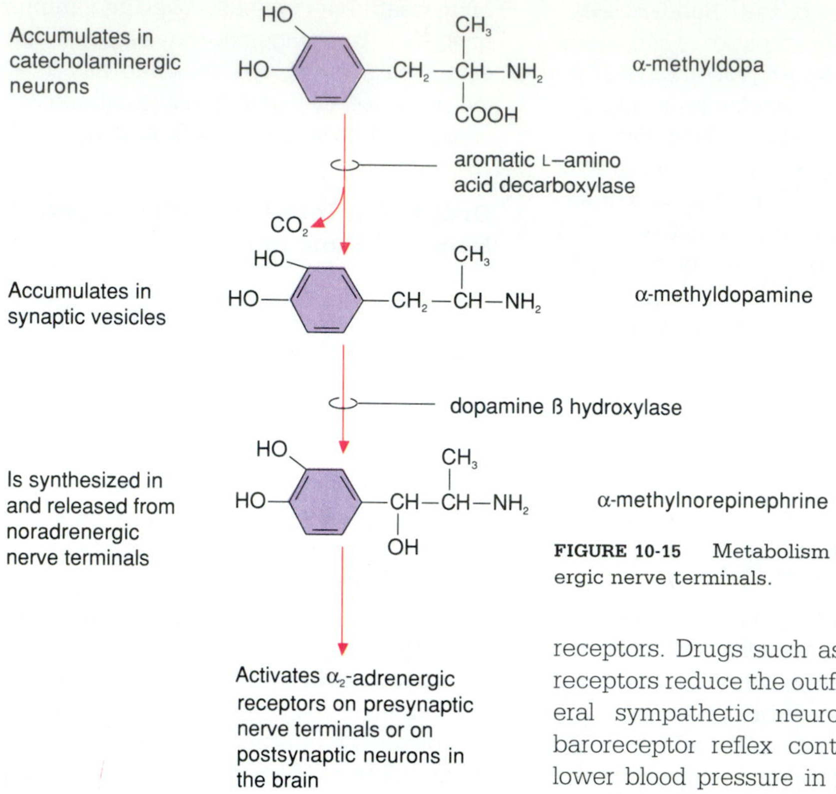

Accumulates in catecholaminergic neurons

α-methyldopa

aromatic L–amino acid decarboxylase

CO_2

Accumulates in synaptic vesicles

α-methyldopamine

dopamine ß hydroxylase

Is synthesized in and released from noradrenergic nerve terminals

α-methylnorepinephrine

Activates α_2-adrenergic receptors on presynaptic nerve terminals or on postsynaptic neurons in the brain

FIGURE 10-15 Metabolism of methyldopa in central noradrenergic nerve terminals.

to guanethidine in that it accumulates in noradrenergic sympathetic neurons and prevents neurogenic release of norepinephrine; it is administered only by IV injection for emergency treatment of ventricular dysrhythmias.

Reserpine depletes neurons of norepinephrine and thereby reduces sympathetic nervous system tone. It disrupts the ability of synaptic vesicles to bind norepinephrine, and so the amine leaks from these vesicles and is oxidatively deaminated by MAO within the sympathetic neuron. Loss of sympathetic tone after reserpine administration results in reduced peripheral resistance, cardiac output, and blood pressure. Only low doses of reserpine are used to treat hypertension, usually with other agents (e.g., thiazide diuretics), and it takes several weeks for the antihypertensive effects to become maximal. Because of its long duration of action, reserpine maintains good control of blood pressure in patients with mild hypertension who have poor drug compliance. Reserpine is no longer widely used.

Drugs That Reduce Central Sympathetic Outflow

The activity of peripheral sympathetic neurons is regulated in a complex manner by neuronal systems located in the hypothalamus and medulla. These central neurons, in turn, are regulated in part by α_2-adrenergic receptors. Drugs such as clonidine that activate these receptors reduce the outflow of impulse traffic in peripheral sympathetic neurons without interfering with baroreceptor reflex control. Accordingly, these drugs lower blood pressure in patients with moderate to severe hypertension and produce less orthostatic hypotension than drugs that act directly on peripheral sympathetic neurons.

Methyldopa is an analog of the catecholamine precursor L-dopa that has hypotensive actions arising from its conversion to a false transmitter, α-methylnorepinephrine. Methyldopa is transported into noradrenergic neurons, where it is converted to α-methyldopamine and then to α-methylnorepinephrine (Figure 10-15). The α-methylnorepinephrine partially displaces norepinephrine in synaptic vesicles, and so, when these neurons are activated, α-methylnorepinephrine is released in place of the normal transmitter. The hypotensive property of methyldopa appears to be attributable to actions of its metabolite α-methylnorepinephrine in the brain, *not in the periphery*. It is believed therefore that α-methylnorepinephrine formed from methyldopa in central noradrenergic neurons is released as a false transmitter to act on presynaptic or postsynaptic α_2-receptors.

Clonidine, like α-methylnorepinephrine, is a potent agonist at α_2-adrenergic receptors. Unlike α-methylnorepinephrine, which must be delivered to the brain as a precursor, clonidine is lipid soluble and penetrates the blood-brain barrier to activate α_2-adrenergic receptors in the hypothalamus and medulla, resulting in diminished sympathetic outflow. Clonidine lowers blood pressure by reducing total peripheral resistance, heart rate, and cardiac output. Like methyldopa, clonidine does not interfere with baroreceptor reflexes and therefore does not produce noticeable orthostatic hypotension. Side effects of clonidine may include dry mouth, sedation, dizziness, nightmares, anxiety, and mental depression. Various symptoms related to sympathetic nervous system overactivity (hypertension, tachycardia, sweating) may occur on withdrawal of long-term clonidine therapy. As a precaution, the dosage of clonidine should be reduced gradually.

Guanabenz and *guanfacine* are recently developed α_2-adrenergic receptor agonists. Like clonidine, they cause central inhibition of sympathetic tone with a relative sparing of cardiovascular reflexes. Guanfacine is longer acting and is less likely to reduce cardiac output and is less sedating than clonidine.

Drugs That Inhibit Catecholamine Synthesis

Metyrosine (α-methyltyrosine) inhibits tyrosine hydroxylase in catecholaminergic neurons in the brain, periphery, and in the adrenal medulla, thereby reducing tissue stores of dopamine, norepinephrine, and epinephrine. Metyrosine is used in the management of patients with pheochromocytoma not amenable to surgery. The most prevalent side effect of metyrosine is sedation.

Carbidopa, a hydrazine derivative of methyldopa, acts like methyldopa to inhibit aromatic L-amino acid decarboxylase. Unlike methyldopa, carbidopa does not penetrate the blood-brain barrier and therefore has no effect in the central nervous system. Because aromatic L-amino acid decarboxylase is ubiquitous, is present in excess, and does not control the rate-limiting step in catecholamine synthesis, clinical doses of carbidopa have no appreciable effect on endogenous synthesis of norepinephrine in sympathetic neurons. They do, however, reduce the conversion of exogenously administered L-dopa to dopamine outside of the brain. Relatively large doses of L-dopa are employed to replace dopamine in the caudate/putamen of patients with Parkinson's disease and thereby reduce some of the motor symp-

TRADE NAMES

In addition to generic and fixed-combination preparations, the following trade-named materials are available in the United States.

SYMPATHOMIMETICS

Nonselective Directly Acting Agonists
- Adrenalin, epinephrine chloride
- Intropin and Dopastat, dopamine HCl
- Isuprel, isoproterenol HCl
- Levophed, norepinephrine bitartrate
- Medihaler, Vaponefrin; epinephrine

α-Agonists
- Neosynephrine, phenylephrine HCl
- Vasoxyl, methoxamine HCl

β_1-Agonists
- Dobutrex, dobutamine HCl

β_2-Agonists
- Brethine, Bricanyl; terbutaline sulfate
- Bronkosol, isoetharine HCl
- Maxair, pirbuterol acetate
- Metaprel, Alupent; metaproterenol sulfate
- Proventil, Ventolin; albuterol sulfate
- Tornalate, bitolterol mesylate
- Yutopar, ritodrine HCl

Nonselective Indirectly Acting
- Biphetamine, amphetamine exchange resin
- Dexedrine, *d*-amphetamine sulfate
- Propagest, phenylpropanolamine

α -Agonists Not Discussed in Text
- Aramine, metaraminol bitartrate
- Wyamine, mephentermine

SYMPATHOLYTICS

α Blockers, Nonselective
- Dibenzyline, phenoxybenzamine HCl
- Regitine, phentolamine mesylate

α_1-Blockers
- Cardura, doxazosin mesylate
- Hytrin, terazosin HCl
- Minipress, prazosin HCl

β-Blockers, Nonselective
- Blocadren, timolol maleate
- Cartrol, carteolol HCl
- Corgard, nadolol
- Inderal, propranolol HCl
- Levatol, penbutolol sulfate
- Visken, pindolol

β_1-Blockers
- Brevibloc, esmolol HCl
- Kerlone, betaxolol HCl
- Lopressor, metoprolol tartrate
- Sectral, acebutolol HCl
- Tenormin, atenolol

Combined α- and β-Blockers
- Trandate, Normodyne; labetalol HCl

Reduce Central Sympathetic Outflow
- Aldomet, methyldopa
- Catapres, clonidine HCl
- Tenex, guanfacine HCl
- Wytensin, guanabenz acetate

Blockers of Norepinephrine Release
- Bretylol, bretylium sulfate
- Hylorel, guanadrel sulfate
- Ismelin, guanethidine sulfate

CLINICAL PROBLEMS

DRUGS THAT INTERFERE WITH SYMPATHETIC NERVOUS SYSTEM NEURONAL FUNCTION

Block norepinephrine release and storage
- Orthostatic hypotension
- Nasal stuffiness
- Impairment of ejaculation
- GI activity increased
- Extrapyramidal effects (reserpine)

Interfere with central sympathetic outflow
- Sedation
- Endocrine problems
- Mild orthostatic hypotension
- Sodium and water retenion
- Rebound hypertension on drug withdrawal

DRUGS THAT BLOCK ADRENERGIC RECEPTORS

α-Adrenergic receptor blockers
- Orthostatic hypotension
- Tachycardia
- Nasal stuffiness
- Impairment of ejaculation
- Sodium and water retention

β-Adrenergic receptor blockers
- Heart failure in patients with cardiac disease
- Increase in airway resistance
- Fatigue and depression
- Rebound hypertension
- Augmentation of hypoglycemia

toms in these patients. When L-dopa is administered with carbidopa, the dose of dopa and the peripheral side effects caused by the actions of its decarboxylated product, dopamine, are reduced (see Chapter 27).

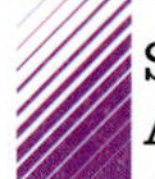

SIDE EFFECTS, CLINICAL PROBLEMS, AND TOXICITY

Major clinical problems are summarized in the box.

NEW DIRECTIONS

For several years after the identification and subsequent clinical use of agonists and antagonists for α- and β-adrenergic receptors, there were relatively few major new developments of drugs that modify functions of the sympathetic nervous system until the combined efforts of pharmacologists and medicinal chemists produced drugs that were selective for interacting with subtypes of the α- and β-adrenergic receptors (e.g., selective agonists included clonidine [α_2], terbutaline [β_2], dobutamine [β_1]; selective antagonists included prazosin [α_1] and atenolol [β_1]). These relatively selective compounds were significant additions to our clinical armamentarium in that the adverse side effects of these newer compounds were reduced when compared with the previously available nonselective α- and β-adrenergic agonists and antagonists. Molecular biological techniques have now characterized several additional adrenergic receptor subtypes ($\alpha_{1A\text{-}C}$; $\alpha_{2A\text{-}D}$; $\beta_{1\text{-}3}$), and it will be a challenge for pharmacologists and medicinal chemists to develop drugs that exert specific agonist or antagonist properties at these newly identified receptors and for the clinical pharmacologists to determine if these compounds have therapeutic potential.

REFERENCES

A symposium: Beta blockade, cardioselectivity and intrinsic sympathomimetic activity, *Am J Cardiol* 59:1F-54F, 1987.

Choice of beta-blocker, Med Lett, 28:20-22, 1987.

Drugs for hypertension, Med Lett; 29:1-6, 1987.

Drugs for ambulatory asthma, Med Lett; 35:11-14, 1993.

Foods interacting with MAO inhibitors, Med Lett; 31:11-12, 1989.

Frishman WH, Furberg CD, Friedewald WT: β-Adrenergic blockade for survivors of acute myocardial infarction, *N Engl J Med* 310:830-837, 1984.

Lasagna L: *Phenylpropanolamine, a review,* New York, 1987, Wiley & Sons.

Summers RJ, McMartin LR: Adrenoceptors and their second messenger systems, *J Neurochem* 60:10-23, 1993.

SELF-ASSESSMENT QUESTIONS

1. Metoprolol would be *most* effective in blocking the ability of epinephrine to:
   a. reduce secretion of insulin from the pancreas.
   b. increase release of renin from juxtaglomerular apparatus.
   c. increase secretion of glucagon from the pancreas.
   d. produce mydriasis (dilatation of pupil).
   e. increase secretion of saliva.
2. Which of the following drugs is *most likely* to produce orthostatic hypotension?
   a. propranolol
   b. dobutamine
   c. labetalol
   d. nadolol
   e. methoxamine
3. Which of the following drugs would be *most likely* to increase airway resistance in a patient with pulmonary obstructive disease?
   a. isoproterenol
   b. atenolol
   c. bitolterol
   d. terbutaline
   e. nadolol
4. Which of the following drugs would *not* be expected to reduce the positive inotropic effects of dopamine on the heart?
   a. propranolol
   b. haloperidol
   c. atenolol
   d. metoprolol
   e. nadolol
5. Which of the following adverse side effects would *not* be experienced by a patient treated with phentolamine?
   a. orthostatic hypotension
   b. impaired ejaculation
   c. nasal stuffiness
   d. bradycardia
   e. sodium and water retention
6. Systemic administration of which of the following drugs would *most likely* cause bradycardia?
   a. dopamine
   b. phentolamine
   c. phenylephrine
   d. prazosin
   e. metaproterenol
7. In a hypertensive patient treated chronically with reserpine, which of the following drugs would be expected to produce the *least* changes in the cardiovascular system?
   a. *d*-amphetamine
   b. phenylephrine
   c. isoproterenol
   d. methoxamine
   e. epinephrine
8. Terbutaline would be expected to cause all of the following effects *except:*
   a. mydriasis.
   b. reduced pulmonary airway resistance.
   c. tachycardia.
   d. hyperglycemia.
   e. increased blood flow in skeletal muscle.
9. The cardiovascular effects of epinephrine in a person treated with phentolamine will most closely resemble the responses after the administration of:
   a. phenylephrine.
   b. terbutaline.
   c. isoproterenol.
   d. norepinephrine.
   e. methoxamine.
10. The pharmacological effects produced by labetalol will resemble most closely those produced by a combination of:
    a. metoprolol and prazosin.
    b. propranolol and phentolamine.
    c. metoprolol and phentolamine.
    d. propranolol and prazosin.
    e. esmolol and phentolamine.
11. After systemic administration, which of the following drugs would *not* act within the central nervous system?
    a. clonidine
    b. α-methylnorepinephrine
    c. ephedrine
    d. methyldopa
    e. reserpine
12. Which of the following actions of ephedrine is blocked by prazosin?
    a. hyperglycemia
    b. relaxation of bronchial smooth muscle
    c. reduced blood flow in the kidney
    d. increased circulating levels of free fatty acids
    e. relaxation of the detrusor muscle in the urinary bladder

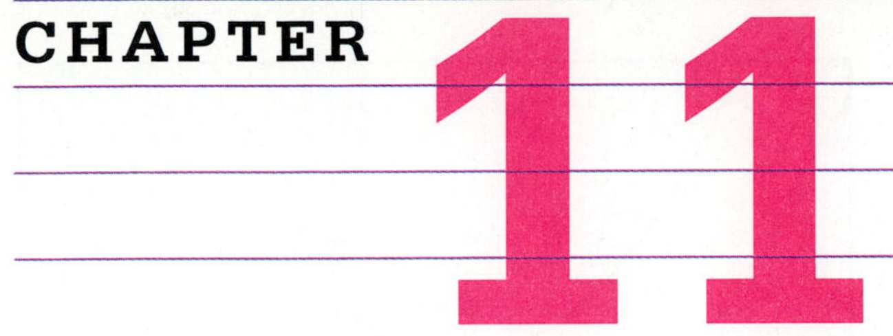

CHAPTER 11 Neuromuscular Blocking Agents

WILLIAM D. ATCHISON

MAJOR DRUGS

Nondepolarizing drugs
Depolarizing agents

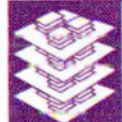

THERAPEUTIC OVERVIEW

Many surgical procedures are performed more safely and rapidly with the aid of drugs that bring about skeletal muscle relaxation. Certain anesthetic agents can produce such relaxation only at high concentrations and therefore are too dangerous to use. Specific skeletal muscle–relaxant drugs are available to reduce the amount of anesthetic agent required during surgery and improve the margin of safety and speed of recovery of the patient from anesthesia.

The muscle-relaxant drugs widely used act by interrupting transmission at the junction between skeletal muscle fibers and the somatic nerves that innervate these fibers. Signal transmission at these junctions occurs by endogenous acetylcholine (ACh) binding to nicotinic cholinergic receptors on the muscle cells. Although the mechanism of these drugs does not involve the autonomic nervous system, some of the side effects do include cholinergic autonomic blockade or stimulation, and so there is a functional, as well as neurotransmitter, commonality between these drugs and drugs acting on the autonomic nervous system.

The neuromuscular blocking agents find widespread use for (1) endotracheal intubation, (2) maintaining controlled ventilation during surgical procedures, (3) reduction of muscle contraction in the region undergoing surgery, and (4) maintaining controlled ventilation over the long term in intensive care units. The neuromuscular blocking agents have the advantage of functioning without producing either analgesia or anesthesia, and for most agents, rapid and effective reversal of the blocking action is accomplished by drugs that increase ACh concentration at the neuromuscular junction. However, the side effects of the blocking agents can be significant, especially at higher concentrations, and so their clinical use is not without problems. In addition, neuromuscular blockers should not be used as alternatives to proper control of consciousness or pain sensation. Newer blocking agents under development are reputed to have fewer side effects.

Additional nonsurgical applications of neuromuscular blocking agents include reduction of laryngeal or general muscle spasms, reduction of spasticity from tetanus in neurological diseases and multiple sclerosis, and prevention of bone fractures during electroconvulsive therapy. These drugs also are used as diagnostic agents for myasthenia gravis and for detecting neurological differences that sometimes develop between spinal and central control of muscle tone.

There are two main classes of neuromuscular blocking agents: competitive antagonists, such as *d*-tubocurarine, atracurium, and vecuronium, and depolarizing agents such as succinylcholine. Therapeutic uses of the neuromuscular blocking agents are summarized in the box.

An additional group of muscle-relaxant drugs that act by different mechanisms and are used primarily for central nervous system (CNS) disorders is discussed in Chapter 27.

ABBREVIATIONS

ACh	Acetylcholine
AChE	Acetylcholinesterase

THERAPEUTIC USE OF NEUROMUSCULAR BLOCKING AGENTS

MUSCLE RELAXATION DURING SURGERY

Inhalational anesthetic agent
- Undesirable side effects (prominent hypotension, cardiac dysrhythmias, myocardial depression, nausea at high concentrations)

Neuromuscular blocking agents
- Allow reduction of anesthetic agent concentration
- Have short (minutes) to long (hours) actions
- Allow endotracheal intubation (surgery)
- Needed for maintaining controlled ventilation (surgery)
- Reduce muscle fasciculations at surgical site
- Side effects must be considered in agent selection
- Action in some cases can be reversed by antagonists
- Patient's age, renal status, and weight must also be considered in the selection of an agent

NONSURGICAL USES
- Intensive care unit use for maintaining controlled respirations
- Reduce muscle spasms
- Myasthenia gravis diagnosis
- Adjunct relaxation during maximal electroshock therapy

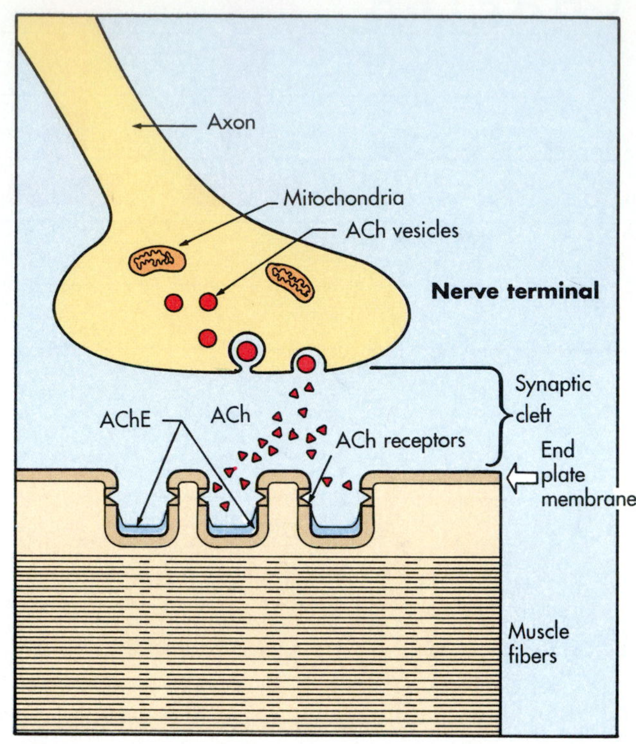

FIGURE 11-1 Acetylcholine *(ACh)* release, diffusion across the synaptic cleft, binding to receptors on end-plate membrane, and hydrolysis by acetylcholinesterase *(AChE)* in the absence of blocking drugs.

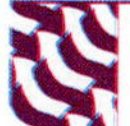

MECHANISMS OF ACTION

Skeletal muscles are innervated by somatic motor nerves that originate in the CNS and terminate at the muscle cell (Chapters 8 and 9). Acetylcholine is the neurotransmitter released from the nerves, and the receptors on the muscle cell endplate are of the nicotinic subtype (different from those at ganglionic sites and in most regions of the brain). At the concentrations of neuromuscular blocking agents used clinically, synaptic transmission is interrupted at the neuromuscular junction. Because cholinergic transmission also occurs at sympathetic and parasympathetic ganglia (Chapters 8 and 9), the ganglionic sites are sources of side effects when concentrations of the neuromuscular blocking agent reach higher values than those needed for neuromuscular blockade. This is discussed in a later section.

In the absence of drug, propagation of an action potential along the somatic nerve fiber results in opening of calcium channels at the nerve terminal. The resulting flux of calcium ions triggers the release of ACh into the synaptic cleft. Diffusion of ACh across the cleft and binding to the nicotinic receptors on the muscle cell end-plate causes the ion channels to open and the end-plate membrane ion permeability to increase. This increase allows a transient flux of Na^+ and K^+ ions, thereby reducing the potential difference across the membrane until a critical value needed to activate muscle contraction is reached. Acetylcholinesterase (AChE) in the vicinity of the muscle end-plate membrane acts quickly to catalyze the hydrolysis and inactivation of unbound ACh. This is described further in Chapters 8 and 9 and is summarized schematically in Figure 11-1. The ACh receptor is described in greater detail in Chapter 2.

Blockade of this process, (1) to inhibit ACh competitively at the receptor site (nondepolarizing) or (2) to maintain end-plate membrane depolarization and thus prevent transmission of another action potential, is the basis by which neuromuscular blocking drugs function. The nondepolarizing and depolarizing agents act by binding to the nicotinic receptor on the muscle cell; however, the detailed mechanisms that cause blockade are different.

The nondepolarizing or competitive blocking agents compete with ACh for unoccupied end-plate receptor sites. The binding of these nondepolarizing agents is reversible, and they occupy the receptor sites without activating the associated cation channel. The structures

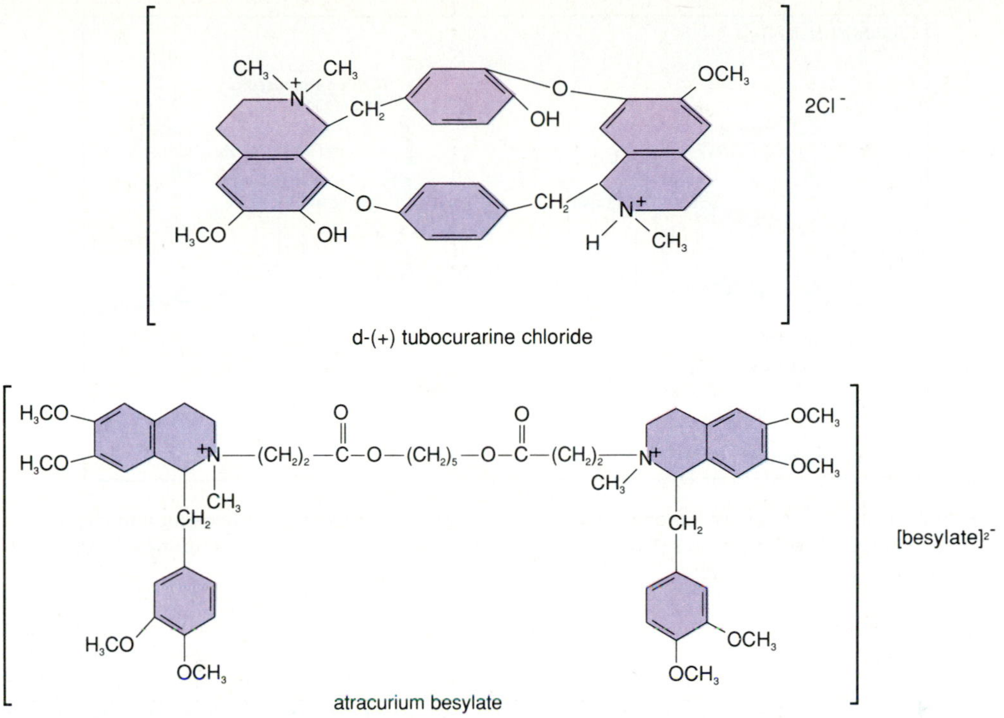

d-(+) tubocurarine chloride

atracurium besylate

FIGURE 11-2 competitive nondepolarizing blocking agents.

of several nondepolarizing blocking drugs are shown in Figure 11-2. Doxacurium, mivacurium, and pipecuronium have been recently approved for clinical use in the United States. Pancuronium, pipecuronium, and vecuronium have similar chemical structures. A second group that includes atracurium, doxacurium, and mivacurium are also structurally related. Gallamine is used only occasionally because of the availability of agents with fewer side effects.

Interference with muscle contraction does not occur until 75% to 80% of the receptors on a muscle cell are occupied by the blocking agent, and complete interruption of contraction requires 90% to 95% occupancy of the receptors. The actual quantities and concentrations of drug required to induce block vary with the agent, the muscle location, and the individual patient. The effects of the blocking agents on the receptor-activated channel are summarized in Figure 11-3.

Additional effects of neuromuscular blocking drugs have been reported. A direct action on the receptor-activated channel may occur at high doses. There also may be a prejunctional effect by which the blocking agent exerts a direct action on the nerve terminal to reduce the amount of ACh released in response to nerve stimulation. This latter mechanism could contribute to reduced muscle contraction through lack of ACh to bind to the receptors, but the mechanism is not well understood. Neither of these actions is likely to contribute substantially to the therapeutic effect.

The blockade caused by the competitive (nondepolarizing) agents can be reversed by increasing the concentration of ACh at the end-plate membrane. The usual method is to inhibit the enzymes that catalyze the hydrolysis of ACh because this endogenous transmitter is still being released and is present in the cleft between the nerve terminal and the muscle end plate. Neostigmine, pyridostigmine, and edrophonium are used clinically to reverse the blockade. Effective chemical reversal, however, requires some degree of spontaneous recovery from neuromuscular block. The chemical structures of these agents are shown in Figure 9-5; the pharmacology of these drugs is discussed in Chapter 9. As with any competitive antagonist, an increase in the concentration of the agonist (in this case, ACh) leads to displacement of the antagonist (the blocking agent) from the receptor. It is also possible, but not demonstrated, that edrophonium and the other enzyme inhibitors may additionally stimulate the prejunctional release of ACh, but this appears to be a secondary effect that is important only with excess edrophonium. When the concentration of the competitive blocking agent in the vicinity of the receptors is greater than the concentration needed for 95% blockade, edrophonium and the other enzyme inhibitors cannot reverse the blockade because the local concentration of ACh is not adequate to overcome the high concentration of the blocking drug.

The mechanism by which depolarizing agents act is different. Among these agents, succinylcholine is the prototype agent in clinical use; decamethonium is still

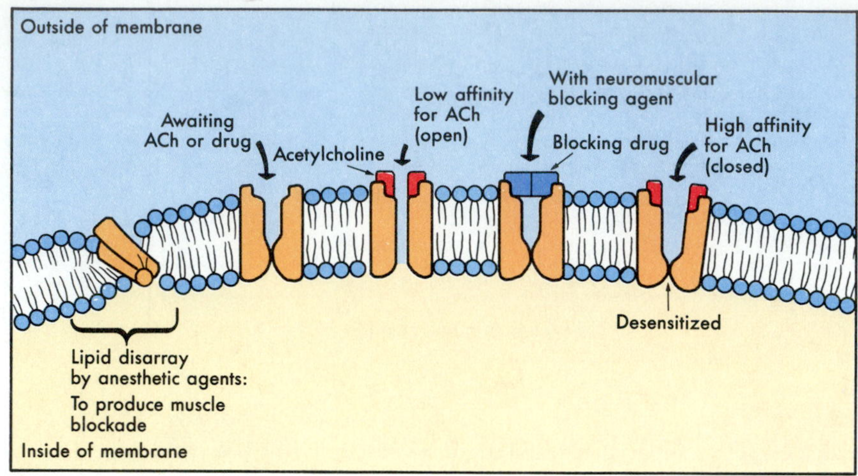

FIGURE 11-3 Summary of ion channel states relevant to neuromuscular blocking agents. *ACh,* Acetylcholine. See Figure 2-11 and Chapter 2 for discussion on low- and high-affinity conformations and desensitized states.

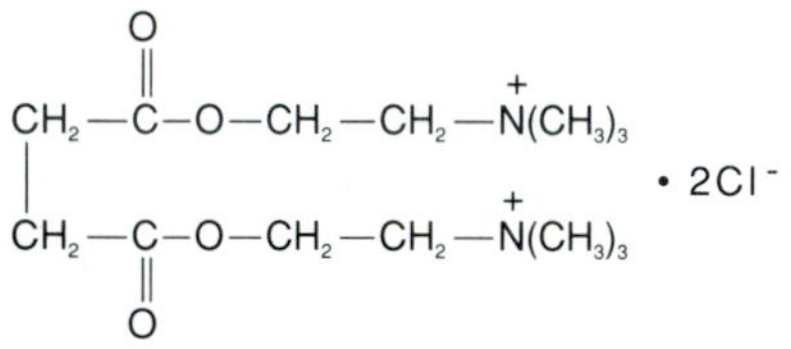

$$\begin{array}{l} CH_2-\overset{\overset{O}{\|}}{C}-O-CH_2-CH_2-\overset{+}{N}(CH_3)_3 \\ | \\ CH_2-\underset{\underset{O}{\|}}{C}-O-CH_2-CH_2-\overset{+}{N}(CH_3)_3 \end{array} \cdot 2Cl^-$$

succinylcholine chloride

FIGURE 11-4 Succinylcholine.

available, but side effects make it much less desirable. Succinylcholine is composed of two molecules of ACh coupled together (Figure 11-4). The binding of succinylcholine to ACh receptors causes opening of ion channels, Na^+ influx, and depolarization of the muscle cell end-plate membrane in the same manner as ACh. However, with succinylcholine, the duration of the depolarization is longer than with ACh because the rate of enzyme-catalyzed hydrolysis (inactivation) is much slower for succinylcholine (0.1 to 2 minutes) than for ACh (turnover time approximately 100 μsec). In fact, ACh and succinylcholine are metabolized by different enzymes. Acetylcholine is hydrolyzed by AChE, and succinylcholine is metabolized primarily by pseudocholinesterase. This enzyme is more widely distributed than AChE but is not present in high concentrations at the neuromuscular junction. The end-plate membrane remains depolarized in the presence of succinylcholine, with the channel presumably remaining open. This occurs at low concentrations of succinylcholine and is termed *phase I block.* Electrical stimulation and muscle-twitch recordings fail to show any drop-off in amplitude (termed *fading*) as the frequency of stimulation is increased. Phase I block can be reversed because the disappearance of the drug is still quite rapid. With repeated dosing of succinylcholine and increased concentration, a more complicated form of blockade, called a *phase II block,* occurs. This type of block behaves similarly to that of nondepolarizing agents but shows fading at higher stimulation frequencies. The details on the state of the ion channels during phase II block (also called *desensitization block*) are controversial; further understanding must await additional research. Cholinesterase inhibitors, such as edrophonium, cannot reverse the effects of succinylcholine or other depolarizing blockers because increasing the synaptic concentration of ACh would only exacerbate the continuing depolarization.

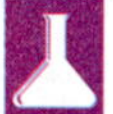

PHARMACOKINETICS

The various neuromuscular blocking drugs differ in pharmacokinetic properties. This is important when choosing an agent for a particular patient. The pharmacokinetic values for the individual drugs are summarized in Table 11-1.

These drugs contain two or three quaternary ammonium nitrogens and are therefore positively charged. As a result, they cross membranes poorly and are generally limited in distribution to the extracellular space. However, the structures of pancuronium, vecuronium, and pipecuronium enable small amounts of these agents to cross membranes. Small amounts of pancuronium cross the placenta, for example, but not in sufficient amounts to cause problems in the fetus when used during a caesarean section.

Use of pancuronium, metocurine, tubocurarine, or

Table 11-1 Pharmacokinetic Parameters

Agent	$t_{1/2}$ (min)	Elimination Route	Protein Binding (%)
succinylcholine	3 (est)	M (100%)	—
mivacurium	2-8	M (100%)	—
atracurium	20	M (100%)	82
vecuronium	54	R (30%)	27
pancuronium	120	M (40%) R (60%)	15
gallamine	134	R (95%)	16
tubocurarine	234	R (60%) B	48*
pipecuronium	~200	n/a	n/a
doxacurium	~200	n/a	n/a
metocurine	280	R (55%) B	55*

M, Metabolism; *R*, renal; *B*, biliary; *n/a*, not available.
*Additional drug binds to cartilage and to connecting tissue; figures are for plasma binding (to albumin, acid glycoproteins, and globulins).

gallamine is influenced by impaired renal function because appreciable fractions of these drugs are cleared by renal filtration. Atracurium is inactivated almost entirely by metabolism, two thirds by enzymatic and one third by spontaneous nonenzymatic breakdown. Vecuronium and pancuronium undergo significant metabolism and the 3-hydroxy metabolite of each has 25% or less neuromuscular blocking activity compared with the parent drugs. Succinylcholine and mivacurium are metabolized by plasma pseudocholinesterase, with minimal hydrolysis by AChE.

The activity of pseudocholinesterase may be abnormal in some patients. This enzyme is synthesized in the liver, and so neuromuscular blockade by succinylcholine may be prolonged in patients with liver dysfunction, decreased hepatic blood flow, or genetic abnormalities. There are two explanations for genetically abnormal pseudocholinesterase activity: lower concentrations of normal enzyme (heterozygous) or an abnormal enzyme (homozygous, 1:2500 frequency; or heterozygous). A clinical dose of 1 to 2 mg/kg succinylcholine in normal patients gives a blockade of <15 minutes. In a deficient patient, the duration may be >2 hours. This is shown over a dosage range in Figure 11-5 with blockade defined as the duration of apnea. Trauma, alcoholism, pregnancy, use of oral contraceptives, and other conditions that can elevate or depress cholinesterase synthesis also can cause prolonged or shortened blockade by these drugs.

The pharmacokinetics for the reversal drugs edrophonium, neostigmine, and pyridostigmine are discussed in Chapter 9. Edrophonium is the most rapid acting of the three.

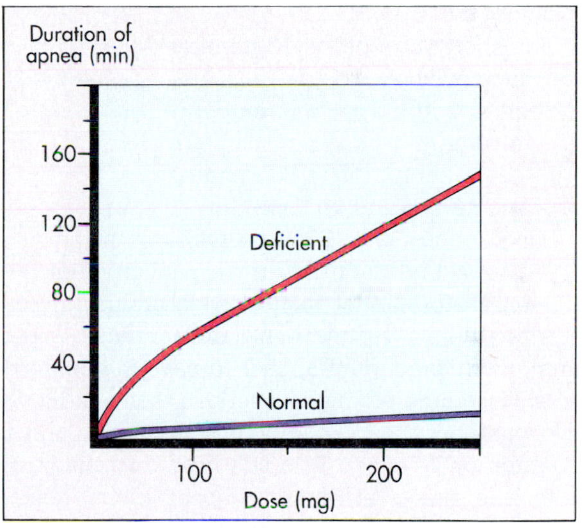

FIGURE 11-5 Length of time patients display apnea after IV dose of succinylcholine. *Normal* and *deficient* refer to the plasma pseudocholinesterase of each patient group.

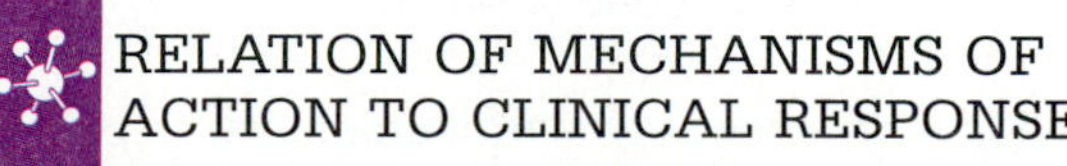

RELATION OF MECHANISMS OF ACTION TO CLINICAL RESPONSE

The choice of neuromuscular blocking agent is based primarily on the duration of the required blockade and the ability to tolerate side effects, though this may become less of a factor as newer blocking agents become available. The duration of blockade required is influenced by the anatomical location of the surgery, the condition of the patient, and the patient's toleration of side effects. The relative potency of the agent is not a principal consideration, despite a 100-fold variation in dose

Table 11-2 Cardiac and Histamine Release Side Effects

Agent	Cardiac Changes		Histamine Release
	Blood Pressure	**Heart Rate**	
succinylcholine	Increased	Increased or decreased	High
mivacurium	Slight transient hypotension	Slight increase	Slight
atracurium	Minimal effect	Minimal effect	Slight
vecuronium	None	None	None
pancuronium	Increased	Increased	Slight
gallamine	Increased	Increased	High dose only
tubocurarine	Decreased	Decreased	High
pipecuronium	None	None	Slight
doxacurium	None	None	Slight
metocurine	Minimal effect	None	Moderate

needed to attain 95% blockade for the clinically used agents.

In terms of duration of action, the following rank order for IV administration of a typical clinically used dose is as follows:

Ultrashort acting (5 to 10 minutes):
succinylcholine
Short acting (10 to 15 minutes):
mivacurium
Medium acting (15 to 30 minutes):
atracurium and vecuronium
Long acting (30 to 120 minutes):
d-tubocurarine, metocurine, pancuronium, pipecuronium, doxacurium, gallamine

Atracurium, vecuronium, mivacurium, pipecuronium, and doxacurium appear to have minimal side effects. Gallamine produces a serious tachycardia. Succinylcholine has the most rapid onset of action and shortest duration of effect. It is still used for intubation despite side effects at higher concentrations. Long-term use of several neuromuscular blockers in the intensive care unit to maintain controlled ventilation has resulted in prolonged periods of paralysis. One of the goals of neuromuscular blocking agent research is the development of a nondepolarizing, ultrashort-acting reversible agent with minimal side effects. Mivacurium may meet this goal.

The major side effects of the neuromuscular blocking drugs are cardiovascular actions and histamine release. The extent to which each agent exhibits these side effects is listed in Table 11-2. Vecuronium is essentially free of cardiac and histamine effects, and the newer drugs mivacurium, pipecuronium, and doxacurium appear to have only minor cardiac effects. Mivacurium has some histamine-like effects. These are discussed in a later section.

Several additional factors such as patient age, weight, and renal function, the presence of anesthetic agents, and the electrolyte content of body fluids can influence the degree of blockade achievable with a given dose. The actions of tubocurarine and atracurium, for example, are potentiated in neonates as compared with children and adults, but succinylcholine is less potent in neonates and requires a dose two to three times greater on a weight basis than that used for children. Pharmacokinetic considerations can explain some of the differences in effectiveness of these drugs between children and elderly adults. The nondepolarizing blocking agents often are potentiated by inhalational anesthetic agents such as halothane, isoflurane, enflurane, or nitrous oxide and also by low concentrations of extracellular potassium or calcium, as may occur after the use of diuretic agents or in renal dysfunction or disease. Elevated potassium or calcium and reduced magnesium concentrations, however, may counter the action of the blocking agents through changes in sensitivity at the muscle end plate.

In most surgical procedures in which neuromuscular blocking agents are used, the drugs enter the systemic circulation and are distributed to all accessible tissues. Spontaneous respiration is usually inhibited, and respiratory support capabilities must be available when these drugs are used. In addition, the fraction of receptors that must be free of blocking agent before recovery occurs varies with different muscles. Typically, muscles recover from blockade in the following order:

1. Respiratory and diaphragm
2. Eyeblink
3. Abdomen, arms, and legs
4. Neck, head, face, hands, and feet
5. Extraocular

It is not practical to attempt selective blockade of one anatomical area for prolonged periods because of the wide distribution of these drugs.

In cases of burns, denervated muscles, spinal cord injury, or other trauma, the sensitivity to neuromuscular

CLINICAL PROBLEMS

OLDER DRUGS

Blood pressure and heart rate changes
Histamine release
Ganglionic effects
Muscarinic effects
Difficulty with controlled reversal (some drugs)
Succinylcholine: hyperkalemia, elevated intraocular or intragastric pressures, muscle pain, induced cardiac dysrhythmias, stimulation of ganglia, block muscarinic receptors, malignant hyperthermia

NEWER DRUGS

Minimal to no cardiac effects
Slight to no histamine release
Easier reversal

blocking drugs may vary. In some burn patients, for example, the doses of atracurium or metocurine may need to be two to three times normal to achieve blockade. The reason for this may be the presence of extra receptors, which are normally not available until trauma brings about their activation, though this is somewhat speculative.

The primary precaution in the use of edrophonium and other enzyme inhibitors for reversal of blockade caused by nondepolarizing neuromuscular blocking drugs is to monitor carefully the dose of the reversal drug. Excessive drug concentrations can lead to excessive ACh and prolongation of channel opening, similar to the action of a depolarizing type of blocker. To avoid this problem, the degree of neuromuscular blockade should be assessed through electrical stimulation and determination of muscle activity, with titration of drug to determine the appropriate end point.

SIDE EFFECTS, CLINICAL PROBLEMS, AND TOXICITY

The strategy in the development of the newer neuromuscular blocking agents is to expand the margin of safety between the concentrations of blocker needed to produce 95% blockade at the neuromuscular junction and those that block transmission at ganglionic nicotinic receptors or at cardiac muscarinic receptors. Parasympathetic and sympathetic ganglia and cardiac parasympathetic neuroeffector junctions are innervated by cholinergic neurons. These junctions are all subject to antagonism by the neuromuscular blocking agents if the concentration of drug is sufficient. Tubocurarine gives a significant degree of ganglionic blockade, with less by metocurine, and essentially none by the other agents at neuromuscular blocking doses. Succinylcholine, because of its similarity in structure to ACh, binds to ganglionic nicotinic and cardiac muscarinic receptors and stimulates cholinergic transmission. Pancuronium exerts a direct blocking effect on muscarinic receptors, but tubocurarine, metocurine, and atracurium show muscarinic blockade only at concentrations much higher than are needed for neuromuscular blockade. Pancuronium, succinylcholine, and gallamine also produce direct muscarinic effects that result in cardiac dysrhythmias. The lack of cardiac effects with the newer agents, if true, will greatly increase the safety in the use of neuromuscular blocking drugs.

Histamine release is a problem with tubocurarine, and to a lesser extent with succinylcholine, metocurine, and mivacurium. Histamine contributes considerably to the cardiovascular side effects of tubocurarine. The release of histamine and the cardiac, respiratory, vascular, and other responses to histamine together with the use of histamine antagonists to offset anticipated histamine response to neuromuscular blocking drugs are discussed in Chapter 59. Some of the newer neuromuscular blocking drugs appear to have little or no histamine-releasing potential, thus minimizing this side effect.

Primary problems in the clinical use of neuromuscular blocking agents are summarized in the box.

With succinylcholine, K^+ efflux is dangerous in patients with extensive soft-tissue damage as occurs with burns. In addition, a succinylcholine-halothane combination may potentiate a malignant hyperthermia syndrome in patients predisposed to this condition (see Chapter 30).

Drug interactions occur with anesthetics, calcium-

TRADE NAMES

In addition to generic and fixed-combination preparations, the following trade-named materials are available in the United States.
Anectine, succinylcholine
Arduan, pipecuronium bromide
Flaxedil, gallamine triethiodide
Metubine, metocurine iodide
Mivacron, mivacurium chloride
Norcuron, vecuronium bromide
Nuromax, doxacurium chloride
Pavulon, pancuronium bromide
Quelicin, succinylcholine
Tracrium, atracurium besylate

channel blockers, and some antibiotics. Many volatile anesthetic agents enhance the action of the nondepolarizing neuromuscular blockers. Isoflurane potentiates the effects of succinylcholine. The local anesthetic bupivacaine potentiates the blockade of both nondepolarizing and depolarizing agents, and both lidocaine and procaine prolong the duration of succinylcholine action through inhibition of pseudocholinesterase.

Calcium-channel blockade, and to a lesser extent β-adrenergic blockers, potentiate neuromuscular blocking drugs. Antibiotics that contribute to drug interactions with the neuromuscular blocking agents are the aminoglycosides, tetracyclines, polymyxin, and clindamycin.

Patients taking phenytoin or carbamazepine chronically have a reduced duration of action of mivacurium.

Neuromuscular blocking agents must be used with caution in patients with underlying neuromuscular or renal disease or electrolyte imbalance (see box).

NEW DIRECTIONS

Neuromuscular blocking drugs are now commonly used on a long-term basis to allow controlled ventilation of patients in intensive care units. This practice is not without problems, including prolonged muscle paralysis after termination of the neuromuscular blocking drug treatment. Agents with potassium channel–blocking actions, such as 2,4-diaminopyridine, are also being used to treat neuromuscular disorders such as the Lambert-Eaton myasthenic syndrome.

REFERENCES

Bevan DR, Bevan JC, Donati F: *Muscle relaxants in clinical anesthesia,* St Louis, 1988, Mosby.

Savarese JJ, Wastila WB: Current research in relaxant development, *Seminars in Anesthesia* V:304-311, 1986.

SELF-ASSESSMENT QUESTIONS:

1. Which of the following neuromuscular blocking drugs cause release of histamine?
   a. vecuronium
   b. metocurine
   c. tubocurarine
   d. b and c are correct.
   e. all of the above are correct.
2. At therapeutic concentrations the primary action of doxacurium is to:
   a. block acetylcholine release.
   b. inhibit acetylcholinesterase.
   c. block muscarinic receptors for acetylcholine.
   d. block the ion channel opened by activation of nicotinic receptors.
   e. block the nicotinic receptor at the motor endplate.
3. Which of the following neuromuscular blocking agents normally has a duration of action greater than 1 hour?
   a. doxacurium
   b. mivacurium
   c. succinylcholine
   d. atracurium
   e. none of the above
4. Metabolism is the main route of elimination for all of the following agents *except:*
   a. gallamine.
   b. succinylcholine.
   c. mivacurium.
   d. atracurium.
   e. pancuronium.
5. Potential therapeutic uses of neuromuscular blockers include:
   a. diagnosis of myasthenia gravis.
   b. control of ventilation during surgery.
   c. endotracheal intubation.
   d. b and c are correct.
   e. all of the above are correct.

PART III

CARDIOVASCULAR SYSTEM: DRUGS AFFECTING CARDIAC FUNCTION, BLOOD PRESSURE, RENAL FUNCTION AND BLOOD COAGULATION

For persons living in industrialized nations, dysfunction of the cardiovascular system is the major cause of mortality. In the United States. about 50% of deaths are attributed to cardiovascular problems.

Included within the functions of the cardiovascular system are:

1. Cardiac pumping ability, including the rhythmic nature of the electrical signals, force of contraction, and magnitude of the discharge pressure.
2. Integrity of the vasculature, including presence of flow-restricting deposits in the arterial lumen, muscular tone and structural integrity of vessel walls, and pressure drops required to pump blood through vascular beds at rates needed to provide nutrients and remove wastes.
3. Blood volume and composition, including water and electrolyte balances, lipid composition, and capabilities for clot formation and lysis.

Many of these functions can be modified therapeutically or prophylactically with drugs. This section describes such drugs, how they act at the molecular level, and their clinical application.

In addressing drug use to modify the pumping ability of the heart, it is necessary to understand physiological and biochemical processes that govern cardiac pacing, the force of cardiac and smooth muscle contraction, and blood pressure. The nervous system plays such a large role in the control of blood pressure that the physiology (Chapter 12) and pharmacology (Chapter 13) of blood pressure control are discussed in separate chapters. For discussions of cardiac pacing (Chapter 14) and cardiac contractile force (Chapter 15) the physiology and pharmacology are described within the same chapters. Another topic that relates to the heart as a pump is that of calcium channel blocking drugs (Chapter 16), that can act at several points of the pump-pacing-pressure control cycle, as well as provide relief in angina pectoris—as can nitrates (Chapter 17).

Pharmacological intervention to assure the integrity of the vasculature is discussed in Chapter 20 in relation to the reduction of deposits that narrow the arterial lumen and cause atherosclerosis. Pharmacological intervention is also included to a lesser extent in Chapter 18, where the prostaglandins are discussed.

Control of water volume and electrolyte content of the blood, primarily through renal mechanisms, is discussed in Chapter 19. The section closes with a discussion of the pharmacological approaches for reduced blood clotting or for stimulation of clot dissolution, especially in conjunction with postmyocardial infarction of a lodged microembolus (Chapter 21).

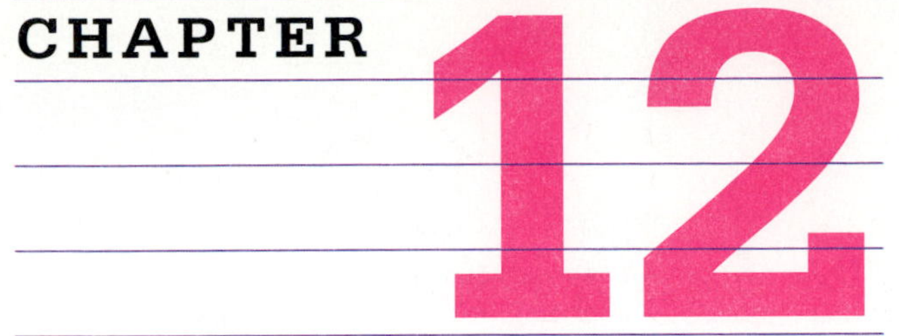

Regulation of Blood Pressure by the Autonomic Nervous System

GREGORY D. FINK

Arterial blood pressure is the product of cardiac output and total peripheral resistance to blood flow through the vascular system. Cardiac output is determined by the rate and efficiency of pumping of the heart. Vascular resistance is directly related to the viscosity of blood and length of blood vessels. Vascular resistance is inversely related to blood vessel luminal diameter (caliber), which normally represents the principal determinant of flow resistance. Cardiac performance and vascular caliber are controlled by several intrinsic regulatory mechanisms. Heart rate is determined by pacemaker cells in the sinoatrial node, and cardiac pumping efficiency is subject to several types of homeostatic regulation. The caliber of most resistance-producing blood vessels is influenced by the normal contractile state of the vessels balanced by release of vasorelaxant substances from the endothelial cell monolayer lining thc vessel lumen.

Superimposed on these intrinsic control processes are extrinsic factors that affect cardiovascular function: tissue metabolic rate and locally produced and blood-borne vasoactive chemicals (autocrine/paracrine/endocrine regulation). Overall coordination and integration of the cardiovascular system, however, is performed primarily by the autonomic nervous system. Through its parasympathetic and sympathetic limbs, the autonomic nervous system has powerful effects on both cardiac performance and blood vessel caliber.

Drugs used to treat hypertension must obviously lower blood pressure. Some drugs act directly on the autonomic nervous system, and others work through other means such as fluid balance or endocrine mechanisms. Reflex reactions of the autonomic nervous system frequently complicate understanding the actions of these drugs. Thus, to appreciate how these drugs alleviate hypertension, it is important to review the function of the autonomic nervous system. This chapter describes some key features of autonomic control of blood pressure to facilitate discussion of the pharmacology of drugs used to treat hypertension (Chapter 13).

ABBREVIATION	
CVO	Circumventricular organ

OVERVIEW OF AUTONOMIC CARDIOVASCULAR REGULATION

The effects of autonomic activity on the mechanisms that control blood pressure are summarized in Figure 12-1. Cardiac performance is influenced by both parasympathetic (vagus) and sympathetic innervation of the heart. Heart rate is decreased by parasympathetic activity and increased by sympathetic activity at the sinoatrial node, but the parasympathetic effect is dominant. Contractile force of the heart is reduced by parasympathetic activity and increased by sympathetic activity to atrial and ventricular muscle, but the sympathetic effect is dominant. Increased sympathetic activity generally reduces vascular caliber by constricting vascular smooth muscle. Although there are parasympathetic influences on a few vascular beds, they contribute little to overall resistance. Constriction of veins in response to sympathetic activity increases cardiac output by augmenting atrial and ventricular filling, whereas sympathetically mediated constriction of arteries reduces cardiac output by increasing afterload. Activation of the sympathetic nervous system can produce more long-term adjustments that can increase blood pressure. For example, increased sympathetic activityl to the kidney increases renin release and causes sodium and water retention. Sympathetic nerves also may exert a trophic effect on blood vessels, resulting in increased "structural" resistance to blood flow. The recep-

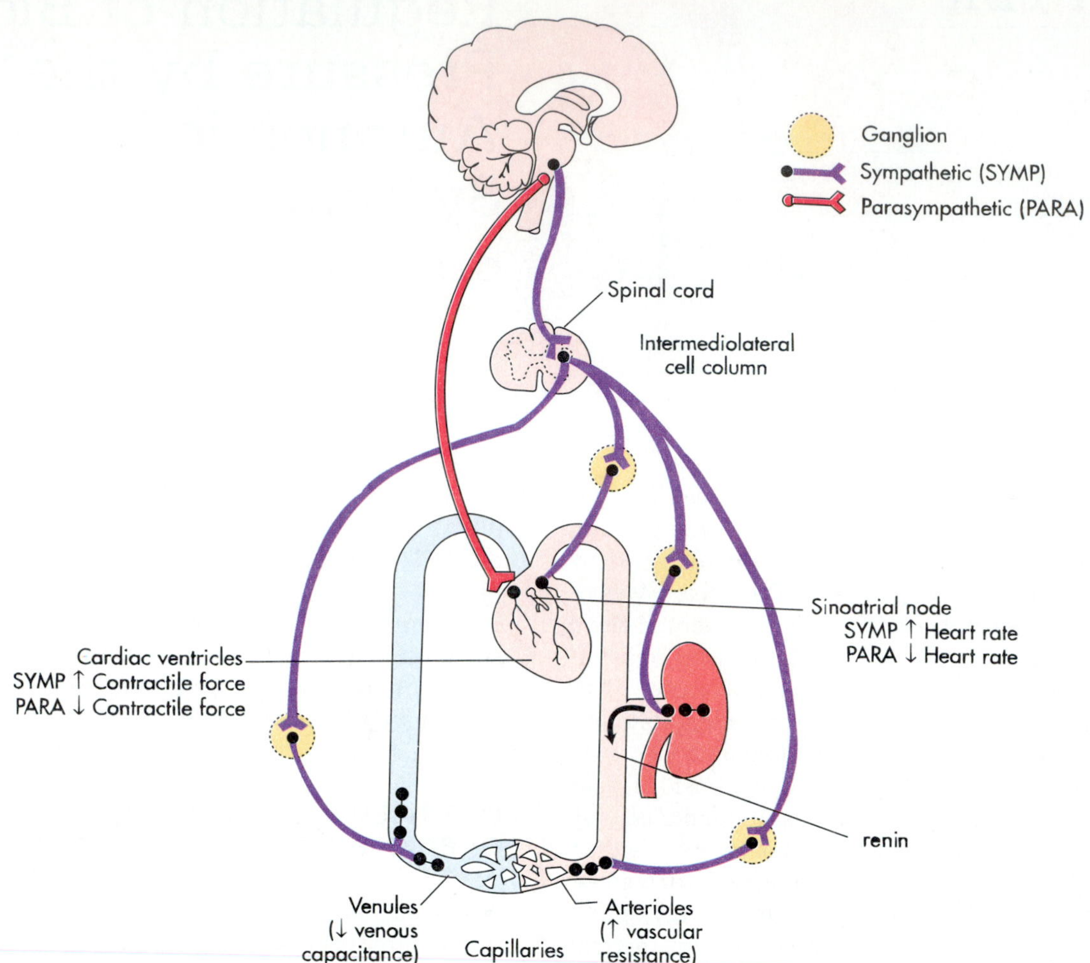

FIGURE 12-1 Effects of autonomic nervous system on blood pressure control. Vascular resistance is affected almost exclusively by the sympathetic nerves, whereas cardiac output is regulated by both sympathetic and parasympathetic influences.

tors and signal pathways involved in these effects are summarized in Chapter 8.

Overall autonomic control of blood pressure is dependent on (1) the rates of firing of sympathetic and parasympathetic nerves; (2) the relationship between nerve firing and neurotransmitter release; and (3) end-organ responsiveness to neurotransmitters. End-organ responsiveness is primarily determined by postjunctional receptors and signaling mechanisms, described in Chapters 8 to 10. This chapter discusses the control of autonomic nerve firing and neurotransmitter concentrations at the neuroeffector junction.

CONTROL OF AUTONOMIC NERVE ACTIVITY

The organization of autonomic cardiovascular control systems is summarized in Figure 12-2. Although autonomic regulation is clearly complex, a hierarchy exists such that only a small number of inputs are important in controlling autonomic activity under normal conditions. The medulla oblongata (brainstem) is the primary site where the rate and pattern of sympathetic and parasympathetic nerve activity is determined.

Origin of Autonomic Activity

Preganglionic neurons providing input to cardiac vagal (parasympathetic) nerves are located in the nucleus ambiguus. These neurons have low levels of spontaneous firing, and their discharge rate is driven mostly by inputs from afferents, particularly arterial baroreceptors. Inputs to spinal sympathetic preganglionic neurons involved in cardiovascular regulation originate in the brainstem, pons, and hypothalamus and can be either excitatory or inhibitory. However, in most cases the activity of sympathetic nerves is primarily controlled by

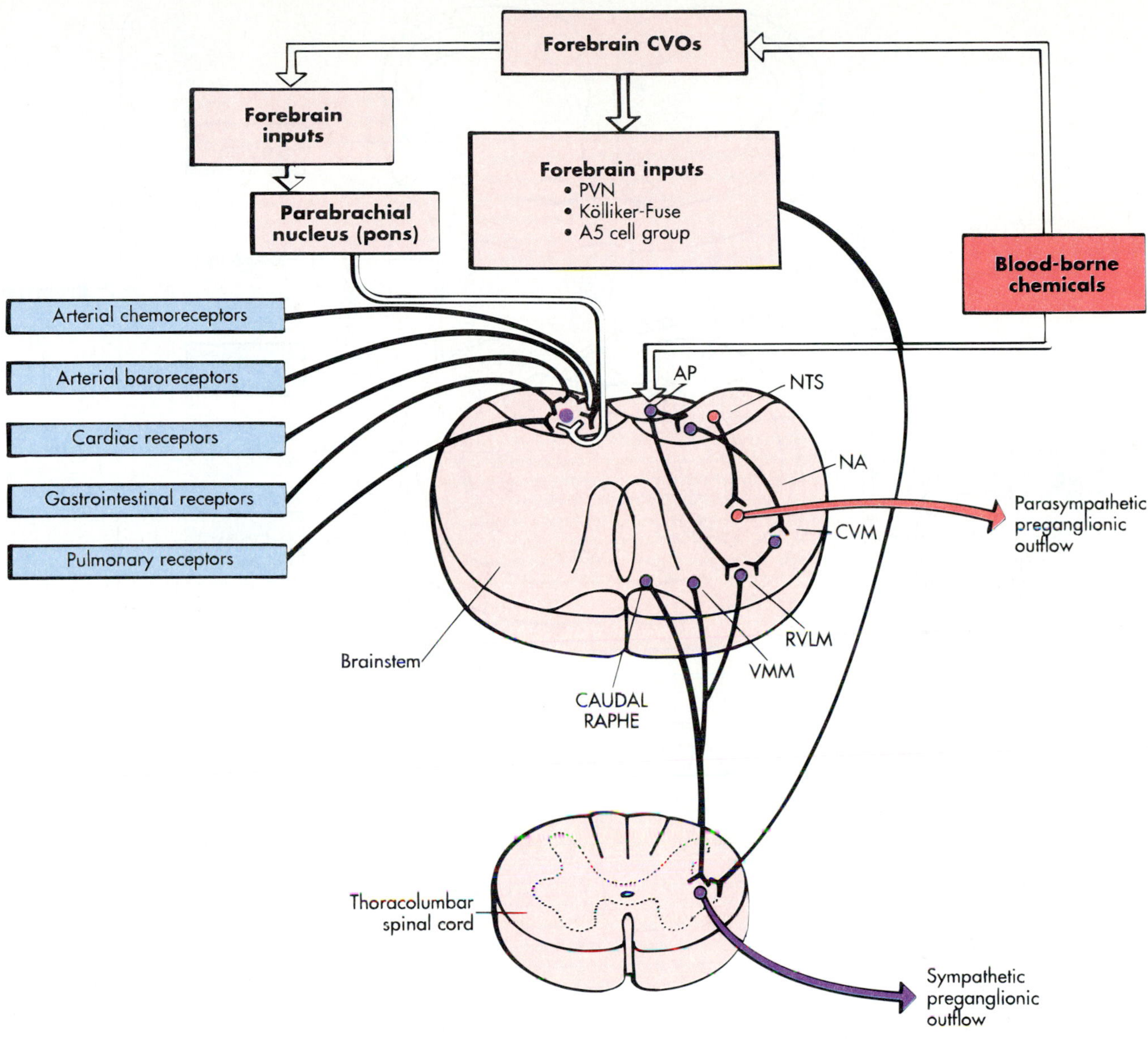

FIGURE 12-2 Organization of autonomic cardiovascular control systems. Major inputs are in boxes. Many reciprocal connections are not illustrated. Somatic afferents enter the brainstem through the spinal cord (not shown). *AP,* Area postrema; *CVM,* caudal ventrolateral medulla; *NA,* nucleus ambiguus; *RVLM,* rostral ventrolateral medulla; *VMM,* ventromedial medulla.

excitatory neurons in the rostral ventrolateral medulla. These neurons can exhibit significant spontaneous firing, possibly because of pacemaker properties or complex integration of inputs from excitatory and inhibitory cells widely distributed throughout the brainstem.

In most situations, however, the activities of both parasympathetic and sympathetic nerves are primarily determined by afferent inputs of two major types. Visceral afferents from receptors located in the cardiovascular system itself provide specific feedback information on arterial pressure (arterial baroreceptors) and cardiac filling (cardiac baroreceptors). Other afferents from lung, gastrointestinal viscera, skeletal muscle, and forebrain serve to coordinate autonomic cardiovascular responses with other bodily functions, such as respiration, digestion, exercise, and temperature regulation. Blood-borne hormones, such as angiotensin II, can also modulate the activity of autonomic nerves by acting on neurons in brain circumventricular organs, brain areas lacking an efficient blood-brain barrier. Within this large variety of feedback mechanisms, the arterial baroreceptors appear to play the most important role in controlling autonomic

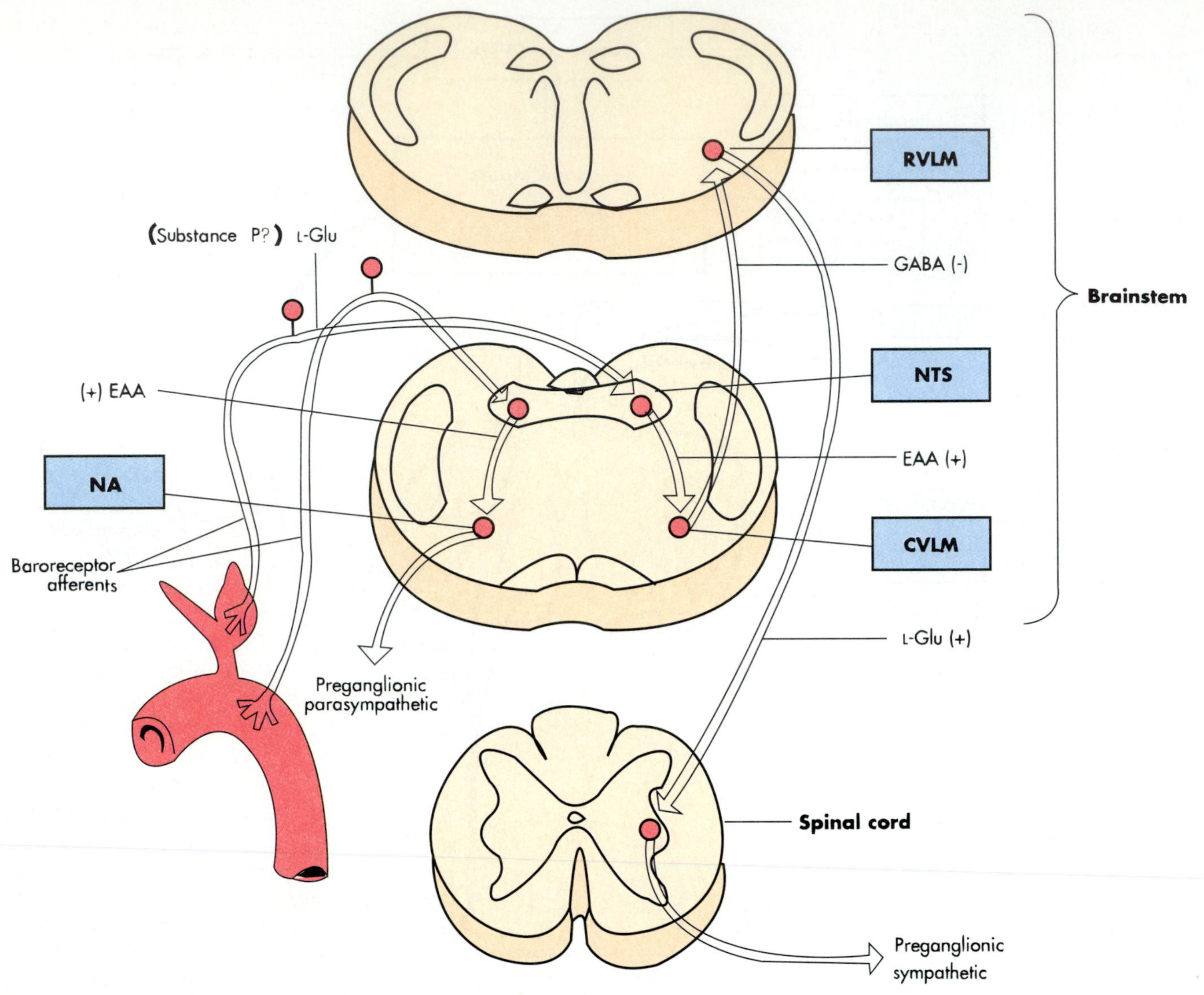

Blood pressure	NORMAL	INCREASED	DECREASED
Baroreceptor afferent activity	NORMAL	↑	↓
Sympathetic activity	NORMAL	↓	↑
Parasympathetic activity	NORMAL	↑	↓

FIGURE 12-3 Brainstem organization of the baroreflex and associated neurotransmitters. Primary pathways only are shown. Other afferents, and interneurons, are omitted. *CVLM,* Caudal ventolateral medulla; *EAA,* excitatory amino acid; *GABA,* γ-aminobutyric acid; *L-GLU,* L-glutamate; *NA,* nucleus ambiguus; *NTS,* nucleus of the solitary tract; *RVLM,* rostral ventrolateral medulla; *SP,* substance P; +, excitatory pathway; −, inhibitory pathway.

nerve activity. This system is therefore described in more detail.

Baroreceptor Reflex

Minute-to-minute control of arterial blood pressure is achieved when small pressure changes are linked to reflex alterations in autonomic nerve activity. Sensory nerve endings embedded in the wall of the carotid sinus and aortic arch (baroreceptors) are activated by wall stretch when arterial pressure increases. Stimulation of these baroreceptors leads within a few seconds to an increase in vagal (parasympathetic) activity and a reduction in sympathetic activity. The parasympathetic activation slows heart rate, and the sympathetic inhibition causes vasodilation, thus tending to return arterial pressure toward the original level. Conversely, a decrease in arterial pressure is rapidly countered by increased sympathetic and decreased parasympathetic activity. This results in vasoconstriction and elevated cardiac rate and force of cardiac contraction. Organization of the baroreceptor reflex is illustrated in Figure 12-3.

The baroreceptor reflex is primarily important in short-term control of blood pressure. When changes in blood pressure persist beyond a few minutes, reflex autonomic responses diminish. This is called **baroreflex adaptation** and involves both peripheral and central components of the reflex. Higher brain centers can also override the baroreflex. During physical exercise, for example, blood pressure increases are accompanied by tachycardia, instead of the anticipated reflex bradycardia. Varying degrees of baroreflex impairment occur with normal aging and in individuals with heart failure or hypertension. These phenomena may help explain why some antihypertensive drugs are more effective in hypertensive than in normotensive patients because the actions of the drugs in normotensive subjects would be opposed by the baroreflex.

The main function of the baroreflex is to stabilize blood pressure in the face of changing physiological conditions. Loss of baroreceptors (experimentally or through disease) may have little effect on daily average blood pressure but is accompanied by wide minute-to-minute swings in pressure. Such episodic hypertension, in the absence of baroreflex control, can occur in response to a variety of environmental stimuli.

The influence of baroreceptors on sympathetic nerve activity can vary greatly in different vascular beds. Some beds, such as the cutaneous vasculature, are largely independent of arterial baroreceptor influence, though such vessels contribute little to total vascular resistance. In contrast, in organs making a major contribution to total resistance such as skeletal muscle and kidney, sympathetic activity is exquisitely sensitive to arterial baroreceptor input. This sensitivity underscores the paramount importance of the arterial baroreflex in blood pressure control. In fact, except under some special circumstances (exercise, sleep, and certain behavioral states), the baroreceptors are able to override all other inputs affecting autonomic blood pressure regulation. This may reflect the evolutionary desirability of the maintenance of a highly stable systemic blood pressure under diverse environmental condition.

Other Factors Involving Autonomic Activity

Complex central integration of sensory information from a variety of sources produces numerous distinct patterns of autonomic outflow to the heart and blood vessels. These patterns of activity are important in generating rapid, specific cardiovascular responses to internal and external stimuli.

The autonomic nervous system is also connected to sensory neurons responding to chemical inputs. Activation of these neurons can cause a more prolonged change in autonomic activity than is usually observed with activation of baroreceptor afferents. A reduction in blood oxygen content activates specialized oxygen-sensing cells (chemoreceptors) in the carotid sinus, aortic arch, and brainstem. Activation of these chemoreceptors leads to coordinated respiratory and cardiovascular responses to restore blood oxygenation.

Changes in blood osmolality and the concentration of certain peptide hormones are sensed by neurons in the circumventricular organs of the brain, where there is an inefficient blood-brain barrier. These include the organum vasculosum of the lamina terminalis (OVLT), subfornical organ, posterior pituitary, median eminence, and area postrema. Circumventricular organs contain receptors for a large variety of biologically active substances (see Box), and have important effects on brain

Endogenous Substances with Receptors in Circumventricular Organs (CVOs)

angiotensin II	endothelin
vasopressin	atrial natriuretic peptide
insulin	somatostatin
opioids	neuropeptide Y
serotonin	bradykinin
histamine	eicosanoids
epinephrine	neurotensin
norepinephrine	bombesin
dopamine	adenosine
acetylcholine	aldosterone
amino acid neurotransmitters	cortisol

Table 12-1 Circulating Substances Known to Affect Autonomic Blood Pressure Regulation through Actions at Circumventricular Organs (CVOs)

Substance	Action
angiotensin II	↑ sympathetic, ↓ parasympathetic activity; inhibit baroreflex
vasopressin	↓ sympathetic, ↑ parasympathetic activity; facilitate baroreflex
insulin	↑ sympathetic activity

regions involved in initiating autonomic outflow. Activation of circumventricular organs produces integrated autonomic, endocrine, and behavioral responses supporting water, electrolyte, and nutrient homeostasis. Table 12-1 lists some substances postulated to affect autonomic blood pressure regulation in this manner. Current evidence indicates that the organum vasculosum of the lamina and area postrema are particularly critical to the pathogenesis of some forms of hypertension.

CONTROL OF NEUROTRANSMITTER CONCENTRATIONS AT THE NEUROEFFECTOR JUNCTION

Neurotransmission at parasympathetic and sympathetic neuroeffector junctions is reviewed in Chapters 9 and 10. The firing rate of postganglionic nerves, the rate of transmitter release, and the removal of transmitter by diffusion, metabolism, and reuptake are important determinants of the neurotransmitter concentration. Postganglionic nerve activity is usually a faithful reproduction of that in preganglionic neurons discussed previously. Neurotransmitter removal can be altered by drugs or disease, but modulation of release is the main mechanism by which junctional transmitter concentration is normally controlled. Increased release of transmitter is caused by elevated nerve-firing frequency but is also controlled by chemicals near the nerve terminal, that is, prejunctional regulation. Because of the importance of the sympathetic nervous system in controlling blood pressure, a summary of prejunctional regulation of norepinephrine secretion is provided.

Sympathetic Neuroeffector Junctions

Axons of postganglionic sympathetic neurons branch repeatedly near effector tissues. The smallest branches arborize extensively and exhibit numerous varicosities containing the transmitter norepinephrine. Neuropeptide Y and adenosine triphosphate are coreleased with norepinephrine at some sympathetic neuroeffector junctions and also exert cardiovascular actions through specific postjunctional receptors.

Transmitter Release Depolarization-induced calcium influx into the varicosities is the main stimulus for exocytotic release of neurotransmitters, though other factors also may modulate release. Although the cellular mechanism of exocytosis is not well understood, it is likely that the entire contents of a secretory vesicle are released in response to depolarization. The probability of release differs among varicosities but on average appears surprisingly low (less than 1/100). Because transmitter is actively reaccumulated in the varicosity, increased nerve firing probably involves only a small number of postjunctional cells exposed to high concentrations of NE from a single varicosity. Coordinated responses then depend on electrical or chemical communication between postjunctional cells and adequate numbers of varicosities releasing transmitter. Therefore prejunctional regulation probably does not involve modulation of the amount of norepinephrine released from a varicosity but rather the probability of transmitter release.

Prejunctional Regulation of Transmitter Release

Receptors in nerve terminal membranes can enhance or inhibit norepinephrine secretion when activated by endogenous chemicals. Such prejunctional receptors are called *autoreceptors* if they are activated by the released transmitter itself and *heteroreceptors* if activated by other transmitters or hormones. Activation of prejunctional receptors does not affect nerve firing rate but increases or decreases the probability of depolarization-induced exocytosis. Several cellular signals may contribute to a change in release probability; altered Ca^{++}, Na^{+}, or K^{+} channel activity; and second messengers like cAMP and inositol trisphosphate. Figure 12-4 illustrates the types of mechanisms that may be involved in prejunctional regulation of released sympathetic transmitter. The probable sources and mechanisms of action of some potential modulators are listed in Table 12-2.

Prejunctional regulation allows fine-tuning of neurotransmitter release. Activation or inhibition of autoreceptors by released transmitters may function at some neuroeffector junctions as a physiological brake on secretion during periods of high-frequency nerve discharge, limiting postjunctional responses. Agonists at heteroreceptors facilitating transmitter release (e.g., angiotensin II) would amplify effects of sympathetic nerve activity, whereas agonists at inhibitory heteroreceptors (e.g., acetylcholine, adenosine) would reduce responses. Thus, similar rates of sympathetic nerve firing might

FIGURE 12-4 Prejunctional regulation at the sympathetic neuroeffector junction. The left varicosity illustrates autoinhibition of neurotransmitter release, including possible "lateral" inhibition (i.e., transmitter from one varicosity inhibiting release from an adjacent varicosity). The right varicosity illustrates prejunctional regulation of transmitter release by tissue and bloodborne chemicals. See Table 12-2 for a list of involved substances. Postjunctional receptors are shown as circles, ○; prejunctional inhibitory autoreceptors are shown as squares, [B]; prejunctional heteroreceptors are shown as triangles, △.

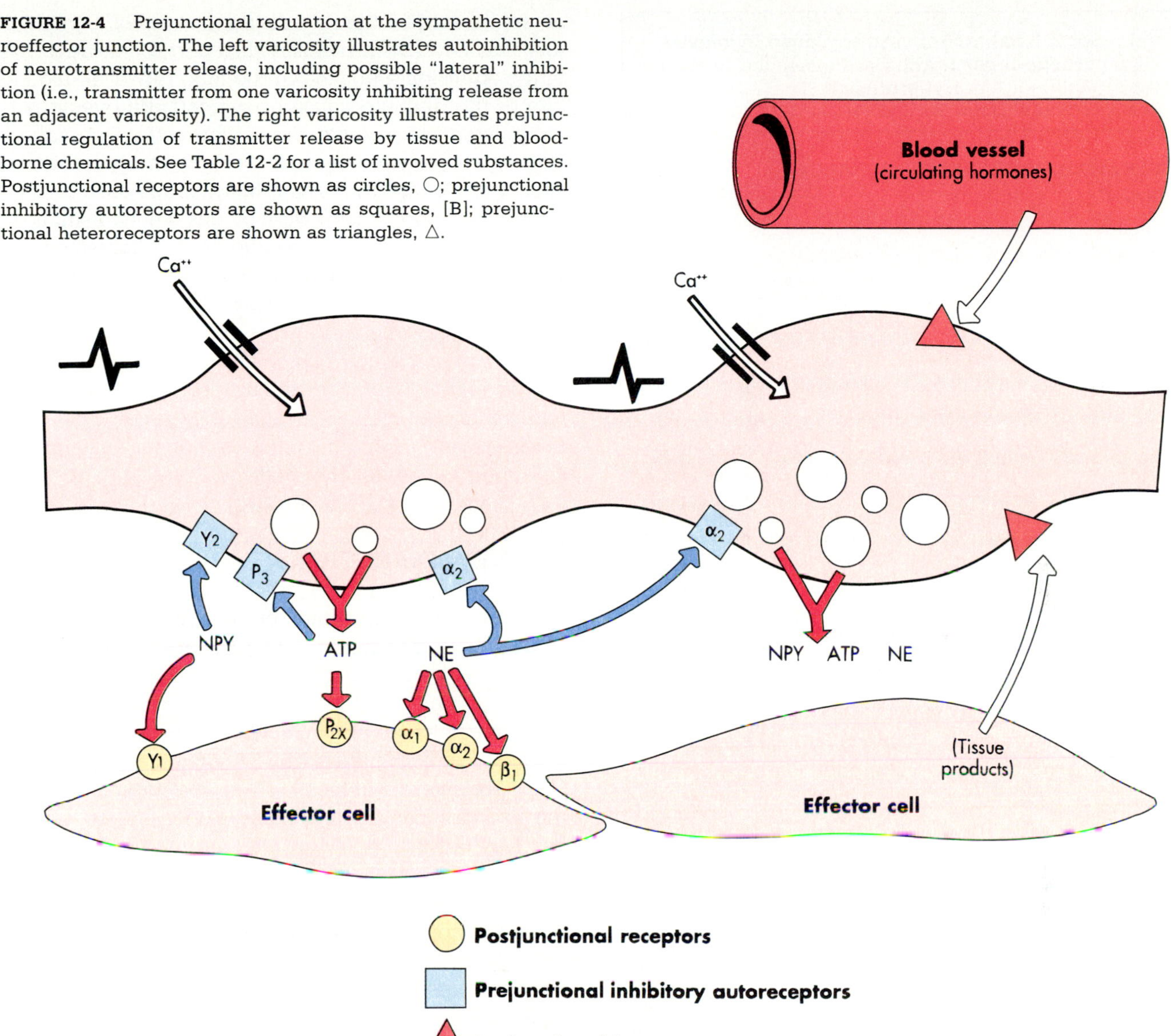

Table 12-2 Prejunctional Modulators of Sympathetic Neurotransmitter Release

Chemical	Source	Receptor	Mechanism	Effect
norepinephrine	SNT	α_2	↓ Ca^{++}	↓
neuropeptide Y	SNT	Y_2	↓ Ca^{++}	↓
ATP	SNT	P_3	↓ Ca^{++}	↓
epinephrine	Blood	β_2	↑ cAMP	↑
angiotensin II	Blood/PJT	AT_1	↑ PLC	↑
prostanoids	PJT	?	↓ Ca^{++}	↓
adenosine	PJT	P_1	↓ Ca^{++}	↓
opioids	Blood	μ, κ, δ	↓ Ca^{++}	↓
acetylcholine	Nerve	M_2	↑ cGMP	↓
dopamine	SNT	D_2	↑ K^+	↓
ANP	Blood	?	↑ cGMP	↓
nitric oxide	EC	?	↑ cGMP	↓

ANP, Atrial natriuretic peptide; *EC,* endothelial cell; *PJT,* postjunctional tissue; *SNT,* sympathetic nerve terminal.

Some Factors Proposed to Cause Increased Sympathetic Input to the Cardiovascular System in Hypertension

ELEVATED SYMPATHETIC DISCHARGE

Neural

Altered "pacemaker" neurons
Impaired baroreflex (arterial or cardiac)
Increased cortical inputs (emotion, stress)

Humoral

Increased plasma insulin
Increased plasma or tissue angiotensin II
Increased extracellular sodium

ENHANCED NOREPINEPHRINE RELEASE

Increased angiotensin II facilitation
Increased β_2-adrenergic facilitation
Decreased neuropeptide Y inhibition

produce different effects in different tissues, depending on the local regulatory mechanisms occurring in the nerve varicosities. The relatively weak contractile response in blood vessels in exercising skeletal muscle in response to high sympathetic discharge, for example, is caused in part by such prejunctional regulatory phenomena.

AUTONOMIC NERVOUS SYSTEM IN HYPERTENSION

One of the causes of hypertension is a relative increase in the balance between sympathetic and parasympathetic control over the heart and blood vessels. Increased sympathetic input can result from changes in neural firing rate, transmitter concentrations at the neuroeffector junction, postjunctional receptors, or signal-transduction pathways. Although there is support for each of these mechanisms, the first two are probably most important. It is clear that control of sympathetic nerve activity and neurotransmitter concentration at the neuroeffector junction is extremely complex. Some factors that have been postulated to play a causative role in hypertension are listed in the Box. However, regardless of the ultimate cause of sympathetic overactivity in hypertensive patients, drugs that inhibit sympathetically mediated cardiovascular effects (sympatholytics) should lower blood pressure. Many drugs used to treat hypertension do, in fact, work by this mechanism; however, other drugs reduce pressure by mechanisms independent of the autonomic nervous system. Such drugs usually result in reflex increases in sympathetic neural activity and decreases in parasympathetic neural activity. This often leads to a diminished antihypertensive response and side effects related to sympathetic overactivity, such as palpitations and tachycardia. This often necessitates concomitant administration of a sympatholytic drug to counter these effects.

NEW DIRECTIONS

Widespread availability of techniques for directly measuring sympathetic nerve discharge (microneurography) now permits detailed examination of autonomic regulation under normal and pathophysiological conditions in conscious human subjects. For example, regulation of sympathetic activity in different vascular beds (e.g., working versus nonworking skeletal muscle) during exercise has been estimated. Autonomic activity has also been assessed in patients with hypertension and in congestive heart failure. Recent studies are focused on distinct patterns of sympathetic nerve discharge as opposed to simple discharge frequency. Studies in patients with autonomic dysfunction have yielded important insights into the role of the autonomic nervous system in cardiovascular homeostasis. Neurotransmitter release studies are attempting to define the importance of autoreceptor activation and underlying actions of drugs and chemicals involved in prejunctional regulation.

SELF-ASSESSMENT QUESTIONS

1. The most important determinant of autonomic neural discharge frequency is:
   a. intrinsic activity of brainstem neurons.
   b. blood oxygen content.
   c. cardiac output.
   d. arterial baroreflex.
   e. cardiac baroreflex.
2. Sympathetic activity to which of the following vascular beds is influenced the least by arterial baroreflexes:
   a. muscle
   b. skin
   c. kidney
   d. heart
   e. splanchic viscera
3. An endogenous chemical that increases norepinephrine release at the neuroeffector junction:
   a. prostaglandin E_2
   b. adenosine
   c. acetylcholine
   d. nitric oxide
   e. angiotensin II
4. The stimulus for exocytotic release of norepinephrine from the sympathetic neuroeffector junction is increased intracellular concentration of:
   a. Ca^{++}.
   b. Na^{+}.
   c. K^{+}.
   d. ATP.
   e. cyclic AMP.
5. A decrease in arterial pressure causes all of the following changes *except:*
   a. decreased baroreceptor afferent activity.
   b. increased sympathetic nerve discharge.
   c. increased heart rate.
   d. increased vagal nerve discharge.
   e. increased release of norepinephrine.

CHAPTER 13 Antihypertensive Drugs

GREGORY D. FINK

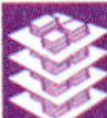

THERAPEUTIC OVERVIEW

Hypertension is defined as an elevation of arterial blood pressure above an arbitrarily defined normal value. This normal value for blood pressure differs according to gender and age; men have higher average pressures than women, and in most populations older individuals have higher pressures than younger subjects. The American Heart Association defines hypertension as arterial blood pressure higher than 140/90 mm Hg, whereas The World Health Organization uses the value 160/95 mm Hg. The prevalence of hypertension varies in different subgroups of the population, but the overall rate in the United States is estimated at approximately 20% of all adults. A physician in general practice can expect to see 20 to 40 patients with hypertension each week.

A small number (<10%) of individuals with hypertension have identifiable causes such as renal disease or endocrine tumors; these are often managed by surgical means. Most patients diagnosed as hypertensive, however, are simply at the upper end of the normal distribution of blood pressure values for their population group. No single mechanism has been identified to explain the higher blood pressure values in such individuals, but it may result from genetic factors, because blood pressure is strongly influenced by inheritance in a polygenetic fashion. This type of hypertension is designated *essential* hypertension, and although usually first diagnosed in middle-aged individuals, it can be found in children and young adults as well.

Hypertension, unless rapid in onset and severe, does not produce noticeable symptoms. However, several cardiovascular diseases are common or more severe in humans with high blood pressure, including atherosclerosis, coronary artery disease, aortic aneurysm, congestive heart failure, stroke, diabetes (with particular reference to insulin resistance), and renal and retinal disease.

DRUGS USED TO TREAT HYPERTENSION

CLASS	DRUGS	
β-adrenergic antagonists (β-blockers)	β_1, β_2	β_1
	propranolol	atenolol
	nadolol	metoprolol
	pindolol	acebutolol
	timolol	betaxolol
	labetalol*	
Centrally acting sympatholytics (α-adrenergic agonists)		clonidine
		guanabenz
		methyldopa
		guanfacine
Sympathetic nerve ending blockers (NE depletors)		reserpine
		guanethidine
		guanadrel
Peripheral α-adrenergic receptor antagonists		prazosin
		terazosin
		doxazosin
Direct vasodilators		hydralazine
		minoxidil
Angiotensin-converting enzyme inhibitors (ACE inhibitors)		captopril
		enalapril
		lisinopril
Diuretics	See page 163 (this chapter) and Chapter 19	
Calcium-channel blockers	See Chapter 16	

*Has α_1-adrenergic blocking action.

ABBREVIATIONS

ACE	Angiotensin-converting enzyme
CO	Cardiac output
TPR	Total peripheral resistance

The presence of diabetes increases the frequency and severity of end-organ damage. The purpose of treatment of hypertension is to prevent these significant cardiovascular complications. Most importantly, effective drug therapy has been shown through controlled clinical trails to reduce the morbidity and mortality associated with high arterial pressure.

The choice of therapy for a patient with hypertension depends on a variety of factors: age, sex, race, body build, and life-style of the patient; cause of the disease; other coexisting diseases; rapidity of onset and severity of the hypertension; and the presence or absence of other risk factors for cardiovascular disease (e.g., smoking, alcohol consumption, obesity, and personality type).

Several nonpharmacological approaches to therapy of hypertension are available. These are listed in the box. Patients differ in their sensitivity to these techniques, but, on the average, only modest reductions (5 to 10 mm Hg) in blood pressure can be achieved. Despite the modest effect of nonpharmacological interventions, when viewed across large populations, specific individuals may be classified based on their sensitivity to these interventions. For example, the "salt-sensitive" individual will have a rapid decrease in blood pressure when placed on a low-sodium diet. The major advantage of nonpharmacological therapies is the relative safety and freedom from side effects, compared with drug therapy. However, most patients with hypertension require drug treatment to achieve an adequate sustained reduction of blood pressure.

Arterial blood pressure is the product of cardiac output (CO) and total peripheral resistance (TPR). Patients with recent-onset essential hypertension tend to have an elevated CO. With chronic sustained hypertension, most patients develop normal or low CO and a fixed elevated peripheral resistance. Drugs currently available lower blood pressure by decreasing either CO or TPR. However, CO and TPR are not independent variables, and changes in one can indirectly affect the other.

Reduction of blood pressure by any means may activate one or more of the physiological mechanisms discussed in the next sections and thereby oppose a drug-induced decrease in blood pressure (Figure 13-1).

NONPHARMACOLOGICAL THERAPY OF HYPERTENSION

- Low sodium chloride diet
- Weight reduction
- Exercise
- Cessation of smoking
- Decrease in excessive (>30 ml of ethanol per day) alcohol consumption
- Psychological methods (relaxation, biofeedback, meditation)
- Dietary decrease in saturated fats

Renin-Angiotensin-Aldosterone System

A decrease in arterial pressure causes release of the enzyme renin from the kidney into the blood. Renin generates angiotensin I from a circulating substrate, angiotensinogen, synthesized in the liver and other tissues. Angiotensin I is converted to angiotensin II by "converting enzyme," found in the endothelial cell membrane, especially in the lung. Angiotensin II constricts blood vessels, enhances sympathetic nervous system activity, and causes renal salt and water retention by direct intrarenal actions, and by stimulating the adrenal gland to release the potent mineralocorticoid aldosterone.

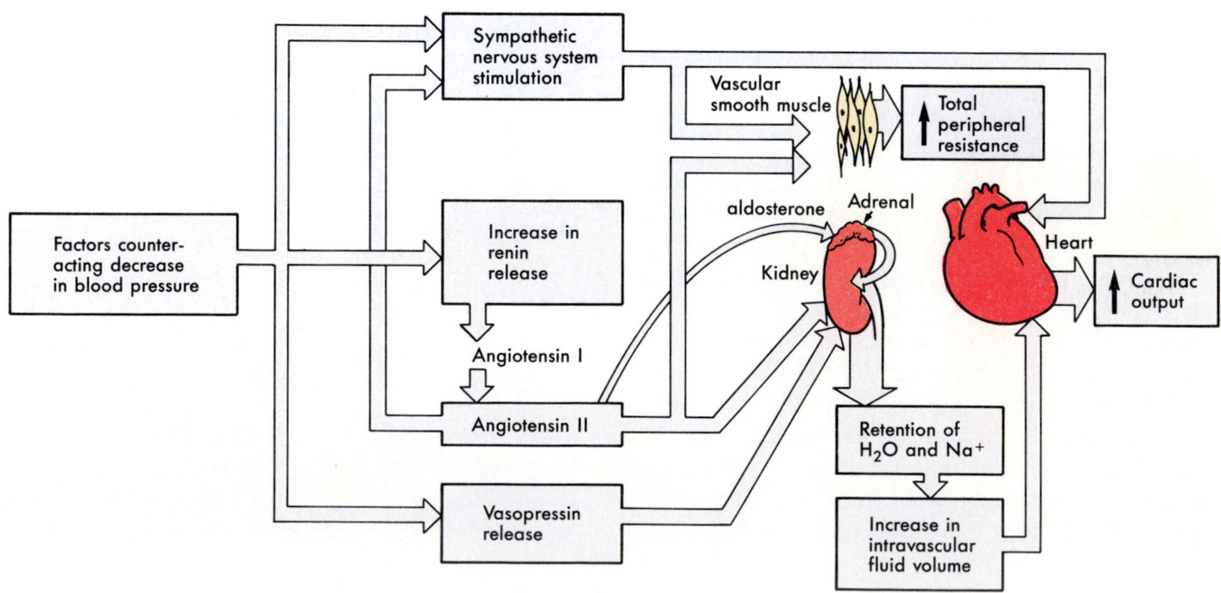

FIGURE 13-1 Processes that occur to counteract a decrease in blood pressure.

Sympathetic Nervous System

A decrease in blood pressure activates the baroreflex, producing increases in sympathetic nervous system activity and leading to (1) increased force and rate of cardiac contraction and enhanced cardiac filling, which combine to elevate CO, (2) constriction of most blood vessels leading to an increase in TPR, and (3) renal retention of sodium chloride and water (by renal sympathetic nerves innervating renal blood vessels and tubules).

Vasopressin System

A decrease in arterial pressure causes baroreflex-mediated release of vasopressin (antidiuretic hormone), which acts on the renal collecting duct to enhance retention of water.

Fluid Retention by the Kidney

A decrease in arterial pressure causes decreased sodium chloride and water excretion by the kidney. This results in part from the direct intrarenal hydraulic effect of reduced renal perfusion pressure and in part from the other mechanisms just listed. The resultant expansion of extracellular fluid and plasma volumes tends to increase CO and arterial pressure and thus reduce the antihypertensive action of the drug.

The most effective and best-tolerated antihypertensive drug regimens impair the operation of one or more of these physiological mechanisms. In addition, drug therapy for hypertension must usually be continued for the lifetime of the patient. Thus, it is imperative that the cost of therapy to the patient be minimized and that the minimum effective dose of drug (or drugs) be employed to reduce the incidence of undesirable side effects.

A summary of therapeutic approaches is given in the box.

THERAPEUTIC OVERVIEW

Hypertension is defined as:	Arterial pressure American Heart Association >140/90 mm Hg World Health Organization >160/95 mm Hg

Exacerbates:
- Atherosclerosis
- Coronary artery diseases
- Congestive heart failure
- Diabetes
- Insulin resistance
- Stroke
- Renal disease
- Retinal disease

Therapy
- Nonpharmacological
  - Dietary: ↓ Na, ↓ alcohol, ↓ weight, ↓ smoking
- Pharmacological: several drug classes
- Physiological counter effects to ↓ blood pressure
  - Fluid retention
  - Release of renin
  - Sympathetic response ↑
  - Baroflex release of vasopressin

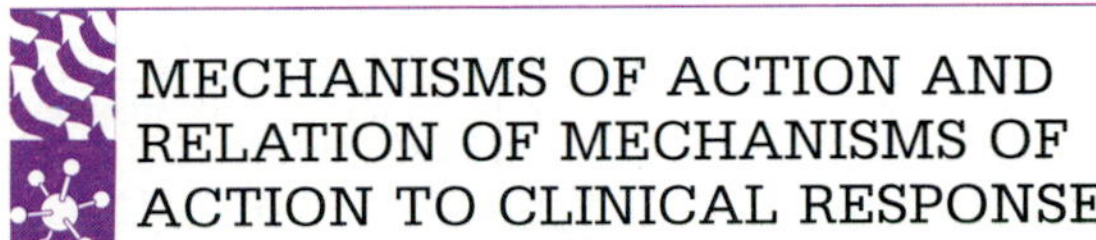

MECHANISMS OF ACTION AND RELATION OF MECHANISMS OF ACTION TO CLINICAL RESPONSE

Antihypertensive drugs can be divided into seven classes, based on mechanisms of action (see box, p. 159, and Figure 13-2). Each of these classes is discussed in

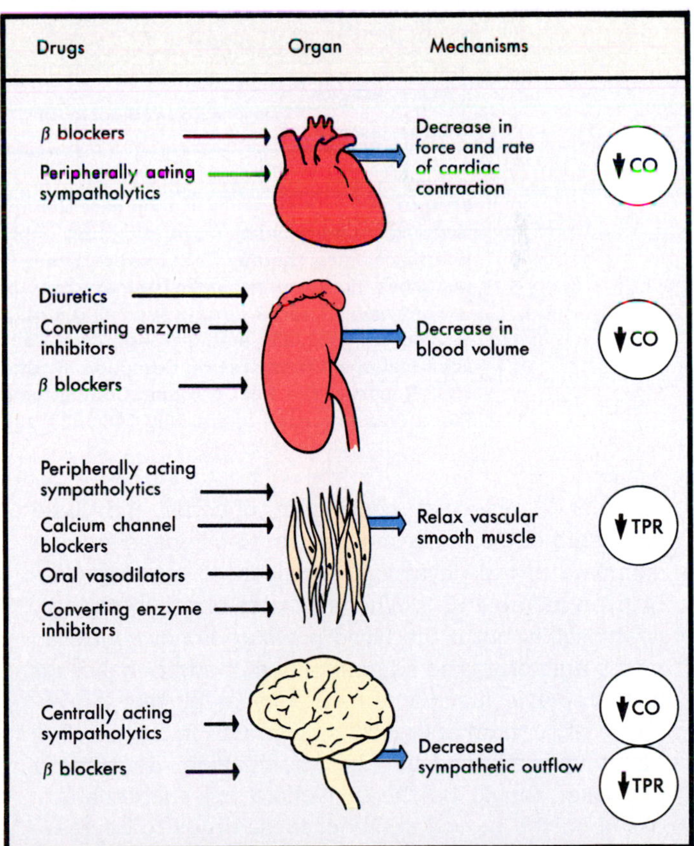

FIGURE 13-2 Summary of sites and mechanisms by which antihypertensive drugs bring about a reduction in blood pressure. *CO*, Cardiac output; *TPR*, total peripheral resistance.

Table 13-1 Physiological Responses to Antihypertensive Drugs

	Plasma Volume	CO	Heart Rate	TPR	Plasma Renin Activity	Sympathetic Nervous System Activity
Diuretics	↓	↓	⇆ ↑	↓	↑	⇆ ↑
β-blockers	⇆	↓	↓	↑ ⇆	↓	⇆ ↓
Centrally acting sympatholytics	↑ ⇆	↓	↓	↓	↓ ⇆	↓
Peripherally acting sympatholytics	⇆ ↑	⇆ ↓	⇆ ↓	↓	⇆	↑
Calcium-channel blockers	⇆	⇆	⇆ ↑	↓	↑ ⇆	⇆ ↑
Orally active vasodilators	↑	⇆ ↑	↑	↓	↑	↑
Converting enzyme inhibitors	⇆	↑ ⇆	⇆	↓	↑	

↑ Increase; ↓ decrease; ⇆ no change.

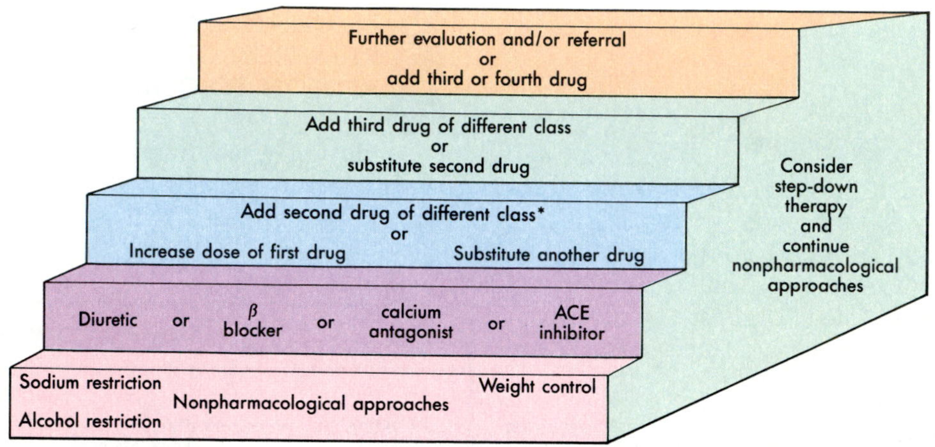

FIGURE 13-3 Individualized step-care therapy for hypertension. For some patients, nonpharmacological therapy should be tried first. If blood pressure reduction goal is not achieved, add pharmacological therapy. Other patients may require pharmacological therapy initially. In these instances, nonpharmacological therapy may be a helpful adjunct. *ACE* , Angiotensin converting enzymes; *Asterisk* , drugs such as diuretics: *β-blockers*, calcium antagonist, ACE inhibitors or blockers, centrally acting α_1-agonists, *Rauwolfia serpentina,* and vasodilators. (From 1988 Joint National Committee on Detection, Evaluation and Treatment of High Blood Pressure: The 1988 Report of the Joint National Committee on Detection, Evaluation, and Treatment of High Blood Pressure, *Arch Intern Med* 148:1023, 1988.)

terms of (1) molecular mechanisms of action and (2) relationship of molecular mechanism to clinical effects. A summary of the physiological responses by drug class is given in Table 13-1. Whenever possible, monotherapy is advisable, but if the blood pressure is not controlled by a single drug, the administration of additional drugs in a stepwise manner is frequently employed. An example of such an approach is illustrated in Figure 13-3. Many experts believe that a thiazide diuretic or β-blocker should be the first choice for monotherapy, based on the proved ability of these drugs to decrease cardiovascular mortality. The pharmacokinetic considerations and clinical problems are discussed in subsequent sections in which the seven classes of drug are considered together.

Diuretics

Diuretics reduce fluid volume by inhibiting electrolyte transport in the renal tubules. Their mechanisms of action on the renal tubule are discussed in Chapter 19.

Various diuretic drugs are used in the therapy of hypertension (see box). Chemical structures are shown in Figure 13-4 and in Chapter 19. However, the complete molecular mechanism of the antihypertensive action of diuretics is not known. Initial administration of a diuretic produces a pronounced increase in urinary water and electrolyte excretion and a reduction in extracellular and plasma volumes. These changes result in a decrease in CO, which is primarily responsible for the decrease in arterial pressure. Some investigators suggest that this initial decrease in extracellular water volume

DIURETIC DRUGS USED TO TREAT HYPERTENSION*	
amiloride†	indapamide
benzothiadiazides (thiazides)	metolazone
bumetanide	spironolactone
chlorthalidone	triamterene†
furosemide	

*See Chapter 19.
†Primarily used as adjunctive therapy to prevent potassium loss caused by other diuretics.

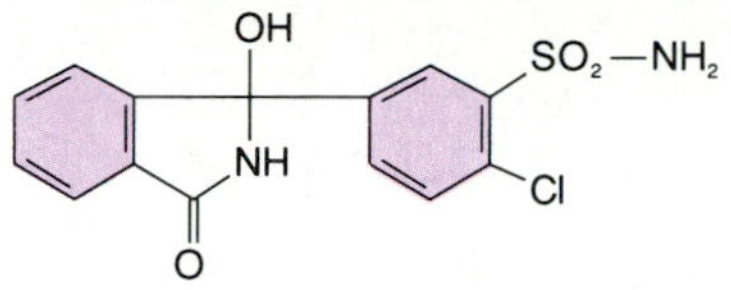

is the full explanation for the antihypertensive effect. After several days the urinary excretion returns to normal, but blood pressure remains at the reduced level. Subsequently, plasma volume and CO also return to, or approximately to, pretreatment values and the TPR decreases, whereas blood pressure remains lowered. The decline in TPR may initially involve autoregulatory vascular adjustments of various tissues to decreased perfusion, but this mechanism would not be expected to remain operative after CO is normalized.

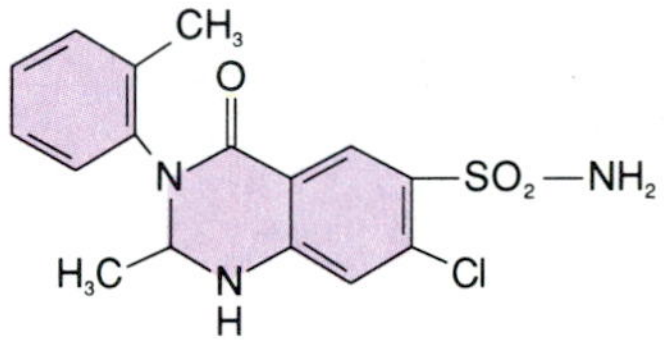

Other possible mechanisms include decreased vascular reactivity to norepinephrine and other endogenous pressor substances, or decreased "structural" vascular resistance secondary to removal of sodium chloride and water from the blood vessel wall. These changes could result directly from the tissue actions of diuretic drugs or indirectly from the generalized loss of sodium chloride and water from the body. The latter possibility seems probable in light of the observation that diuretics fail to lower blood pressure in patients who do not exhibit salt and water loss (i.e., patients on hemodialysis who have had a nephrectomy). However, the antihypertensive actions of diuretics do not parallel their efficacy in causing fluid loss, except in patients with renal insufficiency.

Finally, some diuretics relax vascular smooth muscle directly, but for most agents in this class vasodilation occurs only at doses well above the effective diuretic range. An exception is indapamide, which is a vasodilator at normal therapeutic doses, an action probably producing a major portion of its antihypertensive effect.

chlorthalidone

metolazone

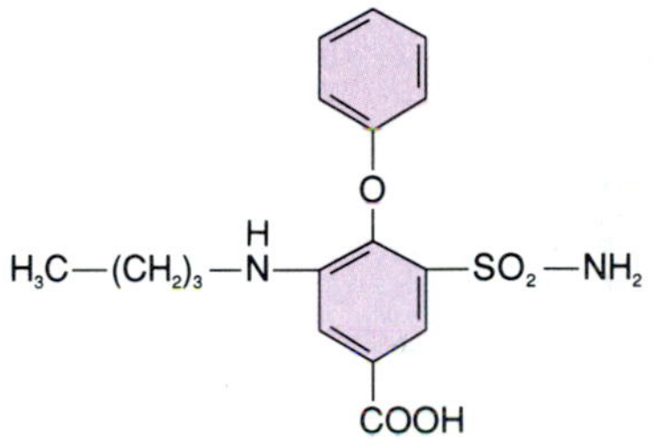

bumetanide

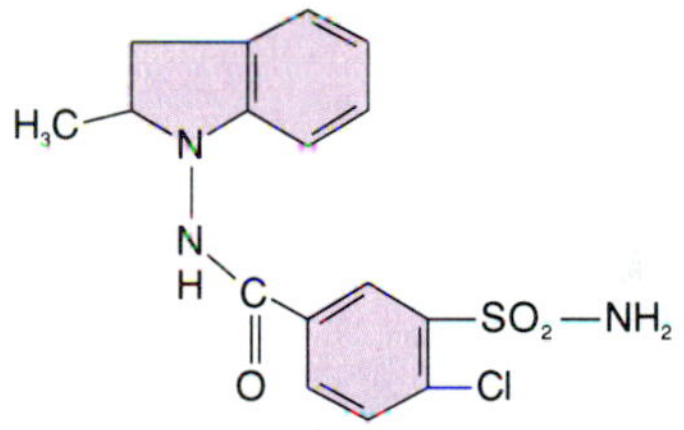

indapamide

FIGURE 13-4 Some of the diuretics used in the treatment of hypertension. See Chapter 19 for structures of additional compounds.

β-Adrenergic Receptor Blockers (β-Blockers)

The common characteristic of β-blockers is their ability to antagonize competitively the effects of the sympathetic effectors norepinephrine and epinephrine on cardiac β-adrenergic receptors. Although many β-adrenergic receptor antagonists have other pharmacological effects, it is clear that blockade of cardiac β-adrenergic receptors is partially responsible for their ability to lower blood pressure. Compounds that exhibit selectivity for the β_1 subtype of adrenergic receptors are effective antihypertensives; thus, one hypothesis is that all drugs in this class exert their effects on blood pressure through β_1-adrenergic receptor blockade.

The chemical structures of some β-blocking drugs used as antihypertensive agents are given in Figure 13-5 and in Chapter 10.

The details of secondary messenger systems of β-adrenergic receptors are given in Chapters 2 and 10.

Numerous reasons have been proposed to explain the antihypertensive response to administration of β block-

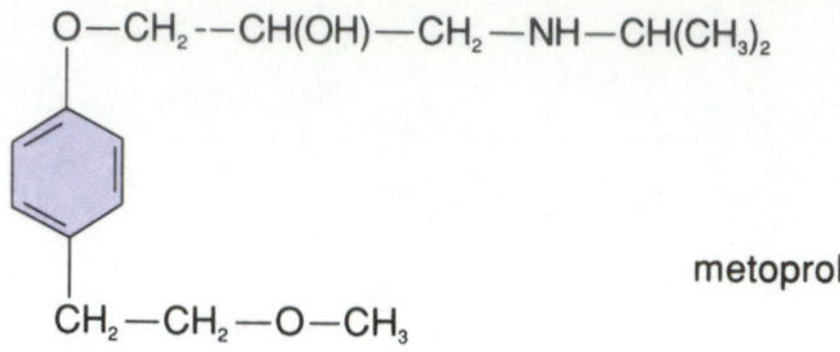

O—CH_2—CH(OH)—CH_2—NH—$CH(CH_3)_2$

CH_2—CH_2—O—CH_3

metoprolol

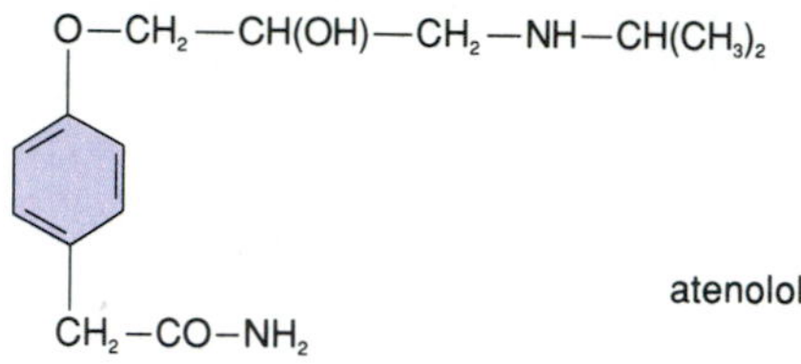

O—CH_2—CH(OH)—CH_2—NH—$CH(CH_3)_2$

CH_2—CO—NH_2

atenolol

CH(OH)—CH_2—NH—$CH(CH_3)$—CH_2—CH_2

—CO—NH_2

OH

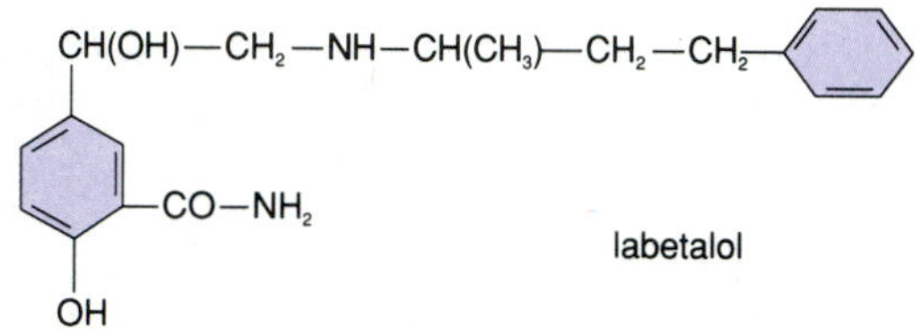

labetalol

FIGURE 13-5 Metoprolol and atenolol are highly selective blockers for β_1-adrenergic receptors. Other β-blockers used in hypertension are not so selective for β_1-receptors; their structures are shown in Chapter 10. Labetalol also acts by blocking α-receptors. Propranolol is not selective for β_1-receptors but is the prototype β-blocker.

ers; none has achieved universal acceptance. In patients with "renin-dependent" hypertension (e.g., renovascular hypertension), a major portion of the blood pressure reduction caused by β-blockers is caused by inhibition of renin release secondary to blockade of β_1-adrenergic receptors present on renin-secreting juxtaglomerular cells in the kidney and innervated by sympathetic nerves. Many hypertensive patients with low or normal plasma renin activity, however, also respond to β-blocker therapy. Thus, therapeutic response cannot be predicted based on pretreatment plasma renin values. Furthermore, β-blockers such as pindolol, which have strong intrinsic sympathomimetic agonist activity, decrease blood pressure without affecting plasma renin activity.

Acute and chronic decreases in CO are observed in most studies employing β-blockers in hypertensive patients, but in some studies CO is reported to return to normal over a period of days to weeks, whereas TPR also declines over the same time. The decrease in TPR may be the result of long-term autoregulatory response to decreased tissue blood flow or to other effects of the drugs. However, some patients exhibit an increase in TPR after β-blockade, which has led to speculation that vascular α-receptors may be activated. For this reason β-blockers are contraindicated in patients with peripheral vascular disease. An initial decrease in CO may therefore be necessary for the antihypertensive action of β-blockers, but it is not sufficient alone because CO declines similarly in patients whose blood pressure does not decrease with administered β-blockers.

The sharp decrease in blood pressure (hours) after β-blockade causes a reflex increase in plasma catecholamines, which is less than that produced by directly acting vasodilators. This fact may reflect an ability of β-blockers to interfere with cardiovascular reflexes, or to inhibit release of norepinephrine from sympathetic nerve terminals by blocking a facilitatory prejunctional β_2-adrenergic receptor. However, not all β-blockers inhibit baroreflexes or sympathetic neurotransmission; all lower blood pressure.

Some evidence such as reduced excretion of catecholamines is suggestive of a CNS-mediated sympathoinhibitory action for β-blockers. Several of these drugs (e.g., propranolol) readily penetrate into the brain, and side effects attributable to perturbation of CNS processes are common with such agents. Studies in experimental animals also indicate that selective administration of β-blockers into the cerebral ventricles lowers blood pressure at doses that are ineffective peripherally. Evidence against the hypothesis is that some drugs in this class do not readily penetrate into the brain after oral administration but retain antihypertensive efficacy. Furthermore, sympathetic neural activity is not reliably reduced by β-blockers at clinically effective doses. It must be understood, however, that although brain penetration is minimal overall, selective access to the CNS at the loci of the circumventricular organs that lack a blood-brain barrier could contribute to the putative central antihypertensive action.

Labetalol is unique among β-blockers in also possessing substantial α-adrenergic receptor blocking properties. This accounts for the greater blood pressure-lowering ability of labetalol compared with other β-blockers.

Centrally Acting Sympatholytics

Sympatholytics with central actions are believed to decrease blood pressure by causing a reduced sympathetic nerve firing rate; the locus of their action is within the CNS. The reduced sympathetic discharge is functionally selective because a hypotensive effect is obtained with only minimal impairment of baroreflexes. Drugs in this class include *methyldopa, clonidine, guanfacine,* and *guanabenz.* Reserpine also may act in part by this mechanism, but it is discussed with the peripherally acting sympatholytics. The chemical structures and mechanism of action of the sympatholytics are discussed further in Chapter 10.

Clonidine, guanfacine, and *guanabenz* are relatively selective agonists at α_2-adrenergic receptors (i.e., their interaction with α_1-adrenergic receptors is minimal, especially in the CNS). These agents readily enter the brain after systemic administration. Evidence that blood pressure reduction occurs as a result of an effect of these substances on α_2-adrenergic receptors in the CNS includes findings that (1) pressure is lowered in experimental animals by low doses injected directly into the cerebral ventricles, into specific brain regions, or selectively into the arterial blood supply of the brain, and (2) the depressor response to peripherally and centrally administered clonidine or guanabenz can be attenuated by intracerebral injection of α_2-adrenergic receptor antagonists. The precise brain site (or sites) where α_2-agonists act to lower blood pressure is controversial, but current evidence favors the ventrolateral medulla.

An endogenous clonidinelike material (clonidine-displacing substance) has been isolated from the brain of experimental animals. The clonidine-displacing substance appears to act in the ventrolateral medulla in a manner similar to clonidine, but at receptors that have high affinity for the imidazole moiety of clonidine. *Guanabenz* and *guanfacine* would not be expected to act at these receptors because they lack an imidazole structure. The relative role of imidazole versus α_2-adrenergic receptors in the antihypertensive response to clonidine is thus unclear, but newly developed drugs selective for imidazoline receptors such as moxonidine and rilmenidine exhibit good antihypertensive activity and may cause fewer side effects than clonidine does. Some studies indicate that the antihypertensive effect of clonidine may involve the release of endogenous opiate peptides. *Clonidine* has reasonable analgesic potency, and the depressor response to clonidine can be inhibited by the opioid antagonist naloxone. Finally, it is possible that under some circumstances activation of α_2-adrenergic receptors located on sympathetic nerve terminals may lead to inhibition of the release of norepinephrine during nerve activity.

Methyldopa is the drug in this class most commonly employed clinically for reductions of blood pressure. Methyldopa (L-isomer) is a prodrug and must be converted in the CNS by dopa decarboxylase and dopamine-β-hydroxylase to active α-methylnorepinephrine to exert an effect on blood pressure. Because α-methylnorepinephrine is a strong agonist at α_2-adrenergic receptors, it may also act at that site. Similar actions are found with the related metabolites α-methylepinephrine and α-methyldopamine. A peripheral action of methyldopa is unlikely because selective blockade of dopa decarboxylase in peripheral noradrenergic nerves does not influence the hypotensive response to methyldopa. As with clonidine, a potential site of action for methyldopa is within the nucleus of the solitary tract. This region contains interneurons that relay inhibitory information from baroreceptor terminals to excitatory vasomotor regions in the rostral ventral medulla. Activation of presynaptic α_2-adrenergic receptors in these interneurons inhibits sympathetic discharge. Noradrenergic innervation of the nucleus of the solitary tract provides the neural substrate for local synthesis and release of α-methylnorepinephrine and related amines.

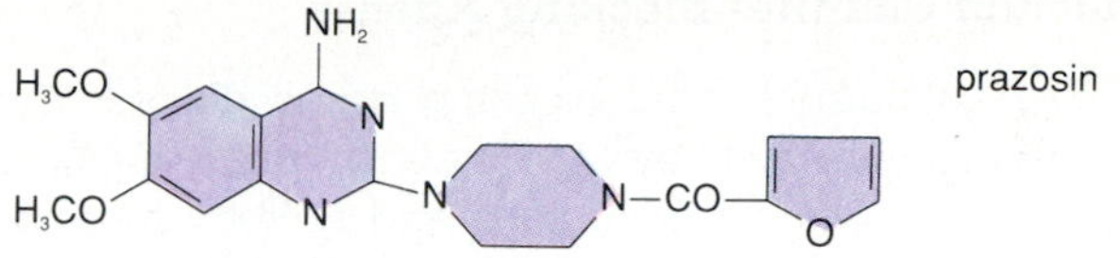

NH₂ H₃CO H₃CO N N N N—CO O prazosin

FIGURE 13-6 A peripherally acting sympatholytic (see Chapter 10 for structures of others).

Peripherally Acting Sympatholytics

Sympatholytics with peripheral action lower blood pressure by interfering with sympathetic neural control of cardiac and peripheral vascular function through effects produced on the sympathetic neuroeffector junction. Reserpine (Figure 13-6) blocks the uptake of dopamine and norepinephrine into storage granules of the sympathetic nerve terminal and subsequently depletes the terminal of neurotransmitter. Thus, a reduced release of transmitter occurs during terminal depolarization. Reserpine also acts centrally to decrease sympathetic outflow by an unknown mechanism. This could be related to depletion of norepinephrine or serotonin in the brain. *Guanethidine* and *guanadrel* inhibit exocytotic release of norepinephrine by a local anesthetic-like action on the nerve terminal. This requires uptake of the drugs by the nerve terminal catecholamine pump. Long-term treatment also results in depletion of transmitter from storage granules in peripheral sympathetic nerves. Guanethidine and guanadrel do not enter the brain.

Unlike the other agents in this class, *prazosin* (see Figure 13-6) acts at the postjunctional side of the sympathetic neuroeffector junction. It occupies α_1-adrenergic receptors selectively and blocks the effects mediated through this receptor of norepinephrine released from sympathetic nerves. Experimental data indicate that prazosin and other α_1-antagonist-like doxazosin or terazosin also can inhibit sympathetic nerve activity through a central mechanism.

The sympatholytic mechanisms are discussed in Chapter 10.

Calcium-Channel Blocking Agents

The calcium-channel blocking drugs decrease calcium entry into cells by binding to proteins of calcium channels in the cell membrane and thereby inhibiting transmembrane calcium movement. The antihypertensive actions of the calcium-channel blockers are discussed in Chapter 16.

Orally Active Direct Vasodilators

Agents in this class (*hydralazine* and *minoxidil*) lower blood pressure by direct relaxation of arterial smooth muscle (see Figure 13-7 for structures). They differ from calcium-channel blockers by different presumed cellular mechanisms of action and by greater selectivity for arterial smooth muscles. Calcium-channel antagonists do not show selectivity, and affect both arterial and venous smooth muscle.

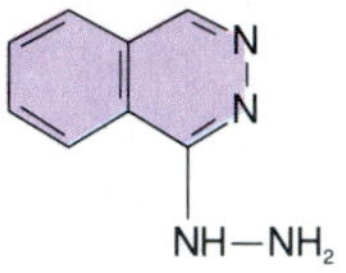

hydralazine

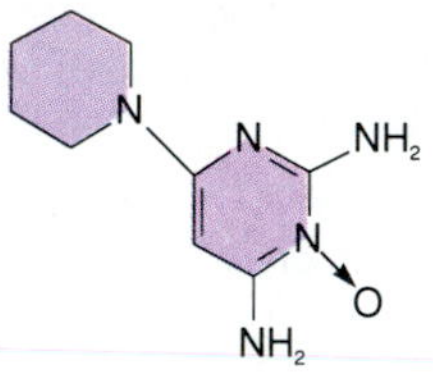

minoxidil

FIGURE 13-7 Structures of antihypertensive drugs that act as direct vasodilators.

The cellular mechanism of vascular relaxation caused by hydralazine is not known but may involve intracellular accumulation of cyclic guanosine monophosphate. Administration of hydralazine to experimental animals also causes release of vasodilator prostaglandins and results in a decreased responsiveness to sympathetic nerve stimulation. It is not known if these effects contribute to the hypotensive action of the drug clinically.

Minoxidil appears to cause vascular relaxation by increasing cellular potassium permeability, thus leading to potassium efflux from the cell, membrane hyperpolarization, and inhibition of stimulated calcium influx through receptor-operated calcium channels. Newer drugs with this mechanism of action are under development.

Angiotensin Converting Enzyme (ACE) Inhibitors

The active component of the renin-angiotensin system, angiotensin II, is generated by the enzymatic conversion from the decapeptide angiotensin I, described earlier in this chapter. The enzyme catalyzing this reaction, converting enzyme (or kininase II), has a wide distribution in the body but is found in highest activity in the endothelium of the pulmonary vasculature, probably because of the large length of the pulmonary capillaries. Converting enzyme inhibitors such as *captopril, enalapril,* and *lisinopril* (Figure 13-8) reversibly inhibit this enzyme. Although converting enzyme has a substantial number of physiological substrates that possess cardiovascular activity (or where the enzymatic products have cardiovascular activity), the hypotensive response to ACE inhibitors is the result of inhibition of

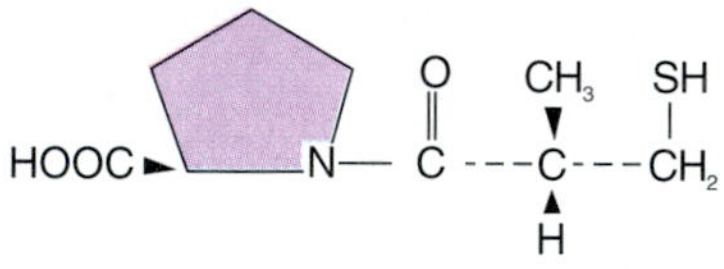

captopril

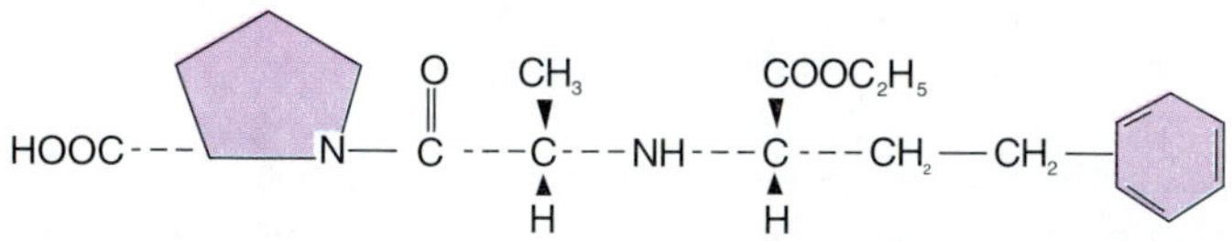

enalapril

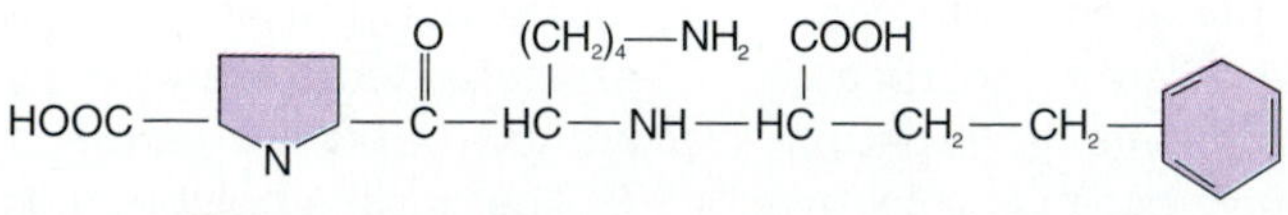

lisinopril

FIGURE 13-8 Converting enzyme inhibitors.

angiotensin II formation, especially in hypertensive patients in whom circulating blood concentrations of this peptide are elevated.

When angiotensin II concentration in the plasma is relatively high (i.e., approximately 100 pg/ml) the peptide causes direct arterial constriction. Inhibition of angiotensin II formation reduces vasoconstriction, and blood pressure decreases. However, hypertensive subjects with lower, or even normal, plasma concentrations of angiotensin II also exhibit a depressor response to converting enzyme inhibition. The mechanism of this effect is less clear. One possibility is that the converting enzyme inhibitors act by blocking local tissue generation of angiotensin II, and some evidence indicates that inhibition of vascular converting enzyme activity correlates temporally with the hypotensive response to ACE inhibitors. Angiotensin II also can be produced by intrarenal renin, where the peptide exerts an antinatriuretic and antidiuretic effect. Inhibition of intrarenal angiotensin II formation by ACE inhibitors could lower blood pressure by promoting salt and water excretion in a manner similar to that of the diuretic agents. A third possibility is that the ACE inhibitors act through inhibition of brain converting enzyme. Brain tissue can generate angiotensin peptides independently, and in experimental animals an increase in intracerebral concentrations of angiotensin II causes an elevation in arterial pressure mediated through activation of the sympathetic nervous system. The ACE inhibitors could decrease blood pressure by reducing the activity of the sympathetic nervous system in a manner similar to that of the centrally acting sympatholytic agents.

A final possibility to explain the depressor response to ACE inhibitors in hypertensive subjects with normal circulating concentrations of angiotensin II is that such individuals are hyperresponsive to circulating angiotensin II. The blood-borne peptide is capable of increasing blood pressure by numerous mechanisms. These include direct vasoconstriction, renal sodium and water retention, release of aldosterone, and peripheral and central augmentation of sympathetic neural input to the cardiovascular system. Although hypertensive patients do not generally exhibit an increased sensitivity to the systemic vasoconstrictor effects of angiotensin II, heightened sensitivity of one or more of the indirect pressor mechanisms previously listed could lead to activation even by normal circulating amounts of angiotensin II.

Drugs for Hypertensive Emergencies

Under some clinical circumstances, blood pressure must be reduced rapidly but in a controlled fashion for a relatively short period (see box). Several of the antihypertensive agents already discussed are given parenterally for this purpose. Other drugs are used exclusively to achieve rapid blood pressure reduction, including the direct-acting vasodilators *nitroprusside* and *diazoxide* (Figure 13-9) and the short-acting ganglionic blocker trimethaphan.

Nitroprusside acts by increasing cGMP concentrations in vascular smooth muscle cells and thereby reducing intracellular calcium-ion concentrations. *Diazoxide,* though related chemically to the thiazide diuretics, produces vasodilatation by an unknown cellular mecha-

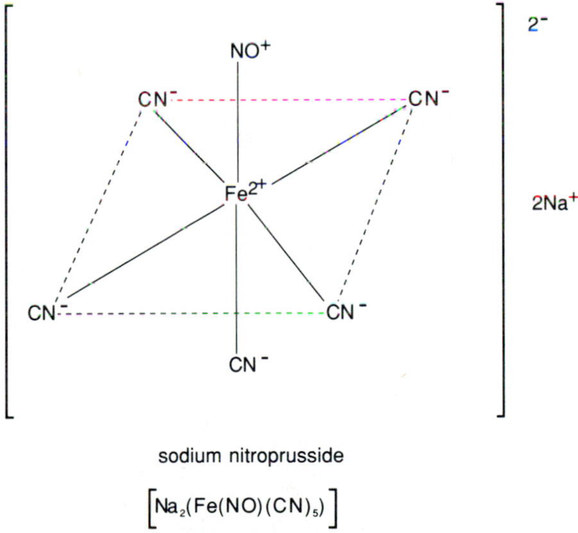

diazoxide

FIGURE 13-9 Rapid-acting antihypertensive drugs for emergency reduction of blood pressure.

CONDITIONS REQUIRING RAPID BLOOD PRESSURE REDUCTION

"Malignant" hypertension
Pheochromocytoma
Hypertensive encephalopathy
Refractory hypertension of pregnancy
Acute left ventricular failure
Aortic dissection
Coronary insufficiency
Intracranial hemorrhage

nism of action. *Trimethaphan* is a reversible nicotinic receptor antagonist that blocks neurotransmission through all autonomic ganglia. Diazoxide is primarily an arterial vasodilator, whereas nitroprusside and trimethaphan produce equivalent relaxation of both arteries and veins.

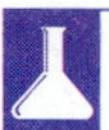

PHARMACOKINETICS

The pharmacokinetic parameters for most of the antihypertensive drugs are summarized in Table 13-2.

The diuretics are generally given orally. The onset of antihypertensive action occurs in 2 to 3 days, with a plateau of action within 2 to 3 weeks. The β-blockers also are administered orally, with labetalol also available for IV use. The antihypertensive effect usually is observed within a few hours.

Dosing schedules typically require more than one dose per day, though the long half-life of some drugs and long-acting preparations require only single-dose-per-day administration.

The sympatholytic agents are administered orally, with a rapid onset of action (few hours) for clonidine, guanabenz, guanadrel, guanfacine, guanethidine, and prazosin. Methyldopa, a prodrug, requires several hours for onset of action because of the need for conversion to the active species; and reserpine requires 2 to 3 weeks of treatment for the full antihypertensive effect to develop.

The oral direct vasodilators hydralazine and minoxidil show a rapid onset of action. Minoxidil, a prodrug, is metabolized to the active form, minoxidil sulfate. The rate of metabolism of hydralazine to form the acetylated amine depends on the patient acetylator phenotype; there being basically two groups, fast and slow acetylators.

With the oral converting enzyme inhibitors, the onset of action is rapid (minutes for captopril and hours for the prodrug enalapril).

Of the drugs used for emergency reduction of hypertensive conditions, diazoxide is usually given in repeated low-dose IV injections to achieve the desire reduction in blood pressure. An effect occurs 1 to 5 minutes after dosing. The duration of effect varies considerably, from hours to a day. Nitroprusside is given by continuous IV infusion; full effects occur in seconds, and recovery takes place within a few minutes of terminating the infusion. Trimethaphan must be administered by continuous IV infusion; full response occurs in seconds and is greater in magnitude when the patient is upright. Recovery of blood pressure after trimethaphan infusion requires 10 to 60 minutes.

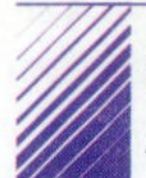

SIDE EFFECTS, CLINICAL PROBLEMS, AND TOXICITY

Diuretics are often used as adjuncts to other antihypertensive agents to prevent fluid retention, and diuretics potentiate the hypotensive effect of most other drugs. They are more effective in black than in white patients, perhaps because there is a high incidence of low renin hypertension among blacks. Lower doses of diuretics are required to treat hypertension than to treat edema. Larger doses do not result in a greater blood pressure reduction but simply increase the incidence and severity of side effects. There is concern that the hypokalemia frequently associated with diuretics may increase the incidence of ventricular arrhythmias. Monitoring of serum potassium concentration and the use of potassium supplements is often recommended. Additional details on the side effects of diuretics are found in Chapter 19.

β-blockers are particularly effective in younger patients and in individuals with high plasma renin activity. White patients respond somewhat better to β-blockers than black patients do. Side effects often observed with β-blocker therapy include nausea, anorexia, fatigue, dizziness, and bradycardia. Selective β_1-antagonists are preferable for use in patients with asthma, but any β-blocker should be used with caution. Abrupt cessation of β-blockers has been associated with tachycardia, angina pectoris, and (rarely) myocardial infarction. This may result from upregulation of β-adrenergic receptors with chronic β-blocker therapy.

Central acting sympatholytics *(clonidine, guanfacine, guanabenz,* or *methyldopa)* can be used alone in the treatment of hypertension but are often used in combination with a diuretic. These drugs are notable for causing less orthostatic hypotension than many other antihypertensive agents. They do not impair renal function and thus are suitable for hypertensive patients with renal insufficiency. Methyldopa is commonly used in pregnant women, in which long-term successful use has been documented. Side effects common to all three drugs are sedation, dry mouth, and dizziness. Methyldopa causes a positive direct Coombs' test in 20% to 30% of patients and frank hemolytic anemia in 1%. The latter, but not the former, requires drug withdrawal. A special problem associated with clonidine (and with other centrally acting α_2-agonists) is a dramatic hypertensive response occurring in some patients after abrupt withdrawal of therapy. It can be counteracted or prevented with the use of peripherally acting sympatholytic agents.

Of the peripheral acting drugs, *prazosin* (or *doxazo-*

Table 13-2 Pharmacokinetic Parameters

Agent	Plasma $t_{1/2}$ (hour)	Disposition	Selectivity	Remarks
B-BLOCKERS				
propranolol	2-3	M (100%)	β_1 β_2	
metoprolol (oral and IV)	3-7	M (90%)	β_1 (first-past effect)	
nadolol	20-24	R (100%)	β_1 β_2	
atenolol	6-7	R (100%)	β_1 (first-pass effect)	
pindolol	3-4	M (60%-65%)	β_1 β_2	
timolol	4	M (80%)	β_1 β_2	
labetalol (oral and IV)	6-8	M (90%)	β_1 β_2 α_1 α_2 (50% plasma protein bound, first-pass effect)	
betaxolal	14-22	M (85%)	β_1	
penbutalol	5	M (90%)	β_1 β_2	ISA
acebutalol	3-4	M (60%)	β_1	ISA
carteolol	6	R (60%)	β_1 β_2	ISA
SYMPATHOLYTICS				
clonidine	12-16	M (45%)		Given as prodrug
methyldopa	2-3	M (30%)		
guanabenz	4-6	M (98%)		
reserpine	33	M		96% bound to plasma protein
prazosin	3-4	M (95%)		Highly bound to plasma protein
guanadrel	12	M (60%), R (40%)		
guanethidine	5 days	M (50%), R (50%)		Strong tissue binding
guanfacine	12-28	M (50%)		
doxazosin	22	M (90%)		
terazosin	12	M (80%)		
DIRECT VASODILATORS				
hydralazine	2-4	M (100%)		Acetylators vary
minoxidil	4-5	M (90%)		Active, eliminated through kidney; given as prodrug
CONVERTING ENZYME INHIBITORS				
captopril	1-2	M (5%), R (50%)		Absorption reduced by food
enalapril*	11	Active metabolite eliminated by kidney		Given as prodrug
lisinopril†	12-24	R (mainly)		Does not require biotransformation to active drug
benazepril*	10-11	R (90%)		
fosinopril*	11-12	M (50%)		
quinapril*	2	R (95%)		
ramipril*	13-17	R (60%)		

ISA, Intrinsic sympathomimetic activity. *M*, metabolism (% of drug disposed of by this route); *R*, renal elimination as unchanged drug (% by this route).
*Metabolized by deesterification to more active diacid.
†Lysine derivative of enalapril.

sin or *terazosin*) is used to treat mild to moderate hypertension, usually in conjunction with a diuretic, guanadrel, and especially guanethidine and reserpine, are seldom used because of the frequent incidence of severe side effects.

Common side effects of *reserpine* are depression (including suicide), increased appetite, weight gain, sedation, and nasal congestion. Dizziness and weakness are side effects of *prazosin* and *guanadrel.* Side effects of *guanethidine* limit it to only occasional use in patients and include fluid retention, dizziness, weakness, retrograde ejaculation, impotence, and diarrhea.

The direct vasodilators *hydralazine* and *minoxidil* are used in combination with other drugs for the treatment of severe or resistant hypertension. Minoxidil is often effective in patients who do not respond to hydralazine. Relatively strong renal vasodilator activity makes these drugs particularly useful in patients with renal insufficiency.

The common side effects with *hydralazine* are headache, palpitations, dizziness, fatigue, tachycardia, and flushing. The incidence and severity of side effects with hydralazine use are greater in slow acetylators (see Chapter 5). A lupuslike syndrome has been observed in some patients taking hydralazine, mostly in slow acetylators taking high doses for long periods. The condition is reversible and necessitates discontinuation of the drug.

Common side effects of *minoxidil* are fluid retention, edema, palpitations, and abnormal hair growth. The latter effect limits compliance in patients and is being exploited to treat male-pattern baldness with topical application of the drug.

The ACE inhibitors *captopril, enalapril,* and *lisinopril* are effective for the treatment of hypertension in patients with normal or high levels of plasma renin. Black subjects thus respond less predictably than white subjects. Combining converting enzyme inhibitors with diuretics, however, lowers blood pressure in most patients and also reduce the incidence of diuretic-induced hypokalemia.

Common side effects observed in patients taking *captopril* are maculopapular rash, angioedema, cough, granulocytopenia, and diminished taste sensation. Similar side effects are observed with enalapril, though at a lower rate of incidence. Administration of converting enzyme inhibitors to patients with significant renal artery stenosis occasionally precipitates acute renal failure.

With drugs used for hypertensive emergencies, side effects can be significant. The usual side effects of diazoxide are fluid retention, tachycardia, and hyperglycemia. Nitroprusside reacts with blood and tissue to release cyanide ion, which is converted to thiocyanate by the liver. Thiocyanate concentrations in blood should be monitored during chronic nitroprusside infusions because this metabolite can cause hypothyroidism or acute toxic psychosis. If liver disease is present, cyanide concentrations should be monitored. Other reversible side effects of nitroprusside include nausea, headache, abdominal cramping, and dizziness. Side effects of *trimethaphan* are those expected from ganglionic blockade, including mydriasis, cycloplegia, constipation, and urinary retention. Tachyphylaxis occurs within a day or two of the development of the hypotensive action of trimethaphan.

Although the goal of antihypertensive therapy is to reduce end-organ damage associated with chronically elevated blood pressure, the effects on other cardiovascular risk factors must be considered. The end-organ damage is not related exclusively to blood pressure level. If an antihypertensive drug effectively lowers blood pressure but increases the influence of other risk factors for cardiovascular disease, the benefit of therapy will be reduced accordingly. This scenario may explain the apparent failure of thiazide diuretics to decrease coronary artery disease in large hypertensive populations, despite their ability to effect a significant reduction in blood pressure. Specifically, potassium-losing diuretics caused increments in total low-density and very-low-density lipoprotein cholesterol, and in total triglyceride content of blood of patients receiving these drugs over the long term. Although a causative relationship between blood lipid changes and the failure of diuretics to decrease coronary artery disease is not estab-

CLINICAL PROBLEMS

METHYLDOPA

Positive direct Coombs' test (usually but not always false)
Accumulates in patients with impaired renal function

Β-BLOCKERS

Use with caution in patients with bronchial asthma
Abrupt withdrawal may precipitate heart failure in patients with limited left ventricular function

CLONIDINE

Sudden withdrawal of drug produces rebound hypertension
CNS side effects

RESERPINE

Interacts with monoamine oxidase inhibitors
Use with caution in patients with peptic ulcers

HYDRALAZINE

Lupuslike syndrome

CAPTOPRIL

Accumulates in patients with impaired renal function
Hyperkalemia
Dry cough

GUANADREL

Interacts with tricyclic antidepressants

THIAZIDE DIURETICS

Potassium and magnesium loss
Increase in cholesterol concentrations
Arrhythmias

TRADE NAMES

In addition to generic and fixed-combination preparations, the following trade-named materials are available in the United States. (See Chapter 19 for diuretics, Chapter 10 for additional β-blockers, and Chapter 16 for calcium-channel blockers.)

SOME Β-BLOCKERS
Cartrol, carteolol
Inderal, propranolol
Kerlone, betaxolol
Levatol, penbutolol
Lopressor, metoprolol
Normodyne, labetalol
Sectral, acebutolol
Tenormin, atenolol
Trandate, labetalol

SYMPATHOLYTICS
Aldomet, methyldopa
Cardua, doxazosin
Catapres, clonidine
Hylorel, guanadrel
Hytrin, terazosin
Ismelin, guanethidine
Minipres, prazosin
Serpasil, reserpine
Tenex, guanfacine
Wytensin, guanabenz

CONVERTING ENZYME INHIBITOR
Accupril, guinapril
Altace, ramipril
Capoten, captopril
Lotensin, benazepril
Monopril, fosinopril
Prinivil, Zestril, lisinopril
Vasotec, enalapril

DIRECT VASODILATORS
Apresoline, hydralazine
Loniten, minoxidil

EMERGENCY TYPES
Arfonad, trimethaphan
Hyperstat, diazoxide

lished, it would seem prudent to consider the influence of antihypertensive agents on the blood lipid profile and other risk factors when one is choosing a drug for the individual patient.

Other cardiovascular risk factors that can be affected by antihypertensive drugs include plasma glucose, potassium, and uric acid concentrations. In particular, insulin resistance is now recognized to be prevalent in patients with hypertension. The resulting high insulin concentration is a risk factor for coronary artery disease. Thus it is noteworthy that thiazides and β-blockers increase, whereas ACE inhibitors and prazosin decrease, insulin resistance. Calcium-channel antagonists do not affect this parameter. There is interpatient variability in the response of these metabolites to antihypertensive drugs, and so therapeutic generalizations are difficult. Nonetheless, thiazide diuretics appear most likely to cause pressure-independent changes in cardiovascular risk, whereas calcium-channel antagonists and ACE inhibitors may actually improve the metabolic risk profile. Nonselective β-adrenergic receptor blockers have been shown to reduce the risk of sudden death during or after myocardial infarction in hypertensive patients. The mechanism is presumed to be a protection against catecholamine-induced ventricular fibrillation. The problems are summarized in the box.

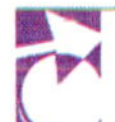

NEW DIRECTIONS

Several new approaches to the pharmacological therapy of hypertension may be available in the United States in the near future. Many that combine two distinct pharmacological activities into one chemical moiety drugs are being evaluated. Examples include (1) urapidil, an α_1-antagonist also having central sympatholytic activity; (2) β-blockers with additional properties such as α_1-antagonism, angiotensin converting enzyme inhibition or direct vasodilatation; and (3) ketanserin, a drug with antagonist activity at α_1-adrenergic and serotonergic (5-HT_2) receptors.

Other new drugs interfere with the renin-angiotensin system in novel ways. Chemicals that selectively block the AT_1 type of angiotensin II receptors and have good oral bioavailability are undergoing extensive laboratory and clinical evaluation as antihypertensives. Losartan is the prototype drug of this class. Progress also has been made in the long search for an orally active agent able to directly inhibit the enzyme renin.

Some currently used antihypertensives increase the open time probability of potassium channels in vascular smooth muscle, and other drugs with this action are being developed (e.g., chromkalim, pinacidil, and nicorandil). A unique approach to blood pressure lowering is an attempt to decrease the metabolism of endogenous vasodilator substances such as atrial natriuretic peptide. Thiorphan and similar drugs, which inhibit neutral endopeptidase 24.11, have shown good antihypertensive activity in early trials. Finally, a particularly promising new avenue for therapy is the discovery of drugs such as rilmenidine, which decrease sympathetic nervous system activity, presumably by activating imidazoline receptors in the brainstem. These agents may cause less sedation and dry mouth than is observed with other centrally acting sympatholytics, which interact with both imidazoline and α_2-adrenergic receptors.

REFERENCES

Harper KJ, Forker AD: Antihypertensive therapy: current issues and challenges, *Postgrad Med* 6:163, 1992.

The Fifth Report of the Joint National Committee on Detection, Evaluation, and Treatment of High Blood Pressure, NIH Publication no. 93-1088, 1993.

SELF-ASSESSMENT QUESTIONS

1. Abrupt cessation of antihypertensive therapy with β-blockers may be associated with all of the following *except:*
   a. salt and water retention.
   b. myocardial infarction.
   c. angina pectoris.
   d. tachycardia.
2. A drug that would be expected to reduce diuretic-induced hypokalemia is:
   a. hydralazine.
   b. captopril.
   c. prazosin.
   d. methyldopa.
   e. chlorthalidone.
3. Black patients respond less predictably to angiotensin converting enzyme inhibitors than white patients do because in general:
   a. they metabolize the drugs faster.
   b. their plasma aldosterone levels are higher.
   c. they have higher vascular resistance.
   d. their converting enzyme activity is higher.
   e. their plasma renin activity is lower.
4. This antihypertensive drug must be chemically modified to have biological activity:
   a. captopril
   b. propranolol
   c. prazosin
   d. clonidine
   e. methyldopa
5. A diuretic drug that also has substantial direct vasodilator effects is:
   a. metolazone.
   b. chlorthalidone.
   c. hydrochlorothiazide.
   d. indapamide.
   e. spironolactone.

CHAPTER 14 Cardiac Electrophysiology and Antiarrhythmic Agents

JOSEPH R. HUME

MAJOR DRUGS

- antiarrhythmics that block myocardial sodium channels
- sympatholytic antiarrhythmic agents (β-adrenergic receptor blockers)
- antiarrhythmics that block myocardial potassium channels
- antiarrhythmics that block myocardial calcium channels

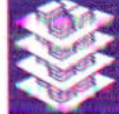

THERAPEUTIC OVERVIEW

Cardiac arrhythmias are disorders of rate, rhythm, impulse generation, or conduction of electrical impulses within the heart. They often are associated with coronary artery disease, including myocardial infarction and atherosclerotic heart disease. Arrhythmias disrupt the normal sequence of myocardial activation and can seriously compromise the mechanical efficiency of the heart, reducing cardiac output. As a result, arrhythmias can be life-threatening events that require immediate intervention.

Since 1949, experimental techniques have allowed investigators to better understand the cellular basis of the electrocardiogram, as well as the basic electrical properties of cardiac cells. These kinds of studies have provided an understanding of the many ionic currents and membrane channels that regulate cell behavior. Studies of the effects of clinically effective antiarrhythmic drugs on these specific membrane channels have led to an understanding of the way in which antiarrhythmic agents interact with individual ionic channels at a molecular level. At a higher organizational level, comprehension of the electrical properties of the different types of cardiac cells that compose the specialized electrical conduction system of the heart and how these are modified by a variety of therapeutic agents is the basis for understanding the normal electrocardiogram and its alterations in disease states or during drug therapy.

The electrical activity of individual cardiac cells depends on the region of the heart from which cells are derived (i.e., sinoatrial, SA, node; atrium; AV, atrioventricular, node; His-Purkinje system; ventricle). In addition, electrical activity may be modified by changes in extracellular pH and ion concentration, as occur during ischemia. Electrical activity arises as a result of differences in ion (Na^+, K^+, Ca^{++}) concentrations across the cell membrane caused by metabolism-dependent processes (e.g., the Na^+, K^+ –ATPase pump). The membrane potential thus established is modulated by ion-selective membrane channels that open and close in a voltage- and time-dependent manner to allow ions to flow through them down their respective electrochemical gradients. As in the other excitable tissues, the action potential thus generated is propagated throughout the myocardium. Arrhythmias result from disorders in impulse formation, its conduction, or both. Many antiarrhythmic drugs act by blocking myocardial Na^+ or Ca^{++} ion channels or by prolonging the time for these channels to recover from activation. Other antiarrhythmic compounds act by modulating the magnitude and course of K^+ currents responsible for action potential repolarization and maintenance of the diastolic membrane potential. These concepts are summarized in the box.

ABBREVIATIONS

AV	atrioventricular
SA	sinoatrial
$\dot{V}_{max}$	maximum rate of depolarization

THERAPEUTIC OVERVIEW

Goal:	To treat abnormal cardial impulse formation or conduction
Effects:	Modify ion fluxes, block Na^+, K^+, or Ca^{++} channels, modify β-adrenergic receptor–activated processes
DRUG CLASSES	USES
IA	Paroxysmal supraventricular tachycardia, atrial fibrillation or flutter, ventricular tachycardia
IB	Ventricular tachycardia, digoxin-induced arrhythmias
IC	Ventricular tachycardia, atrial fibrillation
II	Paroxysmal supraventricular tachycardia, atrial or ventricular premature beats, atrial fibrillation or flutter
III	Ventricular tachycardia, atrial fibrillation or flutter*
IV	Paroxysmal supraventricular tachycardia, atrial fibrillation or flutter
Other:	
Digitalis glycosides	Atrial fibrillation or flutter with increased ventricular rate
Adenosine	Paroxysmal supraventricular tachycardia

*Only amiodarone.

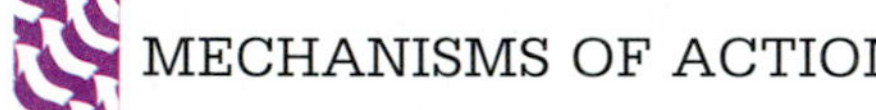

MECHANISMS OF ACTION

Cardiac Electrophysiology

Membrane Potentials An understanding of the molecular mechanisms of antiarrhythmic drugs requires knowledge of cardiac electrophysiology. To accomplish this goal, ionic currents from nonpacemaker type of cardiac cells (ventricular myocardium) and pacemaker type of cardiac cells (sinus node) are considered. Although the sinus node constitutes a dominant pacemaker region of the heart under normal conditions, many other regions are also capable of spontaneous rhythmic activity. An example is the His-Purkinje system, which comprises the specialized ventricular conducting system. Action potentials and ionic currents in these cells can range from similarity to those potentials in sinus node cells or those in other types showing distinctly different properties.

Figure 14-1 illustrates action potentials recorded from a typical nonpacemaker cell and a typical pacemaker cell. In the nonpacemaker cell, the resting membrane potential is usually in the range of −80 to −90 mV with respect to the extracellular medium. There is no spontaneous electrical discharge because the resting potential is stable. Excitation of this cell by intracellular current injection or by local flow from an adjoining cell can elicit a propagating action potential. This action potential is described as having the five following distinct phases:

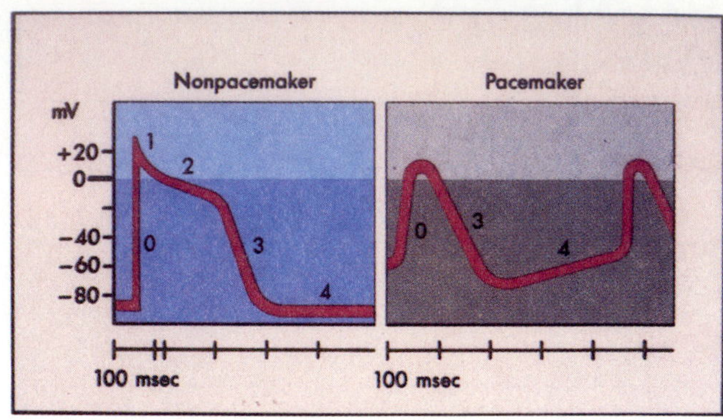

FIGURE 14-1 Phase of action potential (with respect to potential on extracellular side of cell membrane) in a nonpacemaker cell *(NP)* and in a pacemaker cell *(P)*. Numbers refer to phases. **NP cell:** *0*, rapid depolarization; *1*, initial repolarization; *2*, action potential plateau; *3*, repolarization; *4*, resting potential. **P cell:** *0*, rapid depolarization; *3*, plateau and repolarization; *4*, slow diastolic depolarization (pacemaker potential).

Phase 0, rapid depolarization
Phase 1, initial repolarization
Phase 2, action potential plateau
Phase 3, final repolarization
Phase 4, return to a stable diastolic potential

In the pacemaker cell, only three distinct phases of the action potential are described: *phase 0,* rapid depolarization; *phase 3,* plateau and repolarization; and *phase 4,* slow depolarization (often called the *pacemaker potential;* see below), which occurs during diastole and culminates in initiation of another spontaneous depolarization.

Ionic Basis of the Cardiac Resting Membrane Potential The membrane potential of a cardiac cell at any given time is determined by the activity of the electrogenic Na^+,K^+ pump and the permeability of the membrane to various ions (Table 14-1). The permeability involves the diffusion of ions across the membrane through various ion-selective channels. The reader is referred to an appropriate physiology text for the genesis of the resting membrane potential.

Ionic Basis of the Action Potential

Phase 0 Injection of current into a cardiac cell or local current flow from an adjoining cell can cause the membrane potential to depolarize. If the amplitude of depolarization is sufficient, the threshold potential for initiation of an action potential may be achieved. This threshold potential is related to the opening of active membrane channels, which may contribute to further depolarization and initiation of an action potential. This period of rapid depolarization in which the membrane potential changes from negative inside to positive inside relative to the outside is termed *phase 0* of the action potential. Which membrane channels are involved in mediating the depolarization depends on the type of cardiac cell and the level of diastolic potential.

In a nonpacemaker cell, an increase in conductance of Na^+ ions results in phase 0 depolarization. (The opening of membrane channels and the flow of ions through these channels can be described as a conductance change.) Because conductance is the reciprocal of resistance, an increase in membrane conductance is equivalent to a decrease in membrane resistance. The magnitude of the increase in conductance to Na^+ is related to the maximum rate of depolarization (dV/dt_{max}, or $\dot{V}_{max}$) during phase 0. As the membrane is depolarized, there is also increased Ca^{++} conductance during phase 0, normally contributing slightly to $\dot{V}_{max}$. These types of action potentials in nonpacemaker cells are often referred to as **fast responses** because $\dot{V}_{max}$ can be on the order of several hundred volts per second and are primarily due to an increase in Na^+ conductance.

Table 14-1 Typical Ion Concentrations

Ion	Extracellular	Intracellular	Approximate Equilibrium Potential (mV)*
Na^+	145 mM	10 mM	+50
K^+	4	150 mM	−90
Ca^{++}	2 mM	10^{-7} M	+140

*As calculated from Nernst equation.

In pacemaker cells, such as those found in the sinus node, conductance to Na^+ increases very little during phase 0. In these cells, phase 0 is mediated almost entirely by increased conductance of Ca^{++} ions. These types of action potentials are often referred to as **slow responses,** with $\dot{V}_{max}$ in the range of 1 to 20 V/sec.

Ion channels may operate in pacemaker and nonpacemaker cells as a function of membrane voltage and time. The voltage and time dependence of membrane currents through specific populations of ion channels is unique for that particular ion channel. Na^+ channels open at membrane voltages different from those for Ca^{++} channels, and the kinetics of the currents through these two channels are quite different. It is currently believed that physical structures composing portions of the channel protein act as molecular gates to regulate the opening and closing of the channel, as discussed in Chapter 2. In the case of Na^+ channels, an activation gate and an inactivation gate exist to regulate the flow of Na^+ through the channel. As a result of the operation of these gates, Na^+ channels are believed to exist

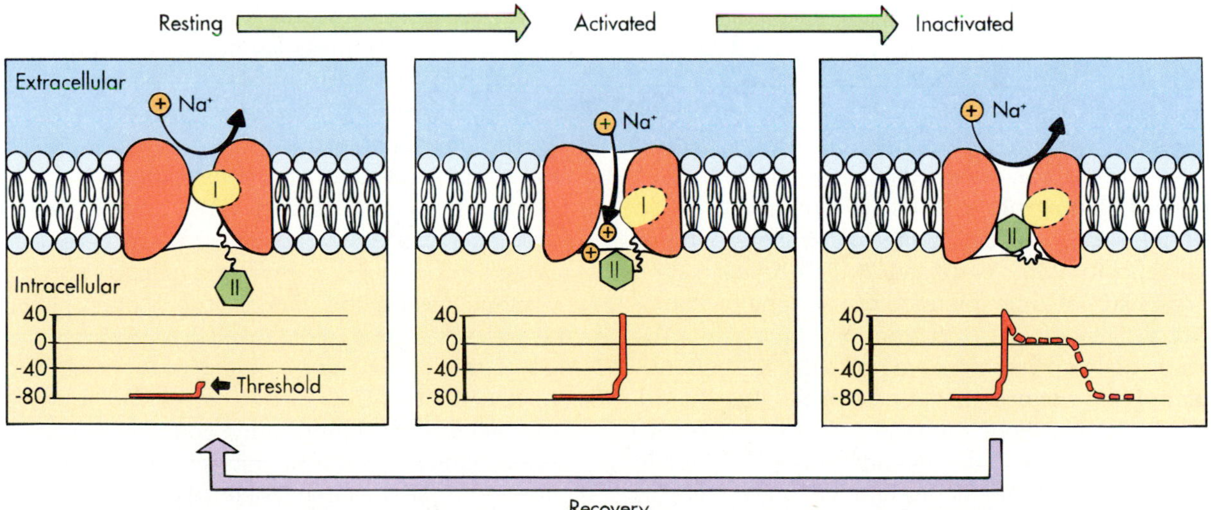

FIGURE 14-2 Postulated conformational arrangements of cardiac Na^+ channels compatible with concept of resting, activated, and inactivated states. Transitions between resting, activated, and inactivated states are dependent on membrane potential and time. Activation gate is shown as I and inactivation gate as II. Potentials typical for each state are shown under each channel schema as a function of time.

in at least three distinct states during the cardiac action potential, as shown in Figure 14-2. At the resting potential, most of the Na^+ channels are in a resting state, available for activation. On depolarization of the membrane potential to a level near the activation threshold for Na^+ channels, most channels become activated (gate I open), allowing Na^+ ions to flow into the cell to cause a rapid depolarization during phase 0. Very quickly, Na^+ channels become inactivated (gate II closes), limiting the time for Na^+ entry to a few milliseconds or less. A discussion of the characteristics of Ca^{++} in contrast to the Na^+ channel can be found in Chapter 16.

Phase 1 Near the end of phase 0, the action potential overshoot occurs. This is the most positive potential achieved during the action potential and represents an abrupt transition between the end of depolarization and the onset of repolarization. This phase of initial repolarization is caused by two factors: the inactivation of the inward Na^+ current and the activation of a transient outward current. The transient outward current is believed to involve activation of chloride and K^+ channels.

Phase 2 The plateau phase of the cardiac action potential is perhaps one of its most distinguishing features. In strong contrast to action potentials recorded in nerves and other types of cells, the cardiac action potential has a relatively long duration of 200 to 500 msec, depending on the type of cell (see Figure 14-1). The plateau results from a voltage-dependent decrease in potassium conductance (the inward rectifier) and is maintained by the influx of Ca^{++} through Ca^{++} channels that inactivate slowly at positive membrane potentials. During this phase there also is slow activation of another outward K^+ current, the plateau-delayed rectifier, which nearly balances the maintained influx of Ca^{++}. As a result of the offsetting effect of these currents, there is only a small change in potential during the plateau because the net conductance change is small.

Phase 3 The slowly increasing magnitude of the plateau-delayed K^+ current begins to dominate, and this triggers repolarization, or phase 3. The repolarization phase results from a combination of two factors: inactivation of the plateau Ca^{++} current and increase in the magnitude of the plateau-delayed rectifier K^+ current.

Phase 4 In a nonpacemaker cell, phase 4 is characterized by return of the membrane potential to the resting potential of the cell. It depends on an increase in the conductance of the potassium channels. At this time during diastole, the potential is relatively stable. In a pacemaker cell, however, there is a slow depolarization during diastole that brings the membrane potential into the threshold range for activation of a regenerative inward current, which will initiate a new action potential (see Figure 14-1). This period of diastolic depolarization is often called *phase 4 depolarization,* or simply the **pacemaker potential.** In a pacemaker cell in the sinus node region, phase 4 depolarization brings the membrane potential to a level near the threshold for activation of the inward Ca^{++} current, as previously discussed.

Phase 4 depolarization is the result of deactivation and activation of several ion-selective channels. The final repolarization phase of the action potential results from deactivation of the outward plateau K^+ current. This current is activated at positive membrane potentials. As repolarization proceeds, this current begins to decline or deactivate. Decline of this outward current is believed to occur during phase 4 and significantly to influence the course of the pacemaker potential. A declining K^+ current in the presence of a background leakage current of Na^+ may account for diastolic depolarization. Activation of the Ca^{++} and a nonselective inward current (I_f) may also play a role.

Mechanisms Underlying Cardiac Arrhythmias

Most arrhythmias are considered to result from disorders of impulse formation, impulse conduction, or a combination of both. Several factors are believed to be involved in precipitating cardiac arrhythmias: ischemia with resulting pH and electrolyte abnormalities, excessive myocardial fiber stretch, excessive discharge of or sensitivity to autonomic transmitters, or exposure to foreign chemicals or toxic substances. There is an 80% to 90% occurrence of arrhythmias associated with myocardial infarction, 20% to 50% with general anesthesia, and 10% to 20% with digitalis therapy.

Disorders of impulse formation can involve (1) no change in pacemaker site (e.g., sinus bradycardia or tachycardia) or (2) a change in pacemaker site involving the development of a ectopic pacemaker. Several factors might lead to the development of an ectopic pacemaker. Ectopic activity might arise because of the emergence of a latent pacemaker. Many cells of the specialized conduction system are capable of rhythmic spontaneous activity. Normally these latent pacemakers are prevented from spontaneously discharging as a result of the dominance of the rapidly firing SA nodal pacemaker cells. Under some conditions, however, a latent pacemaker might become dominant because of abnormal slowing of the SA rate or because of abnormal acceleration of the latent pacemaker rate. Ectopic pacemaker activity might result from a current of injury. Myocardial cells that are damaged by ischemia or hypoxia become depolarized and may affect nearly normally polarized tissue. Two areas of cells with different membrane potentials may therefore cause current to flow be-

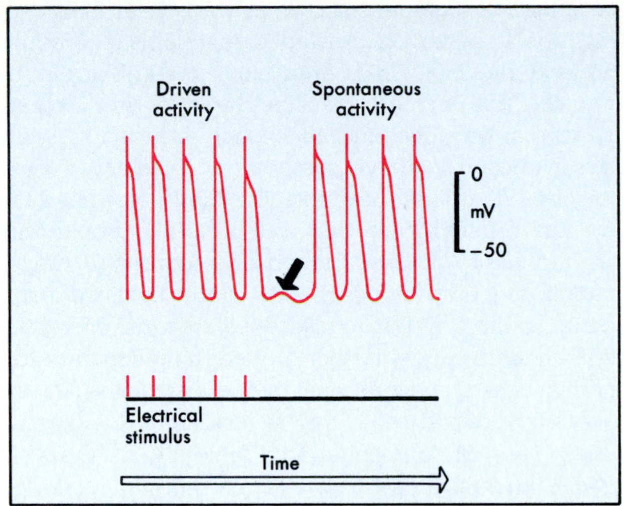

FIGURE 14-3 Development of oscillatory delayed afterdepolarization *(arrow)* that leads to spontaneous activity, as observed with cardiac glycosides. First five action potentials were elicited by electrical stimuli (bottom trace), followed by an afterdepolarization, which was subthreshold initially but attained threshold subsequently, leading to spontaneous discharges.

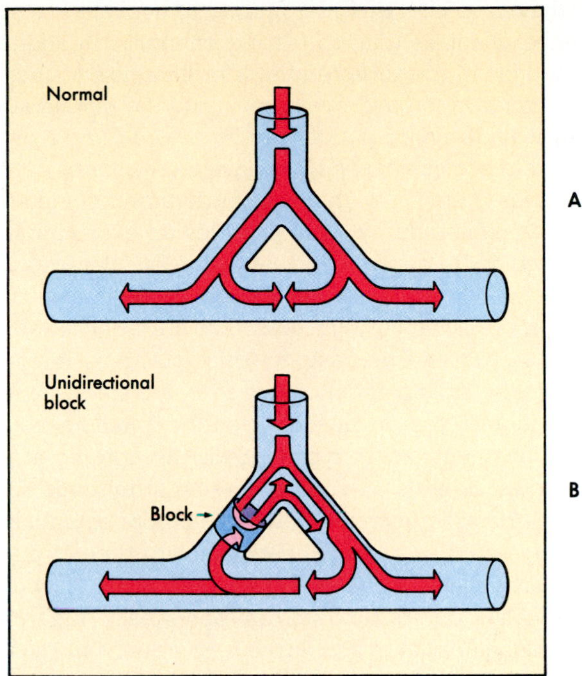

FIGURE 14-4 Hypothetical reentry circuit. **A,** Normally electrical excitation branches around the circuit and becomes extinguished because of collision. **B,** An area of unidirectional block develops in one of the branches, allowing excitation of the blocked area by an impulse traveling from the opposite direction. This can lead to reexcitation and reentry.

tween adjacent regions (injury current), which can depolarize normally quiescent tissue to the point where spontaneous activity is initiated. Finally the development of oscillatory afterdepolarization can initiate spontaneous activity in normally quiescent tissue. These afterdepolarizations can occur at the end of phase 3 (Figure 14-3) and, if large enough in amplitude, reach threshold and initiate a burst of triggered spontaneous activity. Toxic concentrations of digitalis or norepinephrine can initiate this type of activity.

Disorders of impulse conduction can be grouped into those not involving reentry and those involving a reentrant circuit. Differing degrees of nodal block involve slowed conduction, usually without reentry. Slowed conduction with reentry can lead to the development of circus movement within some regions of the heart. Figure 14-4 shows an example of a hypothetical reentry circuit. For circus activity to develop, a region of unidirectional block must exist and the conduction time around the alternative pathway must exceed the effective refractory period of the tissue adjacent to the site of the block. Before the development of unidirectional block (Figure 14-4, *A*), impulse propagation initially branches as a result of the anatomical properties of the circuit. Some of these impulses collide and extinguish around the other side of the branch point. If an area of unidirectional block develops, impulses around the branch do not collide and become extinguished but may reexcite tissue proximal to the site of block, establishing a circular pathway for continuous reentry (Figure 14-4, *B*). A long reentry pathway, slow conduction, and a short effective refractory period are factors that favor the development of reentry circuits.

Specific Antiarrhythmic Drugs

In the normal heart, antiarrhythmic agents have minimal effects on automaticity and conduction velocity at therapeutic concentrations. However, at toxic concentrations, they can depress automaticity and conduction velocity and even be arrhythmogenic. Because arrhythmias usually involve abnormal automaticity or conduction, most antiarrhythmic agents seem to depress selectively areas exhibiting abnormal pacemaker activity or conduction while having minimal effects on normal healthy tissue. Conditions such as hypoxia, metabolic poisoning, ischemia, or abnormal extracellular K^+ are known to precipitate arrhythmias. All of these conditions depolarize myocardial cells. Therefore one possible mechanism for the selectivity of antiarrhythmic agents is that they cause a greater degree of depression in cells that are depolarized, compared with normally polarized cells.

Most antiarrhythmic agents block myocardial Na^+, K^+, or Ca^{++} channels in a state-dependent manner; that is, they bind with a higher affinity to activated or inactivated channels than to resting channels. In addition, they prolong the time required for channels to recover from inactivation and cycle back into the resting state. This is shown schematically in Figure 14-5. As a result, cells that become depolarized have more channels in the inactivated state and bind antiarrhythmic compounds with a higher affinity. This provides an explanation for their ability to depress depolarized cells selectively.

In normally polarized cells, these drugs may also exhibit some selectivity for cells that are firing at abnormally fast rates. The basis for this selectivity might be the prolongation of the recovery of inactivated channels. This is believed to account for the phenomenon of "frequency-dependent block." Cells discharging at normal rates are little affected by an antiarrhythmic agent if the diastolic interval between action potentials is longer than the drug-modified recovery time of inactivated channels (Figure 14-6, *A*). However, for an ectopic pacemaker discharging at an abnormally high rate, channels are selectively blocked, as evidenced by a reduction of $\dot{V}_{max}$, if the diastolic interval between action potentials is shorter than the drug-modified recovery time of inactivated channels (Figure 14-6, *B*).

There is no universally accepted classification scheme for antiarrhythmic agents. One commonly used classification scheme is shown in Table 14-2. This classification is based on presumed mechanism of action and is derived primarily from experimental studies in animals. This scheme classifies agents that depress myocardial Na^+ channels and hence reduce $\dot{V}_{max}$ into class I, those that have sympathetic blocking actions into class II, agents that prolong action potential duration and refractoriness into class III, and agents with Ca^{++}-channel blocking properties into class IV. Classification is complicated by the dose because some agents exhibit multiple classes of action. Moreover, class I agents can be further grouped into separate categories based on additional properties. Class IA are agents that depress $\dot{V}_{max}$, slow conduction, and cause action potential prolongation (Table 14-3). Class IB agents have little effect on $\dot{V}_{max}$ of normal tissue but depress $\dot{V}_{max}$ of abnormal tissue and shorten action potential duration. Class IC agents greatly depress $\dot{V}_{max}$, slow conduction, and have slight effects on action potential duration. Although this classification scheme is useful for learning the properties of antiarrhythmic agents, it must be emphasized that all classification schemes have limited usefulness in the clinical treatment of arrhythmias because of the complex pathophysiology of these events. As new information becomes available on underlying mechanisms of different types of clinical arrhythmias, new classification schemes will emerge.

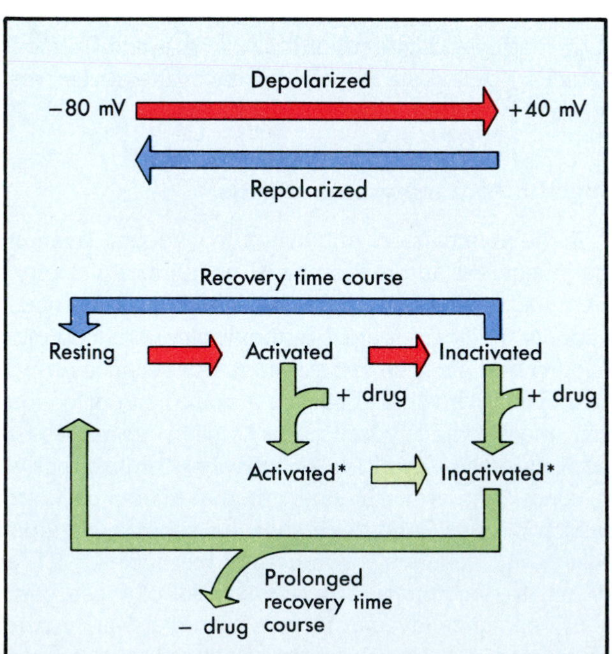

FIGURE 14-5 State-dependent binding of antiarrhythmic drugs to cardiac Na^+ channels. Preferential binding to the activated and inactivated states of the sodium channel occurs, and recovery from inactivation is prolonged in the presence of these drugs.

Class I Antiarrhythmic Agents The structures of these drugs are shown in Figure 14-7.

Quinidine Quinidine (Class IA) is an optical isomer of quinine and is commonly used as an orally active an-

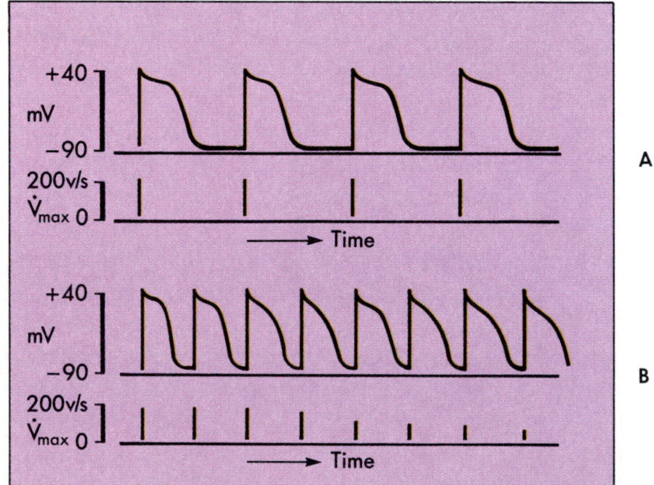

FIGURE 14-6 Frequency-dependent block of $\dot{V}_{max}$ by an antiarrhythmic drug. **A,** Cell is stimulated at relatively low frequency in presence of antiarrhythmic drug and $\dot{V}_{max}$ is not affected (second trace from top). **B,** At faster stimulation frequency, there is a progressive reduction of $\dot{V}_{max}$.

tiarrhythmic agent. It will reduce $\dot{V}_{max}$ of cardiac action potentials in a frequency dependent manner by its ability to preferentially block activated Na^+ channels. This effect can occur for Na^+-dependent action potentials in the atrium, ventricle, and His-Purkinje system. These actions are often described as "local anesthetic properties" of the drug and often manifest as a reduction in membrane responsiveness, which is an alteration in the relationship between $\dot{V}_{max}$ of the action potential and the resting membrane potential. Many other antiarrhythmic agents that block Na^+ channels produce a similar hyperpolarizing shift in the membrane-responsiveness relationship (Figure 14-8).

Quinidine also slows pacemaker activity by depressing the rate of phase 4 depolarization in SA nodal cells and especially in ectopic pacemakers. In addition, repolarization is prolonged, and the effective refractory period is lengthened in the atrium, ventricle, and His-Purkinje system. The effect on action potential duration is probably related to blockade of K^+ channels involved in mediating repolarization. The lengthening of the effective refractory period is caused by a combination of effects on myocardial Na^+ and K^+ channels.

Procainamide and Disopyramide The electrophysiological effects of procainamide and disopyramide are nearly identical to those of quinidine. These agents depress membrane responsiveness of Na^+-dependent action potentials by specifically blocking activated myocardial Na^+ channels.

Lidocaine Lidocaine (Class IB) is a local anesthetic agent that has been used as an antiarrhythmic agent since the late 1940s. It depresses membrane responsiveness primarily in cells in the ventricular myocardium and the His-Purkinje system. Unlike quinidine, lidocaine blocks activated and inactivated Na^+ channels. This additional interaction with the inactivated state of Na^+ channels might explain the relative selectivity of this agent for cells with longer action-potential durations, which are depolarized for longer periods, or depolarized because of ischemia or digitalis toxicity. As a result, atrial cells seem less sensitive to concentrations of lidocaine, which reduce $\dot{V}_{max}$ in ventricular cells of depolarized cells. At therapeutic concentrations, lidocaine has minimal effects on normal ventricular myocardial cells or cells in the specialized conduction system but significantly depresses damaged or depolarized cells.

Mexiletine and tocainide are chemically related derivatives of lidocaine that are orally active. Their electrophysiological effects, antiarrhythmic spectrum, and side effects are similar to lidocaine. They are resistant to the first-pass hepatic metabolism that occurs with lidocaine.

Phenytoin Phenytoin (diphenylhydantoin) was introduced in the 1930s as an anticonvulsive agent and

Table 14-2 Classification of Antiarrhythmic Agents

Class I (blockers of fast Na^+ channel)	Class II (β-blockers)	Class III (blockers of K^+ chaannels)	Class IV (blockers of Ca^{++} channel)
IA (moderate block)	propranolol	bretylium	verapamil
quinidine	metoprolol	amiodarone	diltiazem
procainamide	nadolol	sotalol	
disopyramide	atenolol		
	acebutolol		
IB (weak block)	pindolol		
lidocaine	sotalol		
phenytoin	timolol		
tocainide			
mexiletine			
IC (pronounced block)			
flecainide			
propafenone			

Table 14-3 Differences Among Class I Antiarrhythmic Drugs

	Phase 0 Depression	Repolarization	Action Potential Duration
IA	moderate	prolonged	increased
IB	weak	shortened	decreased
IC	strong	no effect	no effect

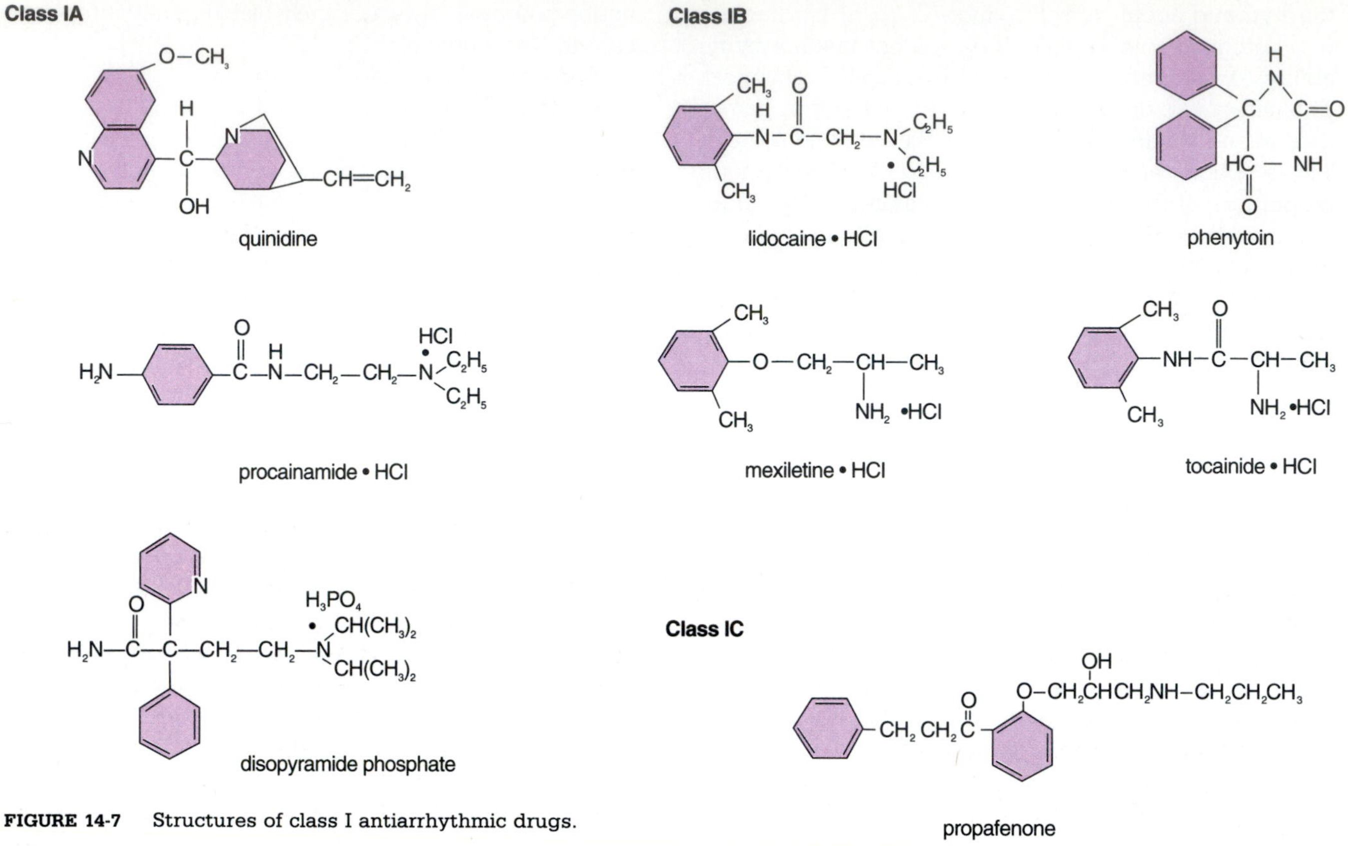

Class IA

quinidine

procainamide • HCl

disopyramide phosphate

Class IB

lidocaine • HCl

phenytoin

mexiletine • HCl

tocainide • HCl

Class IC

propafenone

flecainide

FIGURE 14-7 Structures of class I antiarrhythmic drugs.

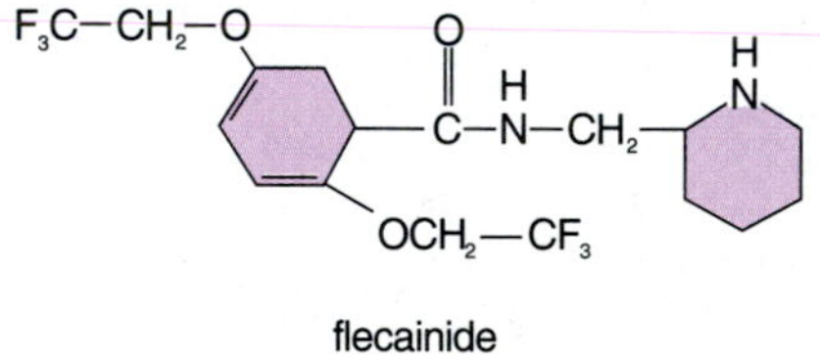

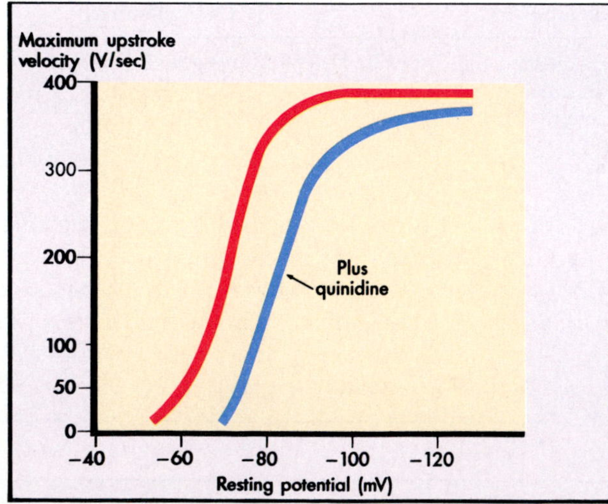

FIGURE 14-8 Maximum upstroke velocity (dV/dt_{max} or $\dot{V}_{max}$) of action potential during phase 0 as influenced by resting membrane potential. This relationship is called *membrane responsiveness.* Plot to the left is in the absence of drugs. Addition of many class I antiarrhythmic agents such as quinidine shifts the curve to more negative membrane potentials (hyperpolarizing direction).

has been used as an antiarrhythmic agent since the 1950s. Many of the electrophysiological actions are similar to those of lidocaine. It depresses membrane responsiveness to a greater extent in ventricular myocardium and the His-Purkinje system than in the atrium. In addition to blocking myocardial Na^+ channels, there is evidence that phenytoin may also block myocardial Ca^{++} channels.

Flecainide and Propafenone (Class IC) With both flecainide and propafenone, conduction velocity is slowed as a result of its ability to depress membrane responsiveness. Propafenone, in addition to blocking Na^+ channels, also has significant sympatholytic activity and has been reported to block Ca^{++} channels also.

Class II Antiarrhythmic Agents (Propranolol and other β-Adrenergic Blockers) The antiarrhythmic properties of β-adrenergic antagonists such as pro-bretylium tosylate

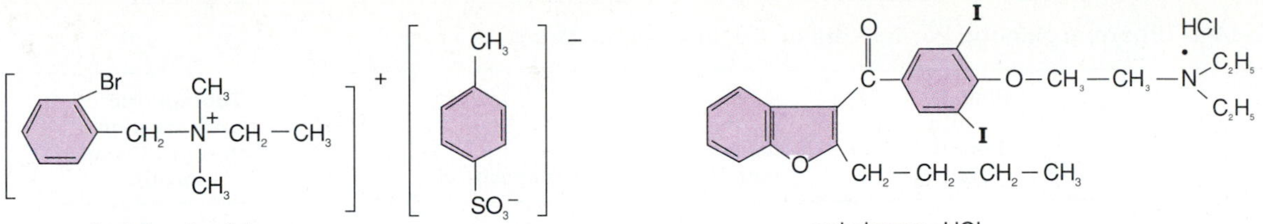

amiodarone • HCl

FIGURE 14-9 Structures of class III antiarrhythmic drugs.

pranolol are caused by two major effects: (1) blockade of myocardial β-adrenergic receptors (β_1-receptors), thereby preventing or antagonizing the actions of endogenous catecholamines, and (2) direct membrane effects, which relate to the ability to block at higher concentrations myocardial Na^+ channels and depress membrane responsiveness "quinidinelike effect." Propranolol exhibits direct membrane effects in atrium, ventricles, and the His-Purkinje system. In addition, it slows SA nodal and ectopic pacemaker automaticity and slows AV nodal conduction velocity by virtue of its ability to block intrinsic sympathetic activity. However, some of these effects may also be caused by direct membrane actions of the drug. Propranolol produces a small prolongation of the action potential duration and refractoriness that is greater in the atrium than in ventricular tissue. The structures of these drugs are described in Chapters 10 and 13.

Class III Antiarrhythmic Agents The structures of some of these agents are shown in Figure 14-9.

Bretylium Bretylium has direct and indirect effects on the heart; the latter include concentration in adrenergic nerve terminals and interference with the release of catecholamines. Initially, release is stimulated but then decreased. Part of bretylium's action in the heart is mediated by release and subsequent block. The major direct effect of bretylium is prolongation of action potential duration and refractoriness in atrium, ventricle, and the His-Purkinje system.

Amiodarone Amiodarone can be classified as a class III agent because of its ability to prolong action potential duration, which can be attributed to block of several different types of myocardial K^+ channels. Like lidocaine, however, amiodarone also preferentially blocks inactivated myocardial Na^+ channels and therefore is more effective in depressing conduction in cells that are depolarized or have a longer action potential duration. It has been reported that amiodarone blocks myocardial Ca^{++} channels and has α- and β-adrenergic blocking activity. It is unclear which action is actually responsible for its antiarrhythmic activity.

Sotalol *d,l*-Sotalol is a potent β-adrenergic receptor blocker with an antiarrhythmic profile similar to that of other class II agents. Additional properties of this compound that contribute to its antiarrhythmic actions include prolongation of action potential duration and refractoriness. These properties are believed to be independent of its β-adrenergic blocking properties, since similar effects are observed with the *d*-isomer, which has less sympatholytic activity. *d*-Sotalol and several newer agents are currently being evaluated as more "pure" class III agents, which may selectively block myocardial K^+ channels involved in initiating action potential repolarization.

Class IV Antiarrhythmic Agents These calcium-channel blocking drugs are discussed in Chapter 16.

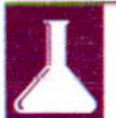

PHARMACOKINETICS

The pharmacokinetic parameters of antiarrhythmic drugs are summarized in Table 14-4. Additional β-blocker pharmacokinetic considerations are discussed in Chapters 10 and 13. Similarly the pharmacokinetics of calcium-channel blocking drugs are found in Chapter 16.

Quinidine is readily absorbed from the gut. Both hepatic and renal functions need to be assessed to prevent the accumulation of toxic concentrations (above 8 μg/ml) in the plasma.

Lidocaine is inactive when administered orally because of the large first-pass metabolism and therefore is usually given only IV for acute treatment of cardiac arrhythmias. Because the majority of the drug is metabolized, liver function is important. The main route of metabolism is by N-dealkylation to produce metabolites that show only mild antiarrhythmic activity.

The large first-pass effect seen with lidocaine is not observed with mexiletine or tocainide, which have similar structures and modes of action. Although mexiletine and tocainamide demonstrate bioavailabilities in the range of 90% to 100%, the half-life of mexiletine is about 35% less for smokers than for nonsmokers. This difference probably results from induction of hepatic enzymes in smokers. Other hepatic enzyme inducers, such as barbiturates, phenytoin, and rifampin, increase the rate of mexiletine metabolism. Antacids, cimetidine, or narcotic analgesics interact with mexiletine to slow its ab-

Table 14-4 Pharmacokinetic Parameters of Antiarrhythmic Drugs

Drug	Plasma Protein Bound (%)	$t_{1/2}$ (hr unless noted)	Disposition	Therapeutic Concentration Range in Plasma (μg/ml)
CLASS IA				
quinidine (O,I)	80	5-7	M/R (50%)	2-5
procainamide (O,I)	15	2.5-5	M (20%)/R (50%)	4-10
disopyramide (O)	35-65	4.5	M (30%)/R (50%)	2-5
CLASS IB				
lidocaine (I)	60	1-2	M (90%)/R (10%)	10-20
mexiletine (O)	50-60	9-11	M/R (20%)	0.5-2
tocainide (O)	50	11-17	M/R (40%)	4-10
phenytoin (O,I)	70-95	22	M (90%)/R	10-20
CLASS IC				
flecainide (O)	40	13	M (60%)/R (30%)	0.2-1
propafenone (O)	—	2-10	M	0.2-1.5
CLASS II				
propranolol (O,I)	90-96	4-6	M	40-100
sotalol (O)	—	10-15	R	—
metoprolol (O,I)	12	3-7	M	—
acebutol (O)	26	8-13	M/R	—
CLASS III				
amiodarone (O,I)	96	20-100 days	M/bile	1-2.5
bretylium (I)	0	8-13	R (100%)	—
CLASS IV				
verapamil (O,I)	90	3-7	M/R	—

O, Oral; *I*, IV; *M*, hepatic metabolism; *R*, renal elimination as unchanged drug (percentage by this pathway, if known).

sorption from the gastrointestinal tract.

The metabolism of procainamide produces the *N*-acetyl derivative, which shows mild antiarrhythmic activity and has a long plasma half-life.

The long plasma half-life (22 hours mean value) of phenytoin shows considerable interpatient variation. Drugs that influence liver microsomal drug metabolism can significantly alter plasma concentrations and thus change the half-life of phenytoin. Considerable interpatient diversity in half-life also is observed with the newer drug flecainide, where metabolism is the major pathway for drug disposition and where one of the metabolites is slightly active.

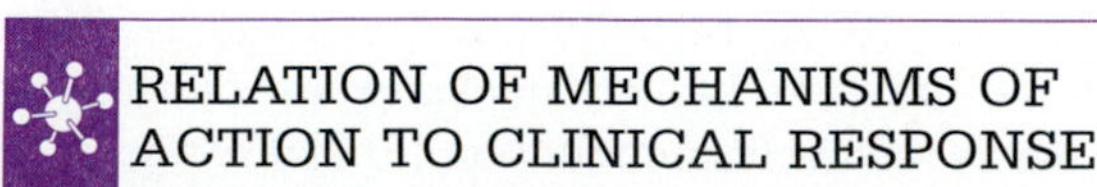

RELATION OF MECHANISMS OF ACTION TO CLINICAL RESPONSE

Antiarrhythmic Agents

A summary of antiarrhythmic drug choice is shown in Table 14-5.

Quinidine Quinidine has potent anticholinergic properties usually manifest by low doses in richly innervated areas of the heart, namely, the SA and AV nodes. These indirect effects are the opposite of the direct effects of this agent in these areas. After initial administration, there may be a small SA nodal tachycardia and an increase in AV nodal conduction velocity (decrease in PR interval) as a result of the indirect, anticholinergic effects of the drug. These initial effects are usually followed by the direct effects of the drug, including a decrease in heart rate and a slowing of AV nodal conduction velocity (increase in PR interval). At therapeutic concentrations, the QRS complex often shows widening as a result of a decrease in ventricular conduction velocity. The QT interval may be lengthened because the prolonged action potential in the ventricular myocardium.

Quinidine is a broad-spectrum antiarrhythmic agent that is effective for nearly all types of cardiac arrhythmias. It is administered for cases of *atrial flutter* or *fibrillation, AV nodal reentry arrhythmias, premature ventricular contractions,* and *ventricular tachycardias.* It

Table 14-5 Summary of Antiarrhythmic Therapy

Arrhythmia	Drug of Choice	Alternative
Atrial fibrillation or flutter	digoxin	verapamil or β-blocker to control rate, procainamide for long-term suppression
Supraventricular tachycardia	adenosine or verapamil IV for termination	β-blocker or digoxin
Ventricular premature complexes (VPCs)	no therapy if patient is asymptomatic	β-blocker if patient is symptomatic
Sustained ventricular tachycardia	lidocaine for acute treatment	procainamide, bretylium; cardioversion safest and most effective
Ventricular fibrillation	lidocaine	procainamide, amiodarone, bretylium
Cardiac glycoside–induced ventricular tachyarrhythmias	lidocaine	phenytoin, procainamide, β-blocker; self-limiting if digitalis stopped; Fab fragments if life threatening; β-blocker or procainamide can worsen heart block
Torsade de pointes	magnesium	cardiac pacing, isoproterenol

Modified from the *Medical Letter on Drugs and Therapeutics,* 33:55-60, 1991.

also is used in the treatment of digitalis-induced arrhythmias but is not the drug of first choice. Quinidine should be administered with caution in patients experiencing atrial flutter or fibrillation because the indirect anticholinergic effects of the drug might exacerbate these conditions by increasing AV nodal conduction velocity. Often quinidine is given with digitalis for treatment of atrial flutter or fibrillation because the vagal enhancing effects of the glycosides tend to offset the anticholinergic properties of quinidine. Because quinidine produces a negative inotropic effect, it should be used cautiously in patients with congestive heart failure or severe hypotension.

Procainamide and Disopyramide Procainamide and disopyramide depress automatically in SA nodal cells, as well as automaticity of ectopic pacemakers. Procainamide, in contrast to quinidine, has much less anticholinergic effect. Therefore, the effects on heart rate and AV nodal conduction velocity are more direct and are usually characterized by a decrease in heart rate and a prolongation of the PR interval. Disopyramide, however, has similar if not more potent anticholinergic properties than quinidine has. Therefore, the same indirect and direct effects on heart rate and AV conduction velocity are observed after administration of this agent. When given for the treatment of *atrial flutter* or *fibrillation,* a digitalis glycoside will very often be coadministered to minimize the anticholinergic properties of disopyramide. Both procainamide and disopyramide prolong action potential duration and effective refractory period in the atrium, ventricle, and the His-Purkinje system. Therefore, a widening of the QRS complex and a lengthening of the QT interval are also observed after administration of these agents. Both compounds are broad-spectrum antiarrhythmics used to treat both *supraventricular* and *ventricular arrhythmias.*

Lidocaine Over a relatively large concentration range, lidocaine has little effect on automaticity of the SA node, and hence heart rate remains relatively normal. Despite this, lidocaine does suppress automaticity of both ectopic ventricular pacemakers and Purkinje fibers. Some shortening of the action potential duration and effective refractory period also is possible; this is more prominent in Purkinje fibers compared with ventricular myocardium. Lidocaine has little effect on AV nodal conduction. At therapeutic concentrations, lidocaine produces minimal changes in the electrocardiogram.

Lidocaine has a narrow antiarrhythmic range compared with quinidine. It is primarily effective in the treatment of *ventricular arrhythmias,* especially those associated with acute myocardial infarction. It has little efficacy for the treatment of supraventricular dysrhythmia such as atrial flutter or fibrillation. Lidocaine is the drug of choice for the treatment of digitalis-induced arrhythmias, of either atrial or ventricular origin. This may be caused by its apparent selectivity for depolarized myocardium.

Phenytoin Unlike lidocaine, phenytoin depresses automaticity of SA nodal cells and ectopic pacemakers. Phenytoin, though devoid of the anticholinergic properties of quinidine and disopyramide, increases AV nodal conduction velocity through some unknown mechanism. The only significant changes observed in the electrocardiogram after administration of phenytoin are a small decrease in the PR and QT intervals. Its antiarrhythmic range is similar to that of lidocaine. It is a second-level drug for the treatment of *ventricular arrhythmias* or *arrhythmias induced by cardiac glycosides* and is often used with other agents.

Flecainide and Propafenone Flecainide may depress sinus node automaticity and slow AV nodal conduction. In patients with preexisting AV nodal conduction disturbances, it may produce conduction block. At therapeutic concentrations, flecainide may prolong the PR interval and widen the QRS complex. It should not be used in patients in heart failure or with drugs that depress cardiac contractility such as β-blockers or Ca^{++}-channel antagonists. Flecainide use is limited to the treatment of life-threatening ventricular arrhythmias that have not responded to other therapies.

Propafenone may depress SA nodal automaticity and lead to SA node block. At therapeutic concentrations, propafenone prolongs PR interval and widens the QRS complex. It is used to suppress *ventricular tachycardias* and *ectopic ventricular rhythms* but should be used with the same reservations as with flecainide.

β-Adrenergic Receptor Blockers At therapeutic doses, the only significant change in the electrocardiogram produced by β-blockers is a prolongation of the PR interval with occasional shortening of the QT interval.

In general, β-adrenergic receptor antagonists have a low efficacy for suppressing ventricular ectopic pacemakers and are not useful for treating most ventricular arrhythmias. They are useful in the treatment of many *supraventricular arrhythmias* because of their ability to slow AV nodal conduction and SA nodal rate and thereby allow stabilization of the ventricular rate. They also are used prophylactically to prevent or reduce the incidence of *recurrent myocardial infarction* in patients.

β-Adrenergic receptor antagonists such as metoprolol or acebutolol (but not propranolol) have a greater selectivity for β_1-receptors than for β_2-receptors. There also are differences between these compounds with regard to their effects on cardiac membrane channels and their intrinsic sympathomimetic activity. Another β-adrenergic receptor antagonist, esmolol, has been approved for emergency control of ventricular rate in patients with *atrial flutter* or *fibrillation*. In contrast to other β-blockers, esmolol has a short duration of action (approximately 10 minutes) when given IV.

Bretylium Bretylium is used in the emergency treatment of *ventricular fibrillation*.

Amiodarone In some antiarrhythmic classifications, amiodarone is considered a class III agent because of its ability to prolong action potential duration and refractoriness. It depresses SA nodal automaticity and automaticity of ectopic pacemakers. Effects on the electrocardiogram include prolongation of the PR and QT intervals and a widening of the QRS complex. It is effective in suppressing *ventricular* and *supraventricular arrhythmias that are refractory to other agents,* but its potential toxicity and long half-life limit its utility.

Sotalol *d*-Sotalol represents the prototype of the newer and more selective class III agents. These agents prolong repolarization and refractoriness uniformly and increase the QT interval. They may slow SA nodal automaticity but usually have minimal effects on cardiac conduction. The antiarrhythmic effects of these agents may be compromised by ischemia or fast heart rates. They are useful in the treatment of *supraventricular arrhythmias* and life-threatening *ventricular arrhythmias*. The ability of these agents to prolong repolarization and refractoriness may be exacerbated at long cycle lengths or hypokalemia. Many agents in this group have proarrhythmic properties, which result in rapid, self-terminating ventricular tachycardias, or a drug-induced *toursade de pointes*.

Calcium-Channel Blockers Calcium-channel blockers are most effective in treating *supraventricular arrhythmias,* which often involve reentry. Their ability to slow AV nodal conduction velocity and refractoriness makes them useful for controlling ventricular rate. They often convert atrial tachycardia to normal sinus rhythm. Calcium-channel blockers have little efficacy in the treatment of most ventricular arrhythmias. They will suppress the development of oscillatory afterdepolarizations induced by cardiac glycosides, but here they are not the drug of first choice (see Chapter 16).

Diltiazem, bepridil, lidoflazine, and flunarizine are other calcium-channel blocking drugs currently under investigation as potential antiarrhythmic agents. The chemical structures, toxicity, and side effects of calcium-channel blockers are described in Chapter 16. These agents' cardiotoxic effects relate to their negative inotropic properties and cardiac depressant effects produced on SA nodal automaticity and AV nodal conduction. They are contraindicated in patients with sick sinus syndrome, AV nodal conduction disturbances, or congestive heart failure. Caution should be exercised when they are administered with other drugs such as digitalis glycosides or β-adrenergic receptor blockers, which also slow AV nodal conduction.

Digitalis Glycosides A predominant effect of the glycosides is their effect on the AV node (see Chapter 15). These drugs slow conduction velocity and increase the refractory period. Thus the cardiac glycosides effectively decrease impulse transmission from atria to ventricles and are therefore useful in supraventricular tachycardias such as atrial flutter and fibrillation. By increasing AV nodal refractoriness, the glycosides are also useful in converting some reentrant arrhythmias such as paroxysmal supraventricular tachycardia to normal. Because the therapeutic index of digitalis is narrow, toxic manifestations are not uncommon and may result in life-threatening arrhythmias. Potential arrhythmogenic actions of the drug are discussed in Chapter 15.

Adenosine Adenosine is useful for termination of paroxysmal ventricular tachycardia. It apparently activates potassium channels and, by increasing the outward potassium current, hyperpolarizes the membrane potential, decreasing spontaneous SA node depolarization. The nucleoside may also decrease the calcium inward current by blocking adenylate cyclase, which normally increases the inward calcium current. The overall action of adenosine is to slow the SA nodal firing rate and decrease AV conduction. Unfortunately, its half-life is very short (in seconds), thereby limiting its clinical usefulness. Dipyridamole can inhibit the metabolism of adenosine and increase its action.

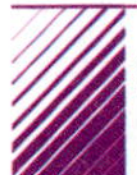

SIDE EFFECTS, CLINICAL PROBLEMS, AND TOXICITY

Major problems associated with use of antiarrhythmic agents are summarized in the box, though information for the β-blockers and calcium-channel blockers is found in Chapters 10 and 16 respectively.

Quinidine is rarely given IV because of its tendency to depress cardiac output and produce hypotension. Side effects observed after oral administration include diarrhea, nausea, and vomiting, as well as a condition known as *cinchonism,* characterized by headaches, dizziness, and tinnitus. In some patients, quinidine syncope where the patient experiences fainting or lightheadedness may develop. Syncope is likely the result of drug-induced ventricular tachycardia, which often subsides spontaneously. Quinidine overdosage can cause severe cardiac depression and precipitate arrhythmias such as ventricular tachycardia, fibrillation, or asystole. Quinidine interacts with a wide range of other drugs.

Lidocaine has minimal toxic effects on the heart. At very high doses it may cause asystole. Most of the toxic side effects associated with lidocaine administration are caused by its local anesthetic effects on the CNS. These include drowsiness, tremor, nausea, hearing disturbances, slurred speech, and, at high doses, psychosis, respiratory depression, and convulsions.

The electrophysiological effects, antiarrhythmic range, and side effects of mexiletine and tocainamide are similar to those of lidocaine, but pharmacokinetic differences allow their oral use.

Procainamide overdose may produce cardiotoxic effects similar to those observed with quinidine. These include severe cardiac depression and the development of arrhythmias. In addition, severe hypotension, caused by procainamide peripheral actions, also may occur at high doses. Side effects observed with therapeutic doses include gastrointestinal disturbances such as diarrhea, nausea, and vomiting. Chronic use of procainamide results in the development of a syndrome similar to systemic lupus erythematosus. Symptoms include arthralgia, skin rash, fever, and hepatomegaly. The development of this syndrome appears to be dose dependent and is readily reversed on cessation of procainamide therapy. These lupuslike effects limit the chronic use of the compound because approximately one third of all patients will exhibit lupuslike symptoms. Granulocytopenia also is observed in some patients.

CLINICAL PROBLEMS

quinidine	GI effects, precipitates arrhythmias, elevates digoxin concentrations, anticholinergic effects
procainamide	Arrhythmias, anticholinergic effects, lupuslike syndrome
disopyramide	Precipitates CHF, anticholinergic effects
lidocaine	CNS effects (dizziness, seizures), first-pass metabolism
phenytoin	CNS and GI effects
tocainamide	CNS and GI effects, blood disorders
mexiletine	CNS and GI effects
flecainide	Negative inotropic effect, proarrhythmogenic, CNS and GI effects
propafenone	CNS effects, proarrhythmogenic
β-blockers	Negative inotropic and chronotropic effects, precipitates CHF, AV conduction block
bretylium	Hypotension, GI effects
amiodarone	Hypotension pneumonitis, bradycardia, *torsade de pointes*, precipitates CHF
sotalol	Modest negative inotropic and chronotropic effects
verapamil	Hypotension, negative inotropic and chronotropic effects

GI, Gastrointestinal; *CHF,* congestive heart failure; *CNS,* central nervous system.

Toxic concentrations of disopyramide may produce electrophysiological disturbances similar to those produced by high doses of quinidine. Disopyramide, in addition, appears to be more cardiodepressant than quinidine, requiring careful monitoring to ensure that cardiac failure does not develop. It should be used with extreme caution in patients with congestive heart failure. Many of the side effects of disopyramide are associated with its anticholinergic properties and include dry mouth, blurred vision, nausea, urinary retention, and constipation.

Oral overdose of phenytoin produces effects related to its interaction with the CNS, including vertigo, nystagmus, ataxia, tremors, slurring of speech, and sedation. Because of its relatively long plasma half-life and the ability of other drugs that influence microsomal metabolism to alter plasma concentrations of phenytoin significantly, considerable patient-to-patient variations in response to a given oral dose typically occur.

Flecainide can potentiate arrhythmias in patients with a history of sustained ventricular tachycardia and severe ventricular dysfunction. Its side effects include dizziness, blurred vision, headache, nausea, and abdominal pain. The compound is orally active but, as noted above, reserved for the treatment of life-threatening ventricular arrhythmias, especially ones that are refractory to more traditional drugs, and is now approved only for the management of life-threatening arrhythmias.

Adverse cardiac effects of amiodarone are significant and include sinus bradycardia and AV conduction block. Other effects observed are anorexia, nausea, vomiting, and clinical hepatitis and cirrhosis. CNS effects include dizziness, ataxia, tremor, and postural instability.

Because of its toxicity and side effects, bretylium is not considered a first-choice antiarrhythmic agent. It is primarily used to stabilize cardiac rhythm in patients with ventricular fibrillation or recurrent tachycardia resistant to other treatment. Its most severe side effect is persistent hypotension caused by peripheral vasodilatation as a result of blockade of peripheral adrenergic nerves. In addition, catecholamine release can transiently enhance ectopic pacemaker activity and cause increases in myocardial oxygen consumption in patients with ischemic heart disease. Nausea and vomiting are also common side effects of bretylium administration.

Caution is indicated when one is administering β-adrenergic antagonists with other drugs that also slow AV nodal conduction velocity because the effects may be synergistic. β-Adrenergic receptor antagonists are generally contraindicated in patients with existing AV nodal conduction disturbances, congestive heart failure, or bronchial asthma. The toxicity and side effects of these drugs are described elsewhere in this book.

NEW DIRECTIONS

Na^+-channel blockade has been considered an important antiarrhythmic mechanism for many years. The ability of drugs that block these channels to suppress premature ventricular complexes has been considered an important property that may be related to reducing risk associated with sudden cardiac death. However, a recent multicenter study, the Cardiac Arrhythmia Suppression Trial, has raised serious questions about the efficacy of several class I agents to improve postinfarction survival of patients with asymptomatic or mildly symptomatic ventricular arrhythmias. Patients treated with encainide and flecainide were found to have a significantly higher risk of cardiac death and nonfatal cardiac arrest than a placebo control group. Encainide is no longer used. Doubts similar to those associated with the use of class IC agents have been raised about the use of all class I agents in postinfarction patients and have stimulated a reevaluation of the survival benefits of suppressing premature ventricular complexes. A recent cumulative metanalysis study of drugs used in the treatment of acute myocardial infarction and also in secondary prevention indicates that a class I agent like lidocaine fails to reduce mortality caused by acute myocardial infarction and only marginally prevents or postpones death after discharge of the patient. The proarrhythmic potential of some class I agents has generally led to more stringent restrictions for their use.

New approaches to antiarrhythmic drug classification are beginning to emerge. Renewed interest has stimulated the development of new class III antiarrhythmic agents, which may produce less cardiac depression than class I agents. Several new agents, some structurally related to sotalol, are presently in various stages of clinical trials and will likely become available in the United States in the near future. Some of these new investigational agents include sematilide, ibutilide, E-4031 (Eisai), UK68, 798 (Pfizer), and RP58866 (Rhône-Poulenc-Rorer).

TRADE NAMES

In addition to generic and fixed-combination preparations, the following trade-named materials are available in the United States. (See Chapter 26 for calcium-channel blockers and Chapters 10 and 23 for β-blockers.)

Bretylol, bretylium
Cordarone, amiodarone
Dilantin, phenytoin
Mexitil, mexiletine
Norpace, disopyramide
Procan SR, procainamide
Pronestyl, procainamide
Quinidex Extentabs, quinidine
Quinora, quinidine
Tambocor, flecainide
Tonocard, tocainide
Xylocaine, lidocaine

REFERENCES

Arnsdorf MF, Wasserstrom JA: Mechanisms of action of antiarrhythmic drugs: a matrical approach. In Fozzard HA, Haber E, Jennings RB, et al, editors: *The heart and cardiovascular system; scientific foundations,* vol 2, New York, 1986, Raven Press.

Cardiac Arrhythmia Suppression Trial (CAST) Investigators. Preliminary report: effect of encainide and flecainide on mortality in a randomized trial of arrhythmia suppression after myocardial infarction. *N Engl J Med* 321:406, 1989.

Colatsky TJ: K^+ channel blockers: synthetic agents and their antiarrhythmic potential. In Weston A, Hamilton T, editors: *Potassium channel modulators: pharmacological, molecular and clinical aspects,* Oxford, 1991, Blackwell Scientific Publications.

Lau J, Elliot EM, Jimenez-Silva J, et al: Cumulative meta-analysis of therapeutic trails for myocardial infarction, *N Engl J Med* 327:248, 1992.

Noble D: Initiation of the heartbeat, Oxford, England, 1979, Oxford University Press.

Reiser HJ, Sullivan ME: Antiarrhythmic drug therapy: new drugs and changing concepts, *Fed Proc* 45:2206, 1986.

Rosen MR, Wit AL: Electropharmacology of antiarrhythmic drugs, *Am Heart J* 106:829, 1983.

Singh BN, Collett JT, Chew CYC: New perspectives in the pharmacological therapy of cardiac arrhythmias, *Prog Cardiovasc Dis* 22(4):243, 1980.

Smith WB, Wallace AG: Drugs used to treat cardiac arrhythmias. In Hurst JW, editor: *The heart,* ed 6, New York, 1986, McGraw-Hill.

Task Force of the Working Group on Arrhythmias of the European Society of Cardiology. The Sicilian Gambit. A new approach to the classification of antiarrhythmic agents based on their actions on arrhythmogenic mechanisms, *Circulation* 84:1831, 1991.

SELF-ASSESSMENT QUESTIONS

1. Quinidine can produce all of the following *except:*
   a. depressed myocardial excitability.
   b. vagal stimulation.
   c. slowed myocardial conduction.
   d. decreased slope of diastolic depolarization of pacemaker cells.
   e. prolonged myocardial refractory period.
2. The antiarrhythmic drug of choice to treat digitalis-induced arrhythmias is:
   a. quinidine.
   b. lidocaine.
   c. procainamide.
   d. verapamil.
   e. propafenone.
3. The plateau of a nonpacemaker cardiac cell is caused by:
   a. an increased conductance to all ions and a delayed efflux of calcium ions, which balances a slowly decreasing efflux of potassium ions.
   b. a reduced conductance to all ions and a delayed influx of calcium ions, which balances a slowly decreasing efflux of potassium ions.
   c. a reduced conductance to all ions and a delayed influx of calcium ions, which balances a slowly increasing efflux of potassium ions.
   d. a reduced conductance to all ions and a delayed influx of calcium ions, which balances a slowly increasing influx of potassium ions.
   e. none of the above.
4. The effectiveness of edrophonium in the treatment of supraventricular arrhythmias is attributable to:
   a. quinidinelike effects.
   b. an increase in AV nodal conduction velocity.
   c. an increase in vagal effects in the heart.
   d. a decrease in vagal effects in the heart.
   e. shortening of the effective refractory period of the atrial action potential.
5. Which of the following agents is *not* orally active?
   a. propranolol
   b. quinidine
   c. licodaine
   d. verapamil
   e. phenytoin
6. The use of propranolol as an antiarrhythmic agent is contraindicated in patients with:
   a. severe AV block.
   b. congestive heart failure.
   c. bronchial asthma.
   d. none of the above.
   e. a, b, and c above.
7. Cinchonism is a syndrome associated with:
   a. digitoxin.
   b. phenytoin.
   c. lidocaine.
   d. propranolol.
   e. quinidine.
8. The effect of a therapeutic dose of quinidine on the normal ECG includes:
   a. an initial decrease in heart rate followed by an increase.
   b. an initial lengthening of the PR interval followed by a shortening.
   c. a widening of the QRS complex.
   d. a shortening of the QT interval.
   e. none of the above.

CHAPTER 15 Drugs Affecting the Force of Cardiac Contraction

TAI AKERA
THEODORE M. BRODY

MAJOR DRUGS
digitalis glycosides
catecholamines
phosphodiesterase inhibitors

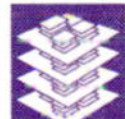

THERAPEUTIC OVERVIEW

Positive inotropic drugs are used to increase the force of myocardial contraction when the heart's ability to pump blood is impaired.

The function of the heart is to pump blood to provide adequate blood flow to various organs in the body and to furnish oxygen and substrates while removing metabolites. For example, skeletal muscle requires as large a blood flow, as does the heart. The need for oxygen and substrates and the removal of metabolites and therefore the demands for blood flow in other organs vary widely depending on the activity of each organ. When the force of cardiac contraction is compromised and the heart cannot meet the prevailing demand for pumping blood, "heart failure" develops.

Several conditions can reduce the force of cardiac contraction. These are (1) myocardial ischemia with subsequent injury to heart muscle, (2) toxic injury caused by chemicals, (3) infections of the heart, and (4) congenital or genetic abnormalities. *If the force of cardiac contraction is reduced only moderately, the heart can meet demand provided that the patient is not subjected to excessive stress or exercise.* This condition is called **compensated heart failure.** Although patients may appear normal, their exercise tolerance is reduced. When the force of contraction is decreased further, pressures in the systemic and pulmonary veins increase even when the patient is at rest. Pressure on the arterial side rarely decreases until the terminal stage of the illness. Congestion of blood in the venous system causes edema, especially of the lower extremities and lungs. Acute pulmonary edema occurs frequently when the patient is recumbent and edematous fluid of the lower extremities returns to the circulating blood. Patients frequently experience shortness of breath or difficulties in breathing. These are typical signs of **congestive** or **chronic (uncompensated) heart failure** (CHF).

ABBREVIATIONS	
ATP	adenosine triphosphate
AV	atrioventricular
cAMP	cyclic adenosine monophosphate
CHF	congestive heart failure
SA	sinoatrial

Arterial blood pressure is well maintained in CHF because (1) sympathetic tone increases and (2) the renin-angiotensin-vasopressin system is activated. These homeostatic mechanisms are brought into play to maintain blood pressure; however, they also increase total peripheral resistance. In addition, (3) circulating blood volume is increased, also contributing to the maintenance of arterial blood pressure. These three mechanisms maintain arterial blood pressures, but place an additional burden on the failing heart. Moreover, increases in peripheral resistance decrease tissue perfusion for a given blood pressure. Because tissue perfusion is more important than blood pressure itself, maintenance of blood pressure by these mechanisms may not be totally advantageous.

Among the pathophysiological changes associated with CHF are increases in end-systolic volume, end-diastolic pressure, and dilation of the ventricle. These changes occur because the compromised heart cannot completely remove the blood returned to it. An increase

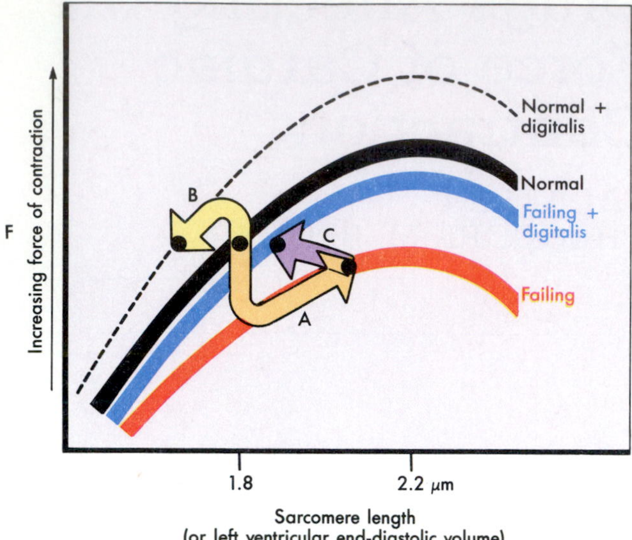

FIGURE 15-1 Frank-Starling ventricular function curve. Force of contraction, expressed as left ventricular dP/dt (rate of pressure development during early systolic phase), is a function of (1) left ventricular volume immediately before the onset of contraction, or (2) sarcomere length. The length of sarcomere, the unit between two Z lines of a myofibril, in the normal heart is 1.7 to 1.8 μm at the endocardial and epicardial layers and 2.0 μm in the middle layer. Reduced force of contraction in a failing heart is partly compensated by stretching of the muscle, which increases the force of contraction, **A,** *arrow.* Positive inotropic interventions in the normal heart are canceled by shortening of the muscle, **B,** *arrow.* The digitalis glycosides shift the ventricular function curve and reduce the end-diastolic volume that is required for the muscle to develop the necessary force of contraction, **C,** *arrow.*

THERAPEUTIC OVERVIEW	
PROBLEM:	Congestive heart failure (CHF) Force of contraction ↓ Ventricular dilation Cardiac output ↓ Total peripheral resistance ↑ Venous pressure ↑ Development of edema Tissue perfusion ↓ Exercise tolerance ↓
GOAL:	Reverse CHF
NONDRUG THERAPY:	Cardiac work reduction through Rest Salt restriction
DRUG THERAPY:	Diuretics Vasodilators (noninotropic) Positive inotropic drugs: Cardiac glycosides Catecholamines Phosphodiesterase inhibitors

in end-diastolic volume increases the force of contraction because developed tension is a function of preload, or stretching of muscle fibers at the onset of contraction. This process is described by the Frank-Starling ventricular function curve (Figure 15-1, *A, arrow*). Stretching of muscle fibers resulting from an adequate increase in end-diastolic volume causes the compromised muscle to develop a greater force. It should be noted, however, that an increase in intraventricular pressure, and not an increase in wall tension itself, causes ejection of blood into the aorta.

The relationship between wall tension and intraventricular pressure is described by the law of Laplace: if one assumes that the cross section of the ventricle is a circle, pressure is proportional to tension divided by the diameter of the ventricle. This means that, for a given aortic pressure, a greater wall tension is required in the dilated heart than in a normal heart to develop a pressure required for moving blood from the left ventricle to the aorta. Therefore, the energetic efficiency is reduced in chronic heart failure because (1) a greater wall tension is required to develop the necessary intraventricular pressure and (2) peripheral resistance is increased. The energetic efficiency decreases further when (3) muscle relaxation is inhibited in the hypertrophied heart and (4) the heart rate is increased by activation of the sympathetic nervous system, resulting in a reduced stroke volume.

Chronic stress causes hypertrophy of cardiac muscle. Stretching of the sarcolemma, the ensuing leak influx of Na^+ ions, and elevated angiotensin II concentration in plasma are possible causes of myocardial hypertrophy. The number of myocardial cells does not increase in the adult heart, though this is observed in the fetal heart (hyperplasia); instead, each cell becomes larger (hypertrophy). Associated with hypertrophy, remodeling of cardiac muscle may occur. Remodeling is a shift of isoforms of various functional proteins such as myosin, creatine kinase, Na^+,K^+-ATPase, etc. It is unknown if these isoform shifts are adaptative events or play a role in causing heart failure. Moreover, the hypertrophied heart loses compliance (i.e., the ability to relax). Inability to relax completely is an early and serious problem of the failing heart. Continued severe heart failure may cause cellular death and complications in other organs from inadequate tissue perfusion.

All these signs of CHF are either direct or indirect consequences of an inadequate force of contraction. Therefore, it is logical to treat these patients with **positive inotropic drugs.** Although digitalis glycosides have been used extensively during the last 200 years, they are not ideal because of their toxic potential and limited ability to increase the force of contraction in certain clinical settings. Moreover, glycosides are incapable of arresting the progress of pathological changes and reversing basic processes that cause heart failure. In fact, glycosides are believed to augment deterioration of the heart in advanced CHF by forcing the damaged heart to work harder. Recent evidence indicates that an alternative and more palliative treatment of the failing heart to reduce the work load may be more beneficial (see also Chapter 17 on vasodilators). The basic problem and therapeutic approaches are summarized in the box.

MECHANISMS OF ACTION

Excitation-contraction coupling

Most positive inotropic drugs increase the force of cardiac contraction by modifying the excitation-contraction coupling mechanism and augmenting Ca^{++} transients. In cardiac muscle cells, the resting state is one of high energy, characterized by steep Na^+,K^+, and Ca^{++} gradients and transmembrane potentials. Among these, K^+ and Na^+ gradients are important for maintenance of transmembrane potential and excitability. Low intracellular Ca^{++} concentration is important for maintaining the relaxed state of resting muscle. The first event in membrane excitation is a sudden opening of Na^+ channels, which causes Na^+ ions, driven by chemical and electrical gradients, to rush into the cell (Figure 15-2). Although Na^+ channels are open for a very short period (typically, 1 to 2 msec), Na^+ ions crossing the sarcolemma during this period are sufficient to depolarize the cell membrane. During the depolarization phase, Ca^{++} channels open and Ca^{++} ions enter the cell driven by the steep Ca^{++} gradient. The inward flow of positively charged Ca^{++} ions keeps the membrane potential depolarized, maintains Ca^{++} channels open, and raises cytoplasmic Ca^{++} concentrations. The latter event triggers the release of Ca^{++} stored in the cisternal area of the sarcoplasmic reticulum. The cytoplasmic Ca^{++} concentration increases transiently (Ca^{++} transients) from approximately 50 nM at rest to approximately 500 nM at the peak Ca^{++} transient.

Typical myocardial cells have mitochondria, contractile proteins, and sarcoplasmic reticulum; this leaves only approximately 10% of the total cell volume as cytoplasmic fluid. Therefore, movements of Ca^{++} into this compartment across the cell membrane and from the

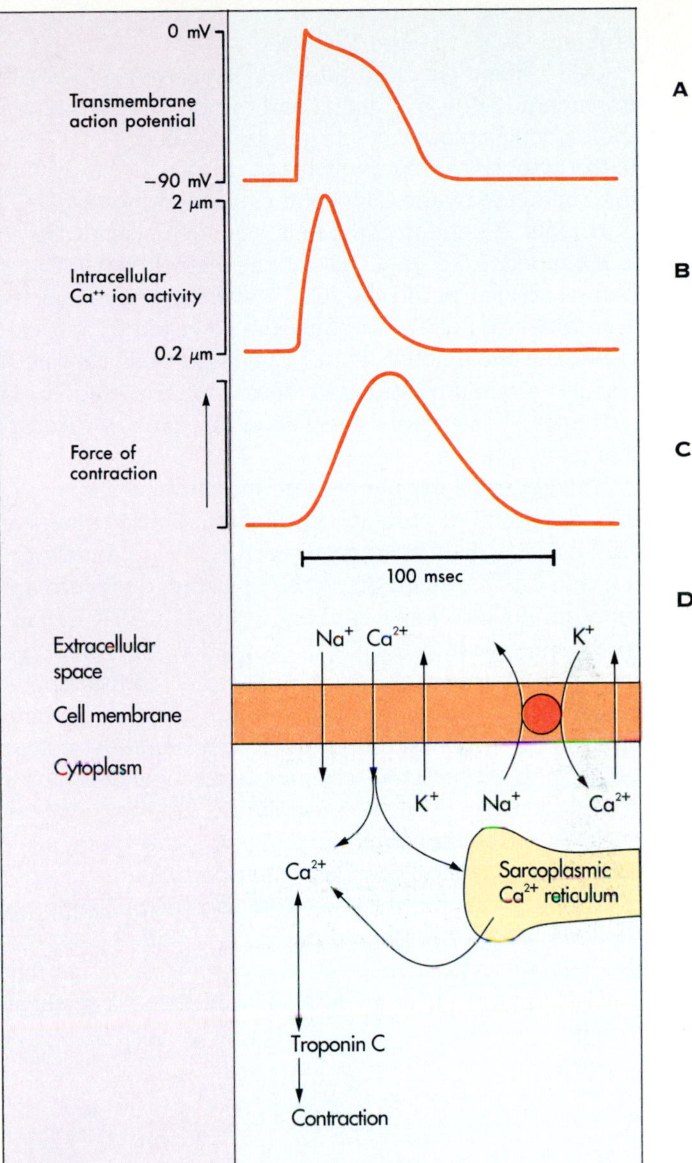

FIGURE 15-2 Time course of events of a single contraction (excitation-contraction coupling). **A,** Transmembrane potential. **B,** Intracellular Ca^{++}-ion activity. **C,** Developed tension. **D,** Biochemical basis for excitation-contraction coupling indicating intracellular ion movements.

sarcoplasmic reticulum significantly affect the free Ca^{++} ion concentration. The sudden and transient increase of cytoplasmic Ca^{++} activates the contractile proteins, causing the muscle to contract (Figure 15-2). Subsequently, K^+ channels open, and K^+ efflux occurs (there is more than one type of K^+ channel) (Chapter 14). The outward movement of positively charged K^+ ions reestablishes the membrane potential (repolarization), which in turn closes the Ca^{++} channels. During membrane depolarization, each Ca^{++} channel may open and close several times; however, a certain percentage of the channels are open at a given moment, allowing Ca^{++} to enter the cell.

Ca^{++} channels close after repolarization. When the transmembrane Ca^{++} influx and the Ca^{++} release from the sarcoplasmic reticulum are terminated, Ca^{++} ions in the cytoplasm are rapidly taken up into the sarcoplasmic reticulum by the Ca^{++} pump, terminating the Ca^{++} transients. A fraction of the increased cytoplasmic Ca^{++} is extruded from the cell by the sarcolemmal Ca^{++} pump and also by the Na^+/Ca^{++}-exchange mechanism. The initial rate of Ca^{++} influx (the so-called trigger calcium) and the amount of Ca^{++} released from the sarcoplasmic reticulum ultimately determine the magnitude of the Ca^{++} transients and hence the force of myocardial contraction.

Theoretically, intervention at any of these steps may alter the force of cardiac contraction. Thus, enhanced Na^+ influx, enhanced opening of the Ca^{++} channels, increased Ca^{++} loading of the sarcoplasmic reticulum, inhibition of Ca^{++} extrusion, and inhibition of K^+ channels, or increasing the Ca^{++} sensitivity of contractile proteins, all increase the force of cardiac contraction.

Calcium entering the cell through the sarcolemma and the Ca^{++} released from the sarcoplasmic reticulum lead to the activation of contractile proteins and hence contraction. The relative contribution of the two sources of Ca^{++} varies depending on the type of muscle. In skeletal muscle, most of the Ca^{++} that participates in contractile activation is released from the sarcoplasmic reticulum, whereas transmembrane Ca^{++} influx plays the predominant role in vascular smooth muscle. In cardiac muscle, trigger calcium derived from the extracellular space and Ca^{++} release from the sarcoplasmic reticulum determine the magnitude of the force of contraction. Therefore, drugs that affect Ca^{++} channels and those that affect the amount of Ca^{++} stored in the sarcoplasmic reticulum affect the force of myocardial contraction.

Mechanism of the Positive Inotropic Action of Digitalis Glycosides

Digitalis glycosides are extracted from the foxglove plant, *Digitalis purpurea,* and other species. Among the cardiac glycosides, digoxin and to a lesser extent digitoxin are clinically used (Figure 15-3). These drugs selectively bind to and inhibit the sarcolemmal sodium pump. Inhibition of the sodium pump leads to an increase in intracellular Na^+ concentration, which in turn affects Na^+/Ca^{++} exchange, leading to an increase in intracellular Ca^{++} and the force of contraction. Thus, direct effects on the Na^+,K^+-ATPase to inhibit sodium-pump activity is the mechanism of the positive inotropic effect of digitalis glycosides.

The primary function of the sodium pump is to exchange three intracellular Na^+ ions for two extracellular K^+ ions (Figure 15-4). Both Na^+ and K^+ ions are moved against their concentration gradients. Moreover, one net

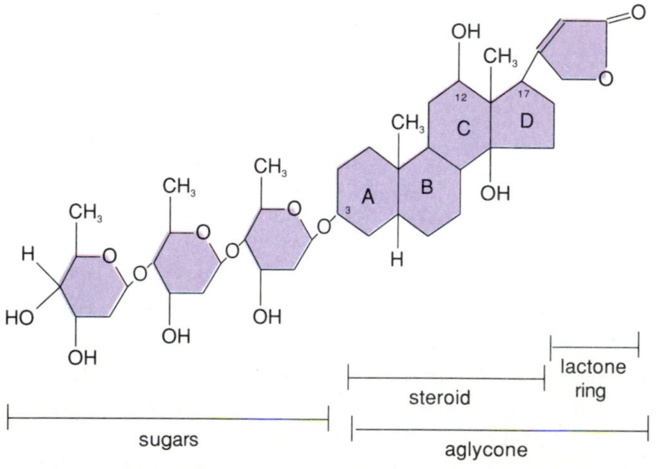

FIGURE 15-3 Chemical structure of digoxin. This molecule consists of an unsaturated lactone ring, a steroid nucleus, and three digitoxose (sugar) groups. The unsaturated lactone ring and the steroid nucleus with the *trans*-C-D fusion are essential for cardiotonic activity, whereas the sugar moiety is not an absolute requirement. Drugs that lack sugars are called *aglycones.* Digitoxin lacks the hydroxyl group at the C-12 position and has a higher lipid solubility.

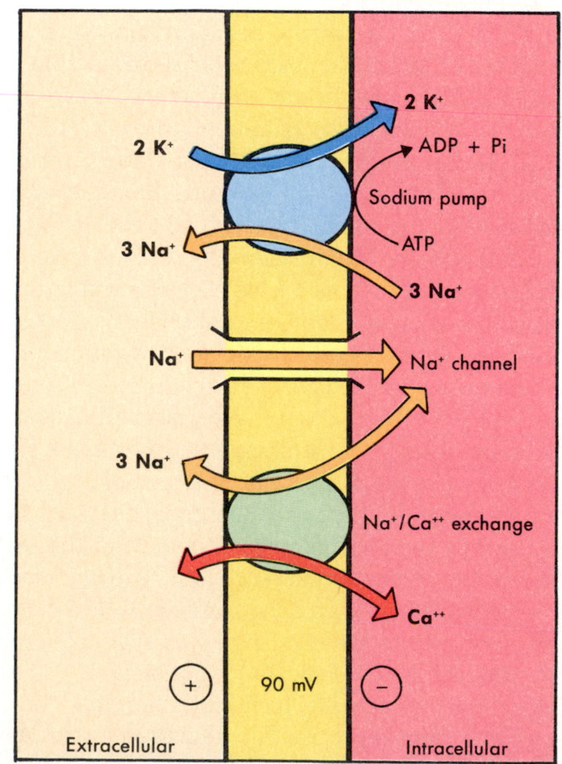

FIGURE 15-4 Membrane ion flux of Na^+ and Ca^{++} in the heart. Glycoside-induced inhibition of Na^+,K^+-ATPase secondarily inhibits Na^+ influx–Ca^{++} efflux exchange reaction.

positive charge is moved from the inside of the cell membrane to the outside against an electrical potential. This chemical and electrical work (active transport) is accomplished by energy supplied by the hydrolysis of adenosine triphosphate (ATP); one molecule of ATP is hydrolyzed to adenosine diphosphate and inorganic phosphate during each cycle of the sodium pump. The sodium pump, which hydrolyses ATP in the presence of Na^+ and K^+, is often referred to as **Na^+,K^+-ATPase.**

The current hypothesis on the mechanism of action of cardiac glycosides is that a slight but significant increase in the intracellular Na^+ concentration (e.g., 1 to 1.5 mM increase over the normal concentration of approximately 8 mM) inhibits Ca^{++} efflux coupled to Na^+ influx and thereby increases Ca^{++} loading of the sarcoplasmic reticulum (Figures 15-2 and 15-4). Unlike the active-transport mechanism of the Na^+ pump that moves Na^+ and K^+ ions against their chemical and electrical gradients at the expense of ATP, the Na^+/Ca^{++}-exchange mechanism mediates a coupled exchange of three Na^+ ions and one Ca^{++} ion. Direction of ion movements is determined by transmembrane Na^+ and Ca^{++} gradients and by the transmembrane potential.

The relationship of intracellular Na^+ to intracellular Ca^{++} is such that a very small increase in Na^+ in terms of percentage increase leads to a large increase in Ca^{++}. The reason is that cardiac intracellular Na^+ is approximately 8 mM whereas intracellular Ca^{++} is less than 100 nM in resting cardiac muscle, and hence a 3-to-1 exchange of Na^+ and Ca^{++} has considerably greater effects on the Ca^{++} concentration than on the Na^+ concentration. Because the sarcoplasmic reticulum has an active Ca^{++} pump, an inhibition of Ca^{++} extrusion from the cell results in a larger fraction of Ca^{++} ions to be taken up by the sarcoplasmic reticulum instead of being extruded. An increase in Ca^{++} uptake by the sarcoplasmic reticulum increases the amount of Ca^{++} to be released from the sarcoplasmic reticulum and thereby augments the Ca^{++} transients, which leads to an enhancement of the force of contraction.

It is also possible that the inhibition of the sodium pump augments Ca^{++} transients by enhancing Ca^{++} influx coupled with Na^+ efflux, which occurs during membrane excitation. In any case, the basic mechanism for the direct positive inotropic action of the cardiac glycoside is an enhancement of the Ca^{++} transient resulting from enhanced Ca^{++} loading of the sarcoplasmic reticulum.

Mechanism of Direct Toxic Effects of Digitalis Glycosides

A moderate inhibition of Na^+,K^+-ATPase causes the positive inotropic (therapeutic) effect of cardiac glyco side, whereas an excessive inhibition produces toxicity. The rate of Na^+ influx is roughly proportional to the frequency of membrane depolarization and hence the heart rate. That the heart rate can be increased to as high as 150 beats per minute without producing arrhythmias indicates that the sodium pump in a heart beating at 60 to 80 beats per minute has a reserve capacity. It may be postulated that an inhibition of the sodium pump that does not deplete the pump reserve capacity produces a therapeutic effect, whereas sodium pump inhibition greater than its reserve capacity produces toxicity.

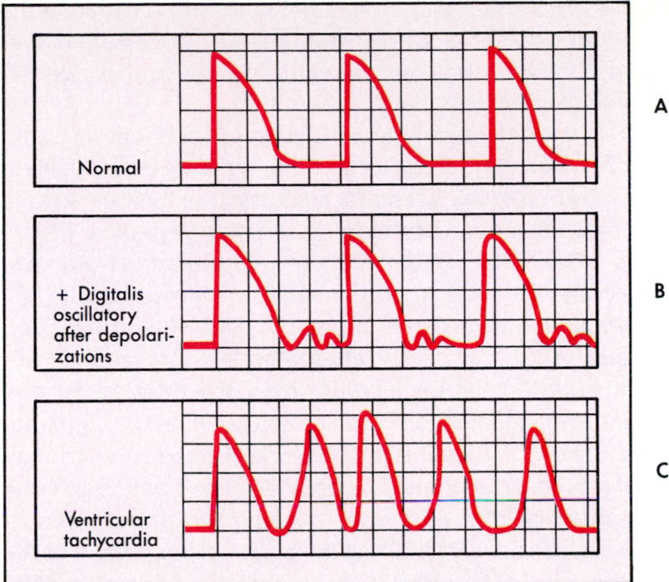

FIGURE 15-5 Normal action potential, **A,** and changes in cardiac action potentials caused by subtoxic, **B,** and toxic, **C,** doses of the cardiac glycosides. **A,** Typical action potential recordings from the cardiac Purkinje fiber cells. Toxic doses produce oscillatory afterdepolarizations, **B,** and ventricular tachycardia, **C.**

When cardiac muscle is exposed to toxic concentrations of a glycoside, sodium pump inhibition and cellular Ca^{++} loading become alarmingly high. The cytoplasmic membrane becomes "unstable" immediately after membrane repolarization. In normal ventricular muscle cells, membrane depolarization is followed by repolarization, in that the membrane potential reaches approximately −90 mV and remains at that level until the next membrane excitation (Figure 15-5, *A*). In digitalis toxicity, however, the permeability of the cell membrane to Na^+, Ca^{++}, and K^+ increases immediately after repolarization; ions flow according to their concentration and electrical gradients, causing the membrane potential to move toward 0mV. The movements of Na^+ and Ca^{++} are particularly prominent because these ions are driven by both chemical and electrical gradients. The movement of K^+ is minimal because the chemical and electrical gradients cancel each other when the transmembrane potential is approximately −90 mV. Therefore, the net movement is the transient inward movement of cations, causing transient inward currents and partial depolarization.

In mild toxicity, the transient inward current subsides, causing the transmembrane potential to return to its resting level. This process may be repeated several times causing oscillatory afterpotentials (see Figure 15-5, *B*). These small oscillatory afterpotentials are most readily observed in cardiac Purkinje fibers and do not propagate beyond the individual cell. When the magnitude of the oscillatory afterpotentials increases in advanced digitalis toxicity, however, the threshold potential is reached causing the cell to fire (i.e., to trigger action potentials; see Figure 15-5, *C*). Such triggered action potentials propagate from Purkinje fiber cells to the ventricular muscle proper, causing the muscle to contract repetitively, and it is no longer under control of the sinoatrial (SA) node. This process may lead to life-threatening ventricular tachycardia and ventricular fibrillation.

Thus, toxicity resulting from direct actions of the glycoside on cardiac muscle is caused by Ca^{++} overload of myocardial cells. Because the therapeutic positive inotropic effect of these drugs is also caused by an enhanced Ca^{++} loading of the cells and in particular the sarcoplasmic reticulum, the therapeutic and toxic effects are inseparable. The small therapeutic index (i.e., the narrow margin of safety) is an inherent property of this class of positive inotropic drugs.

Mechanisms of Extracardiac Effects of Digitalis Glycosides

Most cells in the body have low Na^+ and high K^+ concentrations. This condition is necessary for the function of many intracellular organelles and enzymes, including mitochondrial oxidative phosphorylation. Such intracellular ionic environments are maintained because these cells actively pump Na^+ out and K^+ in by means of the Na^+,K^+-ATPase present in the cell membrane. The Na^+,K^+-ATPases of various human tissues, particularly those that are excitable, have a high affinity for cardiac glycosides. Therefore, the glycosides are capable of influencing the activities of many cells and tissue types. Whether the function of a cell or tissue is affected by the glycoside depends on such diverse factors as the sodium pump reserve, presence or absence of the Na^+/Ca^{++} exchanger, and the role of intracellular Na^+ or Ca^{++} concentrations in the function of that particular cell or tissue.

Neuronal cells of the autonomic nervous system are particularly sensitive to glycoside-induced sodium pump inhibition. Sensitivity of the baroreceptor to blood pressure changes is apparently increased. High doses of glycoside increase parasympathetic discharge to the heart. This decreases SA nodal heart rate and blocks AV conduction. Stimulation of the chemoreceptor trigger zone is responsible for glycoside-induced nausea and vomiting. At sympathetic nerve terminals, inhibition of the sodium pump facilitates neurotransmitter release. Glycoside-induced catecholamine release from sympathetic nerve terminals is responsible for the transient vasoconstriction observed with the intravenous administration of glycoside.

Mechanisms of Action of Catecholamines

Similar to the action of cardiac glycosides, the action of toxic doses of catecholamines results in arrhythmias. Both classes of drugs increase Ca^{++} loading of the sarcoplasmic reticulum, though by different mechanisms. The glycosides inhibit Ca^{++} extrusion and increase cytoplasmic Ca^{++} subsequently taken up by the sarcoplasmic reticulum. Catecholamines enhance Ca^{++} influx through the sarcolemma and also stimulate the Ca^{++} pump of the sarcoplasmic reticulum, resulting in an increase in Ca^{++} uptake by the sarcoplasmic reticulum. Thus, enhancement of the Ca^{++} transients and Ca^{++} overload are common features of the action of both classes of drugs.

Dobutamine, an analog of dopamine, stimulates β_1-β_2-, and α-adrenergic receptors. It does not interact with dopaminergic receptors, nor does it release norepinephrine from sympathetic nerve endings.

Phosphodiesterase Inhibitors

Amrinone and milrinone are bipyridines, chemically unrelated to either digitalis glycosides or catecholamines, that exert their positive inotropic actions by inhibiting cyclic adenosine monophosphate (cAMP) phosphodiesterase, the enzyme that hydrolyzes cAMP. The profile of cardiac effects of these drugs differs from that of the classical phosphodiesterase inhibitors (e.g., caffeine or theophylline). The primary difference is that the bipyridine derivatives are relatively selective inhibitors of a subclass of phosphodiesterases, phosphodiesterase III. In contrast to the classical inhibitors that are nonselective and increase both cAMP and cyclic guanidine monophosphate (c GMP) concentrations in heart muscle inhibitors of phosphodiesterase III increase only tissue cAMP concentrations. Whether a mechanism other than phosphodiesterase inhibition is responsible for the positive inotropic actions remains controversial. The increase in cAMP concentrations promotes cAMP-dependent protein kinase phosphorylation of the Ca^{++} channel, enhancing calcium influx and bringing about

Table 15-1 Pharmacokinetic Parameters

Agent	Route of Administration	Bioavailability (Oral, %)	Peak Effect*	Plasma Protein Binding (% Bound)	Disposition	$T_{1/2}$	Concentration in Plasma (ng/ml)
Digoxin	Oral, IV	45-85	6 hr	25	R(40%-90%)	35 hour	0.5-1.4
Digitoxin	Oral, IV	>90	12 hr	90	M(liver†)	6-7 days	9-30‡
Amrinone	Oral, IV	93	—	14-40	R, M	3.6hr	—
Milrinone	Oral, IV	92	—	—	R, M	0.8 hr	—

M, Metabolized; *R,* Renal clearance as unchanged drug.
*After a single oral dose.
†Large individual variation.
‡Total (free plus bound) drug.

a positive inotropic action by a mechanism similar to that of the catecholamines. A feature of these newer inotropic drugs is that they are reported to produce smaller chronotropic effects compared with catecholamines. This is an important characteristic for positive inotropic agents used to treat chronic heart failure.

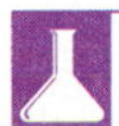

PHARMACOKINETICS

The principal pharmacokinetic parameters of the cardiotonic drugs are presented in Table 15-1. Digoxin and digitoxic are the two most frequently used glycosides, with digoxin being preferentially used in the United States and digitoxin being widely used in Europe.

Tissue binding and the ensuing large apparent volume of distribution for *digitoxin* contributes to its long half-life. The apparent volume of distribution for digoxin is considerably smaller. Because digitoxin has a longer half-life, fluctuation of the drug concentration in plasma during daily dosing is smaller with digitoxin than with digoxin. The absorption of digoxin varies from 45% to 85% when the drug is given as tablets. Digoxin tablets are subjected to a dissolution test to reduce variations in bioavailability; however, even slight differences in dissolution rate and bioavailability may pose serious problems because of the narrow margin of safety inherent with cardiac glycosides. Because bioavailability of digoxin tablets varies widely depending on preparations, patients should be maintained on a specific brand of drug. Bioavailability of digitoxin tablets is consistently high.

The most important factor determining total body elimination of digoxin is renal function, with clearance of digoxin proportional to creatinine clearance. Digitoxin is largely metabolized by the liver, and changes in renal function have minimal effects on its half-life. It is also excreted into bile and undergoes enterohepatic cycling. Because the reabsorbed metabolites are cardioactive, extrahepatic cycling contributes to its extended half-life (Table 15-1).

Large interpatient variations exist in the metabolism of *digitoxin* partly because intestinal flora play a significant role in its overall metabolism. The major pathway of metabolic disposition is a complex hydrolysis of the carbohydrate moiety catalyzed by the mixed function oxidase system followed by conjugation with glucuronic or sulfuric acid. Conversion of digitoxin to digoxin is a minor pathway in humans.

Several factors affect sensitivity of the heart to cardiac glycosides. Binding of the glycoside to the receptor site, Na^+,K^+-ATPase, is slow and is enhanced by high intracellular Na^+ and low extracellular K^+ concentrations. Thus the onset and the magnitude of pharmacological and toxic effects are greater in hypokalemic patients. Tachycardia, which increases Na^+ influx rate (and hence intracellular Na^+), also enhances glycoside actions. Larger doses of cardiac glycoside expressed as milligrams per kilogram of body weight are used in newborn and young infants compared with adults. This is not based on pharmacokinetic differences but is the result of low sensitivity of the infant heart muscle to the glycoside.

Variations in pharmacokinetics may be compensated for by maintenance of a predetermined digoxin or digitoxin concentration in plasma using feedback from assays of serum or plasma glycoside concentrations. This approach, however, does not entirely solve the problem because a given plasma concentration of the glycoside may be therapeutic in some patients and toxic in others resulting from individual differences in glycoside sensitivity of the heart. Because it is impractical to monitor directly the positive inotropic effect of the glycoside, clinical evaluation of the effects of the cardiac glycoside, including an analysis of the electrocardiogram (Table 15-2), is important. A slight (approximately 10%) increase in PR intervals that may be seen in patients receiving therapeutic doses of the glycoside is not alarming; however, a greater delay in AV conduction time and conduction block causing bigeminy or trigeminy herald serious digitalis toxicity.

Table 15-2 Inotropic Drugs

Drug	Mechanism	Use
DIGITALIS GLYCOSIDES		
digoxin, digitoxin	Inhibition of sodium pump (Na^+,K^+-ATPase)	Treatment of congestive heart failure related to ineffective ventricular function
CATECHOLAMINES		
dopamine	Dose-related stimulation of β-adrenergic receptor release of norepinephrine from nerve terminals	Short-term IV therapy in management of cardiogenic traumatic or septic shock in hospital setting
dobutamine	Stimulation of β_1-, β_2-, and α-adrenergic receptors	
PHOSPHODIESTERASE INHIBITORS		
amrinone, milrinone	Increase in concentrations of cAMP, resulting from inhibition of phosphodiesterase III	Weak inotropic drugs, used in hospital setting if all other therapies are not effective

Because digitoxin has a long half-life, it takes more than 20 days for the serum digitoxin concentration to reach a steady state when the treatment is begun without giving a loading dose. Therefore, digitoxin treatment should be started with a digitalizing (loading or priming) dose. Digoxin, which has a shorter half-life, may be given without a loading dose; a steady-state concentration of digoxin being obtained in 3 to 4 days. Special pharmacokinetic considerations are required when the glycosides are switched during chronic treatment. For a patient maintained on digoxin, termination of digoxin treatment and substitution with maintenance doses of digitoxin results in a temporary loss of pharmacological effects. The reason is that digoxin is excreted from the body rapidly whereas the accumulation of digitoxin is slow. Switching from maintenance doses of digitoxin to maintenance doses of digoxin causes a transient overdose because the effect of the rapidly increasing digoxin concentration is superimposed on the effect of a slowly declining digitoxin concentration.

Pharmacokinetic parameters for amrinone and milrinone are also included in Table 15-1. *Milrinone* competes for the same albumin binding sites as iodothyronine and may be a potential source of drug interactions with iodinated compounds.

Dopamine is used only by the intravenous route in patients under intensive care. Because the duration of action is extremely brief, the rate of administration is used to control intensity and duration of action. *Dobutamine* has a half-life of approximately 2 minutes and is administered by continuous intravenous infusion. It is rapidly metabolized in liver to inactive conjugation products with glucuronic acid.

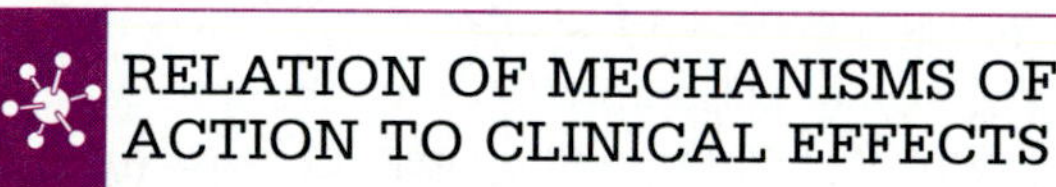

RELATION OF MECHANISMS OF ACTION TO CLINICAL EFFECTS

Digitalis Glycosides

Direct Effects on Na^+,K^+-ATPase Binding of cardiac glycosides to Na^+,K^+-ATPase of the myocardial sarcolemma and the resulting sodium pump inhibition are responsible for both the positive inotropic and toxic effects of the cardiac glycosides. A moderate (20% to 40%) inhibition of Na^+,K^+-ATPase, or the sodium pump, causes a therapeutic effect, whereas a greater sodium pump inhibition elicits toxic reactions. A significant positive inotropic effect of the glycosides requires a dose that is 50% to 60% of the toxic dose. This is the primary reason that all cardiac glycosides have a narrow margin of safety.

When glycosides are used in patients with a normal sinus rhythm to increase force of contraction, the therapeutic end point cannot be readily monitored because it is not possible to estimate the force of cardiac contraction in patients. This is further complicated because the binding of the glycoside to its pharmacological receptor is extremely slow, ordinarily taking several hours to reach equilibrium even when the drug is administered intravenously. Therefore, an immediate change in the force of cardiac contraction or an improvement in the patient's condition does not occur. Moreover, an overdose of glycoside decreases force, making it difficult to determine if the desired effect has not occurred because of an insufficient dose or because too much drug was administered. Finally, the cardiovascular system has multiple homeostatic mechanisms, and drug interventions to alter cardiac function may be counterbalanced by such mechanisms.

Because cardiac glycosides modify basic biochemical mechanisms for excitation-contraction coupling, these drugs are capable of increasing the force of cardiac contraction in either the normal or the failing heart. For a long time, however, the glycosides were believed capable of increasing force only in patients with failing hearts. For example, the administration of glycoside to a normal heart would initially increase the force of contraction and reduce end-diastolic volume. Reduced end-diastolic volume decreases the force of contraction, canceling the positive inotropic effect of the cardiac glycoside (Figure 15-1, *B, arrow*). In the failing dilated heart, however, the glycoside-induced increase in force of contraction and the associated decrease in end-diastolic volume make the heart's operation more nearly normal (Figure 15-1, *C, arrow*). Therefore, hemodynamic improvements can be obtained only in the failing heart even though the glycoside may have a direct positive inotropic effect on both failing and nonfailing cardiac muscle.

Because the systemic circulation is regulated to maintain constant blood pressure, any influence of a reduced force of cardiac contraction to lower the blood pressure triggers regulatory mechanisms. These are increases in sympathetic discharges to the heart and vascular system and activation of the renin-angiotensin-vasopressin system. The volume of circulating blood also may increase. Attempts of the body to increase blood pressure by constricting peripheral blood vessels and thereby increasing total peripheral resistance result in a decreased perfusion of many organs. The positive inotropic effect of cardiac glycoside reverses these changes and improves tissue perfusion. This is the primary beneficial effect of cardiac glycosides.

Cardiac glycosides do not have a direct action to improve energetic efficiency of muscle contraction; increases in force of cardiac contraction are associated with a corresponding increase in energy usage. In the failing heart, however, the glycoside decreases end-diastolic volume and thereby reduces wall tension necessary to develop the required intraventricular systolic pressure. Because the hemodynamic work of blood ejection can be achieved with a smaller wall tension, the net energetic efficiency of hemodynamic work is improved by the cardiac glycosides in patients with CHF.

The cardiac glycosides do not have direct diuretic effects unless injected into the renal artery in high concentrations; however, glycosides do produce notable diuretic effects in edematous patients with CHF. This effect results from improved tissue perfusion and reversal of changes in the renin-angiotensin-vasopressin system.

Indirect Effects Although the cardiac glycosides are capable of increasing the myocardial force of contraction, it has long been debated if the positive inotropic effect of the glycosides is truly the basis for the therapeutic efficacy of these drugs in patients. The glycoside has two clinically useful effects; one is to increase the force of cardiac contraction and the other is to slow the beating of the ventricle in patients with atrial fibrillation or flutter or in patients with chronic heart failure. Negative chronotropic effects of the glycoside results from stimulation of the cardiac parasympathetic (vagus) nerve, suppression of the sympathetic discharge to the heart, and the direct depressant action of the drug on conduction through the atrioventricular (AV) node. Cardiac glycosides do not have significant direct effects on the SA nodal rate. The direct and indirect actions of the glycoside on the AV node prolong its effective refractory period. When the glycosides are used to reduce the frequency of beating of the ventricle in patients with atrial fibrillation or flutter, the therapeutic end point can be clearly defined, and effects are easily evaluated. In this type of arrhythmia, cardiac glycosides are highly effective in reducing ventricular rate and restoring pumping efficiency. Therefore, cardiac glycosides can be used as an efficacious means of treating a patient with certain types of arrhythmias, though the glycosides are themselves arrhythmogenic and an overdose may cause a variety of arrhythmias. Cardiac glycosides, however, are incapable of converting atrial fibrillation or flutter to a normal sinus rhythm and simply reduce the number of depolarizations traversing the AV node and reaching ventricular muscle. The result is a reduction in frequency of ventricular beats in the patient with tachyarrhythmias of supraventricular origin.

The primary mechanism for stimulation of the cardiac parasympathetic nerve and inhibition of the sympathetic nerve is glycoside-induced inhibition of the sodium pump in neuronal cells, especially in pressure-sensitive cells of the baroreceptor. Discharge of the cardiac sympathetic nerve is normally synchronized with systemic blood pressure; during cardiac systole, blood pressure in the carotid artery increases, resulting in suppression of sympathetic outflow. Frequency of cardiac sympathetic discharge is much higher during the diastolic phase, when pressure of the carotid artery is low. This pattern of fluctuating sympathetic discharge is greatly enhanced in patients treated with cardiac glycosides because these drugs sensitize the baroreceptors to changes in blood pressure. Animal experiments indicate that the activity of cardiac sympathetic nerves may

Table 15-3 Effects of the Cardiac Glycosides on the Electrocardiogram

ECG Features	Glycoside-Induced Changes
P wave	Size and shape may change with large doses
PR interval	Prolongation and various degrees of AV block
QRS complex	Widening of abnormal complex in Wolff-Parkinson-White syndrome; however, no widening in normal QRS complex
QT interval	Shortened
ST segment	Depression when QRS complex is upward Elevation when QRS complex is downward
T wave	Diminished amplitude or inversion

be totally inhibited during systole when a toxic dose of glycoside is given. Overall sympathetic discharge is also reduced unless a toxic dose of glycoside causes arrhythmias and thereby greatly decreases systemic blood pressure.

Indirect effects of the glycosides mediated by the parasympathetic system may be eliminated by administration of the cholinergic muscarinic antagonist atropine. The glycosides, however, have a direct action on the AV node in addition to indirect actions through parasympathetic stimulation and sympathetic inhibition. When cardiac glycosides are administered to patients with atrial fibrillation or flutter, the net effect to slow the ventricular rate is caused by a combination of all three actions of the glycoside. Effects of the cardiac glycosides on the electrocardiogram are summarized in Table 15-3.

Because the glycosides do not have significant direct effects on the SA node, they do not alter heart rate in normal subjects. However, the glycosides do reduce the heart rate in patients with chronic heart failure because they decrease the elevated sympathetic influence on the heart, secondary to an improvement of hemodynamics.

Catecholamines

Dopamine and dobutamine are the only sympathomimetic amines used to treat heart failure, and their use is extremely limited. Dopamine's combination of effects on the kidney (vasodilatation) and on β_1-adrenergic receptors make this agent attractive in heart failure where the blood pressure is low and renal perfusion is poor, in such conditions as cardiogenic, traumatic, or hypovolemic shock. Its usefulness is compromised because of its capacity to release norepinephrine from adrenergic nerve terminals.

Dobutamine has a wider spectrum, interacts with β_1-, β_2-, and α-adrenergic receptors and therefore has a lesser tendency to increase peripheral resistance than dopamine does. Like dopamine, it is effective in short-term therapy of cardiogenic or septic shock by IV administration in a hospital setting.

Phosphodiesterase Inhibitors

Milrinone and amrinone have not been shown to be effective in the treatment of heart failure, being weak inotropic drugs and having the potential for inducing dangerous ventricular arrhythmias. Use is limited to hospitalized patients.

Alternative Treatment for Congestive Heart Failure

Because the basic problem of CHF is the relative deficiency in the force of cardiac contraction resulting in failure to meet the demand for blood supply to various body organs, a reduction in demand should be an effective treatment. This may be achieved by nonpharmacological therapies such as reducing physical activity, instituting emotional rest, and restricting salt and water intake. In addition, pharmacological reduction of cardiac work load can be achieved by (1) reduction of afterload and preload of the heart by lowering the systemic blood pressure, (2) dilation of blood vessels to reduce peripheral resistance, and (3) reduction of circulating blood volume. For example, a combination of antihypertensive drug and diuretic is frequently successful in treating patients with CHF. These are usually used in combination with a cardiac glycoside.

The vasodilators for the treatment of chronic heart failure should be used in doses that reduce peripheral resistance but do not cause a sharp decrease in the blood pressure; that is, in doses at which most of blood pressure effects can be compensated by readjustment of homeostatic mechanisms. Moreover, when an angiotensin-converting enzyme inhibitor is used to lower the concentration of angiotensin II, hypertrophy of the heart muscle may be prevented or reversed. Angiotensin II stimulates synthesis of selected proteins, and is believed to cause myocardial hypertrophy in the failing heart.

Angiotensin-converting enzyme inhibitors have been widely used in CHF. They decrease preload and afterload (see Chapter 13) and also increase cardiac output. Blood pressure does not tend to decrease significantly because any decrease in peripheral vascular resistance is counterbalanced by the increase in cardiac output. Because cardiac output increases, there is a tendency for norepinephrine concentrations to decrease. Addi-

Table 15-4 Factors That Affect Digitalis Sensitivity of the Heart

Condition	Glycoside Binding to the Sodium Pump	Reserve Capacity of the Sodium Pump	Glycoside Sensitivity of the Heart	Margin of Safety for the Glycoside
Na^+ influx ↑ or Na^+ efflux ↓	↑	↓	↑	↓
Tachycardia				
Electrical cardioconversion				
Ischemic border zone				
Hypoxemia				
Low plasma K^+	↑	↓	↑	↓
Hypokalemia				
Sodium pump units ↓		↓	No change	↓
Hypothyroidism				
Old age				
Myocardial Ca^{++} loading ↑	No change	No change	↑	↓
Hypercalcemia				
Magnesium depletion				
Altered digitalis sensitivity of the Na^+,K^+-ATPase				
Young children	↓	No change	↓	No change

Glycoside binding to the Na^+,K^+-ATPase (sodium pump) is enhanced by high intracellular Na^+ or low extracellular K^+ concentrations. Resulting inhibition less than prevailing reserve capacity of the sodium pump produces the positive inotropic effect, whereas inhibition exceeding the reserve capacity produces toxicity. Conditions that decrease the reserve capacity, therefore, reduce glycoside tolerance of the heart.

tionally, in contrast to the cardiac glycosides, survival is significantly increased in CHF patients treated with angiotensin-converting enzyme inhibitors.

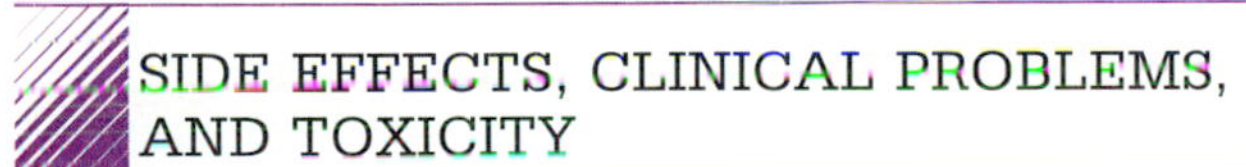

SIDE EFFECTS, CLINICAL PROBLEMS, AND TOXICITY

Two major problems associated with the use of cardiac glycosides are the narrow margin of safety and the inability of these drugs to retard or reverse the basic process that causes the heart to fail. The therapeutic indices of various cardiac glycosides are 1.5 to 3.0, depending on the degree of the positive inotropic effect sought. If a large positive inotropic effect is necessary, the required dose of glycoside is very close to the toxic dose. Therefore, the glycoside concentration in plasma should be kept within a narrow therapeutic window to maintain the drug effect without inducing toxicity.

Individual variation in glycoside sensitivity of the heart makes it difficult to achieve a correct maintenance dose for the patient, especially when drug concentrations approaching toxicity are required to meet the therapeutic need. Several factors affect the tolerance of patients to cardiac glycoside (Table 15-4). Old age and hypoxemia reduce the tolerance of the heart to cardiac glycosides by reducing the reserve capacity of the sodium pump. Hypokalemia, tachycardia and electrical cardioconversion also reduce reserve capacity and in addition promote glycoside binding to Na^+,K^+-ATPase. Under these conditions, the use of cardiac glycosides may not be warranted because a therapeutically useful positive inotropic effect may not be produced before the onset of toxicity. Hypercalcemia and magnesium depletion also reduce tolerance of patients to glycoside toxicity by augmenting Ca^{++} overload. Alternative therapies with vasodilators may be more useful under these conditions.

When treatment of a patient with chronic heart failure and pronounced edema is initiated with a combination of glycoside and diuretic, an initially adequate dose of glycoside will soon become toxic unless the maintenance dose is reduced as K^+ is lost from the body, or the plasma K^+ concentration is maintained by means of potassium supplementation. Because K^+ has a major influence on glycoside action, it is essential to monitor the K^+ concentration as well as the glycoside concentration in plasma during chronic treatment.

Hypokalemia greatly affects digitalis sensitivity of the heart. A lower extracellular K^+ concentration promotes glycoside binding to Na^+,K^+-ATPase and inhibits turnover of the sodium pump. Under these conditions, the sensitivity of the heart to the positive inotropic effect of the glycoside is increased, resulting from enhanced glycoside binding to the sodium pump. The sensitivity of the heart to toxic effects of the glycoside is increased further because toxicity is affected by the reduction in reserve capacity of the sodium pump, in addition to an enhanced glycoside binding. Hypokalemia therefore reduces the therapeutic index of the glycoside.

In patients with acute myocardial infarction, tolerance of the affected area (e.g., ischemic border zone) to digitalis toxicity is greatly reduced because of an elevation in intracellular Na^+; however, the glycoside sensitivity of the nonischemic area, where a positive inotropic effect can be elicited, is not altered. In these patients, the glycoside may fail to produce an adequate positive inotropic effect before the onset of toxicity, and therefore its use in acute heart failure is not recommended.

Toxic manifestations of glycoside overdose may be modified by the sympathetic influence on the heart. Blockade of β-adrenergic receptors increases tolerance of the heart to the arrhythmogenic actions of the glycoside. Animal experiments, however, indicate that β-adrenergic receptor blockade, or surgical removal of sympathetic influence to the heart, does not alter the lethal dose. Therefore, extreme caution is needed when β-adrenergic receptor blockers are used to treat manifestations of digitalis toxicity. With or without β-blockers, death often results from ventricular fibrillation.

Extracardiac manifestations of digitalis toxicity are largely mediated by the actions of the glycoside on neuronal tissues and secretory organs. These include anorexia, nausea, vomiting, excessive salivation, headache, epigastric distress, abdominal pain and diarrhea, yellow or green vision, muscle twitch, fatigue, stupor, visual disturbances, and neurological pain. Psychotomimetic effects including disorientation, confusion, depression, aphasia, delirium, hallucination, and convulsions may also be caused, especially in elderly patients.

Cardiac glycosides may have effects on other organs and tissues. The cardiac glycosides have negligible effects on skeletal muscle because (1) these cells do not have a potent Na^+/Ca^{++} exchanger and (2) transmembrane Ca^{++} does not play an important role in contractile activation. Glycosides have only a minor effect on renal salt and water excretion. It requires a direct infusion of high concentrations of cardiac glycoside into the renal artery to cause diuresis. These results indicate that the sodium pump and the Na^+/Ca^{++} exchanger may not play important roles in renal salt and water excretion, or that the renal sodium pump may have a large reserve capacity. Thus, cardiac glycosides have a principal effect on the heart even though these drugs act on the Na^+,K^+-ATPase that is present and functionally active in these cells.

Ca^{++} ions play an important role as a messenger in neuronal and secretory cells. High doses of cardiac glycosides facilitate neuronal transmission and stimulate secretory cells. Most of the central nervous system, however, is relatively unaffected by digoxin or digitoxin because access to the brain is limited, even though these drugs have a high lipid solubility. Prominent effects of glycosides on the nervous system are observed in neurons that essentially lie outside the blood-brain barrier; such as baroreceptors, chemoreceptors, and cells of the chemoreceptor trigger zone.

SIDE EFFECTS AND CLINICAL PROBLEMS

CARDIAC GLYCOSIDES	
digoxin, digitoxin	CNS: visual problems, fatigue, stupor, neurological pain GI: anorexia, nausea, vomiting cardiac: atrial and ventricular arrhythmias, AV block
CATECHOLAMINES	*hospital setting only*
dopamine	Hypertension, tachyarrhythmias, tolerance
dobutamine	Tachyarrhythmias, tolerance
PHOSPHODIESTERASE INHIBITORS	*hospital setting*
milrinone, amrinone	Weak inotropes, Arrhythmias

The primary signs of digitalis toxicity include arrhythmias caused by suppression of AV conduction. Ventricular premature contractions triggered by oscillatory afterpotentials that originate in Purkinje fibers may also be superimposed. These arrhythmias may be converted to a normal sinus rhythm by K^+ when the plasma K^+ concentration is low or within the normal range. K^+ is often effective against the glycoside-induced arrhythmias because K^+ (1) stimulates sodium pump activity, (2) reduces glycoside binding to Na^+,K^+-ATPase, and (3) probably alters membrane conductance to cations. When plasma K^+ concentration is high, antiarrhythmic drugs such as lidocaine, procainamide, or propranolol can be used. Although phenytoin is reported to be useful in treating arrhythmias, several instances of sudden death have occurred when phenytoin was administered to patients with glycoside overdose. Perhaps the most dramatic treatment for digoxin toxicity is the use of a specific antibody preparation raised against digoxin. The *Fab fragment* of the antibody is administered IV and acts by binding serum digoxin. The complex is excreted rapidly by the kidney.

Pharmacokinetic interactions involving digoxin are serious problems. Quinidine should not be used to treat digoxin-induced arrhythmias because it increases the

TRADE NAMES

In addition to generic and fixed-combination preparations, the following trade-named materials are available in the United States.

Corotrope, milrinone
Crystodigin, digitoxin
Digibind, digoxin immune Fab (ovine)
Dobutrex, dobutamine HCl
Inocor, amrinone
Intropin, dopamine HCl
Lanoxin, digoxin

plasma digoxin concentration. Quinidine reduces the apparent volume of distribution and renal clearance of digoxin. Reduction in the apparent volume of digoxin distribution results from the competitive displacement of the glycoside by quinidine from mutual binding sites. Because of the competitive nature of this interaction, the degree of quinidine-induced increase in digoxin concentration is proportional to the dose of quinidine. These mutual binding sites are not the pharmacological or toxic receptors for the glycoside. Therefore, the therapeutic and toxic effect of the glycoside increases because the displaced glycoside combines with Na^+,K^+-ATPase. Pharmacokinetic interactions between quinidine and digitoxin are less prominent because digitoxin has a large volume of distribution. In addition to quinidine, many drugs have been reported to have pharmacokinetic interactions with digoxin. Significant increases in plasma digoxin concentration may be observed only with high doses of verapamil, nifedipine, amiodarone, or quinine, in contrast to quinidine, which may precipitate digoxin toxicity at relatively low doses.

Other drugs that interact with the cardiac glycoside through various mechanisms are amphotericin B and chlorthalidone. Ethacrynic acid, furosemide, and thiazides increase the therapeutic and toxic effects of the glycoside and reduce the margin of safety by causing K^+ depletion. Large glucose infusions may also reduce serum K^+. Calcium preparations, reserpine, succinylcholine, and sympathomimetics may also precipitate digitalis toxicity. Propranolol may augment bradycardia caused by cardiac glycosides. Barbiturates, phenytoin, and phenylbutazone may enhance metabolism of the glycoside and thereby reduce the therapeutic and toxic effects, whereas the resin cholestyramine combines with digitoxin in the intestine and enhances elimination of glycoside.

The primary side effects and clinical problems are summarized in the box.

NEW DIRECTIONS

Several drugs (sulmazole, pimobendan, DPI-201-106) have been reported to increase Ca^{++} sensitivity of contractile proteins. Their utility as inotropic agents should have the advantage of not causing Ca^{++} overload. These drugs, however, can interfere with rapid and complete relaxation. One new agent that has selective phosphodiesterase inhibitor activity, vesnarinone, has the additional property of increasing action potential duration by depressing a potassium current in a manner similar to that produced by sotalol, a class II antiarrhythmic agent. Thus, this compound would have the advantage of being antiarrhythmic rather than proarrhythmic.

REFERENCES

Akera T: Effects of cardiac glycosides on Na^+,K^+-ATPase. In Greeff K, editor: *Handbook of experimental pharmacology,* 56/1: *Cardiac Glycosides,* Berlin, 1981, Springer-Verlag.

Colucci WS, Wright RF, Braunwald E: New positive inotropic agents in the treatment of congestive heart failure, *N Engl J Med* 314:290; 349, 1986.

Grupp G: Selective updates on mechanisms of action of positive inotropic agents, *Mol Cell Biochem* 76:97, 1987.

Lee CO: 200 years of digitalis: the emerging central role of the sodium ion in the control of cardiac force, *Am J Physiol* 249:C367, 1985.

Marban E, Smith TW: Digitalis. In Fozzard HA, Haber E, Jennings RB, et al., editors: *The heart and cardiovascular system, Scientific Foundation,* vol 2, New York, 1986, Raven Press.

Maskin CS, LeJemtel TH, Sonnenblick EH: Inotropic drugs for the treatment of the failing heart, *Cardiovasc Clin* 14:1, 1984.

SELF-ASSESSMENT QUESTIONS

1. The site responsible for the pharmacological and toxic actions of digitalis glycosides is associated with:
   a. β-adrenergic receptors.
   b. Na^+,K^+-ATPase.
   c. protein kinase C.
   d. cAMP-dependent protein kinase.
   e. Ca^{++} pump.

2. The system or function *not* affected by the cardiac glycosides is:
   a. the sodium channel.
   b. the intracellular Ca^{++} transient.
   c. the sodium pump.
   d. Ca^{++} loading of the sarcoplasmic reticulum.
   e. atrioventricular conduction.
3. The following limit the clinical usefulness of digitalis *except* the
   a. narrow margin of safety.
   b. low potency.
   c. tendency to produce arrhythmias.
   d. variations in bioavailability.
   e. patient-to-patient variability in sensitivity of the heart to digitalis.
4. Which of the following does *not* reduce the tolerance of patients to digital toxicity?
   a. hypokalemia
   b. magnesium ion depletion
   c. hypercalcemia
   d. electrical cardioversion
   e. hyperthyroidism
5. Which of the following can enhance the toxic effects of digitalis if taken concomitantly?
   a. quinidine
   b. lidocaine
   c. nitroglycerin
   d. hydralazine
   e. enalapril

CHAPTER 16

Calcium Antagonists

PAL L. VAGHY

MAJOR DRUGS

nifedipine
verapamil
diltiazem

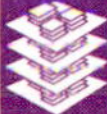

THERAPEUTIC OVERVIEW

It was observed in 1964 that the effects of certain phenylalkylamines such as prenylamine and verapamil on isolated cardiac papillary muscle preparations were indistinguishable from the effects of Ca^{++} removal. These drugs, like Ca^{++} depletion, reduced contractile force without affecting the action potential, thus producing excitation-contraction uncoupling. These drug effects could be reversed by Ca^{++} addition, β-adrenergic agonists, and cardiac glycosides. Verapamil and prenylamine, together with other drugs that inhibit excitation-contraction coupling, were termed **calcium antagonists** by Fleckenstein to indicate that they counteract the effects of Ca^{++} on the cardiac contractile system.

The primary action of these drugs is inhibition of the inward movement of Ca^{++} through the "L type" of voltage-dependent Ca^{++} channels located in cell membranes. To reflect this effect, the terms **calcium channel blockers, slow channel blockers, slow channel inhibitors, calcium channel inhibitors,** and **calcium entry blockers** have been used as alternatives to calcium antagonists.

ABBREVIATIONS

AV	atrioventricular
ECG	electrocardiogram
SA	sinoatrial
CHF	congestive heart failure

Calcium antagonists, encompassing several heterogeneous groups of chemicals are effective in the treatment of several cardiovascular disorders, particularly angina pectoris, supraventricular tachycardias, and hypertension. Several other conditions such as posthemorrhagic cerebral vasospasm and Reynaud's phenomenon appear in some clinical trials to be influenced by calcium antagonists. Therefore, the potential therapeutic range of these drugs is rapidly increasing.

Angina pectoris is the clinical syndrome of transient cardiac ischemia caused by coronary artery disease. It is characterized by severe retrosternal chest pain or pressure that in typical cases radiates to the left shoulder, left arm, or to the back. Exertional (stable), variant (Prinzmetal's), and unstable angina are the clinically recognized forms of this disease. The underlying pathological condition is atherosclerosis, and the related ischemia results from inadequate blood perfusion of an area of the myocardium. Ischemia can also develop from increased metabolic demand. Although angina pectoris is defined primarily as a "supply" defect, an increased metabolic demand is also apparently required.

Exertional (exercise-induced) angina most frequently occurs in patients with atherosclerotic coronary vessels. Typically, these patients are relatively free of symptoms at rest, an indication that the supply of oxygen and nutrients to the heart and removal of the metabolic products by venous blood may be adequate as long as there is no excess load on the heart. On exercise, heart rate and blood pressure increase, which results in increased cardiac work and increased demand for oxygen and nutrients. Blood flow through the narrow, atherosclerotic coronaries to the myocardium becomes limited. When demand exceeds supply, ischemia develops and causes the typical symptoms and signs, including chest pain and depression of the ST segment of the electrocardiogram (ECG). Symptoms can be alleviated by interven-

Table 16-1 Classification of Voltage-dependent Calcium Channels

Channel Type	Conductance	Blockers	Properties	Location/Role
L type	≈25 pS*	Calcium antagonists	Large, long-lasting current with slow inactivation	Cardiac and smooth muscle, neurons/ excitation-contraction and excitation-secretion coupling
T type	≈8 pS*	amiloride, tetramethrin, octanol	Tiny, transient current	Sinoatrial and Purkinje cells/pacemaker activity of the heart
N type	≈12-20 pS*	ω-conotoxin	Neither L or T	Neurons/neurotransmitter release

*Picosiemens.

THERAPEUTIC OVERVIEW

GOALS:	inhibition of Ca^{++} movement into cells through "L type" of voltage-dependent Ca^{++} channels
USES:	Angina pectoris Supraventricular tachycardia Hypertension, including isolated systolic hypertension Posthemorrhagic cerebral vasospasm Reynaud's phenomenon
OTHER NAMES:	Calcium-channel blockers Slow channel blockers Slow channel inhibitors Calcium-channel inhibitors Calcium-entry blocker

tions that either increase the supply of oxygen and nutrients or decrease demand.

Prinzmetal's angina was originally recognized as a variant form, in that it results from a transient narrowing of a large epicardial coronary artery. The vasospasm frequently develops at a sclerotic narrowing but also can occur on a normal segment of the coronary artery. Symptoms occur at rest, typically at night or early morning, and include severe chest pain. Unlike the stable form of angina, elevation of the ST segment of the ECG is recorded during episodes of pain. Focal vasospasm is the hallmark of this form of angina.

Of the three types of angina, *unstable angina* is most difficult to manage; it is characterized by symptomatic episodes that increase in frequency, severity, or duration. Chest pain occurs at rest (day or night) and often is associated with reversible ECG changes. Advanced atherosclerosis and coronary vasospasm may underlie this clinical syndrome.

Supraventricular tachycardias represent another disease group that benefits from treatment with calcium antagonists. Supraventricular tachycardias include *paroxysmal supraventricular tachycardia, atrial fibrillation,* and *atrial flutter.* The pathological mechanisms involved in development of these cardiac rhythmic disorders are described in Chapter 14. The atrioventricular (AV) node, which plays a key role in the mechanism of these arrhythmias, depends on the influx of Ca^{++} through voltage-dependent Ca^{++} channels. Supraventricular tachycardias are therefore sensitive to treatment with calcium antagonists.

The third major condition where calcium antagonists have significant therapeutic value is *hypertension.* The neurohumoral control of blood pressure, the mechanisms involved in hypertension, and drugs used for hypertension treatment are described in Chapters 12 and 13. Several calcium antagonists have been approved and are currently used for the treatment of hypertension.

Calcium antagonists may have an important therapeutic role in some neuropathological conditions, e.g., *posthemorrhagic cerebral vasospasm.* Focal or global cerebral vasospasm is a major implication of stroke. Nimodipine, a calcium antagonist, is used to prevent the vasospasm and related neurologic damage.

Raynaud's phenomenon is a peripheral vascular disease characterized by vasospastic attacks of digital arteries that are frequently precipitated by cold or emotional stress. This disease is reported to be ameliorated by calcium antagonists, particularly dihydropyridines, because of their ability to abolish vasospasm.

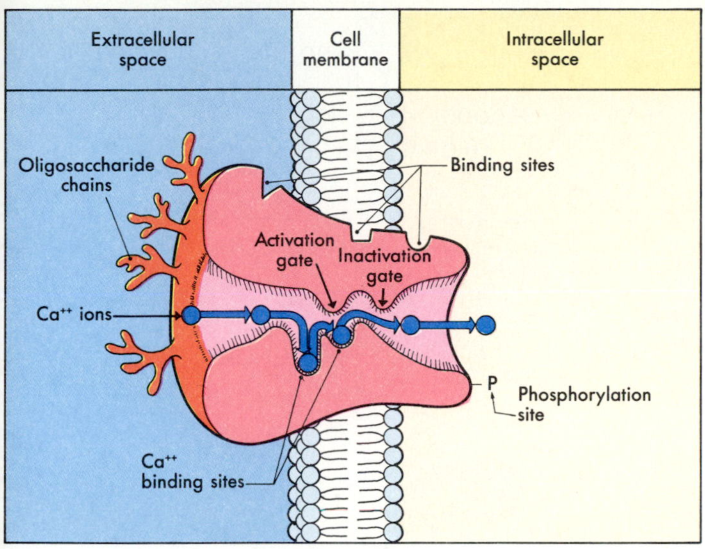

FIGURE 16-1 Schema of calcium-channel glycoprotein positioned in cell membrane. The ion channel is assumed to contain activation *(A)* and inactivation *(I)* gates that are moved or altered by the potential difference across the membrane and by drugs so as to open or close the channel to the transmembrane flux of Ca^{++}. A site of phosphorylation is shown. The detailed configuration and mechanism of the channel are still speculative.

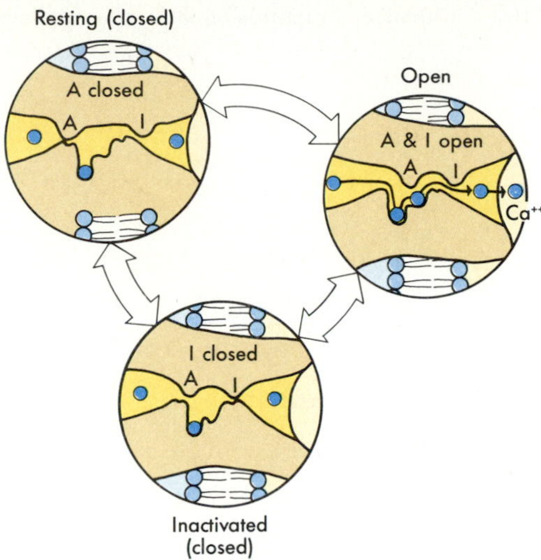

FIGURE 16-2 Three voltage-dependent conformations (states) of calcium channels. The ion channel (pore) is "open" to the transmembrane flux of Ca^{++} only when both the proposed activation *(A)* and inactivation *(I)* sites are open. In the "closed" states, either the *A* or *I* sites are not open. Top view of channel is shown on the left.

MOLECULAR MECHANISMS OF ACTION

Calcium antagonists act by inhibiting the influx of Ca^{++} into cells through specific voltage-dependent calcium channels located in cell membranes. Calcium channels are membrane-spanning, funnel-shaped glycoproteins that function like ion-selective valves (Figure 16-1). They form a water-filled pore and allow Ca^{++} to move in the direction of its electrochemical concentration gradient. When conformational changes in the channel macromolecule occur, the activation and inactivation "gates" move into and out of an occluding position. This determines opening and closing of the channel pore. Ca^{++}-binding sites present in the pore ensure ion selectivity for the channels. Phosphorylation sites of the channel protein apparently also play important roles in regulation of activity of the channel. It should be emphasized that the exact macrostructure of the channel, the spatial location of putative gates, and other regulatory sites are unknown at this time; the structure shown in Figure 16-1 is speculative.

Based on their electrophysiological and pharmacological properties, the voltage-dependent Ca^{++} channels can be divided into different types (Table 16-1). The best characterized are the **L type of channels** (long-lasting, large channels), the **T type of channels** (transient, tiny channels), and the **N type of channels** (found in neuronal tissue and resembling neither of the other two in kinetics and inhibitor sensitivity). Only the L type of Ca^{++} channels are affected by calcium antagonists.

The primary modulator of voltage-dependent Ca^{++} channels is the membrane potential (voltage). The existence of three voltage-dependent conformations is postulated (Figure 16-2): (1) a resting state in which the pore is closed by the A gate, (2) an open state in which both gates are open, and (3) an inactivated state in which the channel is closed by the I gate. Under resting conditions, when the voltage-dependent calcium channels are closed, the membrane potential is -30 to -100 mV (intracellular with reference to extracellular), depending on the cell type. The free intracellular Ca^{++} concentration ($<10^{-7}$M) is more than four orders of magnitude lower than the extracellular free Ca^{++} concentration (1 to 1.5×10^{-3}M). This large concentration gradient represents an enormous driving force for Ca^{++} to enter the cell and can be maintained only by a membrane that is largely impermeable to Ca^{++} and contains active-transport systems that pump Ca^{++} out of the cytosol. The intact cell membrane fulfills these requirements. On excitation, a rapid depolarization of the cell membrane follows, voltage-dependent Ca^{++} channels open and Ca^{++} enters the cell. This is followed by inactivation (closing) of Ca^{++} channels. Before the next depolarization occurs, Ca^{++} channels must recover from

FIGURE 16-3 Chemical structures of calcium antagonists.

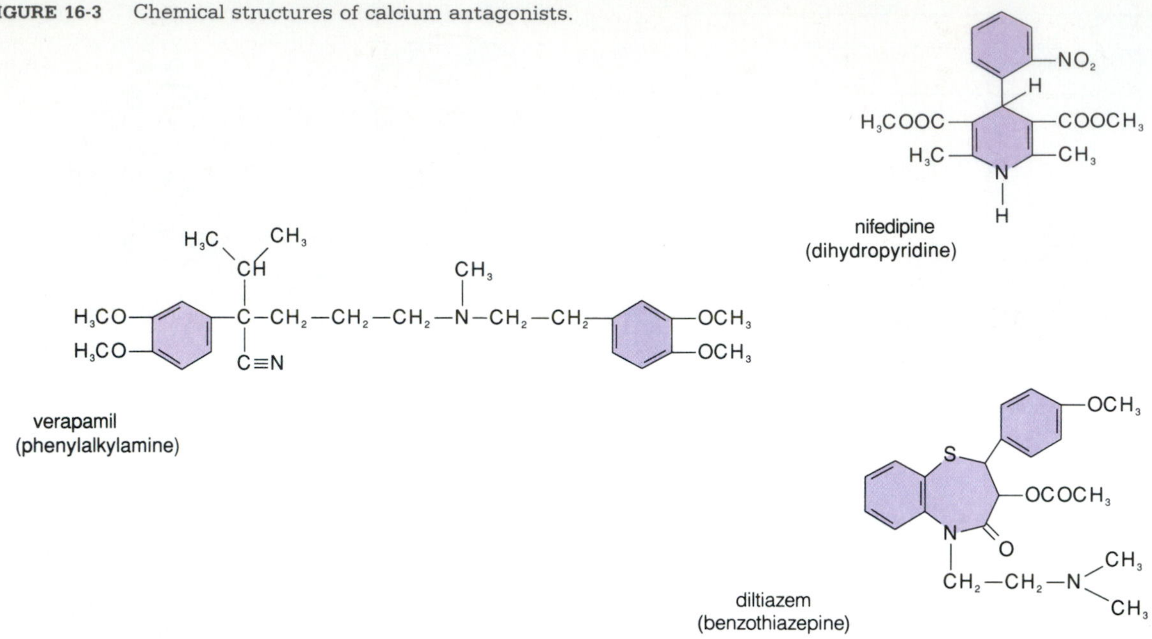

nifedipine
(dihydropyridine)

verapamil
(phenylalkylamine)

diltiazem
(benzothiazepine)

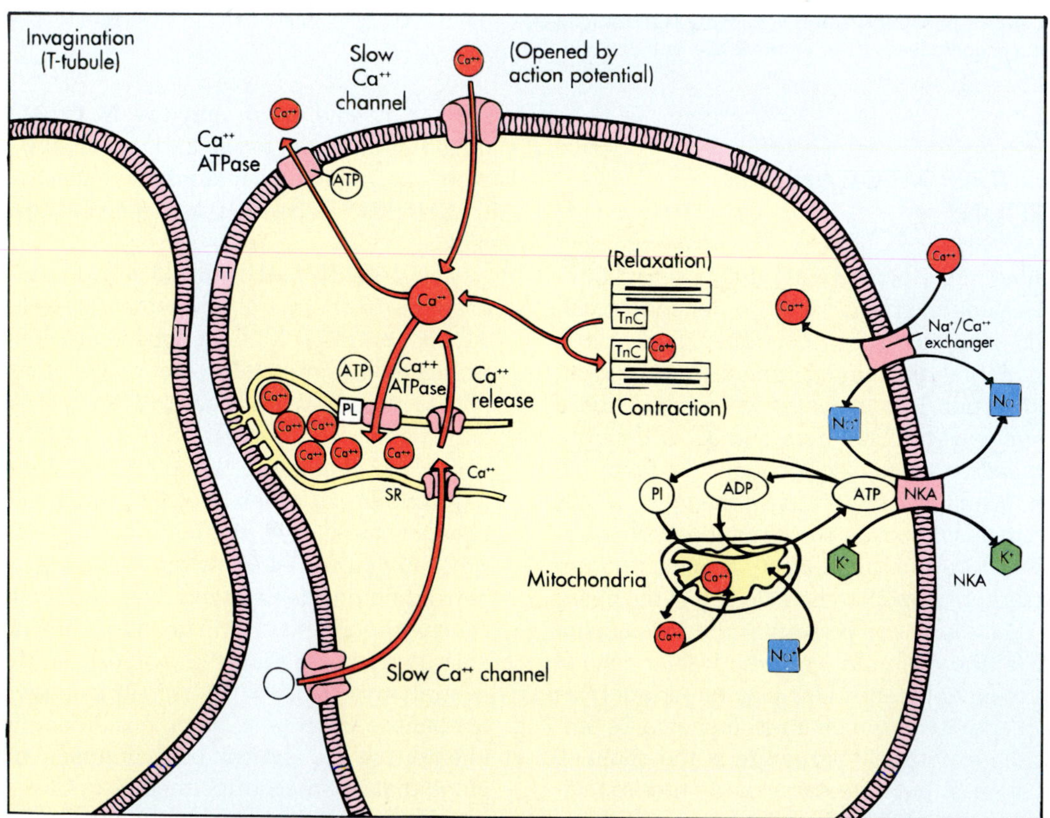

FIGURE 16-4 Excitation-contraction coupling in cardiac cells. *NKA,* Sodium-potassium-ATPase; *PL,* phospholamban; *SR,* sarcoplasmic reticulum; *tt,* T-tubule.

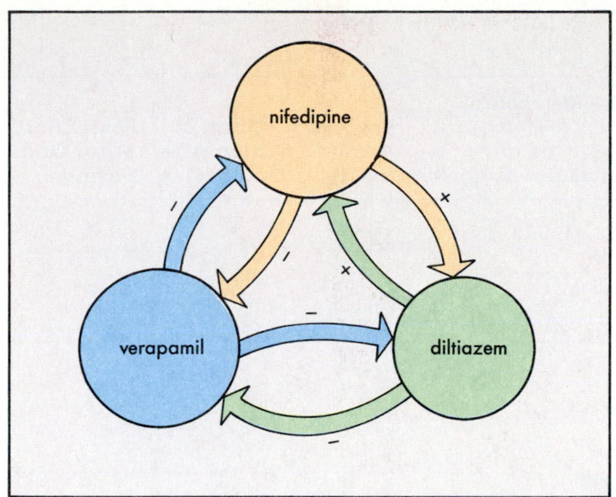

FIGURE 16-5 Allosteric interactions occur among the nifedipine (NIF), verapamil (VER), and diltiazem (DTZ) binding sites of the voltage-dependent Ca^{++} channels. All three binding sites are located on the same subunit.

inactivation and be ready for opening from a resting (closed) conformation.

In addition to the membrane potential, other modulators, both endogenous and exogenous, also affect voltage-dependent Ca^{++} channels. These are hormones, neurotransmitters, and inorganic ions. The drugs that act directly on Ca^{++} channels include both Ca^{++} agonists and Ca^{++} antagonists. Many chemical compounds are known to inhibit voltage-dependent Ca^{++} channels, but only those that have their primary effect on Ca^{++} channels are discussed here. The most selectively acting drugs belong to one of the following chemical groups: 1,4-dihydropyridines, phenylalkylamines, and benzothiazepines. The chemical structures of the representative drugs are completely different, as shown in Figure 16-3; hence one may expect that they bind to distinct sites of the L type of Ca^{++} channel.

Voltage-dependent Ca^{++} channels play a specific role in the excitation-contraction-relaxation cycle (see Chapter 15 and Figure 16-4). Under resting conditions, when the intracellular Ca^{++} concentration is low ($<10^{-7}$M), the regulatory proteins prevent interaction of actin and myosin filaments with each other, and the muscle is relaxed. When the intracellular Ca^{++} concentration increases ($>10^{-7}$M) from the influx of Ca^{++} through Ca^{++} channels and release of Ca^{++} from internal stores, Ca^{++} occupies binding sites on Ca^{++}-binding regulatory proteins such as troponin C (in cardiac and skeletal muscle) and calmodulin (in vascular smooth muscle). These then interact with other regulatory proteins and enzymes (e.g., troponin I in cardiac and skeletal muscle and myosin light-chain kinase in smooth muscle), facilitating cross-bridge formation between actin and myocin and activating contraction. When Ca^{++} channels close and Ca^{++} is pumped out of the cytosol into the sarcoplasmic reticulum and into the extracellular space, the Ca^{++} dissociates from Ca^{++}-binding proteins, activation of contractile proteins is reversed, actin dissociates from myosin, and muscle relaxation occurs.

The interaction of Ca^{++} channel modulators with Ca^{++} channels is complex. Distinct but allosterically interacting receptors exist for the structurally different chemical groups of drugs: 1,4-dihydropyridines (nifedipine-like drugs), phenylalkylamines (verapamil-like drugs), and benzothiazepines (diltiazem-like drugs) bind to different binding sites (Figure 16-5). For example, verapamil inhibits the binding of diltiazem, and diltiazem inhibits verapamil binding. Similar allosteric interactions are shown for the other agents. All these receptors are located on the same α_1 subunit of the L type of voltage-dependent Ca^{++} channels.

The effects of Ca^{++} antagonists are dependent on membrane potential (voltage). This phenomenon can be explained with the **modulated receptor model.** This model, first developed to explain voltage-dependent effects of local anesthetics on the Na^{+} channel, has been extended to explain the voltage-dependent effects of calcium antagonists on Ca^{++} channels. This model postulates that channels are similar to allosteric enzymes that alter their conformations and hence their affinities for substrates. Specifically, the modulated receptor model is an assumption that the channel macromolecule alters its affinity for the drugs when its conformation ("state") is changed by the membrane potential (note resting, open, and inactivated states, Figure 16-2). It is assumed that drugs bind to the inactivated channels with much higher affinity than to the resting and open channels. This may explain why these drugs are more effective on inactivated than on open or resting channels.

The binding and effects of Ca^{++}-channel inhibitors are stereoselective. Generally, stereoisomers of the same compound produce qualitatively the same effects, with one stereoisomer being more effective than the other. In a few special situations, the stereoisomers produce opposite effects. Although the *(R)*-enantiomers act like calcium antagonists, the *(S)*-enantiomers are calcium agonists.

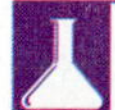 PHARMACOKINETICS

Dosage of different Ca^{++}-channel inhibitors and the mode of administration are determined by several factors, including the nature of the disease state and the

Table 16-2 Pharmacokinetics

Drug	Absorption	Bioavailability	Protein Binding (%)	Volume of Distribution (L/kg)	Active Metabolites	Metabolite Activity (% of parent drug)	$t_{1/2}$ (hr)	Route of Administration	Onset of Action After Oral Dosing	Peak Effect After Oral Dosing
Verapamil	>90%	10%-35%	90%	4	+	20%-30%	5	Oral, IV	<1 hr	1-2 hr
Nifedipine	>90%	60%-70%	95%	1.2	—	0	2	Oral	<20 min (2-3 min)*	30 min
Diltiazem	>80%	40%	75%	5.3	+	25%-50%	3.5	Oral	<1 hr	2-3 hr

*Sublingual.

overall condition of the patient. Therefore, the treatment regimen should always be individualized. A low dose is recommended at the onset of treatment, with subsequent increases to within the normal range until the desired therapeutic effect is reached. For a rapid effect, sublingual or IV administration of the drug may be required. The mode of administration and pharmacokinetic parameters of calcium antagonists are summarized in Table 16-2.

Absorption of *verapamil* from the gastrointestinal tract is effective (>90%), but the bioavailability is very low (≈20%); this results from the extensive first-pass metabolism by the liver. In the systemic circulation, 90% is bound to plasma proteins. The steady-state apparent volume of distribution is 4 L/kg of body weight. Norverapamil, an active metabolite, has a potency approximately 20% to 30% that of verapamil. Metabolites are excreted in the urine, with an elimination half-life of approximately 5 hours. Renal elimination is much longer in patients with hepatic disease.

The gastrointestinal absorption of *nifedipine* is essentially complete (>90%). Because of the first-pass metabolism by the liver, however, only 60% to 70% of the administered drug reaches the systemic circulation. In blood, 95% of nifedipine is bound to plasma proteins. The steady-state apparent volume of distribution is 1.2 L/kg body weight. Nifedipine is metabolized to three inactive metabolites in the liver, and these are excreted in the urine. The elimination half-life is approximately 2 hours but is longer in patients with compromised hepatic function.

Diltiazem is well absorbed from the gastrointestinal tract. Because of first-pass hepatic metabolism, the bioavailability is only 40%. Once absorbed, approximately 75% of diltiazem is bound to plasma proteins. The apparent volume of distribution is approximately 5.3 L/kg. Desacetyl diltiazem is an active metabolite with an activity of approximately 25% to 50% of the parent compound. The elimination half-life of diltiazem is 3.5 hours but is longer in patients with hepatic disease.

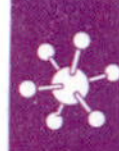

RELATION OF MOLECULAR ACTION TO CLINICAL EFFECTS

In many cardiovascular diseases (i.e., Prinzmetal's angina, hypertension, and Raynaud's phenomenon), constriction of high-resistance vessels occurs, associated with abnormally high cytosolic free Ca^{++} concentrations. It is possible that abnormal contractile proteins, with perhaps increased affinity for calcium, are present, changing endothelial cell function. Elevated cytosolic Ca^{++} may result from either an excessive influx of Ca^{++} or incomplete removal of Ca^{++} by Ca^{++}-ATPase or Na^{+}/Ca^{++} exchange processes. In any event, a rational therapeutic intervention is the inhibition of Ca^{++} influx, which induces vascular smooth muscle relaxation.

Endogenous and exogenous modulators that affect Ca^{++} channels are listed in the box. Drugs such as β-adrenergic agonists act on Ca^{++} channels indirectly, by activating cAMP-dependent protein kinase, which phosphorylates channel subunits and thereby results in an increase in the probability of channel opening. β-Adrenergic blocking agents act by inhibiting the binding of β-agonists, thereby preventing activation of Ca^{++} channels through β-receptors.

All excitable tissues contain voltage-dependent Ca^{++} channels and high-affinity, reversible, and stereospecific binding sites for Ca^{++} antagonists. However, Ca^{++} antagonists do not affect every tissue equally. Some tissues rely primarily on exogenous Ca^{++} (AV node) and are more sensitive to these drugs than other tissues (skeletal muscle) that require little or no external Ca^{++} for function (see box). There are subtypes of voltage-dependent Ca^{++} channels that show different sensitivities for Ca^{++} antagonists. Because the distribution of the channel subtypes differs in various tissues, drug sensitivity of the tissues is also varied. In addition, even the L type of Ca^{++} channels are different in various tissues with respect to their affinities for calcium antagonists. Finally, these drugs bind to the same

CALCIUM-CHANNEL MODULATORS

Membrane potential (voltage)
Hormones and neurotransmitters (e.g., epinephrine) can regulate the channel:
- By activating protein kinases (A or C) that phosphorylate the channel
- Through guanine nucleotide-binding (G) proteins that directly link β-receptors to calcium channels

Inorganic ions; Co^{++}, Ni^{++}, and Cd^{++} are inhibitors

REASONS FOR TISSUE SELECTIVITY OF CALCIUM ANTAGONISTS

Dependence of tissue on external Ca^{++}
Existence of Ca^{++}-channel subtypes
Voltage dependence of binding
Frequency dependence of drug effects

Table 16-3 Pharmacodynamic Effects and Uses of the Calcium Antagonists

	Phenylalkylamines	Dihydropyridines		Benzothiazepines
	A (Verapamil)	**B** (Nifedipine)	**C** (Nimodipine)	**D** (Diltiazem)
Vasodilatation:				
Peripheral	++	+++	+	+
Coronary	++	+++	+	+++
Cerebral	+	+	+++	+
Heart rate	↓	↑*	—	↓
SA node	↓	—	—	↓↓
AV node	↓↓	—	—	↓
Contractility	↓↓	↑*	—	↓

Indications for:
A Prinzmetal's angina; chronic unstable angina (effort-associated); paroxysmal supraventricular tachycardia; atrial flutter; atrial fibrillation; essential hypertension
B Angina pectoris (caused by coronary artery spasm); chronic stable angina (effort-associated); hypertension
C Improvement of neurological deficits caused by spasm after subarachnoid hemorrhage from ruptured congenital intracranial aneurysms
D Prinzmetal's angina; chronic unstable angina (effort associated); hypertension

*Reflex effect; +, mild effect; ++, moderate effect; +++, pronounced effect; ↓, negative effect; —, no change.

receptors with higher affinity under depolarized conditions. Because the resting membrane potential differs in various tissues, the binding and effects of these drugs also vary. Vascular smooth muscle has a more depolarized resting potential (−30 to −40 mV) than that of heart muscle (−70 to −90 mV). This may contribute to the vascular selectivity of many calcium antagonists.

Additionally, frequency dependence indicates that inhibition of channels by these drugs is altered by the rate of stimulation. The underlying mechanism for the frequency dependence appears to be inhibition of recovery of the channel from inactivation (transition from inactivated to resting state), which occurs during the time available between stimuli. Only those channels that have recovered from inactivation can reopen on the next stimulus. At high frequencies, the channels affected by these drugs do not function because they have not recovered from inactivation during the short time available between stimuli. Thus, drugs of this type seem to be very effective at high rates of stimulation. In contrast, at low frequencies, all channels (those affected by the drug and those not affected) may completely recover from inactivation before the next stimulus arrives. Therefore, drug inhibition of Ca^{++} channels is minimal or absent at low stimulation rates. Structurally different drugs show different degrees of frequency dependence. Verapamil shows much more frequency dependence than nifedipine does; diltiazem appears to be intermediate.

The several classes of calcium antagonists possess quite different pharmacological properties, depending on the class. These are discussed below and summarized in Table 16-3.

Verapamil

Verapamil was the first selective Ca^{++}-channel inhibitor available for treatment of cardiovascular disorders. Like nifedipine, verapamil has both coronary and peripheral vasodilatory effects. Verapamil is a more potent negative inotropic agent than nifedipine. This results from nifedipine's more potent activation of the baroreceptor reflex, secondary to the decrease in peripheral resistance. In contrast to nifedipine, verapamil also produces a severe depression of atrioventricular conduction. As a result, verapamil is the drug of choice for treatment of supraventricular tachycardias. Verapamil is also effective for the treatment of angina pectoris and hypertension. The reflex increase in adrenergic tone caused by a sudden decrease in the blood pressure mitigates but does not overcome the strong direct negative inotropic and chronotropic effects of verapamil. Because of these prominent cardiodepressant effects, verapamil is generally contraindicated in CHF. Verapamil is approved for the treatment of all types of angina pectoris, paroxysmal supraventricular tachycardia, atrial flutter, atrial fibrillation, and essential hypertension (Table 16-3).

Nifedipine

This drug has a relatively selective effect on *arterial resistance vessels*. By dilating coronary blood vessels and increasing coronary blood flow, particularly through narrowed coronary arteries (e.g., vasospasm), nifedipine increases oxygen and nutrient supply to the ischemic myocardium. By increasing coronary blood flow, nifedipine also enhances the removal of metabolic end products from the ischemic area. As a result of the dilatation of peripheral arterial resistance vessels, the arterial blood pressure *(afterload)* decreases. Although the decrease is much more significant in hypertensive patients than in normotensive individuals, any sudden decrease in blood pressure in either can result in a reflex increase in the heart rate and contractility. If the reflex increase in contractility is stronger than the direct negative inotropic effect of nifedipine, the overall result observed may be a slight increase or no effect, rather than a decrease in contractility. Pulmonary vascular resistance and the mean pulmonary arterial pressure are also decreased by nifedipine. These effects, together with the previously described effects, produce a favorable hemodynamic condition for patients suffering from angina pectoris and mild CHF simultaneously. However, there is always the potential danger that nifedipine may exacerbate incipient heart failure already present because of the direct cardiac negative inotropic action of the drug.

In contrast to verapamil and diltiazem, which inhibit atrioventricular conduction, nifedipine has no significant effect on atrioventricular nodal conduction in vivo. Nifedipine is preferable to verapamil and diltiazem in those patients who may have an underlying defective atrioventricular conduction problem (e.g., sick sinus syndrome). Nifedipine lowers esophageal sphincter pressure, may inhibit peristalsis, and, by inducing a sympathetic discharge, increases plasma renin activity.

In mild to moderate hypertension, nifedipine has an efficacy equivalent to β-blockers or diuretics. Although it is effective alone, its use in combination with low doses of β-blockers can be particularly efficacious because the reflex increases in heart rate and plasma renin activity produced by nifedipine are attenuated by the β-blocker.

In addition, nifedipine is used in the treatment of Raynaud's phenomenon. It has been employed in some studies in the treatment of ischemic pain immediately after myocardial infarction and for prevention of coronary artery spasm, which frequently occurs during coronary catheterization and coronary artery bypass surgery. Nifedipine is approved for the treatment of vasospastic angina, chronic stable angina (effort associated), and hypertension.

Diltiazem

Diltiazem has some pharmacological effects similar to those of nifedipine but resembles verapamil in its other actions. Like all Ca^{++}-antagonists, diltiazem increases coronary blood flow and decreases elevated blood pressure. Similar to verapamil, diltiazem inhibits atrioventricular conduction, though less effectively than verapamil.

Diltiazem has several therapeutic uses. It is effective in all types of angina, particularly in those forms where coronary vasospasm is involved. Diltiazem has approximately the same efficacy as nifedipine in dilating coronaries but produces fewer side effects. It can be prescribed with sublingual glyceryl trinitrate or with isosorbate trinitrate for treatment of angina pectoris. Diltiazem is effective in decreasing hypertension and has fewer negative inotropic and chronotropic effects than the β-adrenergic blocking drugs have. In paroxysmal supraventricular tachycardia, diltiazem, like verapamil, slows the ventricular response to atrial tachycardia and in many cases restores a regular sinus rhythm. Orally administered diltiazem is useful in preventing the development of paroxysmal supraventricular tachycardia and decreases the ventricular response in atrial fibrillation and flutter by slowing atrioventricular conduction. Other disorders that can be influenced by diltiazem include Raynaud's phenomenon, migraine, and esophageal mobility disorders. Diltiazem is approved by the FDA for the treatment of angina pectoris (caused by coronary artery spasm), chronic stable angina (effort associated), and hypertension (Table 16-3).

Other Calcium Antagonists

Nicardipine is a newer dihydropyridine calcium antagonist and is similar to nifedipine. It increases coronary blood flow in patients with coronary artery disease without causing myocardial depression. Nicardipine also decreases the systemic vascular resistance and has a potent antihypertensive effect. A sudden decrease in blood pressure can result in a reflex increase in heart rate and contractility. Nicardipine, at higher doses, does have a direct negative inotropic effect on the heart and in some patients with severe left ventricular dysfunction can lead to worsened heart failure. Nicardipine has little or no effect on the conduction system. Nicardipine has been approved for treatment of chronic stable angina alone or in combination with nitrates or β-blocker, and for treatment of hypertension alone or in combination with thiazide diuretics or β-blockers.

Isradipine and *felodipine* are other dihydropyridine antagonists used to treat essential hypertension (see New Directions). Isradipine decreases systemic vascular resistance and results in potent antihypertensive effects. A sudden decrease in blood pressure may result in a reflex increase in heart rate. Isradipine, at higher doses, may have a direct negative inotropic effect on the heart, and caution should be exercised in patients with CHF, particularly when used in combination with a β-blocker. Isradipine has no detrimental effects on the conduction system and is indicated for the treatment of hypertension alone or in combination with thiazide diuretics.

Felodipine, in contrast to some of the other calcium antagonists, has very little or no effect on cardiac function. It has a relatively long duration of action and in extended-release formulation is appropriate for treatment of hypertension with a once-daily dose. Reflex increase in heart rate frequently occurs during the first week of therapy, but this increase attenuates over time. The increase in heart rate is inhibited by β-blocking agents.

Amlodipine is a low-clearance, dihydropyridine calcium antagonist that is effective for treatment of hypertension and angina pectoris with once-daily dosing. Good bioavailability (60% to 65%) and slow rate of elimination ($t_{1/2}$ of 45 hours) confer pharmacokinetic characteristics to amlodipine that are not seen with other calcium-antagonist drugs.

Nimodipine is a second-generation dihydropyridine with apparent selectivity for cerebral blood vessels. Nimodipine has been approved for the treatment of neurological complications after subarachnoid hemorrhage. Nimodipine has been used to ameliorate cerebral vasospasm occurring during the prodromal phase of migraine. It has also been approved for treatment of neurological deficits caused by cerebral vasospasm after subarachnoid hemorrhage from ruptured congenital intracranial aneurysms.

Bepridil is a nonselective antianginal agent that is structurally unrelated to the calcium antagonists. It inhibits calcium and sodium channels and interferes with calcium binding to calmodulin and receptor-operated calcium channels in vascular smooth muscle. Bepridil is indicated for treatment of stable chronic angina only after other agents have failed.

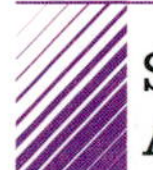

SIDE EFFECTS, CLINICAL PROBLEMS, AND TOXICITY

Problems and side effects are summarized in the box. Most side effects result from excessive vasodilatation or cardiodepression (e.g., negative inotropic and chronotropic effects). Generally, side effects such as dizziness, headache, and flushing decrease or disappear on decreasing the dose. For others, discontinuation of the drug may be necessary. Although true withdrawal symptoms are not observed as such, sudden withdrawal of large doses of calcium antagonists may, rarely, precipitate angina. Neither tachyphylaxis nor tolerance is observed with these drugs.

During *verapamil* treatment, side effects occur in approximately 8% to 10% of patients and may result from

CLINICAL PROBLEMS AND ADVERSE EFFECTS

VERAPAMIL	
Problems in 8% to 10% of patients	
Major	Cardiodepression
Moderate	Hypotension AV block Peripheral edema
Minor	Headache Constipation
NIFEDIPINE	
Problems in 17% to 20% of patients	
Major	Hypotension Headache Peripheral edema
DILTIAZEM	
Problems in 2% to 5% of patients	
Minor	Hypotension Peripheral edema AV block Cardiodepression

Table 16-4 Contraindications of Calcium Antagonists

Generic Name	Contraindications
Verapamil*	Severe left ventricular dysfunction. Hypotension or cardiogenic shock. Sick sinus syndrome or second- or third-degree AV block, except in cases of a functioning artificial ventricular pacemaker. Patients with atrial flutter or atrial fibrillation and an accessory bypass tract. Hypersensitivity.
Nifedipine	Known hypersensitivity reaction to nifedipine.
Diltiazem	Sick sinus syndrome or second- or third-degree AV block, except in the presence of a functioning artificial pacemaker. Hypotension less than 90 mm Hg systolic. Hypersensitivity to the drug. Acute myocardial infarction and pulmonary congestion.

*Verapamil should be avoided in patients with severe left ventricular dysfunction or moderate to severe symptoms of cardiac failure and in patients with any degree of ventricular dysfunction if they are receiving a β-blocker.

excessive vasodilation and blockade of the atrioventricular node. Verapamil (and diltiazem) are contraindicated in the treatment of ventricular arrhythmias or in Wolf-Parkinson, White syndrome. During oral administration, the most frequent side effects are constipation, headache, nausea, dizziness, and ankle edema. Constipation does not appear to be a problem with either nifedipine or diltiazem. Verapamil may produce its side effects by acting on autonomic receptors. Rare side effects are galactorrhea and reversible hepatic damage. Adverse effects with overdoses include hypotension, AV block, bradycardia, CHF, and (rarely) ventricular asystole. Verapamil toxicity, like the effects of all calcium antagonists, may be reversed with isoproterenol alone or in combination with IV calcium gluconate.

With *nifedipine* use, side effects may occur in 17% to 20% of patients, primarily but not exclusively related to excessive vasodilation. Headache, dizziness, flushing, ankle edema, hypotension, and nasal congestion are mitigated by reducing the dose. If this is unsuccessful, discontinuation of drug may be necessary, and substitution with another calcium antagonist may be indicated.

Side effects are rare (2% to 5%) during *diltiazem* treatment and occur mainly with high doses. Headache, flushing, and hypotension occur from excessive vasodilatation and AV block may result from depression of the AV node.

Before the administration of calcium antagonists to patients concurrently on digitalis preparations, two possible drug interactions must be considered. Depression of AV conduction may occur by the combined depressive effects of digitalis and calcium antagonists on the AV node. Digitalis toxicity also may occur if renal clearance of digoxin is reduced by a calcium antagonist.

The combination of nifedipine with β-blocker for treatment of hypertension can be advantageous. Although both drugs directly decrease blood pressure, the reflex effects of nifedipine to increase heart rate and plasma renin activity prevent severe hypotension when the drugs are used in appropriate doses. Nifedipine, although it has no significant effect on AV conduction, produces a small negative inotropic effect in the presence of β-blockade. Therefore, this combined therapy is not recommended in patients with impaired ventricular function. Here, the combination of verapamil and β-blockers may cause severe hypotension, AV block, or heart failure. In several studies, diltiazem and β-blockers have been used safely, but again caution should be observed. Contraindications to calcium-antagonist therapy are found in Table 16-4.

TRADE NAMES

In addition to generic and fixed-combination preparations, the following trade-named materials are available in the United States.

Adalat, nifedipine
Procardia, Procardia XL, nifedipine
Calan, Calan SR, verapamil
Isoptin, verapamil
Cardizem, Cardizem SR, diltiazem
Cardene, Cardene SR, nicardipine
DinaCirc, isradipine
Plendil, felodipine
Norvasc, amlodipine
Nimotop, nimodipine
Vascor, bepridil

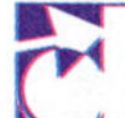

NEW DIRECTIONS

Initially, calcium-channel blockers were indicated for the treatment of angina pectoris and arrhythmias. Only recently have they been introduced for the treatment of hypertension. Many first-generation calcium antagonists have been made available in sustained-release forms to allow once-daily or twice-daily administration. In contrast to multiple daily doses, once- or twice-daily drug administration results in improved patient compliance, and minimal fluctuating in serum drug concentration. This assures a more effective treatment of hypertension. Second-generation calcium antagonists are now also available in the United States. These drugs have a higher selectivity for vascular smooth muscle and therefore have less effect on the heart. These include *nicardipine, isradipine, felodipine,* and *amlodipine* (see above). *Felodipine* and *amlodipine,* because of their favorable pharmacokinetic characteristics (e.g., long elimination half-life) frequently can be used for the management of hypertension at a once-daily dose. .

REFERENCES

Frishman WH, Sonnenblick EH: Principles and practice of calcium-channel blockade. Cardiovascular uses of calcium-channel blockers. In Messerli FH, editor: *Cardiovascular drug therapy,* Philadelphia, 1990, WB Saunders.

Janis RA, Triggle DJ: Drugs acting on calcium channels. In Hurwitz L, Partridge LD, Leach JK, editors: *Calcium channels: their properties, functions, regulation, and clinical relevance,* Boca Raton, Fl, 1991, CRC Press.

SELF-ASSESSMENT QUESTIONS

1. All of the following statements about calcium antagonist are true *except* that:
   a. they decrease peripheral vascular resistance.
   b. they increase coronary blood flow.
   c. they decrease cardiac afterload.
   d. they decrease serum Ca^{++} concentration.
   e. they may cause hypotension.
2. All of the following untoward effects are correctly matched with the therapeutic agents *except:*
   a. cardiodepression—verapamil.
   b. hypotension—nifedipine.
   c. atrioventricular block—diltiazem.
   d. cardiodepression—felodipine.
3. All of the following contraindications are correctly matched with the therapeutic agents *except:*
   a. heart failure—verapamil.
   b. second- or third-degree AV block—diltiazem.
   c. advanced aortic stenosis—nicardipine.
   d. ventricular arrhythmias—bepridil.
   e. essential hypertension—verapamil
4. All of the following statements about verapamil are true *except* that:
   a. it can be administered safely with β-adrenergic receptor blocking agents.
   b. it is useful for the treatment of atrial flutter.
   c. it is useful for the treatment of atrial fibrillation.
   d. negative inotropic action limits its use in a damaged heart.
   e. it is useful for the treatment of paroxysmal supraventricular tachycardia.
5. True statements about the use of calcium antagonists in the treatment of paroxysmal supraventricular tachycardia include which of the following?
   a. All are equally effective.
   b. Only nifedipine can be used.
   c. Verapamil is the drug of choice.
   d. The second-generation calcium antagonists must be tried first.
   e. Calcium antagonist can be used only if other drugs have failed.
6. Calcium antagonists act by inhibiting:
   a. Ca^{++} influx into the cells through "L type" of voltage-dependent Ca^{++} channels.
   b. Ca^{++} influx into the cells through "T type" of voltage-dependent Ca^{++} channels.
   c. Ca^{++} influx into the cells through "N type" of voltage-dependent Ca^{++} channels.
   d. Ca^{++} influx into the cells through "P type" of voltage-dependent Ca^{++} channels.
   e. Ca^{++} influx into the cells through receptor-operated Ca^{++} channels.
7. The reason for tissue selectivity of calcium antagonists may include all *except:*
   a. dependence of the tissue on external Ca^{++}.
   b. existence of Ca^{++}-channel subtypes.
   c. voltage dependence of binding and effects.
   d. frequency dependence of effects.
   e. differential metabolism of different drugs in different tissues.

CHAPTER 17 Vasodilators

DAVID WESTFALL
WILLIAM T. GERTHOFFER

MAJOR DRUGS

ACE inhibitors
hydralazine
minoxidil
nitroglycerin and nitrates
prazosin
sodium nitroprusside

THERAPEUTIC OVERVIEW

Ischemic heart disease is characterized by angina pectoris, chest pain that arises generally midsternally but also may radiate along the inner portion of one or both arms or to the back. Vasodilators, specifically the nitrates, are mainstays in management. There are several different types of angina, depending on whether the disease is atherosclerotic in origin, the result of coronary artery spasm, or a combination of both. Angina also may be classified according to whether the pain is exertional or occurs more frequently at rest. These differences are discussed in Chapter 16. However, irrespective of the type of angina, the purpose of pharmacological intervention is to bring about vasodilatation of the coronary arteries or redistribution of blood flow in the heart or a reduction in the oxygen demands of the heart. Vasodilators, such as the nitrates, provide no permanent beneficial effect on the underlying pathological condition but merely afford temporary symptomatic relief.

Vasodilator drugs have important uses in the management of coronary artery disease, hypertension, and congestive heart failure (CHF). Some modest success in preventing vasospasm or peripheral vascular disease also has been achieved with vasodilators. A minor role for these agents is the lowering of blood pressure to reduce bleeding into a surgical field.

Recent studies indicate that vasodilator therapy is extremely effective in the treatment of CHF. Drugs used more frequently for treating CHF are those that increase the force of cardiac contraction (digitalis glycosides) and minimize sodium and water retention (diuretics). Cardiac glycosides affect only two of the several determinants of cardiac function—contractility and heart rate. Vasodilators can be useful in the treatment of CHF, reducing either preload, afterload, or both. Whether preload or afterload is affected depends on the specific action of the vasodilator on the arteriolar and venous vessels. Patients who are refractory to cardiac glycosides frequently do well if treated with vasodilators. Among the direct-acting vasodilators used to treat CHF are the nitrates, hydralazine, minoxidil, and sodium nitroprusside. Angiotensin converting enzyme (ACE) inhibitors are also of proved effectiveness in the treatment of CHF.

Vasodilators are also used to treat certain peripheral vascular disorders. Direct-acting vasodilators, α-adrenergic blockers, calcium-channel blocking drugs, and ACE inhibitors are used to treat Raynaud's phenomenon. Vasodilators do not appear to be effective in increasing blood flow when organic obstruction is sig-

ABBREVIATIONS

ACE	angiotensin converting enzyme
ADP	adenosine diphosphate
ATP	adenosine triphosphate
cAMP	cyclic adenosine monophosphate
cGMP	cyclic guanosine monophosphate
CHF	congestive heart failure
EDRF	endothelium-derived relaxing factor
IP_3	inositol 1,4,5-trisphosphate
NO	nitric oxide

nificant. In some instances, the use of vasodilator therapy may actually be harmful in that blood is shunted away from diseased areas (see below).

Although vasodilators have actions that make them valuable therapeutic agents, they are not without some problems. One major problem with the use of vasodilators is the "steal" phenomenon. Some data indicate that the use of vasodilator drugs to promote blood flow to ischemic or diseased tissue is limited. It appears that the small blood vessels around the ischemic area are already significantly dilated. Thus the vasodilators may do little to enhance flow in the ischemic region. However, in the normal nonischemic areas where the small blood vessels are not dilated, there is an increase in blood flow with vasodilator therapy. By shunting blood to these areas, vasodilators may actually be reducing flow to the ischemic region by the "steal" mechanism.

Another concern with vasodilators is that, by decreasing peripheral vascular resistance, the sympathetic nervous system is reflexly activated. Enhanced sympathetic activity can lead to unwanted cardiac effects. The release of renin from renal juxtaglomerular cells is also enhanced by sympathetic nerve stimulation caused by baroreflex effects. To counteract this action, β-adrenergic receptor antagonists (e.g., propranolol) are frequently administered in conjunction with the direct-acting vasodilator.

A further issue is the potential of these vasodilators to cause dilation of smooth muscles other than vascular smooth muscle. Although not common, there are circumstances in which this is a significant problem, as in the treatment of hypertension associated with the toxemia of pregnancy. In this case the presence of vasodilators might interrupt labor by relaxation of uterine smooth muscle.

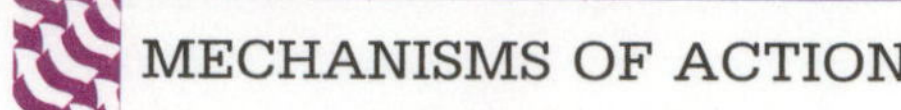

MECHANISMS OF ACTION

The commonly used vasodilators are listed in Table 17-1.

Control of Vascular Smooth Muscle Tone by Vasodilators

Vasodilators act at different sites in the cascade of events that couple excitation of vascular smooth muscle with contraction. Vascular smooth muscle contraction, similar to contraction of other smooth muscle, is ultimately regulated by the intracellular calcium concentra-

THERAPEUTIC OVERVIEW

CLINICAL PROBLEM	GOAL OF DRUG INTERVENTION
Hypertension	Decrease blood pressure
Congestive heart failure	Increase cardiac output and decrease oxygen consumption
Coronary artery insufficiency	Increase effective flow through coronary arteries and decrease oxygen consumption by the heart
Peripheral vascular disease	Increase blood flow to the ischemic area
Hemostasis	Slow bleeding into surgical field

Table 17-1 Mechanisms, Sites of Action, and Uses of Selected Vasodilator Drugs

Drug	Mechanism	Vessels Affected	Uses
nitroglycerin and nitrates	Direct effect, conversion to NO, increase in cGMP	Venous	Angina pectoris (coronary artery disease), CHF, Raynaud's disease
hydralazine	Direct effect, partially EDRF-dependent formation of NO*, increase in cGMP; possible K^+-channel agonist	Arteriolar	Hypertension, CHF (with nitrate)
sodium nitroprusside	Direct effect, conversion to NO*, increase in cGMP	Arteriolar and venous	Hypertensive emergencies, acute CHF
captopril, enalapril, and lisinopril	Inhibition of angiotensin converting enzyme	Arteriolar and venous	Hypertension, CHF
minoxidil	Direct effect, K^+-channel agonist	Arteriolar	Refractory hypertension
prazosin	Blockade of α-adrenergic receptor	Arteriolar and venous	Hypertension, Raynaud's disease,

See Chapter 14 for calcium channel blockers.
*May be nitric oxide (NO) or a chemically related unstable nitroso compound.

tion $[Ca^{++}]_i$. Excitation-contraction coupling occurs by several mechanisms. Depolarization of the vascular smooth muscle cell membrane allows Ca^{++} entry through potential- (or voltage-) operated channels. When potential-operated channels open, Ca^{++} flows into the cell along its concentration gradient. Activation of membrane receptors for certain vasoconstrictor substances can open calcium channels. In addition to elevating $[Ca^{++}]_i$ by channel opening, receptor activation can increase $[Ca^{++}]_i$ by activation of phospholipase C, which hydrolyzes phosphatidyl-inositol 4,5-bisphosphate to diacylglycerol and inositol 1,4,5-trisphosphate (IP_3). Both substances participate in intracellular events related to contraction (see also Chapters 2 and 8). IP_3, for example, releases calcium from bound sites in the sarcoplasmic reticulum.

When Ca^{++} enters the smooth muscle cell through the voltage-operated calcium channel or is released from intracellular sites by IP_3, it combines with calmodulin. The Ca^{++}-calmodulin complex activates myosin light-chain kinase, which in turn phosphorylates the myosin light chain. It is this phosphorylation of the myosin light chain that promotes the interaction of myosin and actin and cross-bridge formation, leading to vascular smooth muscle contraction (Figure 17-1).

The sites of action of vasodilators are shown in Figure 17-1. Calcium-channel antagonists block or limit the entry of calcium through channels in membranes of vascular smooth muscle cells. These calcium-channel blockers will therefore limit the amount of $[Ca^{++}]_i$ available to interact with contractile proteins. Thus, these agents dilate blood vessels that exhibit some degree of vasoconstrictor-tone or limit the vasoconstriction caused by endogenous or exogenous vasoactive stimulants (Chapter 14).

Agents such as minoxidil cause vasodilatation by activating potassium channels in vascular smooth muscle. The increase in potassium conductance results in hyperpolarization of the cell membrane associated with relaxation of smooth muscle. The hyperpolarizing effect of an increase in potassium conductance also offsets the influence of stimulants that act by depolarizing the membrane and promoting calcium entry.

Nitrovasodilators activate a soluble guanylate cyclase in vascular smooth muscle, causing an increase in intracellular cyclic guanosine monophosphate (cGMP). cGMP in turn activates a cGMP-dependent protein kinase. The mechanism by which cGMP-dependent protein kinase leads to smooth muscle relaxation is not entirely clear but may include a decrease in $[Ca^{++}]_i$ as a result of several actions, including a modification of calcium entry through membrane channels. Other actions that could potentially contribute to this effect would be a cGMP-dependent protein kinase–induced inhibition of phosphoinositol hydrolysis, or stimulation of calcium pumps, resulting in extrusion or sequestration of calcium. Another possible action is that cGMP-dependent protein kinase may directly decrease the sensitivity of the contractile proteins to calcium. Regardless of the specific mechanism or mechanisms, it is clear that increases in cGMP are associated with vascular smooth muscle relaxation.

The action of nitrovasodilators appears to be quite similar to that of endothelium-derived relaxing factor (EDRF). EDRF is formed in and released from endothelial cells of blood vessels. EDRF has recently been shown to be nitric oxide (NO) or a closely related nitrosothiol compound. NO stimulates guanylate cyclase in smooth muscle. That nitrovasodilators generate NO in vivo indicates that this substance may be the final common mediator for several vascular smooth muscle relaxants. In addition to nitrovasodilators, which may form nitric oxide or a related molecule, some endogenous agents that cause vasodilatation do so in whole or in part by releasing EDRF from endothelial cells. Included among these are bradykinin, histamine, adenosine triphosphate (ATP), adenosine diphosphate (ADP), substance P, and acetylcholine (Figure 17-2).

Increases in cyclic adenosine monophosphate (cAMP) are also associated with smooth muscle relaxation. When cAMP is elevated, cAMP-dependent protein kinase is activated. The exact mechanism of vasodilatation produced by this second messenger pathway is not known but may include decreased $[Ca^{++}]_i$ secondary to reduced influx of calcium, enhanced calcium uptake into the sarcoplasmic reticulum, or enhanced calcium extrusion through the cell membrane. cAMP-dependent protein kinase may also phosphorylate and inhibit myosin light-chain kinase, thus inhibiting contraction, though the relative importance of this pathway is not clear. The relaxation of smooth muscle produced by β-adrenergic receptor agonists, such as isoproterenol, is dependent on the formation of cAMP. Stimulation of β-receptors activates adenylate cyclase, which catalyzes the generation of cAMP from ATP. Drugs that inhibit phosphodiesterases, enzymes that metabolize cAMP and cGMP, can promote smooth muscle relaxation by elevating concentrations of these second messengers. Thus, drugs such as papaverine may act by this mechanism. Phosphodiesterases exist in several isoforms, and there is considerable interest for developing agents with specificity for these several isoforms. This may lead to the development of new vasodilators.

Vasodilator Drugs

The organic nitrate vasodilator drugs include the prototype nitroglycerin plus isosorbide dinitrate, erythrityl

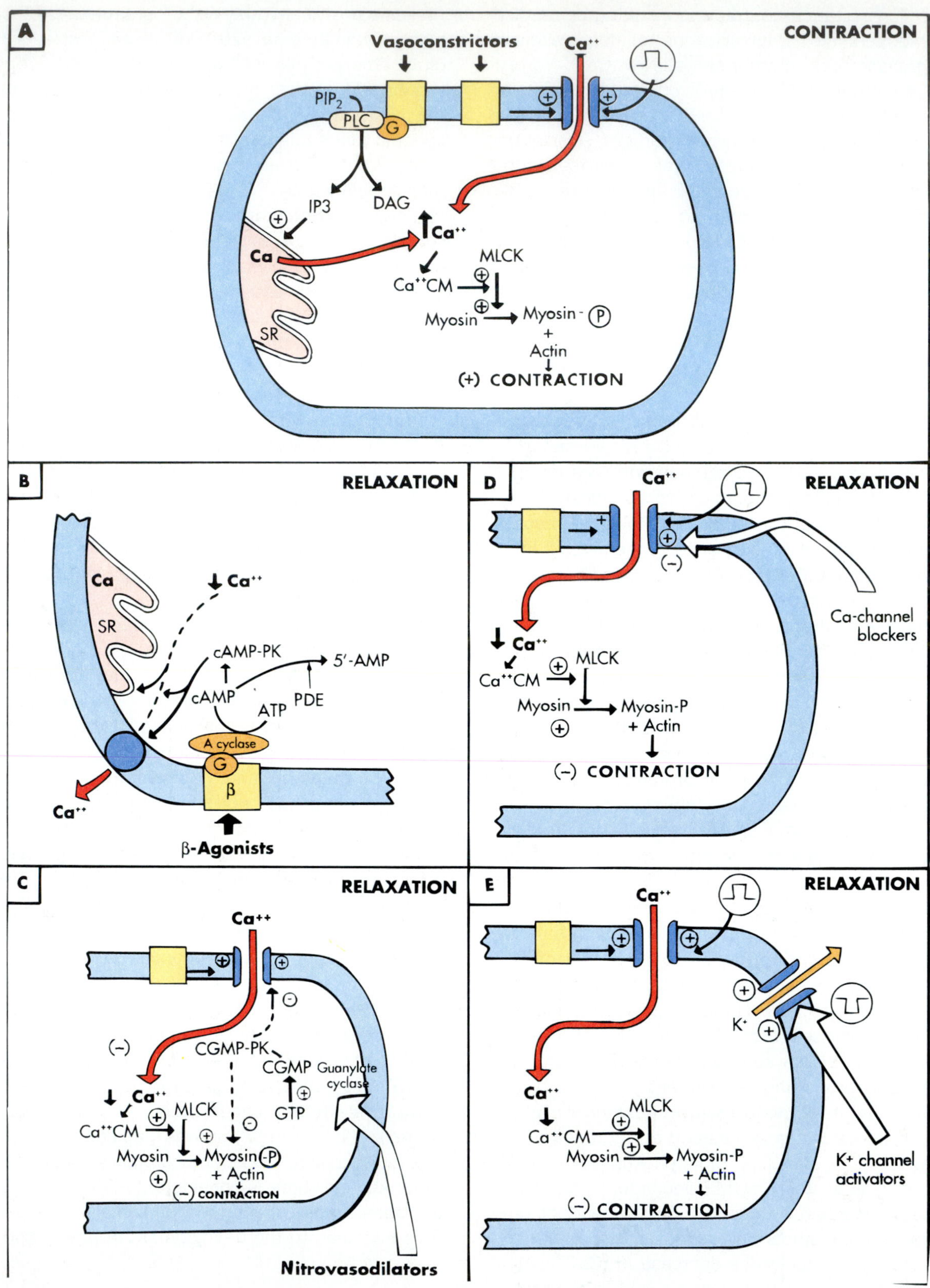

FIGURE 17-1 For legend see opposite page.

FIGURE 17-1 Schema of mechanisms of contraction of a vascular smooth muscle cell, **A,** and possible mechanisms of relaxation by β-adrenergic agonists, **B,** nitrovasodilators, **C,** Ca^{++}-channel blockers, **D,** and K^{+}-channel activators, **E.** Elevations in $[Ca^{++}]_i$ can occur by calcium entry through channels opened by a change in potential, by receptor activation, or by calcium release from sarcoplasmic reticulum (SR), an event triggered by IP_3. IP_3 is formed by the hydrolysis of phosphatidylinositol 4,5-bisphosphate (PIP_2) through the action of phospholipase C (PLC). Calcium interacts with calmodulin, which activates myosin light-chain kinase (MLCK). The latter phosphorylates myosin, which interacts with actin, resulting in contraction. Calcium-channel blockers, **D,** act by limiting calcium entry through membrane channels, promoting relaxation. K^{+}-channel activators increase K^{+} conductance, which hyperpolarizes the cell, **E,** causing relaxation. Nitrovasodilators, **C,** activate soluble guanylate cyclase, leading to an increase in cGMP and subsequently an activation of cGMP-dependent protein kinase. This substance may influence contractility in several ways, including limiting Ca^{++} entry through channels or a direct decrease in the sensitivity of contractile proteins to Ca^{++}. β-Agonists, **B,** cause relaxation by stimulating the formation of cAMP, which activates protein kinase, which decreases $[Ca^{++}]_i$. This may occur by activating calcium pumps in the sarcoplasmic reticulum membrane or cell membrane to either sequester Ca^{++} in the sarcoplasmic reticulum or pump it from the cell.

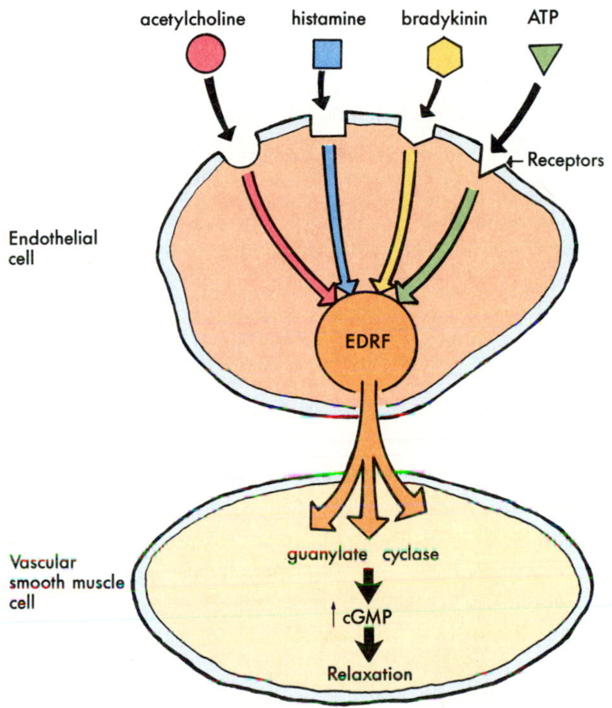

FIGURE 17-2 Endothelium-dependent relaxation produced by vasodilators. These substances act on the endothelial cell at their respective receptors to release EDRF or nitric oxide (see text). The latter diffuses into the vascular smooth muscle cell, increases guanylate cyclase activity and cGMP, and promotes relaxation.

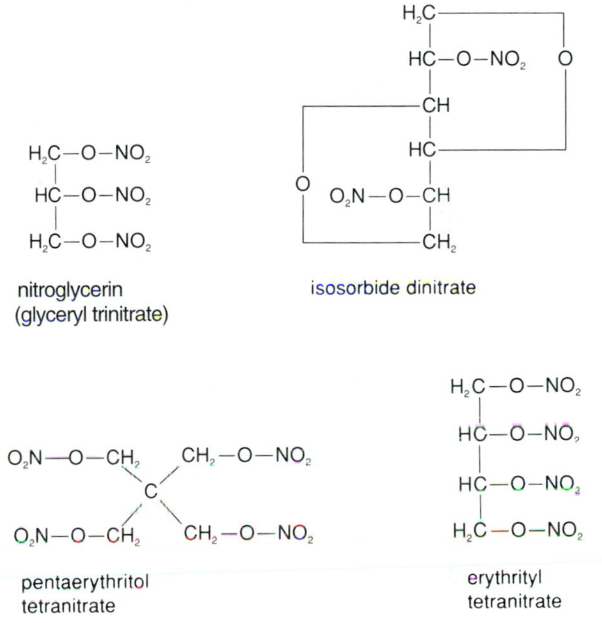

nitroglycerin (glyceryl trinitrate)

isosorbide dinitrate

pentaerythritol tetranitrate

erythrityl tetranitrate

FIGURE 17-3 Structures of some commonly used nitrates. See the text for further information.

tetranitrate, and pentaerythritol tetranitrate. The chemical structures are shown in Figure 17-3. Structures of other vasodilators (hydralazine, minoxidil, enalapril, prazosin, and captopril) are shown in Chapter 13.

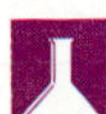

PHARMACOKINETICS

The pharmacokinetic parameter values for nitrate vasodilators are summarized in Table 17-2.

Organic nitrates are almost completely absorbed from the gastrointestinal tract and fairly completely from the buccal mucosa. After sublingual administration, peak plasma concentrations are achieved in 1 to 2 minutes. Absorption is much slower with topical ointments and transdermal patches, and plasma concentrations attained with transdermal preparations are lower and more variable than those obtained with ointment. The nitrates are metabolized in liver by glutathione nitrate reductase (e.g., nitroglycerin is rapidly converted to inorganic nitrite and to denitrated metabolites). Isosorbide dinitrate is also metabolized by hepatic glutathione reductase and converted to inactive products, as well as to an active metabolite, 5-isosorbide mononitrate. This may account for its longer duration of antianginal activity. Isosorbide dinitrate is also used in therapy of intractable chronic congestive heart failure, frequently in combination with other vasodilators that cause relaxation of resistance vessels.

Table 17-2 Pharmacokinetic Parameters

Drug	Route of Administration	Remarks
Nitroglycerin	Sublingual	Onset 2-4 min, duration 30-60 min depending on patient activity, minimal first pass effect, all organic nitrates metabolized by liver
	Oral	Onset 10-20 minutes, duration 2-3 hours, significant first pass effect
	IV	Immediate onset, used to maintain stable blood concentration
	Transdermal	Discs or patches: slower onset, 10-18 hr variable duration; ointment less variable, duration 20-24 hr, for nocturnal angina
	Aerosol	Rapid onset, difficult to control
Isosorbide dinitrate*	Sublingual	Similar in onset to nitroglycerin, longer duration (2-4 hr)
	Oral	Onset 10-20 min, duration 4-8 hours
Erythrityl tetranitrate	Sublingual	Onset 3-5 min, duration 1-2 hr
Pentaerythrityl tetranitrate	Oral	Onset 15-30 min, duration 4-8 hr

*active metabolite; oral preparations: onset varies with dose, and duration depends on extent of first pass metabolism; nitric oxide early reactive intermediate responsible for effects of all parent drugs

Sublingual nitroglycerin is the mainstay of therapy in anginal attacks and is also used prophylactically. It is rapid in onset and inexpensive. Sublingual isosorbide dinitrate is also available and has a longer duration of action than nitroglycerin. The nitroglycerin aerosol spray appears to be as effective as the sublingual tablets. The transdermal patches are not as effective as the oral, timed-release preparations, largely because of the variable absorption through the skin. As a result of tolerance development, those transdermal patches that are left in place for 24 hours are ultimately ineffective for the treatment of angina, even if the dosage is increased. However, patches that deliver 10 mg or more nitroglycerin can be effective if the patches are removed for a 10- to 12-hour period daily.

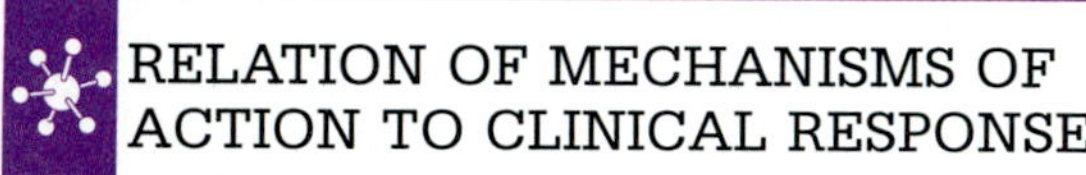

RELATION OF MECHANISMS OF ACTION TO CLINICAL RESPONSE

Vasodilators in Angina

The goal of therapy in coronary artery disease is to reduce pain and to increase the patient's exercise tolerance. This can be accomplished by administration of organic nitrates, the prototype of which is nitroglycerin. Organic nitrates are the mainstay of antianginal therapy used effectively for this purpose for approximately 100 years.

The pharmacological properties of the organic nitrates that make them useful depend on the underlying cause of the angina. If pain is associated with atherosclerosis, the chief benefit arises from actions of nitrates on the peripheral circulation and not on coronary vessels. Nitrates produce a vasodilation of the venous vasculature. Dilatation of venous capacitance vessels diminishes venous return to the heart, reducing ventricular volume and pressure. This decreases ventricular wall tension, a major contributor to the oxygen demands of the heart (Figure 17-4). Thus, by decreasing preload on the heart, oxygen needs of the heart diminish and demand is consistent with supply.

Other consequences of nitroglycerin administration also contribute to its beneficial effect in angina. For example, nitrates cause relaxation of resistance vessels of the arterial circulation. This action decreases afterload placed on the heart, or the impedance against which the heart must pump. Reducing afterload decreases oxygen demands of the heart, just as reducing preload does. The nitrate effect on resistance vessels generally requires somewhat higher concentrations than those needed for venodilatation.

Another feature of organic nitrate action of benefit in angina pectoris is redistribution of blood flow to the subendocardial areas of the heart, which are especially vulnerable to ischemia. Perfusion of the subendocardial region occurs most prominently during early diastole. Later in diastole, as the ventricle fills, subendocardial arteries are constricted because of pressure in the ventricles, with the subsequent decrease in perfusion of these arteries. By decreasing preload, nitrates reduce ventricular filling pressure and increase the time available for endocardial perfusion.

In management of angina pectoris caused by coronary artery spasm, the organic nitrates, in addition to effects described above, are useful because they can dilate constricted coronary vessels. Nitrates are available in many dosage forms, including sublingual, transdermal, and longer-acting oral preparations (Table 17-2). The choice of nitrate preparation depends on the ne-

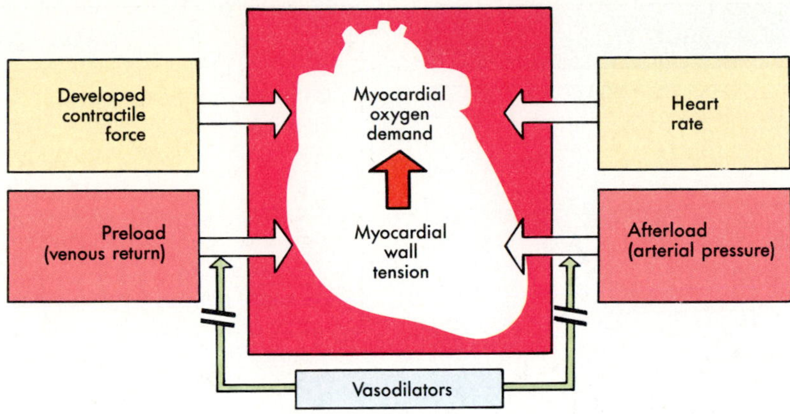

FIGURE 17-4 Mechanism of vasodilator action in the therapy of CHF. The four main determinants of cardiac function act to determine the myocardial oxygen demand. Nitrates decrease preload and afterload but do not effect contractile force, thereby decreasing oxygen demand. Heart rate may increase slightly as a result of the baroreceptor reflex.

cessity for a rapid onset or a longer duration of action.

Other drugs used in the treatment of angina pectoris are β-*adrenergic receptor antagonists* and *calcium-channel blocking drugs* (Chapter 14). The beneficial effect of β-blockers in angina is their ability to decrease oxygen demands of the heart. Beta-blockers decrease heart rate and ventricular contractile force (Chapter 13). Heart rate and contractile force, together with ventricular wall tension, are major determinants of myocardial oxygen demand (Figure 17-4). In addition, chronic therapy with β-blockers reduces blood pressure. Thus, these drugs also decrease afterload. Unlike organic nitrates, β-blockers are not used to terminate an acute attack of angina pectoris but rather to increase exercise tolerance of the patient and to reduce the frequency of anginal attacks.

Vasodilators in CHF

Vasodilator therapy is now widely used for the treatment of chronic CHF, particularly when the patient has not responded adequately to drugs that increase the force of cardiac contraction or to diuretics. Increased survival of patients under a vasodilator regimen has been demonstrated. As previously described, the determinants of cardiac function are preload, afterload, contractility, and heart rate (Figure 17-4). Among the major mechanisms by which vasodilators increase cardiac performance are afterload reduction, preload reduction, and the resulting increased left ventricular diastolic compliance. Afterload reduction, by use of other vasodilators and *high* concentrations of nitrates, is accomplished by dilating arterioles and thereby decreasing systemic vascular resistance. This increases cardiac output and tissue perfusion. Venodilators, including low doses of nitrates, predominantly decrease preload, reducing systemic and pulmonary venous pressures. Ventricular volume is also affected by the decreasing preload. The venodilators do not increase the force of contraction, and the heart rate is generally unchanged, so that the work of the heart remains the same. The overall effect, therefore, is a reduction in myocardial oxygen consumption and demand on the heart. The vasodilator drugs may also improve left ventricular diastolic performance by shifting the diastolic pressure-volume curve to the left (i.e., to pump the same volume at a lower pressure). This shift also moves the ventricular function curve to the left, demonstrating an improvement in left ventricular performance.

Vasodilators used to treat CHF influence preload, afterload, or both. Among the agents used are the direct-acting agents (nitrates, hydralazine, and nitroprusside), the α-adrenergic receptor blocker (prazosin), and the angiotensin converting enzyme inhibitors (captopril, enalapril, and lisinopril). Long-term treatment with hydralazine alone is only minimally effective in treatment of CHF, but the combination of hydralazine with a nitrate, isosorbide dinitrate, effectively decreases mortality. Minoxidil is also generally not very effective when used alone.

Vasodilators in Peripheral Vascular Disease

Peripheral vascular diseases are either vasospastic or occlusive. In Raynaud's disease, a vasospastic disorder, blood flow to the extremities is reduced as a result of a reversible vasoconstriction. Therefore vasodilators may be helpful to these patients by dilating the blood vessels of the skin. Vasodilators are of limited usefulness in occlusive disease with a physical obstruction, however,

CLINICAL PROBLEMS

VASODILATORS IN GENERAL

Orthostatic hypotension
Tachycardia

NITRATE VASODILATORS

Headache
Tolerance

HYDRALAZINE

Lupus-like effect

SODIUM NITROPRUSSIDE

Thiocyanate accumulation

MINOXIDIL

Sodium retention
Hypertrichosis

TRADE NAMES

Cardilate, erythrityl tetranitrate
Isordil, Sorbitrate, Dilatrate; isosorbide dinitrate
Nitrobid, Nitrospan, Nitrolingual; nitroglycerin sublingual
Nitrol, nitroglycerin ointment
Nitrodisc, Transderm-Nitro, Nitro-Dur: nitroglycerin transdermal
Peritrate, Pentitrol; pentaerythrityl tetranitrate

and they do not generally improve flow to either skeletal muscle or skin. A wide variety of drug classes has been used in the treatment of peripheral vascular diseases, including α-adrenergic blockers, calcium-channel blockers, prostaglandins, β-adrenergic agonists, and direct-acting vasodilators. Nitroglycerin ointment may be helpful as an adjunctive agent in Raynaud's phenomenon. Other nonspecific vascular smooth muscle vasodilators such as cyclandalate, papaverine, ethaverine, and nicotinyl tartrate have been used but are of questionable efficacy in the treatment of peripheral vascular disorders.

Vasodilators in Hemostasis

Vasodilators may be used as aids during surgical procedures. They can be used to provide a more satisfactory surgical field, to minimize large blood volume losses, and to improve cardiac performance by reducing preload or afterload.

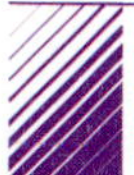

SIDE EFFECTS, CLINICAL PROBLEMS, AND TOXICITY

As with all vasodilators, orthostatic hypotension and tachycardia are adverse effects of nitrate therapy. Vascular headache is quite common but rapidly disappears on continued nitrate use. Tolerance to the vascular effects of nitrate does occur; however, this is not of great clinical significance, except possibly in the treatment of chronic CHF. Cross-tolerance exists between nitroglycerin and the other nitrate esters, but this and other nitrate tolerance can be reduced by only a short period of nitrate abstention. Orthostatic hypotension can be minimized by careful adjustment of the dose and by having the patient avoid the upright position when taking the rapid-acting preparations. Physical dependence to the nitrates has been observed in munitions workers exposed continuously to very high concentrations. In these individuals, withdrawal from the industrial environment may result in angina. This phenomenon is not observed in patients normally taking therapeutic doses of nitrates but can occur in individuals who have been taking large doses for a long time.

Nitrates can be reduced to nitrites, which in turn can oxidize the ferrous iron of hemoglobin, converting it to methemoglobin. The latter reduces oxygen delivery to tissues. Methemoglobinemia is not a problem with normal nitrate therapy but may be observed in accidental poisoning or overdose.

Problems associated with nitroprusside, prazosin, hydralazine, the ACE inhibitors, and minoxidil are discussed in Chapter 13 and the clinical problems caused by the vasodilators are summarized in the box.

NEW DIRECTIONS

In addition to nitric oxide (NO), several products of endothelial cells, called **endothelins,** have been isolated from various tissues. The most prominent and well studied is a 2′-amino acid peptide, endothelin-1. This compound is released from endothelial cells in response to physiological challenges such as hypoxia or stress, or by endogenous hormones such as angiotensin. Endothelin-1 initially dilates smooth muscle but subsequently produces an intense, long-lasting vasoconstriction. Although specific receptors for the endothelins have been identified in smooth muscle cells, no role has been attributed to them at this time.

New functions for NO continue to appear with increasing frequency. Nitric acid is now reported to have regulatory functions, both beneficial and detrimental, in many tissues other than smooth muscle.

REFERENCES

Cook NS: The pharmacology of potassium channels and their therapeutic potential, *Trends Pharmacol Sci* 9:21, 1988.

Furchgott RF, Zawadzki JV: The obligatory role of endothelial cells in the relaxation of arterial smooth muscle by acetylcholine, *Nature* 288:373, 1980.

Ignarro LJ: Biological actions and properties of endothelium-derived nitric oxide formed and released from artery and vein, *Circ Res* 65:1, 1989.

Needleman P, Jakschik B, Johnson EM: Sulfhydryl requirement for relaxation of vascular smooth muscle, *J Pharmacol Exp Ther* 187:324, 1973.

Nishimura J, van Breemen C: Direct regulation of smooth muscle contractile elements by second messenger, *Biochem Biophys Res Commun* 163:929, 1989.

Palmer RMJ, Ferrige AG, Moncada S: Nitric oxide release accounts for the biological activity of endothelium derived relaxing factor, Nature 327:524, 1987.

Peach MJ, Loeb AL, Singer HA, et al: Endothelium derived vascular relaxing factor, *Hypertension* 7:I-94, 1985.

Rapoport RM, Murad F: Agonist-induced endothelium dependent relaxation in rat thoracic aorta may be mediated through cGMP, *Circ Res* 52:352, 1983.

Rüegg JC, Pfitzer G: Contractile protein interactions in smooth muscle, *Blood Vessels* 28:159, 1991.

Schocken DD, Hollaway JD: Vasodilators in the treatment of congestive heart failure, *Rational Drug Ther* 22:1, 1988.

Schwartz AB, Chatterjee K: Vasodilator therapy in chronic congestive heart failure, *Drugs* 26:148, 1983.

Vanhoutte PM, Rubanyi GM, Miller VM, et al.: Modulation of vascular smooth muscle contraction by the endothelium, *Annu Rev Physiol* 48:307, 1986.

Waldman SA, Murad F: Cyclic GMP synthesis and function, *Pharmacol Rev* 39:163, 1987.

SELF-ASSESSMENT QUESTIONS

1. All of the following are side effects of nitrovasodilators *except:*
   a. hypotension.
   b. reflex tachycardia.
   c. headache.
   d. lupuslike syndrome.
   e. tolerance.
2. Which of the following is a mixed (venous and arteriolar) dilator?
   a. hydralazine
   b. minoxidil
   c. nitrates
   d. prazosin
   e. captopril
3. In the vascular smooth muscle cell:
   a. depolarization of the membrane allows calcium entry via voltage-operated channels.
   b. IP_3, a product of phospholipase C activation, increases $[Ca^{++}]$ by stimulating receptor-operated membrane channels
   c. calcium combines with calmodulin to activate myosin light-chain kinase.
   d. a and c are correct.
   e. all are correct.
4. All of the following actions of nitrovasodilators are correct *except* that:
   a. they inhibit phosphodiesterase.
   b. they generate nitric oxide.
   c. they increase cGMP.
   d. they are similar to EDRF.
   e. all are correct.
5. All of the following can be used to treat chronic congestive heart failure *except:*
   a. nitrovasodilators.
   b. ACE inhibitors.
   c. minoxidil.
   d. hydralazine.
   e. prazosin.

CHAPTER 18

Prostaglandins and Related Autoacoids

BARRIE ASHBY

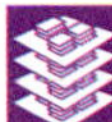

THERAPEUTIC OVERVIEW

Prostaglandins form one branch of a larger family of endogenous compounds known as **eicosanoids,** which constitute a diverse group of oxygenated unsaturated 20-carbon fatty acids. The eicosanoids exert profound effects on practically all cells and tissues and thus provide potential targets for pharmacological intervention in the treatments of several disease states.

The chemical classification of the major eicosanoids, including the prostaglandins, is summarized in Figure 18-1.

Most of the eicosanoid biochemical pathways of pharmacological interest originate with arachidonic acid, the parent compound, a major component of mammalian membrane phospholipids. Because of the diversity of in vivo biochemical and physiological actions attributed to the prostaglandins and other eicosanoids, numerous therapeutic applications for these agents are anticipated (see box). Unfortunately actual clinical applications are fewer than expected, though continued research into their mechanisms of action may result in additional uses of analogs of therapeutic value.

The principal circumstances or organs in which therapy with prostaglandins (and related leukotrienes) is available or may be possible are summarized in the box, p. 231, with chapters noted in which the clinical applications are discussed. This chapter presents an overview of the pharmacological implications of prostaglandins and a summary of their clinical applications.

ABBREVIATIONS

ADH	antidiuretic hormone
AVP	vasopressin
cAMP	cyclic adenosine monophosphate
EPA	eicosapentaenoic acid
FLAP	5-lipoxygenase activating protein
HETE	hydroxyeicosatetraenoic acid
HPETE	hydroxyperoxyeicosatetraenoic acid
LTA, LTB, LTC	leukotrienes
PGD, PGE, PGF, PGG, PGH, PGI_2	prostaglandins
PLC	phospholipase C
TXA_2	thromboxane A_2

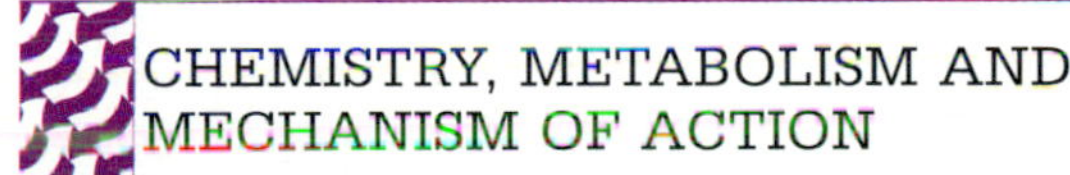

CHEMISTRY, METABOLISM AND MECHANISM OF ACTION

Chemical Structures and Nomenclature

The structures and biosynthesis of the prostaglandins are summarized in Figure 18-2. The relatively stable prostaglandins, PGD_2, PGE_2, and $PGF_{2\alpha}$, are unsaturated fatty acid derivatives that contain 20 carbon atoms, five of which are present as a cyclopentane ring; they originate from common intermediates, the cyclic endoperoxides, PGG_2 and PGH_2. The nature of the substitution on the pentane ring is denoted by a capital letter (e.g., D, E, F). The endoperoxide PGH_2 is also metabolized into two unstable and highly biologically active compounds: (1) thromboxane A_2 (TxA_2), distinguished by a six-membered oxane ring instead of the pentane ring, and (2) prostacyclin (PGI_2), containing the pentane ring and also a second ring system closed by an oxygen bridge between carbons 6 and 9. TxA_2 has a short chemical half-life, less than 1 minute at body temperature, whereas that of PGI_2 is approximately 5 minutes. The inactive hydrolysis products, TxB_2 and 6-keto-$PGF_{1\alpha}$ arise nonenzymatically from TxA_2 and PGI_2, respectively. All of these products (thromboxanes, prostaglandins, and prostacyclin) are derived from

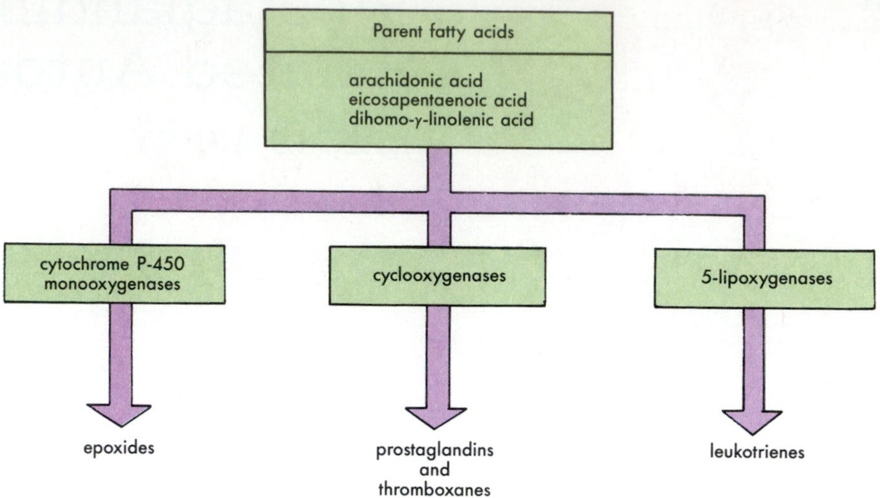

FIGURE 18-1 Classification of the major eicosanoids of pharmacological interest.

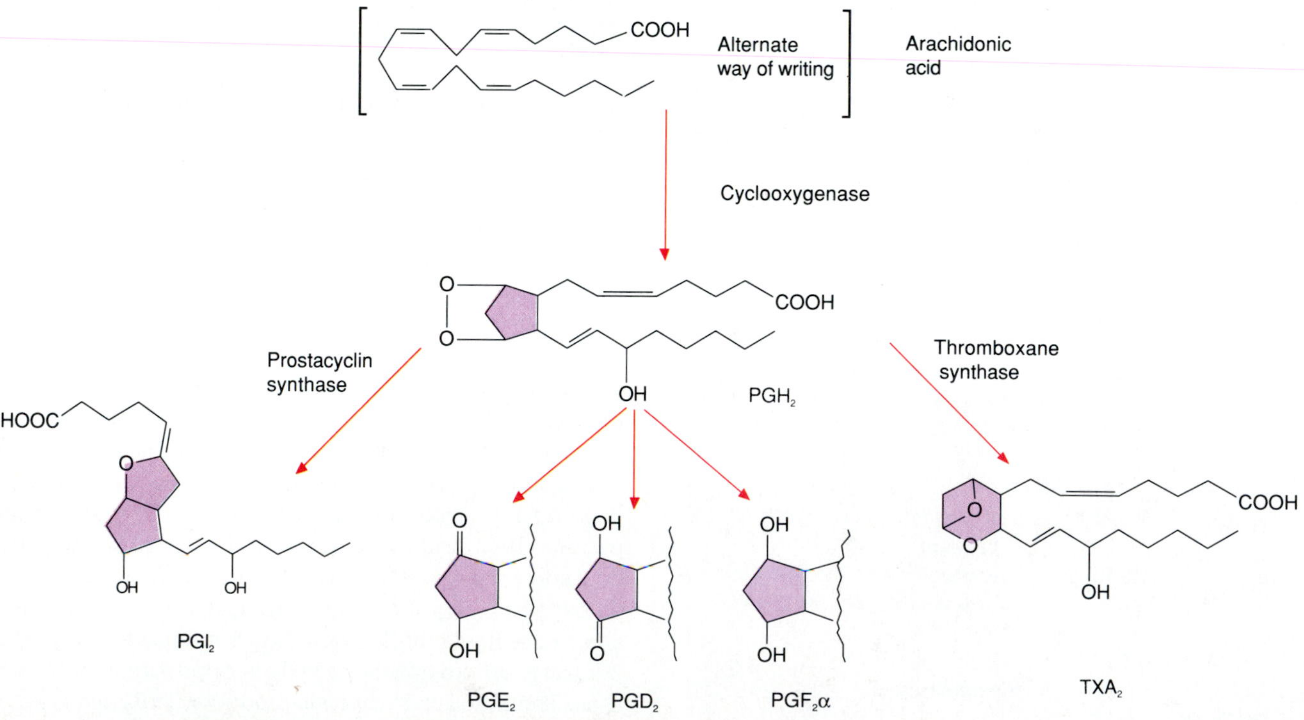

FIGURE 18-2 Chemical structures and biosynthesis of principal prostaglandins. *PG*, Prostaglandin; *Tx*, thromboxane; *PGI₂*, prostacyclin, *PGE₂*, *PGD₂*, and *PGF₂α* differ from endoperoxide PGH₂ as indicated.

THERAPEUTIC OVERVIEW

DRUG	EFFECT	USE
Alprostadil PGE_1	Increased blood flow and oxygenation by vessel relaxation	Neonatal defects; interruption of aortic arch, pulmonary stenosis
Dinoprostone PGE_2	Increase uterine contraction	Abortifacient
Carboprost 15-methyl $PGE_{2\alpha}$		
Iloprost PGI_2 derivative (prostacyclin)	Reduce platelet hyperaggregation	Peripheral vascular disease

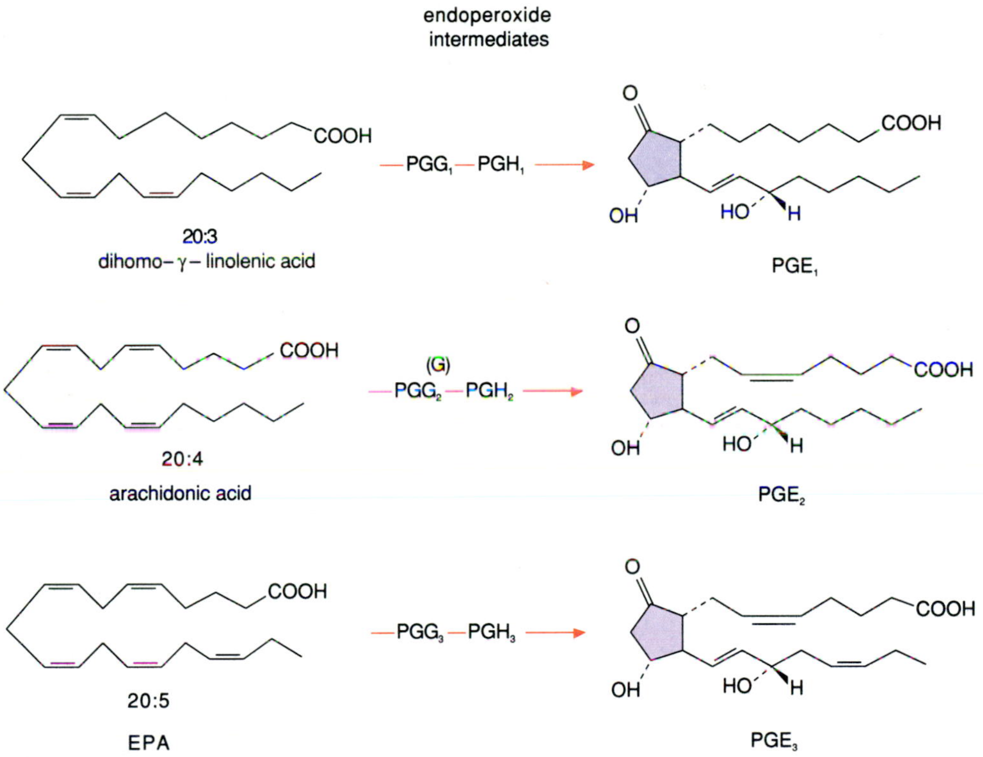

FIGURE 18-3 Nomenclature for prostaglandins originating from the parent compounds. *EPA,* eicosapentaenoic acid (*Eicosa*-'containing 20 carbon atoms.')

unsaturated 20-carbon essential fatty acids, primarily arachidonic acid, a major component of membrane phospholipids. The numbering designation of arachidonic acid, 20:4, indicates 20 carbon atoms and four double bonds. The compounds that retain two double bonds in their alkyl side chains are denoted by the subscript 2, and those that retain three double bonds by the subscript 3.

Examples of prostaglandins derived from the three known parent compounds (see Figure 18-1) are shown in Figure 18-3. Several products generated from eicosapentaenoic acid (EPA) are less potent than corresponding products derived from arachidonic acid. The number of double bonds in the side chains usually does not fundamentally alter the biological properties of prostaglandins; for example, prostaglandins E_1, E_2, and E_3 have similar effects on smooth muscle. However, some differences in potency are noted; for example, TxA_3 is less potent than TxA_2 relative to aggregation of platelets and constriction of blood vessels. Furthermore, PGE_1 resembles PGI_2 in its ability to inhibit platelet aggregation, a property not shared with PGE_2.

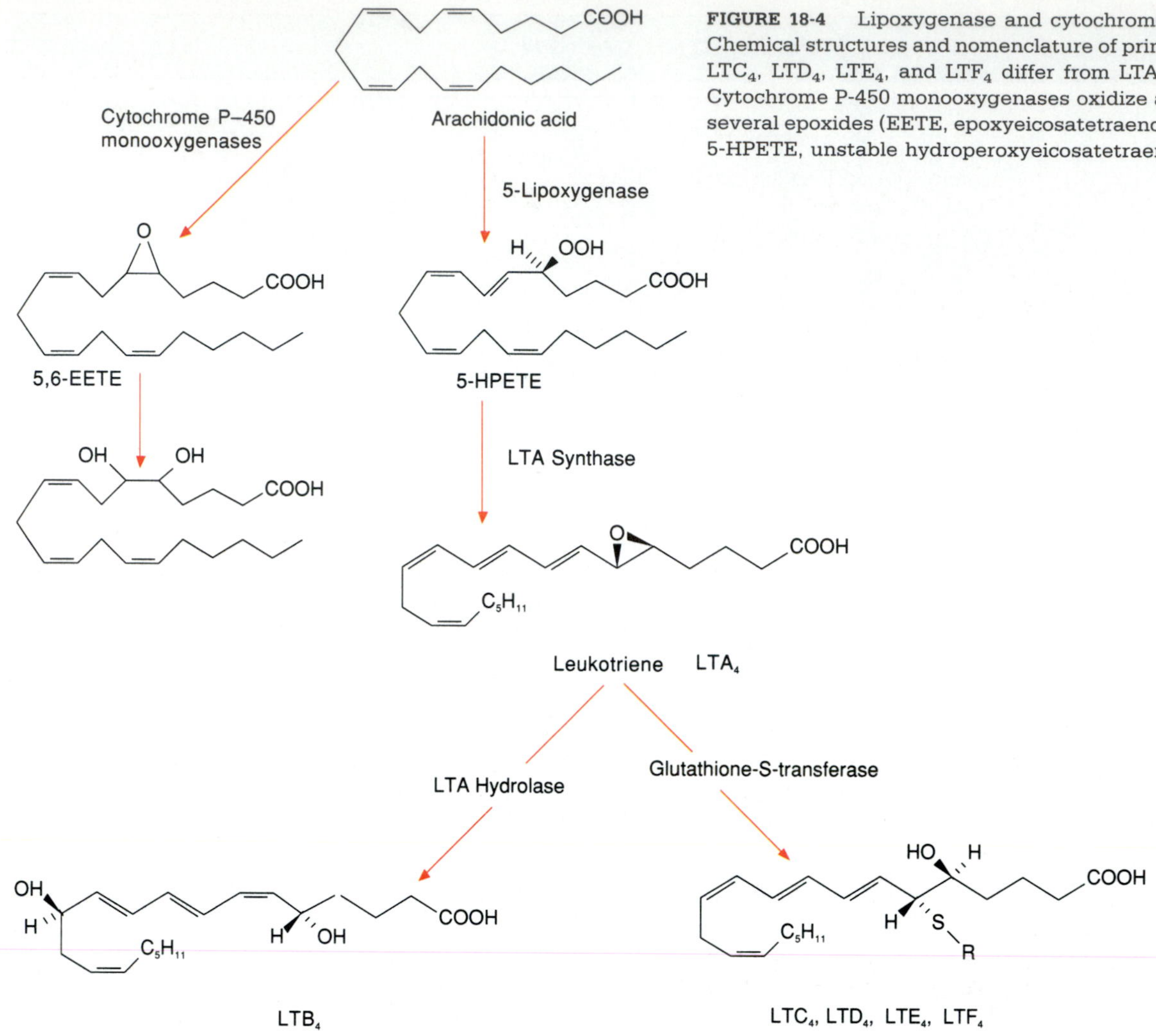

Cytochrome P–450 monooxygenases

Arachidonic acid

5-Lipoxygenase

5,6-EETE

5-HPETE

LTA Synthase

Leukotriene LTA_4

LTA Hydrolase

Glutathione-S-transferase

LTB_4

LTC_4, LTD_4, LTE_4, LTF_4

FIGURE 18-4 Lipoxygenase and cytochrome P-450 pathways. Chemical structures and nomenclature of principal leukotrienes. LTC_4, LTD_4, LTE_4, and LTF_4 differ from LTA_4 in the R-groups. Cytochrome P-450 monooxygenases oxidize arachidonic acid to several epoxides (EETE, epoxyeicosatetraenoic acids) and diols. 5-HPETE, unstable hydroperoxyeicosatetraenoic acid.

The lipoxygenase and cytochrome P-450 pathways are summarized in Figure 18-4.

Synthesis of Prostaglandins and Other Eicosanoids

Three pathways for the enzymatic conversion of arachidonic acid have been identified: cyclooxygenases, lipoxygenases, and cytochrome P-450–dependent monooxygenases. These pathways are shown schematically in Figure 18-1.

Two distinct cyclooxygenases have been cloned. One of them is inducible during inflammation and corticosteroids suppress induction of this form, an indication of probable complex control of prostaglandin synthesis and a mechanism for the antiinflammatory action of corticosteroids (see New Directions, p. 399).

Three major lipoxygenases have been discovered so far, catalyzing incorporation of a molecule of oxygen into the 5-, 12-, or 15-positions of arachidonic acid with formation of the corresponding 5-, 12-, or 15-hydroperoxyeicosatetraenoic acids (HPETEs). 5- and 15-lipoxygenases give rise to the leukotrienes. The lipoxygenases are cytoplasmic and are almost entirely restricted to white blood cells. Platelets contain 12-lipoxygenase, which gives rise to 12-HPETE and its reduction product 12-hydroxyeicosatetraenoic acid (HETE), which have no known function. 5-lipoxygenase activating protein (FLAP) is an 18,000-dalton protein with three putative transmembrane domains that is responsible for translocation of 5-lipoxygenase from the cytoplasm to the membrane.

Metabolism and Concentrations of Prostaglandins

Prostaglandins are not stored but are synthesized in response to diverse stimuli and enter the extracellular space. Prostaglandins and TxA_2 act primarily as local hormones (autacoids), with their biological activities

Table 18-1 Subtypes of Prostaglandin Receptors

Receptor Type	Endogenous Agonist	Rank Order of Potency	Signal Transduction
DP	PGD_2	$D_2 > E_2, F_{2\alpha}, I_2, TXA_2$	cAMP ↑
EP	PGE_2	$E_2 > I_2 \geq F_{2a} > D_2$	
EP_1			PLC
EP_2			cAMP ↑
EP_3			cAMP ↓
FP	$PGF_{2\alpha}$	$F_{2\alpha} > D_2 > E_2 > I_2$	PLC
IP	PGI_2	$I_2 > D_2, E_2, F_{2\alpha}, TXA_2$	cAMP ↑
TP	TXA_2	$TXA_2 > D_2 > F_{2\alpha}, I_2, E_2$	PLC

usually being restricted to the cell, tissue, or structure where they are synthesized. Concentrations of PGE_2 and $PGF_{2\alpha}$ in arterial blood are very low because of pulmonary degradation, which normally removes more than 90% of these prostaglandins from the venous blood as it passes through the lungs. The initial and most important step in the breakdown of prostaglandins results in their rapid inactivation through oxidation of the 15-OH group catalyzed by 15-OH prostaglandin dehydrogenase, an enzyme widely distributed in the body.

Not all cells synthesize prostaglandins; for example, there are segments of the nephron that lack cyclooxygenase or show negligible capacity to transform added arachidonic acid to prostaglandin. In contrast, within the vasculature, cyclooxygenase is found in abundance, though the principal products vary longitudinally along the vasculature and cross-sectionally within the blood vessel wall (e.g., endothelium versus vascular smooth muscle). Within the coronary circulation the larger blood vessels synthesize principally PGI_2, whereas in microvessels PGE_2 predominates.

Prostaglandins are usually released in bursts into the extracellular space immediately after synthesis in response to a stimulus. Under unusual circumstances, prostaglandins may achieve relatively high concentrations in circulating blood; PGD_2 in human mastocytosis, PGE_2 in some solid tumors with metastases to bone, and PGI_2 in pregnancy. In a small group of patients having solid tumors that metastasize to bone, the associated hypercalcemia, related to elevated PGE_2 concentrations, responds to treatment with aspirin-like drugs. In late pregnancy, the gravid uterus may serve as a reservoir of prostacyclin, which is released into the systemic circulation. In addition, diseases of the lung associated with the shunting of blood to the systemic circulation, thereby bypassing the lungs, can result in elevated prostaglandin concentrations in arterial blood.

Under basal conditions, PGI_2 concentrations in blood are less than 5 pg/ml ($\sim 10^{-11}$ M), well below the threshold that produces vasoactive and myotropic effects. The minimum prostaglandin concentration that elicits biological effects in most instances approaches 10^{-9} M, a value identical to the reported dissociation constant (K_d) of prostaglandin receptors. Whether the pulmonary vascular bed can act as a reservoir for release of prostacyclin into the systemic circulation, as proposed, is not established but remains a possibility.

Mechanisms of Prostaglandin Action

Prostaglandins exert their effects by binding to specific membrane receptors. Prostaglandin receptors have been pharmacologically subdivided into subtypes that differ in their potency toward different prostaglandins and in the signal transduction system to which they are coupled. Prostaglandins may cause stimulation or inhibition of adenylate cyclase, or stimulation of phospholipase C leading to formation of diacylglycerol and inositol trisphosphate (which itself stimulates Ca^{++} mobilization). The subtypes are indicated in Table 18-1.

A human thromboxane receptor and a mouse prostaglandin receptor of the EP_3 subtype (coupled to inhibition of adenylate cyclase) have been cloned and sequenced. They possess seven putative transmembrane domains typical of guanine nucleotide–binding regulatory (G) protein–linked receptors. G proteins mediate transmembrane signaling and are specific for each transduction system; G_s couples receptors to stimulation of adenylate cyclase; G_i couples receptors to inhibition of adenylate cyclase. The platelet TXA_2 receptor has been shown to couple to the G protein G_q, which is in turn couples to phospholipase C, (PLC). The relationship between receptor G protein and target enzyme is indicated in Figure 18-5.

TXA_2 receptors have been identified on the plasma membranes of platelets, blood vessels, bronchial smooth muscle, and mesangial cells of glomeruli. The prostaglandin endoperoxides, PGG_2 and PGH_2, also bind to thromboxane receptors. PGI_2 produces effects by interacting with high-affinity cell surface receptors with wide distribution. PGI_2 binding is linked through a G_s protein to stimulation of adenylate cyclase, increased

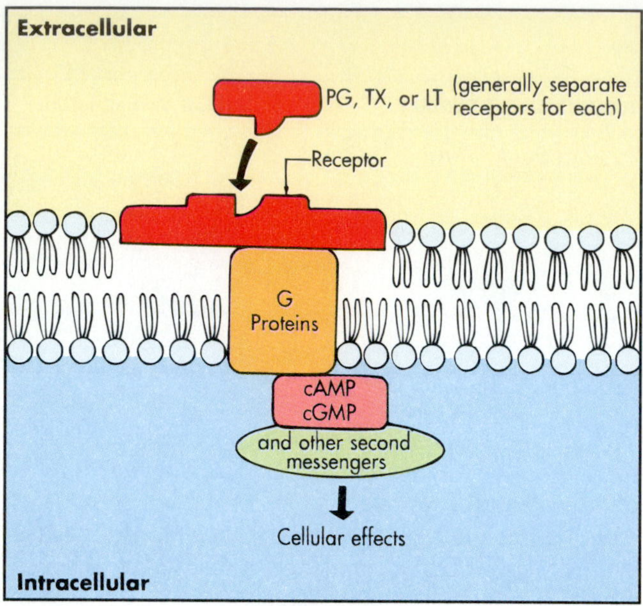

FIGURE 18-5 Eicosanoids act through specific membrane receptors, mainly G-protein types with various second-messenger systems. *PG,* Prostaglandins; *Tx,* thromboxanes; *LT,* leukotrienes.

cAMP concentrations, and inhibition of platelet aggregation. The high density of PGI_2 receptors in the vasculature is reflected in the vasodilator potency of PGI_2, an effect related to elevation of cyclic adenosine monophosphate (cAMP) concentrations in vascular smooth muscle. The tissue-specific functional changes induced by PGE_2 include vasodilatation, bronchodilatation, promotion of salt and water excretion, inhibition of lipolysis, glycogenolysis, and fatty acid oxidation.

There is evidence that many cell types possess several of the prostaglandin receptor subtypes and respond in a variety of ways to prostaglandins. For example, renal tubules appear to possess prostaglandin receptors coupled to both stimulation and inhibition of adenylate cyclase. This belief is based on the observation that low concentrations of PGE_1 inhibit arginine-vasopressin–induced water reabsorption through G_i-mediated inhibition of adenylate cyclase, whereas higher concentrations of PGE_1 cause G_s-mediated activation of adenylate cyclase, presumably causing water reabsorption.

Prostaglandins, after release, are usually denied entrance into cells, presumably because the lipid bilayer is impermeable to prostaglandins. In the lung, renal proximal tubules, thyroid plexus, and ciliary body of the eye, an active transport system that demonstrates saturation kinetics is responsible for the rapid uptake of prostaglandins from extracellular fluids. Prostaglandins differ in their affinity for this transport system. PGE_2 and $PGF_{2\alpha}$ have high affinity, thus accounting for removal and subsequent metabolism of PGE_2 and $PGF_{2\alpha}$ within the lung. In contrast, PGI_2 passes intact through the pulmonary circulation. It is possible to inhibit this transport system, which resembles the organic acid secretory system of the renal proximal tubules, with probenicid, the prototypical inhibitor of proximal tubular secretion. The diuretic drug furosemide and other organic acids also inhibit this uptake in the lung, kidney, and possibly in the brain and eye. One effect of diuretics is to increase prostaglandin concentrations in blood, urine, and perhaps spinal fluid.

A practical therapeutic application of suppressing the effects of PGE_2 on adenylate cyclase can be demonstrated in Bartter's syndrome, a disease characterized by excessive renal prostaglandin production associated with diuresis, kaliuresis, natriuresis, and hyperreninemia. Inhibition of cyclooxygenase activity with nonsteroidal antiinflammatory drugs results in improvement in these patients by allowing expression of salt- and water-retaining hormonal influences, chiefly those of angiotensin II and vasopressin (AVP). The effect of these pressor peptides is blunted by high prostaglandin concentrations intrarenally, particularly PGE_2. For example, by inhibiting the action of antidiuretic hormone (ADH) on adenylate cyclase in the collecting tubules, elevated PGE_2 concentrations prevent water retention by ADH. Further, PGE_2 promotes salt excretion (presumably through an adenylate cyclase–related mechanism) by inhibiting Na^+ and Cl^- cotransport in the thick ascending limb of the loop of Henle. Suppression of prostaglandin synthesis with a nonsteroidal antiinflammatory agent partially corrects the depletion of extracellular fluid volume in these patients.

In contrast to PGE_2-induced relaxation of vascular smooth muscle, the less frequently encountered contraction of smooth muscle produced by PGE_2 is probably linked to Ca^{++} mobilization consequent to stimulating PLC. This mechanism is also considered to be the principal one involved in the actions of $PGF_{2\alpha}$, leading to contraction of smooth muscle through the 5-lipoxygenase receptor.

Prolonged infusion of prostacyclin or a stable prostacyclin analog (e.g., iloprost) in patients with peripheral vascular disease produces decreased platelet sensitivity to these agonists (Figure 18-6). The production of platelet desensitization by infusion of prostacyclin or a PGI_2 analog limits the therapeutic benefit obtained from this group of agents because, in most conditions in which PGI_2 is given, one of the purposes of therapy is to reduce vascular complications resulting from enhanced platelet aggregation. However, when the infusion is stopped, platelets demonstrate increased tendency to clump (hyperaggregatory ability), a potentially dangerous side effect in patients who are at risk be-

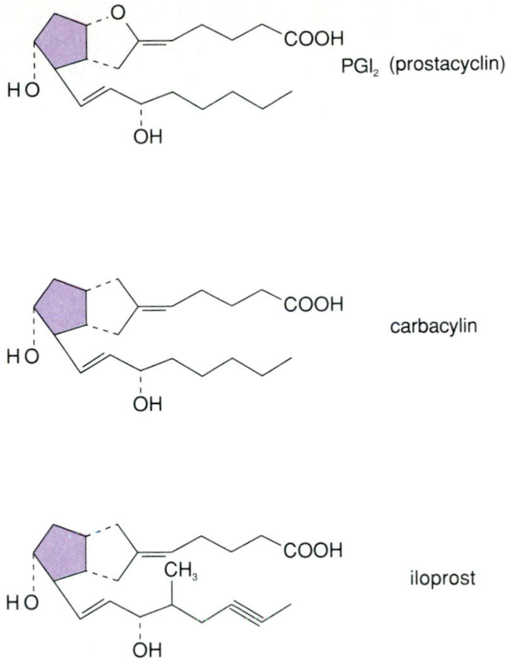

PGI$_2$ (prostacyclin)

carbacylin

iloprost

FIGURE 18-6 Chemical structures for prostacyclin and its analogs.

THERAPEUTIC AREAS OF PROSTAGLANDIN AND OTHER EICOSANOID INTERVENTION	
PROSTAGLANDINS	
Platelet aggregation	Chapter 21
Uterine motility	Chapter 40
Cardiac arterial insufficiency	Chapter 15
Vasoconstriction	Chapter 13
Bronchodilatation/ bronchoconstriction	Chapter 58
Renal tubule stimulation	Chapter 19
Inflammation	Chapter 29
Gastric ulcers	Chapters 59, 60
Myocardial infarction prophylaxis	Chapters 20, 29
LEUKOTRIENES	
Allergy response (anaphylaxis)	Chapter 45

cause of underlying cardiovascular disease.

Prostaglandins and other eicosanoids act at or near their sites of synthesis to "coordinate net biological responses" of a tissue. As coordinators of cellular and tissue function, a major biological activity of prostaglandins is to modulate the activity of hormones and neurotransmitters. The concept that eicosanoids act locally as modulators of peptide hormones and neurotransmitters aids in understanding the multiple and overlapping spheres of biological activity and diverse effects of prostaglandins and other arachidonic acid metabolites. For example, peptide-induced metabolism of arachidonic acid by cells within a segment of the nephron or the vasculature results in changes in the intensity and range of activities of the peptide.

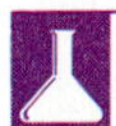

PHARMACOKINETICS

Prostaglandins and their pharmacokinetics and side effects are discussed in the individual chapters noted in the box.

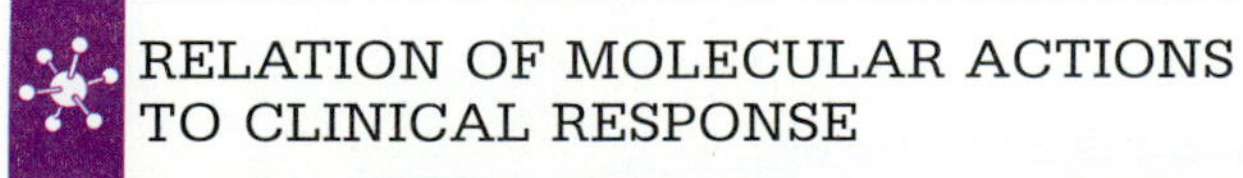

RELATION OF MOLECULAR ACTIONS TO CLINICAL RESPONSE

Therapeutic applications of the eicosanoids have failed to meet the high expectations of more than a decade ago, when PGI$_2$ was discovered and synthesized. However, the ubiquity of prostaglandins is reflected in the number of organ systems that can be modulated to some degree by clinical use of prostaglandins.

Potential targets for prostaglandin therapy are summarized in the box, p. 231, with chapters noted in which the clinical applications are discussed. Following is a summary of prostaglandin and other eicosanoid effects on organ systems and their uses in therapeutic intervention. The box on p. 231 shows some current applications of eicosanoids or their derivatives.

Blood Flow Regulation

PGE$_1$, PGE$_2$, and PGI$_2$ are all potent vasodilators, and endogenously produced PGE$_2$, and PGI$_2$ may be local regulators in many vascular beds. Attempts to use authentic PGI$_2$ or its stable analogs to forestall or ameliorate myocardial infarction, cerebral ischemia, and other manifestations of arterial insufficiency are restricted by the hypotension, headache, and flushing attendant with its administration by IV infusion. Nonetheless, patients with peripheral vascular disease benefit from PGI$_2$ infusions of several hours into the femoral artery of the involved leg. Close arterial infusion of PGI$_2$ is associated with less troublesome side effects because of the selective route of administration and the consequently smaller dose of prostacyclin required to achieve therapeutic goals. However, because its use is restricted to patients under direct medical supervision, it has limited therapeutic application.

TXA_2 is a potent constrictor of cerebral and coronary arteries, and $PGF_{2\alpha}$ constricts superficial veins in the hands. Prinzmetal's angina, a vasoconstrictive problem in coronary arteries, may be partly caused by TXA_2 released from platelets. The peptide leukotrienes LTC_4 and LTD_4 also constrict coronary arteries.

Platelet Aggregation

The dynamic interplay at the platelet-endothelium interface between proaggregatory vasoconstrictor and antiaggregatory vasodilator mediators influences the outcome of arterial insufficiency, thrombosis, and ischemia. The key components are TXA_2 and PGI_2, with those interventions that favor PGI_2, with those interventions that favor PGI_2 production while lowering formation of TXA_2 having the greatest benefit. Aspirin inhibits cyclooxygenase irreversibly by covalent acetylation of a serine residue at position 530. Thus, therapeutic strategies strive to maximize the effect of aspirin on platelet cyclooxygenase while sparing as much as possible the effect of cyclooxygenase on endothelial cells. Unlike the endothelium, platelets lack nuclei and cannot synthesize new cyclooxygenase to replace that inactivated by aspirin. The effects of aspirin therefore continue for the life of the platelet, more than 10 days. Thus, deficient platelet production of thromboxane cannot be corrected until new platelets are formed. In contrast, vascular cyclooxygenase, after inhibition, can be replaced by new cyclooxygenase, reflecting the synthetic capacity of the endothelial cell.

The resulting low-dose aspirin strategy limits the opportunity for aspirin to enter the systemic circulation to inhibit vascular cyclooxygenase but still allows aspirin to act on platelet cyclooxygenase in the portal circulation (from the site of absorption of aspirin to its metabolism by the liver).

Differences in platelet aggregatory potency between the thromboxanes, TXA_2 versus TXA_3, and in chemotactic activity between the leukotrienes, LTB_4 versus LTB_5, constitute part of the rationale for dietary supplementation with eicosapentaenoic acid (EPA). EPA is found primarily in marine animals residing in cold waters. The addition of EPA to the human diet either in purified form or by consumption of coldwater fish has been suggested as a novel therapeutic strategy in the prevention of thrombosis (reduces formation of TXA_2) and of other vascular complications as well as moderating the inflammatory response (reduces formation of LTB_4).

Ductus Arteriosus

The ductus arteriosus generally closes spontaneously at birth, but in some cases, especially premature deliveries, it remains patent (open) so that 90% of cardiac output is shunted away from the lungs. The patency is probably attributable to high production of PGI_2 after delivery. Indomethacin inhibits prostaglandin production and closes the ductus arteriosus.

On the other hand, neonates with certain congenital heart defects depend on an open ductus arteriosus for survival until corrective surgery can be performed. The defects include interruption of the aortic arch, transposition of the great vessels, and pulmonary atresia or stenosis. PGE_1 (alprostadil) is used therapeutically to dilate the ductus by continuous intravenous infusion or by catheter through the umbilical vein.

The Gastrointestinal Tract

PGE_1 and PGE_2 inhibit basal, as well as stimulated, gastric acid production and pepsin secretion in response to feeding, vagal stimulation, or administration of histamine or pentagastrin. These antiulcer properties of E series prostaglandins have been exploited in the development of analogs that are active orally. One analog, the methylester prodrug misoprostol has proved useful for the treatment of peptic ulcers. Misoprostol, a 15-deoxy-16 hydroxy-16-methyl PGE, resists degradation by the principal catabolizing enzyme, the 15-OH prostaglandin dehydrogenase. Misoprostol must first be deesterified to the active acidic form. An unwanted side effect of PGE (and $PGF_{2\alpha}$) analogs is gastrointestinal (GI) hypermotility and associated diarrhea, consequences of the contractile effects of E series prostaglandins on GI smooth muscle. However, in appropriate dosage misoprostol is usually devoid of major side effects. The antiulcer properties of PGE analogs are related to stereospecific binding to a PGE type of receptor located on the plasma membrane of gastric parietal cells.

In addition to the treatment of peptic ulcer disease, PGE analogs can prevent gastric ulcers and promote healing of those caused by nonsteroidal antiinflammatory drugs. The propensity of aspirin-like drugs to cause GI ulcers is a consequence of eliminating the prostaglandin contribution to maintenance of mucosal integrity. That prostaglandins have protective actions on the gut mucosa distinct from their ability to inhibit secretory activity has occasioned the assignment of a "cytoprotective" action to prostaglandins and their analogs. This action of prostaglandins is manifest in their protecting the gastric mucosa from damage after topical application of injurious compounds.

Immune Responses

There is one type of inhibitory activity of PGE analogs that must be monitored closely because it can affect the immune response, that is, suppression of cells participating in inflammation and immune responses. PGE_2 and by extension its analogs can influence the inflammatory and immune responses by affecting activation, mobilization, and secretion of neutrophils, basophils, mast cells, and lymphocytes. For example, the inhibitory effect of PGE_2 on LTB_4 release from activated neutrophils has been linked to stimulation of neutrophil adenylate cyclase by the prostaglandin. A similar mechanism operating through adenylate cyclase is believed to serve as the basis for PGE modulation of the activity of other cells involved in either the immune or inflammatory response.

The Reproductive System

Human semen contains large (microgram) amounts PGE_1, PGE_2, $PGF_{2\alpha}$, and $PGF_{2\alpha}$. Prostaglandins may serve to stimulate smooth muscle contraction necessary for ejaculation and to contract the myometrium and oviducts after being absorbed by the vagina. However, the requirement for prostaglandins in these processes does not appear to be absolute, and their precise role remains to be determined. Both PGE_2 and $PGF_{2\alpha}$ cause contraction of uterine smooth muscle and may modulate menstruation. Consequently, nonsteroidal antiinflammatory drugs such as ibuprofen are prescribed for relieving menstrual cramps.

Elevated levels of prostaglandins have been measured in the circulating blood of women during labor or spontaneous abortion, an indication that initiation and maintenance of uterine contractions may be caused by increased synthesis of prostaglandins. In fact, labor can be induced by PGE_2 given orally (0.5 mg/hr); if labor does not occur after 12 hours, intravenous oxytocin is substituted. Use of PGE_2 to induce labor is accompanied by uterine hypertonus and fetal bradycardia, and so the main use of prostaglandins in gynecological practice has been as abortifacients. In contrast to oxytocin, prostaglandins will induce uterine contractions at all stages of pregnancy. PGE_2, $PGF_{2\alpha}$, and 15-methyl $PGF_{2\alpha}$ are used as abortifacients generically as dinoprostone, dinoprost, and carboprost respectively.

Bronchoconstriction

The lungs produce PGE_2, PGI_2, PGD_2, $PGF_{2\alpha}$, TXA_2, LTC_4, and LTD_4. Mast cells lining the respiratory passages are the likely source of leukotrienes and PGD_2. Overproduction of these substances leads to bronchoconstriction, and so they are potential mediators of asthma. $PGF_{2\alpha}$ and TXA_2 are also potent bronchoconstrictors, whereas PGE_1, PGE_2, and PGI_2 are potent vasodilators. However, inhaled prostaglandins irritate the airways and are not suitable as antiasthmatic drugs.

Nerve Transmission

There is evidence that eicosanoid-dependent mechanisms act within the neuron of origin and externally at nerve endings to modulate autonomic transmission. It therefore seems likely that eicosanoids have intracellular actions in addition to the effects that register at the cell membrane.

NEW DIRECTIONS

As with many aspects of pharmacology, techniques of molecular biology will greatly advance knowledge of prostaglandin synthesis and function. Detailed knowledge of the regulation of genes such as those for cyclooxygenases is already being used to define the antiinflammatory role of steroids. Steroids may also decrease the synthesis of phospholipase A_2 in cells, and regulation of this type is readily accessible by current technology.

Prostaglandin receptors have resisted purification, but the structure of several receptors has been elucidated by cloning techniques. Knowledge of receptor structures may lead to rational drug design but, more immediately, knowledge of gene sequences will allow detailed analysis of the distribution of receptor subtypes among tissues. For example, studies with certain agonists indicate that platelets and vascular endothelial cells possess different receptors coupled to stimulation of adenylate cyclase. The ability to screen for receptors by Northern blot analysis or by cloning and sequencing the receptors from platelets and vascular cells will resolve this question.

Detailed information on control of eicosanoid synthesis will open up new targets for drugs intervention. For example, there has been discovered a novel class of inhibitors of leukotriene biosynthesis that have no effect on 5-lipoxygenase itself but interact with FLAP, a novel membrane protein that regulates 5-lipoxygenase.

REFERENCES

FitzGerald GA, Murray R, Moran N, et al: Mechanisms of eicosanoid action, *Advances In Prostaglandin, Thromboxane, & Leukotriene Research* 21B:577, 1991.

Nicosia S, Patrona C: Eicosanoid biosynthesis and action: novel opportunities for pharmacological intervention, *FASEB J* 3:1941, 1989.

Smith WL: The eicosanoids and their biochemical mechanisms of action, *Biochem J* 259:315, 1989.

SELF-ASSESSMENT QUESTIONS

1. Which one of the following statements about eicosanoids is *not* true?
   a. Eicosanoids are unsaturated fatty acids.
   b. Eicosanoids all contain a pentane ring.
   c. Eicosanoids originate primarily from arachidonic acid.
   d. Eicosanoids may act through several second messengers.
   e. Eicosanoid synthesis results from activation of phospholipase A_2.
2. Which one of the following statements about prostaglandins is *not* true?
   a. Prostaglandin synthesis is inhibited by aspirin.
   b. Prostaglandins play an important role in inflammation.
   c. Prostaglandins are products of cyclooxygenase activity.
   d. Prostaglandins act exclusively to stimulate adenylate cyclase.
   e. Either prostaglandin E_2 or oxytocin can be used to induce labor.
3. All of the following possess vasoconstrictor activity *except:*
   a. thromboxane A_2.
   b. prostaglandin I_2.
   c. prostaglandin $F_{2\alpha}$.
   d. leukotriene LTD_4.
   e. leukotriene LTC_4.
4. Which one of the following statements is *not* true?
   a. Leukotrienes are products of lipoxygenases.
   b. Prostaglandins act through G protein–linked receptors.
   c. Thromboxane A_2 is a stable metabolite of arachidonic acid.
   d. Prostaglandin synthesis can be inhibited by corticosteroids.
   e. Prostaglandins act primarily as local hormones (autoacoids).
5. All of the following are actions of thromboxane A_2 *except:*
   a. bronchoconstriction.
   b. constriction of cerebral arteries.
   c. constriction of coronary arteries.
   d. contraction of uterine smooth muscle.
   e. activation of platelet aggregation.
6. Clinical indications for eicosanoids or their inhibitors include all of the following *except:*
   a. transposition of the great arteries.
   b. hypertension
   c. patent ductus arteriosus.
   d. abortion.
   e. treatment of peptic ulcers.

CHAPTER 19

Diuretics: Drugs That Increase Excretion of Water and Electrolytes

EDWARD J. CAFRUNY
THEODORE M. BRODY

MAJOR DRUGS

- osmotic diuretics
- carbonic anhydrase inhibitors
- thiazides and thiazide-related agents
- loop diuretics, types I and II
- potassium-sparing agents
  - aldosterone antagonists
  - pteridines
  - pyrazinoyl guanidines

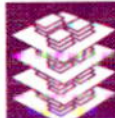 THERAPEUTIC OVERVIEW

The term *diuretic* classically denotes an agent that increases the rate of urine flow. By this definition, water is a diuretic because its ingestion is followed by an enhancement of the rate of urine production. However, the diuresis induced by ingestion of water is not accompanied by a substantial increase in excretion of electrolytes, and this factor separates the effect of water ingestion from the effects of agents described in this chapter. The primary effect of diuretics is an increase in solute excretion, mainly sodium salts. The increase in urine flow is secondary to the increase in solute excretion, a response to the osmotic force of the additional solute. Drugs that increase the net urinary excretion of sodium salts are often called **natriuretics.**

ABBREVIATIONS

ATP	adenosine triphosphate
ECF	extracellular fluid
GFR	glomerular filtration rate
PAH	*p*-aminohippuric acid
pH	logarithm of the reciprocal of the H-ion concentration

A deleterious expansion of the volume of the extracellular fluid (ECF) is characteristic of diseases such as congestive heart failure, cirrhosis of the liver, and nephrosis. The classic use of diuretic drugs is to effect a reduction in ECF by enhancing the excretion of salts (mainly NaCl) and water. In addition, one or another of these drugs has therapeutic efficacy in hypertension, nephrogenic diabetes insipidus, hypercalcuria, hypercalcemia, hypokalemia, and glaucoma. The major classes of drugs are listed in the box on this page, and their therapeutic applications in the box on the next page. In all cases, the drugs inhibit the tubular absorption of sodium ions either directly or indirectly. Thiazides, loop diuretics, pteridines, and pyrazinoyl guanidines directly attack specific transport mechanisms. Osmotic diuretics, carbonic anhydrase inhibitors and aldosterone act by mechanisms that are described later.

Response to diuretics is moderated by internal homeostatic mechanisms sensitive to body fluid volumes and osmolar concentrations. Magnitude of the diuretic response depends on the preexisting physiological status and the type and severity of the disorder. For example, individuals who take a thiazide daily for even a short period may develop a relative refractoriness that is not a true tolerance to the drug but rather originates from activation of compensatory salt-retaining mechanisms. Similarly, cirrhotic patients with ascites often do not respond at all to a diuretic because homeostatic mechanisms for adjusting salt and water balance apparently signal the existence of depleted ECF when, in fact, the tissues are water logged.

The purpose of diuretic intervention in the treatment of edema is to normalize the volume of the ECF compartment without distorting electrolyte concentrations. The size of the ECF compartment is largely determined by the body's total content of dissolved sodium. There are two reasons for this: (1) sodium is the predominant cation of the ECF and thus is available in quantities sufficient to influence the osmotic distribution or redistri-

THERAPEUTIC OVERVIEW

GOALS	Generally to increase excretion of salt and water and to treat several diseases and conditions:
USE:	
Thiazide diuretics	Hypertension Congestive heart failure Renal calculi Diabetes insipidus Chronic renal failure (as adjunct to loop diuretic)
Loop diuretics	Hypertension, in patients with impaired renal function or for immediate effect Congestive heart failure in patients with impaired renal function Acute pulmonary edema Chronic or acute renal failure Nephrotic syndrome In chemical intoxication (to increase urine flow)
Potassium-sparing diuretics	Chronic liver failure Congestive heart failure, when hypokalemia is a problem
Carbonic anhydrase inhibitors	Cystinuria (to alkalinize tubular urine) Glaucoma (to decrease intraocular pressure by lowering bicarbonate) Periodic paralysis that affects muscle membrane function Acute mountain sickness (to counteract respiratory alkalosis)
Osmotic diuretics	Acute or incipient renal failure, reduce intraocular or intracranial pressure (presurgical)

bution of large amounts of water, and (2) movements of sodium between the extracellular and intracellular compartments are controlled by active-transport mechanisms that are regulated in turn by a variety of integrating mechanisms. The existence of multiple points of control ensures that blockade or failure of one mechanism evokes compensatory responses in others.

To maintain electrolyte and water balance, the urinary excretion of sodium and water must equal intake minus the sum of all losses through other routes. This requirement could not be met if the periodic fluctuations in blood pressure, which occur in all humans, produced equivalent changes in blood flow to the kidneys. It is necessary therefore that wide swings in renal blood flow be dampened when blood pressure fluctuates. In addition, adjustments in the renal tubular handling of sodium and fluid should come into play as rapidly as the need arises.

To achieve the first requirement, an intrarenal autoregulatory mechanism controls arteriolar resistance and the glomerular capillary pressure, thereby preventing wide swings in renal blood flow and glomerular filtration rate. Adjustments in sodium transport rates, both short term and long term, are achieved through the integrated activity of renal mechanisms and extrarenal factors discussed in the next section.

To achieve the second requirement in the control of sodium, potassium, and passive water transport in nephrons, the dominant factors are aldosterone, antidiuretic hormone, and atrial natriuretic hormone. These hormones are discussed in a later section.

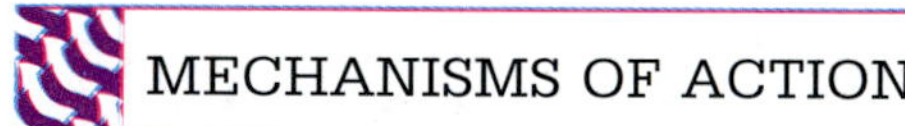

MECHANISMS OF ACTION

Renal Transport

The names of the parts of the nephron, as used in this discussion, are based primarily on functional properties (Figure 19-1). Because diuretic agents often influence the rates of transport of sodium (Na^+), potassium (K^+), hydrogen (H^+), chloride (Cl^-), bicarbonate (HCO_3^-), and urate, the renal mechanisms of transport of these ions are reviewed before discussion of the mechanisms of action of the diuretic agents.

Tubular Reabsorption: Proximal Transport The glomerular filtration rate of healthy human adults is usually in the range of 1.7 to 1.8 ml/min/kg. At least 99% of this filtrate must be transferred from tubular lumen back to the blood. Although paracellular (between cells) reabsorption of fluid and electrolytes takes place, the primary pathway is lumen to cell to interstitial fluid to capillary. In the process, two membranes, both permeable to water, must be traversed. The process is initiated in the proximal tubule by the active transport of sodium ions. Passage of filtered sodium into the cell generates an osmotic gradient for the nearly simultaneous movement of water. Because anions, chiefly but not exclusively chloride (see below), follow the same route as so-

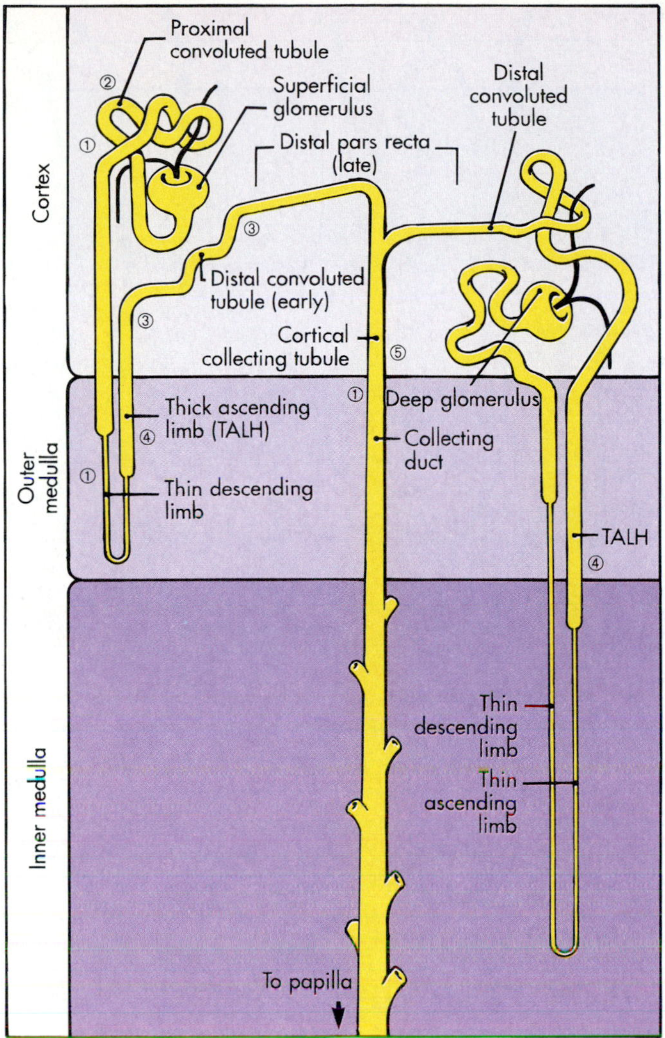

FIGURE 19-1 Renal tubular segments. Distal convoluted tubule: early distal tubule; late distal pars recta; distal tubule and cortical collecting tubule. *TALH,* Thick ascending loop of Henle. Sites of action of diuretics: (1) osmotic; (2) carbonic anhydrase inhibitors; (3) thiazides; (4) loop diuretics; (5) K^- sparing agents.

dium, charge separation is minimal and electroneutrality of the reabsorbate is maintained. This efficient operation is responsible for the reabsorption of two thirds or more of the Na^+ filtered and, because it is accomplished isosmotically, the reabsorption of the same fraction of glomerular fluid. When glomerular filtration rate increases, excretion of salt and water also increases, but fractional reabsorption in the proximal tubule does not change. This phenomenon is called **glomerulotubular balance.** Glomerulotubular balance moderates but does not entirely eliminate the effects of alterations in the glomerular filtration rate (GFR) on salt and water excretion.

The essential elements of sodium translocation are shown diagrammatically in Figure 19-2. Two steps are involved: entry across the luminal membrane and egress across the basolateral membrane. The latter process is the crucial one, for it not only involves the expenditure of metabolically derived energy but also governs entry into the cell from the lumen. Egress is an active process (i.e., movement is "uphill" or against the prevailing electrochemical gradient), fueled by the energy released when adenosine triphosphate (ATP) is converted to adenosine triphosphate by a Na^+,K^+-dependent ATPase located in the basolateral membrane. As shown in panel *A* of Figure 19-2, three Na^+ ions are ejected from the cell into the interstitial space; simultaneously, two K^+ ions gain entry. The resultant change in the cellular concentration of Na^+ and the loss of one positive charge create a favorable electrochemical gradient for the passive entry of Na^+ across the apical membrane.

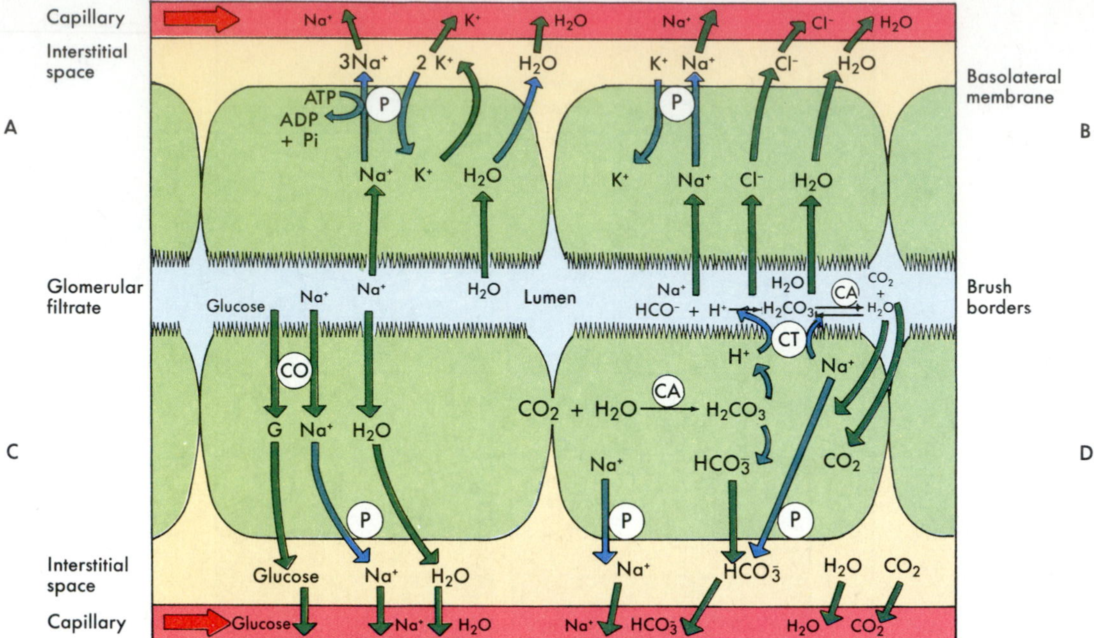

FIGURE 19-2 Transport in the proximal tubule. *P,* Sodium pump; *CO,* cotransport; *CT,* countertransport; *CA,* carbonic anhydrase, in cytoplasm and brush border, ATPase only in basolateral membrane.

The electronegative cell attracts positively charged sodium ions from the lumen (electrical gradient), and the low concentration of cellular sodium resulting from its active egress promotes continual entry (chemical or concentration gradient). The process is self-sustaining and proceeds as long as ATP and enzyme are available. It should be understood that the charge separation created when an extra Na^+ ion leaves the cell is largely dissipated by flow of other positive and negative ions in the vicinity. Healthy proximal tubular cells, however, remain slightly electronegative with respect to the lumen.

The concentration gradient favors the passive return of the potassium ions, which were initially countertransported (see below) by the ATPase pump from interstitial fluid into the cell, back to the interstitial space. There are approximately 35 times as many Na^+ ions in extracellular fluid as there are K^+ ions. Obviously, the supply of potassium needed for the operation of the sodium pump would be inadequate if recycling of potassium between cell and interstitial fluid did not take place.

Because electrical and concentration gradients for passage of luminal sodium into proximal tubular cells are favorable, entry is essentially passive. It is facilitated, however, by attachment to or interaction with unidentified channel or carrier-protein receptors. Three types of entry mechanisms are recognized: diffusion with chloride, cotransport with uncharged molecules or acidic anions, and countertransport with hydrogen ion.

Diffusion with chloride, quantitatively the most important, is depicted in Figure 19-2, *B.* Movement of both ions into the cell is downhill. The osmotic transfer of fluid from the lumen into the cell and thence into the interstitial space increases the concentration of chloride in the lumen, thereby accelerating both its diffusive entry across the luminal membrane against the small electrical gradient and its egress through the basolateral membrane. Chloride is also cotransported with sodium. Finally, it appears that in the inner cortical straight portion of the proximal tubule at least, chloride ions can penetrate the tight junctions between cells, traveling from lumen to interstitial space without entering the cell.

Cotransport with uncharged molecules or acidic anions is illustrated in panel C. This type of transport involves the joint, unidirectional passage of two chemical species, one "downhill" and one "uphill." In the proximal tubule, a variety of substances may be cotransported with sodium. The list includes glucose, phosphate, amino acids, and urate.

The last mechanism, countertransport with hydrogen ion, important in acid-base regulation, is shown in Figure 19-2, *D.* It is operative not only in the proximal tubule but also in the late portion of the distal segment and is located in the luminal membrane. Sodium ions enter the cell from the lumen in exchange for hydrogen

Table 19-1 Summary of Reabsorption in the Proximal Tubule*

Component	Filtered	Reabsorbed	Entering Loop
	mEq/24 hr		
Na^+	25,200	17,640	7560
Cl^-	19,440	13,414	6026
K^+	810	405	405
HCO_3^-	4320	3825	648
H_2O	180 liters	126 liters	54 liters

*Representative values for a 70-kg human.

ions originating in the cell. Because the concentration of cellular H^+ is low, the reaction proceeds in the direction: $CO_2 + H_2O \rightarrow H_2CO_3^- \rightarrow H^+ + HCO_3^-$. Thus a constant supply of hydrogen ions is furnished for countertransport with sodium. Dissociation of the carbonic acid formed by intracellular hydration of carbon dioxide provides both hydrogen ions and bicarbonate anions. The HCO_3^- ions are cotransported with Na^+ across the basolateral membrane into interstitial fluid and subsequently back into the bloodstream. The cytoplasmic hydration reaction occurs spontaneously but at a rate too slow to accomplish the reabsorption of the massive load of bicarbonate filtered (normally more than 4000 mEq/24 hr). The catalyst, carbonic anhydrase, ensures that little or none of the filtered bicarbonate will be excreted. The result of coupling of Na-H countertransport to carbonic anhydrate–mediated hydration and rehydration of CO_2 is the preservation of body bicarbonate. Each HCO_3^- ion saved can buffer one H^+. The Na^+ ions exchanged for H^+ are removed from the cell by the sodium pump.

The final step is transfer from the interstitial fluid into peritubular capillaries. Reabsorptive transport systems of the proximal tubule deposit large amounts of fluid and solutes in the interstitial space. This deposit tends to raise pressure in the interstitium and must be removed if reabsorption is to continue. Theoretically, the sodium can reenter the sodium-depleted cell, pulling anions and water with it. When this occurs, the active transport mechanism reextrudes it. The permeable peritubular capillary can easily carry away reabsorbed fluids and solutes. Pushed by interstitial pressure and pulled by the oncotic pressure of intracapillary proteins (higher in postglomerular than in preglomerular capillaries), filtered fluid and solutes return to the bloodstream.

In summary, the convoluted and straight portions of the proximal tubule reabsorb approximately 70% of the filtered water and sodium, 69% of the chloride, 85% of the bicarbonate, and 50% of the potassium filtered through the glomerular membranes (Table 19-1). These percentages are relatively constant, even when filtered quantities increase or decrease. As a result, minor fluctuations in GFR do not influence fluid and electrolyte excretion very much. The driving force for reabsorption of water and electrolytes is the sodium pump. Passive movements of the other ions and of water are initiated and sustained by the active transport of sodium across the basolateral membranes. Osmotic equilibrium with plasma is maintained to the end of the proximal tubule. Most of the filtered bicarbonate is not actually reabsorbed from the lumen; it is converted to carbon dioxide and water in the vicinity of the brush border membranes within which large concentrations of the catalyst, carbonic anhydrase, are found. The direction of this reaction is $H_2CO_3 \rightarrow CO_2 + H_2O$ (established by the high concentration of carbonic acid in luminal fluid resulting from secretion of hydrogen ion). A carbonic anhydrase isoenzyme in the cellular cytoplasm catalyzes the formation of carbonic acid, the source of the cellular hydrogen ion exchanged for luminal sodium and of the bicarbonate ion, which leaves with sodium across the basolateral membranes (see Figure 19-2, *D*). Thus, newly formed bicarbonate replaces the bicarbonate removed from plasma through glomerular filtration.

Tubular Reabsorption: Transport in the Loop of Henle Diuretic agents exert no discernible action in the descending limb of the loop of Henle. The cells of this portion of the renal tubule are probably not equipped with specialized transporting systems. They are relatively impermeable to sodium and chloride but do permit water to diffuse easily from the lumen to the medullary interstitium, where higher osmotic pressures are encountered. The following segment discusses the transporting functions of the ascending limb, an important site of action of the "loop" (also called high-ceiling) diuretics.

In contrast to the proximal tubule, the ascending limb of the loop of Henle transports chloride uphill, the intracellular chloride concentration exceeding that predicted by the Nernst equation. The system, present in a variety of transporting epithelia, is aptly called $Na^+,K^+,2Cl^-$ cotransport. Its activity depends on the simultaneous presence of these three ions in luminal fluid. A schematic model of the system is presented in Figure 19-3. The major source of energy required to drive it is the Na^+,K^+-ATPase of the peritubular membrane. A favorable electrochemical gradient (with the lumen positive) prompts the "downhill" entry of a sodium ion into the cell, and a transporter in the membrane facilitates the cotransport of a potassium ion and two chloride anions "uphill." The cell, now overloaded with chloride, releases the ion into the interstitium. Potassium passively reenters the lumen, shuttling back and forth. The ascending limb is highly permeable to the three cotransported ions but not to water. Accordingly, the fluid in

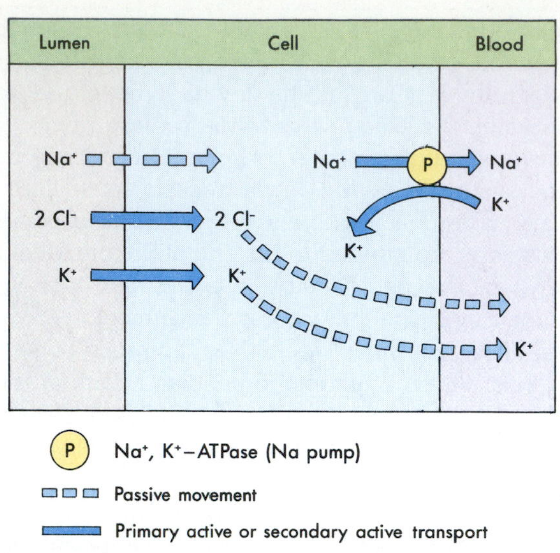

FIGURE 19-3 The Na^+,K^+, $2Cl^-$ cotransport system in cells of the ascending limb of the loop of of Henle.

Table 19-2 Summary of Reabsorption in the Loop of Henle*

Component	Entering Loop	Reabsorbed	Entering Distal Tubule
	mEq/24 hr		
Na^+	7560	6300	1260
Cl^-	6026	4860	1166
K^+	405	324	81
HCO_3^-	648	little	<648
H_2O	54 liters	27 liters	27 liters

*Representative values for a 70 kg human

the ascending limb remains in the lumen and is progressively diluted. The countercurrent mechanism in the renal medulla depends on the activity of this cotransport system, and drugs that block cotransport diminish the ability of the kidney to excrete urine that is either more concentrated or more dilute than plasma.

In summary, fluid is reabsorbed from the lumen of the descending limb as it pushes progressively deeper into medullary areas of higher osmotic pressure. Electrolyte concentrations increase to a maximum at the bend and then gradually decrease as the Na^+,K^+, $2Cl^-$ cotransport mechanism and sodium pump, working in tandem, achieve the reabsorption of sodium and potassium chloride. The quantitative relationships are shown in Table 19-2. Thick ascending limb cells reabsorb about 25% of the filtered NaCl and 40% of the potassium, whereas the entire loop reabsorbs only 15% of the fluid. Loop cells do not exchange H^+ for luminal Na^+ and thus probably process only small quantities of HCO_3^-, if any.

Tubular Reabsorption: Distal Tubule and Collecting Duct Transport In contradistinction to the proximal tubule and loop of Henle, quantitative reabsorption of water and electrolytes in the distal tubule and collecting ducts is much less and quite variable. NaCl is reabsorbed against an electrochemical gradient. Because the early distal tubule is relatively impermeable to water, removal of NaCl amplifies an already unfavorable concentration gradient and probably limits the effectiveness of the sodium pump.

The amount of sodium and potassium present in the final urine is tightly controlled by aldosterone released from the adrenal cortex. The hormone penetrates cells

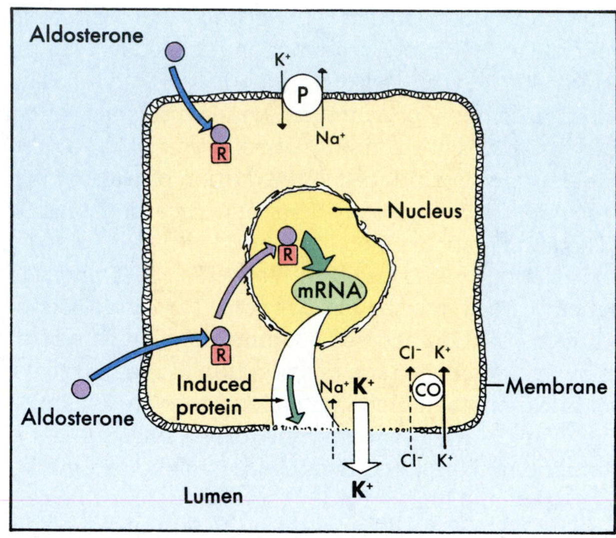

FIGURE 19-4 Cellular action of aldosterone. *CO,* Cotransport.

of the late distal segment and attaches to a cytosolic receptor (Figure 19-4). The hormone-receptor complex then migrates to the nucleus, where it induces the formation of a specific messenger RNA (mRNA). The newly formed mRNA leaves the nucleus to direct the production of a protein that enhances the permeability of the apical (luminal) membrane of the cell to Na^+ and K^+. Increased entry of substrate feeds the sodium pump and thus speeds reabsorption.

Because the pump simultaneously carries interstitial K^+ across the basolateral membrane, the cellular concentration of this ion increases. This is the first step in the secretion of potassium. But potassium is also actively transported inward, across the apical membrane, by a cotransport system. Thus it is free to move passively down its concentration gradient through either membrane. Because sodium entry from the lumen is electrogenic, the resultant electrical negativity attracts potassium (i.e., completes the final secretory step). Predominance of secretion or reabsorption generally depends on the dietary intake of potassium, the principal determinant of plasma concentration. When plasma K^+ is high, basolateral entry increases and net secretion is demonstrable; when it is low, the basolateral pump is less effective and reabsorption predominates. By indirectly rousing the activity of the sodium pump, aldosterone promotes sodium retention and potassium loss.

The final equilibratory steps take place in medullary collecting ducts. Small amounts of NaCl and potassium are reabsorbed. In the presence of antidiuretic hormone, water moves out of the lumen, following the medullary osmotic gradient established by ion transport in the ascending limb. A quantitative summary of fractional reabsorption of water and sodium of each tubular segment is shown in Figure 19-5. The data are based on average values for a 70 kg adult in good health living in a moderate climate. Plasma sodium concentration is 140 mEq/L and glomerular filtration rate is 125 ml/min. The proximal tubule reabsorbs more sodium than water; the entire distal tubule and medullary collecting system extract less than 5% of filtered sodium.

Tubular Secretion and Bidirectional Transport of Organic Acids and Bases Except for two classes, osmotic agents and competitive inhibitors of aldosterone, all the diuretics in clinical use release or accept a proton at the pH of body fluids. Thus these drugs exist in the body both as uncharged molecules and as charged organic ions. In large measure, this duality of chemical form determines transport of the drugs in the body, how quickly they undergo transport from a particular site, and what actions they exert in the kidney and other organs.

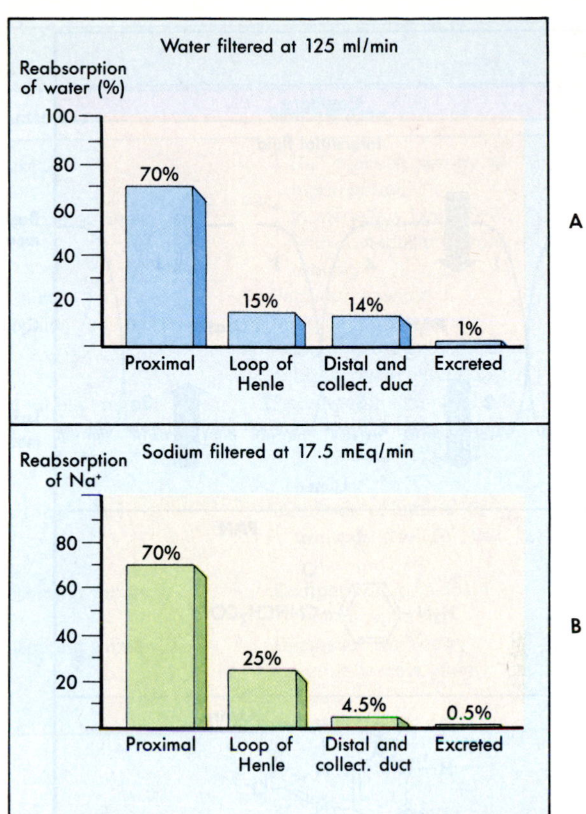

FIGURE 19-5 Summary of renal reabsorption of filtered water (**A**) and sodium (**B**) for a 70 kg human.

Proximal tubular secretion of diuretic anions and cations illustrates the profound influence of electrical charge on the delivery of drugs to renal receptors and on their rapid decline in plasma. Two generic secretory systems that transport organic ions from blood to urine reside in the proximal tubule. One handles organic acids (anions as A^- form of acid HA), and the second transports organic bases (cations as BH^+ form) of base B (see Chapter 5). The chief characteristics of these systems are as follows:

1. At least one step in the transport process is active (uphill) and against the concentration gradient, though metabolic energy is furnished indirectly
2. The systems are saturable (fixed number of carriers)
3. The systems are susceptible to competitive inhibition by other transported organic ions bearing the charge

The lack of any specific structural requirement supports the conjecture that these two secretory mechanisms serve primarily as "glomerular backups" for the urinary excretion of a large number of endogenous and environmental chemicals, especially but not exclusively, solutes of low molecular weight that bind to plasma proteins and thus are not freely filtered through glomerular membranes. In addition to most of the diuretics, organic acids and bases that are secreted include acetylcholine and choline, bile acids, uric acid, *p*-aminohippuric acid (PAH), epinephrine, norepinephrine, histamine, and morphine.

The tubular transport of two major acids, PAH and uric acid, is summarized in Figure 19-6. Step 1 is the same for both acids. A membrane transporter carries Na^+ downhill and PAH or urate uphill in the same direction across the basolateral membrane into the cells. Step 1 may also be accomplished by an exchange (countertransport) for a cellular anion. The cell, now loaded with PAH or urate, readily loses these substances to the urine as they move downhill to complete step 2 with the help of a transporter in the brush border. Step 3, movement back into the cell by exchange with a cellular anion, is either insignificant for PAH or is prevented by the large concentration gradient favoring movement of that organic anion into the urine. Although reabsorption is demonstrable in some species and can be inhib-

acetazolamide

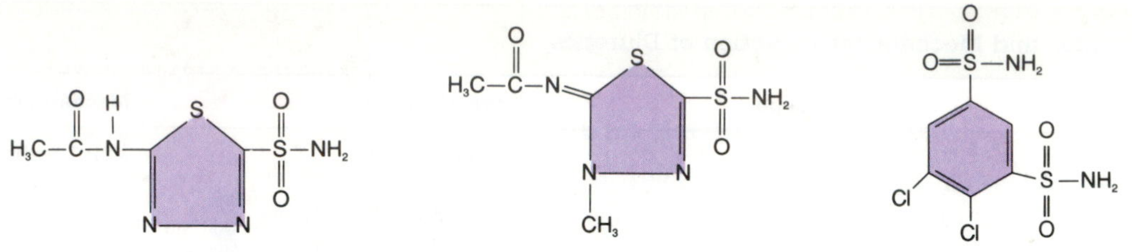

methazolamide

dichlorphenamide

FIGURE 19-8 Carbonic anhydrase inhibitors.

ion decreases when sodium is transported and water does not follow the sodium. This results in a change in the sodium-concentration gradient and leads to a return flux of sodium chloride into the lumen, and ultimately to a small increase (relative to water) in the excretion of sodium. Urinary loss of sodium is dependent on dosage but is invariably less than the fractional excretion of water. The initial dilution of plasma electrolytes induced by acute expansion of the ECF volume reverses when renal excretion of water catches up. Overzealous administration of mannitol may result in hypernatremia, hyperkalemia, and volume depletion.

Under normal circumstances, reabsorption of NaCl in the thick ascending limb increases when proximal tubular reabsorption is repressed. This compensatory response fails to occur during osmotic diuresis, possibly because mannitol increases medullary blood flow, an action that washes out the countercurrent gradient. The NaCl concentration of fluid in the thick ascending limb is much reduced, and this indirectly diminishes the efficiency of the Na^+,K^+, $2Cl^-$ cotransport system. Transport of sodium and water is decreased. Ascending limb cells are thus an important site of natriuretic action. Distal segments and medullary collecting ducts, responsible for transport of only a small fraction of filtered sodium, are unable to cope with the large salt and water loads presented during osmotic diuresis. (Fig. 19-1)

Carbonic Anhydrase Inhibitors Acetazolamide, the prototypical carbonic anhydrase inhibitor, has limited use as a diuretic; it is used to reduce intraocular pressure in glaucoma.

Carbonic anhydrase is a metalloenzyme containing one zinc atom per molecule. High concentrations are found in renal proximal tubular cells, ciliary processes of the eye, red blood cells, choroid plexes, intestine, and pancreas. There are five major isozymes in mammalian tissues. Carbonic anhydrase catalyzes the hydration of carbon dioxide (reaction 1) and the dehydration of carbonic acid (reaction 2) according to the following:

$$H_2O + CO_2 \underset{2}{\overset{1}{\leftrightharpoons}} H_2CO_3 \leftrightharpoons HCO_3^- + H^+$$

The prevailing direction of the reaction is established by the pH; normally hydration of carbon dioxide occurs, resulting in H^+ generation. The latter exchanges for sodium, which enters the renal tubular cell.

Acetazolamide inhibition of the enzyme reduces the hydrogen-ion concentration in the tubular lumen and decreases the availability of H^+ for the H^+/Na^+ exchange. As a result, there is an increase in bicarbonate in the proximal portion of the tubular lumen along with sodium. Although some bicarbonate is reabsorbed at other tubular sites, ultimately approximately 50% of the bicarbonate normally reabsorbed is eliminated in the urine. A hyperchloremic metabolic acidosis results from the bicarbonate depletion, which renders ineffective subsequent doses of acetazolamide.

The sulfanilamide type of compounds such as acetazolamide, methazolamide, and dichlorphenamide reversibly inhibit carbonic anhydrase, resulting in increased urine flow and sodium bicarbonate excretion. The chemical structures of these drugs are shown in Figure 19-8.

Thiazide Diuretics This type of diuretic drug was discovered from attempts to find compounds that increase the excretion of NaCl rather than $NaHCO_3^-$, as occurs with the carbonic anhydrase inhibition. The basic structure (Figure 19-9) comprises a heterocyclic (benzothiadiazide) ring and an unsubstituted sulfamyl ($-SO_2$ NH_2) group. Thiazide-related diuretics are formed by alteration of the ring structure. Hydrochlorothiazide is formed by addition of hydrogen at positions 3 and 4. This minor change improves oral absorption, increased diuretic potency, and substantially reduced inhibitory carbonic anhydrase activity.

The major site of action of thiazides is the early distal portion of the tubule. (Fig. 19-1) They also act in the cortical thick ascending limb of the loop of Henle. Suppression of sodium and chloride transport at this locus increases the delivery of these two ions, along with fluid attracted osmotically, to the later portions of the nephron. There, a small fraction of the excess sodium ion in excess is reabsorbed and replaced with potassium. Because only 15% or less of the glomerular filtrate

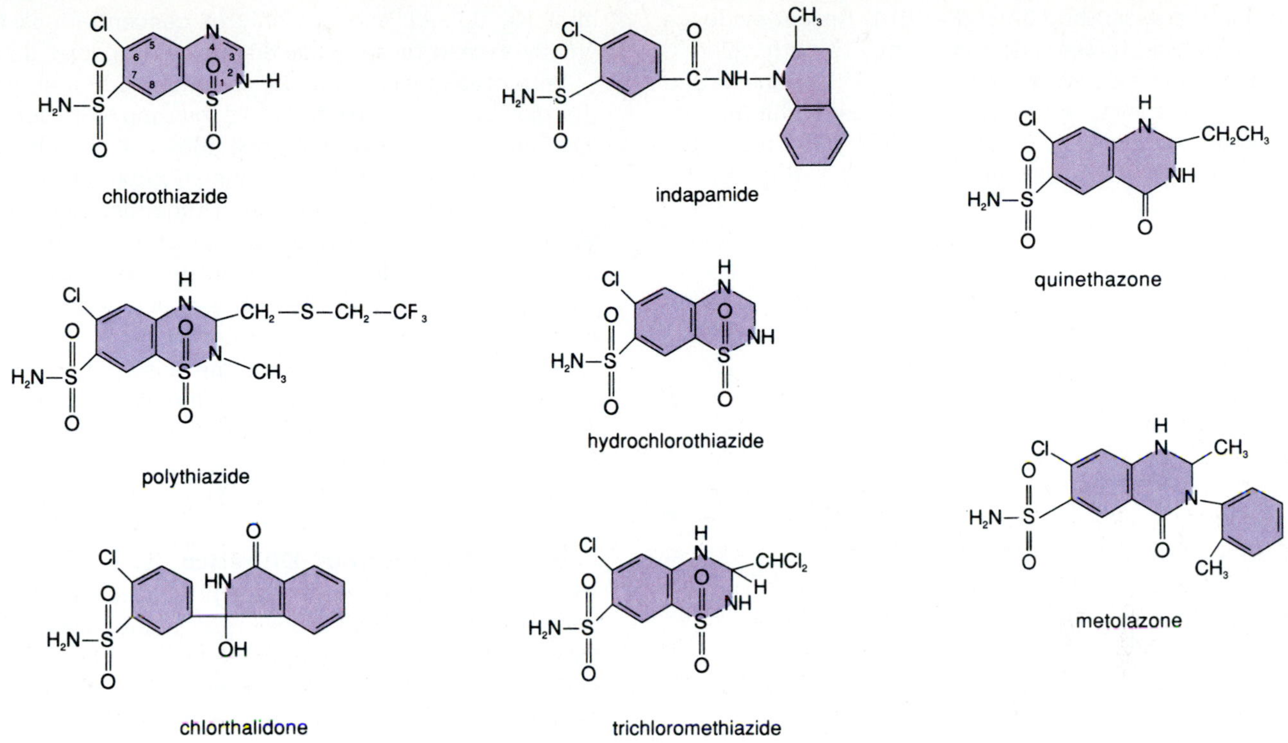

FIGURE 19-9 Thiazide diuretics.

reaches the early distal segment, the magnitude of the diuretic effect is more limited than that induced by agents that act earlier (e.g., in the ascending loop of Henle). Thiazides interfere with the electroneutral passage of NaCl from lumen to cells.

Chlorothiazide in recommended doses may inhibit bicarbonate transport in the proximal tubule, but most of the thiazides and thiazide-related drugs are weaker inhibitors of carbonic anhydrase and do not affect bicarbonate at usual therapeutic doses.

Loop Diuretics Loop diuretics satisfy the need for agents capable of generating larger responses than those produced by thiazides. Acting on the ascending limb, loop diuretics can inhibit the reabsorption of as much as 25% of the glomerular filtrate (Figure 19-10) and are often effective when thiazides do not suffice. Greater efficacy confers greater ability to distort fluid and electrolyte balance. Overdoses of thiazides are usually tolerated, but overdoses of loop agents may evoke serious consequences. Nevertheless, loop diuretics are remarkably safe when used properly.

Three loop diuretics are available in the United States (Figure 19-11). Ethacrynic acid and furosemide are prototypes of loop I and II drugs, respectively. Bumetanide, of the same class as furosemide, is considerably more potent and differs pharmacokinetically but otherwise is similar to the older drug. Ethacrynic acid attaches to

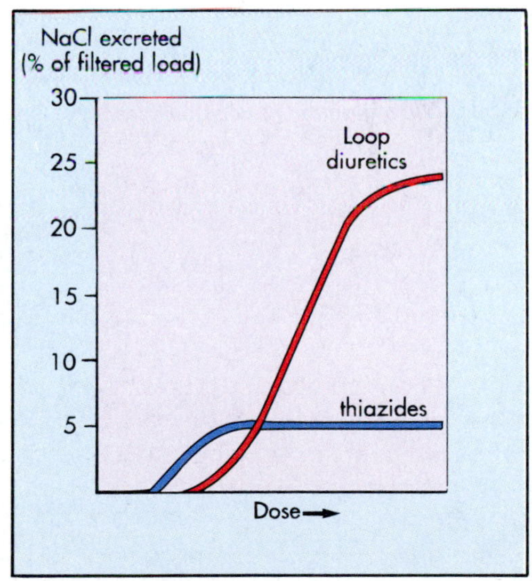

FIGURE 19-10 Schematic dose-response curves comparing thiazides with loop diuretics.

sulfhydryl groups in vivo, a reaction formerly considered the antecedent of diuresis. This opinion no longer prevails, because several natriuretic compounds with related structures do not react chemically with sulfhydryl groups in vitro. Loop diuretics suppress reabsorption of

NaCl in the ascending limb. (Fig 19-1) Recent evidence indicates that furosemide may compete with chloride for a binding site on the Na^+,K^+, $2Cl^-$ cotransporting system. Although ethacrynic acid also inhibits this transport mechanism, efforts to identify the molecular mechanism have been unsuccessful. The drug can inhibit Na^+,K^+-ATPase but only at concentrations that greatly exceed those achieved with therapeutic doses.

Both drugs reach their site of action by first entering the glomerulas filtrate and then passing with luminal flow into the loop and thence into cell membranes. Proximal tubular secretion is thus an important component of the delivery mechanism. Drugs that block tubular secretion (e.g., probenecid) influence the temporal response to loop diuretics but do not abolish their effects. Evidence that ancillary sites of action are present in segments of the nephron other than the ascending limb is largely discounted on the assumption that a proximal tubular action would be annulled downstream and a distal action, in any event, would be trivial. This overlooks the fact that loop diuretics interfere with reabsorptive transport in the loop. Thus full compensation may not be possible.

Potassium-Sparing Diuretics The potassium-sparing diuretics comprise three pharmacologically distinct groups: steroidal aldosterone antagonists, pteridines, and pyrazinoylguanidines. One drug from each group is available in the United States. Locus of action for all is the late distal segment, in which they interfere with sodium reabsorption and potassium secretion, though each operates through a different molecular mechanism. Diuretic activity is weak because fractional sodium reabsorption in the late distal segment usually

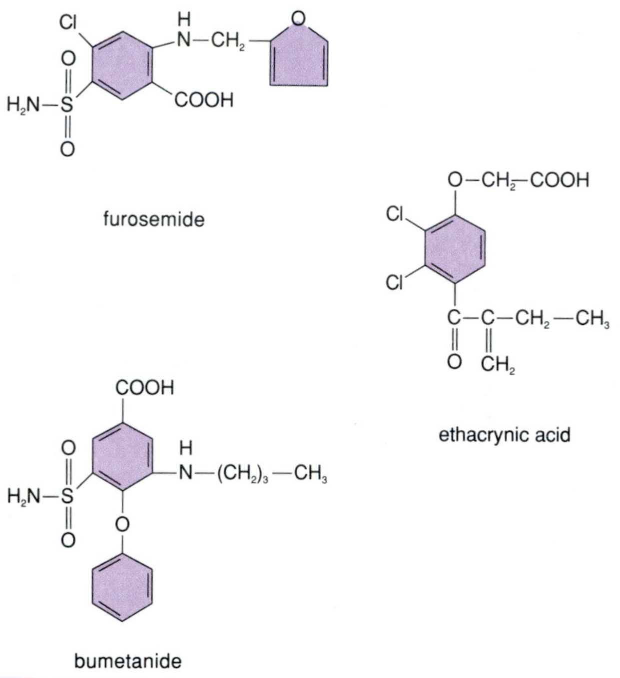

furosemide

ethacrynic acid

bumetanide

FIGURE 19-11 Loop diuretics.

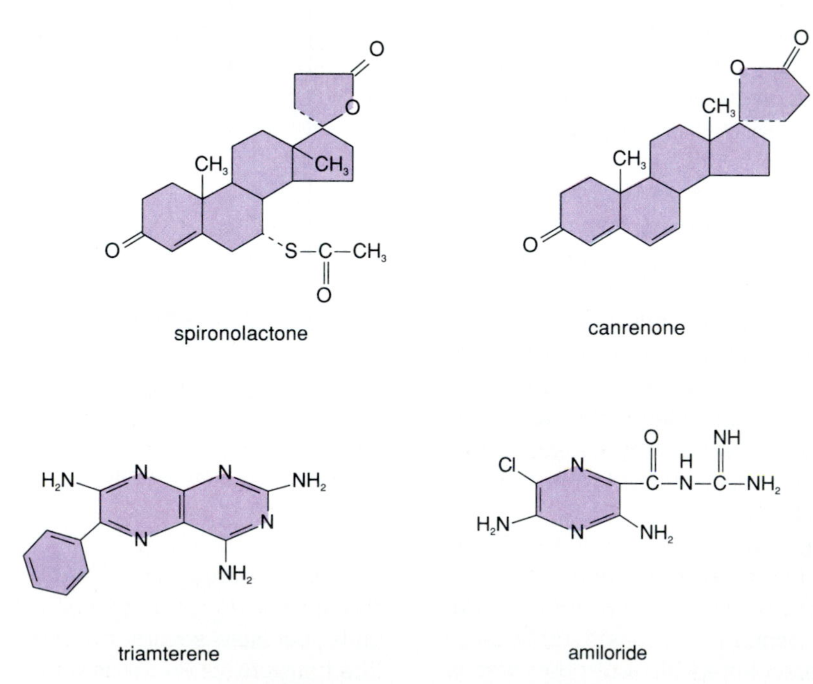

FIGURE 19-12 K^+-sparing diuretics.

does not exceed 3% of the filtered load. For this reason, potassium-sparing drugs are ordinarily used in combination with thiazides or loop diuretics, often in a single preparation, to restrict potassium losses and sometimes to augment diuretic action. Use as single agents is infrequent.

Spironolactone (Figure 19-12) is an analog of aldosterone. Spironolactone and its major metabolite, canrenone, attach to aldosterone receptors in the kidney and elsewhere and act as competitive inhibitors of the endogenous hormone, resulting in a longer duration of action.

Triamterene and amiloride (see Figure 19-12) are structurally diverse but use the same primary site of action. The molecular mechanisms of action probably differ somewhat, but the results are virtually identical. Triamterene is an aminopteridine chemically related to folic acid. Amiloride is a pyrazinoylguanidine. Both are organic bases secreted in the proximal tubule. Prevailing evidence indicates that basolateral movement into the cell is downhill and egress through the luminal membrane is uphill, with transporters involved in both cases. Triamterene and amiloride prevent entry of luminal sodium into cells of the late distal tubule. The molecular mechanism of this action is unknown. It may involve closure of sodium channels, which produces a selective reduction in permeability of the membranes to sodium. Because sodium transport at this site is electrogenic, failure of entry dispels the electrical gradient between cell and lumen, and thus cancels a critical force that draws intracellular potassium into the urine. Although the drugs are weak diuretics and natriuretics, potassium is conserved and chloride is excreted with sodium. These two agents may also increase bicarbonate excretion and interfere with urinary acidification. Amiloride can reduce sodium-hydrogen exchange in the proximal tubule and possibly also downstream. Some investigators believe that a portion of the natriuretic response to triamterene is related to inhibition of Na^+,K^+-ATPase. Amiloride also depresses the renal clearance of calcium, an action that is coupled with the inhibition of sodium reabsorption in the late distal segment. In contrast to spironolactone, triamterene and amiloride are active in the presence or in the absence of circulating aldosterone.

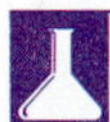

PHARMACOKINETICS

The pharmacokinetic parameters for diuretic agents are summarized in Table 19-4.

Because *mannitol* is not readily absorbed from the intestine and large doses are required to produce a significant effect, it is administered IV as a bolus or by drip over an extended period. It distributes in extracellular fluid. Excretion is almost entirely by glomerular filtration, with approximately 90% appearing in the urine within 24 hours. Less than 10% is reabsorbed in the renal tubule, and a similar quantity is metabolized, probably in the liver. The plasma half-life is approximately 15 to 20 minutes.

Isosorbide and *glycerol* are administered orally to reduce intraocular pressure before ophthalmological surgery. Urea is rarely given by mouth because it induces nausea and emesis. It is administered IV as an aqueous solution containing dextrose, or invert sugar. Urea, glycerol, and isosorbide are metabolized extensively.

Acetazolamide is well absorbed from the gastrointestinal (GI) tract. More than 90% of the drug is plasma protein bound. Because it is relatively insoluble in lipid, it does not readily penetrate cellular membranes or cross the blood-brain barrier. The highest concentrations are found in tissues that contain large amounts of carbonic anhydrase (e.g., renal cortex, red blood cells). Renal effects are noticeable within 30 minutes and are usually maximal at 2 hours. Acetazolamide is not metabolized but is excreted rapidly by glomerular filtration and proximal tubular secretion. The half-life is approximately 5 hours and renal excretion is essentially complete in 24 hours. In comparison, methazolamide is absorbed more slowly from the gastrointestinal (GI) tract, and its duration of action is long, with a half-life of approximately 14 hours.

Individually, the thiazides differ considerably with respect to pharmacokinetic properties. Plasma protein binding varies from 10% to 95%, but extensive binding does not prevent access to the site of action. Free drug enters the lumen by filtration and by organic acid secretion and subsequently diffuses or is transported to its site of action.

Each thiazide and thiazide-related drug possesses singular attributes with respect to potency, onset, and duration of action. For example, the diuretic action of chlorthalidone, a thiazide-related drug, is slow in onset but remains for 24 hours or more. The course of action and potency are manifestations of solubility in lipid, with highly soluble members of the thiazide family possessing larger apparent volumes of distribution and lower renal clearances. All the agents, however, appear to share the same mechanism of action. Dose-response curves are parallel, and maximal responses (efficacy) are similar. The thiazides are not metabolized. The major route of disappearance is renal, with elimination by glomerular filtration and proximal tubular secretion. Biliary excretion is a second less prominent route.

Although *chlorothiazide* has adequate bioavailability

Table 19-4 Pharmacokinetic Parameters

Drug	Administration	Onset (hours)	t½ (hours)	Disposition
THIAZIDES				
Chlorthiazide	oral	1-3	6-12	R (main) B
	IV	0.25	2	R (main) B
Hydrochlorthiazide	oral	1	8-12	R (main) B
Chlorthalidone	oral	2-4	24	R (main) B
Metazolone	oral	1	12-24	R (main) B
Indapamide	oral	1-2	18-36	R (main) B
LOOP DIURETICS				
Furosemide	oral	1	6	R (40%) M
	IV	5-10 min	2	R (40%) M
Ethacrynic acid	IV	0.25	3	R (main) M*
Bumetamide	oral	0.5-1	4-6	M*
	IV	0.25	0.5-1	M*
CARBONIC ANHYDRASE INHIBITORS				
Acetazolamide	oral	1	5	R
Methazolamide	oral	2-3	14	R
POTASSIUM-SPARING DIURETICS				
Spironolactone	oral	1-2 days	2-3 days	RMB
Triamterine	oral	2hr	12-16	RMB
Amiloride	oral	2 hr	24 hr	RMB

R, renal excretion (parent drug); *M*, metabolized; *B*, biliary excretion; *active metabolite

when given orally, it is not extensively absorbed from the GI tract. Absorption is dose dependent in the therapeutic range; approximately 20% of a 250 mg dose enters the systemic circulation, but only 10% of a 500 mg dose is absorbed. Either the absorptive site is easily saturated or poor water solubility interferes. Hydrochlorothiazide is approximately 70% bioavailable and its fractional absorption is not dose-dependent. This drug has a large apparent volume of distribution, and the plasma concentration provides a rapid (1-hour) onset of action. The half-life is 8 to 10 hours.

Ethacrynic acid is administered intraveneously, has a rapid onset of action, and is rapidly excreted. Ethacrynic acid is conjugated with glutathione, which subsequently forms an ethacrynic acid–cysteine adduct that is more potent than the parent drug. Because ethacrynic acid is poorly soluble in lipid, the apparent volume of distribution is small. Plasma protein binding is extensive and the compound and its metabolites are excreted in the urine by filtration and proximal tubular secretion. Elimination by the intestine is augmented through biliary transport and accounts for approximately one third of the administered dose. Ototoxicity limits its use.

Furosemide is practically insoluble in lipid and almost totally bound to plasma protein (>95%). Well absorbed from the GI tract, its onset and duration of action match those of ethacrynic acid, and it is excreted by the same routes. The average therapeutic dose excreted unchanged is 30% to 50%, and the elimination half-life is approximately 1 hour. Half-life increases in patients with renal insufficiency or cirrhosis. The liver forms an inactive glucuronide.

Spironolactone is poorly soluble in aqueous fluids. Bioavailability of an oral dose is approximately 90% in some but not all commercial preparations. The drug is rapidly metabolized in the liver. Canrenone, the predominant metabolite, is responsible for roughly 80% of the potassium-sparing effect. Canrenone binds extensively to plasma protein (98%). Its half-life varies from 10 to 35 hours, and it is excreted in urine and bile along with smaller quantities of additional metabolites. Tubular secretion of canrenone has been reported but unmetabolized drug is not detectable in urine. The onset of action is extremely slow, with peak response sometimes occurring 48 hours or more after the first dose; effects gradually wane over a period of 48 to 72 hours.

Oral absorption of *triamterene* in humans is rapid and almost complete in healthy subjects. Half-life is approximately 2 hours. Approximately 60% of the parent drug and 90% of the major metabolite, a sulfate conjugate, are bound to plasma proteins. Up to 70% is excreted in the urine, but only a small fraction is unchanged. A considerable quantity is metabolized in the liver, and biliary excretion is significant. Most patients respond during the first day of treatment but the maximum is not reached for several days.

When *amiloride* is administered orally, approximately 50% of the dose is recovered in the urine and 40% in the feces. The half-life is 6 hours, with action usually beginning in 2 hours and lasting about 24 hours. Amiloride is not metabolized.

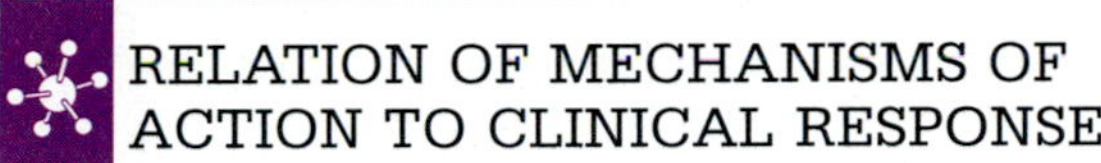

RELATION OF MECHANISMS OF ACTION TO CLINICAL RESPONSE

Osmotic Diuretics

Mannitol is usually the drug of choice among osmotic agents because its properties best satisfy the requirements for an efficient osmotic diuretic. It is inherently nontoxic, freely filtered through glomeruli, essentially nonreabsorbable from tubular fluid, and not readily metabolized. Urea, glycerol, and isosorbide are less efficient as osmotic agents because they penetrate cellular membranes. As drug molecules are reabsorbed, luminal concentration decreases and the tendency to retain filtered fluid diminishes. Patients treated with mannitol may develop mild hyperkalemia acutely. Although the origin of this action is not firmly established, it is likely that bulk flow of potassium accompanies the osmotic-induced discharge of water from cells into the interstitium. Mannitol increases the excretion of many important ions. The list includes potassium, bicarbonate, phosphate, calcium, and magnesium. Losses are usually modest and clinically unimportant. Nevertheless, it is prudent to be aware of the potential imbalances that may be induced in patients receiving prolonged therapy or in those in whom concentrations of these electrolytes are already distorted.

It is a common clinical impression that mannitol improves renal hemodynamics in a variety of situations of impending or incipient renal failure. There is supporting evidence in some clinical studies, but dissenting reports abound and the topic is controversial. Mannitol does not increase glomerular filtration rate or renal blood flow in humans, as it clearly does in some laboratory species.

Because they penetrate into the aqueous compartment in trace amounts only, osmotic drugs reduce the volume and pressure of the aqueous humor by extracting fluid from it. Hence, they may be used for the short-term treatment of acute glaucoma. Similarly, infusions of mannitol are used to lower the elevated intracranial pressure of cerebral edema associated with tumors, neurosurgical procedures, or other conditions. Osmotic agents cause the redistribution of body fluid, increase urine flow rate, and accelerate the renal elimination of filtered solutes. These effects are often sought in the treatment of many clinical disorders.

These drugs are also administered prophylactically to prevent the development of renal failure associated with severe traumatic injury; cardiovascular and other complicated surgical procedures, or therapy with cisplatin and other renotoxic drugs. Efficacy and mechanism of action in such instances are not well established. Based on studies in experimental animal models, many investigators claim that mannitol dilates renal blood vessels that are in the constricted state and, by causing the rate of urine flow to increase, prevents obstruction of the renal tubules and further reduction in glomerular filtration.

Mannitol is occasionally used to promote renal extraction of bromides, barbiturates, salicylates, or other drugs in overdosed individuals.

Carbonic Anhydrase Inhibitors

Acetazolamide is used effectively in the prevention and treatment of acute mountain sickness and to alkalinize the urine. All three of the carbonic anhydrase inhibitors (see Figure 19-8) can be used to treat epilepsy.

The popularity of carbonic anhydrase inhibitors as diuretics has waned because of (1) rapid tolerance development, (2) increased urinary excretion of bicarbonate with inevitable acidotic manifestations when these drugs are given daily, and, most importantly, (3) because of the advent of more suitable agents. Nevertheless, acetazolamide can be administered for short-term therapy, especially in combination with other diuretics to patients who are resistant or who do not respond adequately to other agents. The rationale for using a combination is based on summation of sites of action. It is occasionally used in the treatment of chronic open-angle glaucoma. Since the aqueous humor has a high bicarbonate concentration, these drugs can be used to reduce aqueous humor formation.

Thiazide Diuretics

The development of chlorothiazide offered the opportunity, for the first time, to treat edematous patients with a diuretic agent that was orally effective, well tolerated, and relatively safe. Also, it was discovered that chlorothiazide potentiates the antihypertensive response to ganglionic blocking agents and is mildly antihypertensive when used alone. This drug, however, has largely been supplanted by hydrochlorothiazide, a much weaker carbonic anhydrase inhibitor but a more potent chloruretic agent, and by other newer compounds. All of the thiazides act in the same way, with the differences among them attributable largely to pharmacokinetic characteristics and inherent carbonic anhydrase inhibitory activity.

The renal effects of thiazides are dependent in large measure on (1) the physiological state of water and electrolyte balance at the time they are administered and (2) the functional status of the kidneys, cardiovascular system, and liver. A large dose may be ineffective in a patient with severe renal hepatic disease, whereas a standard dose can produce a tremendous diuretic response in a severely edematous patient whose renal and hepatic functions are relatively normal.

Effects on Potassium and Magnesium When the natriuretic action of a diuretic is exerted proximally to the late portion of the distal segment (i.e., in advance of the site where aldosterone action is prominent), the agent increases the excretion of potassium. Such is the case for thiazides and for loop diuretics (discussed later). There are three cogent reasons for this increase: (1) more sodium and water delivered to the aldosterone exchange site, where reabsorption of larger amounts of sodium and dilution of luminal fluid enhance the secretion of potassium; (2) contraction of the ECF, causing an increase in secretion of aldosterone; and (3) hypochloremic alkalosis induced by diuretics promoting potassium excretion. The fraction of patients who develop hypokalemia or display evidence of potassium depletion while receiving long-term thiazide dosing is quite variable. Young people with hypertension treated with thiazides may have no effects or become only slightly hypokalemic. Others develop clear signs of deficiency. That hypokalemia generated by thiazides results in increased ventricular ectopy has been questioned by some investigators. The Medical Research Council trial found no difference in mortalities and cardiac events between hypertensive patients who take thiazides and those who are undergoing β-blocker therapy. Nevertheless, even mild hypokalemia should be avoided, especially in cirrhotic patients, those taking cardiac glycosides, patients with diabetes, and the elderly. Disturbances in insulin and glucose metabolism can often be prevented if potassium depletion is avoided. Measures for preventing or correcting potassium deficiency are discussed in a later section.

Although reabsorption of magnesium takes place primarily in the proximal tubule, thiazides and loop diuretics can accelerate its excretion. Magnesium depletion in patients on chronic diuretic therapy is occasionally reported and is considered by some clinicians to be a risk factor in the development of ventricular dysrhythmias. The addition of potassium-sparing diuretics reportedly prevents magnesium loss.

Effects on Calcium Under most conditions, a parallel relationship exists between sodium and calcium excretion in the urine. Measures that alter the elimination of one of these ions alter the second similarly. However, this association does not exist when thiazides are used. Paradoxically, sodium reabsorption is reduced while calcium reabsorption is increased. The underlying mechanism involves contraction of the ECF volume. Acutely, thiazides do not enhance calcium reabsorption. When administered repeatedly, however, they display a hypocalciuric action. This action can be overcome merely by restoration of salt and water losses. Thus dissociation between sodium and calcium transport begins only when volume contraction opposes the natriuretic response.

Thiazides are now widely used to prevent the formation of recurrent calcium stones. The serum calcium concentration often increases, but the rise is modest and rarely causes a problem.

Effects on Uric Acid Thiazides increase the serum concentration of urate. Two mechanisms are involved: increased proximal tubular reabsorption and reduced tubular secretion of urate. The former, like calcium reabsorption, depends on contraction of the ECF volume. Volume reduction enhances fractional sodium reabsorption, and sodium carries urate with it (cotransport). Depletion of ECF volume alone elevates serum urate concentration. Replacement of thiazide-induced salt and water loss lessens the effect of thiazides on serum urate. The extent to which suppression of urate secretion contributes to urate retention is not defined.

More than 50% of patients on long-term thiazide therapy develop hyperuricemia. In the majority, elevation of urate is modest and does not precipitate gout unless the patient is afflicted with the primary disease or possesses a gouty diathesis. Currently, there is no reason to believe that the risk of hyperuricemia outweighs the benefits of thiazide therapy in patients who do not have a history of gout.

Other Effects Carbohydrate intolerance may develop in nondiabetics and usually worsens in diabetic patients on chronic thiazide therapy. The cause is not established but has variously been attributed to such factors as suppression of insulin secretion, resistance to insulin action, or increased glycogen breakdown. In most instances, carbohydrate tolerance returns to the predrug levels within a year after the thiazide is withdrawn. Another disturbance associated with chronic thiazide therapy is a small increase in serum lipids and lipoproteins. Low-density lipoprotein-cholesterol and triglyceride concentrations may increase during short-term therapy, but total cholesterol and triglyceride concentrations usually return to base-line values in studies of more than 1 year in duration. It has been suggested that this action on lipids is linked to glucose intolerance and that both of these metabolic disturbances are, in part, consequences of potassium depletion.

Clinical Indications and Uses The primary indications for thiazides are listed in the box on p. 252. In general, these agents are used in the treatment of hypertension and CHF and in other conditions when reduction of ECF volume is beneficial. Reduction of blood pressure in patients with hypertension results, in part, from contraction of ECF volume (see Chapter 13). This occurs acutely, leading to a decrease in cardiac output with compensatory elevation of peripheral resistance. Vasoconstriction then subsides enabling cardiac output to return to normal values. Augmented synthesis of vasodilator prostaglandins is reported and may be a crucial factor for long-term maintenance of a lower pressure, even though ECF volume tends to return toward normal (see Chapter 18).

Thiazides also are employed in the treatment of vasopressin-resistant diabetes insipidus. In these patients, urine is copious and dilute, and plasma is hyperosmotic. Chronic administration of thiazides increases the osmolarity and reduces urine flow in this condition. The mechanism hinges on the removal of sodium from the ECF, an action that inevitably contracts ECF volume. The proximal tubule then overreabsorbs sodium. Urine flow rate diminishes and urine osmolality rises when sodium transport in the early distal segment is inhibited by the diuretic. Drug therapy in this instance is most effective in combination with dietary salt restriction.

Loop Diuretics

Loop agents are extremely efficacious at the low end of the dosage spectrum. NaCl losses are equivalent to those obtained with thiazides; at high doses, massive amounts of salt are excreted. Two decisive factors adjust the magnitude of the response: (1) the existing status of the salt and water balances and (2) the delivery of drug to the site of action. Contraction of ECF volume is an example of the first factor. Salt and water depletion invariably lessens the diuretic response by enhancing proximal and distal tubular reabsorption of sodium. Renal insufficiency is an example of the second. Less drug reaches critical receptors when some of the pathways (glomeruli or proximal tubules) are destroyed. Loop diuretics also increase the excretion of potassium, calcium, magnesium, and protons, and all the electrolyte depletion phenomena associated with thiazides may occur. Similarly, carbohydrate intolerance and hyperlipidemia have been reported.

Loop diuretics initially produce a slight increase in the excretion of urate. On continued administration, however, this effect is reversed and retention of urate becomes evident. The second event undoubtedly depends on contraction of the ECF volume (discussed under thiazides). *Furosemide* and *ethacrynic acid* may increase renal blood flow for brief intervals during which urinary excretion of prostaglandin E is elevated. IV injections of furosemide reduce pulmonary arterial pressure and peripheral venous compliance. *Indomethacin,* an inhibitor of prostaglandin synthesis, interferes with all these actions. Vascular phenomena of this sort occurring in the kidney and elsewhere precede the onset of diuresis. The therapeutic value of loop diuretics in pulmonary edema may be attributable in part to stimulation of prostaglandin synthesis in the lung.

Common clinical indications for loop diuretics are listed in the box. In most cases, their employment overlaps that of thiazides, but there are some major differences. The greater efficacy of loop agents often enables their successful use in evoking diuresis in edematous patients with disturbances of cardiovascular, renal, or hepatic origin. For example, an oliguric patient whose GFR is only 10% of normal derives no benefit from a thiazide but may respond well to a large dose of a loop diuretic. In addition, furosemide is an important adjunct in the treatment of acute pulmonary edema. The drug increases pulmonary and peripheral venous compliance, thereby affording rapid relief, and then maintains these beneficial effects by reducing the plasma volume. The initial vascular effects are not linked to actions on the renal tubule (venodilatation occurs in anephric patients).

Many investigators report that thiazides or related drugs, especially longer-acting members of each group, are more effective than loop agents for reducing blood pressure. Others, citing evidence of lesser effects on carbohydrate metabolism and plasma lipids, prefer furosemide. The 1988 Report of the Joint National Committee on Detection, Evaluation, and Treatment of High Blood Pressure does not address this question. Loop diuretics are used to lower serum calcium concentrations of patients with hypercalcemia. Isotonic saline is often coadministered to maintain the glomerular filtration rate.

Potassium-Sparing Diuretics

Depletion of body potassium with or without significant lowering of serum K^+ concentration (only 2% of total body potassium is present in ECF) is probably the most common side effect of diuretic therapy. Hypokalemia of sufficient magnitude creates many problems and may be life threatening. These problems may include impairment of neuromuscular function, cardiac

CLINICAL PROBLEMS

THIAZIDES

Depletion phenomena (hypokalemia, dilutional hyponatremia, hypochloremic alkalosis, hypomagnesemia), retention phenomena (hyperuricemia, hypercalcemia), metabolic changes (hyperglycemia, hyperlipidemia, insulin resistance), hypersensitivity (fever, rash, purpura, anaphylaxis), and (azotemia in patients with poor renal function.

LOOP DIURETICS

Hypokalemia, hyperuricemia; metabolic alkalosis; hyponatremia; hearing deficits particularly with ethacrynic acid, watery diarrhea with ethacrynic acid

CARBONIC ANHYDRASE INHIBITORS

Metabolic acidosis, tolerance, drowsiness, fatigue, CNS depression, paresthesias, hypersensitivity to thiazides and thiazide-related agents

POTASSIUM-SPARING DIURETICS

aidosterone inhibitors: hyperkalemia, gynecomastia, hirsutism, menstrual irregularities
triamterene: hyperkalemia, megaloblastic anemia in patients with cirrhosis
amiloride: hyperkalemia, increase in blood urea nitrogen, glucose intolerance in diabetes mellitus

OSMOTIC DIURETICS

Acute increase in ECF volume and serum potassium concentration, nausea and vomiting, headache

dysrhythmia, intestinal disturbances, and partial loss of the ability to concentrate urine. Predisposition of diuretics to potassium wasting is especially worrisome during the treatment of CHF. In patients receiving digitalis preparations and a diuretic, diuretic-induced hypokalemia can ensue and sensitize the heart to the toxic effects of the cardiac glycoside.

Measures to elude the hazards of potassium deficit or to correct an established deficit are plentiful, but success is not guaranteed. The first steps are precautionary: dietary intake of large amounts of potassium, avoidance of excessive NaCl intake, and monitoring of serum K^+ concentrations. If serum potassium concentrations do not stabilize at an acceptable value, supplements of KCl may be prescribed; however, compliance may be a problem. The most effective therapeutic measure is to add a potassium-sparing diuretic to the therapeutic regimen, but KCl supplements should be *discontinued* if a K^+-sparing agent is used.

Spironolactone Uses Spironolactone is most effective in patients with primary or secondary hyperaldosteronism and is ineffective in patients with nonfunctional adrenal glands. The drug prevents the attachment of aldosterone to a cytosolic receptor in the late distal segment of the nephron (see Figure 19-4). Consequently, the hormonal stimulus to formation of new protein ceases. In the absence or reduction in amount of this protein, the permeability of the luminal membrane to sodium and potassium decreases, with the result that sodium excretion is enhanced and potassium secretion is diminished. Entry of potassium across the basolateral membrane also abates. Additional actions in both the proximal and distal tubule have been reported. These involve the transport of protons and bicarbonate anions and appear to depend on the hormonal status of the recipient. They may be related to intrinsic glucocorticoid activity or to one of the implicit steroidal effects of spironolactone.

Spironolactone is used for correction of hypokalemia. The drug is also administered alone, with thiazides, or a loop diuretic, to reduce the ECF volume without causing potassium depletion or hypokalemia. The drug is especially appropriate for the treatment of cirrhosis with ascites, a condition invariably associated with secondary hyperaldosteronism. It is also employed to boost natriuresis when the response to agents acting on the ascending limb or early distal tubule is inadequate. Although its natriuretic action is weak, spironolactone lowers blood pressure in patients with mild or moderate hypertension and is frequently prescribed for this purpose.

Triamterene and Amiloride Use Triamterene or amiloride is generally used in combination with potassium-wasting diuretics, especially when maintenance of normal serum potassium concentrations is clinically important (e.g., patients with dysrhythmias, receiving a cardiac glycoside, or with low serum potassium concentrations). Fixed-combination preparations are generally not appropriate for initial therapy but may be more expedient when the dosage schedule is demonstrated to be correct. Because these drugs possess a different site and mechanism of action from those of thiazides or loop agents, they are sometimes administered together to increase the response in patients who are refractory to a single agent.

SIDE EFFECTS, CLINICAL PROBLEMS, AND TOXICITY

Effective diuretic therapy alters the volume and composition of the extracellular fluid compartment—the reason for using the drugs. However, it is difficult to achieve the desired objectives entirely, and the volume and composition changes are often not attained or are exceeded. Moreover, it is not possible to restrict the effects of these drugs only to those desired for the therapeutic purposes. Accordingly, the repeated use of diuretics is frequently associated with shifts in acid-base balance and changes in serum electrolyte concentrations. Two shifts frequently encountered when diuretics are administered continuously include potassium depletion and hyperuricemia. Because these changes are manifestations of the molecular mechanism of action of the drugs, they are difficult to avoid in most patients unless counteractive measures are taken. It is best to anticipate the occurrence of such side effects. Patients at risk include the elderly, those with severe disease of any kind, individuals taking cardiac glycosides, and the malnourished. Supplemental intake of potassium (dietary or oral KCl) or the concomitant use of potassium-sparing diuretics with thiazides or loop diuretics is often successful. Elevation of urate rarely, if ever, precipitates an attack of gout in patients who are not disposed to the disease.

Paradoxical diuretic-induced edema may be observed in patients with hypertension when abrupt withdrawal of diuretics is initiated after a period of chronic use. Similarly, "idiopathic edema" appears to be associated with irregular use or abuse of diuretics among women who are concerned with their weight and appearance. It is probable that the edema in these instances is also caused by sudden withdrawal after a period of use. The designation "idiopathic" is incorrect because the subjects lose all traces of edema when they are weaned from salt-losing drugs. These findings are not surprising. Chronic use of diuretics results in a persistent elevation of plasma renin activity and the development of secondary aldosteronism. When it is necessary to discontinue diuretic therapy, stepwise reduction over a period of a few weeks combined with reduction of sodium intake is recommended. The main problems are summarized in the box.

Osmotic Diuretics

Acute expansion of the ECF engendered by osmotic diuretics increases the work load of the heart. Patients already in cardiac failure are especially susceptible and may develop pulmonary edema. They should not be treated with these drugs. Underlying heart disease in the absence of frank congestive failure, though not an absolute contraindication, is a serious risk factor. Rapid expansion of the plasma volume can precipitate congestive failure and pulmonary congestion. *Mannitol* is sometimes given to restore urine flow in oliguric or anuric states induced by extrarenal factors (e.g., hypovolemia, hypotension). In these cases, the response to a test dose should be evaluated before therapeutic quantities are administered.

Severe volume depletion and hypernatremia may result from the prolonged administration of mannitol unless sodium and water losses are replaced. Mild hyperkalemia is often observed, but intolerable elevations of potassium are not likely to occur except in patients with diabetes, patients with adrenal insufficiency, or those whose renal function is severely impaired.

Carbonic Anhydrase Inhibitors

Among the side effects of carbonic anhydrase inhibitors are metabolic acidosis, drowsiness, fatigue, CNS depression, and parathesias. Hypersensitivity reactions are rare.

Thiazides

Because most complications of thiazide therapy are direct manifestations of their pharmacological effects, adverse events are usually predictable. The list in the box includes adventitious hazards that have no apparent relationship to the descriptive pharmacology of the drugs. Although relatively uncommon, the latter are usually more serious. Thiazides should be used cautiously in patients with renal insufficiency. Alterations in fluid and electrolyte balance may precipitate hepatic coma in such patients. Thiazides reduce the clearance of lithium and, as a rule, should not be administered concomitantly. Although not an absolute contraindication, the drugs are not recommended during pregnancy unless the anticipated benefit justifies the risk. Thiazides cross the placenta and appear in breast milk. Anuria and precedent hypersensitivity to sulfonamides are absolute contraindications.

Loop Diuretics

The depletion phenomena and metabolic derangements occur also with loop diuretics; azotemia may be observed in conjunction with disturbances in electrolyte balance. Normal serum calcium concentrations are usually maintained even though urinary excretion of the ion increases initially; losses of calcium are not sustained during long-term therapy, probably because the ECF

TRADE NAMES

In addition to generic and fixed-combination preparations, the following trade-named materials are available in the United States.

Aldactone, spironolactone
Anhydron, cyclothiazide
Aquatag, benzthiazide
Bumex, bumetanide
Diamox, acetazolamide
Diucardin, hydroflumethiazide
Diulo, metolazone
Diuril, chlorothiazide
Dyrenium, triamterene
Edecrin, ethacrynic acid
Enduron, methyclothiazide
Esidrix, hydrochlorothiazide
Exna, benzthiazide
Hydrodiuril, hydrochlorothiazide
Hydromox, quinethazone
Hygroton, chlorthalidone
Lasix, furosemide
Lozol, indapamide
Metahydrin, trichlormethiazide
Midamor, amiloride hydrochloride
Naqua, trichlormethiazide
Naturetin, bendroflumethiazide
Neptazane, methazolamide
Proaqua, benzthiazide
Renese, polythiazide
Saluron, hydroflumethiazide
Zaroxolyn, metolazone

volume undergoes contraction. Nevertheless, hypocalcemia and rare cases of tetany are documented. Hypersensitivity reactions of the sulfonamide variety may be seen with furosemide.

Vertigo and deafness sometimes develop in individuals receiving large IV doses of loop diuretics, but coadministration of an aminoglycoside antibiotic (known to be ototoxic) and impaired renal function may also need to be present for this toxic reaction to occur. It is prudent to avoid concurrent use of ototoxic antibiotics and loop agents. Additional drug interactions occur with indomethacin (decreased activity of the loop diuretic), warfarin (displacement of the anticoagulant from plasma protein), and lithium (decreased clearance and increased risk of lithium toxicity).

All diuretics are contraindicated in anuric patients.

Table 19-5 Potential Drug Interactions

Drug Class or Agent	Diuretic	Problem
β-Adrenergic blockers	Thiazides	Increase in blood glucose urates and lipids
Digitalis glycosides	Thiazides, loop diuretics	Hypokalemia resulting in increased digitalis binding and toxicity
Angiotensin converting enzyme inhibitors	K^+-sparing diuretics	Hyperkalemia, cardiac effects
Aminoglycosides	Loop diuretics	Ototoxicity, nephrotoxicity
Adrenal steroids	Thiazides, loop diuretics	Enhanced hypokalemia
Chlorpropamide	Thiazides	Hyponatremia

Potassium-Sparing Diuretics

The most serious adverse reaction encountered during therapy with spironolactone is hyperkalemia. Serum potassium should be monitored periodically even when the drug is administered with a potassium-wasting diuretic. Patients at highest risk are those with low glomerular filtration rates and any individuals who take potassium supplements concurrently. Simultaneous use of supplements and a potassium-sparing agent is contraindicated.

Gynecomastia may occur in men, possibly as a consequence of binding of canrenone to androgen receptors; decreased libido and impotence have also been reported. These actions are dose related. Women may develop menstrual irregularities, hirsutism, or swelling and tenderness of the breast. Triamterene and amiloride may cause hyperkalemia, even when a potassium-wasting diuretic is part of the therapeutic program. This risk is highest in patients with limited renal function (e.g., renal insufficiency, diabetes, and elderly patients). Additional complications included elevated serum blood urea nitrogen and uric acid, glucose intolerance, and GI disturbances. Triamterene may contribute to or initiate formation of renal stones, and hypersensitivity reactions may occur but are rare. The drugs are contraindicated in patients with hyperkalemia, individuals taking potassium supplements in any form, and in patients with severe renal failure with progressive oliguria. Anuria is always a contraindication for diuretics. Some drug-drug interactions involving diuretics are indicated in Table 19-5.

NEW DIRECTIONS

Among the several metabolic changes that occur during therapy with the thiazide diuretics is the development of insulin resistance. This is a significant clinical problem and has led to the search for new chemical entities that are effective diuretics but might be devoid of this undesirable side effect. Such compounds would be particularly important in the therapy of hypertension, for which the thiazides are widely prescribed and for which the patient takes the drug over a lifetime.

REFERENCES

Brater DC: Resistance to loop diuretics, *Drugs* 30:427, 1985.

Cragoe EJ Jr, editor: *Diuretics: chemistry, pharmacology, and medicine,* New York, 1983, John Wiley.

Lant A: Clinical pharmacology and therapeutic use, *Drugs* 29; Part I, 57; Part II, 162, 1985.

Shackleton R, Wong NLM, Sutton RAL: Distal (potassium-sparing) diuretics. In Dirks JH, Sutton RAL, editors: *Diuretics: physiology, pharmacology, and clinical use,* Philadelphia, 1986, Saunders.

Weiner IM: General pharmacologic aspects of diuretics. In Dirks JH, Sutton RAL, editors: *Diuretics: physiology, pharmacology, and clinical use,* Philadelphia, 1986, Saunders.

SELF-ASSESSMENT QUESTIONS

1. The loop diuretics have their principal diuretic effect on the:
   a. ascending limb of loop of Henle.
   b. distal convoluted tubule.
   c. proximal convoluted tubule.
   d. distal pars recta.
   e. collecting duct.
2. Quantitative reabsorption of water and electrolytes:
   a. is greatest in the loop of Henle.
   b. particularly NaCl is against an electrochemical gradient.
   c. is driven by the sodium pump.
   d. b and c are correct.
   e. all of the above are correct.
3. Spironolactone:
   a. competes for aldosterone receptors.
   b. inhibits the excretion of potassium.
   c. acts at the late distal tubule.
   d. a and c are correct.
   e. all of the above are correct.
4. The following are potential side effects of the thiazide diuretics:
   a. hypokalemia, hyperglycemia, hyperlipidemia
   b. hypokalemia, ototoxicity, hyperuricemia
   c. hyperkalemia, alkalosis, nausea/vomiting
   d. increase in blood urea nitrogen, hyperkalemia, metabolic acidosis
   e. hypermagnesemia, hypercalcemia, fever

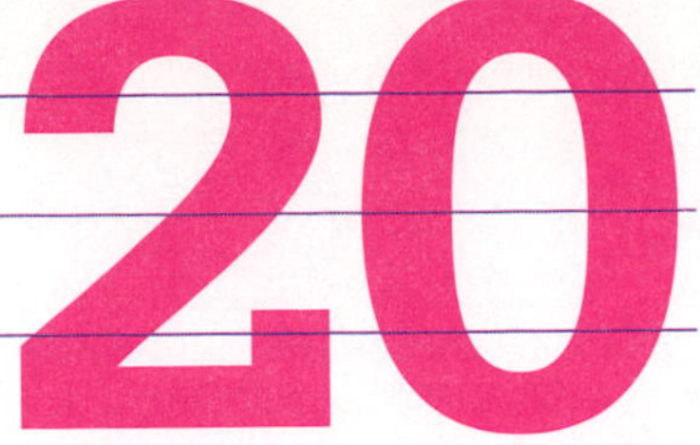

CHAPTER 20 Lipid-Lowering Drugs and Atherosclerosis

ROBERT H. MCDONALD, JR.

MAJOR DRUGS

- bile acid ion-exchange resins
- cholesterol synthesis inhibitors
- fibric acid derivatives
- probucol
- nicotinic acid
- other agents : neomycin and sitosterol

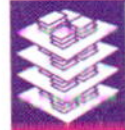

THERAPEUTIC OVERVIEW

Diseases of the heart and blood vessels are the principal causes of death in industrialized countries of the world. In the United States, more people die of such diseases than of cancer or any other illness. Of deaths resulting from cardiovascular disease, more than three fourths can be attributed to atherosclerosis and its complications. Atherosclerosis is a generalized disease of the arterial tree that usually develops in a symptom-free manner over many years. The most common manifestation of atherosclerosis is coronary heart disease, followed by stroke and peripheral vascular disease. Because it is a slowly developing disorder, to be effective treatment must be directed at causative factors and at prevention rather than reversal (Figure 20-1). In primates, actual reversal of lipid deposits in the arterial wall and a regression of the attendant fibrous tissue has been demonstrated. Therefore, there is the potential for clinical reversal in humans. Several studies now show either slower progression or regression of atherosclerotic lesions in coronary artery disease, with very vigorous drug therapy.

ABBREVIATIONS

acetyl CoA	acetylcoenzyme A
Apo proteins	apoproteins A, B, E, CII, and CIII
HDL	high-density lipoprotein
HMG-CoA	hydroxy-3-methyl-glutaryl coenzyme A
IDL	intermediate-density lipoprotein
LDL	low-density lipoprotein
VLDL	very low-density lipoprotein

Elevated cholesterol concentrations are a major contributing factor in the development of atherosclerosis. Cholesterol enters the circulation from two major sources, absorption from food (exogenous pathway) and synthesis by the liver (endogenous pathway). Under most circumstances, the latter pathway is the most significant. Cholesterol is taken up by the liver from the circulation to form bile acids or is taken up by other cells, either to form steroid hormones or to be inserted into and be a part of membranes. When present in excess, it is taken up by fibroblasts and scavenger cells in regenerating tissues and in fat cells. Transport of cholesterol in the plasma is by way of lipoprotein particles.

Currently, smoking cessation, blood pressure normalization, maintenance of normal plasma glucose concentrations, aspirin, and lowering of plasma concentrations of cholesterol and its associated lipids are the only proved approaches to reduction of the risk for atherosclerosis-related disorders. Clinical studies demonstrate the feasibility of lowering cholesterol with diet and treatment with drugs such as niacin, clofibrate, bile-acid binding resins, gemfibrozil, and the hydroxy-3-methyl-glutaryl coenzyme A (HMG-CoA) reductase inhibitors (Figure 20-1). These trials have demonstrated that a reduction in total cholesterol and low-density lipoprotein or elevation in high-density lipoprotein fractions is clearly associated with a lower rate of coronary artery diseases (angina, myocardial infarction, need for coronary bypass surgery). In general, for every percentage point that the total cholesterol concentration is low-

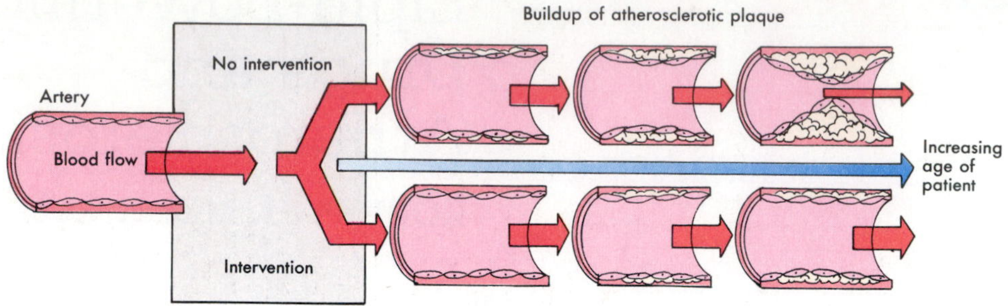

FIGURE 20-1 Atherosclerosis prevention. Intervention (treatment) involves (1) diet to decrease cholesterol and lipids, (2) cessation of smoking, (3) drugs to reduce plasma cholesterol, (4) control of blood pressure, and (5) control of diabetes.

THERAPEUTIC OVERVIEW

ANTILIPID DRUGS

Goal: prevention of myocardial infarction and other atherosclerotic disorders such as stroke and peripheral vascular disease

Approach: prophylactic use to reduce formation of atherosclerotic plaque and subsequent narrowing of lumen in cardiac arteries

Primary risk factors:
- High blood cholesterol and certain lipids
- High blood pressure
- Smoking
- Overweight
- Sedentary life-style

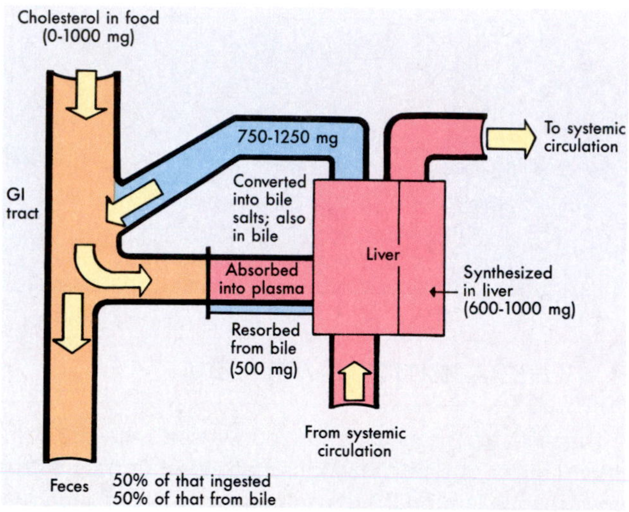

FIGURE 20-2 Total body balance of cholesterol, showing input by ingestion and liver synthesis, output by nonabsorption into feces, conversion into bile salts, delivery in bile salts to small intestine, partial reabsorption from bile, and delivery as lipoproteins into systemic circulation. Quantities shown are approximate daily amounts.

ered, there is a 2% lowering of the risk of coronary heart disease.

The metabolism of cholesterol and fatty acids and the associated lipid-transport particles (the lipoproteins) takes place in the gut, liver, and peripheral tissues. Drugs reduce cholesterol concentrations by altering the kinetics of one or more aspects of the metabolic cycle. Production and secretion of bile formed from cholesterol by liver cells is necessary for emulsification of dietary fat and cholesterol before absorption. Most secreted bile is reabsorbed during the digestive process and recycled with approximately one third lost in the stool. Interruption of this cycle by bile-acid binding resins such as cholestyramine, colestipol, and neomycin, results in reduced gastrointestinal absorption of cholesterol and dietary fats. Prevention of the reabsorption of bile acids secondarily causes hepatocyte synthesis of increased amounts of bile. Because cholesterol is a necessary precursor for bile formation, the increased cholesterol usage reduces the total body pool of cholesterol by promoting an increase in low-density lipoprotein receptors on the hepatocyte, which facilitates removal of that fraction of cholesterol binding to these receptors.

Therapeutic uses of lipid-lowering drugs are summarized in the box.

Cholesterol Balance

The dynamics of cholesterol ingestion, synthesis, metabolism, and elimination are summarized in Figure 20-2. Dietary intake can vary from 0 to 1000 mg/day, and usually between 30% and 75% of the total is absorbed. Normal endogenous synthesis varies between 600 and

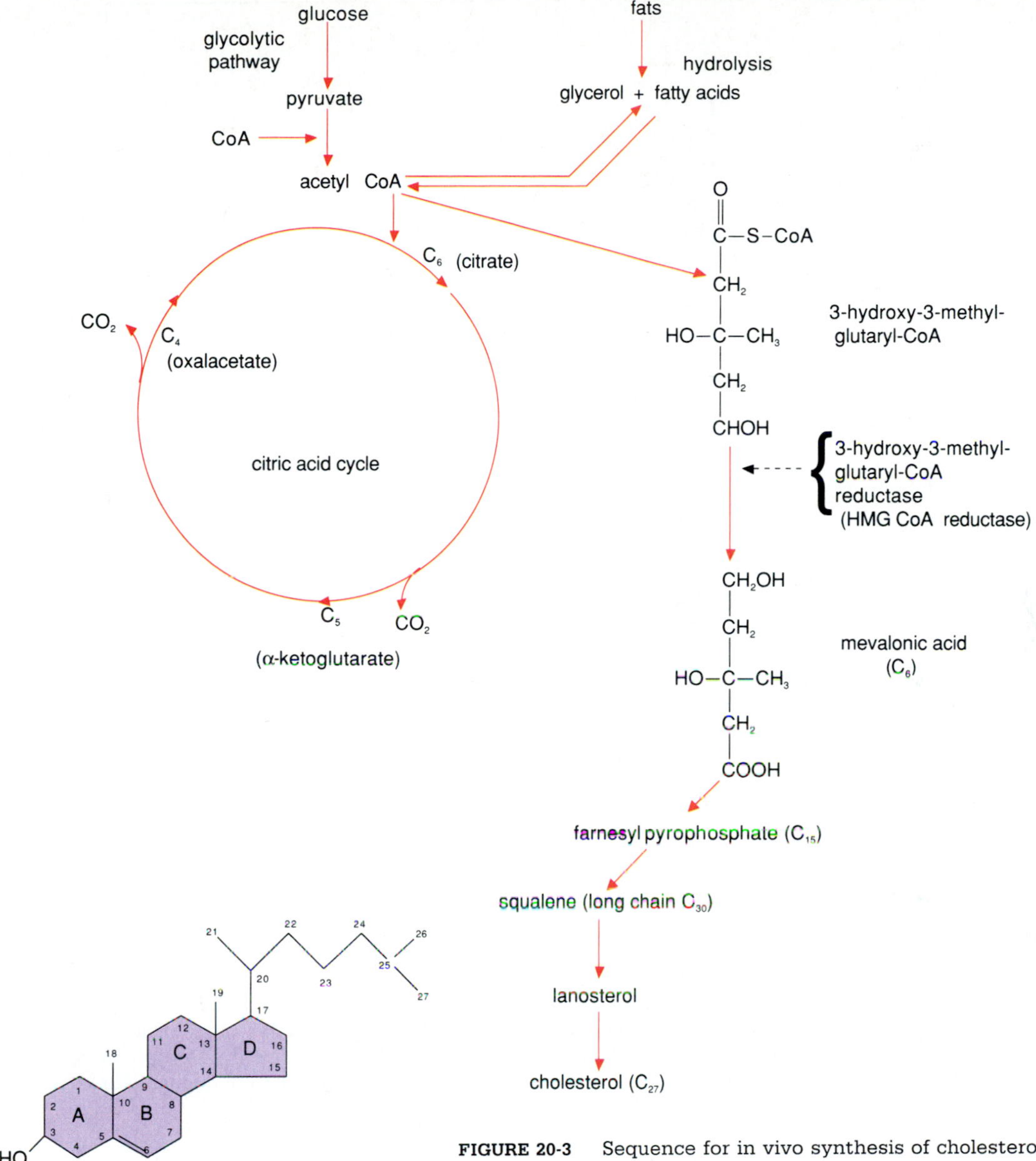

FIGURE 20-3 Sequence for in vivo synthesis of cholesterol.

1000 mg/day. Approximately 750 to 1250 mg is secreted in the bile daily. Of the total secreted in bile, approximately half is reabsorbed and the remainder is excreted in the stool. The total body pool of cholesterol is estimated to be in excess of 125 g, of which at least 90% is a part of cell membranes.

De novo synthesis of cholesterol is the major source of cholesterol. Although cholesterol can be synthesized in most body cells, cells most active in the synthesis of cholesterol are in the adrenal glands and the liver. Because liver mass is much greater, synthesis in the liver is critical to the total body burden of cholesterol. The synthesis of cholesterol originates with acetylcoenzyme A (acetyl CoA), a key intermediate for glycolysis, the citric acid cycle, and fatty acid degradation. In vivo synthesis of cholesterol from acetyl CoA involves a large number of steps and is summarized in Figure 20-3. The first, the irreversible conversion of HMG-CoA to mevalonic acid, is rate limiting. The rate of synthesis is influenced by several factors, including time of day, diet composition, fasting, excessive food intake, or obesity. Diets rich in saturated fats result in an increase in serum cholesterol, whereas substitution of either unsaturated fats or carbohydrates generally is accompanied by decreases in serum cholesterol.

In addition to effects of diet, a variety of cellular factors affect the rate of cholesterol synthesis. Cellular concentrations of cholesterol are in dynamic equilibrium

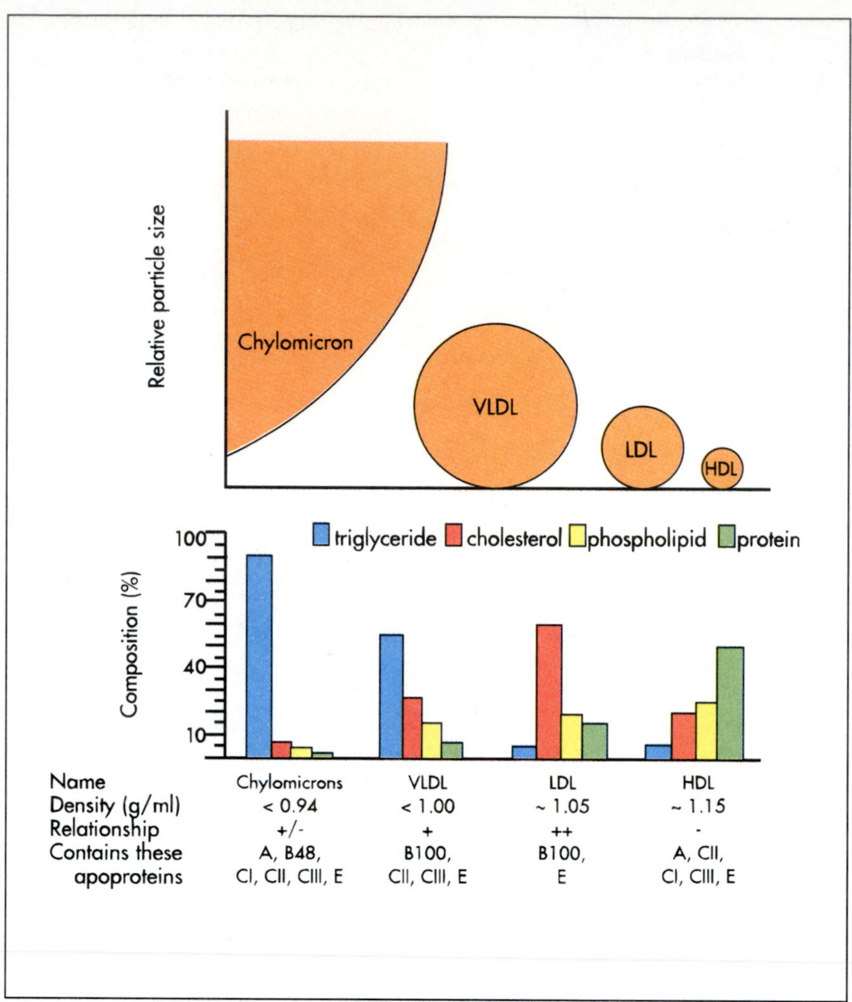

FIGURE 20-4 Summary of nomenclature, approximate composition, size, and relative atherogenic potential of lipoprotein particles, which serve as transport vehicles for cholesterol and triglycerides. *VLDL,* Very low-density lipoproteins; *LDL,* low-density proteins; *HDL,* high-density lipoproteins; +, definite relationship; −, no relationship (+ and − refer to relationship of concentration to atherogenic potential).

with the concentrations of certain lipoproteins (see below).

The liver is the primary organ for cholesterol uptake and degradation. Most cholesterol is converted to bile acids, which in turn are secreted into the intestine to emulsify ingested fats. The bile acids are then reabsorbed and recycled. The total bile pool mass is estimated at 2 to 3 g and is recycled about six times per day. Approximately 50% of the cholesterol secreted in the bile is reabsorbed as part of chylomicrons and the remainder is excreted in feces. Rapid recycling normally limits the need for high rates of synthesis of bile acids. Cholesterol is also secreted in bile as free cholesterol. Because cholesterol is fairly insoluble, large amounts of bile are required for solubilization. The enhanced synthesis and increased excretion of cholesterol in bile is a probable cause of cholesterol-containing gallstones in obesity. Similarly, the increased ratio of cholesterol to bile in patients on clofibrate therapy makes them more likely to develop gallbladder disease.

Transport of cholesterol and other lipids in plasma and other body fluids is accomplished by encasement of the lipid in protein coats to form lipoprotein particles. The nomenclature and characteristics of the lipoprotein particles are summarized in Figure 20-4. Larger lipoprotein particles undergo size reduction through the action of lipoprotein lipases. Delivery of smaller particles to specific cells for the use of cholesterol or triglycerides occurs through the binding of lipoprotein particle components to receptors on the cell walls.

The largest of the lipoprotein particles is the chylomicron, composed of approximately 85% to 95% triglyceride and 3% to 6% cholesterol (Figure 20-4). The shell is composed of phospholipid, cholesterol, and several apoproteins (A, B48, CI, CII, CIII, and E). The chylomicron is formed in the gut wall and ranges in size from 200 to 500 nm. Its principal role is transport of absorbed fats to adipose tissue. As the chylomicron leaves the gut, it acquires the apoprotein CII, the presence of which triggers the enzyme lipoprotein lipase in the capillary wall. Triglyceride is released from the chylomicron and cleaved into free fatty acids and glycerol. The chylomicron remnants, containing apoprotein A (Apo A), apoprotein B (Apo B), and apoprotein E (Apo E) but having lost Apo CII and Apo CIII, return to the venous blood and are eventually removed by specific receptors on hepatic cells. This route is the principal method of transport of dietary fat and is referred to as the exogenous pathway (Figure 20-5).

Endogenous transport of triglycerides is by very low-density lipoprotein (VLDL). Synthesized principally by the liver and to a lesser extent by the gut, these particles are approximately 1/100 of the volume (50 to 80 nm diameter) of chylomicrons. In contrast to chylomicrons, the source of triglyceride in the VLDL is from fatty acids synthesized by the liver or released by adipose tissue. In addition to cholesterol and phospholipid, the wall of VLDL particles contains apoproteins B 100, CII, CIII, and E. The internal composition is approximately 50% to 60% triglyceride and 20% to 30% cholesterol. The presence of the Apo CII in the VLDL particle again activates lipoprotein lipase; the presence of Apo E allows the VLDL fragments, after lipolysis, to be bound by the same hepatic receptors that bind chylomicron fragments.

As the VLDL particles are reduced by lipoprotein lipase cleavage, a substantial percentage of the particles are transformed to a size and density classified as intermediate-density lipoprotein (IDL) and are approximately 6% of the volume of the VLDL particle. IDL particles follow two routes. Significant amounts of IDL particles are bound to receptors on hepatocytes, which recognize Apo E; the remainder also lose Apo E as the particles lose further triglyceride. The contracted particles are known as low-density lipoprotein (LDL) and have a size approximately 2% of the VLDL particle or 1/5000 the volume of a chylomicron. LDL particles contain approximately 50% to 60% cholesterol, less than 10% triglyceride, and have one molecule of Apo B 100 on their surfaces.

Apo B 100 is recognized by the LDL receptors located in pits on the cell walls of hepatocytes and peripheral cells. When the LDL particle binds to the receptor, the LDL particle and the associated receptor are transported into the cytoplasm by receptor-mediated endocytosis. The LDL particle is then incorporated into lysosomes and separated from the receptor, which is recycled. The coating of the particle is removed, and the esterified cholesterol is hydrolyzed and released as free cholesterol.

The released cholesterol has the following three major effects on cholesterol metabolism:

1. The intracellular concentration of cholesterol affects the cellular content of HMG-CoA reductase. Thus, as cholesterol concentrations increase, the internal synthesis of cholesterol decreases.
2. Increasing concentrations of cholesterol stimulate the activation of the enzyme acyl CoA: cholesterol acyl transferase.
3. Increasing concentrations of cholesterol lower the transcription of LDL receptor onto messenger RNA, whereas decreasing concentrations increase transcription.

This third effect enables cells to adjust their cholesterol concentrations according to need. For example, dividing fibroblasts, which require new membranes, have up to 40,000 receptors per cell, whereas quiescent fibroblasts appear to have only one tenth as many. Decrease in the number of LDL receptors is the basis for familial hypercholesterolemia. The heterozygous form appears in about 1 in 500 individuals, whereas the homozygous form is rare (1 in 1,000,000). Actually various genetic defects impair the generation of LDL receptor, but the result is the same. Heterozygotes have serum cholesterol concentrations approximately two times normal and account for about 5% of those individuals who have heart attacks before 60 years of age. Homozygotes have cholesterol concentrations six times normal, and they may show evidence of coronary artery disease at a very early age. Many homozygotes die before 10 to 12 years of age, and almost all experience a myocardial infarction by 20 years of age. The elevated blood cholesterol concentrations can be directly related to a reduction in the number of LDL receptors. Roughly 25% of the cholesterol is removed by the scavenger pathway.

The remaining type of lipoprotein particle is the high-density lipoprotein (HDL). This particle is relatively small, approximately 8 nm in diameter and has a volume of approximately 0.12% of the VLDL particle. HDL contains Apo A and Apo CII; however, smaller amounts of Apo CI, Apo CIII, and Apo E are also present. It is formed from nascent HDL synthesized in the liver or as a "spin-off" fragment during the lipolysis of chylomicrons or VLDL fragments (Figure 20-5). HDL is the major vehicle for the transport of cholesterol from the peripheral tissues to the liver for use or excretion.

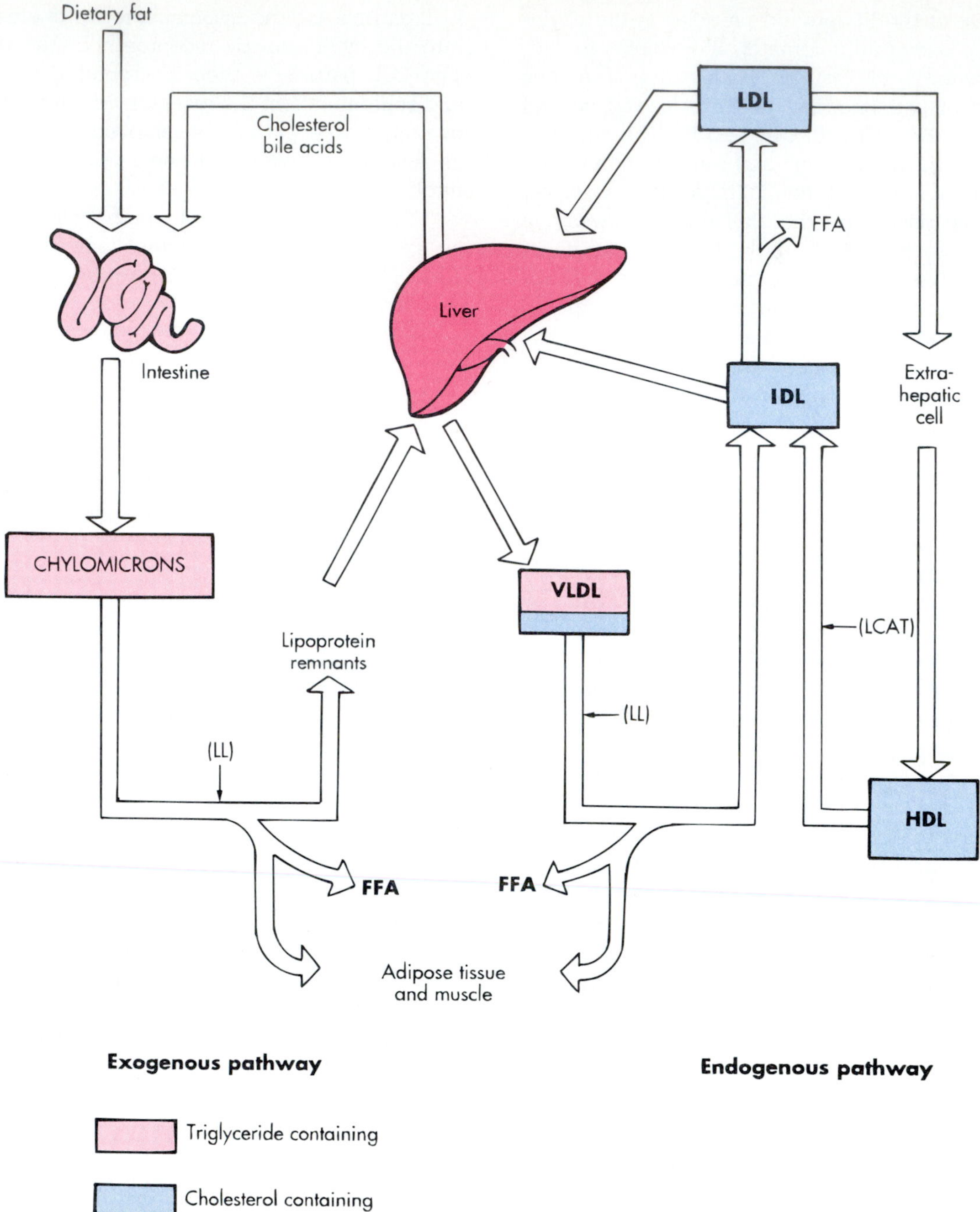

FIGURE 20-5 Lipoprotein-transport system. *Exogenous pathway:* Fats are incorporated into chylomicrons in the intestine and enter the circulation through the lymphatics. As the chylomicron leaves the intestine, it acquires apoprotein CII, triggering lipoprotein lipase *(LL)* in the capillary. Triglyceride is released and cleaved into free fatty acid *(FFA)* and glycerol. Chylomicron remnants are removed by the liver, where the cholesterol lipoproteins are used for other processes. Cholesterol bile acids promote the emulsification and the intestinal absorption of fats. *Endogenous pathway:* Transport of triglycerides, and some cholesterol, is by very low-density lipoprotein (VLDL) synthesized in liver. FFA from VLDL is deposited in adipose tissue and muscle after lipolysis by lipoprotein lipase. The resultant intermediate-density lipoprotein (IDL) takes two routes. Most is taken up by hepatocytes; the remainder loses more triglyceride and also apoprotein E and becomes contracted as low-density lipoprotein (LDL), the major transport lipoprotein for cholesterol. Low-density lipoprotein enters hepatic and extrahepatic cells by receptor-mediated exocytosis and is incorporated into lysosomes. The coating of the particle is removed, and the esterified cholesterol is hydrolyzed and released as free cholesterol. Cholesterol is taken up and transported as high-density lipoprotein (HDL), which is then converted to IDL by lecithin-cholesterol acyltransferase, and returned to the liver. *FFA,* free fatty acid; *HDL,* high density lipoprotein; *IDL,* intermediate density lipoprotein; *LCAT,* lecithin cholesterol acyl transferase; *LDL,* low density lipoprotein; *LL,* lipoprotein lipase, *TG,* triglyceride; *VLDL,* very low density lipoprotein. (Modified from Brown MS, Goldstein JL, in Harrison's Principles of Internal Medicine, 12th Ed, New York McGraw Hill, 1991.)

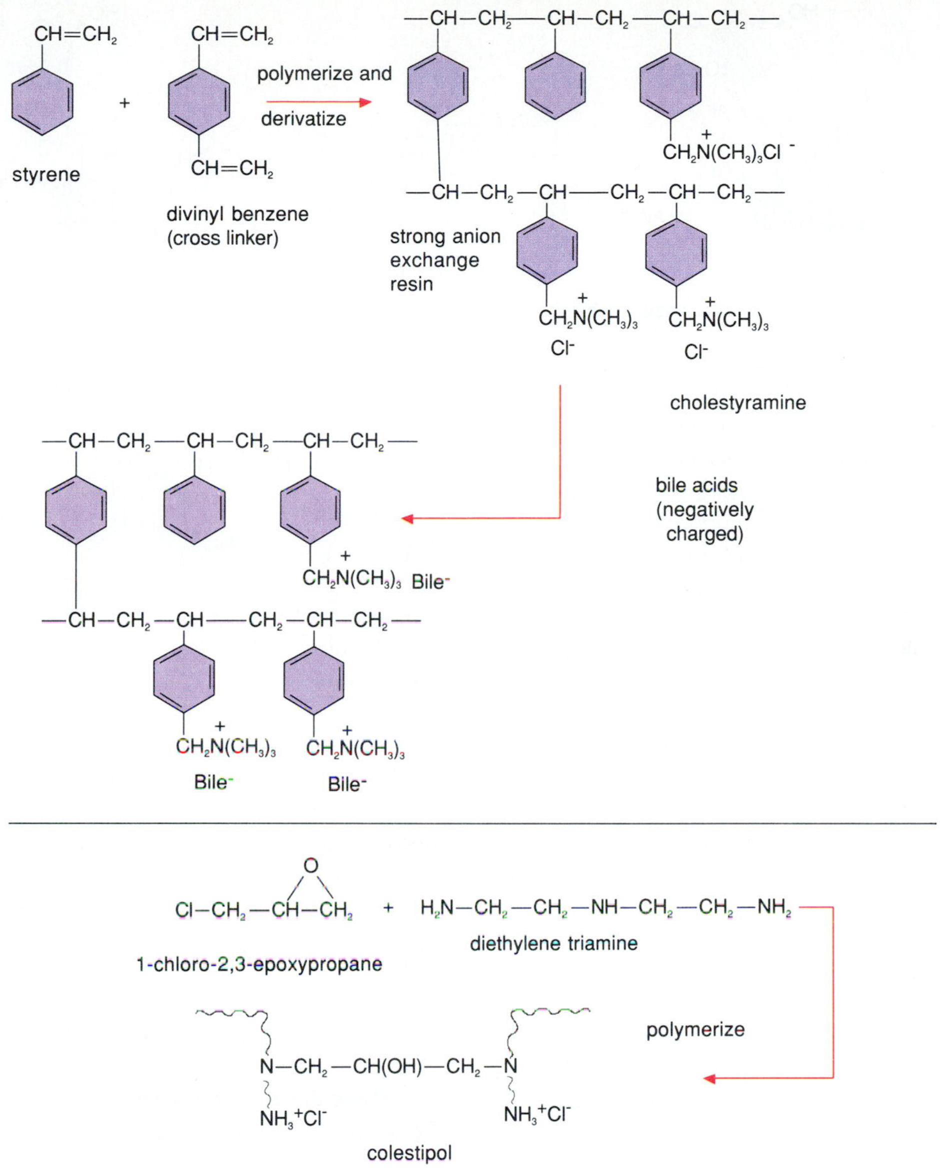

CH=CH2 styrene + CH=CH2 CH=CH2 divinyl benzene (cross linker) polymerize and derivatize strong anion exchange resin cholestyramine bile acids (negatively charged) 1-chloro-2,3-epoxypropane + diethylene triamine polymerize colestipol

FIGURE 20-6 Anion-exchange resins for ingestion to remove bile acids. Resins act by exchanging Cl^- for negatively charged bile salt anion and passing out the gut with the stool.

MECHANISMS OF ACTION

Bile Acid Sequestrants If the predominant source of excess cholesterol is dietary, alteration of the digestion and absorption of cholesterol-rich fatty foods is an approach to decreasing cholesterol concentrations and lipoprotein metabolism. As previously noted, bile acids and cholesterol are secreted into the gastrointestinal tract, and bile acids play a critical role in emulsification of ingested fats.

Cholestyramine and *colestipol* are the two bile acid ion-exchange resins approved for use in the treatment of hypercholesteremia. Cholestyramine is a large copolymer of styrene and divinyl benzene, with fixed cationic sites provided by trimethylbenzylammonium groups. It is administered as the chloride salt, with the anion exchange of bile acids for chloride occurring in the gut (Figure 20-6). Colestipol is also a copolymer formed from dimethylenetriamine and chlorepoxypropane, with fixed cation sites available for exchange of chloride and ionized bile acids. Both resins are insoluble and are administered as suspensions that are indigestible and pass unchanged in the stool, bound to bile acids. As previously noted, the usual bile acid pool is 2 to 3 g but is recycled up to six times per day. When bile acids are

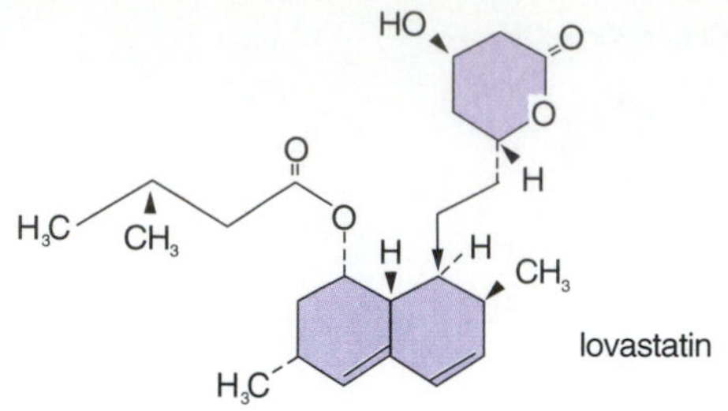

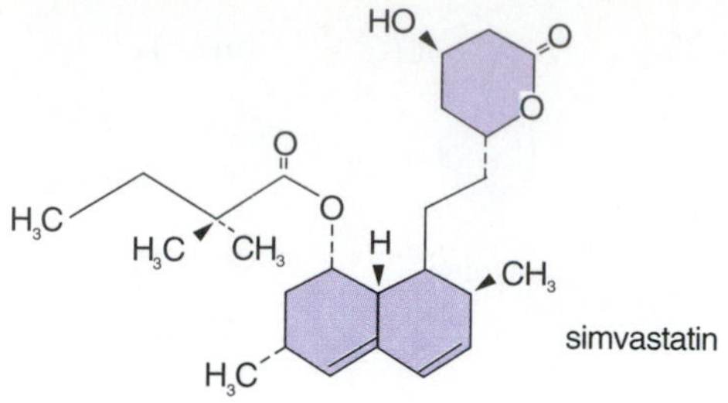

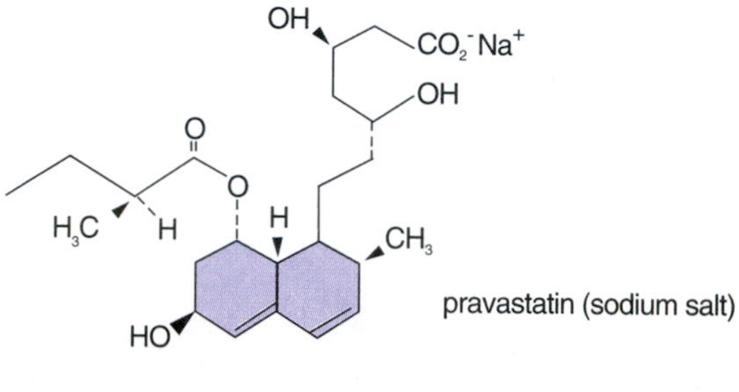

FIGURE 20-7 Structures of HMG-CoA reductase inhibitors.

removed from the enterohepatic recirculation, the liver synthesis of bile acids is increased. The resultant increase in cholesterol synthesis by hepatic cells also results in an increase in LDL receptors and greater hepatic uptake of LDL. Circulating concentrations of LDL are reduced by 20% to 35% with maximum doses of bile acid sequestrants; at the same time VLDL and plasma triglyceride concentrations may increase as much as 20%. Usually this latter effect disappears within 2 to 3 months, but changes are not predictable. In some subjects in whom triglyceride elevation is a major finding, resins are contraindicated. There is no consistent effect on HDL concentrations with resin administration; however, they often rise slightly.

Inhibitors of Cholesterol Synthesis A series of related compounds, *lovastatin, pravastatin,* and *simvastatin,* inhibit the enzyme HMG-CoA reductase, the initial rate-limiting step in cholesterol synthesis (see Figure 20-3). The inhibition of cholesterol synthesis, particularly in the hepatocyte, results in an increased need for exogenous (extracellular) cholesterol. This need is met by an increased uptake of LDL particles, which are rich in cholesterol. As increased catabolism of LDL cholesterol occurs, plasma concentrations of LDL decrease, and less LDL is available to react with cellular elements in the blood and blood vessel walls.

The structures of lovastatin, pravastatin, and simvastatin are shown in Figure 20-7. Although pravastatin is administered as the sodium salt, the other agents are prodrugs that are administered as inactive tricyclic lactone derivatives and are rapidly converted to an active form in the liver. They act as competitive inhibitors for the active site on the reductase enzyme, with a much higher affinity than HMG-CoA.

These agents are more effective than all other drugs (except niacin) in lowering total cholesterol and LDL cholesterol, VLDL cholesterol, apolipoprotein B, and triglycerides. They are effective in most patients with hypercholesteremia, except those who are homozygous for LDL-receptor absence.

The HMG-CoA inhibitors varies in LDL-receptor affinity. Pravastatin has 1500, lovastatin 6250, and simvastatin 13,000 times the affinity for the receptor compared with the natural substrate, HMG-CoA. Because all have at least 1000 times the affinity of the natural substrate, these differences probably do not affect the relative drug efficacies.

The effects of these drugs are seen within days. In addition to lowering both total cholesterol and LDL-cholesterol, HDL-cholesterol generally increases. The effect on triglycerides and Apo B varies.

Pravastatin is more hydrophilic than the other two agents, but all are rapidly taken up by the liver, which is the principal site of action.

Table 20-1 compares reported effects of 20 mg/day doses of the three currently available HMG-CoA reductase inhibitors.

Fibric Acid Derivatives Phenoxyisobutyric acid, or fibric acid, is the parent compound for several drugs that lower plasma cholesterol and triglyceride concentrations. Clofibrate and gemfibrozil are two currently available drugs of this class (Structures are shown in Figure 20-8.) These drugs have multiple sites of action. Clofibrate and, to a lesser degree, gemfibrozil increase the amount of cholesterol secreted into bile and thereby increase the amount of bile lost in the feces. Lipoprotein lipase activity is also increased, accelerating the peripheral mobilization of fats and thereby facilitating their return to the liver. These agents alter the rate of synthesis of several apoprotein components that form the receptor recognition site on the surface of lipoprotein particles, thus facilitating the uptake of these particles by the liver.

Clofibrate, the original fibric acid derivative for the treatment of dysbetalipoproteinemias, was first tested in 1962. Early metabolic balance studies indicated a significant increase of neutral sterols but a decrease in acid

Table 20-1 Estimated Cholesterol Reductions After Therapy

	Lovastatin (20 mg after 12 weeks)	Simvastatin (20 mg after 8 weeks)	Pravastatin (20 mg after 8 weeks)
Total cholesterol	−27%	−25%	−24%
LDL-cholesterol	−32%	−33%	−32%
HDL-cholesterol	+9%	+11%	+2%
Triglycerides	−21%	−19%	−11%

With cessation of therapy, *lipids* return to pretreatment concentrations within 4 weeks. The effects can be enhanced by combination with a resin and dietary restriction.

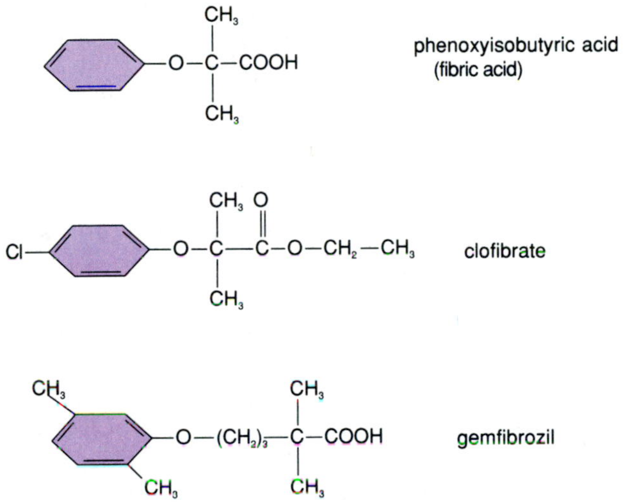

phenoxyisobutyric acid (fibric acid)

clofibrate

gemfibrozil

FIGURE 20-8 Fibric acid–based compounds that lower plasma cholesterol and triglycerides.

sterols in the feces of patients on clofibrate. These findings indicate a probable increased fecal excretion of cholesterol and a decline in bile acid excretion. This hypothesis is confirmed by the increased cholesterol in bile.

Recent work demonstrates that clofibrate uniformly increases extrahepatic lipoprotein lipase activity but not hepatic lipase activity. Thus the triglyceride-lowering effect of clofibrate may be caused by increased efficiency of removal of VLDL, as well as by reduced VLDL secretion by the liver.

Clofibrate has been used in several clinical trials in which long-term changes in cholesterol and triglycerides were noted. Significant side effects, including an increase in cholelithiasis (gallstones), cardiac arrhythmias, and a possible increase in malignancies in subjects actively receiving drug compared to placebo, have caused the drug to fall from favor.

Gemfibrozil is a newer fibric acid derivative. Although the full range of activity and its underlying mechanism of action are not known, gemfibrozil causes (1) alteration of the rates of synthesis of apoproteins CII and CIII, with increases in CII compared with CIII resulting in activation of extrahepatic lipoprotein lipase and (2) increased rate of synthesis of Apo AI and AII and thus increased formation of HDL particles. However, these effects do not explain the increased cholesterol content in the bile and the decreased reabsorption of cholesterol from the small intestine.

In several clinical trials, gemfibrozil lowered serum concentrations of triglycerides and cholesterol. It is currently approved for treatment of persons with very high concentrations of serum triglycerides (>750 mg/dl). Such concentrations pose a risk not only for atherogenesis but more frequently in the occurrence of episodes of abdominal pain and pancreatitis. In a recent Finnish study, 4081 asymptomatic men (40 to 55 years of age) with primary dyslipidemia (non-HDL cholesterol greater than 200 mg/dl and triglyceride concentrations up to 700 mg/dl) received 600 mg of gemfibrozil or placebos. The group (2051) who received gemfibrozil showed a 10% increase in HDL, a decline of non-HDL cholesterol by 14%, and a decline of triglycerides by 43% in the first 2 years of the study. In the final 3 years of the study, there was a 2% decline in HDL and a slight increase in triglycerides (12%) and in non-HDL cholesterol (0.4%). The dropout rate of subjects was 29.9%. The total number of cardiovascular problems in the gemfibrozil group was 56 (27.3/1000) compared with 84 in the placebo group (41.4/1000). This overall reduction difference of 34% is statistically significant. It should be noted that although there was a significant decrease in both mortality and morbidity with respect to cardiovascular events in the treated group the rate of death from carcinoma was the same in the two groups. The all-cause mortality in the two groups also remained the same. Similar discrepancies in mortality change have been reported in other trials of lipid-lowering agents as well. Based on several cholesterol-lowering trials, a metanalysis (a cumulative analysis of several trials) showed increases in violent deaths in subjects receiving active drugs. No basis for this finding has been suggested.

Other fibric acid derivatives such as finofibrate and bezafibrate are currently under investigation. Although

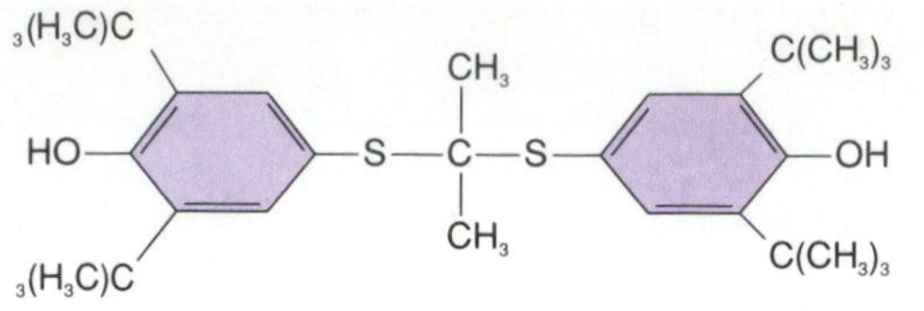

FIGURE 20-9 Probucol.

their overall mechanisms of action appear similar, there are some differences in their effect on various lipoprotein fractions.

Probucol Probucol is a unique antilipidemic compound unrelated in structure to any other lipid-lowering drug (Figure 20-9). Its effect on atherosclerotic lesions and decreases in peripheral accumulations of cholesterol are independent of changes in total serum cholesterol concentrations. Based on animal and clinical studies, two mechanisms of action are suggested. Enhanced synthesis of Apo E messenger RNA in peripheral tissues by probucol appears to play a significant role. Apo E seems to be critical for the peripheral mobilization of cholesterol, its movement to the liver, increased catabolism in the liver, and increased elimination in bile. More recent work indicates that probucol may be incorporated in LDL particles, where it functions as an antioxidant. Its presence inhibits formation of pathogenic cholesterol esters and the conversion of tissue macrophages to foam cells when they incorporate LDL particles. In most studies, probucol lowers plasma cholesterol by 10% to 25%.

Nicotinic Acid Nicotinic acid, or niacin, was found in the mid-1950s to lower triglycerides and serum cholesterol. It was successfully used as one treatment arm of coronary drug trials to reduce the rate of myocardial reinfarction.

Hepatic uptake of released free fatty acids and also the synthesis of VLDL are reduced by nicotinic acid. In addition, the clearance of chylomicrons and VLDL from the plasma is enhanced. The mechanism for these phenomena in humans is not clear. In rats, lipoprotein lipase activity is increased, but such increases in activity have not been demonstrated in humans. The increased catabolism of VLDL results in a decrease in LDL and an increase in the HDL particles containing Apo A. Central to the action of niacin is its inhibition of the release of free fatty acids from tissue fat stores. The effect of niacin on cholesterol lowering can be enhanced by coadministration of it with resins. A full dose of niacin reduces LDL concentrations by 10% to 15%; when taken in combination with resins, however, a 60% to 70% reduction is often reported. Side effects, including intense flushing and pruritus, limit the acceptance and usefulness of this drug as a cholesterol-lowering agent.

Other Agents *Neomycin* and *sitosterol* have been used to lower plasma cholesterol by effects on the gastrointestinal tract. Neomycin, a poorly absorbed aminoglycoside antibiotic, lowers plasma cholesterol by an average of 22% in clinical studies. The mechanism is unclear. Binding of exogenous and bile-secreted cholesterol; precipitation of fatty acids, cholesterol, and bile acids; and alteration of gastrointestinal bacterial flora all are proposed as possible mechanisms of action.

It is claimed that side effects of administered 0.5 to 1.0 g doses of neomycin per day dissipate within several weeks of therapy. However, 14% of patients discontinue neomycin because of troublesome diarrhea. Larger doses of neomycin (>20 g/day) are associated with steatorrhea, deafness, and impairment of renal function. Pretreatment auditory testing and use only in patients without compromised renal function is indicated.

Because doses of neomycin greater than 1.0 g/day have been associated with interference with digoxin absorption, it is necessary to monitor plasma concentrations of digoxin when it is taken concurrently with neomycin.

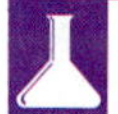

PHARMACOKINETICS

HMG-CoA Reductase Inhibitors

Lovastatin and simvastatin are both β-lactones that are readily hydrolyzed to the corresponding β-hydroxyacids. The three HMG-CoA reductase inhibitors differ in their bioavailability and in the effect of food on their absorption. Lovastatin absorption is enhanced by food, pravastatin absorption is reduced by food, and simvastatin absorption is unaffected. All three are subject to high extraction (approximately 60%) by the liver on the first circulation.

When radioactive-labeled doses of these drugs were administered to humans, between 10% and 20% of the label appears in the urine and 60% to 83% appears in the feces, which at least in part represents unabsorbed drug. Pravastatin has a half-life of 77 hours, compared with half-lives of less than 24 hours for the other agents. Efficacy in lowering LDL is marginally improved with a single evening dose of either of these agents when compared with the same total dose, taken as two doses daily.

Other Agents

Both clofibrate and gemfibrizol (fibric acid derivates) show nearly complete absorption. Gemfibrizol is the active form, whereas clofibrate is a prodrug that is rapidly

Table 20-2 Pharmacokinetic Parameters

lovastatin	Administered orally as prodrug. Peak plasma concentrations occur within 2 hours of dose and decline to 10% by 24 hours. 95% bound to plasma proteins. High first-pass extraction by liver; 85% of administered dose (including metabolites) in feces. Administration with food enhances bioavailability.
pravastatin	Administered orally as active drug, rapidly absorbed (34%) Food reduces bioavailability but not effect Excretion: 70% feces, 20% urine Major degradation product: 3α-hydroxy isomer, which has some activity 50% bound to plasma proteins First-pass extraction by liver very high
simvastatin	Administered orally as prodrug, 85% absorbed Peak plasma concentrations are seen at about 2 hours after dose. Plasma concentration decline to 10% of peak within 12 hours. 95% bound to plasma proteins. First-pass extraction by the liver very high.
gemfibrozil	Administered orally Disposition: 90% metabolized, $t_{1/2}$ 1.5 hr
probucol	Administered orally, 10% absorbed, remains in fatty tissue for months
cholestyramine	Administered orally, not absorbed
colestipol	Administered orally, not absorbed
niacin	Administered orally Disposition: metabolized
neomycin	See Chapter 47

hydrolyzed to its active form, chlorophenoxyisobutyric acid. Both are excreted in the urine, primarily as glucuronides. Although the plasma half-life of clofibrate is about 15 hours, that of gemfibrizol is less than 2 hours.

Because probucol is hydrophobic, only about 10% of the administered dose is absorbed, and significant amounts of the drug persist in fatty tissues after cessation of therapy. Absorption can be enhanced by administration of the drug with meals. The average total decline in concentration of serum cholesterol with probucol is 10% to 25%. However, the full magnitude of decline in blood lipid concentrations is not seen immediately, with about 60% of the decline seen within 6 weeks. A maximum effect may take from 6 to 12 months.

The half-life of niacin in plasma is approximately 1 hour. It is rapidly converted to nicotinamide, which has no effect on lipid metabolism. When given by mouth, peak concentrations are achieved within 1 hour.

Pharmacokinetic parameters are summarized in Table 20-2.

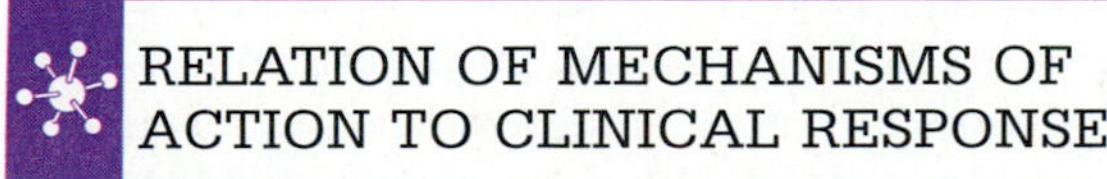

RELATION OF MECHANISMS OF ACTION TO CLINICAL RESPONSE

Pathophysiology of Lipid Metabolism and Development of Atherosclerosis

To rationally use drugs that potentially alter the development and course of atherosclerosis, an understanding of the current concepts of atherogenesis is necessary. Current theory states that atheromatous plaques develop in arteries as a "response to injury." The exact nature of the injury may be obscure, but certain areas in arteries, such as branching sites, which are subject to turbulent rather than laminar flow appear more susceptible to plaque development than other sites. Factors contributing to the development of atherosclerotic lesions include elevated blood pressure, elevated cholesterol concentrations, elevated plasma transport lipid concentrations, and cigarette smoking. The discussion that follows focuses on cholesterol and the plasma lipids.

The "response-to-injury" hypothesis is a proposition that the initial event is a form of damage or disruption of the endothelial lining of arteries. High concentrations of plasma lipid, particularly LDL cholesterol, are considered to be deleterious to the vascular endothelium, but other factors such as oxidation of LDL particles and formation of antibodies also may be involved. Fatty streaks are the initial manifestation of intimal injury. They can often be seen at autopsy in the arteries of children and young adults who have died suddenly. With time, the fatty streak progresses and is converted to a fibrous plaque. The fibrous plaque consists of a fibrous matrix of intimal smooth muscle cells surrounded by large amounts of both intracellular and extracellular lipids. Coronary and other vascular disease occurs when the plaque becomes large enough to compromise the flow of blood through the vessel. Plaque formation is illustrated in Figure 20-10.

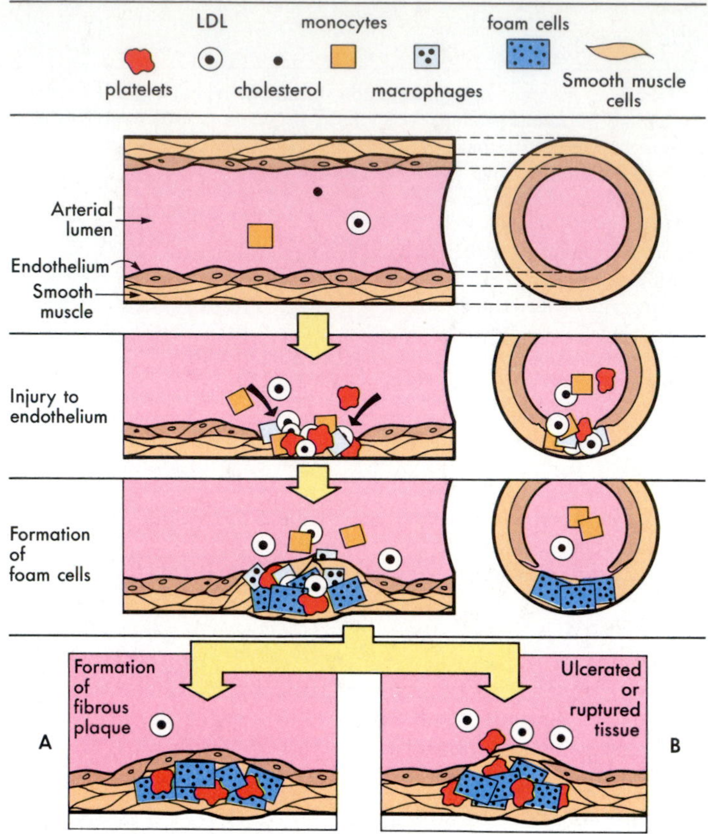

FIGURE 20-10 Development of an atheromatous plaque. An injury to the endothelial lining allows LDL particles, monocytes, and platelets to enter the smooth muscle tissue. Inflammation at the injury site triggers the conversion of monocytes to macrophages, which scavenge the LDL particles and cholesterol to form enlarged foam cells (xanthoma cells). Smooth muscle cells, foam cells, platelets, and LDL particles form fibrous plaques. The plaques form in two way: **A,** at the interface between the endothelium and the smooth muscle tissue, leaving an elevation in the repaired endothelium, or **B,** as an ulcerated, or ruptured lesion in the endothelium that protrudes into the lumen. Both types of plaque result in narrowing of the lumen and restricted blood flow.

In monkeys, pigs, dogs, rabbits, and pigeons fed a lipid-rich diet, lesions similar to those seen in humans are observed. Because it is not possible to determine the progression of atherosclerotic lesions in humans accurately, most of our current knowledge of plaque formation is based on animal models.

In monkeys fed a high-fat, high-cholesterol diet, the following sequence occurs:

1. After 2 weeks, clusters of leukocytes (principally monocytes) can be seen attached to the arterial endothelium or lining cells of arteries, especially at or near branching points of vessels.
2. On tissue cross section, an inward migration of monocytes from the lumen to the smooth muscle layers is observed.
3. Large amounts of lipid accumulate, and the monocytes take on the appearance of foam cells.
4. Over the following weeks to months, there is continuing attachment of monocytes and continued migration into the vessel wall.
5. The fatty streak enlarges as a result of continued inward migration and accumulation of smooth muscle cells, which migrate and grow from their origin in the muscularis layer of the vessel (see Figure 20-10).

As this heterogeneous group of cells of various origins increases in number, the previously intact junctions between endothelial lining cells begin to separate and retract. As a result, the early plaque is exposed to the circulating blood and its contents. These exposed cells represent a disruption of normal vessel endothelium and thus provide an opportunity for platelet adherence, aggregation, and development of mural thrombi. Increased lipid concentrations also enhance platelet adhesiveness.

In animals, it is established that the rate of formation and growth of atherosclerotic lesions depends on the rate of increase of the cholesterol concentration in plasma, the total circulating cholesterol concentration, and the duration of that elevation. The invasion of smooth muscle cells and their conversion into other cell types appear to be key steps that determine the rate of growth and extent of the fatty streak and subsequently the development of the fibrous plaque. Thus, the intensity of the smooth muscle cell response ultimately determines whether clinical sequelae develop. These cells form the fibrous matrix of the plaque and also assume the appearance of foam cells with an intracellular collection of cholesterol and lipid.

The smooth muscle response is determined by several factors. It is known that smooth muscle cells respond to chemotactic and mitogenic factors (i.e., stimuli to move and reproduce). The vascular endothelium and circulating platelets are the sources of these factors. The role of platelet aggregation and release of the granular contents of platelets as a major component of the response to endothelial injury is recognized, and modifiers of platelet response, such as aspirin, play a significant role in the treatment of atherosclerotic disease.

When the endothelium is intact, it prevents adherence of platelets to the vessel by the formation and release of antithrombogenic substances such as heparin and prostacyclin. Disruption of endothelial continuity or endothelial injury alters the formation and release of these substances, and in their absence the attachment of platelets with resultant aggregation or clumping may occur. Among materials released when platelets clump are epidermal growth factor and platelet-derived growth factor. The latter may be most critical in plaque formation because it is mitogenic and chemotactic to smooth muscle cells, thus causing their replication and luminal migration.

The third significant cell type that contributes to development of the atherosclerotic plaque is the circulating monocyte. These cells are the source of histiocytes and macrophages in tissue. Indeed, subendothelial migration of monocytes is the initial step in fatty streak formation. Monocytes and their transformation product, macrophages, have multiple receptors on their cellular surfaces. Most important, they have receptors for LDL that are rich in cholesterol. Macrophages accumulate LDL and cholesterol. They also secrete superoxide anions, lysosomal hydroxylases, and fibroblast growth factors and esterify cholesterol.

Although the cellular factors critical to development of the atherosclerotic plaque are present in animals and in humans, development of fatty streaks and atheromatous plaques is not a universal finding. Unknown factors apparently determine whether some animals and humans develop atherosclerosis, whereas others do not.

Chronically elevated concentrations of plasma lipoprotein, particularly LDL and VLDL, have long been associated with an increased incidence of atherosclerosis. Atherosclerosis can be induced in experimental animals by elevation of concentrations of these lipoproteins. Normally the incorporation of these lipoproteins into cells is controlled by the number of cellular receptors. At higher lipoprotein concentrations, other modes of entrance of lipids into the cell occur. Receptor number is controlled by the need of the cell for cholesterol and also by certain genetic factors. The critical mechanisms that link excess LDL and VLDL cholesterol and the development of atherosclerosis are not well established, but various contributory factors are recognized. First, it appears that alterations in the ratio of cholesterol to phospholipid in the cell membrane will alter membrane viscosity. Thus, endothelial malleability may be distorted, particularly at sites of intravascular stress or turbulence. If true, this is a partial explanation for the early attachment of lymphocytes and platelets at these sites, as well as a cause for retraction of the endothelium over fatty streaks. Second, the presence of excess lipoprotein in macrophages may result in oxidation products that are toxic to the endothelium. Furthermore, the recruitment of antibodies may be another factor. In summary, although atherosclerosis is described as a "response to injury," the exact nature of the injury, or in fact if any injury is necessary, is still debatable.

The strongest positive correlations between lipoproteins and atherosclerosis exist for LDL. Impressive evidence derives from studies from lipid research clinics that have completed an integrated series of epidemiological community-based studies, as well as primary prevention trials. When total and LDL cholesterol concentrations are compared, there is a consistent increase in both concentrations during adulthood. Total cholesterol and LDL concentrations gradually increase in women until 70 years of age. In men, concentrations increase until 50 years, with a subsequent plateau until 70 and then a modest decline. The pattern, however, is not one of a simple constant increase; thus ratios between various fractions continuously change. Because HDL and LDL cholesterol concentrations are independent of each other, information derived from the measurement of each has additive value in the prediction of future coronary heart disease. Strong quantitative clinical data provide a relationship between serum cholesterol and coronary heart disease mortality, shown in Figure 20-11. These studies also demonstrate that the major determinants of lipoprotein concentrations are dietary and genetic factors. The major factors affecting lipoprotein concentrations are shown in the box.

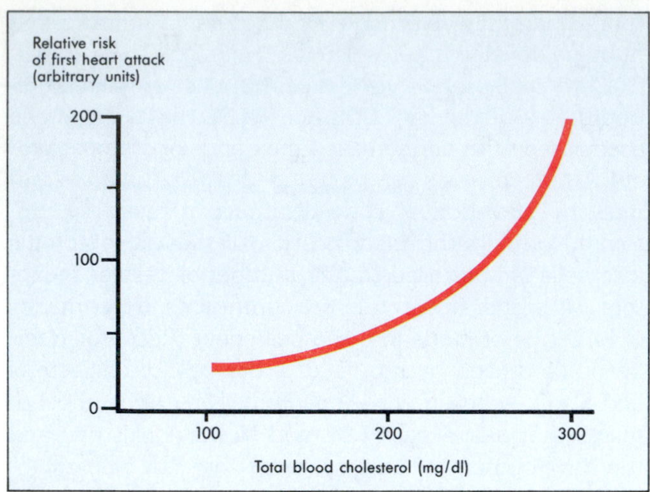

FIGURE 20-11 Summary of relationship between blood cholesterol concentrations and relative risk of initial heart attack.

In contrast to a positive correlation between LDL concentrations and the development of atherosclerotic disease, epidemiological studies demonstrate an inverse relationship between HDL concentrations and the risk of atherosclerotic disease. However, although several studies show that lowering LDL concentrations reduces the incidence of atherosclerotic disease, it has not been demonstrated that elevation of HDL concentrations alone will reduce the risk of cardiovascular disease. Many of the dietary changes, such as reducing the total fat in the diet, consuming a greater percentage of polyunsaturated fats, and increasing the fraction of total calories obtained from carbohydrates, all recommended to reduce LDL concentrations, will enhance HDL turnover.

Drug and Dietary Interventions

Some drugs that increase HDL concentrations have adverse effects that preclude their use. Estrogens increase HDL concentrations, but when they are used in men after a first myocardial infarction, there is an increased incidence of recurrent infarction. Drugs such as barbiturates induce hepatic microsomal enzyme activity and also enhance HDL concentrations, but their central nervous system actions preclude their usefulness in treating this disease.

The administration of probucol, which apparently enhances reverse cholesterol transport, results in decreased concentrations of HDL cholesterol. Use of nicotinic acid and fibric acid derivatives results in increased HDL concentrations. Cholestyramine and colestipol appear to have little or no effect on HDL cholesterol concentrations. The HMG-CoA reductase inhibitors seem to have a variable effect, but increases between 2% and 12% are frequently seen.

There are several forms of HDL, and the confusion generated by these divergent findings may be related to the type of HDL present and the relative content of various apoproteins. As knowledge of lipoprotein transport and metabolism increases, it is clear that many of the apparent defects in the system, as well as the mechanism of action of several of the drugs mentioned, depend on the rate of synthesis and catabolism of several apoproteins. Measurement of various apoprotein concentrations may ultimately be superior in allowing prediction of atherosclerotic disease and drug effects. Because techniques for measuring apoproteins are still too complex for routine use, the critical epidemiological studies have not been completed at this time.

The best treatment for atherosclerosis appears to be that directed at altering the major risk factors associated with its development. Lowering lipid concentrations should be accompanied by weight control, smoking cessation, and blood pressure control.

Because most individuals with elevated cholesterol concentrations acquired those increases as a result of diet, a basic recommendation for reduction of cholesterol is decreasing calories and lowering the proportion of the diet composed of saturated fat. Current recommendations of the American Heart Association and the National Heart, Lung, and Blood Institute are summarized in Table 20-3.

The effect of dietary intervention varies widely in the population. However, dietary intervention enhances the effectiveness of concurrent drug therapy. If diet alter-

FACTORS AFFECTING LIPOPROTEIN CONCENTRATIONS

- Dietary*
  - Total calories
  - Calories from fat
  - Cholesterol intake
- Anthropometric*
  - Weight-to-height ratio (obesity)
- Behavioral*
  - Smoking
  - Exercise
  - Alcohol intake
- Race
- Genetic
- Sex
  - Estrogen concentrations (endogenous and exogenous)*
- Other diseases, including diabetes*

*Modifiable factors.

Table 20-3 Summary of Dietary Recommendations

Phase	Typical American Diet	Phase I Modification of AHA	Phase II Modification of AHA
Fat (% calories)	40	30	25
Saturated fats (% calories)	17	10	7
Protein (% of calories)	15	15	15
Carbohydrates (% of calories)	45	55	60
Cholesterol (mg)	500	300	200
U/S (ratio of unsaturated to saturated)	1.5:1	2:1	2.5:1
CLASSIFICATION OF CHOLESTEROL CONCENTRATIONS			
Total blood cholesterol:	<200 mg/dl	Desirable	
	200-239 mg/dl	Borderline	
	≥240 mg/dl	High	
LDL cholesterol (blood):	<130 mg/dl	Desirable	
	130-159 mg/dl	Borderline	
	≥160 mg/dl	High risk	
HDL cholesterol (blood):	>35 mg/dl	Desirable	

ation is attempted first and fails to lower cholesterol to acceptable concentrations, various pharmacological interventions are available. The argument for dietary change as the initial step is based on the following four considerations:

1. It is the most physiologic approach.
2. The change should be lifelong.
3. No drugs are without known or potential side effects.
4. Drug therapy is relatively expensive, costing 1 to 2 dollars per day.

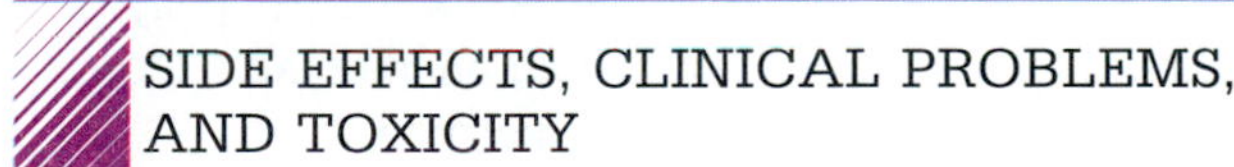

SIDE EFFECTS, CLINICAL PROBLEMS, AND TOXICITY

Clinical problems are summarized in the box.

Resin Therapy

Resin therapy is not without problems. Resins are insoluble, have the consistency of fine sand, and must be mixed with fluids to be ingested. They tend to cause GI bloating, excess flatus, and constipation with associated nausea and indigestion. A diet high in fluids and fiber is necessary to minimize these effects and prevent impaction.

Because of the exchange of chloride ion for bile acids, excess chloride absorption may result in a hyperchloremic metabolic acidosis. Transient rises in alkaline phosphatase and transaminase also have been reported.

Because of the binding of bile acids by resins and

CLINICAL PROBLEMS

HMG-COA REDUCTASE INHIBITORS

Increases serum transaminase; produces some increase in creatine phosphokinase and GI distress

RESINS

Lead to bloating and constipation; produce unwanted removal of chloride ions, dietary components, and drugs

PROBUCOL

Causes GI distress; prolongs Q-T interval

CLOFIBRATE

Produces cholelithiasis; possibly carries a carcinoma risk

GEMFIBROZIL

Possibly produces same problems as clofibrate; interacts with oral anticoagulants

NIACIN

May exacerbate cardiac dysrhythmias, gout, gallbladder disease, and liver disease; causes GI distress and intense flushing and pruritus

NEOMYCIN

Shows poor absorption, produces diarrhea, impairs renal function, interferes with digoxin absorption the loss of their emulsifying action, excess fat may appear in the stool. Although the potential for interfering with fat-soluble vitamins exists, experts disagree as to whether supplementation of fat-soluble vitamins is indicated. The binding properties of the resins may also interfere with the intestinal absorption of thiazide diuretics, phenobarbital, thyroxine, warfarin, and digitalis preparations that undergo enterohepatic circulation. It is advisable not to coadminister these resins with other therapeutic agents. A time differential of several hours is recommended. The use of resins in persons with elevated concentrations of cholesterol and particularly LDL lowers the risk of coronary heart disease.

HMG-CoA Reductase Inhibitors

Myalgias and transient elevations of creatine phosphokinase have been reported as side effects in patients on HMG-CoA reductase inhibitor therapy. In cardiac transplant patients receiving immunosuppressive drugs such as cyclosporin, 30% develop myositis within 1 year of initiating lovastatin administration. In a few of these patients, the myositis progressed to severe rhabdomyolysis and acute renal failure. Approximately 5% of patients taking gemfibrozil and immunosuppressives exhibit similar reactions. In early studies with gemfibrozil approximately 11% of patients had creatine phosphokinase concentrations that were twice normal, and in comparative trials, 9% of patients on cholestyramine and 2% of patients on probucol showed similar increases. It has been suggested that the creatine phosphokinase elevations may be related to exercise. Pronounced and persistent increases in serum transaminase occur in nearly 2% of adult patients who receive lovastatin for longer than 12 months, and such changes in transaminase concentrations are frequent reasons for drug cessation. Such enzyme increases usually appear between 3 and 12 months of therapy. With cessation of therapy, the elevated transaminase concentrations gradually return to normal. Patients on lovastatin should have their transaminase concentrations monitored at 3-month intervals for the first 15 months of therapy.

Discontinuation of drug is recommended in a patient who develops risk factors that may lead to renal failure secondary to rhabdomyolysis (i.e., severe infection, hypotension, major surgery, trauma, or uncontrolled seizures).

Up to 10% of patients have gastrointestinal symptoms, including diarrhea, constipation, dyspepsia, excess flatus, abdominal pain or cramps, and nausea. In double-blind trials, headache was twice as frequent in patients receiving lovastatin as in those given a placebo.

Because these drugs inhibit cholesterol synthesis, the potential exists for inhibition of the synthesis of adrenal and gonadal steroid hormones and bile acids. However, substantial evidence indicates that such inhibition does not occur. Other end products of mevalonic metabolism such as dolichol, required for glycoprotein synthesis, or ubiquinone, used for mitochondrial electron transport, do not appear to be significantly affected by cholesterol synthesis inhibitors. Because HMG-CoA reductase inhibitors reduce serum cholesterol by increasing receptor-mediated uptake of LDL, they are of little use in patients with homozygous familial hypercholesterolemia because such patients lack LDL receptors. Other than the adverse reactions described, there are few interactions of HMG-CoA reductase inhibitors with other drugs.

Fibric Acid Derivatives

Clofibrate use has diminished because of the increased incidence of cholelithiasis and a possible increased incidence of carcinoma. In a study by the World Health Organization, there was a significantly higher (36%) mortality from all causes in patients on clofibrate compared with those taking a placebo. In the Coronary Drug Project study, there was no difference in mortality between those taking a placebo and those taking clofibrate. These studies also suggested an increased incidence of thrombosis and the development of claudication in patients taking clofibrate. Studies of gemfibrozil in Finland failed to indicate the same associations.

Both agents enhance the anticoagulant effect of warfarin and associated compounds. Thus, doses of warfarin often must be reduced by as much as 50% when a fibric acid derivative is added to the patient's treatment. Other side effects with these drugs are principally gastrointestinal and consist of abdominal pain and, less frequently nausea, vomiting, and diarrhea.

Probucol

Side effects of probucol include dyspepsia, abdominal pain, nausea, vomiting, flatulence, and diarrhea. The last two are probably caused by increased bile flow. Prolongation of the Q-T interval on the electrocardiogram is seen in a significant number of patients. In monkeys fed atherogenic high-cholesterol diets and probucol, an increased incidence of sudden death was reported. In dogs given high doses of probucol, sensitization of the myocardium to epinephrine and resultant ventricular fibrillation are observed. These effects appear to be species specific and have not been reported in humans or in other animal species.

Drug interactions appear to be minimal. There is little advantage in using this agent in conjunction with clo-

TRADE NAMES

In addition to generic and fixed-combination preparations, the following trade-named materials are available in the United States.

Atromid-S, clofibrate
Colestid, colestipol
Lescol, fluvastatin
Lopid, gemfibrozil
Lorelco, probucol
Mevacor, lovastatin
Nicolar, niacin*
Pravachol, pravastatin
Questran, cholestyramine
Zocor, simvastatin

*Niacin preparations also are available as vitamin supplements. (See Chapter 48 for neomycin.)

fibrate because further lowering of serum cholesterol does not occur.

Niacin

Side effects are generally noted within 30 minutes of niacin ingestion. Intense flushing and pruritus of the trunk, face, and arms generally occurs. This probably is caused by prostaglandin E_1 release and can be partially inhibited by the ingestion of 325 mg of aspirin 60 minutes before niacin. In addition, there are gastrointestinal side effects, including vomiting, diarrhea, and dyspepsia. Elevations of transaminases as well as creatine phosphokinase concentrations are common. Serum uric acid increases, and there is an increased incidence of gouty arthritis in patients treated with niacin. Based on several studies there appears to be an increased incidence of cardiac arrhythmias, including but not limited to atrial fibrillation. These side effects limit the usefulness of niacin as a cholesterol-lowering drug.

NEW DIRECTIONS

Other new HMG-CoA reductase inhibitors can be expected to be introduced in the coming years. However, the major advances in the treatment of dyslipidemia will come with the demonstration that lowering of LDL cholesterol results in the lessening of cardiovascular risk. Elucidation of the role of free radicals as a cause of oxidation of cholesterol and the latter deposit in the vascular wall may offer new strategies for halting the progression of atherosclerotic lesions. Some preliminary studies have indicated that certain antihypertensive agents may also effect regression. With the advent of noninvasive imaging techniques, the ability to follow change in atherosclerotic lesions in patients under study is enhanced. The critical question at this time is determining whether cholesterol lowering truly improves life expectancy. Most trials reported up until the present have shown reduction in cardiovascular events but had no significant effect on overall mortality.

REFERENCES

Brown G, Albers JJ, Fisher LD, et al: Regression of coronary artery disease as a result of intensive lipid-lowering therapy in men with high levels of apolipoprotein B, *N Engl J Med* 323(19):1289-1298, 1990.

Brown MS, Goldstein JL: How LDL receptors influence cholesterol and atherosclerosis, *Sci Am* 251(5):58, Nov 1984.

Green MS, Heiss G, Rifkind MB, et al: The ratio of plasma high-density lipoprotein cholesterol: age-related changes and race and sex differences in selected North American populations, *Circulation* 72(1):93, 1985.

Grundy SM: HMG-CoA reductase inhibitors for treatment of hypercholesterolemia, *N Engl J Med* 319(1):24, 1988.

Johnson WJ, Bamberger MJ, Latta RA, et al: The bidirectional flux of cholesterol between cells and lipoproteins, *J Biochem* 26(13):5766, 1986.

Manninen V, Elo MO, Frick HM, et al: Lipid alterations and decline in the incidence of coronary heart disease in the Helsinki heart study, *JAMA* 260(5):641, 1988.

Muldoon MF, Manuck SB, Matthews KA: Lowering cholesterol concentrations and mortality: a quantitative review of primary prevention trials, *Br Med J* 301:309-314, 1990.

Oster G, Epstein AM: Cost-effectiveness of antihyperlipemic therapy in the prevention of coronary heart disease, *JAMA* 258(17):2381, 1987.

Report of the national cholesterol education program expert panel on detection, evaluation, and treatment of high blood cholesterol in adults, *Arch Intern Med* 148:36, 1988.

Steinberg D, Parthasarathy S, Carew TE, et al: Beyond cholesterol: modifications of low-density lipoprotein that increase its atherogenicity, *N Engl J Med* 323(14):915-924, 1989.

Strandberg TE, Van Hanen H, Miettinen TA: Probucol in long-term treatment of hypercholesterolemia, *Gen Pharmacol* 19(3):317, 1988.

Zilversmit DB: Atherogenesis: a postprandial phenomenon, *Circulation* 60(3):473, 1979.

SELF-ASSESSMENT QUESTIONS

1. Which of the following statements for cholesterol and cholesterol metabolism is not true?
   a. The liver is the primary organ for cholesterol uptake and degradation.
   b. Most cholesterol is converted into bile acids.
   c. The transport of cholesterol is primarily accomplished by encasement by protein to form lipoprotein particles.
   d. The major source of cholesterol is dietary intake.
2. HMG-CoA reductase inhibitors:
   a. are effective in reducing cholesterol concentrations in patients with hypercholesterolemia, including those who are homozygous for low-density lipoprotein absence.
   b. have a high affinity for the LDL cholesterol receptor.
   c. are all pro-drugs.
   d. result in a decreased need for exogenous cholesterol.
3. A variety of epidemiological studies have shown a negative correlation between the levels of high-density lipoproteins (HDL) and the risk of cardiovascular disease. Agents that increase HDL levels include all but:
   a. fibric acid.
   b. estrogens.
   c. probucol.
   d. nicotinic acid.
4. Epidemiological studies on the incidence of atherosclerosis indicate that:
   a. the greatest correlation exists for LDL cholesterol.
   b. there is an inverse correlation between LDL and HDL cholesterol concentrations.
   c. there is usually a consistent increase in LDL cholesterol and total cholesterol concentrations.
   d. all of the above are correct.

CHAPTER 21 Drugs Affecting Coagulation, Fibrinolysis, and Platelet Aggregation

J. BRYAN SMITH
DAVID C. B. MILLS

MAJOR DRUGS

anticoagulants
fibrinolytics
platelet function inhibitors

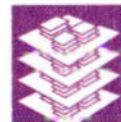

THERAPEUTIC OVERVIEW

Normally, the system of hemostasis functions so that neither excessive bleeding nor the formation of unwanted thrombi are a problem. However, in a significant number of patients (particularly those undergoing surgery or with cardiovascular diseases), therapeutic approaches modifying pathways involved in coagulation, fibrinolysis, or platelet aggregation are useful. Events that lead to arterial thrombosis (usually involving a platelet thrombus) or venous thrombosis (usually involving a fibrin clot) or that cause clot lysis are activated and inhibited by numerous endogenous blood and tissue components as well as by exogenous materials. Although the total range of activators and inhibitors and how they interact to stimulate or modify platelet aggregation, coagulation, or fibrinolysis in a variety of disease states is still not fully understood, much progress has been made. Greater appreciation is being given to the role of vascular endothelial cells and other blood cells and how they modulate the activation, inhibition, and storage of proteins involved in hemostasis. This highlights the importance of understanding in vivo as well as in vitro events in the management of clot-forming and clot-dissolution systems.

ABBREVIATIONS

ADP	adenosine diphosphate
APTT	activated partial thromboplastin test
AT-III	antithrombin III
cAMP	cyclic adenosine monophosphate
PT	prothrombin time
t-PA	tissue plasminogen activator
TXA_2	thromboxane A_2
u-PA	urokinase plasminogen activator
vWF	von Willebrand factor

The main reasons for therapeutic intervention into the hemostatic mechanism are (1) to inhibit blood coagulation, (2) to stimulate lysis of an already formed but unwanted thrombus, or (3) to inhibit platelet function. Certain surgical procedures such as hip-joint replacement or cardiopulmonary bypass, in which whole blood comes into contact with foreign materials, result in initiation of blood coagulation and thrombus formation. Here, prophylactic administration of anticoagulants, usually heparin or coumarin, is effective in diminishing unwanted thrombus formation. In clinical situations such as deep vein thrombosis, acute myocardial infarction, or pulmonary embolism where a thrombus already has formed, rapid activation of the fibrinolytic system to obtain lysis of the thrombus and initiation of anticoagulation to minimize further clot formation are effective. Clinical trials support the use of drugs that inhibit platelet function in the management of cardiovascular disease and stroke.

Therapeutic uses of anticoagulant, fibrinolytic, and antiplatelet drugs are summarized in the box.

MECHANISMS OF ACTION

The interactions of the coagulation, fibrinolytic, and platelet systems are summarized in Figure 21-1. Blood vessels are lined with endothelial cells, which present a nonthrombogenic surface. When blood comes into con-

THERAPEUTIC OVERVIEW	
Anticoagulation	
heparin, coumarins	Arterial thrombosis
	Atrial fibrillation
	Cardiomyopathy
	Cerebral emboli
	Hip surgery
	Vascular prostheses
	Heart valve disease
	Venous thromboembolism
Fibrinolysis	
streptokinase, urokinase, tissue plasminogen activator	Acute myocardial infarction
	Deep vein thrombosis
	Pulmonary embolism
Platelet aggregation inhibition	
aspirin	Cerebrovascular accident, stroke
	After coronary bypass surgery
	Restenosis after angioplasty or thrombolysis
	Myocardial infarction
	Transient ischemic attack
ticlopidine	Cerebrovascular accident, stroke

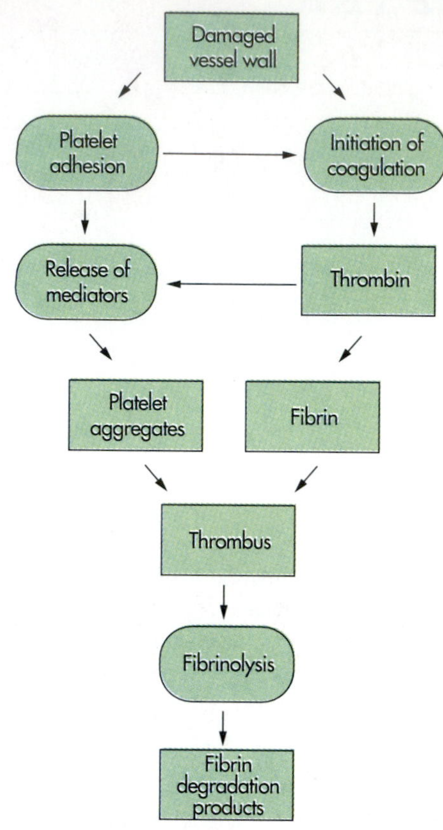

FIGURE 21-1 Involvement of thrombin and platelets and their interaction in thrombosis.

tact with other tissues or foreign surfaces, platelets are activated by exposed collagen and blood coagulation is initiated by tissue factor. These two processes are intimately related. The removal of thrombi by the fibrinolytic system is dependent on the generation of plasmin.

Coagulation

Blood coagulation is propagated by the sequential conversion of a series of inactive proteins into catalytically active protease enzymes (Figure 21-2). After damage to the endothelium, blood comes into contact with cells that express tissue factor, a membrane lipoprotein. A catalytically active complex of tissue factor with plasma factor VII is produced. This then converts plasma factor X to its enzymatically active form, factor X_a. In turn, factor X_a, in the presence of cofactor V_a and activated platelets, converts prothombin to thrombin. Thrombin then removes small peptides from fibrinogen, converting it to fibrin monomer, which spontaneously polymerizes to give the fibrin clot.

In addition to clotting fibrinogen, thrombin activates platelets and converts factors V and VIII to their active forms (factors V_a and VIII_a). Factor VIIIa participates as a cofactor with activated platelets in the generation of factor X_a by an alternative route (the so-called intrinsic pathway). This involves factor IX, which is activated by the factor VII_a–tissue factor complex or by factor XI_a. In vitro, on contact of blood with a glass surface, the "contact phase" of blood coagulation involving factor XII, prekallikrein, and high molecular weight kininogen leads to the activation of factor XI. The relevance of this pathway to the initiation of coagulation in vivo is brought into question by the failure of defects in these contact-phase proteins to cause bleeding.

The final events in the coagulation process are fibrin cross-linking and fibrinolysis (Figure 21-3). Fibrin is stabilized by the action of factor XIII_a (transglutaminase), which introduces covalent bonds between adjacent fibrin molecules. Factor XIII occurs in plasma as a precursor that is activated by thrombin. Fibrinolysis, catalysed by plasmin, eventually removes the clot (see below).

Most enzymes involved in coagulation belong to the family of trypsinlike serine proteases and share considerable structural homology (Figure 21-4). The vitamin

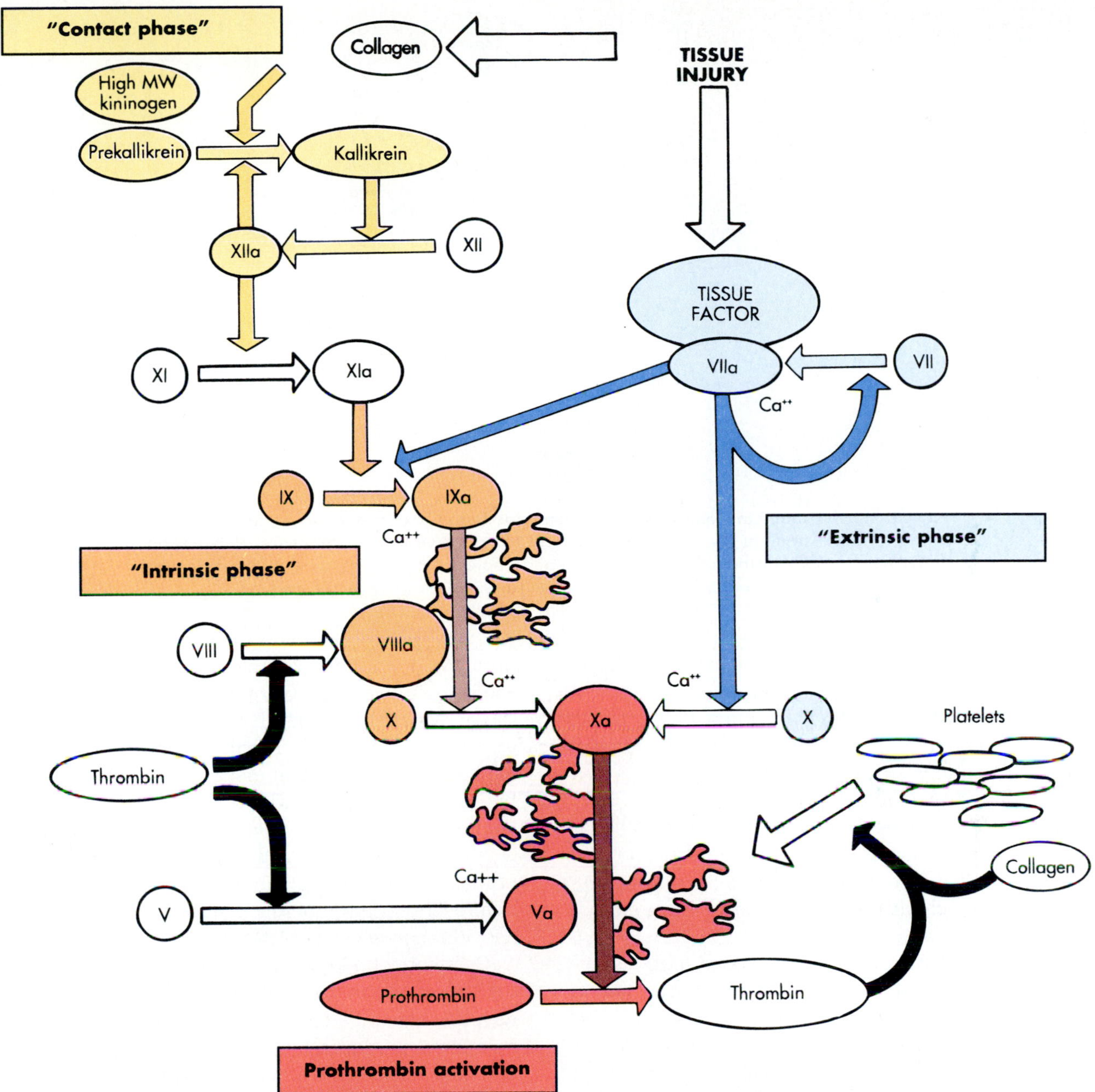

FIGURE 21-2 A simplified model for thrombin generation. Reactions fall into four phases, which occur preferentially on surfaces. Activated platelets provide the surface for two of these phases; nonvascular tissue provides the surface for the "extrinsic" phase, and foreign surfaces such as glass and collagen activate the "contact" phase. In each, a multicomponent complex is assembled comprising an enzyme, its substrate (a proenzyme), and a cofactor. This complex affects conversion of proenzyme to its active form at a rate thousands of times faster than that of the enzyme alone.

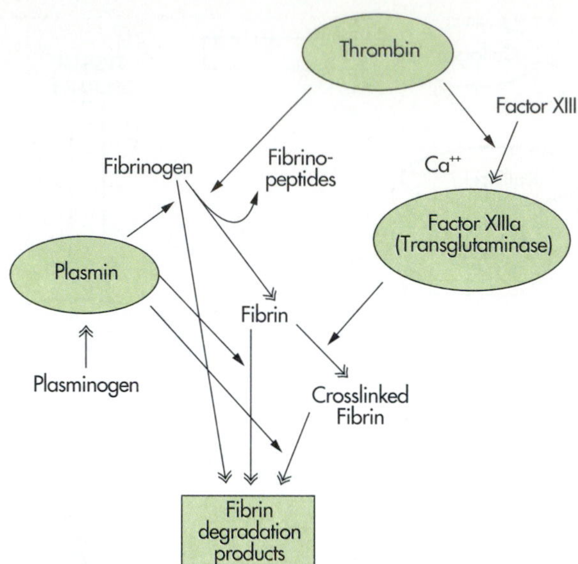

FIGURE 21-3 Thrombin cleaves two small peptides from fibrinogen, allowing its polymerization to fibrin. Thrombin also converts factor XIII to an active transglutaminase. This enzyme stabilizes fibrin by introducing Glu-Lys isopeptide bonds between adjacent fibrin molecules. Fibrin and fibrinogen are both substrates for the thrombolytic enzyme plasmin.

K–dependent factors, in addition, share a specific calcium-binding domain containing several γ-carboxyglutamic acid (GLA) residues that interact with phospholipid on the activated platelet surface. Plasma also contains a variety of protease inhibitors that regulate the coagulation cascade (Table 21-1).

The two major types of clinically useful anticoagulants, heparin and coumarins, inhibit coagulation to give the same result (i.e., a reduction in fibrin deposition). However, the mechanisms of blockade by these anticoagulants differ greatly.

Heparin Commercial heparin obtained from hog intestinal mucosa or beef lung is a linear polysaccharide composed of alternating residues of glucosamine and glucuronic or iduronic acid. The amino group of glucosamine is either acetylated or sulfated, whereas a variable degree of sulfation (up to 40%) occurs on other hydroxyl groups (Figure 21-5). It has an average molecular weight of approximately 15 kDa (5 to 30 kDa).

Heparin acts by binding to a plasma glycoprotein antithrombin III (AT-III), which serves as a major inhibitor of serine protease clotting enzymes. AT-III inhibits these enzymes by forming a stable 1:1 molar complex by association between an arginine reactive site in AT-III and the active center serine in the enzyme. Heparin binds to a lysine-rich site in AT-III, leading to a greatly enhanced rate of inhibition, particularly of X_a and thrombin, but also of IX_a and XI_a; heparin dissociates from the complex and can then interact with another molecule of AT-III (Figure 21-6). Although low-dose heparin acts primarily by neutralizing factor X_a, at high doses it acts by preventing thrombin-induced activation of factors V and VIII, as well as of platelets.

Commercial heparin is heterogeneous; fractions that bind most tightly to AT-III are responsible for most of its anticoagulant effects. Low molecular weight heparin fragments, produced by enzymatic or chemical hydrolysis, may have increased anti–factor X_a activity and a longer half-life than standard heparin, which may promote convenience of use.

Coumarins Coumarins, typified by warfarin (Figure 21-7), make up the second major type of clinically used anticoagulants. They resemble vitamin K in structure and act by blocking vitamin K regeneration during the

FIGURE 21-4 Proposed linear structures for five vitamin K–dependent plasma proenzymes, drawn to show the similarities between them. Cys-Cys bridges within the proteins are indicated by ○=○, and the point or points of cleavage that lead to conversion to the active enzyme are shown by *arrows*. The amino acids at these points are indicated by the standard single-letter code. *D-OH* indicates the unusual amino acid, β-hydroxy-aspartate; γ-carboxyglutamate *(GLA)* residues are indicated by *o*. The active site region of these enzymes is composed of three amino acids: serine *(S)*, histidine *(H)*, and aspartate *(D)*, indicated in the catalytic domain. Points at which the proteins have carbohydrate side chains are shown by ◇.

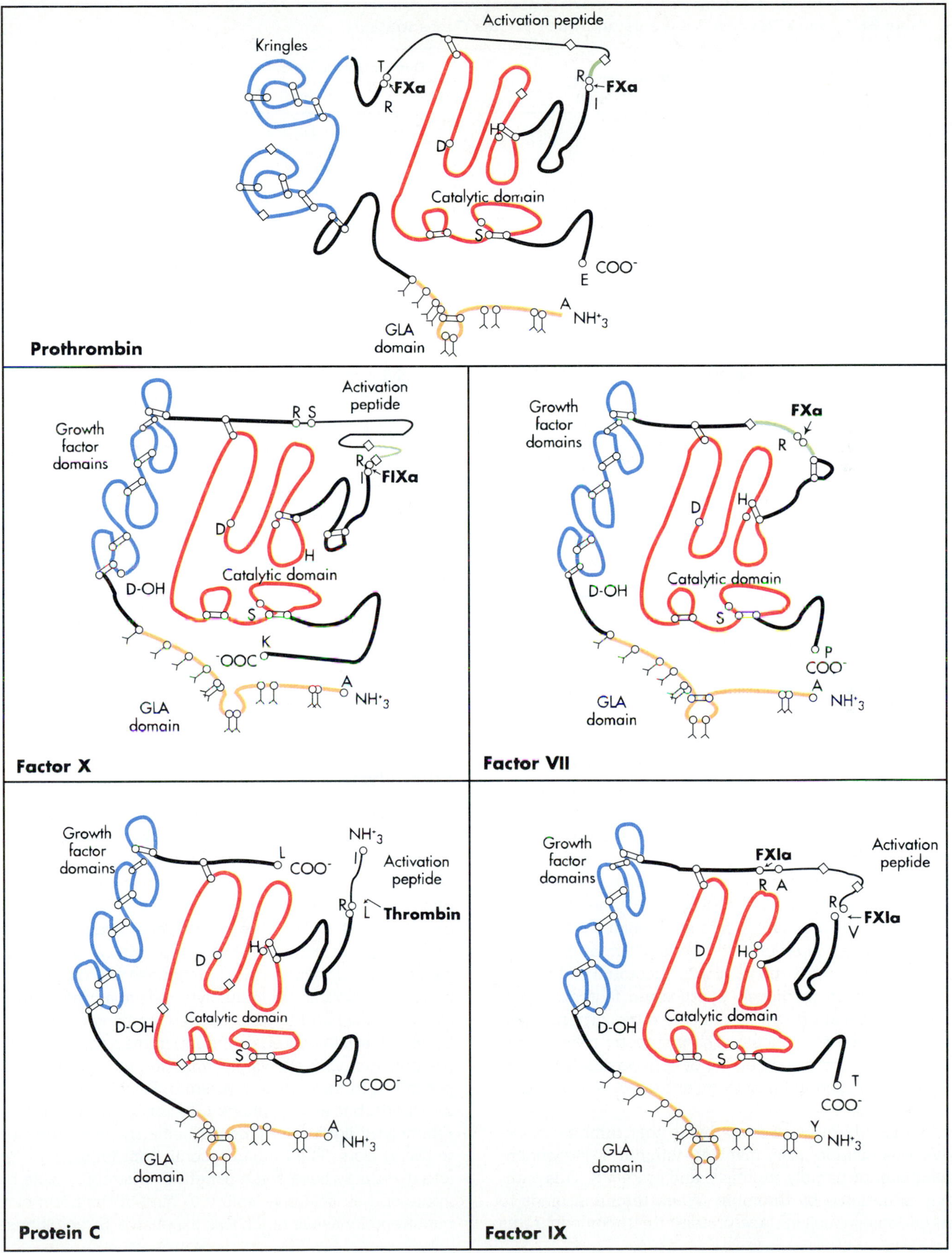

FIGURE 21-4 For legend see opposite page.

Table 21-1 Some Protease Inhibitors with their Plasma Concentrations

Name	Molecular Wt (kilodaltons)	Concentration (g/L)	Concentration (nM)	Principal Target
α_1-Protease inhibitor	55	1.3	23.6	Elastase
α_1-Antichymotrypsin	69	0.5	7.2	
Antithrombin III	62	0.3	4.8	Thrombin, X_a, IX_a, VII_a
α_2-Macroglobulin	725	2.5	3.4	Nonspecific
Inter-α-trypsin inhibitor	160	0.5	3.1	
C1 inhibitor	105	0.2	1.9	Complement, XII_a
α_2-Plasmin inhibitor	67	0.1	1.5	Plasmin
Heparin cofactor II	66			Thrombin, X_a

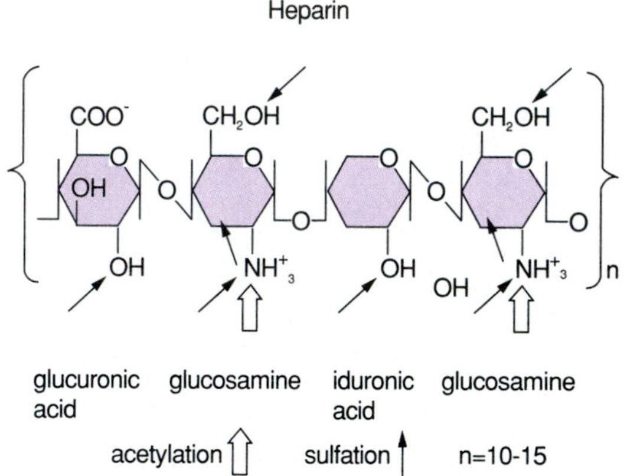

FIGURE 21-5 Proposed structure of a repeating unit in heparin that has high affinity for antithrombin III. There is considerable variation in extent of sulfation of different hydroxyl groups.

posttranslational modification of several endogenous clotting proteins (Figure 21-8). These vitamin K–dependent proteins include clotting factors VII, IX, X and prothrombin and the anticoagulant proteins, protein C and protein S. These six proteins in their amino terminal region have several glutamic acid residues (see Figure 21-4) that undergo liver microsomal enzyme carboxylation to form γ-carboxyglutamic acid residues that function as binding sites for Ca^{++} ions. Coumarins inhibit the synthesis of functional clotting factors but have no direct effect on previously synthesized factors. Therefore, a significant delay occurs before the anticoagulant effect is observed clinically. The first factor to decline is factor VII, which has a half-life of approximately 5 hours (Table 21-2). The full anticoagulant effect is reached in 2 to 3 days.

A recently discovered pathway that inhibits excessive coagulation also involves vitamin K–dependent components, namely, protein C and protein S. This pathway is initiated by thrombin. When thrombin binds to an endothelial cell surface protein, thrombomodulin, its proteolytic specificity is altered. In this state thrombin no longer cleaves fibrinogen but instead becomes an activator of protein C. Activated protein C, in combination with protein S, destroys the essential clotting cofactors V_a and VIII_a (Figure 21-9). Genetic deficiency of protein C is associated with a high incidence of thromboembolic disease.

Because of the slow onset of anticoagulation with warfarin therapy, heparin treatment is used for the first 5 days. This obviates the possibility of a transient hypercoagulable state caused by suppression of functional protein C synthesis. Abruptly ending heparin treatment can be hazardous because of reduced levels of antithrombin III. If heparin is terminated too early when one is switching from heparin to warfarin, rethrombosis may occur.

Fibrinolysis

The major route of fibrin clot lysis results from the proteolytic action of plasmin, the enzyme produced by the activation of plasminogen, a single-chain protein of 94 kDa (Figure 21-10). A minor component of clot lysis may be caused by the release of proteolytic enzymes from leukocytes. The three principal activators of plasminogen are urokinase (u-PA), streptokinase, and tissue plasminogen activator (t-PA). Urokinase and tissue plasminogen activator are proteolytic enzymes that cleave a susceptible bond in plasminogen to generate plasmin. Streptokinase (a bacterial product) forms a complex with plasminogen that allows plasminogen to activate other plasminogen molecules to plasmin. Plasmin attacks not only fibrin but also fibrinogen, factor V, and factor VIII. Fibrinolytic agents may cause hemorrhage in addition to lysing clots. The human recombinant proteins ru-PA and rt-PA may have some benefit over streptokinase by virtue of their selective ability to bind to the fibrin clot, but streptokinase is much less expensive. Streptokinase

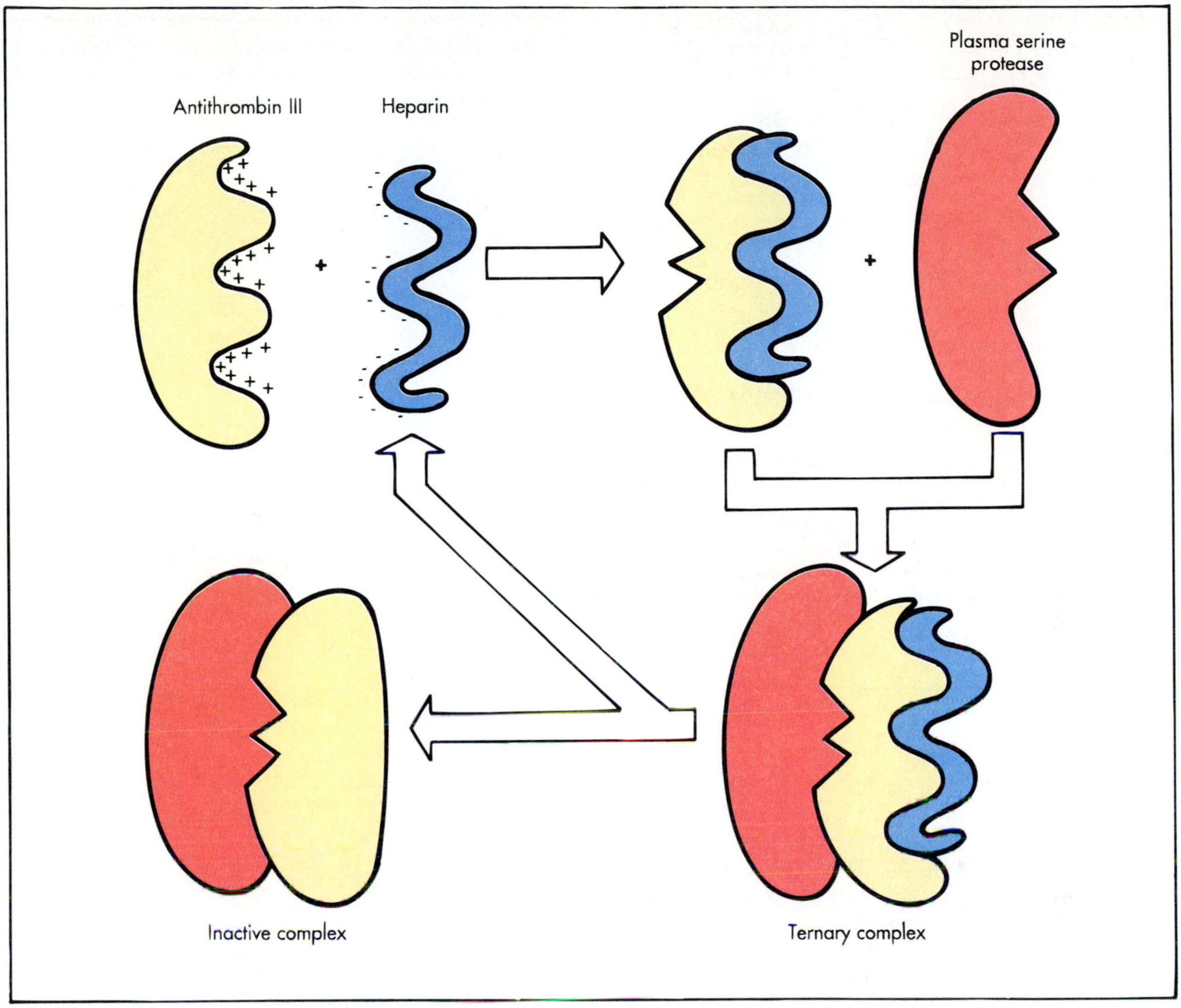

Plasma serine protease
Antithrombin III
Heparin
Inactive complex
Ternary complex

FIGURE 21-6 Heparin binds to a positively charged region of antithrombin III (AT-III) and greatly increases the rate at which AT-III interacts with plasma serine proteases. Heparin then dissociates from the ternary complex and can interact with more AT-III. This gives heparin the quality of a nonprotein enzyme. AT-III can inactivate thrombin and factors X_a, VII_a, and IX_a.

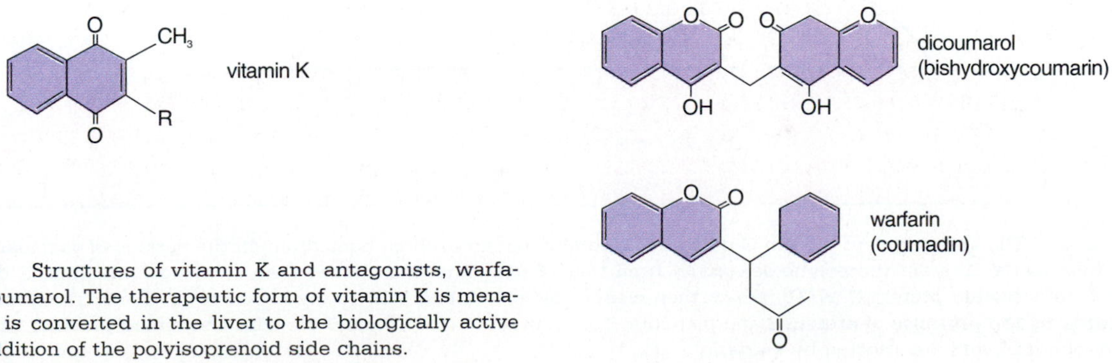

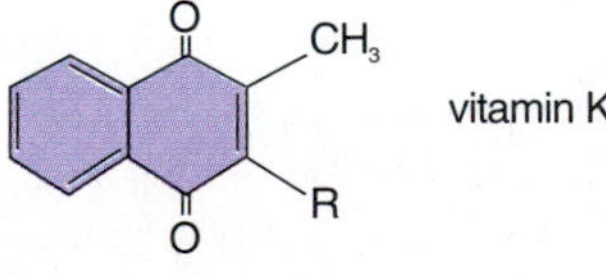

dicoumarol
(bishydroxycoumarin)

warfarin
(coumadin)

FIGURE 21-7 Structures of vitamin K and antagonists, warfarin and dicoumarol. The therapeutic form of vitamin K is menadione. This is converted in the liver to the biologically active forms by addition of the polyisoprenoid side chains.

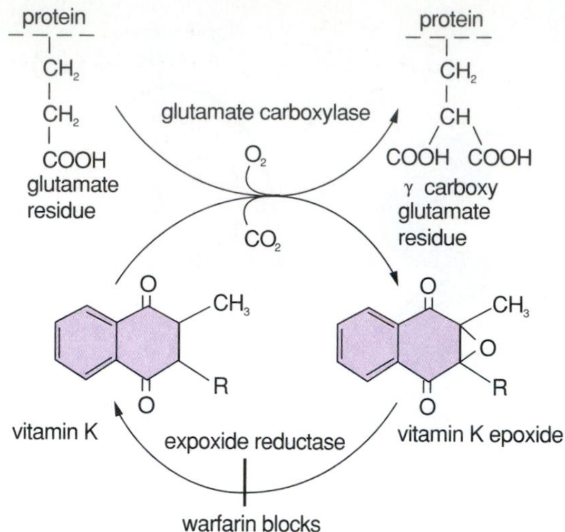

FIGURE 21-8 The role of vitamin K in the conversion of glutamate residues in certain plasma proteins to γ-carboxyglutamate *(GLA)* residues in the liver. Warfarin and other coumarin derivatives block the reduction of vitamin K epoxide formed in this reaction to its active form.

Table 21-2 Rates of Disappearance of Vitamin K–Dependent Proteins from Blood

Protein	Time
Coagulation factors	
Factor VII	5 hours
Factor IX	15 hours
Factor X	1 day
Prothrombin	2-3 days
Anticoagulant proteins	
Protein C	6 hours
Protein S	10 hours

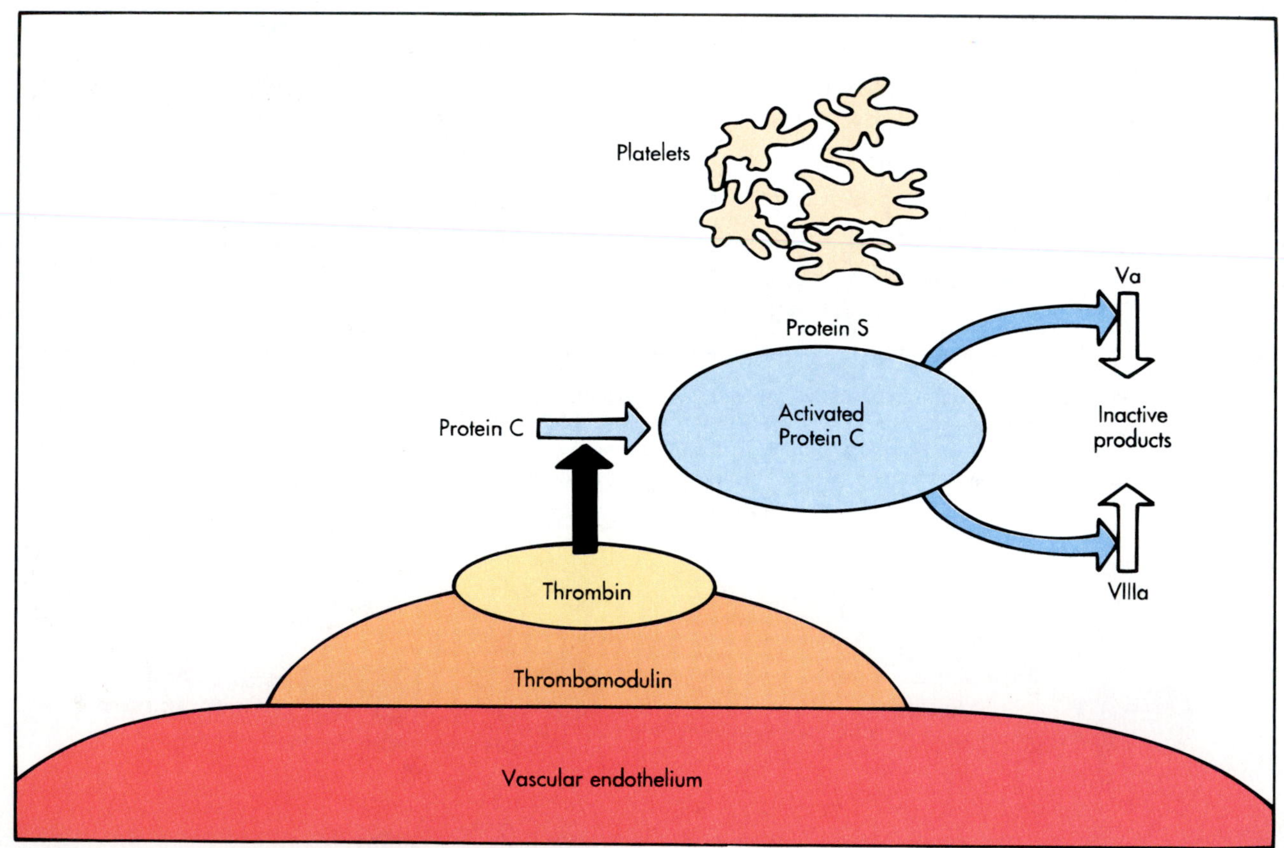

FIGURE 21-9 The anticoagulant protein C pathway. Thrombin bound to thrombomodulin on the surface of vascular endothelial cells has a different proteolytic selectivity from that of free thrombin. Rather than cleaving fibrinogen, it cleaves protein C to activated protein C *(APC)*, which then cleaves factors V_a and VIII_a to give inactive products. This process is accelerated by the presence of protein S and platelets. Both protein C and protein S are GLA-containing proteins, are vitamin K dependent, and are affected by warfarin.

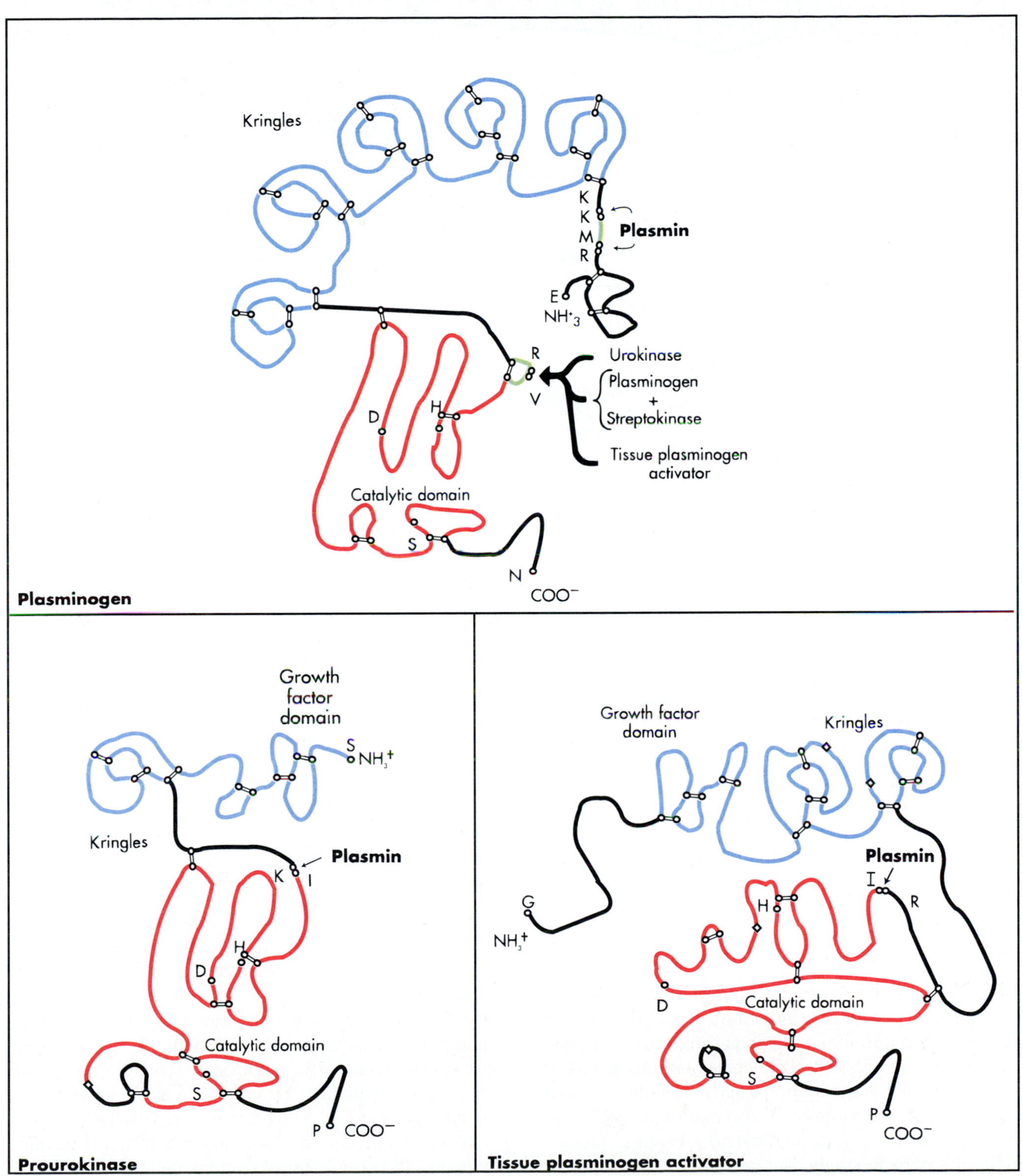

FIGURE 21-10 Proposed linear structures for plasminogen and for two plasminogen activators drawn to show their similarities, and to vitamin K–dependent factors (Figure 21-4). Disulfide bridges, points of cleavage, and glycosylation sites are indicated as in Figure 21-4.

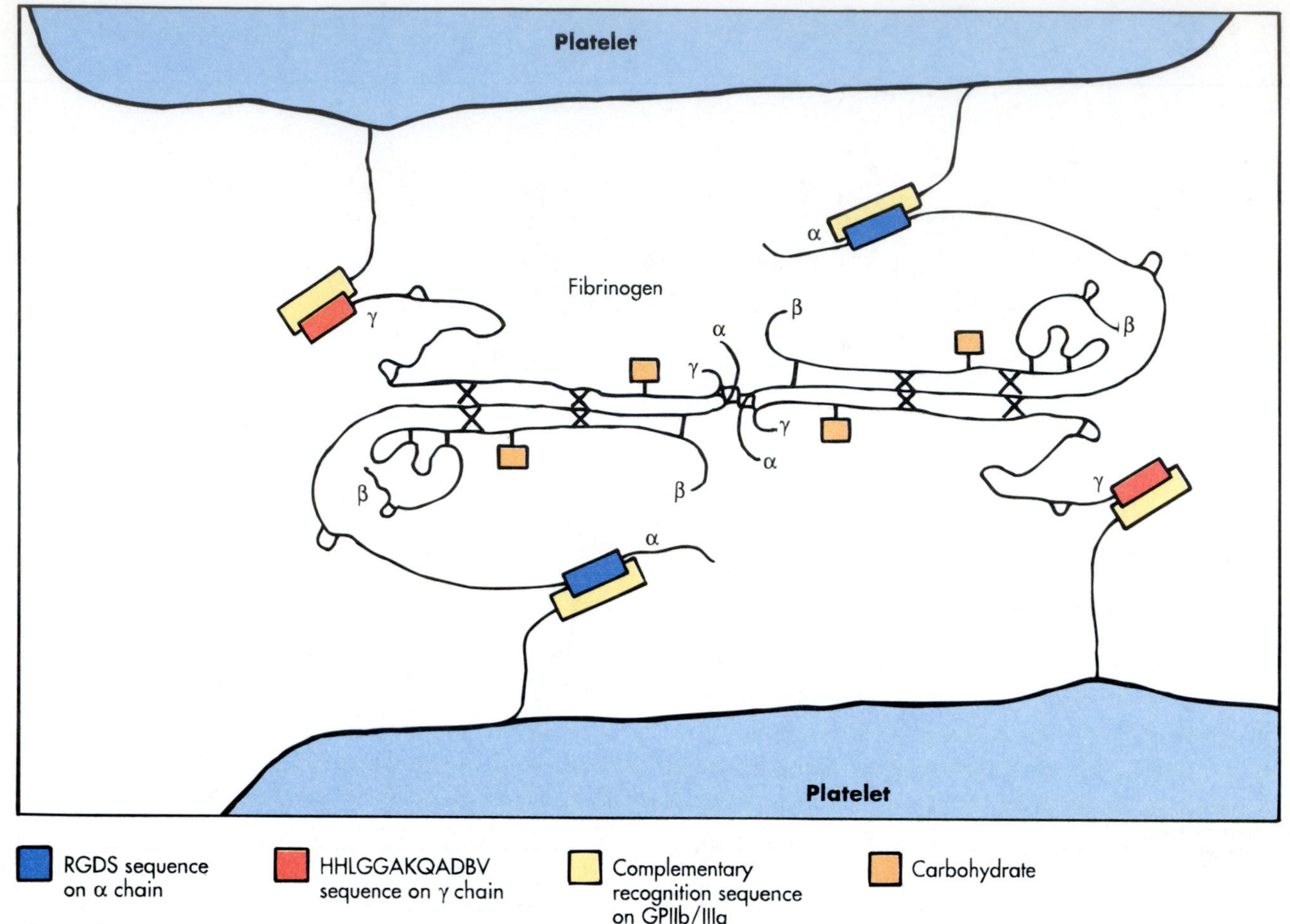

FIGURE 21-11 Fibrinogen is a symmetrical dimeric structure containing three chains (Aα, Bβ, and γ). Both the monomeric units and the individual chains are linked by multiple disulfide bonds indicated by X. Fibrinogen mediates aggregation of stimulated platelets through binding sites on the Aα and γ chains.

is highly immunogenic, and care should be taken if this agent is used repeatedly for clot lysis.

Platelet Aggregation

Activation and subsequent aggregation of platelets is a major component of arterial thrombosis and may be involved in the initiation of venous thrombosis. Interaction of platelets with vessel wall collagen appears to be the first step in platelet aggregation. Activation of these platelets leads to the formation and release of thromboxane A_2 (TXA_2) from arachidonic acid present in platelet membrane phospholipids. Thromboxane A_2 is a potent aggregating agent and vasoconstrictor. Platelet activation also causes the secretion of adenosine diphosphate (ADP) from platelet storage granules. Both TXA_2 and ADP, acting through specific receptors, cause the appearance of binding sites on the platelet membrane for fibrinogen (Figure 21-11) and for other adhesive proteins, including von Willebrand factor (vWF). Fibrinogen is involved in platelet-to-platelet adhesion (aggregation), whereas vWF is important in adhesion of platelets to other tissues. Thrombin generated locally on the surface of activated platelets greatly amplifies the response by causing further platelet activation (aggregation and secretion of mediators). Although both TXA_2 and thrombin cause increases in cytoplasmic calcium concentrations, the mechanism by which thrombin activates its receptor is unique. Thrombin cleaves its receptor, removing 15 amino acids from the extracellular N-terminal domain. The new N-terminus forms a "tethered ligand" that is the true agonist (Figure 21-12).

Platelet activation is inhibited by elevation of platelet cyclic adenosine monophosphate (cAMP). Thus agents that lead to increased platelet cAMP inhibit platelet aggregation. The most active agent is prosta-

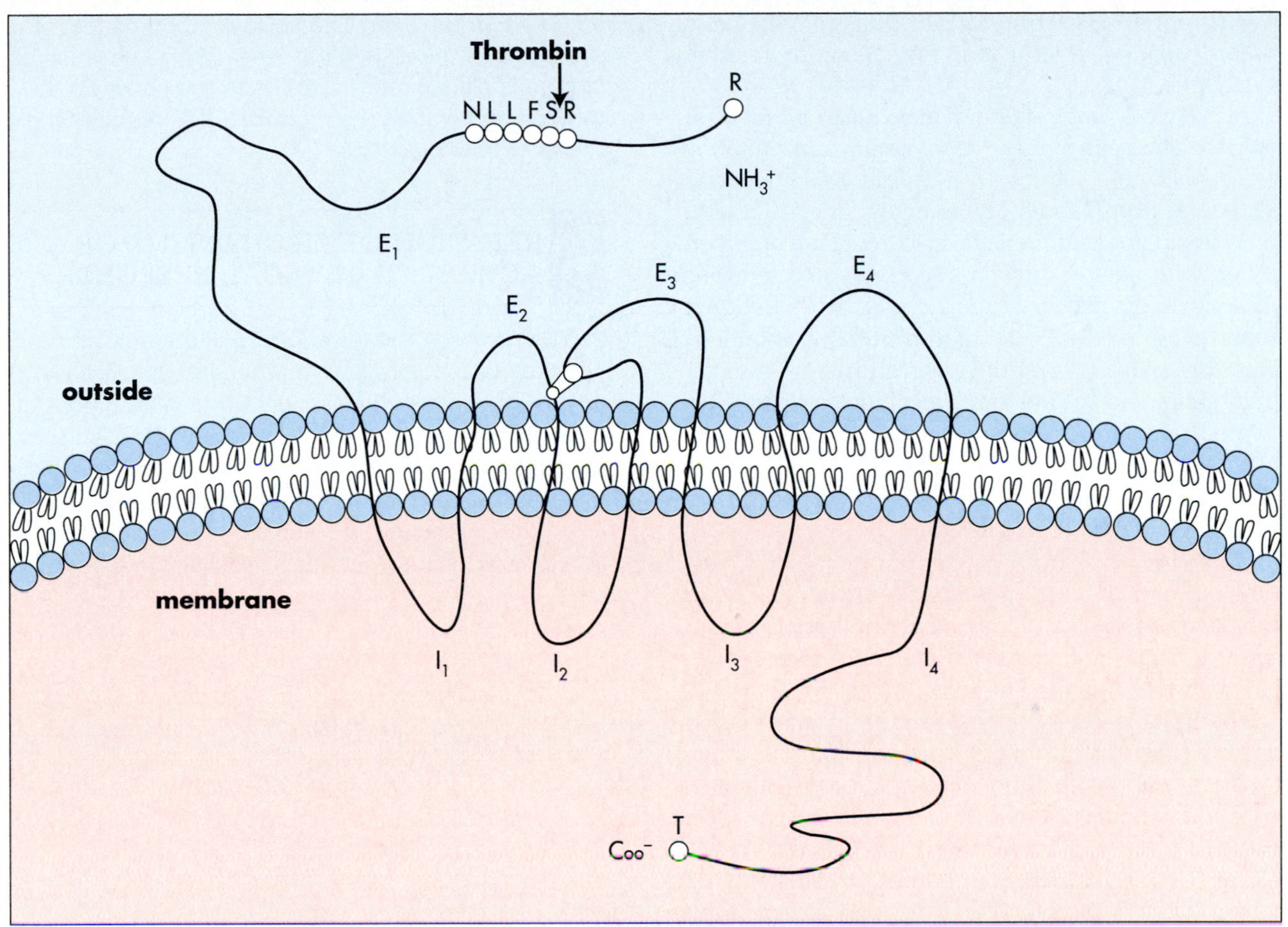

FIGURE 21-12 Proposed linear structure of the platelet thrombin receptor. The protein contains seven hydrophobic regions that are highly homologous to similar regions in other members of the rhodopsin family of receptors. They are believed to form seven helical membrane-spanning domains and are probably arranged in a tight group rather than strung out, as shown here for clarity. The second and third extracellular domains (E_2 and E_3) contain Cys residues, which are believed to be joined by a disulfide bridge. Thrombin acts by cleaving the N-terminal extracellular tail of the receptor protein between arginine *(R)* and serine *(S)* residues, leaving the new N-terminal sequence: Ser· Phe· Lys· Lys· Arg· . This sequence acts as a "tethered ligand," which activates the receptor. The oligopeptide with this sequence is a powerful aggregating agent. The intracellular domains (I_1 to I_4) are believed to be involved in signal transduction.

cyclin (PGI_2), released by cells of the vessel wall. Nitric oxide is released by endothelial cells and may also raise platelet cAMP concentrations.

The major therapeutic approach to reducing platelet aggregation is through inhibition of cyclooxygenase. Aspirin irreversibly inhibits platelet cyclooxygenase by acetylation of a serine residue near the active site of the enzyme, thereby blocking TXA_2 formation. The nonsteroidal antiinflammatory drugs ibuprofen and indomethacin inhibit this enzyme competitively. Sulfinpyrazone is metabolized to a product that can also inhibit this enzyme. Aspirin also blocks the synthesis of the endogenous aggregation inhibitor prostacyclin (PGI_2). Although it has been suggested that a lower dose of aspirin might be less effective in inhibiting PGI_2 biosynthesis, this question is still open.

Clinical trials have shown that aspirin reduces by 30% to 50% the incidence of myocardial infarction and death from cardiac causes in people with unstable angina. Aspirin also significantly reduces the incidence of a first myocardial infarction in men with stable angina and is effective as an antithrombotic agent in patients undergoing coronary angioplasty or bypass grafting. Aspirin also is recommended for use in patients with transient ischemic attacks. It is less clear whether aspirin is beneficial in survivors of myocardial infarction. There is a substantial dose-related risk of gastrointestinal ulceration associated with long-term aspirin treatment (see Chapter 29).

Dipyridamole was originally introduced as a vasodilator and has been widely used as an antithrombotic agent, usually in company with aspirin. Despite encouraging data from laboratory animals models, neither dipyridamole nor sulfinpyrazone, either alone or in combination with aspirin, proved superior to aspirin alone.

The use of ticlopidine (Figure 21-13) for the treatment of recurrent stroke in patients intolerant to aspirin represents an alternative antiplatelet strategy. This compound appears to act by selectively blocking platelet responses to ADP.

PHARMACOKINETICS

The principal pharmacokinetic parameters of the anticoagulants, fibrinolytic activators, and antiplatelet aggregation drugs are given in Table 21-3. Warfarin is typical of orally administered anticoagulants (see Figure 21-7). Heparin is given by intravenous infusion or subcutaneously. Because of different mechanisms of action, the maximum heparin anticoagulant effect after a single dose is immediate, whereas that of warfarin is observed in 36 to 48 hours in humans. Warfarin is metabolized in the liver. Warfarin is strongly bound to plasma albumin, whereas heparin is not. The half-life of low molecular weight heparin is longer than that of the natural compound. Thus low molecular weight heparin is effective when administered once daily by subcutaneous injection.

Aspirin is hydrolyzed in plasma to salicylic acid, with a half-life of 15 to 20 minutes. Salicylic acid is further degraded in the liver. The antithrombotic effect of aspirin, however, persists for at least 2 days because circulating platelets cannot synthesize cyclooxygenase. Restoration of the ability to produce TXA_2 requires the synthesis of new platelets.

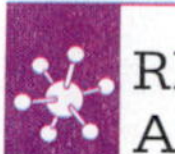

RELATION OF MECHANISMS OF ACTION TO CLINICAL RESPONSE

The common use of anticoagulants and antiplatelet compounds is to prevent thromboembolic disease. Heparin is effective in the prevention and treatment of venous thrombosis and pulmonary embolism and related events and can be used either for prophylaxis or treatment. In the former case, referred to as "minidose heparin," the compound is given by continuous IV infusion at a dose that does not affect clotting time in vitro. For

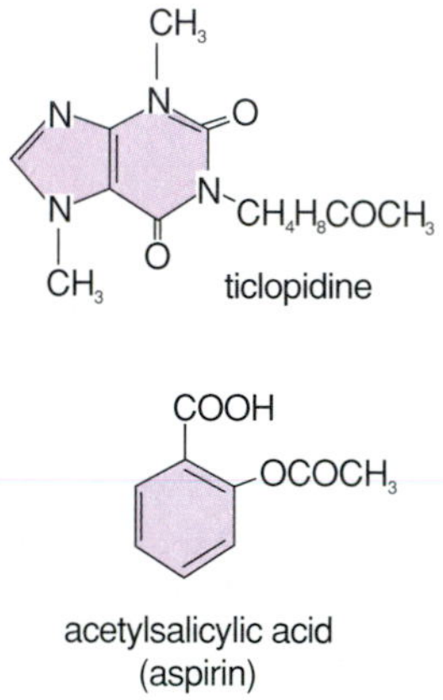

FIGURE 21-13 Chemical structures of aspirin and ticlopidine.

Table 21-3 Pharmacokinetic Parameters

Drug	Administration	$t_{1/2}$ (hours)	Disposition	Plasma Protein Binding (%)
Heparin	IV	1		Trace
	SC	3		
Low molecular weight heparin	IV	2	R	Trace
	SC	4		
Warfarin	Oral	40	M, (R)	97
Aspirin	Oral	2-3	M, R	50-70
Ticlopidine	Oral	30	M, R	?
Streptokinase	IV	0.3	M	
Urokinase	IV	0.3	M	
rt-PA*	IV	0.2	M	

M, Metabolism; *R*, renal Excretion.
*Recombinant DNA–derived t-PA.

treatment of ongoing thrombotic processes, a higher dose is required, and this must be monitored by a suitable clotting time test. The anticoagulant response to heparin varies widely among patients with thromboembolic disease. Clinical efficacy is optimized when the anticoagulant effect is maintained above a defined minimum level. The risk of bleeding is increased as the dose of heparin increases. For this reason, the activated partial thromboplastin time (APTT) is used to monitor the degree of anticoagulation. One performs this test by mixing patient plasma (citrated to chelate calcium) with a commercial tissue extract that restores calcium and certain clotting factors and measuring the time in seconds for a clot to form. Anticoagulation prolongs this time. Because the degree of anticoagulation observed in vitro varies depending on the specific APTT reagents, heparin treatment is monitored to maintain the ratio of the patients' APTT to mean control APTT within a defined range of 1.5 to 2.5, referred to as the therapeutic range. This range usually corresponds to a heparin concentration of 0.2 to 0.4 U/ml.

Oral anticoagulants are effective in primary and secondary prevention of venous thromboembolism. The one-stage prothrombin time (PT) is used to measure the anticoagulant effect of coumarins. As with the APTT, the PT test result depends greatly on the reagents (particularly the thromboplastin) used and is maintained to two to three times the time set for normals using the same reagents.

Platelet function is assessed by measurement of the bleeding time, a test that involves incising the forearm skin under standardized conditions. Platelet aggregation responses are monitored optically using an aggregometer.

SIDE EFFECTS, CLINICAL PROBLEMS, AND TOXICITY

The major problem with all antithrombotic agents is bleeding, even when used in therapeutic doses. Thrombocytopenia (heparin), drug interactions (warfarin), and platelet aggregation by other drugs also pose significant problems (see box).

The anticoagulant effect of heparin can be reversed rapidly with protamine sulfate. Protamine sulfate itself is an anticoagulant, and the dose used should be based on the calculated amount of heparin remaining in the circulation. Protamine sulfate also can cause damage to to the vessel wall and is immunogenic. Rapid reversal of the effect of warfarin can be achieved only by transfusion of plasma containing the clotting factors.

Bleeding caused by warfarin can be treated only by transfusion of plasma containing active clotting factors. Bleeding as a consequence of excessive fibrinolysis can be treated with ε-aminocaproic acid (Amicar), which is a both competitive inhibitors of plasmin.

Transient thrombocytopenia is a well-recognized, usually asymptomatic complication of heparin therapy. The reported incidence of heparin-associated thrombocytopenia varies widely, from 1% to up to 15% in various studies. It is more common with heparin derived from bovine lung than that from porcine gut. It is associated with arterial or venous thrombosis in approximately 0.4% of patients and occasionally can be extremely serious and even fatal. Platelet counts may decrease well below 100,000 platelets/mm^3, with the decrease most evident 3 to 15 days after the initiation of heparin therapy. The mechanism appears to involve formation of an immune complex consisting of heparin and both the Fab and Fc portions of the IgG molecule. The usual treatment is to discontinue the use of heparin, whereupon the platelet count usually returns to normal within 4 days. So far, no guidelines are available to predict which patients are most likely to have this complication.

CLINICAL PROBLEMS

HEPARIN

Causes bleeding, thrombocytopenia, hypersensitivity, transient hypercoagulability when discontinued

WARFARIN

Causes bleeeding, drug interactions, induction of drug metabolizing enzymes; some subjects are resistant

STREPTOKINASE

Causes bleeding by attacking fibrinogen and factors V and VIII, immunogenic

UROKINASE

Causes bleeding by attacking fibrinogen and factors V and VIII, expensive

RT-PA*

Causes bleeding by attacking fibrinogen and factors V and VIII, expensive

ASPIRIN

Dose-dependent gastrointestinal irritation, hypersensitivity, Reye's syndrome in children

TICLOPIDINE

Reversible neutropenia, skin rashes

*Recombinant DNA–derived t-PA.

DRUG INTERACTIONS WITH WARFARIN

DECREASED ANTICOAGULATION

Increased warfarin metabolism by cytochrome P-450: barbiturates, carbamazepine, griseofulvin, rifampin
Reduced warfarin absorption: cholestyramine
Unknown mechanism: penicillins

INCREASED ANTICOAGULATION

Inhibition of warfarin clearance: disulfiram, amiodarone, metronidazole, sulfinpyrazone
Displacement of warfarin from plasma albumin: salicylates, chloral hydrate
Increased clearance of clotting factors: thyroid hormones
Unknown mechanism: erythromycin, anabolic steroids

FUNCTIONAL SYNERGISM

Inhibition of coagulation: heparin, thrombolytic agents
Inhibition of platelet function: aspirin, other nonsteroidal antiinflammatories, ticlopidine

TRADE NAMES

In addition to generic and fixed-combination preparations, the following trade-named materials are available in the United States.

ANTICOAGULATION

Aquamephyton, vitamin K, menadione
Calciparine, heparin calcium
Coumadin, warfarin sodium

FIBRINOLYSIS

Abbokinase, urokinase
Activase, recombinant tissue plasminogen activator, rt-PA
Streptase
Kabikinase, streptokinase

PLATELET AGGREGATION INHIBITION

Aspirin—many brands
Ticlid, ticlopidine

Heparin is the anticoagulant of choice in pregnancy and during lactation because it does not cross the placenta and therefore does not produce untoward effects in the fetus or newborn. Orally administered anticoagulant drugs cross the placenta and can produce central nervous system abnormalities or fetal bleeding.

Because chronic warfarin administration often extends over many months or years, the likelihood of drug-drug interactions is very high. The reason is primarily attributable to warfarin's high degree of binding to plasma albumin and its mode of elimination. The box lists the potential drug-drug interactions. Hereditary resistance to warfarin has been described, and the affected individuals require 5 to 20 times the average normal dose.

Several drugs used therapeutically for the treatment of other disease states also influence the anticoagulant, fibrinolytic, or platelet systems. The most common example is aspirin, which when used as an antipyretic or analgesic drug, is also an antithrombotic agent.

NEW DIRECTIONS

Low molecular weight heparin is currently being evaluated in the United States for the prevention of venous thromboembolism in surgical and medical patients who are high risk because of its longer persistence compared with standard heparin.

An interesting new concept is to replace protamine sulfate with recombinant platelet factor 4 for the neutralization of heparin, thus avoiding the serious side effects encountered with protamine.

Several protein anticoagulants are produced by predatory species that feed on blood, as well some poisonous reptiles. These agents have the advantage over heparin in not requiring a plasma cofactor. They include hirudin from the medicinal leach *Hirudo medicinalis* and several agents produced by ticks, insects, and bats. The production of these proteins by genetic engineering makes them available for clinical use. In addition, genetically engineered modifications of these proteins are being studied.

Other recently discovered synthetic thrombin inhibitors also have been reported to be superior to heparin. One such agent, argatroban, has been studied in clinical trials in Japan. These thrombin-specific inhibitors appear to inhibit platelet-arterial wall interaction, an indication that thrombin is a major mediator of platelet-dependent thrombosis.

A wide variety of antiplatelet drugs have been developed, including inhibitors of the TXA_2 receptor, the thrombin receptor, the fibrinogen receptor and the von Willebrand factor receptor. These agents have not been tested in clinical trials.

REFERENCES

Coller BS: Antiplatelet agents in the prevention and therapy of thrombosis, *Annu Rev Med* 42:171-180, 1992.

Esmon CT: The regulation of natural anticoagulant pathways, *Science* 235:1348-1352, 1987.

Freedman M: Oral anticoagulants: pharmacodynamics, clinical indications and adverse effects, *J Clin Pharmacol* 32:196-206, 1992.

Hirsh J: Heparin, *N Engl J Med,* 324:1565-1574, 1992.

Hirsh J: Oral anticoagulant drugs, *N Engl J Med* 324:1865-1875, 1992.

Hirsh J, Levine MN: *Blood,* 79:1-17, 1992.

Marder VJ, Sherry S: Thrombolytic therapy: current status, *N Engl J Med* (Part 1): 318:1512-1520, (Part 2): 318:1585-1595, 1988.

TIMI Study Group: Comparison of invasive and conservative strategies after treatment with intravenous tissue plasminogen activator in acute myocardial infarction, *N Engl J Med* 320:618-627, 1989.

Willard JE, Lange RA, Hillis LD: The use of aspirin in ischaemic heart disease, *N Engl J Med* 327:175-181, 1992.

SELF-ASSESSMENT QUESTIONS

1. Heparin:
   a. has thrombolytic activity.
   b. has most prolonged activity when given orally.
   c. acts by binding to antithrombin III.
   d. inhibits the aggregation of platelets caused by thromboxane A_2.
   e. acts by blocking hepatic vitamin K regeneration.
2. Warfarin:
   a. acts rapidly when given orally.
   b. is potentiated by barbiturates.
   c. is antagonized by protamine sulfate.
   d. affects the activity of clotting factors.
   e. is potentiated by platelet factor 4
3. Warfarin is *not* used in the treatment of:
   a. unstable angina after myocardial infarction.
   b. embolism after hip surgery.
   c. arterial rethrombosis after thrombolysis.
   d. pulmonary embolism in pregnancy.
   e. disseminated intravascular coagulation.
4. The risk of bleeding in patients receiving heparin is increased by aspirin because aspirin:
   a. inhibits heparin anticoagulant activity.
   b. inhibits platelet function.
   c. displaces heparin from plasma protein binding sites.
   d. inhibits prothrombin formation.
   e. causes thrombocytopenia.
5. The risk of bleeding in patients taking warfarin is:
   a. reduced when the drug is displaced from albumin with chloral hydrate.
   b. increased when the drug is used with heparin.
   c. reduced when the drug is used with aspirin.
   d. increased when the drug is used with barbiturates.
   e. increased when the drug is used with cholestyramine.
6. Aspirin can:
   a. inhibit endothelial cell prostacyclin synthesis.
   b. prolong the whole blood clotting time.
   c. shorten the bleeding time.
   d. inhibit fibrinolysis.
   e. potentiate the effects of dipyridamole.
7. Which of the following may cause increased bleeding as a serious unwanted side effect?
   a. warfarin
   b. heparin
   c. aspirin
   d. tissue plasminogen activator
   e. all of the above

PART IV

CNS: DRUGS AFFECTING BEHAVIOR, PSYCHOTIC STATE, PAIN SENSATION, MUSCLE CONTROL, AND SLEEP

Drugs affecting the central nervous system (CNS) play an increasingly important role in the modern world. Mankind has experienced the effects of mind-altering drugs throughout recorded history, and a large number of compounds with specific and therapeutically useful effects on brain and behavior have been discovered and characterized over the last half century (Table IV-1). Drugs acting on the CNS are now among the most widely used of all drugs. These drugs have dramatically improved the quality of life for many people with diverse medical problems. Discovery of the general anesthetics was an absolute prerequisite for the development of surgery, and continued advances in the development of anesthetics, sedatives, narcotics, and muscle relaxants have made possible the complex microsurgical procedures in common use today. Discovery of antipsychotic drugs in the 1950s revolutionized the treatment of schizophrenia and other psychiatric disorders. Although they possess many potentially serious side effects, the well-regulated use of antipsychotic drugs allows many people to lead happy and productive lives in society instead of being confined to mental institutions. Other drugs act on the CNS to reduce pain or fever, relieve seizures and movement disorders associated with neurological diseases, or control mood and motivational states such as depression, mania, anxiety, arousal, or appetite. Proper use of such compounds results in dramatic increases in the quality of health care.

Both the therapeutic utility of drugs affecting the CNS and the nonmedical use of these compounds have increased dramatically. Historically, alcohol, caffeine, and nicotine have been used to alter mood and behavior and are still widely used. However, increasing awareness of the addictive and potential toxic effects of alcohol and nicotine has led to legal restrictions on their marketing and use. Many stimulants, depressants, and antianxiety agents intended for medical use are obtained illicitly and used for their mood-altering effects. Although the short-term effects of these drugs may be useful, exciting, or pleasurable, excessive use often leads to physical dependence or toxic effects that result in long-term problems. Illicit "recreational drugs" such as heroin and cocaine are major problems in society. The extremely high abuse liability of these drugs often results in physiological or psychological addiction, with their severe attendant social problems.

The increasing use and abuse of centrally acting drugs prompts the intense interest in the mechanisms by which these drugs act. It is useful to understand the specific molecular targets on which these drugs act, the physiological processes affected by the interactions of these drugs with their target molecules, and the relationship of such physiological changes to the complex mood and behavioral effects caused by these drugs. Such information is valuable in maximizing the therapeutic efficacy of centrally acting drugs, while minimizing their toxic effects, addiction liability, and abuse potential.

Table IV-1 Drugs That Act on the CNS and Are Commonly Used in Medical Practice, Arranged by Their Approximate Period of Introduction

Period of Drug Introduction	Indication for Use
BEFORE 1900	
morphine	Pain
caffeine	Drowsiness
nitrous oxide	Surgery
aspirin	Pain, fever, inflammation
1900 TO 1950	
barbiturates	Epilepsy
phenytoin	Epilepsy
meperidine and analogs	Pain
antihistamines	Wakefulness
SINCE 1950	
halothane and related fluorocarbons	Surgery
lithium carbonate	Bipolar affective disorders
chlorpromazine and related phenothiazines	Psychoses
chlorprothixene and related thioxanthines	Psychoses
haloperidol and related butyrophenones	Psychoses
monoamine oxidase inhibitors	Depression
tricyclic antidepressants	Depression
mixed agonist/antagonist opioids	Pain
methadone	Opiate dependence
opioid antagonists	Opiate overdoses
clonidine and related imidazolines	Hypertension
diazepam and related benzodiazepines	Anxiety
primidone, ethosuximide, carbamazepine and valproic acid	Epilepsy
most nonsteroidal anti-inflammatory agents	Pain, inflammation
L-dopa	Parkinson's disease
amantadine	Parkinson's disease
"second-generation" antidepressants	Depression
bromocriptine and other dopamine agonists	Parkinson's disease
baclofen and related drugs	Spasticity

Because of the complexity of the brain, the molecular targets through which various drugs alter function are often poorly understood. Much of what is known about the mechanisms by which drugs affect the CNS relates observed actions on specific molecular processes to known mood-altering or behavioral actions of drugs. Studies on the mechanism of actions of these drugs often follow the pattern outlined in Figure IV-1. Drugs with demonstrated behavioral actions are examined to determine if they have specific cellular or biochemical actions. When a biochemical effect is identified, other drugs with similar behavioral profiles are also studied. If they cause similar biochemical actions with potencies similar to their behavioral potencies, this action is postulated to be involved in the behavioral actions of the drug. This hypothesis is then tested with other compounds and experimental approaches. Clearly, this type of approach results in only correlative information and cannot prove that a drug acts by a particular mechanism. In many cases, this is the best approach currently available for studying the mechanisms of action of centrally acting drugs.

Chapters in this section describe drugs used for the therapeutic modification of behavior (psychoses, Chapter 23; mood, Chapter 24; and anxiety, Chapter 25), control of epilepsy (Chapter 26) and movement disorders (Chapter 27), diminish pain sensations (Chapters 28 to 30), control inflammation (Chapter 29), and provide relief for sleep disorders (Chapter 33). The nontherapeutic role of alcohol (Chapter 31) and mind-altering often addictive abused drugs (Chapter 32) are also described.

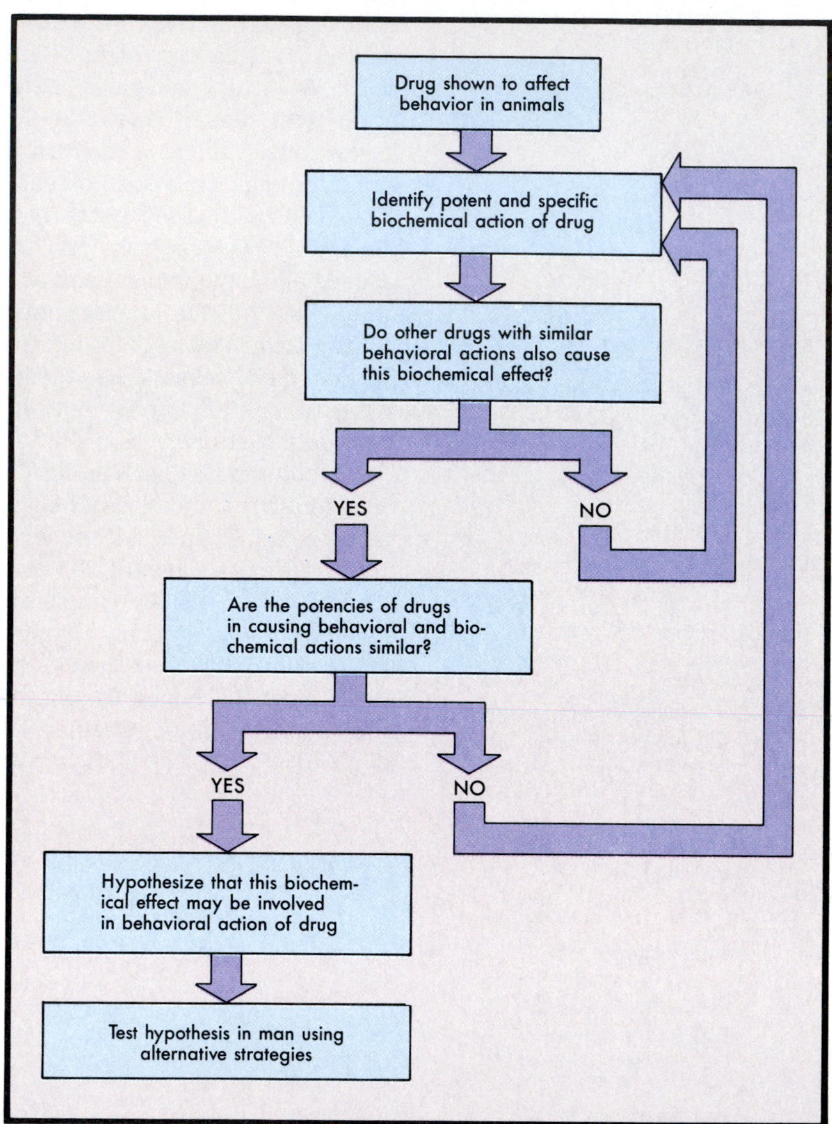

FIGURE IV-1 How the mechanisms of action of mood-altering drugs are studied.

CHAPTER 22 Pharmacological Organization of the CNS

KENNETH P. MINNEMAN

To understand the effects of drugs on the central nervous system (CNS), it is important to have a basic understanding of the cellular physiology and biochemistry of the brain. A review of the basic biology of the CNS is provided in this chapter, with an emphasis on the molecular processes believed to be specific targets for drug actions. Although drugs act at many sites in the brain, many of the most selective and useful drugs appear to act specifically at chemical synapses. Because this is the predominant site of information transfer and integration, it is also an ideal target for affecting specific brain functions. For this reason, the chemistry and physiology of synaptic transmission are heavily emphasized.

CELLULAR BUILDING BLOCKS

Cell Types

The two major classes of cells in the CNS are neurons and glia. Each has many morphologically and functionally diverse subclasses (Figure 22-1). Neurons exhibit many different shapes but have four general morphological regions: the cell body, dendrites, axon, and axon terminals. The cell body (or **soma**) is the region surrounding the nucleus, where the main organelles of the cytoplasm are grouped to perform the basic processes necessary to maintain the cell. Arising from the cell body are elaborate branching processes, **dendrites,** the parts of the neuron where incoming messages from other neurons are usually received. The cell body also gives rise to an elongated tube called an **axon,** a cable-like process that can be very long (up to 1 meter). Near its termination, the axon has characteristic structural features, often dividing into many fine branches, each of which terminates in a specialized ending called an **axon terminal** or **synaptic bouton.** Other types of axons exhibit multiple dilated regions **(varicosities)** near the termination point. These presynaptic structures are the sites where electrical signals passing down axons are converted into chemical messages for transmission to nearby cells.

Although most neurons have these four characteristic features, their relative prominence varies dramatically in different cells (see Figure 22-1). Some neurons have only a single major process extending from the cell body (which may, however, branch) and are thus called **unipolar neurons.** Others have two **(bipolar)** or more **(multipolar)** major processes arising from the cell body. Although most neurons have one axon, a few have more than one, and some function without any axon. The largest variability occurs in the length of the axon and the number and branching of the dendrites. Classification by shape, number of processes, arborization, or similar anatomical criteria can give only limited insight into neuronal function. Therefore neurons are usually classified by their localization and functional properties and the types of neurotransmitters that they synthesize and to which they respond.

Although glial cells outnumber neurons in the CNS, their functions are poorly understood. It is thought that glial cells provide various passive support services for the neurons, the major components involved in information transfer and integration. This is analogous to the role played by connective tissue in other parts of the body. However, recent evidence indicates that glial cells may contain many types of neurotransmitter receptors and ion channels, and the possibility that glial cells are

ABBREVIATIONS	
ATP	adenosine triphosphate
cAMP	cyclic adenosine monophosphate
GABA	γ-aminobutyric acid

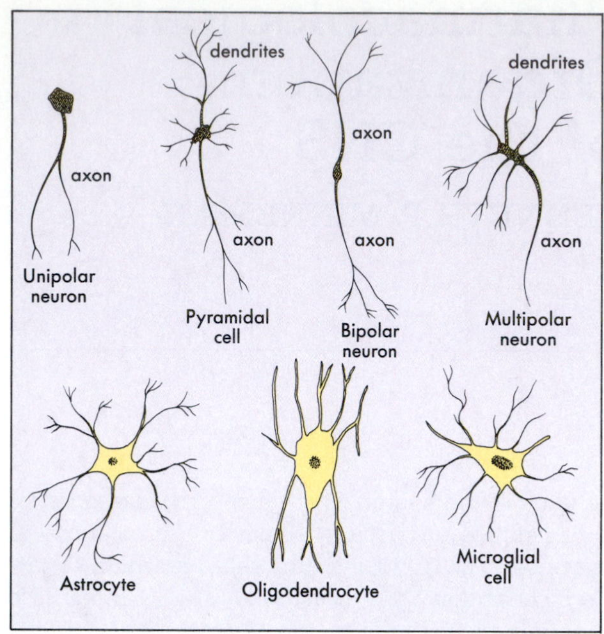

FIGURE 22-1 Types of cells in the CNS: selected examples.

also actively involved in information transfer and integration is increasingly likely.

The glial cells in the CNS are the astrocytes, oligodendrocytes, and microglia (see Figure 22-1). There are at least two main types of **astrocytes,** distinguished by morphology and surface antigens. The main functions of astrocytes appear to be (1) the physical separation of different nerves and nerve pathways from each other, (2) assistance in repairing nerve injury, and (3) modulation of the metabolic and ionic microenvironment of nerve cells. **Oligodendrocytes** generally have fewer and thinner branches than astrocytes and are responsible for formation of the myelin sheath around axons in the CNS. **Microglia** are small cells scattered throughout the nervous system that proliferate after injury or degeneration. These cells move to the site of injury and transform into large macrophages (phagocytes), which remove the debris.

It is tempting to think simplistically of a network of information-processing neurons embedded in a matrix of inert glial cells, much as patterns of semiconductor material are etched on a background of inert substrate in the manufacture of integrated circuits. It is now clear, however, that glial cells help control the environment of neurons and may play an essential role in many of their functions.

Functional Compartmentalization of Neurons

The complex structures of neurons (and to a lesser extent glial cells) indicate that there must be substantial compartmentalization of function, also reflected in a compartmentalization of intracellular organelles (Figure 22-2). The organelles necessary for synthesis of macromolecules and general cell maintenance are mainly in the cell body, though they can also be in dendrites. These include the nucleus, the ribosomes, Nissl substance, endoplasmic reticulum, the Golgi complex, and mitochondria. The axon contains a large number of neurofilaments and microtubules, which also extend into dendrites and cell bodies. These play a major role in transporting substances between the different parts of nerve cells. Dendrites also contain mitochondria for energy production, as well as some neurotransmitter-containing vesicles. The nerve terminals and varicosities are specialized for neurotransmitter release and mainly contain mitochondria and large numbers of synaptic vesicles containing neurotransmitter.

Such anatomical compartmentation has major implications for nerve cell function. The most obvious is the need for transport of macromolecules from their sites of synthesis in the cell body to the specific parts of neurons in which they perform their functions. For example, proteins essential for the function of synaptic vesicles must be synthesized in the ribosomes of the cell body and transported to axon terminals. This is accomplished by the microtubules and neurofilaments extending throughout the neuron in a process called **axonal** or **axoplasmic transport.** Axonal transport can be "slow" (1 mm/day) or "fast" (>100 mm/day). Fast and slow are used in a relative sense here; fast axonal transport could still take many days to transport a substance from the cell body to the end of a long axon. Similar types of transport processes also occur in highly branched dendrites.

Neurons must fire rapidly and repetitively to transmit information, and it is important that supplies of neurotransmitter at the axon terminals be readily replenished. Fast axonal transport is an inefficient way to ensure a constant supply of transmitter in the terminals of a rapidly firing neuron. Neurons circumvent this problem by synthesizing most neurotransmitters locally in the nerve terminals. The major exception to this generalization are peptide neurotransmitters, which require ribosomes for synthesis. The peptides are synthesized as larger precursor molecules in the cell body and must be transported to the axon terminals. This is only one of the fundamental differences between peptide and other neurotransmitters, which will be discussed further.

Another consequence of the complicated morphology of neurons is in their response to incoming signals. Integration of these messages occurs mainly at the **axon hillock.** This is the area where the axon arises from the cell body and where action potentials that will traverse down the axon are generated. Small changes in membrane potential occurring in the distal parts of highly ar-

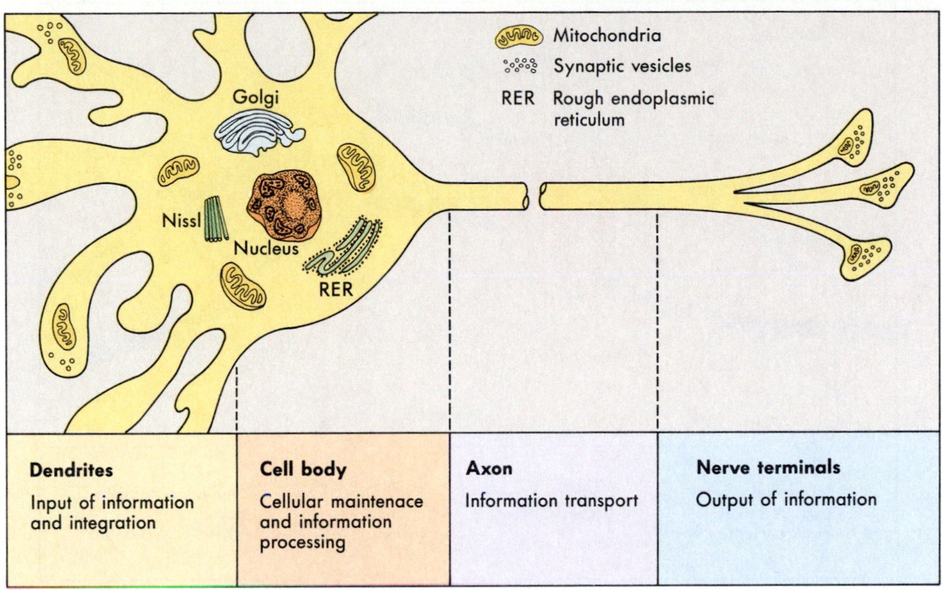

FIGURE 22-2 Structural components of nerve cells.

borized dendrites have a smaller effect on the membrane potential of the axon hillock than have similar changes occurring more proximally. The extensive branching of the dendrites confers a spatial aspect to all incoming signals, which, in addition to the temporal and quantitative aspects of the signal, forms part of the message received by the neuron.

Clearly, neurons are extremely complex cells that have evolved highly specialized subcellular regions for performing specific tasks. The complicated morphology of neurons is an important aspect of their role in the input, processing, and output of information. A neuron by any other shape would probably not function nearly as well.

ELECTRICAL PROPERTIES OF NEURONS

Most information transfer and processing in the CNS is accomplished by alterations in electrical currents flowing across neuronal membranes. It is therefore important to have a firm understanding of how charge differences across nerve cell membranes are controlled.

Pumps, Channels, and the Resting Membrane Potential

Similar to other biological membranes, the membranes of nerve cells are composed of lipid bilayers stabilized by hydrophobic interactions. As such, they present physical barriers to free diffusion of water-soluble molecules between the intracellular and extracellular compartments. The electrical properties of nerve cells are generated by the ability of their surface membranes to control the movement of charged molecules (ions) and to selectively concentrate them on only one side of the membrane. The resulting ion gradients result in a charge difference (voltage) across the membrane, referred to as a potential difference or **membrane potential.** The membrane potential is one of the major mechanisms by which information is stored and processed in the CNS.

There are two classes of protein molecules spanning the cell membrane whose primary functions are to control ion movement. **"Pumps"** actively move charged ions from one side of the membrane to the other, selectively concentrating them against their concentration gradient in a manner that requires energy. **"Channels,"** as described in Chapter 2, are molecular pores in the membrane that allow specific species of ions to pass. Channels can exist in two states—open or closed—although some investigators suggest the existence of a third state in which the channel cannot be activated. Ions generally traverse a channel from high to low concentration. In addition to pumps and channels, there is a constant relatively small permeability of the cell membrane to ions, referred to as the **leak current.**

The relative distribution of three ions, sodium, potassium, and chloride, is the primary determinant of the membrane potential of nerve cells. Although the total concentrations of these three ions are similar, their distribution across the membrane is different. Sodium and chloride are found in high concentration outside the cell, whereas potassium is in high concentration inside the cell. These concentration gradients constantly encour-

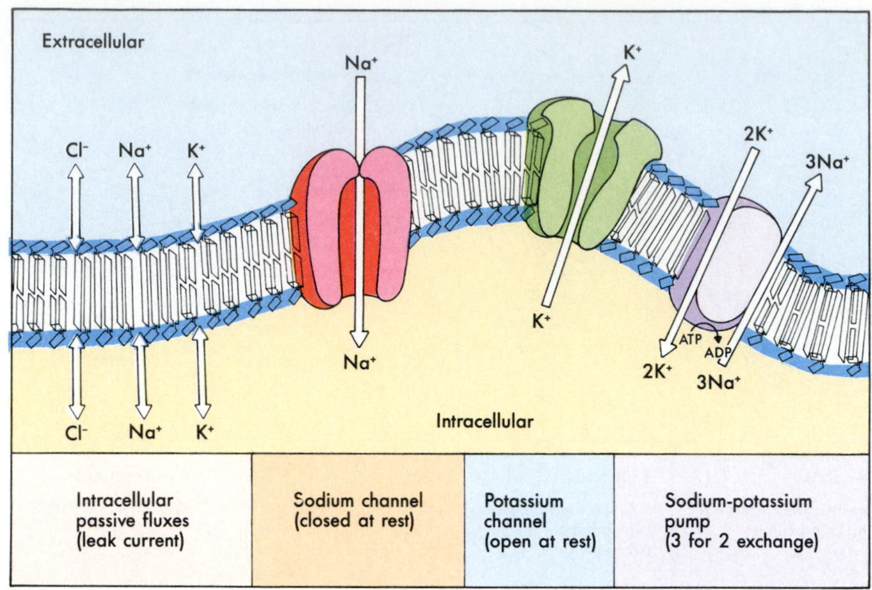

FIGURE 22-3 Primary determinants of resting membrane potential in nerve cells. *ADP,* Adenosine diphosphate.

age sodium to leak into the cell, and potassium to leak out. The gradients are supported by continuous exchange of sodium and potassium by Na^+,K^+-ATPase. This membrane-spanning enzyme pump exchanges three sodium ions from the intracellular fluid for two potassium ions from the extracellular fluid using energy obtained from hydrolysis of adenosine triphosphate (ATP). Because the ions exchanged by this enzyme are positively charged, the activity of this pump generates a small unequal charge distribution across the membrane and sets the stage for the resting membrane potential.

The presence of ion channels selectively permeable to sodium or potassium causes an unequal distribution of charge across the membrane (Figure 22-3). Chloride ions are distributed passively across most nerve cell membranes and contribute little to resting membrane potential, though they can be important in determining electrical responses to incoming signals. At rest, the nerve cell membrane is most permeable to potassium because most sodium channels are closed but many potassium channels are open. Positively charged potassium ions flow down their concentration gradient out of the cell, leaving behind a relative negative charge as a result of the large nonpermeant anionic proteins inside the cell. As the inside of the cell becomes increasingly negative, it is more difficult for a positive charge to leave the cell, and potassium outflow slows. Eventually the concentration gradient and the electrical potential difference balance, and there is no further net ionic movement.

Because potassium is selectively allowed to flow out, the inside of the neuron is negative with respect to the outside. Although this **"resting membrane potential"** is attributable mainly to selective permeability to potassium, some sodium channels are also open at rest. This allows some sodium to enter and reduce the magnitude of the resting membrane potential. In practice, the resting membrane potential of different cells ranges between −90 and −40 mV, depending on the relative activity of various pumps and channels.

Action Potentials

Nerve cells can carry electrical signals over long distances without any loss of signal strength. This is accomplished by the **action potential**—a regenerative, all-or-none phenomenon that actively propagates electrical impulses rapidly down axons to their nerve terminals.

Inputs to nerve cells consist of graded changes in membrane potential caused by the actions of neurotransmitters and modulators. Such "synaptic potentials" are spatially and temporally summated in the cell body. When the strength of these inputs is sufficient to cause a substantial reduction in membrane potential at the base of the axon (axon hillock), an action potential is generated. This is caused by a complex sequence of events initiated by the change in membrane voltage, which is summarized in Figure 22-4.

The primary components in the generation and form of an action potential are ion channels in the cell mem-

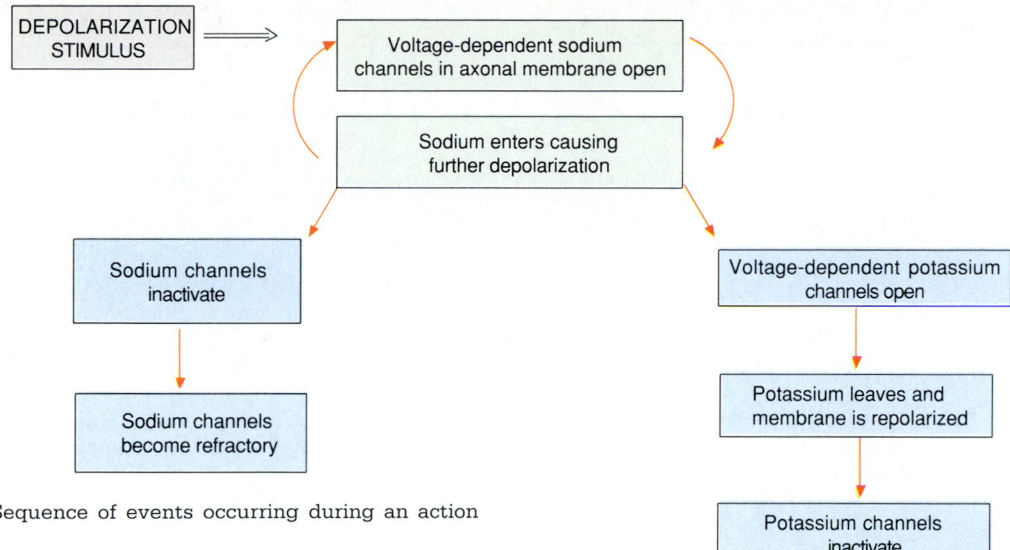

FIGURE 22-4 Sequence of events occurring during an action potential.

brane whose permeability changes when the transmembrane electrical potential is altered. Such channels are called **voltage-dependent,** or **voltage-gated,** as described in Chapter 2, because the change in transmembrane voltage can be thought of as opening or closing a "gate" over the pore.

Initiation of the action potential is caused by opening of voltage-dependent sodium channels at the axon hillock. These channels are usually closed at the normal resting membrane potential, preventing the high concentration of sodium in the extracellular fluid from entering the cell. When the membrane is partially depolarized, these channels open and allow sodium to flow into the cell down its concentration gradient. This influx of positive charge depolarizes the cell further, opening more voltage-dependent sodium channels. This is the self-regenerating part of an action potential because opening sodium channels causes further depolarization, resulting in opening of more sodium channels. These channels are the site of action of local anesthetics that, by blocking sodium influx, prevent regenerative action potentials and conduction of nerve impulses.

If sodium influx continues, the cell becomes completely depolarized. However, sustained depolarization causes an automatic inactivation of the voltage-dependent sodium channels, shutting off sodium influx. The channels not only close, but also become temporarily refractory to reopening. There is also a concurrent but independent opening of voltage-dependent potassium channels, allowing an increased outflow of potassium ions to counterbalance the inflow of sodium ions. Potassium channels become inactivated very slowly and often remain open as long as the membrane is depolarized. Potassium efflux causes the membrane potential to return to its normal resting value when the sodium channels are inactivated.

The temporary inactivation of voltage-dependent sodium channels results in impulse conduction that is unidirectional (Figure 22-5). When the newly opened channels are inactivated and become refractory, they form an effective block to further depolarization. Therefore, depolarization can proceed only in a forward direction, toward resting channels that have not recently been opened. The inactivated refractory channels are eventually returned to their normal resting state and can participate in subsequent action potentials.

The voltage-dependent sodium and potassium channels involved in the action potential are proteins whose structures have recently been determined by gene cloning and sequencing techniques as described in Chapter 2.

Speed of Axonal Conduction

In many situations messages must be sent quickly along long axons. The speed of conduction of the action potential is controlled by the passive spread of changes in membrane potential into adjacent regions of the axon, causing the opening of more voltage-gated sodium channels. This spread of depolarization is the rate-limiting factor in action potential propagation.

One way to increase the speed of conduction of action potentials is to increase the diameter of the axon. Because internal resistance to current flow decreases as the axon diameter increases, axons with a larger diameter conduct impulses more rapidly than those with a smaller diameter. Increasing the axon diameter also causes an increase in the membrane capacitance (abil-

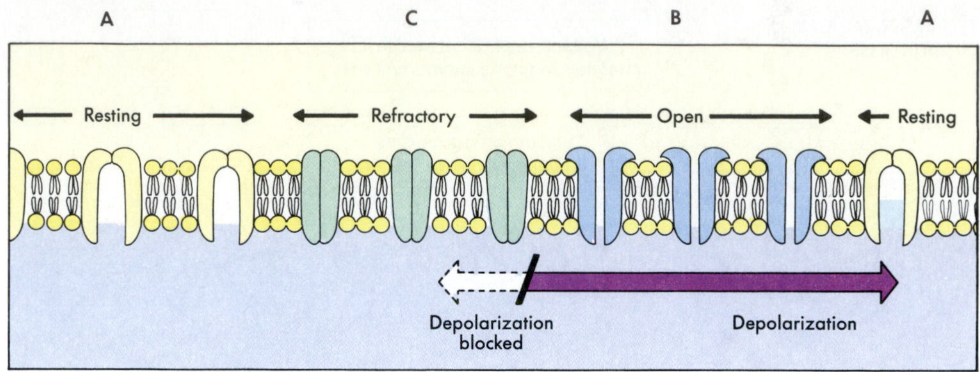

FIGURE 22-5 Unidirectional nature of axonal impulse conduction. Sodium channels are depicted as being in the resting **(A)**, open **(B)**, or refractory **(C)** state. The refractory channels prevent the depolarization from proceeding in more than one direction.

ity to separate and store charge), thus further facilitating the spread of depolarization down the axon.

There are practical limitations to axon size, and myelination also increases the speed of action potential propagation. **Myelination** is the process of wrapping a surface membrane of oligodendrocytes (or Schwann cells in peripheral nerves) around nerve axons in tight concentric layers. The number of layers can be very high (20 to 300) and provides a dramatic increase in membrane resistance to current flow. The myelination is interrupted every 1 to 2 mm by bare stretches of axon, called **nodes of Ranvier.** These nodes contain very high densities of voltage-dependent sodium channels (up to 12,000 per square micrometer), whereas the axon under the myelin contains few, if any, of these channels. The myelin provides a very effective insulator with a high resistance and low capacitance, and current can flow only at the myelin-free nodes of Ranvier. Current, therefore, tends to flow along the fiber to the next node rather than leak back across the membrane. Each node responds with an active regenerative depolarization to the spread of depolarization from the preceding node. The impulse essentially jumps from node to node (Figure 22-6), rapidly speeding up impulse conduction. Such conduction is very efficient; because less active membrane is required, fibers can be smaller, and less energy is required to restore the ionic gradients. Myelination is common in higher organisms, where it plays an important role in facilitating high-speed conduction.

The presence and characteristics of voltage-dependent ion channels make the axon uniquely suited for long-distance transmission of information. The next step to be considered is the transmission of information between neurons and their target cells.

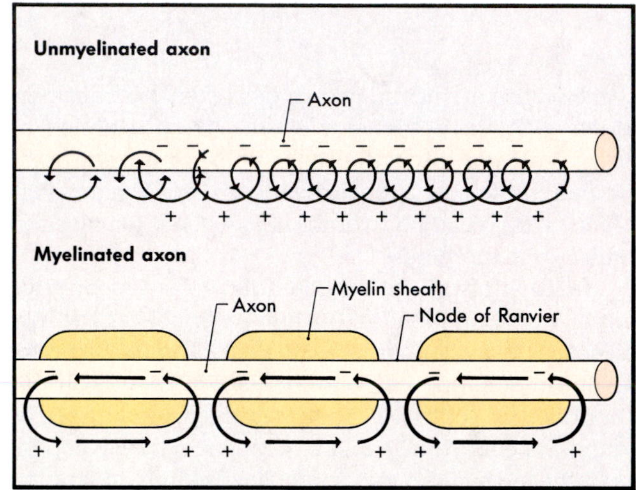

FIGURE 22-6 Spread of current in unmyelinated and myelinated axons.

SYNAPTIC TRANSMISSION

Effective transfer and integration of information in the CNS requires that neurons pass information encoded by action potential frequency to adjacent neurons or other target cells. Because the axon terminal is usually separated from adjacent cells by an intercellular gap of 20 nm or more, there must be some way for the signal to cross this gap. This is usually accomplished by specialized areas of communication around axon terminals, referred to as **synapses.**

Synapses

As the axon approaches its point of termination it exhibits a variety of subcellular specializations, previously

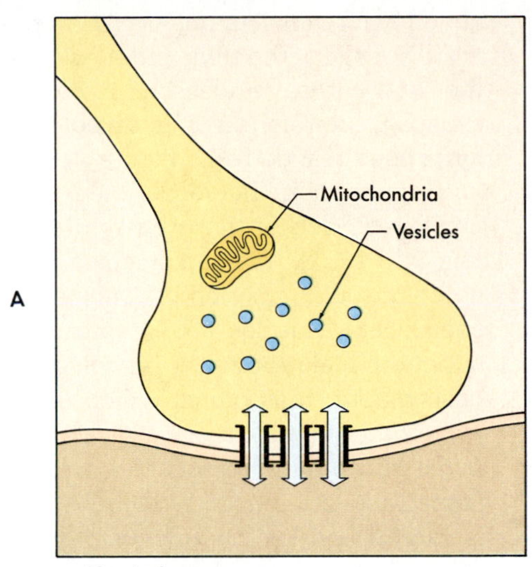

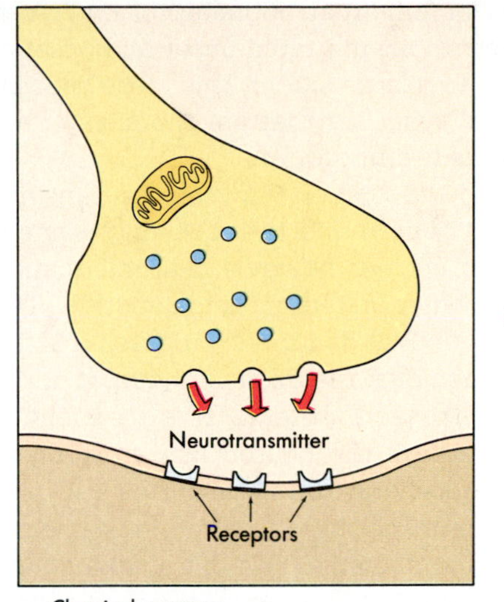

FIGURE 22-7 Electrical and chemical synapses. **A,** Electrical synapses have channels bridging the gap between presynaptic and postsynaptic neurons. These "gap junctions" allow free, bidirectional passage of ions and small molecules. **B,** Chemical synapses do not have gap junctions and rely on chemical mediators to transfer information.

discussed. Most prominent are the appearance of varicosities and synaptic boutons filled with mitochondria and large numbers of synaptic vesicles. These are referred to as **synaptic terminals** because they form the transmitting portion of the synapse. The synaptic terminals usually form a specialized contact zone with the adjacent cell, referred to as the **postsynaptic cell** because it forms the receiving portion of the synapse. It is across this junction, between a synaptic terminal filled with vesicles and a postsynaptic specialization on the adjacent cell, that information must be transmitted.

It was originally believed that the depolarization of the axon terminal might, through passive electrical influences, directly affect the membrane potential of the postsynaptic cell. It rapidly became clear, however, that nerves could also release chemical messengers conveying messages to postsynaptic cells. It is now known that there are two different and apparently unrelated types of synapses: electrical and chemical. Electrical synapses are common in invertebrates and lower vertebrates, and chemical synapses predominate in higher organisms.

A comparison of electrical and chemical synapses is shown in Figure 22-7. In electrical synapses, large protein channels physically bridge the gap between the presynaptic and postsynaptic membrane, thereby connecting the cytosol of the two cells. These channels are similar to the gap junctions often found connecting epithelial cells in the body. They allow free passage of ions and other small molecules from the interior of one cell to the interior of another cell, in either a forward or a reverse direction. When an action potential invades an electrical synapse, the resulting influx of positive charge in the presynaptic terminal can flow directly into the postsynaptic cell and cause a local depolarization in the postsynaptic cell.

The configuration of most synapses in the mammalian CNS indicates that electrical communication is not of prime importance. A very small presynaptic terminal with a high resistance could not deliver enough current to depolarize a large postsynaptic cell, even with essentially no resistance at the synaptic junction. In fact, most synapses in the human brain use chemical messengers to transfer messages across the synaptic junction (see Chapter 2). Depolarization of the presynaptic terminal causes release of a chemical mediator **(neurotransmitter)** into the extracellular fluid between the presynaptic and postsynaptic cells (the **synaptic cleft**). The neurotransmitter then diffuses across the synaptic cleft to act on the postsynaptic cell membrane to deliver its message. The postsynaptic cell must then respond in some appropriate fashion to the received message.

Chemical synapses require a greater degree of specialization than electrical synapses. The presynaptic terminal must have mechanisms for storing neurotransmitters and releasing them in response to a depolarization stimulus. The postsynaptic cell must have receptors for detecting the presence and identity of different neurotransmitters and initiating appropriate changes in cell physiology or metabolism. Finally, there must be efficient mechanisms for formation, degradation, and reuse of neurotransmitters to ensure rapid onset and offset of arriving messages. To a large extent, it is these specializations of chemical synapses that are the sites of action for many centrally acting drugs.

A synapse is the juxtaposition between the transmitting element of one neuron and the receiving element of another neuron. It is clear, however, that information does not pass only from axon terminals to dendrites. The classical concept of input at dendrites, processing in the cell body, transmission over the axon, and output at the presynaptic terminals (see Figure 22-2) is too simplistic. In fact, most parts of the neuron may function in both sending and receiving roles. Dendrites can also store neurotransmitters and release them in response to changes in membrane potential, and therefore function as a "presynaptic" element. Targets for released neurotransmitters include not only dendrites, but also the cell soma, the initial segment of the axon, and the axon terminals. Examples of possible types of synaptic connections between neurons are illustrated in Figure 22-8. Communication from an axon to a dendrite is referred to as an **axodendritic** synapse, from a dendrite to an axon as **dendroaxonic,** and between two axons as **axoaxonic.** Other combinations are possible (Figure 22-8). In some "reciprocal" synapses, there can be impulse traffic in both directions when appropriate synaptic specializations are present.

Other criteria by which synapses can be classified include the distance between the presynaptic terminal and the postsynaptic target (i.e., the distance the released neurotransmitter must diffuse to its site of action). If the terminal is closely apposed to the postsynaptic membrane, the transmitter will be released at its site of action, have little opportunity to diffuse, and thus act on only a small target area. However, if the terminal is farther away, the transmitter will have to diffuse farther and will have access to a wider target area. Such synapses are referred to as **directed** and **nondirected synapses** respectively (Figure 22-9).

The peripheral nervous system contains extreme examples of each of these types of synapses (see Chapters 8 to 11). A directed synapse is exemplified by the neuromuscular junction between somatic motor nerves and skeletal muscles (see Chapter 11). Here, the presynaptic terminal terminates very close (20 to 30 nm) to the postsynaptic membrane, which sends out extensively invaginated ramifications that almost surround the terminal and greatly restrict the diffusion of the released neurotransmitter, acetylcholine. A nondirected synapse is exemplified by the junction between postganglionic sympathetic nerves and their target organs in the autonomic nervous system (see Chapter 10). Here, the neu-

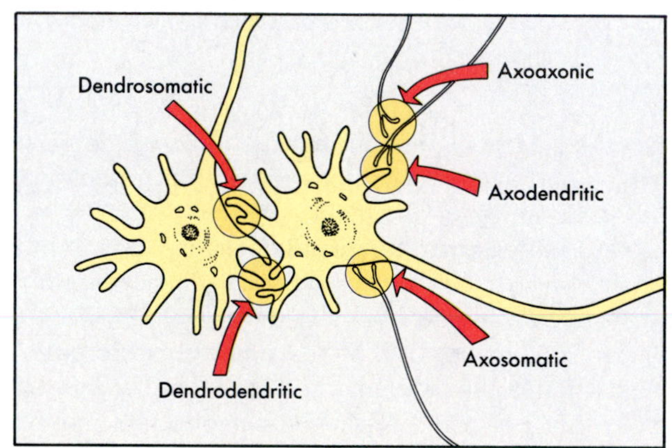

FIGURE 22-8 Types of synaptic connections in the CNS.

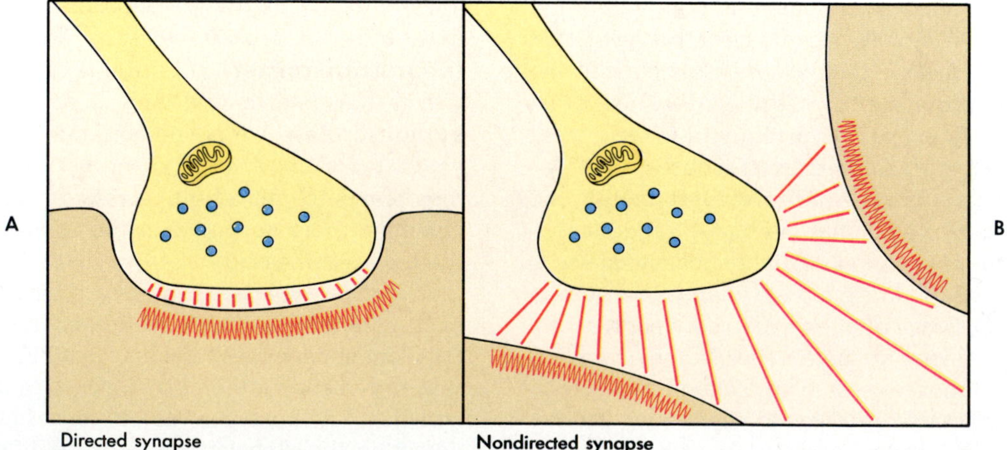

FIGURE 22-9 **A,** In directed synapses, the site of transmitter action is spatially restricted. **B,** In nondirected synapses, the transmitter can diffuse over a much wider target area.

rotransmitter (norepinephrine) is released from varicosities relatively distant (up to 400 nm) from the nearest cell. Few, if any, postsynaptic specializations are observed, and the released neurotransmitter appears to act on a relatively large target area.

Most synapses in the CNS lie somewhere between these two extremes. Synaptic clefts are usually relatively narrow (20 to 30 nm), but there is a large heterogeneity in the postjunctional area and the postsynaptic specializations on the target cells. There are various types of synaptic vesicles in neurons, ranging from 30 to 400 nm diameter, with different shapes and electron densities. Although these different types of vesicles probably contain different types of transmitters, it is not yet possible to determine the neurotransmitter based on the type of vesicles contained in neurons. Clearly, synapses are heterogeneous; however, the functional implications of such heterogeneity have not been determined.

Neurotransmitters

Neurotransmitters are the substances nerve cells use to communicate with each other. Although this is a simple definition, it is remarkable how much disagreement there is over which substances function as neurotransmitters in the CNS. Part of the controversy is caused by the methodological difficulties involved in isolating and identifying neurotransmitter substances. However, there is also substantial discussion about the directedness and specificity of synaptic communication and the types of messages encoded by specific intercellular mediators.

The chemical messengers that are released by cells to send signals to other cells vary between two extremes. Hormones are secreted into the blood, diffuse throughout the body, and act on many different target cells. Neurotransmitters at "directed" synapses are secreted into the extracellular space, act solely on the patch of postsynaptic membrane surrounding the nerve terminal, and are inactivated before they can diffuse further. In such cases, the distinction between hormones and neurotransmitters is obvious.

However, some substances are not easily classified. Antigen-stimulated histamine release from mast cells can be highly localized to the area immediately adjacent to the immune insult. Prostaglandins released locally from platelets may have short-lived effects on nearby vascular smooth muscle contractility before being rapidly inactivated. Similarly, some neurotransmitters have larger or more diverse target areas, such as in the "nondirected" synapses discussed previously. These examples do not fall clearly into hormone or neurotransmitter categories.

The dilemma has no obvious solution. Classification of intracellular messengers is based primarily on the type of cell from which they are released. Neurons secrete neurotransmitters; other cells secrete hormones. Further subclassification might be based on the relative speed, duration, specificity of action, or distance traveled by the released messenger. Neurotransmitters may have highly localized action, neuromodulators slightly larger target areas, and neurohormones diffuse to still more distant sites. However, the net result is that the terms *neurotransmitter, neuromodulator,* and *neurohormone* are used interchangeably. For simplicity, the term *neurotransmitter* is used here to indicate any messenger substance released from neurons, regardless of its specificity or localization of action.

Identification of Neurotransmitters The following common sense criteria are necessary to establish whether a particular substance is responsible for conduction of an impulse across an identified synapse:

1. The suspected neurotransmitter substance must be present in the nerve terminals, and the cell must be capable of making or accumulating the substance and inactivating it
2. The substance must be released on nerve stimulation, and exogenous application of the substance must mimic nerve stimulation
3. Drugs with known effects on enzymes and receptors for the proposed transmitter must affect the nerve-stimulated response in a predictable manner

Unfortunately, it is impossible to fulfill all these criteria for most synapses. Particularly in the CNS, where various heterogenous cells are closely apposed and intermingled, such specific information is often unavailable. Because of these complicating factors, there is little direct information about the identities of the neurotransmitters at the large majority of synapses in the mammalian brain. A few compounds have been unequivocally identified, particularly in the peripheral nervous system. There is also substantial evidence for a large number of other compounds that are believed to play a neurotransmitter role in the brain.

Classes of Neurotransmitters Substances believed to be neurotransmitters at various synapses in the mammalian brain are an extremely heterogeneous group of compounds. They range from the small two-carbon amino acid glycine to large peptides composed of 30 to 40 covalently bonded amino acids (see box), with subclassification on the basis of chemical structure. Examples of structures from each class are shown in Figure 22-10.

Interestingly, neurotransmitters can also be subdivided on the basis of their functional roles in other cells. First, there are the substances that have no other known function in mammalian physiology. These include three of the biogenic amines (acetylcholine, norepinephrine, and dopamine), one amino acid (γ-aminobutyric acid, GABA), and a few of the peptides (e.g., neuropeptide Y, calcitonin-gene–related peptide, and substance P). There is a large second class of substances that function as hormones in other tissues but also serve as neurotransmitters. These include three other biogenic amines (epinephrine, histamine, serotonin) and all the remaining peptides. The third class includes the three remaining amino acids, which are important building blocks in the formation of peptides and proteins (glutamate, glycine, aspartate). Finally, there are the nucleotides (adenosine and ATP) which serve prominent roles in energy metabolism. Clearly, neurons co-opt a variety of compounds to serve as intercellular messengers, involving some unique structures but making use of many compounds with other important functional roles.

It is believed that a single neuron will release the same neurotransmitter from all of its synapses. This concept is based on the assumption that during development some process of differentiation determines the type of neurotransmitter that a given neuron will synthesize, store, and release. This implies that if the identity of a neurotransmitter can be ascertained at one synapse, one can assume that the same neurotransmitter is released at all of the potentially thousands of synapses that neuron might form with different target cells.

Cotransmitters It was assumed for many years that a single neuron would synthesize and release only *one* neurotransmitter. We now know that this is not true. Advances in neurotransmitter localization by immunocytochemical techniques and microchemical analysis of released substances indicate that some neurons can synthesize, store, and release more than one neurotransmitter. As far as we know, however, whichever transmitters are released at one synapse will be released at all synapses made by a single neuron. Although this phenomenon was first identified in developing neurons, it is also observed in an increasing variety of mature, fully differentiated neurons. Two or more proposed neurotransmitter substances are often localized to the same presynaptic terminal, and up to four neuropeptides have been localized to a single neuron.

Two transmitter substances colocalized in a single neuron are shown, in some instances, to be coreleased in response to depolarization of the neuron. In some cases, both substances cause identifiable physiological effects when applied to the postsynaptic cell, though this can be difficult to demonstrate. These observations necessitate major revisions in the classical concept of chemical synaptic transmission. Instead of thinking about a single chemical signal being responsible for transmitting a single message from the presynaptic nerve terminal to the postsynaptic cell, the possibility of multiple signals carrying independent, complementary, or mutually reinforcing messages must be considered. These multiple signals are referred to as **cotransmitters.**

SUBSTANCES BELIEVED TO PLAY A NEUROTRANSMITTER ROLE IN MAMMALIAN BRAIN

BIOGENIC AMINES
acetylcholine
dopamine
norepinephrine
epinephrine
histamine
serotonin

AMINO ACIDS
GABA
glutamate
glycine
aspartate

NUCLEOTIDES AND NUCLEOSIDES
adenosine
ATP

PEPTIDES
carnosine
thyrotropin-releasing hormone
enkephalins
angiotensin II
cholecystokinin
oxytocin
vasopressin
bradykinin
dynorphin
luteinizing hormone-releasing hormone
substance P
substance K
neurotensin
α-melanocyte stimulating hormone
bombesin
somatostatin
secretin
vasoactive intestinal peptide
β-endorphin
glucagon
calcitonin-gene–related peptide
neuropeptide Y
adrenocorticotropic hormone (ACTH)
corticotropin-releasing factor
insulin

Several ramifications to the concept of cotransmitters have implications for pharmacology. Would the cotransmitters be stored in the same, or different, vesicles? If they are stored in different vesicles, one transmitter could be released preferentially in response to low-frequency nerve impulses, whereas the other could require a higher frequency to cause release (Figure 22-11). The two substances might then convey different messages to the postsynaptic cell. In fact, supposed cotransmitters are sometimes found stored in separate vesicles and sometimes in the same vesicles, an indication that both types of situations may exist in the brain.

There are similar questions about the targets of the

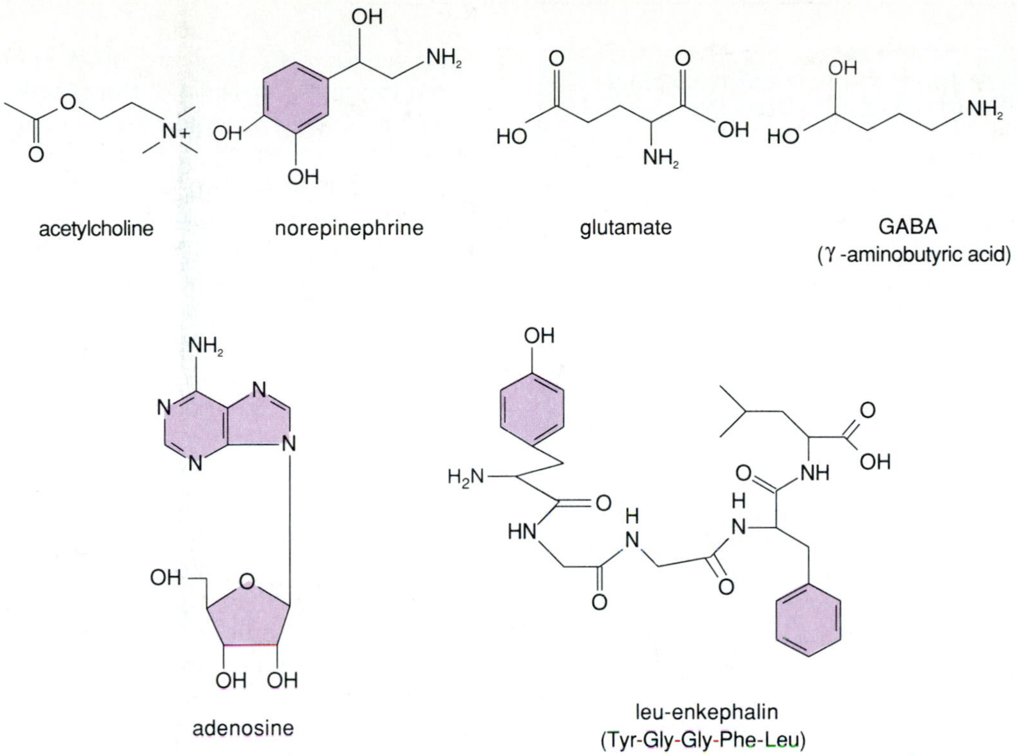

OH
NH_2
O
O
OH
NH_2
O
N+
OH
HO
OH
HO
O
OH
NH_2
acetylcholine
norepinephrine
glutamate
GABA
(γ -aminobutyric acid)
NH_2
OH
N
N
N
N
O
H_2N
O
NH
OH
O
H
HN
H
N
N
OH
O
O
O
OH OH
adenosine
leu-enkephalin
(Tyr-Gly-Gly-Phe-Leu)

FIGURE 22-10 Structures of selected neurotransmitter candidates.

Stimulation
frequency
Separate
storage
vesicles
Co-stored
in same
vesicles

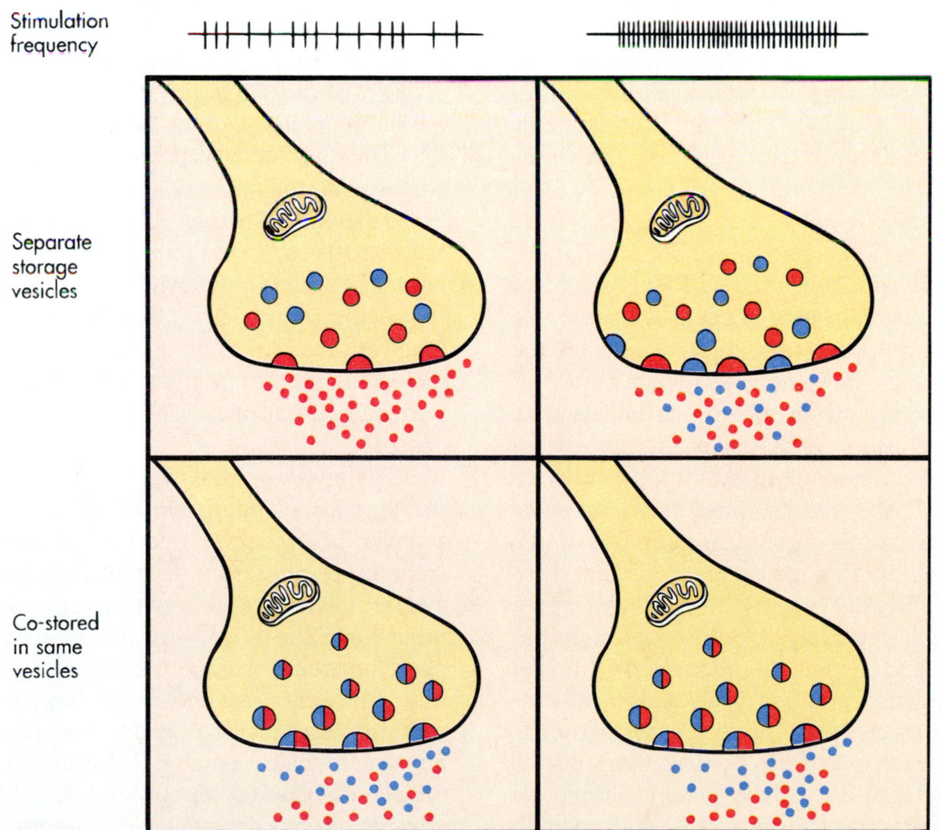

FIGURE 22-11 Release patterns for cotransmitters stored in the same or different vesicles. Notice that the frequency of release will be the same if the two substances are stored in the same vesicles but can be different if they are stored in different vesicles.

COEXISTENCE OF NEUROTRANSMITTERS (FOUND EXPERIMENTALLY)

acetylcholine/vasoactive intestinal peptide
acetylcholine/substance P
norepinephrine/somatostatin
norepinephrine/enkephalins
norepinephrine/neurotensin
norepinephrine/neuropeptide Y
norepinephrine/ATP
dopamine/cholecystokinin
dopamine/neurotensin
epinephrine/neuropeptide Y
epinephrine/enkephalin
epinephrine/neurotensin
serotonin/substance P
serotonin/thyrotropin-releasing hormone
serotonin/enkephalin
vasopressin/cholecystokinin
vasopressin/dynorphin
oxytocin/enkephalin

cotransmitters. In a directed synapse, one might expect that both substances would be directed to the same restricted postsynaptic target area. However, in a less-directed synapse, each substance might have an anatomically distinct target. One substance might transfer messages to adjacent neurons, while the other controls local metabolic processes and activities of nearby glial cells.

Analysis of the presence of cotransmitters in a wide variety of individual neurons discloses a definite pattern (see box). With few exceptions, one member of each pair of cotransmitters appears to be a peptide. This fact and several unique features of neuropeptides indicate the possibility that the large variety of peptides in nerve terminals may not be neurotransmitters in the classical sense, that is, transmitting messages to the postsynaptic cell based on the frequency of action potentials arriving from the cell body. Rather, they may play some more subtle, long-term role in such information transfer, possibly enhancing the message of another "primary" transmitter.

Several features of peptides seem to make them unsuitable for rapid and reversible information transfer known to occur between neurons. First and most obvious, peptides cannot be synthesized locally in the region in which they are released because there are no ribosomes in nerve terminals. This prevents rapid replenishment of peptide transmitters and would seem to be an inefficient mechanism for providing transmitter to the nerve terminals. Second, peptides are usually at least 1000 times more potent in causing effects on postsynaptic cells than are other transmitters. This raises the question whether the effects of such potent compounds could be rapidly reversed. In fact, the effects of peptides are usually much longer lasting and much more difficult to reverse than are the effects of other transmitter substances. So far, it is difficult to identify specific and rapid mechanisms for terminating the actions of peptides after synaptic release, and it appears that simple diffusion from the site of action plays a major role (see below). This also argues against a role in rapid synaptic communication.

All these considerations raise the question as to whether peptides are really neurotransmitters. Many of the established criteria for neurotransmitters are met by some peptides, but no peptide has met them all for a given synapse. On the other hand, several other transmitters (including acetylcholine, norepinephrine, GABA, and glutamate) fulfill all the criteria necessary to be regarded as neurotransmitters at particular synapses.

In considering the possibility of cotransmitters, however, the criteria for identification of neurotransmitters must be revised. Obviously, if a neuron is releasing more than one neurotransmitter, the application of a single substance cannot be expected to mimic the postsynaptic effects of nerve stimulation. Rather it is necessary to isolate and apply all the substances released by the neuron at the same time. Similarly, pharmacological modification of the effects of a single substance might not have the same effect on the response to nerve stimulation because other substances might also be released that would cancel out the pharmacological intervention.

Synthesis, Storage, and Inactivation of Neurotransmitters Several centrally acting drugs exert their effects by altering the synthesis, storage, or inactivation of specific neurotransmitters. Although the mechanisms involved are almost as varied as the diverse types of molecules that function as neurotransmitters, a few important generalizations can be made about these processes.

The nerve terminal must be able to rapidly replenish its supplies of neurotransmitter to enable continuous transfer of incoming information across the synaptic cleft, even after high-frequency stimulation. The enzymes necessary for synthesizing neurotransmitters must be made on the ribosomes in the cell body and are then transported and concentrated in nerve terminals. The precursor molecules from which neurotransmitters are made are usually common molecules such as amino acids, sugars, and nucleotides, which are widely distributed throughout the body. These substances are readily available to nerve terminals and are often actively concentrated there to facilitate transmitter synthesis. Finally, the neurotransmitter itself or one of its major breakdown products is often effectively recaptured after release, thus allowing efficient reutilization of the available raw material. The major exception to these generalizations are the peptides, as discussed previously.

To ensure accurate transfer of information across the synapse, neurons have complex mechanisms for regulating the synthesis and concentrations of neurotransmitter within the nerve terminal. Synthesis of neurotransmitters is controlled by the amount and activity of enzymes of synthesis, the availability of substrates, and the presence of catalytic cofactors necessary for optimal enzyme activity. One of these three factors is usually responsible for controlling the synthesis of a single type of transmitter. Synthesis of acetylcholine is regulated mainly by the availability of the substrate choline. On the other hand, synthesis of norepinephrine is regulated mainly by the activity of the first (of four) enzymes in the synthetic pathway, tyrosine hydroxylase (see Chapters 8 and 10).

Most neurotransmitters are stored in the synaptic vesicles, which are prominent features of nerve terminals. Concentration into vesicles appears to be responsible for maintaining a ready supply of transmitter in a convenient ready-to-use packet and for protecting transmitters from breakdown by intracellular enzymes. These vesicular packets are then available for exocytotic release. Recent discussion includes the possibility of nonvesicular release of some neurotransmitters (see Chapter 9) (possibly by opening of channels in the terminal membrane). However, there is good evidence that vesicles are actively involved in storage and release of most transmitters, and the vesicle hypothesis is still generally accepted.

After release, the transmitter acts on its target to cause a response. To ensure reversibility of action and allow for further information transfer across the synapse, the transmitter must be rapidly inactivated. The two highly effective ways of terminating the actions of neurotransmitters are (1) rapid enzymatic breakdown by extracellular degradative enzymes in the synaptic cleft and (2) rapid reuptake into the nerve terminal by specific, high-affinity pumps in the plasma membrane. Both mechanisms provide rapid and efficient termination of transmitter action. An effective but much slower way of terminating the action of transmitter is by simple diffusion from the site of action. Diffusion is more effective in nondirected synapses than in highly directed synapses because diffusion in directed synapses is greatly reduced by morphological barriers. Transmitter can also be removed by nonspecific absorption into tissues (i.e., partitioning into neuronal or glial structures caused by the chemical properties of the transmitter—without involvement of specific energy-requiring uptake pumps). This process, though effective, can be slow. If a released transmitter persists in the synapse for a long time, a new signal cannot get through. Therefore, the slow processes of diffusion and nonspecific uptake are believed to be generally less important methods of transmitter inactivation than are the more rapid processes of degradation and active reuptake.

Released neurotransmitters are usually reused in some form. This helps replenish transmitter concentrations and prevents local depletion of substrates or cofactors in nerve terminals. The most efficient mechanism is the rapid reuptake of the neurotransmitter itself and subsequent reuptake into synaptic vesicles. Norepinephrine and dopamine appear to be directly reused in this efficient manner, removing the necessity for further synthesis and reducing the amount of energy required. Other transmitters are degraded by enzymes in the synaptic cleft and the breakdown products are subsequently reused for further transmitter synthesis. For example, acetylcholine is hydrolyzed into choline and acetate in the synaptic cleft, and the choline is actively reconcentrated into the cell.

Information on the synthesis, storage, and degradation of many of the heterogeneous group of compounds serving as neurotransmitters in the brain (see box) is presented in the chapters in this section and in Chapter 8 for acetylcholine and norepinephrine. However, some differences in neurotransmitter life cycles are illustrated schematically in Figure 22-12, using acetylcholine, norepinephrine, GABA, and a peptide transmitter as representative examples. The major differences include the following:

1. Synthesis in the cell soma (peptide), nerve terminal cytosol (acetylcholine, GABA), or vesicle (norepinephrine)
2. Uptake of transmitter (acetylcholine, GABA, peptide) or precursor (norepinephrine) into vesicles
3. Inactivation by enzymatic hydrolysis (acetylcholine), active reuptake (norepinephrine), nonspecific uptake (GABA), or diffusion (peptide)
4. Reuse of transmitter (norepinephrine, GABA) or hydrolysis product (acetylcholine), or neither (peptide) for further transmitter synthesis
5. Control of synthesis by substrate availability (acetylcholine) or enzyme activity (norepinephrine, GABA, peptide)

Release of Neurotransmitters The arrival of an action potential at a nerve terminal causes a depolarization of the terminal membrane, resulting in exocytotic release of neurotransmitter from synaptic vesicles.

Calcium provides the essential link between depolarization and transmitter release. Calcium therefore must be added to the list of ions (sodium, potassium, and chloride) that are critical to the function of neurons. However, calcium often plays a fundamentally different

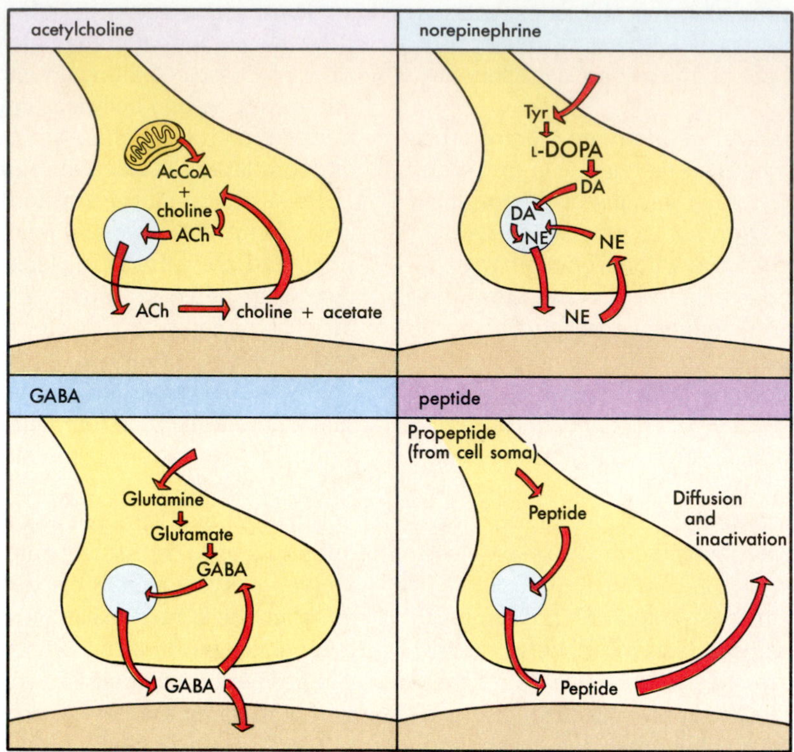

FIGURE 22-12 Synthesis, inactivation, and reutilization of selected neurotransmitters. *AcCoA,* Acetyl coenzyme A; *ACh,* Acetylcholine *DA,* dopamine; *GABA,* γ-aminobutyric acid; *NE,* norepinephrine; *Tyr,* tyrosine.

role from that of the other three ions, which function mainly as charge carriers. Although calcium can also function as an important charge carrier (i.e., in cardiac action potentials), it plays a more important role in regulating metabolic activity. The reason is that the total concentration of calcium in the central nervous system (1 to 2 mM), is much lower than that of either sodium, potassium, or chloride (100 to 150 mM). The latter are therefore more likely to contribute significantly to total charge distribution.

Similar to that of sodium, the concentration of calcium is much higher in the extracellular fluid surrounding neurons than in the cytoplasm. This gradient is maintained by continuous extrusion of calcium by energy-requiring pumps in the plasma membrane and also by active sequestration of calcium by intracellular organelles, particularly the mitochondria. The net result is a calcium concentration gradient substantially larger than that of sodium and potassium, a concentration about 10,000 times higher in the extracellular than in the intracellular fluid.

When the resting membrane of the nerve terminal is depolarized by arrival of an action potential, there is a large influx of free calcium. This is caused by the opening of voltage-dependent calcium channels concentrated in the membrane of the nerve terminal. At the normal resting potential, the channels are mainly closed and impermeable to calcium; however, depolarization causes them to open (probably by some rearrangement of charge in the channel protein, as with sodium channels). When open, they selectively permit passage of calcium down its concentration gradient into the cell.

The influx of calcium into the nerve terminal initiates processes that result in exocytosis of synaptic vesicles and release of neurotransmitters. However, the molecular mechanisms by which calcium influx promotes exocytosis of synaptic vesicles are poorly understood. The increase in intraterminal calcium probably alters the conformation of certain enzymes or structural proteins in the synaptic vesicle or the plasma membrane, which eventually causes fusion of these two structures.

After exocytosis, the terminal must decrease the high concentration of calcium to prevent continued release of neurotransmitter and allow incoming signals to initiate additional transmitter release. This is accomplished by inactivation of the voltage-dependent calcium channels in response to continued depolarization. After the channels close, the active processes normally responsible for keeping calcium concentrations low within the cell again come into play.

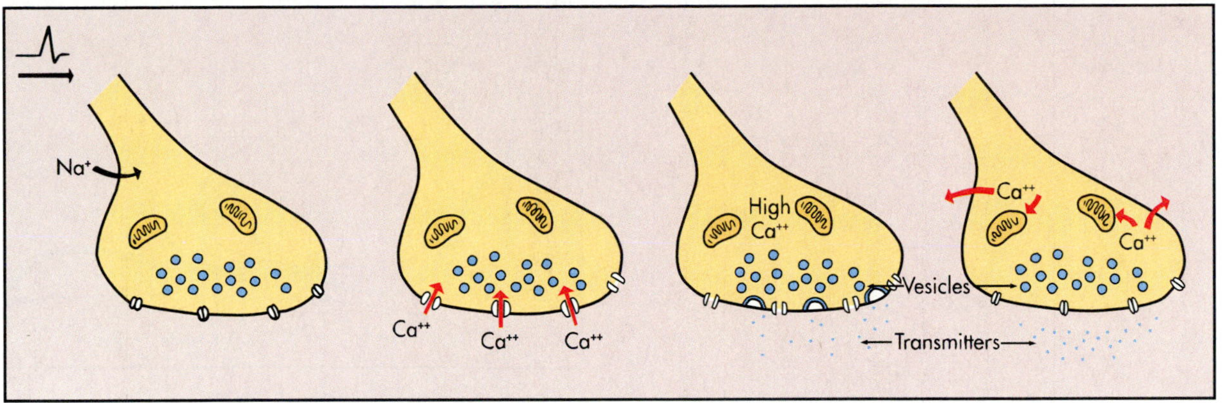

FIGURE 22-13 Sequence of events linking depolarization of a nerve terminal to release of neurotransmitter. **A,** Action potential arrives at nerve terminal and depolarizes resting membrane potential. **B,** Voltage-gated calcium channels open, allowing influx of calcium down the concentration gradient. **C,** The increased intracellular calcium promotes fusion of transmitter-containing synaptic vesicles with plasma membrane, resulting in exocytosis of vesicular contents. **D,** Calcium channels rapidly inactivate and the intracellular calcium is returned to normal by sequestration into mitochondria and active extrusion from the cell.

The steps linking arrival of an action potential to neurotransmitter release from nerve terminals are summarized in Figure 22-13. It is important to understand that voltage-dependent calcium channels in nerve terminals are different from those in other tissues. The calcium-channel antagonists are an important class of drugs whose primary mechanism of action is a use-dependent blockade of voltage-dependent calcium channels in cardiac and smooth muscle (see Chapter 16). However, there are distinct subtypes of these channels that can be distinguished by their electrical and pharmacological properties. The calcium-channel antagonists that effectively block the channels most often found in cardiac and smooth muscle (L type) have no effect on most of the voltage-dependent calcium channels found in nerve terminals (N type). This is fortunate because if calcium-channel antagonists also blocked neurotransmitter release, their toxicity would undoubtedly prevent them from being therapeutically useful.

POSTSYNAPTIC ACTIONS OF NEUROTRANSMITTERS

When released, neurotransmitters are effective only if they interact with receptors on their target cells. The specificity of neuronal interactions is based on the type of transmitter released and on the types of receptors that are present for the transmitter to activate.

Receptors

Receptors are the sensors by which cells detect incoming messages. Progress has been made in the identification and characterization of neurotransmitter receptors over the past two decades, as discussed in detail in Chapters 2 and 34. Here, emphasis is placed on the functional actions and interactions of receptors that are of special interest to the CNS.

Receptors have highly specialized recognition sites with rigid structural requirements for binding transmitter. They usually bind only one type of transmitter, though other natural and synthetic substances also may bind to the receptor with high affinity. Because they are recognition molecules, receptors are named by the type of neurotransmitter that activates them. Although most receptors recognize only a single transmitter, each transmitter can activate more than one subtype of receptor. As more specific and selective drugs are developed, it becomes clear that each transmitter probably acts on a (sometimes large) family of different receptor subtypes.

The rank order of potencies of a series of structurally diverse compounds for activating a receptor (agonists) or inhibiting the response to receptor activation (antagonists) is considered to be diagnostic of the receptor subtype. If a receptor in another cell or tissue shows a similar order of potencies, it is probably of the same subtype. However, if the order of potencies is different, the subtypes must be different. As more and more

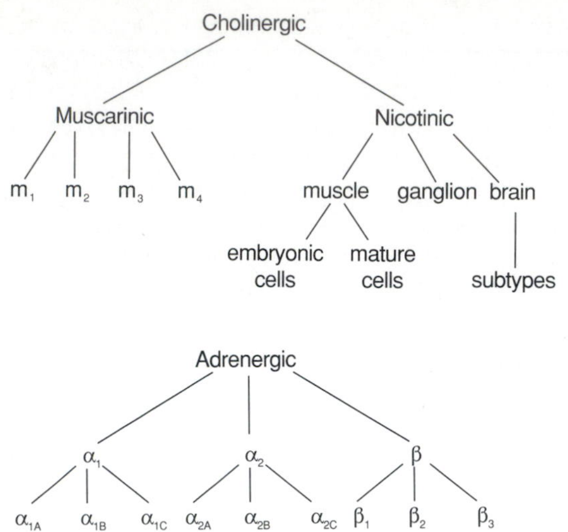

FIGURE 22-14 Families of cholinergic and adrenergic receptors.

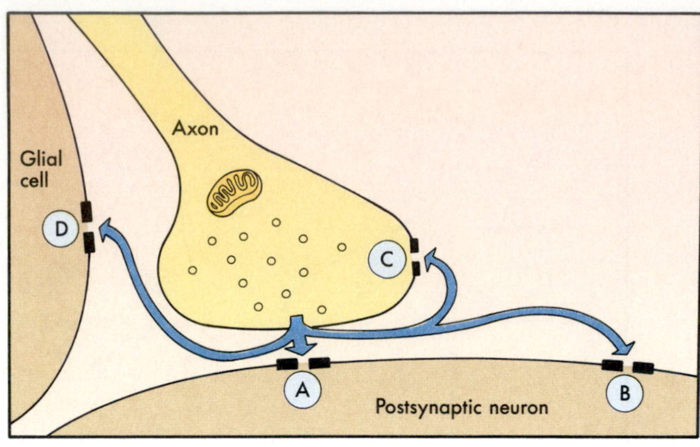

FIGURE 22-15 Potential targets for transmitter released from nerve terminal. Transmitter can activate receptors on a postsynaptic cell adjacent to the release site *(A)* or at some distance away *(B)*, on its own presynaptic nerve terminal *(C)*, or on adjacent neurons or glial cells *(D)*.-

closely related subtypes are distinguished, the differences between their binding properties sometimes become very subtle and difficult to distinguish. There is no uniform nomenclature for receptor subtypes. Each of the subtypes can often be further subdivided. For example, there are at least eight subtypes of cholinergic and nine subtypes of adrenergic receptors identified so far (Figure 22-14).

Localization and Coexistence of Receptor Subtypes

The presence or absence of appropriate receptors determines whether a particular cell or area of cell membrane responds to transmitter. Neurotransmitter receptors are almost always located in the external plasma membrane, ensuring rapid onset of incoming messages, as well as rapid removal of transmitter. This allows rapid and repetitive information transfer.

In some directed synapses such as the neuromuscular junction, receptors are highly clustered in the areas of postsynaptic membrane surrounding the nerve terminal. This is unusual, however, and receptors are usually less highly localized. In neurons, receptors are often diffusely spread over the dendrites, cell soma, and axon terminals. Functional receptors on axons removed from cell bodies or nerve terminals have not been demonstrated, though receptor molecules undergoing transport to nerve terminals can be identified in axons. Receptors are also commonly found on glial cells, an indication that these cells also respond to released neurotransmitters.

Thus transmitter released from a nerve terminal can have several targets (Figure 22-15). It obviously can act on the immediately adjacent postsynaptic membrane. However, depending on its rate of inactivation it can also diffuse relatively far from the synapse and act on an "extrasynaptic" area of the cell, or of adjacent neurons or glial cells. In addition, many transmitters also activate receptors on the nerve terminals from which they are released. These are called **autoreceptors** because they respond to the transmitter released from the cell on which they are located. Activation of autoreceptors provides feedback about the quantity of transmitter in the synaptic cleft and regulates further synthesis and release of transmitter.

Many different types of receptors can coexist on a single cell. This includes multiple receptors for different transmitters, as well as multiple subtypes of receptors for a single transmitter. The types of receptors on particular neurons or glial cells obviously is determined by which receptor genes are expressed by that cell. This is another of the differentiated characteristics of brain cells, which, as usual, is highly variable but has important implications for neurotransmitter actions.

Responses to Receptor Activation

The response of a particular neuron to released neurotransmitter depends as much on the type of receptors available as on the type of transmitter released. It is important to realize that *a given neurotransmitter does not always cause the same postsynaptic effect.* An example of this is found in the peripheral nervous system, where neuronally released acetylcholine causes relaxation of cardiac muscle and contraction of skeletal muscle through different receptor subtypes. Similarly, release of a given transmitter in the CNS can cause different postsynaptic effects, depending on the type of receptors available for it to activate.

Receptors initiate signals in neuronal and glial cells by the types of signal transduction mechanisms outlined in Chapters 2 and 34. In the CNS, however, the most important signal transduction mechanisms are those occurring in the external cell membrane. Thus the primary effect of receptor activation is usually a direct influence on an ion channel or activation of one of the large family of guanine nucleotide regulatory proteins (G proteins) (see Chapter 2). Ion channels controlled directly by transmitters are usually referred to as **chemically gated (or ligand-gated) channels** because the channel permeability is altered by direct binding of the transmitter to the channel protein. Activation of different G proteins may activate specific ion channels or, more generally, alter the activity of a membrane-bound enzyme that synthesizes or releases a second messenger inside the cell (cyclic adenosine 3′, 5′ monophosphate [cAMP], inositol trisphosphate, diacylglycerol, and arachidonic acid). These second messengers produce metabolic effects on the cell, prominent among which are activation of protein phosphorylation by protein kinase activation and release of intracellular calcium.

Because much information in the nervous system is encoded electrically, released transmitters usually alter the membrane potential of their postsynaptic targets. These local alterations in membrane potential are called **synaptic potentials.** It is obvious how activation of chemically gated channels, where the channel is an integral part of the receptor protein, can produce synaptic potentials. However, the mechanisms by which activation of receptors linked to G proteins can produce synaptic potentials are less intuitively evident because channels that are not part of the receptor protein may be involved. The general mechanisms by which receptor activation can result in synaptic potentials are diagrammed schematically in Figure 22-16. Regardless of the intermediary steps, receptor activation eventually alters charge distribution across the membrane by altering ion-channel permeability.

Comparison of the direct and relatively circuitous routes by which receptor activation can alter permeability of ion channels in the nervous system (Figure 22-16) raises another interesting aspect of transmitter action. This is the speed with which the signal is initiated and terminated. Opening of channels in response to direct binding of transmitters on the channel molecule is clearly much faster than the cascade of events including G protein activation, enzyme activation, formation of a second messenger, protein kinase activation, and phosphorylation of a channel. It is consequently suggested that receptors mediating synaptic responses can be divided into two general classes based on the time latency of their synaptic potentials. Chemically gated channels would be responsible for "fast" information transfer, whereas receptors stimulating second messenger formation would take longer to initiate signals. Termination of the signals is also different. Chemically gated channels rapidly close when transmitter is removed, whereas the biochemical events caused by activation of G protein–linked receptors might persist for substantially longer periods after removal of transmitter. Figure 22-16 also shows that the number of intermediate reactions linking G-protein activation to channel permeability alterations varies greatly with different transduction mechanisms, an indication that responses should not be classified as simply fast or slow, but with various gradations of latency.

As previously mentioned, the availability of specific receptors determines the type and magnitude of response caused by release of a given transmitter. Because each transmitter can activate a family of different receptors associated with distinct signal transduction mechanisms, a single transmitter may cause completely different effects on different cells. Figure 22-17 illustrates one example. Acetylcholine causes depolarization of the resting membrane potential in one cell through activation of nicotinic receptors gating sodium influx. In a separate cell, acetylcholine causes hyperpolarization through activation of muscarinic receptors gating a potassium channel through an intermediary G protein. Thus a synaptic connection cannot be classified as excitatory or inhibitory based solely on the identity of the released transmitter but must include the type of receptor that it activates.

The situation is complicated further by the fact that multiple receptor subtypes for one transmitter can coexist on a single cell. This raises the possibility that one transmitter can deliver multiple messages to the same cell. These messages may be opposing, complementary, or independent. For example, in Figure 22-18 various combinations of adrenergic receptors can be present on the same cell. The β_1 subtype activates adenylate cyclase through a G protein (G_s). Because the α_2 subtype inhibits adenylate cyclase through a different G protein (G_i), the presence of both subtypes will result in mutually antagonistic signals caused by the neurotransmitter norepinephrine. In a like manner, additive signals can be generated by the copresence of the β_2 subtype, which also activates adenylate cyclase through G_s, or independent signals can be generated by the copresence of the α_1 subtype which activates phospholipase C (see Figure 22-18). Obviously, the response of a cell to a single transmitter depends on the types and relative proportions of receptor subtypes present in the target membrane.

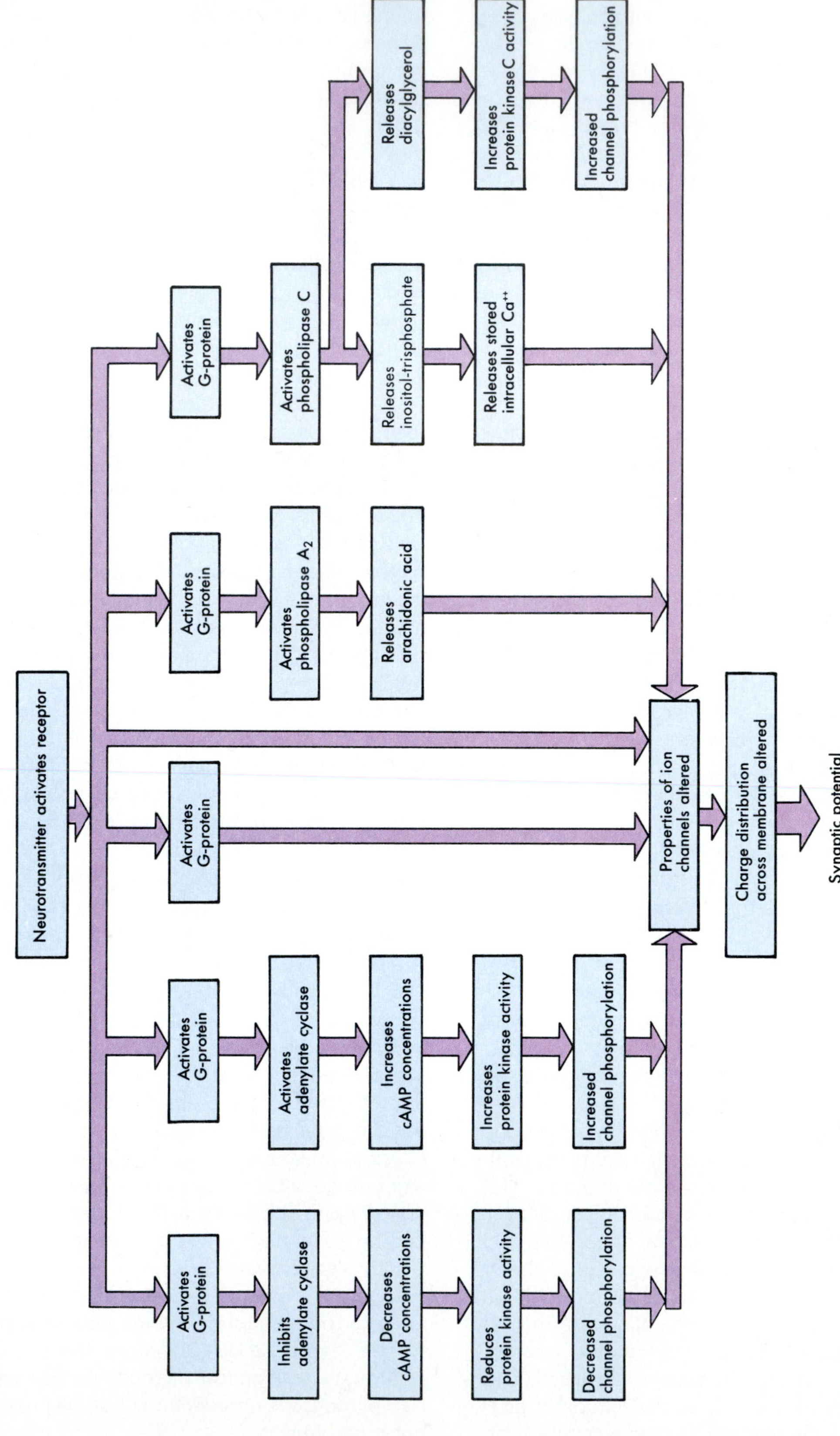

FIGURE 22-16 Mechanisms by which transmitter-receptor interactions can result in synaptic potentials. Ion channels may be of two types: (1) those that are part of the receptor protein and activated by chemical gating and (2) those that are located elsewhere and activated through G proteins.

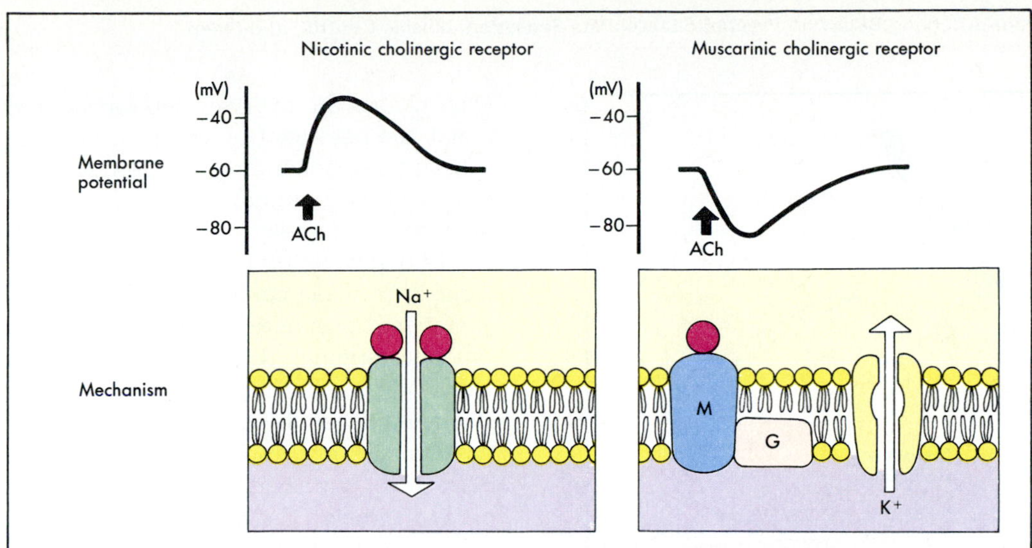

FIGURE 22-17 Activation of different receptors by acetylcholine can cause opposite effects on resting membrane potential. Activation of the nicotinic subtype *(left)* opens a chemically gated channel to allow sodium to enter and depolarize the cell. Activation of the muscarinic subtype *(right)* activates a G protein, which in turn opens a potassium channel, leading to potassium efflux and hyperpolarization of the cell.

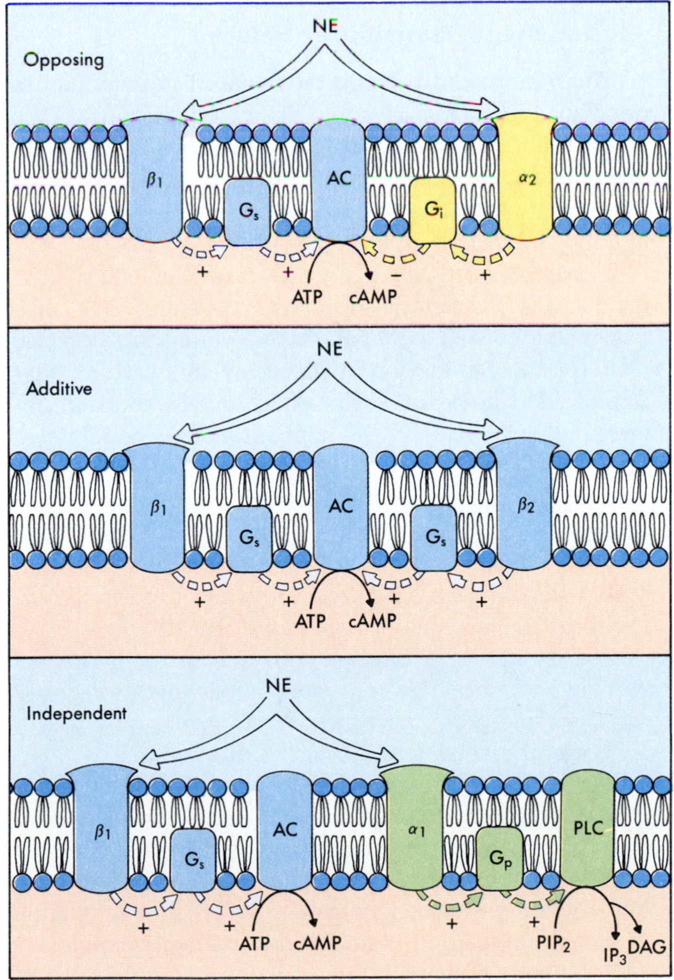

FIGURE 22-18 Activation of multiple receptors by a single transmitter: effects on signal transduction. Coactivation of more than one receptor subtype for norepinephrine can result in second-messenger responses, which are opposing, additive, or independent. G proteins shown for stimulatory (G_s), inhibitory (G_i), and phospholipase (G_p) NE, norepinephrine; *AC,* Adenylate cyclase; *ATP,* adenosine triphosphate; *cAMP,* cyclic adenosine monophosphate; *PLC,* phospholipase C. *PIP_2,* phosphatidylinositol 4,5-bisphosphate; *IP_3* inositol 1,4,5-trisphosphate; *DAG,* 1,2-diacylglycerol.

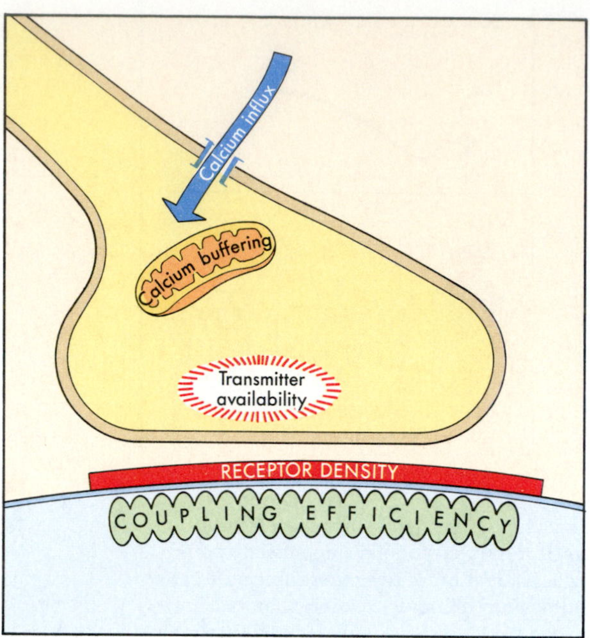

FIGURE 22-19 Major factors controlling efficiency of synaptic transmission.

Similar situations can arise when different types of transmitters act on specific receptors in the same cell. Incoming messages may be opposing, complementary, or independent, and each released transmitter can cause excitatory or inhibitory potentials, or both, depending on the receptors present. The function of the neuron is to integrate all these multiple messages, from a single transmitter or from multiple transmitters, to control the impulse activity of its own axon.

ALTERATIONS IN SYNAPTIC EFFICIENCY

The information output of a neuron is encoded in the rate at which it initiates action potentials at the axon hillock. Because action potentials are an all-or-none phenomenon, their quantitative and temporal characteristics usually do not vary. Degree of depolarization and length of time necessary for repolarization are similar for all action potentials in a particular axon. Therefore a uniform depolarization may cause a uniform release of neurotransmitter quanta, and activation of a given terminal may always result in the same postsynaptic response. In this case, a particular synapse could be thought of as a simple on/off circuit, like a switch. The terminal could be either active or inactive, but when active it would always send the same message to the postsynaptic cell.

However, this is not the case. The strength of a synaptic connection is not uniform and can be altered by a variety of mechanisms. Although an action potential always causes an invariant depolarization of a nerve terminal, the net effect on the postsynaptic cell can vary substantially depending on the recent and long-term history of the terminal. In fact, a nerve terminal might be more accurately compared to a rheostat than a simple on/off switch because its output is continuously variable between certain upper and lower limits. Such alterations in synaptic efficiency can occur in either the synaptic terminal, the postsynaptic cell, or both, by a variety of mechanisms. The most important of these are illustrated schematically in Figure 22-19. In the synaptic terminal, alterations in depolarization-evoked calcium influx, intracellular buffering of calcium, or transmitter synthesis and availability can result in changes in the amount of neurotransmitter released by nerve terminal depolarization. On the postsynaptic side, changes in receptor density or coupling efficiency can alter the response to a given concentration of released transmitter. These modifications may form the cellular basis of learning and memory and also play an important role in the tolerance and dependence that are observed on chronic administration of many centrally acting drugs.

Alterations in Transmitter Release

The quantity of transmitter released in response to depolarization is mainly controlled by two factors: (1) the concentration of intracellular calcium and (2) the availability of transmitter. Each of these is carefully regulated by the neuron and can be increased or decreased as the situation warrants.

Transmitter synthesis must be carefully controlled to ensure that a constant supply of messenger molecules is available to transport information across the synaptic cleft. Synthesis must be increased when nerve activity is high, and decreased when it is low. In addition, increasing or decreasing the concentration of transmitter might alter the amount released in response to depolarization and consequently alter the postsynaptic response.

The factors controlling transmitter synthesis are diagrammed in Figure 22-20 and are subject to the following three major types of regulatory control:

1. The amount of synthetic enzyme can be increased by induction. This is a slow process, requiring new enzyme protein synthesis in the cell soma, which then must be transported to the terminal.
2. Activity of already existing enzymes can be regulated by several mechanisms, including activation or inhibition by covalent modifications such as phosphorylation, or allosteric "feedback" inhibition by increased concentrations of product (transmitter). Regulation is rapid and rapidly reversible.
3. Substrate availability regulates the synthesis of

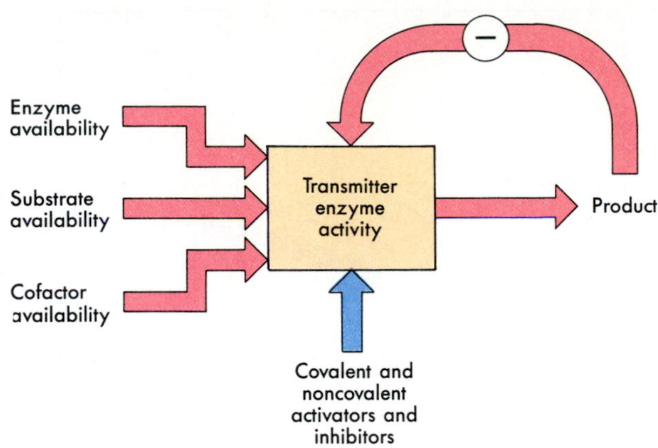

FIGURE 22-20 Factors controlling transmitter synthesis.

several transmitters. This type of regulation is also rapid in onset, though the rate of reversal depends on the rapidity with which substrate concentrations can be normalized.

Although a nerve terminal is usually depolarized to a constant potential by an incoming impulse, the magnitude of the resulting increase in cytosolic calcium can vary. Several factors control depolarization evoked increases in cytosolic calcium. These include the resting membrane potential, the density and state of calcium channels, and the ability of the cell to sequester or extrude the incoming calcium. Variations in calcium concentrations often are directly reflected in variations in transmitter release.

One way of altering depolarization-evoked transmitter release from a nerve terminal is through axoaxonic synapses (see Figure 22-8). Axoaxonic synapses that increase transmitter release are called **sensitizing synapses** and those that decrease transmitter release **inhibitory synapses.** There are various mechanisms by which activation of receptors on the nerve terminal can alter transmitter release. A common mechanism is through alterations in resting membrane potential in the nerve terminal, which affects the concentration of calcium attained in response to an action potential. When the membrane is slightly depolarized, resting calcium influx is increased and normal cytosolic concentrations are higher. Action potentials then result in a higher cytosolic calcium concentration and greater transmitter release. Opposite effects are observed with hyperpolarization, in which the resulting calcium concentrations in response to action potentials are lower, and less transmitter is released.

Another mechanism by which activation of receptors on presynaptic terminals can alter transmitter release is by alteration of the properties of the voltage-dependent channels in the terminal membrane. Phosphorylation of calcium and potassium channels has been shown to alter their gating characteristics. If the number of functional voltage-dependent calcium channels is reduced, depolarization opens fewer channels and causes a smaller increase in calcium and less transmitter release. If the number of functional voltage-dependent potassium channels is reduced, it is harder to repolarize the membrane and depolarization causes a greater increase in calcium and more transmitter release.

Alterations in the strength of a synaptic connection can also occur based on the recent history of the cell. One of the best studied of such alterations is the process called **habituation,** in which repetitive stimulations of a single synaptic connection cause progressively smaller postsynaptic potentials. This is the classic dilemma in which an initial stimulus results in a large behavioral response, but repetitive stimulations cause increasingly smaller responses. In neurons, such habituation appears to be caused by a progressive inactivation of the voltage-dependent calcium channels of the nerve terminals caused by the persistent activation. This results in a decrease in calcium influx and a decreased release of transmitter.

The other mechanism by which transmitter release is often controlled is the rate at which calcium is removed from the cell or sequestered into intracellular sinks, particularly the mitochondria. In situations of intense nerve stimulation, so much calcium flows into the cell that the mechanisms for extruding and sequestering calcium become overloaded. The sinks become "full," and the cell is less able to reduce cytosolic calcium to its normal resting concentration. The resting calcium concentration increases greatly, causing an increase in basal and depolarization-evoked transmitter release. This phenomena is referred to as **facilitation** and is often observed after a train of high-frequency impulses. A similar phenomenon occurs in skeletal muscle, where it is referred to as **posttetanic potentiation.** Facilitation can also be caused by other mechanisms such as slow inactivation of potassium channels, leading to slower repolarization and increased transmitter release.

Alterations in Postsynaptic Sensitivity

Alterations in transmitter availability and calcium homeostasis occur in the presynaptic terminal to change the amount of transmitter released in response to depolarization. Other modifications can occur in the target cell to alter the postsynaptic response to a given concentration of transmitter. The clearest example is when multiple inputs converge on a single postsynaptic target and initiate competing signals. Transmitter released from one terminal may cause an inhibitory postsynaptic potential, whereas transmitter released from an adjacent terminal may cause an excitatory postsynaptic potential. The effect of activation of one input reduces or cancels out the effect of activation of the other input. Such synaptically induced hyperpolarizations that reduce the magnitude of excitatory postsynaptic potentials are referred to as **postsynaptic inhibition.**

The postsynaptic response to a single input can also be varied independently by adaptational responses of the postsynaptic cell. The cell can increase or decrease its response to transmitter in response to changes in synaptic input, much like increasing or decreasing the gain on an amplifier. If an incoming nerve fires more rapidly than normal, the postsynaptic cell receives more transmitter and often decreases its responsiveness to further input. This phenomenon is called **desensitization** or **subsensitivity** and protects the cell from excessive stimulation. Conversely, reductions in the normal impulse traffic tend to increase cellular responsiveness; a phenomenon called **supersensitivity.** This magnifies the effect of incoming signals and is useful for amplifying available information when signal traffic is reduced.

Desensitization and supersensitivity can be caused by changes in the density of receptors for transmitter in the postsynaptic membrane or the efficiency with which these receptors are coupled to changes in cell function. Chronic activation of a synaptic connection can decrease the density of receptors in the postsynaptic cell membrane, whereas chronic decreases in synaptic activation can result in increases in receptor density. Similar effects can be observed when the postsynaptic receptors are continuously activated or inhibited by chronic agonist or antagonist treatment (Figure 22-21). Such changes in receptor density are usually relatively slow in onset and only slowly reversible. For example, increasing receptor density requires importing new receptor protein from the cell body, and reversing such an increase would necessitate degrading these newly acquired receptors. Thus, changing receptor density is usually a long-term (days-to-weeks) adaptive response to changes in synaptic input.

Probably of more importance, the postsynaptic cell can regulate the efficiency with which receptor activation is coupled to changes in cell physiology. These changes usually occur at the level of the coupling of the receptor to channel opening or second-messenger production and can be extremely rapid in onset and termination of activation. This makes them ideal for rapid control of the efficiency of synaptic transmission. Often these changes in coupling efficiency are caused by increases or decreases in covalent modifications of the receptors, G proteins, channels, or enzymes responsible for second-messenger synthesis. Some of these are discussed in Chapter 34.

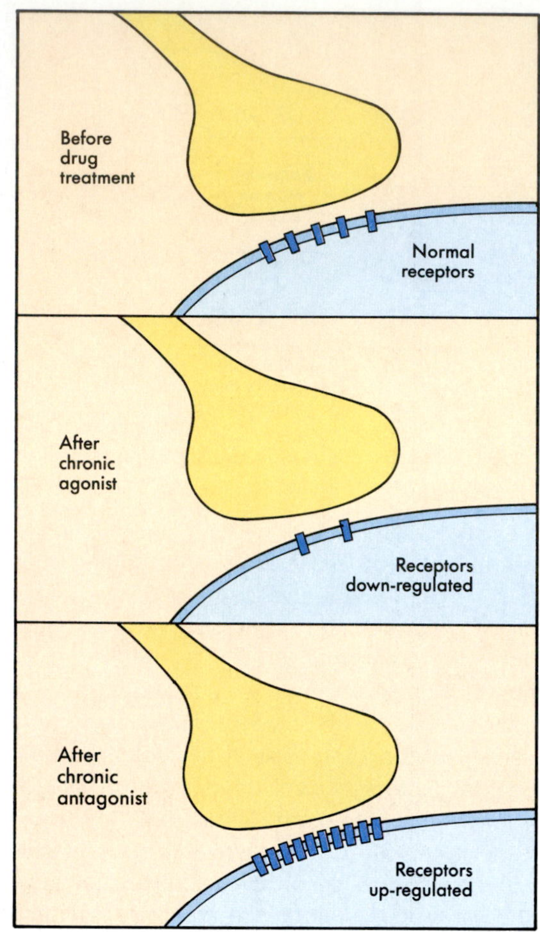

FIGURE 22-21 Chronic treatment with agonists or antagonists can alter postsynaptic receptor density or responsiveness.

As mentioned previously, alterations in synaptic efficiency are probably responsible for many types of learning and memory and are also responsible for the adaptive responses to chronic drug administration. The characteristics of presynaptic and postsynaptic alterations indicate that they might result in different patterns of adaptive responses. For example, depletion of a transmitter from the presynaptic terminal reduces the effect of a drug whose actions require release of that transmitter. This effect could not be overcome no matter how intense the stimulus. On the other hand, postsynaptic reductions in receptor coupling efficiency might cause a reduced responsiveness to that drug, though a high-enough concentration of drug might still be able to initiate a full response. Such "insurmountable" and "surmountable" types of tolerance to drug action are illustrated in Figure 22-22. Understanding the mechanisms by which synaptic efficiency is altered can be useful in predicting the types of adaptive responses that might occur.

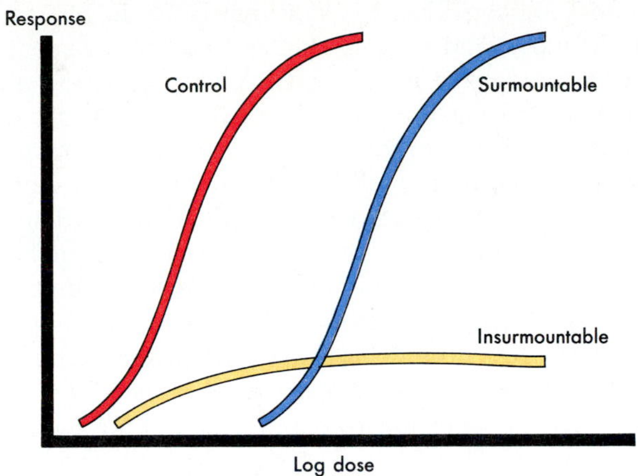

FIGURE 22-22 Types of tolerance. Insurmountable tolerance is often caused by presynaptic depletion of transmitter. Surmountable tolerance is often caused by a decrease in postsynaptic receptor density or coupling efficiency.

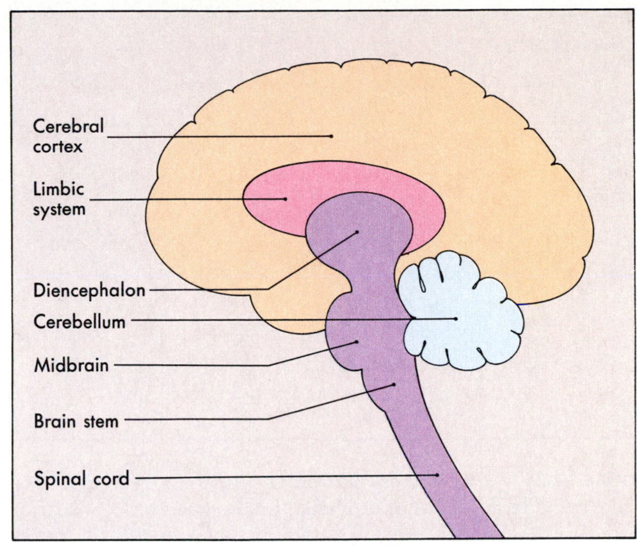

FIGURE 22-23 Major brain regions.

ORGANIZATION OF THE CNS

The individual cells in the CNS are organized into circuits of varying sizes and complexities. These circuits control the processes necessary for survival of the organism and coordination of function. Such circuits range from simple two-neuron rapid reflex arcs to enormous networks of cells controlling complex functions such as sensation, motor activity, mood, and motivation. Although the relationship between individual cells and the complex functions mediated by large neural systems are not well understood, some general principles of organization have been identified and are useful when one is thinking about the mechanisms by which drugs affect the CNS.

Major Subdivisions

Specialized areas of the brain have evolved to perform particular functions in higher vertebrates. This localization of function can be appreciated by a quick review of the major subdivisions of the CNS (Figure 22-23). The cerebral cortex is the largest region of the brain where most sensory, motor, and associational information is processed, and where integration of many somatic and vegetative functions occurs. The limbic system consists in a variety of structures lying beneath the neocortex that integrate emotional state with motor and visceral activities. The cerebellum, which resides behind the cerebral hemispheres, provides complex sensorimotor coordination. The midbrain and brainstem relay information from the cerebral hemispheres and limbic system to the spinal cord and provide central integration of essential reflexive acts. The spinal cord extends caudally from the brainstem and receives, sends, and integrates sensory and motor information.

Each of these regions is heterogeneous and can be subdivided into many smaller regions and groups of cells with diverse functions, many of which have been extensively studied. Although obviously interesting and important, the gross anatomy of the brain does not shed much light on the mechanisms by which drugs affect the brain. The effects of drugs are determined more by the phenotype and activity of the individual cells in which their molecular targets are located, and the types of neural relays in which those cells participate, than in the particular brain region in which the cells are located.

Types of Circuits

Neuronal systems are usually subdivided into two major types, hierarchical and diffuse. **Hierarchical systems** transmit information in a sequential manner from one neuron to the next, providing a highly directed and precise flow of information. **Diffuse systems,** as the name implies, are less directed and extend many divergent connections to a variety of target cells. Activation of diffuse systems affects large areas of the CNS simultaneously, often in a relatively uniform manner. Conceptually, hierarchical and diffuse systems can be thought of as multicellular analogs of directed and nondirected synapses (see Figure 22-9). Hierarchical systems provide a highly specific and directed flow of information, whereas diffuse systems blanket a much wider target area; much like serial and parallel information processing (Figure 22-24). These represent two extremes, and

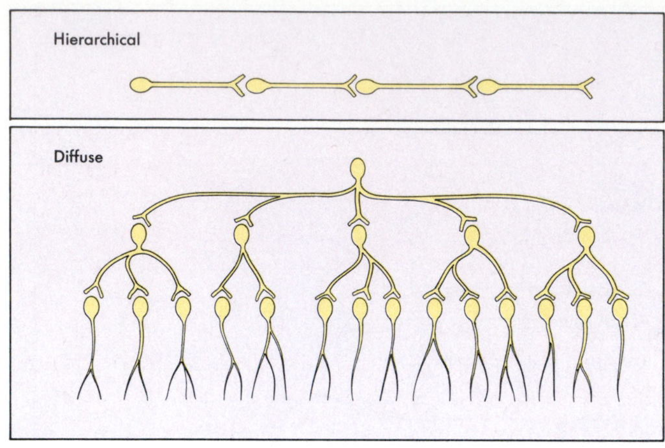

FIGURE 22-24 Hierarchical and diffuse systems of neural networks provide for serial and parallel information processing.

many neuronal systems combine aspects of both types of information processing.

Many of the pathways involved in sensory perception and motor control involve hierarchical and diffuse processing. In hierarchical pathways, information is detected in sensory cells, transmitted to relay cells, and finally to sensory fields in the cerebral cortex. Motor information is output from the motor cortex through intermediate relays to the spinal motor neurons controlling muscles. The neurotransmitters involved have not been clearly identified; however, excitatory amino acids, acetylcholine, and certain peptides have been implicated at specific synapses. The sequential nature of these connections results in highly orderly information transfer, though interruption at any point in the sequential pathway causes complete interruption of the system.

As might be expected, diffuse systems have less well-defined and specific functions. They appear to have major importance in many integrated functions of the brain, such as mood, arousal, emotion, and motivational states. Certain of the biogenic amines (norepinephrine, serotonin, and dopamine) and some peptides are implicated as neurotransmitters in diffuse systems. These neurons extend multiple branching axons to many target cells and can affect many brain regions in a simultaneous and relatively uniform manner. Interference with diffuse systems does not result in the dramatic loss of information transfer observed when hierarchical systems are interrupted. Interruption of diffuse systems results in more subtle changes in brain activity, consistent with modulatory roles in more global aspects of CNS function.

Drugs can interact with hierarchical and diffuse systems in specific ways. Actions on hierarchical systems usually result in highly specific and defined effects. For example, anticonvulsants specifically block the hyperactivity of motor and sensory systems, analgesics specifically block transduction of sensory pain information, and antiemetics block vomiting reflexes. The actions of each of these classes of drugs are caused by interruption of highly directed and specialized information flow. Drugs acting on diffuse systems cause effects that, although specific, are more difficult to define. These include drugs for treatment of depression, psychoses, anxiety, and sleep disorders. Although the actions of these drugs are specific, they are not caused simply by interruption of information flow. They appear to be caused by subtle modifications occurring throughout the entire system, rather than by blockade of transmission at particular synapses.

Tonic Activity

Another important characteristic of neuronal systems is their level of tonic activity. In the absence of synaptic input, neurons can exist in either of two states. They can be totally quiescent by maintaining a constant and uniform depolarization of their cell membrane, or they can initiate action potentials at uniform intervals by spontaneous graded depolarizations. Neurons that automatically generate action potentials are called **pacemaker cells** (such as those in the sinoatrial node of the heart) and their spontaneous activity is often caused by a constant inward leakage of sodium greater than that extruded by the sodium-potassium pump. The ability of neurons to generate their own rhythmic impulse activity is another area that functionally distinguishes them from electrical circuits, which always require external input for activity. Thus neurons can require external drivers or they can generate their own patterns of impulse activity.

In a similar manner, systems of neurons can require external stimuli for activity or demonstrate spontaneous activity, depending on the pacemaker activity of their individual components. Clearly, a system with an intrinsic spontaneous activity has different characteristics from a quiescent system. Although both can be activated, only a spontaneously active system can be inhibited. Drugs that inhibit neuronal function (e.g., anesthetics and other CNS depressants) may have quite different effects, depending on the pattern of activity of the neuronal system involved. Any system with a constant level of activity (either intrinsic or externally driven) will be inhibited by such drugs, whereas the activity of a quiescent system will be unaffected.

Excitatory and Inhibitory Systems

The net effect of activation of one neuronal system generally will be to increase or decrease information out-

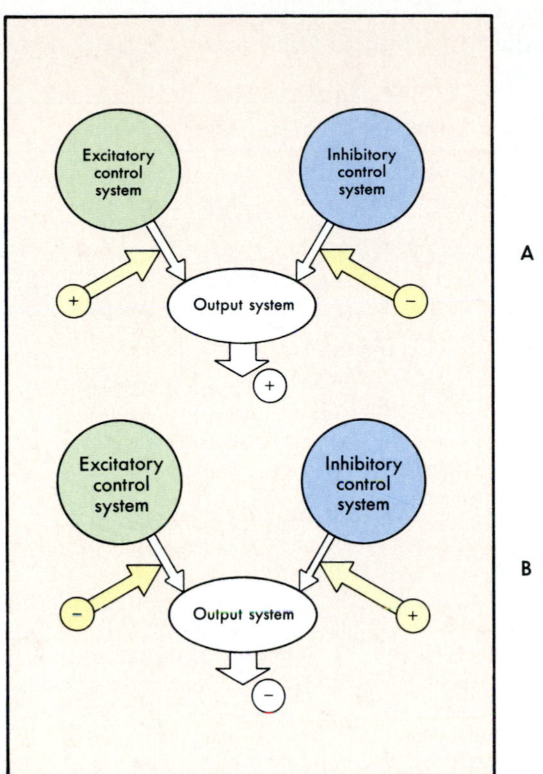

FIGURE 22-25 **A,** Neuronal output can be increased by increasing a tonic excitatory control or decreasing a tonic inhibitory control. **B,** Output can be reduced by decreasing tonic excitatory control or increasing tonic inhibitory control.

flow from the CNS or increase or decrease the activity of another neuronal system in the brain. Whether activation of a particular neural system is excitatory or inhibitory depends primarily on the neurotransmitters released at the output synapse or synapses and the types of receptors on the target cells (discussed previously). This has important consequences for drug action.

As discussed, any tonically active neural network can have its activity increased or decreased by excitatory or inhibitory control systems respectively. This type of bidirectional regulation means that the effect of a drug cannot necessarily be predicted based solely on its effect on isolated neurons. A drug that reduces neuronal firing can activate a neural system by reducing a tonically active inhibitory input. Conversely, a drug that increases neuronal firing can inhibit by activating an inhibitory input (Figure 22-25). Thus a "depressant" drug may in some circumstances cause excitation, and a "stimulant" drug may in some cases cause sedation. A well-known example of this is the stimulant phase that is frequently observed after ingestion of ethyl alcohol. Ethanol is a general neuronal depressant, and the initial stimulation is attributable to depression of an inhibitory control system. This effect occurs only at low concentrations of ethanol; higher concentrations cause a uniform depression of nerve activity. A similar "stage of excitement" can sometimes be observed during induction of general anesthesia, which is also caused by the removal of tonically active inhibitory control systems.

Normal physiological variations in this activity of neuronal systems can also alter the effects of centrally acting drugs. Anesthetics are generally less effective in hyperexcitable patients, and stimulants are less effective in more sedate patients. This is probably attributable to the presence of varying levels of excitatory and inhibitory control systems, which alter sensitivity to drug-induced manipulation. The effects of other stimulant and depressant drugs administered concurrently also alter responses to centrally acting drugs. Depressants are generally additive with depressants, and stimulants are additive with stimulants. For example, ingestion of ethanol potentiates the depression caused by barbiturates and can be fatal. However, the interactions between stimulant and depressant drugs are more variable. Stimulant drugs usually physiologically antagonize the effects of depressant drugs, and vice versa. Because such antagonism is caused by activation or inhibition of competing control systems and not by neutralization of the effect of the drugs on their target molecules, concurrently administered stimulants and depressants usually do not completely cancel the effects of the other drug.

SITES OF DRUG ACTION

Almost all drugs with primary actions on the CNS cause their effects by modifying some aspect of chemical synaptic transmission. Thus, a "pharmacologist's view of the brain" is much like the famous "New Yorker's view of the United States," in which New York and surrounding boroughs dominate the landscape, with the rest of the country squeezed into a small area as an unimportant afterthought. Similarly, pharmacologists magnify the importance of chemical synapses and relegate the remainder of the brain to supporting status (Figure 22-26).

Target Molecules

Drugs act on specific molecular targets to alter cell function. The distribution of these targets determines which cells are affected by a particular drug and is the primary determinant of the specificity of drug action.

Drugs acting on the CNS can be divided into several major classes, based on the distribution of their specific target molecules (Table 22-1). Drugs that act on molecules expressed by all types of cells (DNA, lipids, and structural proteins) are said to have "general" actions. Other drugs act on molecules that are expressed in es-

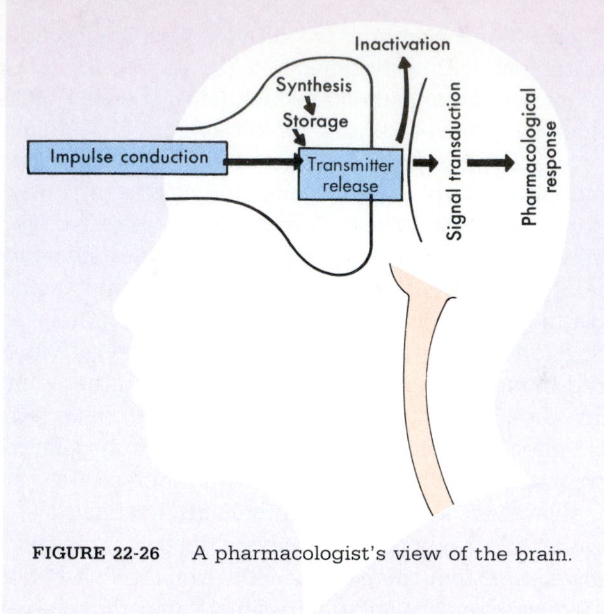

FIGURE 22-26 A pharmacologist's view of the brain.

sentially all neurons but not in other cell types. These drugs are called **neuron specific** and usually interact with the pumps and channels that maintain the electrical properties of neurons. Some drugs interact specifically with the macromolecules involved in synthesis, storage, release, actions, and inactivation processes associated with particular neurotransmitters. The targets for these **transmitter-specific** drugs will be expressed only by neurons synthesizing or responding to certain neurotransmitters; consequently these drugs have more discrete and limited actions. The various targets for transmitter-specific drugs can be any of the large variety of macromolecules involved in the life cycle of different transmitter molecules (see Figure 22-26). Finally, some drugs mimic or interfere with specific signal transduction systems shared by a variety of different receptors. Such **signal-specific** drugs affect responses to activation of various different receptors that use the same pathway for initiating signals in their target cells.

Although examples of these four drug categories are found in clinical practice, the transmitter-specific drugs are clearly the largest class. Some of the known and suspected target molecules for centrally acting drugs are listed in Table 22-1. The transmitter-specific drugs are most common, probably because their specific target molecules have a more limited distribution than those of the general, neuron-specific, or even the signal-specific, classes. The more limited distribution of target molecules for transmitter-specific drugs often results in a greater specificity of drug action and is reflected clinically by a lower incidence of unwanted side effects.

Table 22-1 Targets for Selected Centrally Acting Drugs

Cellular Target	Class of Drugs
membrane lipid	general anesthetic drugs
cyclooxygenase	nonsteroidal antiinflammatory drugs
voltage-dependent sodium channels	local anesthetics
L-type of voltage-dependent calcium channels	calcium-channel blockers
opioid receptors	opioid analgesics
opioid receptors	opioid antagonists
GABA receptors	benzodiazepines
GABA receptors	barbiturates
adrenergic receptors	clonidine
histamine receptors	antihistamines
dopamine receptors	antipsychotic drugs
adenosine receptors	caffeine
monoamine oxidase	monoamine oxidase inhibitors
dopamine synthesis	L-dihydroxyphenylalanine
norepinephrine reuptake	tricyclic antidepressants
serotonin reuptake	tricyclic antidepressants
dopamine reuptake	amantidine
phosphatidylinositol breakdown	lithium carbonate
cAMP breakdown	caffeine (?)

Specificity

Although drugs exert their primary actions by interacting with the specific target molecules previously discussed, they also have other actions. No drug causes only a single specific effect because few if any drugs bind to only a single molecular target. At higher concentrations, most drugs can interact with a wide variety of biological molecules, often resulting in functional alterations to the cell.

To be therapeutically useful, drugs must specifically interact with their target molecules without disrupting normal cellular activity. There is usually a range of concentrations in which a drug affects its specific target molecule without affecting other cellular processes. However, higher drug concentrations always have other effects, and the size of the "window of selectivity" is variable with different drugs (see Therapeutic Index, Chapter 1). Sometimes it can be fairly large (e.g., benzodiazepines), and other times it is quite small (e.g., barbiturates). Such selectivity is always relative, however, and it is important to remember that all drugs also have other "nonspecific" actions, particularly at higher concentrations.

Some drugs have potent actions on so many different processes in the CNS that it is difficult to identify

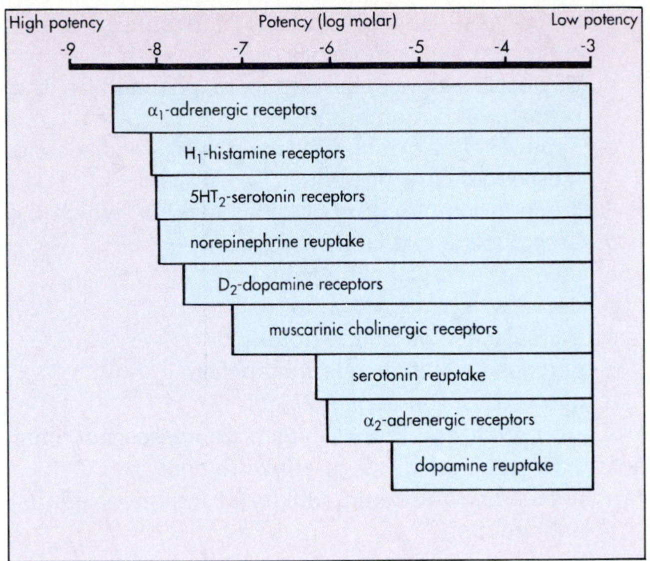

FIGURE 22-27 Potency of chlorpromazine in inhibiting various receptors and reuptake pumps. Notice that this drug has multiple actions at low concentrations.

their primary molecular targets. Some of these drugs may cause their therapeutic effects by combinations of specific effects on multiple cellular processes. Others may exert their primary actions through interaction with a single cellular target, and the simultaneous interaction with other targets does not influence the primary effect of the drug. For such drugs, the window of selectivity is very small, and use of these compounds is often associated with a wide range of unwanted side effects. For example, the antipsychotic drug chlorpromazine is believed to exert its beneficial effects on schizophrenia by blocking D_2 dopamine receptors. However, chlorpromazine blocks many different monoamine receptors and uptake pumps with various potencies (Figure 22-27). Some of the molecular effects of chlorpromazine occur in concentrations lower than those required to block D_2 dopamine receptors, whereas some occur at higher concentrations. Figure 22-27 clearly illustrates that the window of selectivity of chlorpromazine is essentially nonexistent. This is one of the reasons why the use of chlorpromazine (similar to many other antipsychotic drugs) is associated with a wide range of unwanted side effects, including drowsiness (histamine receptor blockade), dry mouth and blurred vision (muscarinic cholinergic receptor blockade), and orthostatic hypotension (α-adrenergic receptor blockade). Also, the fact that any administered dose of chlorpromazine affects multiple molecular targets makes it difficult to separate which effects are important for its therapeutic actions.

This example demonstrates some of the difficulties involved in determining the mechanisms by which drugs affect CNS function. As discussed in the introduction to this section, it is challenging enough to attempt to relate specific biochemical actions of drugs to observed changes in mood or behavior. To this challenge must be added an appreciation for the cellular and molecular complexity of neurons and their transmitters, a recognition of the plasticity of synaptic connections, and the likelihood of multiple targets for drug action within the brain. Clearly, how psychoactive drugs exert their effects on a molecular level are only beginning to be understood.

Despite these obstacles, important discoveries about how centrally acting drugs work continue. Manipulating brain biochemistry and physiology with specific drugs and observing the effects on integrated behavioral parameters is one of the few approaches currently available for relating the function of brain cells with complex integrated behaviors. Increased understanding results in an increasingly sophisticated appreciation of the relationship between the cellular components of the brain and its global functions. Such information will be useful in the future for rational design of drugs for various diseases of the CNS. Another result will be the intrinsic satisfaction of understanding more about the genesis and control of human thought and emotion. Although understanding the actions of drugs on the CNS poses a great challenge, it also promises great rewards.

REFERENCES

Cooper JR, Bloom FE, Roth RH: *The biochemical basis of neuropharmacology,* New York, 1991, Oxford University Press.

Kandel ER, Schwartz JH, Jessell TM: *Principles of neural science,* New York, 1991, Elsevier Science Publishing.

SELF-ASSESSMENT QUESTIONS

1. Most centrally acting drugs were discovered
   a. before 1900.
   b. between 1900 and 1920.
   c. between 1920 and 1940.
   d. between 1940 and 1950.
   e. after 1950.
2. Local anesthetic drugs, which block voltage-gated sodium channels, will
   a. hyperpolarize a nerve cell at rest.
   b. depolarize a nerve cell at rest
   c. block neurotransmitter-induced synaptic potentials.
   d. block depolarization-induced initiation of action potentials.
   e. prevent action potential repolarization by blocking potassium efflux.

3. Most neurotransmitters
   a. are synthesized in the cell body.
   b. are released in an exocytotic process dependent on Na^+.
   c. are rapidly inactivated following release from presynaptic terminals.
   d. diffuse many centimeters before reaching their sites of action.
   e. are compounds with unique structures, which have no other role in non-neuronal cells.
4. An antidepressant drug that inhibits reuptake of norepinephrine, such as desipramine, will
   a. prolong the action of released norepinephrine.
   b. increase the amount of norepinephrine released in response to presynaptic depolarization.
   c. reduce the enzymatic breakdown of norepinephrine in presynaptic terminals.
   d. do none of the above.
5. The effects of acetylcholine released onto a postsynaptic cell membrane will be
   a. to cause hyperpolarization.
   b. to cause depolarization.
   c. to increase phosphorylation of channels in the postsynaptic membrane.
   d. to decrease phosphorylation of channels in the postsynaptic membrane.
   e. dependent on which type of receptors and second messengers are present.
6. Administration of a drug, such as lecithin, which increases choline availability might
   a. increase acetylcholine synthesis.
   b. decrease acetylcholine release.
   c. increase acetylcholine uptake.
   d. decrease acetylcholine metabolism.
   e. cause all of the above effects.
7. A drug such as ethanol, which depresses neuronal firing, can cause a "stage of excitement" by
   a. decreasing the tonic activity of inhibitory neuronal circuits.
   b. stimulating excitatory neuronal circuits.
   c. decreasing the tonic activity of excitatory neuronal circuits.
   d. stimulating inhibitory neuronal circuits.
   e. any of the above mechanisms.

CHAPTER 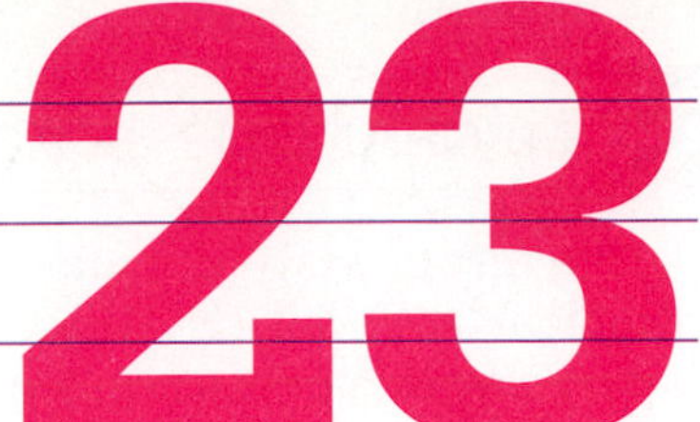

Antipsychotic Agents

JAMES P. BENNETT, JR.

MAJOR DRUGS

phenothiazines
thioxanthenes
butyrophenones

THERAPEUTIC OVERVIEW

Psychosis is a severe disturbance of reality perception that may have many underlying causes. Psychotic individuals may exhibit many signs and symptoms, including impairment of cognitive function, hallucinations, feelings of persecution or thought control, extreme fear, agitation, emotional lability or flatness, or extensive social withdrawal and apathy. For a diagnosis of psychosis, it is important to rule out medical causes, such as drug intoxication or withdrawal, CNS infection or inflammation, brain structural lesions, metabolic abnormalities or nutritional deficiencies, and medical illnesses such as cardiac disease or pneumonia. Psychosis attributable to these "organic" causes is part of the clinical syndrome of **delirium** and should be viewed as a medical emergency requiring prompt diagnosis and management. A significant proportion of patients with dementias, most having Alzheimer's type of disorder also develop psychoses of varying intensity during their illness. In both delirium and psychosis associated with dementia, antipsychotic therapy may be necessary to control disruptive or dangerous behavior until the underlying cause or causes can be discerned and treated.

The majority of antipsychotic drugs are used to treat schizophrenia and other mood disorders, including psychosis associated with depression and bipolar illness. These psychoses respond to antipsychotic drug treatment, which usually must be combined with additional therapy directed at the mood disorder. Schizophrenia affects about 1% of adults worldwide, is generally a progressive, life-long illness beginning in adolescence or young adulthood, and is the cause of most chronic antipsychotic drug use. Schizophrenia is often refractory to treatment and disabling for about half its victims. In a typical patient the first "psychotic break" occurs in the teens or twenties, following a decline in social interactions and academic or job performance. Then appear several "positive" symptoms that dramatically define the onset of the illness. These include auditory, more often than visual, hallucinations, agitation, suspiciousness, feelings of persecution, ideas of reference (attaching unrealistic personal significance to trivial events), and intrusion of unwanted thoughts. However, often the illness evolves more insidiously, with "negative" symptoms, such as emotional apathy or flatness (anhedonia), extreme inattentiveness, and social withdrawal evolving for months or years before "positive" symptoms appear. Successful control of "positive" symptoms with medical therapy may return the individual to nearly normal functioning. However, the "negative" symptoms may predominate at some point in the illness and limit functional recovery. For most patients, schizophrenia is characterized by a failure to return completely to premorbid base-line functioning, despite medical control of "positive" symptoms. Recurrence of multiple psychotic breaks may worsen the ultimate outcome, and efforts must be made to maintain medication compliance. Noncompliance is the leading cause of recurrent positive

ABBREVIATIONS

GABA	γ-aminobutyric acid
VTA	Ventral tegmental area

THERAPEUTIC OVERVIEW

PSYCHOSES IN WHICH DRUGS ARE USED EFFECTIVELY

Schizophrenia
Affective disorders
Acute idiopathic psychoses
Certain drug-induced psychoses

THERAPY APPROACHES

Symptomatic treatment
Positive symptoms (schizophrenia, affective disorders) respond to medication
Negative symptoms often do not respond to medication

psychotic symptoms in those who initially responded to neuroleptic treatment.

Available evidence indicates but is not yet conclusive that schizophrenia has a strong genetic component and may occur as a pathological reaction to stress by an individual with disordered integration between the limbic system and overlying cerebral cortex. This evidence includes:

1. An increased risk among first-degree relatives of schizophrenics (identical twins > fraternal twins or siblings), independent of the environment in which the individual was raised.
2. Neuroradiological abnormalities, including increased lateral ventricle size and atrophy of temporal or medial frontal cortex, greater than that seen in age-matched controls or non-afflicted sibs.
3. Decreased average frontal lobe electroencephalographic background frequencies and frontal cortical glucose metabolic rate, though these decreases are not specific to schizophrenia.
4. Disordered neuronal structure and lamination in the frontal and temporal cortex, suggestive of a developmental abnormality rather than a postnatal insult.

Certain drugs also can produce altered states that appear similar but not identical to endogenous psychoses. These drugs include the hallucinogens such as natural and man-made amphetamines (mescaline), substituted indoles (dimethyltryptamine), and lysergic acid derivatives. These drugs produce intense visual hallucinations, depersonalization, and altered perception of the environment. Some of these symptoms can be alleviated by treatment with antipsychotic drugs.

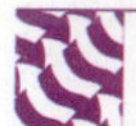

MECHANISMS OF ACTION

The first antipsychotic drug that relieved signs and symptoms of psychosis rather than merely provided sedation was chlorpromazine, a member of the phenothiazine family (Figure 23-1). Its antipsychotic activity was discovered by chance, and the efficacy of this drug was not generally accepted until large clinical trials had been conducted. Other phenothiazines were developed later and shown to be equally effective with chlorpromazine in relieving psychotic signs and symptoms. Additional nonphenothiazine neuroleptic (*lēptos* = 'taken hold of, seized") drug classes were developed later, including diphenylbutylpiperidine (pimozide), thioxanthene (thiothixene), dibenzoxazepine (loxapine), dihydroindole (molindone), butyrophenone (haloperidol), and the dibenzodiazepine atypical drug clozapine (Figures 23-1 and 23-2).

Neuroleptic drugs have been found to interact with multiple neurotransmitter systems, but clinical antipsychotic potency correlates only with their affinity for forebrain D_2 dopamine receptors (Figure 23-3). Multiple lines of investigation indicate that the unifying principle of antipsychotic action of these drugs may be the reduction of dopamine synaptic activity in the limbic forebrain. The efficacy of neuroleptics in relieving positive schizophrenic symptoms, psychotic symptoms in other neuropsychiatric diseases, and psychosis associated with amphetamine and cocaine toxicity appears to be associated with this mechanism.

Pharmacology of Dopamine Receptors

Postsynaptic receptors for dopamine are of two major classes, D_1 and D_2, defined functionally by degree of coupling to second-messenger systems and pharmacologically by interaction with selective agonists and antagonists. D_1 dopamine receptors are characterized by positive coupling through a stimulatory guanine nucleotide protein, Gs, to activation of adenylate cyclase and intracellular production of cyclic adenosine monophosphate (cAMP). D_2 -receptors in certain tissues are coupled through an inhibitory guanine nucleotide protein G_i or G_o to adenylate cyclase; activation of D_2 -receptors in some cases inhibits D_1-induced increase in cAMP synthesis.

Dopamine, the naturally occurring agonist, interacts with D_1- and D_2-receptors, and both receptors are found in high density in the corpus striatum and the nucleus accumbens. Most striatal neurons have D_1 responses and most accumbens neurons have D_2 responses.

Dopamine postsynaptic responses can be mediated by either D_1- or D_2-receptors, whereas presynaptic re-phenothiazine nucleus

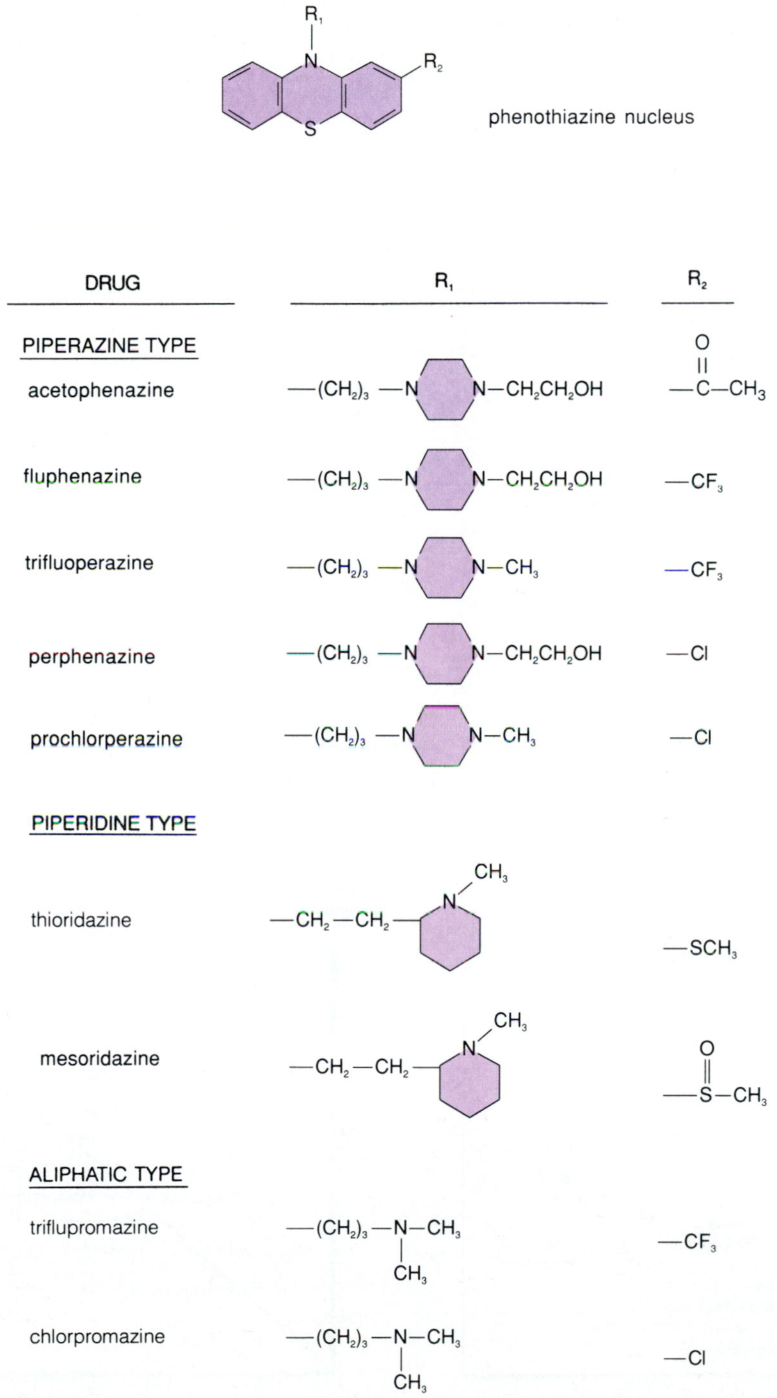

DRUG	R_1	R_2
PIPERAZINE TYPE		
acetophenazine	$—(CH_2)_3—N$ (piperazine) $N—CH_2CH_2OH$	$—C(=O)—CH_3$
fluphenazine	$—(CH_2)_3—N$ (piperazine) $N—CH_2CH_2OH$	$—CF_3$
trifluoperazine	$—(CH_2)_3—N$ (piperazine) $N—CH_3$	$—CF_3$
perphenazine	$—(CH_2)_3—N$ (piperazine) $N—CH_2CH_2OH$	—Cl
prochlorperazine	$—(CH_2)_3—N$ (piperazine) $N—CH_3$	—Cl
PIPERIDINE TYPE		
thioridazine	$—CH_2—CH_2—$ (N-CH_3 piperidine)	$—SCH_3$
mesoridazine	$—CH_2—CH_2—$ (N-CH_3 piperidine)	$—S(=O)—CH_3$
ALIPHATIC TYPE		
triflupromazine	$—(CH_2)_3—N(CH_3)—CH_3$	$—CF_3$
chlorpromazine	$—(CH_2)_3—N(CH_3)—CH_3$	—Cl

FIGURE 23-1 Structures of selected phenothiazine antipsychotic agents.

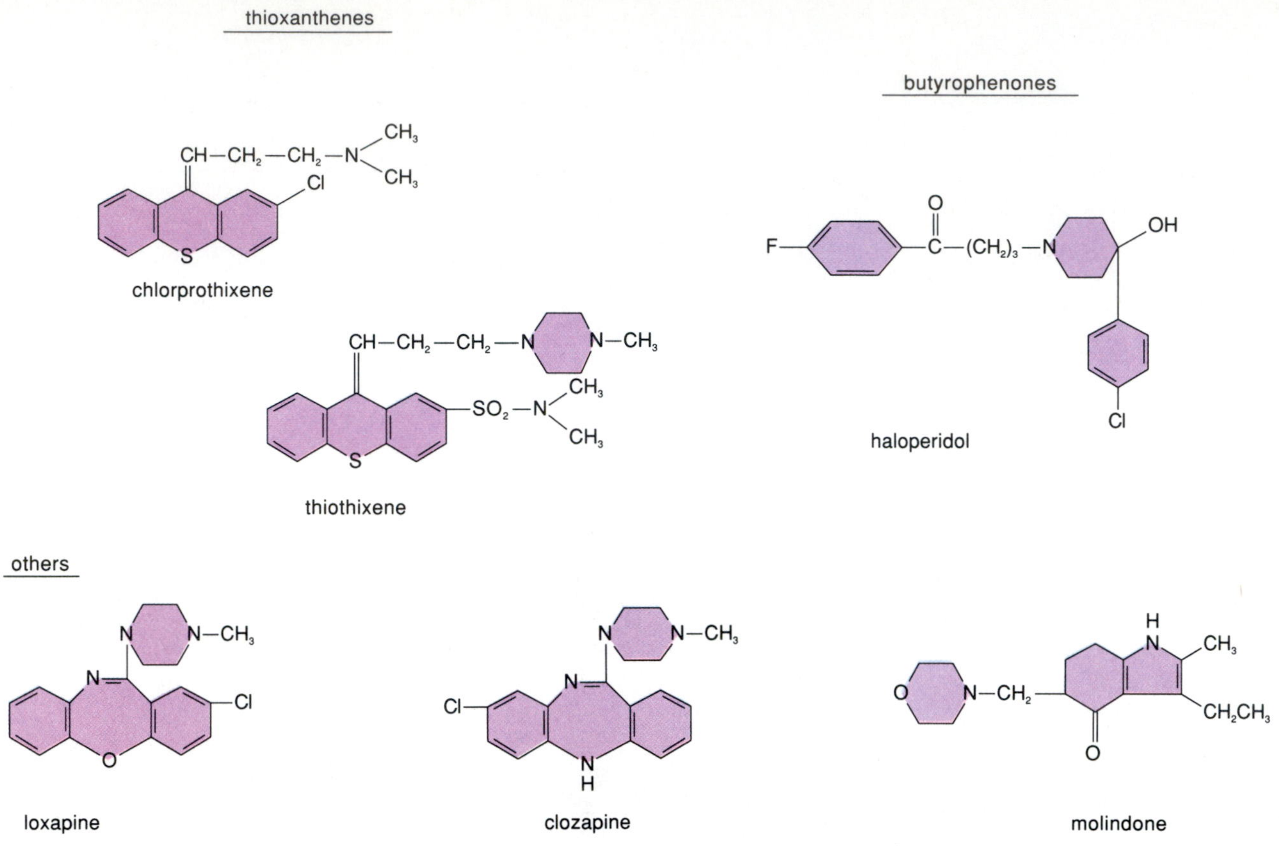

thioxanthenes
chlorprothixene
thiothixene
butyrophenones
haloperidol
others
loxapine
clozapine
molindone

FIGURE 23-2 Structures of nonphenothiazine antipsychotic agents.

KD (mol/L) on 3H-SCH23390 binding
A
Clebopride
Molindone
Sulpiride
Spiperone
Chlorpromazine
Clozapine
Haloperidol
Thioridazine
Fluphenazine
Trifluperazine
Flupenthixol
Range and average clinical dose for controlling schizophrenia (mg/dl)
KD (mol/L) on 3H-haloperidol binding
B
Promazine
Chlorpromazine
Trazodone
Clozapine
Molindone
Thioridazine
Prochlorperazine
Moperone
Trifluoperazine
Thiothixene
Droperidol
Haloperidol
Fluphenazine
Trifluperidol
Pimozide
Benperidol
Spiroperidol
Range and average clinical dose for controlling schizophrenia (mg/dl)

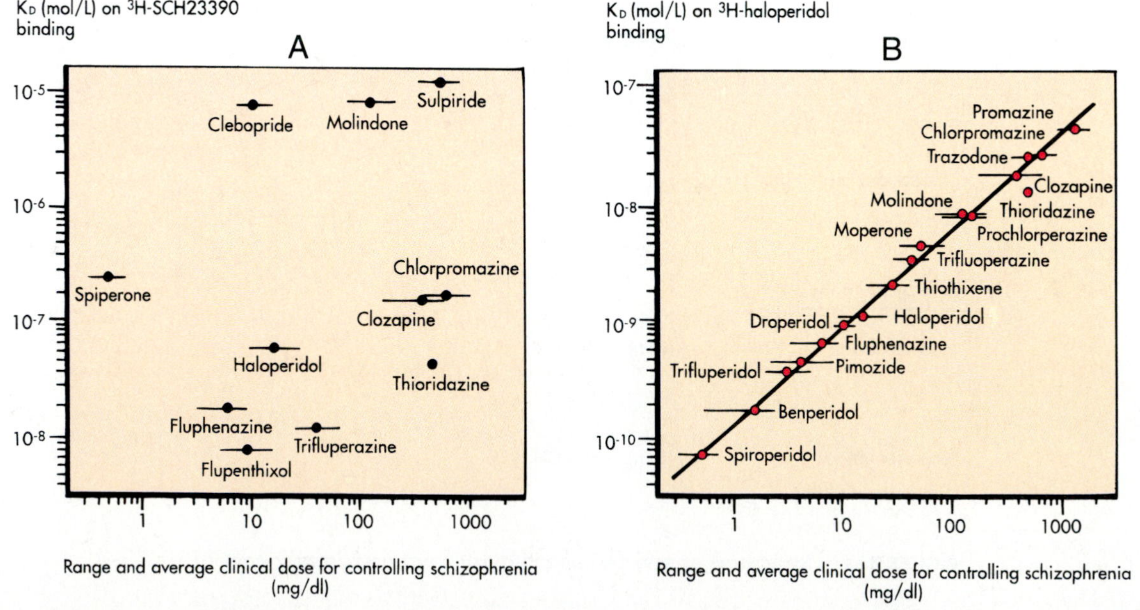

FIGURE 23-3 Correlation among affinities of neuroleptic drugs to bind to D_2-dopamine receptors and average daily clinical dose necessary to treat psychosis **(A)**. Notice lack of correlation with affinity of binding to D_1 -receptors **(B)**. (Adapted from Seeman P. *Synapse* 1:133-152, 1987.)

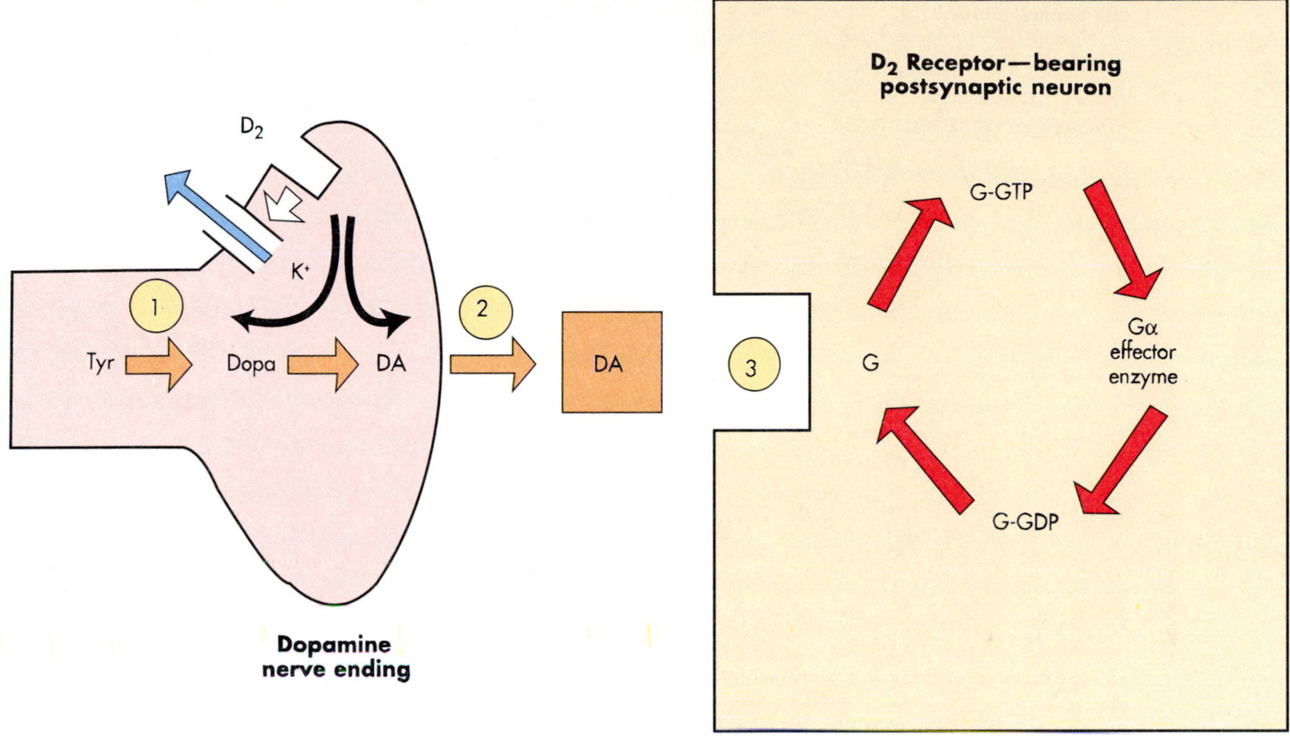

FIGURE 23-4 Sites of action of many antipsychotic drugs on dopamine neurotransmission. Blockade of presynaptic receptors increases dopamine *(DA)* synthesis *(1)* and release *(2)* and can reduce passage of K^+ through an ion channel. Classic antipsychotic drugs also block postsynaptic dopamine receptors *(3)*. D_2, Dopamine receptor; G-guanine nucleotide binding protein (G protein). G-GDP and G-GTP reqresent G protein bound to either guanosine diphosphate or guanosine triphosphate, respectively.

ceptors appear to be exclusively the D_2 subtype. In addition, D_2-receptors on midbrain dopamine neurons (i.e., presynaptic receptors) and on striatal neurons (i.e., postsynaptic receptors) open a potassium channel and would be expected to hyperpolarize neurons and slow firing rates. Ionic responses to activation of D_1-receptors are not yet known (Figure 23-4).

Recent cloning experiments have expanded the family of dopamine receptor subtypes. The mRNAs coding for the new subtype receptor proteins (D_3, D_4, D_5) are found primarily in limbic areas (D_3), medulla and frontal cortex (D_4), or hippocampus (D_5). All expressed receptors bind neuroleptic drugs, but the D_4-receptor has a notably high affinity for clozapine. Their restricted localization to limbic and frontal cortical areas and the unusual affinity of D_4 for clozapine indicate the possible involvement of one or more of the new subtypes in antipsychotic drug action and perhaps in the cause of schizophrenia. However, little is presently known about their normal physiological function.

A remarkable property of all "classical" neuroleptic drugs (phenothiazines, thioxanthines, butyrophenones) is that their binding affinity to brain D_2-receptors correlates closely with their clinical potency as antipsychotics. Although all these drugs also bind to D_1-receptors, there is no demonstrable association between D_1-receptor binding and clinical potencies.

Effects of Antipsychotic Drugs

After acute administration, antipsychotic drugs produce catalepsy (a state of immobilized inactivity not primarily attributable to sedation). They also increase the rate of synthesis and breakdown of dopamine in forebrain limbic structures, such as the nucleus accumbens. Drugs with a higher risk of causing parkinsonism as a side effect also increase dopamine turnover in the corpus striatum. Increases in dopamine turnover are now known to be primarily the result of blockade of presynaptic D_2-receptors ("autoreceptors") on dopamine neurons and nerve endings, whereas catalepsy arises primarily from acute blockade of postsynaptic D_2-receptors.

The chemical potency of neuroleptics acting at D_2-receptors, coupled with the observations of paranoid psychosis produced either by the abuse of amphetamine or cocaine or by the use of levodopa/dopamine in Parkinson's disease, led to the formulation of the "do-

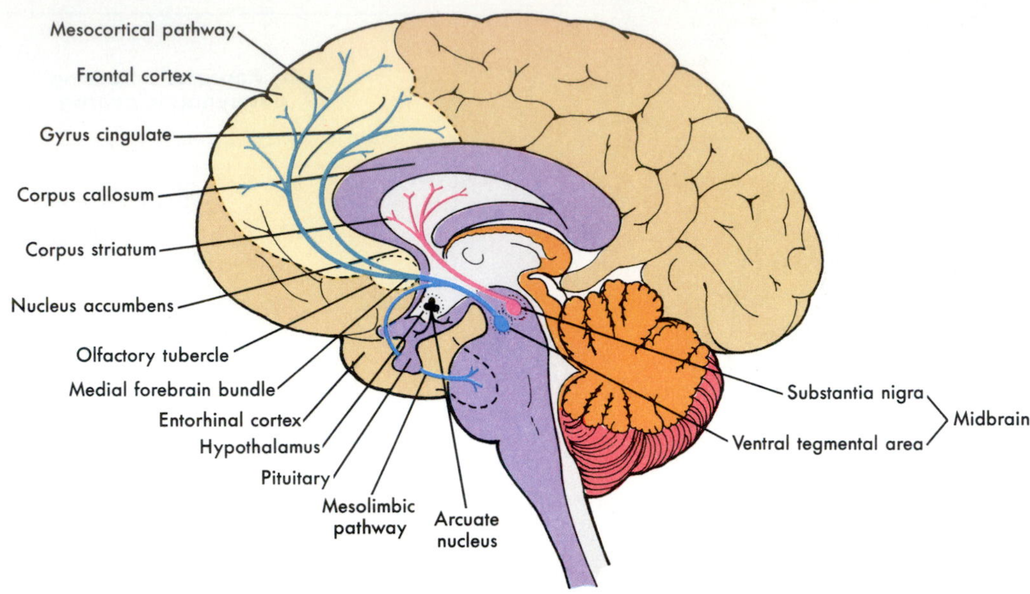

FIGURE 23-5 Anatomy relevant to dopamine neurons believed to be involved in actions of antipsychotic agents. Dopamine neurons in substantia nigra and ventral tegmental areas lead to ascending nigrostriatal and mesolimbic/mesocortical pathways, respectively, which ascend in medial forebrain bundle to their forebrain targets. The nigrostriatal pathway terminates in the corpus striatum (caudate/putamen). Major mesolimbic targets are the nucleus accumbens, olfactory tubercle, and entorhinal cortex. Mesocortical innervation is primarily to the medial frontal cortex and cingulate gyrus. Tuberoinfundibular dopamine neurons in the arcuate nucleus project to the median eminence (pituitary stalk).

pamine hypothesis" of psychosis. This hypothesis states that the positive signs and symptoms of psychosis derive from overactivity of dopamine at forebrain synapses, especially those in limbic structures. Antipsychotic drugs block dopamine receptors and thus relieve the signs and symptoms.

Although conceptually appealing, the above formulation is inconsistent with several observations:

1. Blockade of D_2 dopamine receptors by antipsychotic drugs occurs rapidly, yet clinical antipsychotic activity is apparent only after at least 3 to 6 weeks, particularly in schizophrenia. However, responses to antipsychotic drug treatment are quicker in amphetamine or cocaine abuse or in levodopa intoxication, where the improvement can be demonstrated within days.
2. The antipsychotic-induced increase in forebrain dopamine turnover lasts for several injections and then fades. The dopamine terminals "adapt" and become resistant to the effects of chronic blockade of their dopamine receptors when signs and symptoms of psychosis are usually improving.
3. Atypical neuroleptics, such as clozapine, have weak affinity for dopamine receptors and little selectivity for D_2 over other subtypes. Yet clozapine is helpful in about one third of schizophrenic patients resistant to traditional D_2-receptor blocking drugs.

Anatomy and Physiology of Dopamine Pathways

Although acute blockade of dopamine receptors does not completely explain the antipsychotic effect of neuroleptic drugs, midbrain dopamine neurons remain the most likely targets of these agents. There are three major dopamine pathways that can be affected (Figure 23-5). Dopamine-containing nerve cell bodies of these pathways are clustered in nuclei in the rostral midbrain, with the borders between the nuclei not always well defined. Anatomically, the most distinctive nuclei are the paired substantia nigra neurons, whose axons ascend rostrally in the nigrostriatal pathway to provide dopaminergic innervation of the corpus striatum (caudate and putamen). The substantia nigra neurons selectively degenerate in Parkinson's disease (Chapter 27). Impairment of nigrostriatal dopaminergic transmission by certain neuroleptic drugs is thus responsible for parkinsonian side effects. One population of dopamine neurons in the more medially placed ventral tegmental area (VTA) innervates limbic forebrain targets, such as the nucleus accumbens (mesolimbic pathway), and a separate population of VTA dopamine neurons innervates "limbic" cortex, such as the medial frontal cortex and the cingulate gyrus (mesocortical pathway). Another dopamine nucleus, the arcuate, is in the hypothalamus, projects to the median eminence, and releases dopamine directly into the hypophyseal portal circulation. Dopamine is then carried to the anterior lobe of the pituitary where it inhibits prolactin release.

Midbrain dopamine neurons have similarities and differences in their firing properties and in regulation of transmitter synthesis and release. Many dopamine neurons have the same type of slow regular discharge, but others fire in bursts of higher frequency. In particular, mesocortical neurons fire faster and with greater bursting than most substantia nigra and mesolimbic neurons. In addition, the regulation and effects of neuroleptics on the firing rates of these midbrain dopamine cells differ. Acute, behaviorally active doses of all classes of neuroleptics increase the firing rates of some neurons, though not those that make up the mesocortical pathway. The latter neurons normally fire at elevated rates at base-line value compared to the former group and are relatively insensitive to neuroleptics. This is caused by the presence of somatic autoreceptors for dopamine, activation of which decreases cell firing. Acute blockade of these autoreceptors by neuroleptics increases firing.

Nerve terminals of both substantia nigra and VTA neurons regulate dopamine synthesis and release by D_2-"autoreceptors" on the presynaptic nerve terminal, and regulate dopamine release by presynaptic excitatory amino acid receptors, especially those of the *N*-methyl-D-aspartate (NMDA) subtype. The excitatory transmitter, glutamic acid, is released from terminals of overlying cortical neurons, which project to the corpus striatum and the nucleus accumbens. Thus, two independent mechanisms regulate synaptic dopamine concentrations in striatal and limbic forebrain, impulse flow along mesostriatal and mesolimbic pathways, and terminal autoreceptor/glutamate receptor activity.

Daily treatment with neuroleptics for several weeks produces a reversible cessation of firing of midbrain dopamine neurons. These inactivated neurons are said to be in a state of "depolarization block," and can be induced to fire again by local application of inhibitory transmitters such as γ-aminobutyric acid (GABA). Depolarization block blunts stress-induced increases in midbrain dopamine neuronal firing but does not substantially alter base-line dopamine release. Traditional neuroleptic agents, such as haloperidol, have a significant propensity to cause parkinsonism as a side effect and produce depolarization block of both substantia nigra and VTA neurons. Clozapine, which has no parkinsonian side effects, produces depolarization block only in VTA neurons. It is now regarded that the ability of a drug to induce depolarization block predicts both its antipsychotic activity (VTA neurons) and its propensity to cause parkinsonian side effects (substantia nigra neurons). The molecular mechanism underlying production of depolarization block of midbrain dopamine neurons is unknown, but the block is presently the most cohesive explanation of antipsychotic action.

Thus mesolimbic dopamine neurons and associated nerve endings possess impulse-, release-, and synthesis-modulating presynaptic dopamine receptors. The neurons are capable of monitoring synaptic dopamine concentrations and fine-tuning firing rates, depolarization-release coupling, and synthesis of dopamine to meet demands.

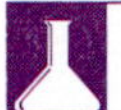

PHARMACOKINETICS

Most neuroleptic drugs are highly lipophilic, bind avidly to proteins, and tend to accumulate in highly perfused tissues. Oral absorption is often incomplete and erratic, whereas IM injection is more reliable. With repeated administration, variable accumulation occurs in body fat and possibly in brain myelin. Half-lives are generally long, and so a single daily dose is effective. An esterified derivative of fluphenazine requires dosing only once every few weeks. After long-term treatment and drug administration is stopped, therapeutic effects may outlast significant blood concentrations by days or weeks. This may result from tight binding of parent drug or active metabolites in the brain.

Metabolism of antipsychotic drugs usually starts with oxidation by hepatic microsomal enzymes, followed by glucuronidation and excretion in the urine. After long-term use, the rate of conversion of the parent drug increases slightly, causing a mild metabolic tolerance; however, monitoring the blood concentration of drug is generally not useful in preventing this problem. In individual patients, very wide variations in blood concentrations of antipsychotic agent can still achieve control of symptoms. Thioridazine because of its prominent anticholinergic activity in the gastrointestinal tract, may display erratic absorption after oral administration. Even with regular dosing, especially in older patients, periods of inadequate or excessive blood concentrations of drug may result. The pharmacokinetic parameters for the antipsychotic agents are listed in Table 23-1.

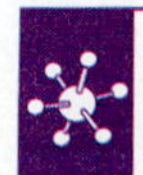

RELATION OF MECHANISM OF ACTION TO CLINICAL RESPONSE

Although the underlying cause of psychosis is unknown, treatment with neuroleptic drugs usually results

Table 23-1 Pharmacokinetic Parameters

Drug	Administration	$t_{1/2}$ (hr)	Disposition	Active Metabolite
acetophenazine				
fluphenazine HCl	Oral, IM	20	M	
trifluoperazine HCl				
perphenazine HCl	Oral, IM			
prochlorperazine	Oral, IM, IV			
thioridazine HCl	Oral			
mesoridazine				
triflupromazine				
chlorpromazine	Oral, IM, IV	30	M	+
chlorprothixene				
thiothixene	Oral, IM			
haloperidol	Oral, IM	18 (decanoate 3 wks)	M	
loxapine	Oral		R	
molindone HCl	Oral		M (95%)	
clozapine	Oral	24	M	

M, Metabolized; *R,* renal.

in a specific improvement in psychotic signs and symptoms and does not simply cause sedation or reduce agitation. Modern antipsychotic drugs allow many schizophrenics to lead productive lives outside hospitals or less restrictive lives within hospitals. Unfortunately, for about half of patients with schizophrenia, classical neuroleptics are not completely effective in controlling positive symptoms. The progression of negative symptoms can lead to progressive deterioration.

Until the introduction of clozapine, the unifying hypothesis of D_2-dopamine receptor blockade as the mechanism of action of antipsychotic drugs seemed secure. However, the course of receptor blockade and its therapeutic benefit were not consistent, and the efficacy of clozapine and newer experimental drugs more active at other neurotransmitter receptors (i.e., serotonin type 2) have brought about a rethinking of the original hypothesis. One view is that a final common pathway is the production of a depolarization block of midbrain dopamine neurons and that this block can be brought about by manipulation of other neurotransmitter systems. A second view is that neuroleptic drugs primarily interact with "sigma opiate" receptors. A third is that interaction with one or more of the newer dopamine receptor subtypes explains the actions of these drugs. Whatever the underlying mechanism, acute blockade of any known receptor population is not, in isolation, a sufficient explanation for antipsychotic action.

In schizophrenia, negative signs and symptoms are generally more resistant to antipsychotic drug therapy and are commonly the cause of chronic disability. It is likely that negative signs and symptoms have a pathophysiological description different from that of positive signs and symptoms and are associated more with decreased frontal lobe metabolic rate. In some patients, negative signs and symptoms may worsen with neuroleptic treatment. The increased efficacy of clozapine compared to traditional neuroleptics derives primarily from its greater efficacy in improving negative signs and symptoms.

All antipsychotic drugs are equally efficacious but differ dramatically in potency and side effects. Treatment choices are empiric, and there is no scientific rationale for having a patient take more than one neuroleptic at a time, except during drug changeover.

The schedule for antipsychotic administration is dependent on the clinical situation. A severely agitated, violent patient poses an immediate challenge different from that of a quiet and withdrawn catatonic. One may reduce agitation by inducing catalepsy either with large neuroleptic doses, or by using neuroleptic doses combined with a parenteral sedative-hypnotic (e.g., lorazepam). Because initiation of therapy with large neuroleptic doses may increase the risk of acute dystonic reactions, it is preferable to attempt management of agitated, psychotic patients initially with the neuroleptic sedative–hypnotic strategy. Agitation may be rapidly controlled either way, but the true antipsychotic effect will require weeks of treatment.

Neuroleptic choice is dictated by desirability or undesirability of side effects, prior history of side effects and responses, and other individual circumstances. For example, drugs with significant anticholinergic side effects should be avoided in the elderly, those with narrow-angle glaucoma or prostatic hypertrophy, and in patients with a history of psychosis caused by drug intoxication. Patients with low blood pressure or histories of orthostatic hypotension symptoms should avoid agents with significant α-adrenergic receptor antagonist activity.

The common cause of relapse of psychotic signs and symptoms is noncompliance with medication, and there is the suggestion that the ultimate outcome in schizophrenia varies inversely with the number of psychotic breaks. Maintaining drug compliance is a major challenge in the chronically psychotic population. Long-duration depot-injection preparations of fluphenazine and haloperidol are available for treating individuals who are unable to maintain compliance with oral medication. Maintenance dose requirements must be empirically determined, and the introduction of depot injections is sometimes accompanied by dystonic reactions. Lifelong psychological and social support contributes greatly to quality of life and may influence the frequency or severity of psychotic episodes.

SIDE EFFECTS, CLINICAL PROBLEMS, AND TOXICITY

Neuroleptic drugs are replete with side effects. Many side effects occur early during treatment and result from neuroleptic blockade of receptors in the central and peripheral nervous systems; others appear later in the course of treatment.

Many of the side effects of individual neuroleptic drugs can be understood on the basis of their ability to block specific receptor types. Prominent among these interactions are α-adrenergic (causing orthostatic hypotension, reflex tachycardia), anticholinergic (dry mouth, difficulty in focusing the eyes, memory impairment, constipation, tachycardia), and antihistaminergic (sedation, weight gain). Occasionally, side effects are desirable. Examples include the use of anticholinergic neuroleptics to reduce parkinsonian side effects, or use of neuroleptics with antihistamine activity in an individual requiring sedation. Usually side effects are troubling, need to be anticipated, and are a common cause of drug changes.

Blockade of D_2-receptors on pituitary lactotroph cells leads to increased serum prolactin concentrations in both males and females, with the increase in females sufficient to produce breast engorgement and galactorrhea.

Neuroleptic drug therapy is usually well tolerated, even in surprisingly high doses (100 mg/day of haloperidol or equivalent). Several neuroleptic-specific side effects are as follows.

"Extrapyramidal" Reactions

Extrapyramidal reactions include parkinsonism, which can mimic idiopathic Parkinson's disease but is usually of a mild degree. It responds to anticholinergic drugs or amantadine. More severe parkinsonism is seen in older individuals who have age-related nigral dopamine neuron deficiency and may necessitate discontinuation of neuroleptic drug, change to clozapine, or careful addition of levodopa. The most severe parkinsonian side effect is neuroleptic malignant syndrome. This is a life-threatening medical emergency and can appear in any patient at any age taking any neuroleptic drug for any period of time. Signs and symptoms include fever, confusion, depressed level of consciousness, autonomic instability, muscular rigidity, and elevated white blood cell count and serum creatine kinase. Treatment (in an intensive care unit) includes discontinuation of the neuroleptic and a search for other causes, particularly infection. If no other causes are found, neuroleptic malignant syndrome requires aggressive physiological support and may respond to specific measures. These include dopamine agonists or levodopa/carbidopa in high doses, dantrolene to lessen muscular rigidity, or even neuromuscular blockade.

Akathisia is a subjective sense of restlessness usually accompanied by mild to moderate motor hyperactivity. It is among the most common of side effects and usually responds to β-adrenergic receptor antagonists, anticholinergics, antihistamines, or amantadine. Akathisia is sometimes misinterpreted as increased agitation, leading to increased neuroleptic dosing, resulting in greater akathisia.

Acute dystonic reactions usually appear within a few days of starting neuroleptic treatment and can appear as **oculogyric crisis** (dystonic posturing of neck, face, and eyes) or any combination of focal dystonias. They are frightening but also very responsive to injected anticholinergic or antihistamine drugs. They do not tend to recur during neuroleptic treatment.

Tardive movement disorders appear late in the course of neuroleptic treatment, usually after at least 6 months of continuous drug administration. Their true incidence is unknown, with estimates of 15% to 50% of chronic psychiatric patients experiencing some type of tardive disorder. The most common is **tardive dyskinesia,** which clinically resembles other hyperkinetic choreoathetotic disorders but also has several unique characteristics. In older patients tardive dyskinesia commonly presents in and remains localized to the mouth, face, and tongue muscles. Excessive involuntary movement produces a rhythmic lip puckering, chewing, and tongue-protrusion pattern, referred to as "oral-buccal-lingual dyskinesia." In younger patients hyperkinetic limb and trunk movements are more likely. Tardive dyskinesia is frequently embarrassing and benign in terms of intensity but can be disabling and interfere with speaking, eating, or regular breathing (if diaphragmatic muscles are involved).

Initial formulations of tardive dyskinesia considered it to be the result of dopamine released onto receptors made supersensitive by chronic neuroleptic antagonism. Dopamine receptor hypersensitivity can be produced experimentally after 2 weeks of daily neuroleptic treatment but does not increase with longer periods of neuroleptic use. Tardive dyskinesia clinically requires longer neuroleptic exposure to appear.

Oral dyskinetic movements similar to tardive dyskinesia in humans can be produced in primates by neuroleptic treatment for 1 to 2 years. Brains from these animals and from humans suffering from tardive dyskinesia at death show significant reductions in markers for GABA neuron functioning in certain basal ganglia regions, compared to neuroleptic-treated primates without dyskinesia or age-matched human controls, respectively. Because acute blockade of GABA-A receptors in these same basal ganglia regions of primates produces dyskinesia, a more cogent mechanism is that chronic neuroleptic treatment leads to a functional reduction in GABA activity in selected brain regions, which in turn produces dyskinesia. The capacity of dopamine receptor blockade to alter transcription of the gene for the GABA-synthesizing enzyme glutamate decarboxylase provides a possible mechanism for functional loss of GABA activity with chronic neuroleptic use.

Intact nigrostriatal dopamine functioning is required for production of tardive dyskinesia movements. These movements may be temporarily suppressed by increased neuroleptic dose or by addition of reserpine. The reserpine dose usually required for long-term dyskinesia suppression is in the 2 to 5 mg/day range and carries a high risk of depression as a side effect.

Appearance of tardive dyskinesia must always prompt a reevaluation of the necessity for continuation of the neuroleptic. If continued therapy is desirable, a change to clozapine is reasonable. Clozapine not only has no reported risk of causing tardive dyskinesia but also can suppress movements in preexisting tardive dyskinesia.

Other tardive ("late-appearing") disorders include **tardive dystonia,** which is rare but unfortunately more severe than most cases of tardive dyskinesia. Response of tardive dystonia to clozapine has not yet been systematically examined. Scattered reports of **tardive akathisia** indicate that this subjective discomfort can appear much later in neuroleptic treatment than initially believed.

Seizures

Many neuroleptics lower experimental seizure thresholds, and their use in humans with known seizure disorders must be attempted cautiously. Clozapine has been shown to cause a dose-related increase in seizure production, independent of any prior seizure history in an individual patient. The reported risk of seizures increases at doses above 600 mg/day.

CLINICAL PROBLEMS WITH ANTIPSYCHOTIC DRUGS

- Failure to control negative effects
- Significant toxicity
  - Parkinsonian-like syndrome
  - Akathisia
  - Tardive dyskinesia
  - Autonomic, endocrine, and cardiac effects
  - Neuroleptic malignant syndrome (NMS)
- Poor concentration or dose-effect relationship
- Drug treatment choices are empiric

Toxicity to Other Organs

Chronic neuroleptic therapy is usually well tolerated with rare organ toxicity. Among the more notable toxicities is a 2% incidence of bone marrow suppression, particularly white blood cell count, with clozapine use. This problem is not dose related, tends to appear within the first year of treatment, was initially unrecognized, and resulted in several deaths attributable to agranulocytosis. Weekly blood counts are presently required when a patient is taking clozapine. Otherwise, regular monitoring of hepatic, renal, or marrow function is not normally required during neuroleptic treatment but should be part of quality primary medical care of these patients. Routine laboratory surveillance cannot substitute for good clinical judgment about emergence of possible rare side effects (anorexia or jaundice caused by allergic hepatitis, a high fever, and a sore throat caused by agranulocytosis).

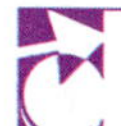

NEW DIRECTIONS

Additional atypical neuroleptic drugs, following the lead of clozapine, should provide improved symptom control with reduced risk of long-term side effects. A unifying pathophysiology of psychosis is evolving, which states that defective cortical control of limbic outflow is responsible for positive symptoms. In schizophrenia, the defect is believed to be in development of cortical input to limbic forebrain, which in humans is not complete until early adulthood. In dementia, the previously intact cortical neurons degenerate. If this hypothesis is correct, primary pharmacological control of signs

TRADE NAMES

In addition to generic and fixed combination preparations, the following trade-named materials are available in the United States.

PHENOTHIAZINES

Compazine, prochlorperazine
Mellaril, thioridazine
Permitil, fluphenazine
Serentil, mesoridazine
Stelazine, trifluoperazine
Thorazine, chlorpromazine
Tindal, acetophenazine
Trilafon, perphenazine
Vesprin, triflupromazine

OTHERS

Haldol, haloperidol
Leponex, clozapine
Loxitane, loxapine
Moban, molindone
Navane, thiothixene
Taractan, chlorprothixene

and symptoms will depend on reduction of limbic outflow, which is a GABA/neuropeptide–mediated process. Improved control of negative signs and symptoms is more problematic and will depend on improved understanding of neurotransmitters involved in frontal cortical synaptic activity.

REFERENCES

Hollister LE: Drug treatment of schizophrenia, *Psychiat Clin North Am* 7:435, 1984.

Kaplan HI, Saddock BJ: Synopsis of Psychiatry, Baltimore, 1991, Williams & Wilkins.

Meltzer H, editor: Psychopharmacology: the third generation of progress, New York, 1987, Raven Press.

Nasrallah HE, Weinberger DR, editors: The Neurology of Schizophrenia. New York, 1986, Elsevier.

Seiden LS, Balster RL, editors: Behavioral pharmacology: the current status, New York, 1985, Alan R. Liss, Inc.

Trimble MR, Zarifian E, editors: Psychopharmacology of the limbic system, New York, 1985, Oxford University Press.

SELF-ASSESSMENT QUESTIONS

1. Which of the following recognized side effects of antipsychotic drugs should be treated immediately?
   a. Gradual appearance of repetitive puckering mouth movements.
   b. Rapidly worsening rigidity, with elevated white blood cell count and serum creatine kinase activity.
   c. Production of breast milk in a non-nursing female.
   d. Mild slowing of gait.
2. Which of the following is not a consistent property of antipsychotic drugs?
   a. Reduction of firing of ventral tegmental area dopamine neurons with chronic administration.
   b. Reduction of "positive" psychosis symptoms within a few weeks of treatment.
   c. Blockade of non-dopamine biogenic amine receptors.
   d. Variable efficacy in treating "negative" symptoms of schizophrenia.
3. Which of the following statements is true about brain dopamine receptors?
   a. All appear to belong to the same gene superfamily with similar 7-transmembrane loop structures.
   b. They are found on the nerve cell body, terminals, and postsynaptic membranes.
   c. They are coupled to second messenger systems or ion channels through interactions with guanine nucleotide binding proteins (G-proteins).
   d. Blockade of the D_2 subtype by antipsychotic drugs generally correlates with clinical potency in treating psychosis.
   e. All of the above.

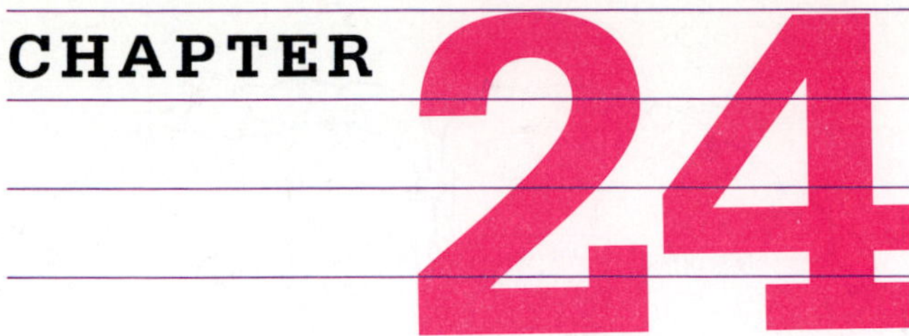

Drugs for Affective (Mood) Disorders

JAMES P. BENNETT, JR.

MAJOR DRUGS

Tricyclic antidepressants
Monoamine oxidase inhibitors
Fluoxetine
Trazodone

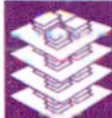 THERAPEUTIC OVERVIEW

Mood disorders are serious disturbances of the internal emotional state. They should be distinguished from alterations of affect, which is the external manifestation of an internal emotional state. The most prevalent and disabling mood disorders are **unipolar depression** and **bipolar illness,** which was previously called *manic-depressive,* or *bipolar affective, illness.*

Unipolar depression is the most common disabling psychiatric illness in the adult population, with about 6% to 10% of the population being affected at some time during their lives. Depression frequently leads to somatic complaints, is routinely underdiagnosed, and may complicate or be secondary to other illness or side effects of drugs. It is life-threatening because 15% to 20% of depressed patients attempt (and may complete) suicide. The depressed patient has a negative attitude, loses interest in activities (anhedonia), ruminates about the impossibility of improvement in life circumstances, and is frequently convinced that one or more body parts is severely diseased or "rotting." Depressed patients assume a characteristic body posture, avoid direct eye contact, and exhibit a pronounced slowness in voluntary movements and responses to questions ("psychomotor retardation"). Paradoxical agitation is also seen in the elderly, and cognitive impairment ("pseudodementia") and isolated recurrent somatic complaints also can occur. Unless comprehensive histories are obtained and questions designed to determine mood are asked, the presence of unipolar depression can be overlooked.

Biological ("vegetative") signs of unipolar depression are helpful in diagnosis, though they are not present in all patients. These include weight loss, a characteristic sleep disturbance with early morning awakening and difficulty returning to sleep, changes in bowel habits (usually constipation), and loss of libido. Opposite signs such as weight gain and excessive sleeping are also observed in some cases. Depressed patients sometimes exhibit disturbed pituitary-adrenal axis function, particularly in the feedback regulation of cortisol in the morning, or other neuroendocrine abnormalities.

Patients with mania exhibit symptoms that are exactly the opposite. These individuals have seemingly endless energy, are excessively talkative, and possess grandiose schemes for achieving personal success. They typically experience a decreased need for sleep, increased libido, and surges of creativity. Examination often reveals several of the following: inflated self-opinion, pressured speech, a subjective sense that thoughts are racing ("flight of ideas"), easy distractibility, preoccupation with pleasure-giving behaviors, even if dangerous, and excessive goal-directed behavior. Impaired insight and lack of judgment lead to faulty and destructive decisions about financial and personal behavior. Prolonged periods of sleep deprivation and excessive activity can cause physiological exhaustion. Bipolar illness involves cycling between depression and mania with an individually consistent cycle length, usually measured in months. Rare individuals have much shorter cycle lengths. Repeated episodes of mania without depression ("unipolar mania") are less common than bipolar illness.

ABBREVIATIONS

MAO	monoamine oxidase

THERAPEUTIC OVERVIEW

AFFECTIVE DISORDERS

Unipolar
- Depression or mania (not both)

Bipolar
- Recurring depression and mania (both)

THERAPY

Act on biogenic amines to inhibit amine transport or degradation and reduce density of amine receptors
Several mechanisms involved
Successful therapy requires several months
Produce significant side effects

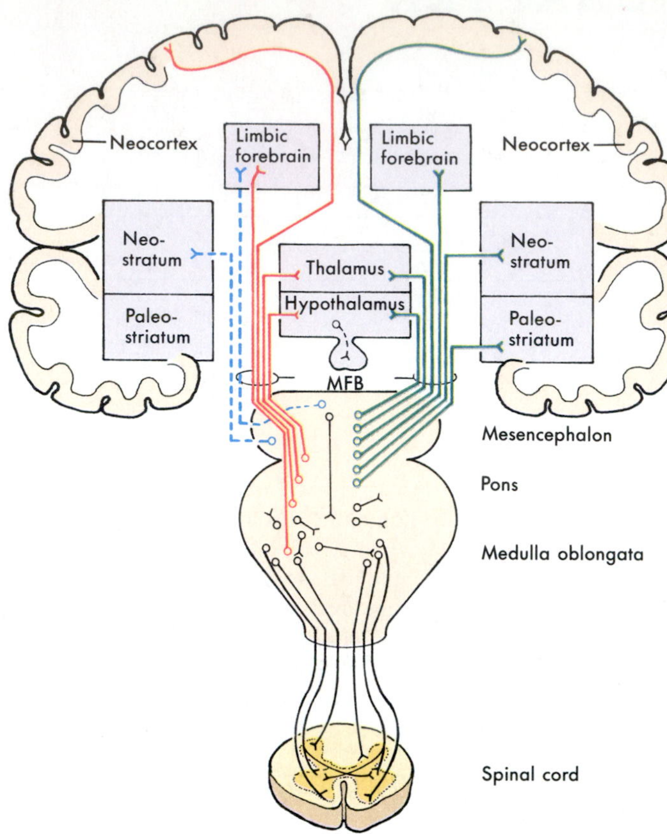

FIGURE 24-1 Organization of norepinephrine (NE) *(red)* and serotonin (5-HT) *(green)* pathways in the mammalian brain. Cell bodies of NE neurons are localized in the pons medulla. NE-containing axons ascend in dorsal and ventral pathways, project diffusely to the forebrain, and descend to the spinal cord. Cell bodies of the 5-HT neurons are located in the raphe nuclei in the midbrain (mesencephalon) and also project diffusely to the forebrain *(green)* and spinal cord. Ascending NE and 5-HT fibers travel near each other in the medial forebrain bundle *(MFB)*. Dopamine (DA) *(blue)* pathways also are shown for reference.

Unipolar depression and bipolar illness should not be viewed simply as extreme examples of normal variations in mood. Both illnesses have significant genetic risk factors and respond to specific somatic therapies. Like all illnesses, depression and mania can be precipitated or worsened by concomitant environmental stress. Drug treatment alone is unlikely to produce a good long-term outcome and is usually combined with supportive psychotherapy.

Mood disorders are lifelong diseases though the number of occurrences and intervals between occurrences vary. Unipolar depression is twice as common in women as in men, has a mean age of onset around 40 years, and an untreated duration of symptoms of 6 to 12 months. The major effect of drug therapy in unipolar depression is to prevent suicide, shorten the duration of symptoms, and lessen the risk of recurrence.

Patients with unipolar depression or bipolar illness can also develop a psychotic disorder of their perception of reality, in addition to disturbance of mood (see Chapter 23). In such cases, antipsychotic therapy also becomes necessary as an adjunct to treatment of the underlying mood disorder. However, it is difficult to diagnose mood disorders when schizophrenia or other chronic psychosis is present.

Drugs can be used to treat depression, control manic symptoms, and prevent relapse into mania or depression. Chronic use of certain drugs such as opiates and sedative-hypnotics can lead to depression.

MECHANISMS OF ACTION

Antidepressant Drugs

Although the precise causes of mood disorders remain elusive, several observations indicate that they may be primarily attributable to alterations in firing patterns of certain subsets of biogenic amine–containing neurons in the CNS (Fig. 24-1). For example, reserpine was once a mainstay of therapy for hypertension, probably because it inhibited storage of norepinephrine in sympathetic nerve terminals. However, chronic reserpine use was associated with about a 25% risk of depression, clinically indistinguishable from unipolar depression. Thus reserpine is used very little today. Its depressive effect probably results from depletion of one or more biogenic amines (serotonin, dopamine, norepinephrine) from the brain. In addition, the antituberculosis drug isoniazid was found to relieve depression in patients with chronic tuberculosis. These antidepressant effects appear to be attributable to the ability of isoniazid to inhibit biogenic amine degradation by monoamine oxidase (MAO), leading to increased brain bio-tricyclic

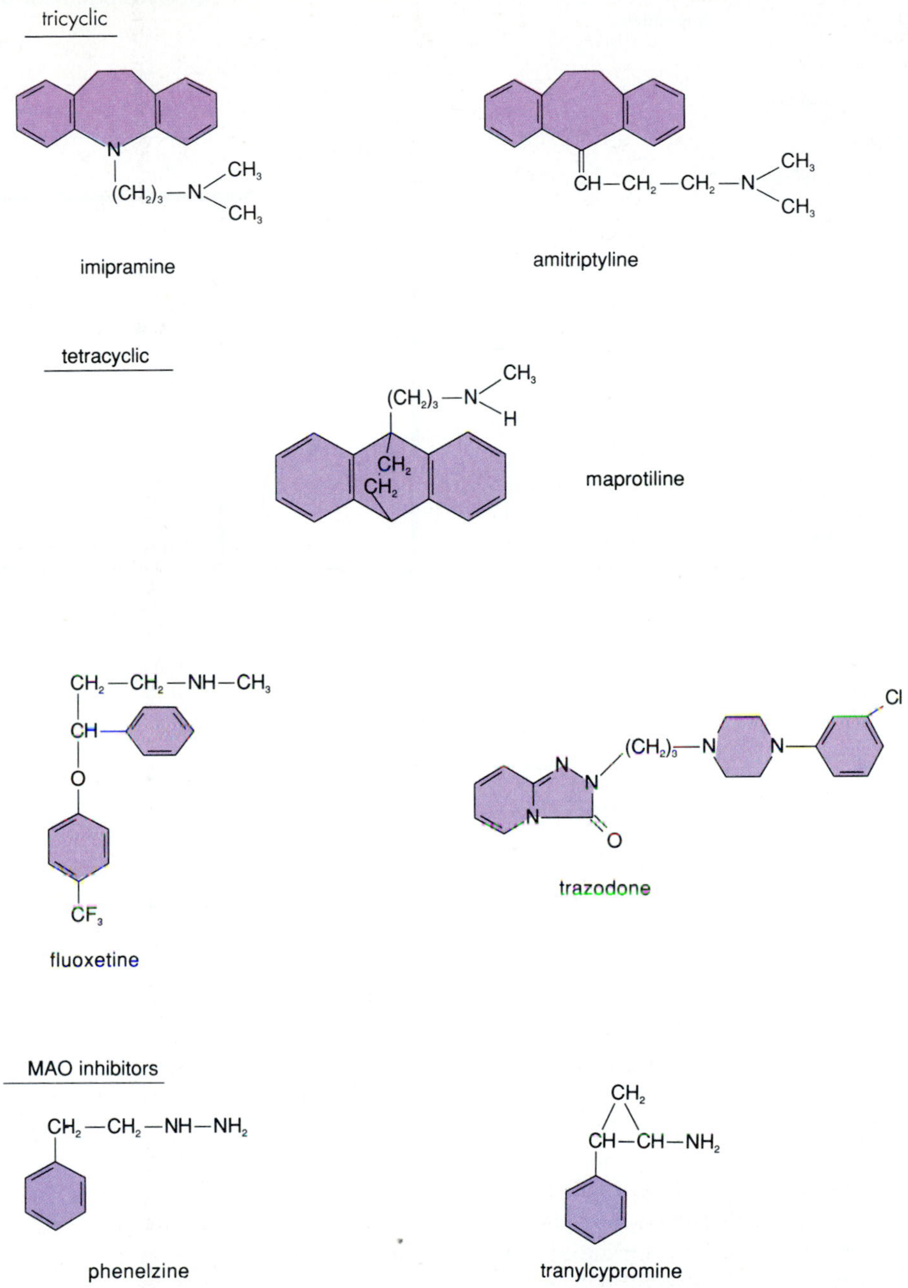

imipramine

amitriptyline

tetracyclic

maprotiline

fluoxetine

trazodone

MAO inhibitors

phenelzine

tranylcypromine

FIGURE 24-2 Chemical structure of selected examples of the major classes of antidepressant drugs.

genic amine concentrations. Finally, clinically effective antidepressant drugs can reverse reserpine-induced catalepsy in experimental animals, an effect caused by depletion of biogenic amines. These observations indicate that depression may involve deficits in brain biogenic amines and raise the possibility that increased catecholamine function is one mechanism by which antidepressant drugs may alleviate depression.

Antidepressant drugs can be classified into tricyclics, tetracyclics, monoamine oxidase inhibitors, and "atypical" antidepressants (Figure 24-2). All these drugs appear to increase biogenic amine availability in the brain. Tricyclic and tetracyclic drugs specifically block reuptake of the neurotransmitters norepinephrine and serotonin into nerve terminals after exocytotic release. Since reuptake is the primary mechanism for terminat-

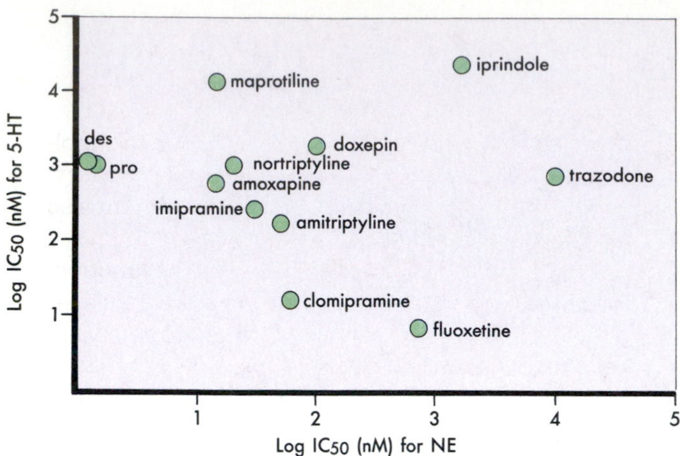

FIGURE 24-3 Relative potencies of antidepressants to inhibit norepinephrine (NE) and serotonin (5-HT) uptake into nerve terminals. An IC_{50} value is the concentration of drug that blocks 50% of the high-affinity uptake of NE or 5-HT into nerve terminals measured in vitro. A smaller IC_{50} means the drug is more potent in inhibition of uptake. *des,* Desipramine; *pro,* protriptyline.

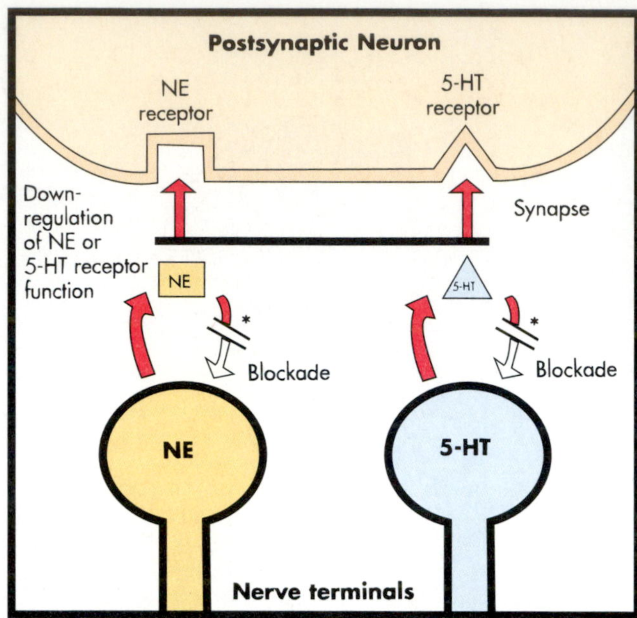

FIGURE 24-4 Effects of antidepressant drugs on biogenic amine neurotransmission. Blockade of reuptake into nerve terminals of norepinephrine *(NE)* or serotonin *(5-HT)* will increase synaptic levels and result in downregulation of postsynaptic receptor function

ing the actions of these compounds, tricyclic and tetracyclic drugs increase the concentrations of these transmitters at their postsynaptic effector sites. Tetracyclics are more potent at blocking norepinephrine uptake, and "atypical" antidepressant drugs have a wide variation in their effects on the uptake of both norepinephrine and serotonin (Figure 24-3).

MAO is a mitochondrial enzyme that breaks down norepinephrine and serotonin, as well as dopamine. There are two isozymes, designated *A* and *B,* both of which oxidatively inactivate these neurotransmitters. The available MAO inhibitors for treatment of depression nonselectively inhibit both enzyme types, though it has been determined experimentally that inhibition of the A subtype is responsible for antidepressant activity. Phenelzine and isocarboxazid irreversibly bind to and inactivate MAO, whereas tranylcypromine is a reversible inhibitor. Since new enzyme is synthesized only slowly, complete and continuous inhibition of MAO is possible.

An understanding of the mechanisms by which antidepressant drugs act must take into account the delay of several weeks that is observed before mood begins to improve. It is clear that potentiation of aminergic transmission by blockade of reuptake or inhibition of MAO will occur quickly after drug administration (Fig. 24-4) and therefore cannot solely be responsible for the therapeutic effects of these compounds. Animal studies have found that chronic administration of antidepressant drugs reduces the density of postsynaptic receptors for norepinephrine (particularly of the β subtype) and serotonin (particularly the 5-HT_2 subtype) in brain tissue after several weeks. It is believed that this **receptor downregulation** may be an adaptive response to the chronic increases in norepinephrine and serotonin caused by these drugs and may be involved in their therapeutic effects.

Obviously, no single biochemical effect can explain the mechanism of action of antidepressant drugs. It is unlikely that inhibition of biogenic amine uptake or degradation, in isolation, can correct the fundamental chemical abnormalities of depression. However, the available data indicate that manipulation of biogenic amine synaptic transmission may be involved in antidepressant action.

Antimanic Drugs

Acute manic episodes are managed with lithium salts, alone or in combination with carbamazepine, valproic acid, or calcium-channel blockers. Concomitant psychosis or agitation may require temporary use of antipsychotic drugs (see Chapter 23).

Lithium remains the drug of choice for the treatment and prophylaxis of mania. Lithium is a small monovalent cation, intermediate in size between hydrogen and sodium ion, which gets distributed throughout total body water (similar to sodium ion). Lithium is adminis-

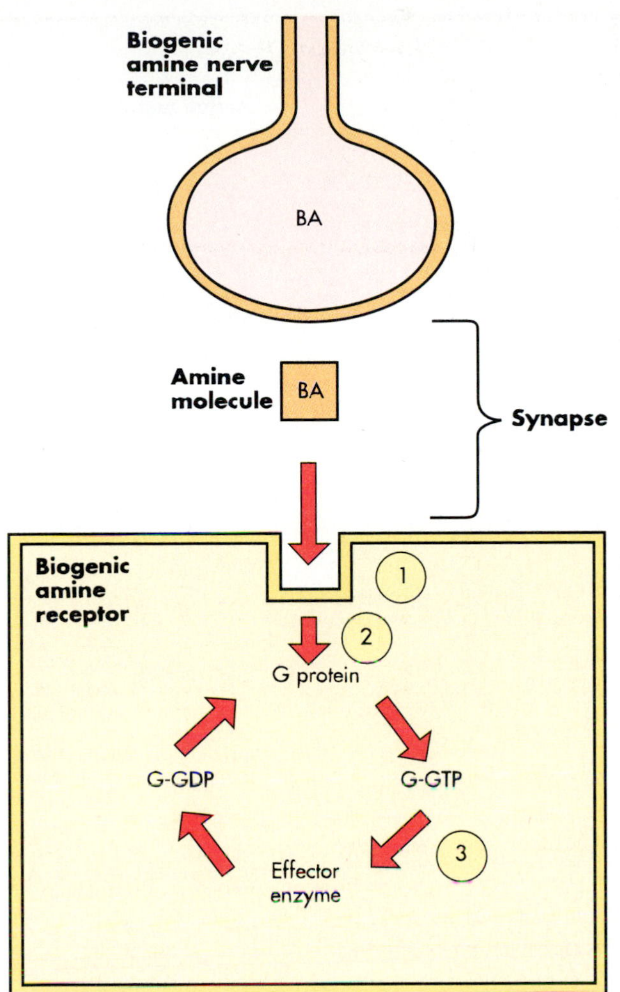

FIGURE 24-5 Potential sites for lithium action on *BA*, biogenic amine *(NE, 5-HT)*, synapses. Lithium can reduce affinity of binding to receptor *(1)*, reduce coupling to G protein *(2)*, or lower stimulation of effect or enzyme system (i.e., adenylate cyclase, phospholipase C) by activated G protein *(3)*. *GDP,* Guanosine diphosphate; *GTP,* guanosine triphosphate.

tered as the carbonate or citrate salt. Although the antimanic effects require weeks or months to develop, lithium administration has clearly been shown to prevent or reduce the intensity of additional manic episodes. Lithium also helps to alleviate the depressive phase of bipolar illness but is not so effective as antidepressant drugs in relieving established depressive symptoms.

Unlike antidepressant drugs, long-term administration of lithium does not produce consistent alterations in aminergic receptor density but does alter the coupling of receptors to their signaling pathways. Lithium acutely inhibits the breakdown of inositol 1-phosphate, preventing the recycling of inositol (see Chapter 2). This may lead to a long-term depletion in inositol polyphosphates in the brain, which play an important role in controlling cellular calcium concentrations in response to cell surface receptor activation. Lithium has been suggested to prevent development of the supersensitivity of amine receptors that normally occurs after denervation, leading to alterations in important signaling molecules such as adenylate cyclase or phospholipase C (Figure 24-5). Therapeutic concentrations of lithium also reduce the formation of certain second messengers, perhaps by direct alterations of G-protein levels or function.

Carbamazepine and valproic acid are anticonvulsant drugs used in treating mania in patients refractory to, or unable to tolerate, lithium. Carbamazepine is often as effective as lithium but has no advantages over lithium and may cause more serious side effects. The mechanisms of action of these drugs in treating seizures is discussed in Chapter 26. The mechanisms by which they reduce mania are not clear. Carbamazepine is structurally similar to tricyclics but does not block amine uptake or downregulate adrenergic receptors.

Several antagonists of L-type voltage-dependent calcium channels (nifedipine, diltiazem, verapamil) are effective in the treatment of bipolar illness. These drugs can exert significant cardiovascular effects, and their use in bipolar illness is usually restricted to those who cannot tolerate or do not respond to lithium or carbamazepine. The mechanism by which they alleviate bipolar illness is not clear.

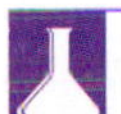

PHARMACOKINETICS

Antidepressant drugs

Tricyclics and tetracyclics are lipophilic, well absorbed after oral administration, and are distributed widely in body tissues (Table 24-1). The oral bioavailability of most antidepressants is reduced by first-pass metabolism by the liver. Drug disposition is predominantly by metabolism. Some tricyclic tertiary amines undergo demethylation to yield active secondary amines. The degree of demethylation varies widely among patients, tends to stabilize for a given patient, and necessitates assay of plasma concentrations of both parent drug and active metabolites. The anticholinergic activity of many of these drugs can delay gastrointestinal absorption of the tricyclic and other drugs administered at the same time.

Tricyclics and tetracyclics have long half-lives, frequently more than 24 hours, and such a characteristic allows once a day dosing. This can improve compliance, which is a major factor in achieving therapeutic success. The atypical antidepressant fluoxetine is notable for having a half-life of 2 to 3 days for the parent drug and 7 to 9 days for the active metabolite, norfluoxetine.

Table 24-1 Pharmacokinetic Parameter Values

Drug*	$T_{1/2}$*	Disposition	Bioavailability (%)	Active metabolites
TRICYCLICS				
amitriptyline	10-30	M	30-60	nortriptyline
amoxapine	8	M	—	7.8-OH
clomipramine	20-40	M	—	desmethyl
desipramine	15-60	M	60-70	—
doxepin	8-25	M	15-45	desmethyl
imipramine	10-25	M	30-75	desipramine
nortriptyline	15-55	M	50-80	10-OH
protriptyline	55-124	M	75-95	—
TETRACYCLIC				
maprotiline	25-60	M	40-75	desmethyl
ANTIMANIC				
carbamazepine	10-20	—	70	—
lithium salts	8-40	R (95%)	100	none
ATYPICAL				
bupropion	8-16	M	—	yes
fluoxetine	24-72	M	—	norfluoxetine
mianserin	10-27	—	30-75	—
nomifensine	2-4	—	—	—
trazodone	6-11	M	—	*m*-chlorophenylpiperazine
sertraline	26-100	M	—	N-desmethyl
MAO INHIBITORS†				
phenelzine	—	M	—	—
tranylcypromine	—	M	—	—
isocarboxazid	—	M	—	—

M, Metabolized; *R*, renal.
*Oral administration.
†Little information is available on the pharmacokinetics of MAO inhibitors, though their therapeutic effects are often long lasting. This is partly attributable to the irreversible inhibition caused by phenelzine and isocarboxazid.

Sertraline, a newer atypical antidepressant, has an average half-life of 26 hours for the parent drug and 60 to 100 hours for the much less active metabolite *N*-desmethylsertraline. Both fluoxetine and sertraline can be administered once a day, and steady-state concentrations of the parent drugs are not reached for at least 5 to 7 days.

MAO inhibitors are well absorbed after oral administration. Those that produce irreversible inhibition have long biological half-lives because of the slow turnover of this enzyme. Drug abstinence for a minimum of 2 to 3 weeks is necessary for MAO activity to return to near normal and is necessary before one introduces other drugs, which may have adverse interactions, particularly other antidepressants. Some MAO inhibitors are inactivated by hepatic acetylation, the rate of which is under genetic control. Adequacy of dosing can be assessed by measurement of platelet MAO activity (which is mostly of the B subtype), with greater than 65% inhibition associated with improved therapeutic response.

Antimanic Drugs

Lithium salts are rapidly and completely absorbed from the intestinal tract, are distributed within a few hours to extracellular water, and finally are distributed into total body water. Lithium concentrations in brain extracellular space are about half the serum concentrations. Lithium is filtered by the glomerulus and extensively reabsorbed (about 80%) in the tubules, where it competes with sodium ion for reabsorption. Lithium excretion is enhanced by sodium loading and inhibited by sodium depletion. Conditions that increase sodium reabsorption, such as congestive heart failure, ascites, or cirrhosis, can increase lithium reabsorption and lead to toxic concentrations. Diuretics that inhibit distal sodium reabsorption can increase lithium reabsorption and produce toxicity. In general, patients receiving lithium should avoid situations or drugs that produce alterations in salt and water metabolism.

Serum lithium concentrations peak within a few hours of each dose and then decline in a biphasic elimi-

Table 24-2 Relative Potencies of Antidepressants on Amine Receptors

Drug	ACh	α_1-Adrenergic	α_2-Adrenergic	H_1
amitriptyline	high	high	high	medium
protriptyline	medium	low	low	very low
doxepin	medium	high	high	high
imipramine	low	medium	medium	very low
clomipramine	low	medium	medium	—
nortriptyline	low	medium	medium	very low
maprotiline	low	medium	low	—
amoxapine	low	medium	medium	—
desipramine	low	low	low	very low
iprindole	very low	very low	low	very low
fluoxetine	very low	very low	low	—
trazodone	very low	medium	high	very low

ACh, Muscarinic cholinergic receptor; H_1, histamine receptor.

nation pattern. Individual pharmacokinetics vary among patients but tend to be constant for a given person. The pharmacokinetics of carbamazepine and sodium valproate are discussed in Chapter 26 (Drugs for Seizure Disorders) and those of calcium-channel blockers in Chapter 16 (Calcium Antagonists).

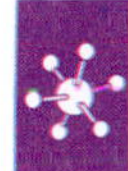

RELATION OF MECHANISMS OF ACTION TO CLINICAL RESPONSE

The therapeutic efficacy of atypical antidepressant drugs, some of which do not significantly block amine transport or inhibit MAO, indicates that neither of these biochemical actions may be ultimately responsible for antidepressant efficacy. Although depression encompasses a reproducible core of clinical symptoms, individual patients may be biochemically or "synaptically" heterogeneous and more responsive to particular antidepressants. All antidepressant drugs have about equal efficacy in treating depressive symptoms and differ primarily in side effects. The antidepressant efficacy of fluoxetine and sertraline, which specifically block serotonin reuptake and interact very little with other transport systems or receptors, demonstrates that isolated manipulation of one biogenic amine system is sufficient for antidepressant action.

The site or sites of action for lithium's antimanic and mood-stabilizing activity remain elusive, but it is likely that interference with receptor-effector coupling, possibly at the level of G-protein functioning, is the major mechanism. Specific mechanisms for antimanic efficacy of carbamazepine, sodium valproate, and calcium-channel antagonists are less clear.

Because of the cardiac toxicity and anticholinergic side effects of typical tricyclic antidepressants, atypical antidepressants are used increasingly as first-line drugs for unipolar illness. As a result, at the time of this writing fluoxetine is the most commonly prescribed antidepressant in the United States.

The major cause of treatment failure is inadequate dosing for too short a period of time. Serum drug concentrations are useful as guidelines for adequacy of dosing. Response times for improvement of affect vary among individuals but usually are in the range of 3 to 6 weeks.

Patients with mania (bipolar) are at risk of physiological exhaustion and require hospitalization to initiate drug therapy and attend to nutrition, hydration, and rest. Treatment is initiated with lithium carbonate in divided daily doses and a neuroleptic or a sedative-hypnotic (usually benzodiazepine), depending on the presence of psychosis or severity of agitation. Lithium exerts an antimanic effect, but the delay in onset of this effect necessitates initiating therapy to provide rapid sedation and rest.

Patients with documented bipolar disease usually require maintenance therapy with lithium to prevent relapse into mania or depression. Patients refractory to lithium often respond to carbamazepine, with the latter begun at low doses and increased slowly to maintenance. Frequent monitoring of serum concentrations ensures adequate dosing and prevention of toxic side effects.

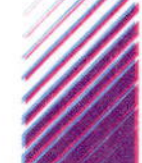

SIDE EFFECTS, CLINICAL PROBLEMS, AND TOXICITY

Tricyclic and Tetracyclic Antidepressants

Most of the side effects of tricyclic and tetracyclic antidepressants derive from interactions with central and peripheral neurotransmitter receptors (Table 24-2). Typical side effects from antagonism of muscarinic receptors include dry mouth, blurred vision, urinary retention, reduced sweating, constipation, and recent memory impairment. The incidence and severity of these side effects, coupled with the very slow development of the antidepressant effect, give rise to the widely noted "patients feel worst at first" phenomenon. With overdosage, generalized life-threatening seizures can occur, but they are responsive to inhibition of brain acetylcholinesterase with physostigmine. Sedation is principally caused by histamine (H_1) blocking activity and is prominent with doxepin. Orthostatic hypotension is the result of antagonism of α-adrenergic receptors. The atypical agents trazodone, fluoxetine, and sertraline are less potent in blocking these receptors and cause fewer side effects.

An important side effect not related to specific receptor antagonism is cardiac toxicity. Tricyclics should be used cautiously if at all in patients with cardiac conduction defects, particularly those in acute myocardial infarction. Cardiac toxicity is the most serious side effect of tricyclic drugs. This toxicity results in part from the quinidine-like actions of tricyclic drugs on cardiac muscle.

The increased suicide risk in depression, combined with the toxicity of antidepressant drugs, necessitates careful attention to the amounts of drug available at any given time to a seriously depressed patient. Obvious suicidal risk necessitates inpatient treatment, where access to these potentially lethal drugs can be restricted. In outpatient treatment, no more than 1 week's worth of medicine should generally be dispensed at one time. Paradoxically, most suicide attempts occur as the patient is beginning to emerge from depression. Overdosage with tricyclic and tetracyclic antidepressants must be managed in an intensive care unit, with particular attention paid to cardiac and CNS toxicity of these drugs.

Patients with known seizure disorders may have seizure recurrence when tricyclics are given. Seizures may occur from lowering of the seizure threshold and alteration of metabolism of anticonvulsant drugs by tricyclics. Tricyclic drugs potentiate the sedative actions of other central nervous system (CNS) depressants such as alcohol, barbiturates, and benzodiazepines. Finally, tricyclic drug administration to a patient with bipolar illness, usually presenting as depression without a history of mania, can precipitate acute mania or rapid cycling.

MAO Inhibitors

Therapy with MAO inhibitors usually proceeds without significant side effects. However, this is a deceptive situation because the catabolic capacity of the body to deaminate a wide variety of drugs and natural products is severely impaired. This diminished catabolic capacity is dramatically demonstrated by the appearance of a hypertensive crisis. This occurs after ingestion of foods that contain tyramine, such as pickled fish, aged cheeses, and red wines. Tyramine is a naturally occurring amine that potently releases norepinephrine from sympathetic nerve endings. Dietary tyramine is normally deaminated by gastrointestinal MAO-A, but in the presence of MAO inhibitors dietary tyramine is rapidly absorbed into the circulation. The resulting hypertensive crisis can be severe, and lead to intracranial bleeding or other organ damage. Selective MAO-B inhibitors do not cause this problem but also do not relieve depression.

MAO inhibitors should not be administered along with tricyclic-tetracyclic antidepressants because the drug combination may provide a "central hyperexcitation syndrome." This consists of high fever, delirium, and hypertension, though the mechanisms involved are obscure. Other reported adverse interactions of MAO inhibitors with opiates, anesthetics, sedatives, and sympathomimetic amines limit the use of these compounds in the United States.

Depression that is refractory to standard treatments

CLINICAL PROBLEMS

TRICYCLIC ANTIDEPRESSANTS

Autonomic and Cardiovascular Side Effects

Hypotension
Tremors
Blurred vision
Cardiac dysrhythmias

Toxic Overdoses: Problem With Long-Term Therapy

Loss of consciousness
Acidosis
Hypotension
Cardiac dysrhythmias

MAO INHIBITORS

Hypotension
Side effects similar to those of tricyclics
Hypertensive crisis with tyramine-containing foods

LITHIUM

Small therapeutic index
GI upset
Toxicity serious
Renal damage

> **TRADE NAMES**
>
> In addition to generic and fixed-combination preparations, the following trade-named materials are available in the United States.
>
> **TRICYCLIC ANTIDEPRESSANTS**
>
> Anafranil, clomipramine
> Asendin, amoxapine
> Aventyl, nortriptyline
> Elavil, amitriptyline
> Norpramin, desipramine
> Sinequan, doxepin
> Tofranil, imipramine
> Vivactil, protriptyline
>
> **MAO INHIBITORS**
>
> Marplan, isocarboxazid
> Nardil, phenelzine sulfate
> Parnate, tranylcypromine sulfate
>
> **OTHERS**
>
> Desyrel, trazodone
> Ludiomil, maprotiline
> Prozac, fluoxetine

can be treated with lithium salts or carbamazepine in addition to tricyclic and tetracyclic therapy or coadministration of an MAO inhibitor and a tricyclic or tetracyclic drug. This latter combination should be undertaken only by physicians experienced in this type of potentially dangerous therapy. Failure of drug therapy can be followed by electroconvulsive therapy. In fact, electroconvulsive therapy consistently produces the fastest improvement in the greatest percentage of patients and is now the treatment of first choice for many depressed elderly.

Selective Serotonin Reuptake Inhibitors (SSRI)

This class of antidepressants has very few serious direct side effects, but certain pharmacokinetic interactions are important. Most of the side effects reported involve anxiety with or without insomnia or mild gastrointestinal complaints (nausea, anorexia, diarrhea). Initial concerns about increased suicide risk with SSRIs have not been confirmed with larger clinical trials.

As is the case with multiple drug classes, age influences metabolism of two of the three available SSRIs. Compared with younger individuals given equal oral doses, elderly patients will achieve higher blood concentrations of fluoxetine (and its major metabolite norfluoxetine) and paroxetine. Both groups achieve equal blood concentrations of sertraline.

All of the available SSRIs can inhibit the hepatic drug metabolizing enzyme P450 IID6, with sertraline being the weakest inhibitor of this system. Inhibition of the P450 system by SSRIs can alter the metabolism of other drugs, including tricyclic antidepressants, phenothiazenes, quinidine, and certain type Ic antiarrhythmics (flecainide, encainide). SSRIs can also have a potentially fatal interaction with MAOI. Coadministration of SSRIs with other drugs must take place with attention to these potential adverse interactions.

Lithium

Use of lithium is complicated by its low therapeutic index, which usually necessitates frequent checking of serum concentrations. Many patients receiving lithium develop a fine tremor, similar to essential tremor. If troubling, this tremor can be reduced by addition of β-adrenergic receptor antagonists. Toxic concentrations of lithium in serum progressively impair CNS functioning, first causing ataxia and confusion (1.5 to 2.0 mEq/L), followed by delirium, myoclonus, and seizures (2.0 to 2.5 mEq/L), and leading to renal failure, refractory seizures, coma, and death (>2.5 mEq/L).

The most common problems associated with use of lithium are gastrointestinal (nausea, vomiting, diarrhea) and may be alleviated by use of a different lithium salt. About one third of patients chronically using lithium develop elevated serum concentrations of thyroid-stimulating hormone, and around 5% develop nontoxic goiter. Around 20% to 25% of lithium-treated individuals experience polyuria with elevated excretion of antidiuretic hormone. True nephrogenic diabetes insipidus (resistant to antidiuretic hormone) as a side effect of lithium administration is rare. Toxic doses of lithium cause permanent renal damage in animals, but permanent renal impairment as a result of lithium therapy in humans has not been unequivocally demonstrated. Cardiac side effects are similar to those caused by hypokalemia and include benign repolarization changes (t wave flattening) and impairment of sinoatrial node functioning or cardiac conduction. The potential multiplicity of organ side effects with lithium therapy necessitate frequent monitoring of serum lithium concentrations, thyroid and renal function, urine volumes, and electrocardiograms.

Finally, lithium has potential fetal toxicity and its use in pregnancy must be questioned and closely regulated.

NEW DIRECTIONS

Additional atypical antidepressants are being developed, and the use of such compounds will likely increase. The term "atypical" is rapidly becoming an anachronism and soon will no longer be in clinical usage. Drugs with biochemical actions similar to lithium, but that are not monovalent cations and therefore not as toxic as lithium, are being actively developed for use in bipolar illness. Advances in understanding of the genetic components of mood disorders may lead to increased understanding of the biochemical deficits, which, one would hope, will guide more specific treatments. Multiple drug regimens have received increasing attention and will be more thoroughly tested for treatment of refractory bipolar illness.

REFERENCES

Mendels J: The acute and long-term treatment of major depression. *Int Clin Psychopharmacol* 7(Suppl 2):21-29, 1992.

Potter WZ, Rudorfer MV, Manji H: The pharmacologic treatment of depression. *New Engl J Med* 325:633-642, 1991.

Pinder RM, Wieringa JH: Third-generation antidepressants. *Medicinal Res Rev* 13:259-325, 1993.

Preskorn SH: Recent pharmacologic advances in antidepressant therapy for the elderly. *Am J Med 94* (Suppl 5A):2S-12S, 1993.

SELF-ASSESSMENT QUESTIONS

1. A patient diagnosed with unipolar depression should *not* receive which of the following?
   a. isoniazid
   b. reserpine
   c. fluoxetine
   d. tyramine
   e. amitriptyline
2. Which of the following would be preferred for initial treatment of a patient with bipolar disease?
   a. carbamazepine
   b. lithium carbonate
   c. valproic acid
   d. carbamazepine and lithium carbonate
   e. lithium carbonate and valproic acid
3. Tricyclic and tetracyclic antidepressants often cause:
   a. sedation by blocking histamine H_1-receptors.
   b. dry mouth by blocking muscarinic cholinergic receptors.
   c. orthostatic hypotension by blocking α_1-adrenergic receptors.
   d. a and c are correct
   e. all are correct
4. Therapy with MAO inhibitors:
   a. usually proceeds without significant side effects.
   b. is often combined with therapy with tricyclic antidepressants.
   c. can cause orthostatic hypotension if the patient ingests cheese or red wine.
   d. is often first-choice therapy for treatment of unipolar depression.
   e. all of the above

CHAPTER 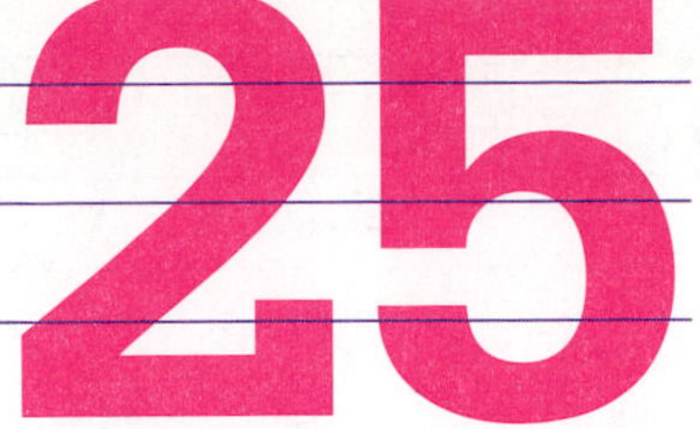

Drugs to Treat Anxieties and Related Disorders

RICHARD H. RECH

MAJOR DRUGS

benzodiazepines
buspirone

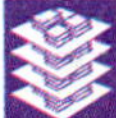

THERAPEUTIC OVERVIEW

Anxiety is the most commonly observed symptom in mental illness but also occurs in normal individuals. Normal anxiety is of short duration, usually event related, not under conscious control, and is characterized by dissatisfaction, somatic complaints, or apprehension. Some research indicates that anxiety is a conditioned fear response. Severe stress often induces increased muscle tension, autonomic nervous system dysfunction, irritability, and fatigue. When these symptoms persist and impair normal activities, they are considered pathological and require treatment. Patients suffering significant anxiety over extended periods may have an inherited predisposition.

Most types of anxiety are relieved by alcohol, opiates, or barbiturates and similar sedative-hypnotic drugs (see Chapter 33) but usually at the expense of prominent sedation and some motor incoordination. *Benzodiazepines,* introduced in the 1960s, are often **anxiolytic** (reduce anxiety) in doses causing little sedation. In addition, benzodiazepines have muscle-relaxant (Chapter 27), sedative-hypnotic (Chapter 33), anticonvulsant (Chapter 26), and amnestic (memory-disturbing) activities. *Buspirone* is a recently developed anxiolytic with minor sedative actions. In contrast to other drugs in this class, buspirone causes no potentiation of the effects of alcohol and does not have anticonvulsant or muscle relaxant activity.

Psychotherapy is generally conceded to be the most effective long-term treatment for anxiety. However, benzodiazepines are usually effective in relieving acute anxiety states, and judicious use of these drugs along with psychotherapeutic management may afford the best outcome. β-Adrenergic receptor antagonists may also be effective against some types of anxiety, especially in reducing autonomic symptoms in some phobias, as in "stage fright."

ABBREVIATIONS

GABA	γ-aminobutyric acid
5-HT	5-hydroxytryptamine

MECHANISMS OF ACTION

The benzodiazepines are the primary agents for the treatment of anxiety. *Chlordiazepoxide, diazepam, oxazepam, lorazepam, clorazepate, halazepam, prazepam,* and *alprazolam* are used for this purpose in the United States. Benzodiazepines have virtually replaced barbiturates, meprobamate, and other sedative-hypnotic drugs previously used. Buspirone is a recently developed antianxiety drug with minimal sedative effects (Table 25-1). Chemical structures of several prototype benzodiazepines and a nonbenzodiazepine, buspirone, are shown in Figure 25-1.

The binding sites for benzodiazepines and barbiturates (formerly widely used for anxiety) are intimately linked with the γ-aminobutyric acid (GABA) receptor, which has a major role in inhibitory mechanisms in brain functions. Molecular cloning has shown that both benzodiazepine and barbiturate binding sites are contained within the multisubunit $GABA_A$ receptor ion chloride-channel complex in central nervous system (CNS) neurons. $GABA_B$ receptors, in contrast, recognize different agonist and antagonist drugs and are important in controlling skeletal muscle spasticity (see Chap-

Table 25-1 Comparison of Anxiolytic Drugs

Drug	CNS Effects	Mechanism	Uses	Comments
alprazolam	Forebrain depression Dependence	GABA enhancement	Anxiolytic, antipanic	Short duration
diazepam	Broad CNS depression Dependence	GABA enhancement	Anxiolytic, sedative, muscle relaxant	Long duration
buspirone	Little sedation No dependence	5-HT effect	Anxiolytic	Delayed onset

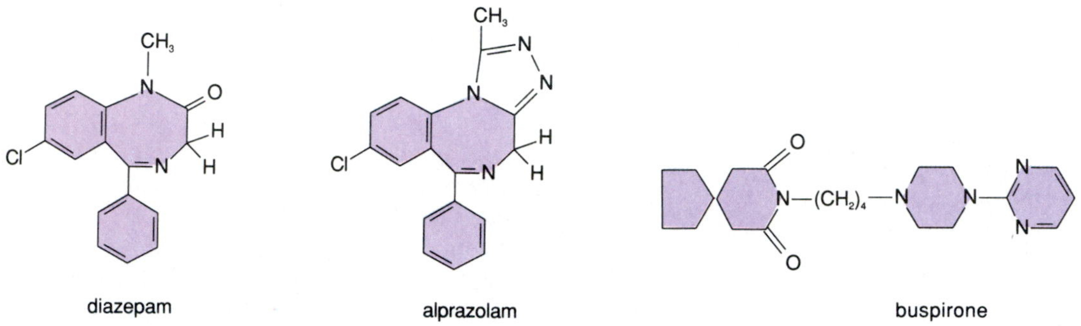

FIGURE 25-1 Chemical structures of representative anxiolytic benzodiazepines and buspirone.

THERAPEUTIC OVERVIEW

GOAL

Effective safe relief of clinical anxiety

CLINICAL APPLICATIONS

Nondrug: Psychotherapy for long-term treatment

Drug

- Benzodiazepines for short-term treatment
- Buspirone for extended treatment

ter 27). The $GABA_A$ receptor is a complex glycoprotein, related in structure to the nicotinic acetylcholine receptor cation channel (Chapter 2). The benzodiazepines bind to an allosteric site distinct from the GABA-binding site but require integrity of the GABA receptor function to increase inhibitory synaptic activity (Figure 25-2). Barbiturates bind to a separate site closer to the chloride channel and, at least in part, can increase chloride-ion conductance (increased inhibition) independent of activity at the GABA site.

Slight variations in receptor structure occur in different brain regions and account for differences in efficacies of individual benzodiazepines as to sedative, anticonvulsant, and anxiolytic effects. GABA-gated chloride-ion channels are found in most postsynaptic membranes of brain neurons, usually innervated by short-axon GABA interneurons. Nerve terminal depolarization by an invading action potential releases Ca^{++}, which in turn promotes exocytosis of GABA neurotransmitter vesicles. GABA released into the synaptic cleft acts on the postsynaptic receptor to open the chloride-ion channel, resulting in influx of chloride ions and hyperpolarization of the membrane. There are also presynaptic GABA-inhibitory functions, but these appear not to relate to benzodiazepine receptors or anxiety.

Binding of a barbiturate or a benzodiazepine to the GABA receptor complex (Figure 25-2) allosterically facilitates the activity of GABA to open the chloride-ion channel (Chapter 2). Larger doses of barbiturates but not benzodiazepines increase chloride-ion conductance even when GABA receptor binding is compromised. Further definition of the GABA and barbiturate binding sites is seen in the activities of the experimental convulsant agents bicuculline and picrotoxin. *Bicuculline* binds selectively to the GABA site, whereas *picrotoxin* is more specific for the barbiturate site. Both bicuculline and picrotoxin block opening of the chloride channel.

Another class of compounds, the β-carbolines, bind to the benzodiazepine site of the GABA receptor complex but allosterically reduce rather than increase chloride-ion conductance by decreasing the affinity of

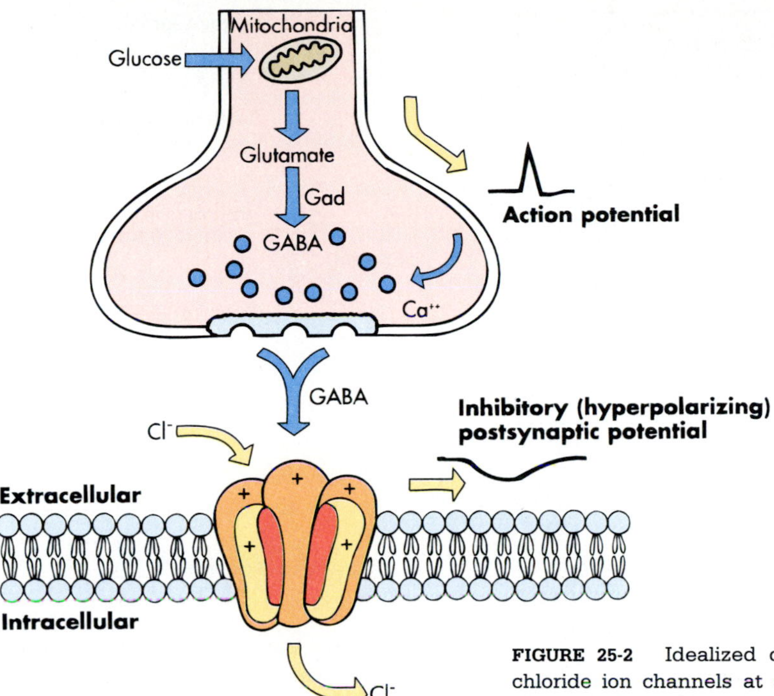

FIGURE 25-2 Idealized depiction of GABA–benzodiazepine–chloride ion channels at axosomatic (postsynaptic) inhibitory synapses. *Gad,* Glutamic acid decarboxylase.

GABA at its receptor site. Thus, β-carbolines (and certain other experimental compounds) are called *inverse agonists* and increase CNS excitability and irritability. They have no therapeutic use and may actually precipitate panic attacks.

Flumazenil is another benzodiazepine agent recently introduced as an antagonist. This drug occupies the benzodiazepine site with high affinity but has little intrinsic activity. However, flumazenil can block the activity of either direct benzodiazepine agonists (diazepam) or inverse agonists (β-carbolines) and has therapeutic utility in treating benzodiazepine overdose. The mechanisms of action of several important drugs and experimental agents are summarized in Table 25-2 (see also Chapter 2).

Despite the preponderance of evidence for mediation of benzodiazepine effects through GABA neuronal systems, alternative mechanisms have been proposed. For example, larger doses of some benzodiazepines inhibit adenosine uptake and potentiate its CNS-depressant effects. Some investigators have suggested that benzodiazepines may exert anxiolytic effects by acting on brain 5-hydroxytryptamine (5-HT) systems. In addition, benzodiazepines modify the activity of glycine, acetylcholine (muscarinic), dopamine, and norepinephrine neurotransmitter systems in the brain. Whether these are direct effects or mediated indirectly through GABA remains unclear. There are also nonneuronal benzodiazepine receptors in peripheral organs not involved in the antianxiety effects. Endogenous benzodiazepine-like anxiolytic or anxiogenic substances have been postulated to exist in the brain and to have a role in normal brain function. However, evidence for such a role is still preliminary.

Table 25-2 Agents Affecting GABA-Linked Inhibitory Chloride Channel

Drug	Mechanism
GABA	Endogenous agonist, binds to $GABA_A$ receptor to promote chloride-ion flux
muscimol	Agonist at GABA site
benzodiazepine	Allosteric agonist
barbiturate	Allosteric agonist at site distinct from benzodiazepine
β-carboline	Allosteric antagonist ("inverse agonist") at benzodiazepine site
flumazenil	Allosteric blocker at benzodiazepine site, no intrinsic activity
bicuculline	Competitive antagonist to GABA
picrotoxin	Blocks channel noncompetitively

Although rapid and extensive tolerance to the sedative and anticonvulsant activity of benzodiazepines has been observed during chronic administration (Chapters 26 and 33), it is generally accepted that minimal tolerance develops to the anxiolytic effects of these compounds. The most widely used drugs have active metabolites with long half-lives (see page 54), which may mask both development of tolerance and signs and

Table 25-3 Pharmacokinetic Values for Representative Benzodiazepines and Buspirone

Drug	$t_{1/2}$ (hours)	Disposition
chlordiazepoxide	5-30	M*
clorazepate	30-200	M*
prazepam	48-80	M*
lorazepam	10-20	M
oxazepam	5-15	M
diazepam	20-70	M*
alprazolam	8-20	M*
clonazepam	15-50	M
buspirone	2-3	M*

M, Metabolized; *M**, active metabolite(s). The active metabolites of alprazolam and buspirone are of little significance in humans.

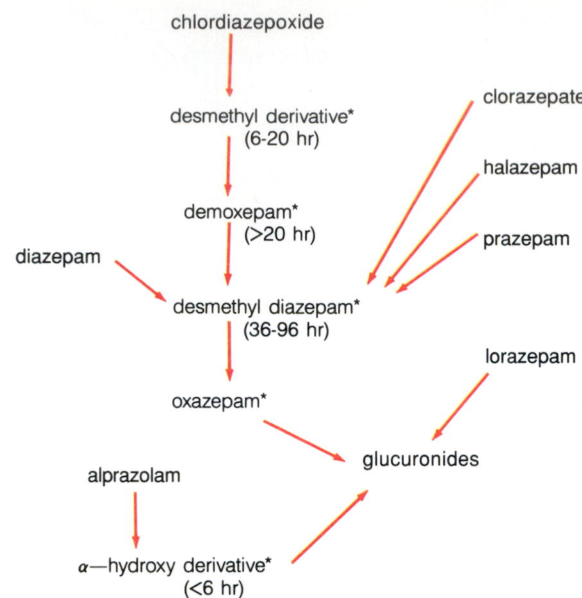

FIGURE 25-3 Metabolism pathways for anxiolytic benzodiazepines. Numbers in ( ) are disposition half-lives. *Active metabolite.

symptoms of withdrawal. Clinical experience with a potent short-acting benzodiazepine, alprazolam, indicates that sudden withdrawal after chronic use frequently induces rebound anxiety.

Certain second-generation anxiolytics (buspirone and others) are partial agonists at the 5-HT_{1A} receptor and have a weak affinity for dopamine receptors but have no activity on benzodiazepine or GABA receptors. The anxiolytic effects of these compounds are characterized by minimal sedation and muscle relaxation.

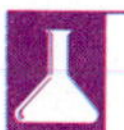

PHARMACOKINETICS

Pharmacokinetic parameters for anxiolytic benzodiazepines and buspirone are summarized in Table 25-3.

The benzodiazepines are very lipid soluble and are rapidly absorbed after oral administration, with a few exceptions. Many are converted to active metabolites, the most significant of which is *N*-desmethyldiazepam (Figure 25-3). Several compounds (clorazepate and prazepam) are prodrugs, having no biological activity and requiring metabolism to be activated. The maintenance dosage of these agents is determined by elimination times of both the parent drug and the active metabolites. Benzodiazepines bind to plasma proteins with variable affinities; less than 2% of diazepam but about 30% of alprazolam remains unbound. Diazepam enters the brain rapidly after a single IV administration and is redistributed rapidly into peripheral tissues, providing CNS depression for less than 2 hours. This is similar to the kinetics observed with the short-acting barbiturate thiopental. In contrast, lorazepam, which is less lipid soluble, depresses brain function for as long as 8 hours after an IV dose.

When administered chronically, diazepam and its active metabolites accumulate in plasma, with the active metabolites having long half-lives. Sudden termination after long-term treatment with diazepam usually results in a gradual and mild withdrawal as the active metabolites (especially *N*-desmethyldiazepam) dissipate slowly. Lorazepam and alprazolam are metabolized more rapidly to inactive products, have a shorter half-life than diazepam, and are less likely to cause cumulative toxicity during chronic administration. After development of tolerance to the sedative effects, however, sudden withdrawal of lorazepam or alprazolam can result in "breakthrough" rebound anxiety. This indicates that some degree of tolerance and dependence can develop with the anxiolytic effect of these drugs. Other withdrawal signs also occur more rapidly and intensively when long-term treatment with benzodiazepines having short elimination times is discontinued. With these drugs it may be advisable to substitute the longer-acting diazepam or chlordiazepoxide and then gradually reduce dosage.

Some benzodiazepines are metabolized by hydroxylation in the liver, whereas others are converted to inactive glucuronides (Figure 25-3). However, clonazepam is detoxified primarily by reduction of the 7-nitro constituent. In the elderly, in patients with liver disease, or in those concomitantly taking cimetidine or estrogens, for example, hepatic oxidative processes may be greatly compromised. Conjugating mechanisms are spared, however, and drugs such as oxazepam or lorazepam, which are biotransformed by glucuronidation, would seem to be the preferred agents in these conditions.

RELATION OF MECHANISMS OF ACTION TO CLINICAL RESPONSE

Since anxiety is characterized by a variety of symptoms and is widespread, it is frequently difficult to define therapeutic treatment. Anxiety is identified with stressful experiences, and normally the individual adjusts to resolve the stress. However, anxiety can become a psychiatric problem for some patients by disrupting normal behavioral patterns. Sensitization to the anxiogenic influence of stress can occur in patients with a history of earlier trauma and neurotic manifestations. Anxiety has also been associated with depression, and more recent evidence points to a neurobiological basis of anxiety. Clinical anxieties include the following:

1. Panic disorders with or without agoraphobia (fear of being alone in open spaces)
2. Simple phobias
3. Social phobias
4. Obsessive-compulsive disorders
5. Generalized or less specific anxiety disorders

Posttraumatic stress disorder has been included in some more recent classifications because research indicates a closer relationship of it to anxiety disorders than to depression. Most authorities recognize that psychotherapeutic, cognitive, and behavioral interventions continue to be the mainstay of long-term management, particularly of phobias and obsessive-compulsive states.

Generalized anxiety disorders are most common and more difficult to manage in many instances. Somatic complaints of muscle pain, epigastric distress, respiratory distress, and insomnia may have an organic basis, especially in the elderly. It is therefore often difficult to decide whether the anxiety that accompanies these symptoms is primary or secondary. Nevertheless, studies have not indicated a genetic predisposition for generalized anxiety disorders, and both these disorders and panic disorder are related to depression. A primary diagnosis of generalized anxiety disorder requires that symptoms persist for at least 6 months. Diagnosis and treatment of these disorders are further complicated by spontaneous remissions and simultaneous or sequential occurrence of several types of anxiety in a particular patient. Furthermore, patients with other psychiatric disorders may exhibit anxiety symptoms. For example, more than 20% of alcoholics are estimated to have preexisting anxiety disorders, and 10% of the general population may manifest clinically significant anxiety.

Although there is a high incidence of disabling anxiety in the population and the prescribing of anxiolytic drugs is common, most individuals experiencing severe anxiety receive no prescribed medication. Serious concerns raised in the past about excessive use of benzodiazepines and their abuse potential have been countered by recent surveys showing that patients have a much lower tendency to abuse this class of drugs than previously assumed. Certain benzodiazepines *(diazepam, alprazolam)* are still the most effective drugs for the symptomatic treatment of more generalized anxiety disorders. Intermittent use for acute attacks or limited chronic use (4 to 8 weeks) for recurring symptoms is often beneficial. A debilitating anxiety secondary to another illness can be effectively controlled by short-term treatment with anxiolytic drugs while treatment for the primary condition is being implemented. Care should be exercised in prescribing for elderly patients, especially regarding agents metabolized to long half-life intermediates *(chlordiazepoxide, diazepam)*. Patients with a history of addiction or more chronic and severe emotional disturbances should be administered benzodiazepines cautiously, particularly the more potent anxiolytics such as *diazepam* and *alprazolam*.

Panic attacks appear to be most effectively controlled with *tricyclic antidepressants* or *monoamine oxidase inhibitors* (see Chapter 24); benzodiazepines are generally not effective except to relieve associated generalized anxiety symptoms. *Alprazolam* may be an exception and have a specific efficacy in treating panic attacks. This drug (see Figure 25-1) has greater anxiolytic and less sedative activity than other benzodiazepines and may also possess some antidepressant activity. Thus alprazolam may be an effective substitute in controlling depression associated with anxiety when tricyclic antidepressants or monoamine oxidase inhibitors are contraindicated because of unacceptable side effects.

The recent introduction of buspirone offers an attractive alternative to benzodiazepines for long-term therapy of certain forms of anxiety (see box). *Buspirone*, chemically distinct from benzodiazepines (see Figure 25-1), is a partial agonist at 5-HT_{1A} receptors without activity at the benzodiazepine–GABA–chloride ion channel receptor complex. This drug produces little sedation or effect on motor functions and appears to be devoid of significant physical or psychological depen-

BENZODIAZEPINES (BZD) VERSUS BUSPIRONE (BUS)

Relief of generalized anxiety—Bzd and Bus
Addiction liability—Bzd
Rebound anxiety—Bzd
Physical dependence—Bzd
Delay in anxiolytic effects—Bus
Relief of somatic symptoms—Bzd
Potentiates alcohol intoxication—Bzd

3. A large overdose of which of the following is least likely to result in lethality?
   a. lorazepam
   b. pentobarbital
   c. alcohol
   d. meprobamate
   e. imipramine
4. The most valid use of diazepam in anxiety disorders is/are:
   a. in controlling anxiety associated with psychosis.
   b. in managing acute and intermittent attacks of severe generalized anxiety associated with nonpsychotic disorders.
   c. in the prophylaxis of panic attacks.
   d. in the long-term management of obsessive-compulsive disorders.
   e. Choices a and c are correct.
5. Which of the following is least sedative, will not potentiate the effects of alcohol, and has no appreciable dependence liability?
   a. chlordiazepoxide
   b. amobarbital
   c. alprazolam
   d. meprobamate
   e. buspirone
6. The pharmacology of alprazolam differs from that of diazepam or chlordiazepoxide in that:
   a. alprazolam has little effect in attenuating acute anxiety attacks.
   b. alprazolam has specific antipanic activity.
   c. alprazolam has a short duration and is more likely to promote rebound anxiety.
   d. Choices a and b are correct.
   e. Choices b and c are correct.
7. The mechanism of anxiolytic activity of buspirone is proposed to relate to:
   a. a direct action on chloride-ion channels to enhance hyperpolarizing effects at brain inhibitory synapses.
   b. a decrease in muscarinic cholinergic function in the brain "punishment" regions.
   c. an agonist activity at brain 5-HT_{1A} receptors.
   d. an agonist activity at brain noradrenergic receptors.
   e. an antagonist activity at brain dopaminergic receptors.
8. Besides anxiolytic activity, benzodiazepines are useful as:
   a. hypnotics.
   b. anticonvulsants.
   c. muscle relaxants.
   d. All of the above are correct.
   e. Only choices a and b are correct.
9. Diazepam resembles other general CNS-depressant drugs in:
   a. promoting psychological dependence.
   b. development of seizures on sudden withdrawal after chronic treatment with large doses.
   c. demonstrating a cross-dependence pattern to alcohol.
   d. All of the above are correct.
   e. Only choices a and c are correct.
10. Tolerance develops fairly rapidly to most effects of the benzodiazepines, except for:
    a. anxiety.
    b. anticonvulsant activity.
    c. sedation.
    d. motor relaxation.
    e. none of the above.

CHAPTER 26

Drugs for Seizure Disorders (Epilepsies)

JANET L. STRINGER

MAJOR ANTIEPILEPTIC DRUGS

carbamazepine
phenytoin
valproate
ethosuximide
phenobarbital
primidone
clonazepam

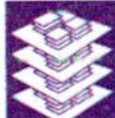

THERAPEUTIC OVERVIEW

Epilepsy is a chronic disorder characterized by recurrent self-limited seizures in which the brain is subject to abnormal, excessive discharges synchronized throughout a localized or generalized population of neurons. About 0.5% of the population suffers from epilepsy. Seventy-five percent of these individuals have their first seizure before 18 years of age. Recurrent seizures, if frequent, interfere with a patient's ability to carry out day-to-day activities. However, judicious use of antiepileptic medications allows about 75% of epileptic patients to remain seizure free.

Identification of seizure type is important because antiepileptic medication is selected accordingly. The current classification of seizure types is listed in Table 26-1. The classification recognizes two broad categories of seizures: those that arise in part of one cerebral hemisphere and are accompanied by focal electroencephalographic abnormalities **(partial,** or **focal, seizures)** and those with clinical and electroencephalographic manifestations that indicate essentially simultaneous involvement of all or large parts of both cerebral hemispheres from the beginning **(generalized onset seizures).** Partial seizures are termed **simple** if no alteration of consciousness occurs and **complex** if consciousness is impaired or lost. In partial complex seizures, motor activity often appears as nonreflex actions that can be complicated and seemingly purposeful. Partial seizures can secondarily generalize to involve the entire brain. Generalized seizures are also subclassified, mainly by the presence or absence of certain patterns of motor convulsions. They may range from **absence seizures,** characterized by only impaired consciousness, to **generalized tonic-clonic seizures** in which widespread convulsive activity takes place.

Often an epileptic syndrome can be classified by the type of seizure; cause of seizure; natural history, including certain clinical findings and age of onset; family history; and prognosis. Recognition of a syndrome will help determine whether medication is necessary and, if so, how long it should be continued. In addition, identification of the syndrome has genetic implications. Juvenile myoclonic epilepsy (Janz's syndrome) is an example of an epileptic syndrome that is characterized by generalized tonic-clonic seizures, usually occurring on awakening, that first develop in adolescence. The patient often has early morning myoclonus as well. Consideration of the type of seizure alone could lead to selection of a specific drug; however, identification of the syndrome indicates the use of a different drug.

All individuals can experience seizures. Brain insults such as fever, hypoglycemia, hyponatremia, and extreme acidosis or alkalosis can result in a seizure, but if the condition is corrected, the seizure does not recur. The causes of isolated seizures and **epilepsy** (recurrent seizures) are summarized in the box on p. 352.

The occurrence of a single seizure requires a decision as to whether to treat the patient. Factors associ-

ABBREVIATIONS

GABA	γ-aminobutyric acid
NMDA	*N*-methyl-D-aspartate

Table 26-1 Classification of Seizures, Frequency, and Clinical Manifestations

Seizure type	Frequency (%)	Clinical Manifestations
PARTIAL (FOCAL) SEIZURES		
Simple partial	10	No impairment of consciousness; focal motor, sensory, or speech disturbance
Complex partial (temporal lobe)	35	Impaired consciousness; dreamy dysaffective state, with or without automatisms
Partial seizures, secondarily generalized	10	
GENERAL SEIZURES		
Tonic-clonic (grand mal)	30	Loss of consciousness, falling Rigid extension of trunk and limbs (tonic phase) Rhythmic contraction of arms and legs (clonic phase)
Absence (petit mal)	10	Impaired consciousness with staring spells, with or without eye blinks
Others including myoclonic, atonic (atypical)	4	Myoclonic jerks (shocklike contractions), loss of muscle tone, falling, "drop attacks"
UNCLASSIFIED EPILEPTIC SEIZURES	1-8	Includes all other seizures

CAUSES AND THERAPY OF SEIZURES

CAUSES

- Birth and perinatal injuries
- Vascular insults
- Head trauma
- Congenital malformations
- Metabolic disturbances (e.g., serum sodium, glucose, calcium, urea)
- Drugs or alcohol, including withdrawals from barbiturates and other CNS depressants
- Neoplasia
- Infection
- Genetic
- Idiopathic
- Hyperthermia in children

THERAPY

- Monodrug therapy is preferable to polydrug therapy because of
  - Lower incidence of adverse effects
  - Avoidance of drug interactions
  - Improved patient compliance
  - Lower medication costs
- Success with monodrug therapy depends on:
  - Correct seizure classification and diagnosis
  - Appropriate drug choice for seizure type
  - Optimal drug administration and serum monitoring

ated with a higher risk of seizure recurrence include neurological deficits, an abnormal electroencephalogram, abnormal neuroimaging studies, or a family history showing epilepsy. If any predisposing factors are present, treatment with antiepileptic drugs should be considered. Otherwise it may be appropriate to wait until a second seizure occurs.

An example of a single seizure occurrence is the febrile convulsion. This seizure occurs in up to 5% of children, constitutes a relatively benign disorder of early childhood, and is characterized by general convulsive seizures occurring during an acute febrile illness. The majority of febrile convulsions are brief and uncomplicated. The overall risk of developing epilepsy after a febrile convulsion is less than 4%; the majority of children do not require drug treatment. However, if there are neurological abnormalities, the febrile seizure is longer than 15 minutes, or there is a history of nonfebrile convulsions in parents or siblings, then a limited period of treatment with antiepileptic drugs may be warranted.

The goal of antiepileptic drug therapy (see the box at left) is to prevent seizures while minimizing side effects, using the simplest drug regimen. After initiation of therapy, if seizures continue and further increases in dosage are inadvisable because of dose-related side effects, one should try at least one and sometimes another alternative drug as monodrug therapy before considering the use of two drugs simultaneously. Discontinuation of antiepileptic medication after several seizure-free

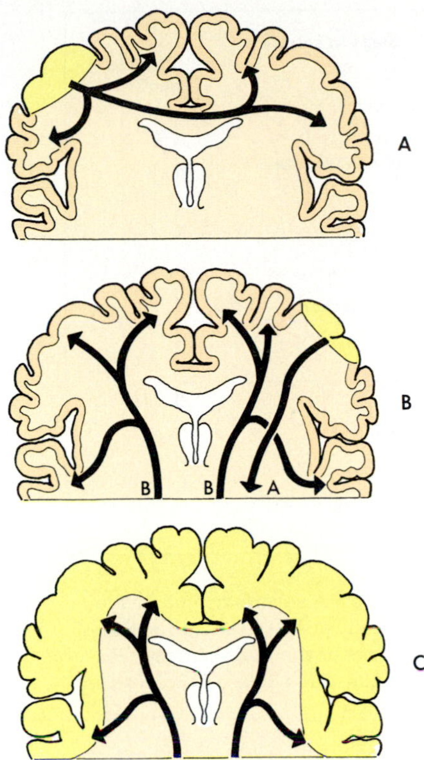

FIGURE 26-1 Schema of seizure spread. *A*, Focal seizure with spread to adjacent and contralateral cortical regions. *B*, Focal seizure with secondary generalization. Seizure discharge activated subcortical centers, *A*, which then activate entire cortex, *B*. *C*, Primary generalized absence seizure in which thalamocortical relays are believed to act on a diffusely hyperexcitable cortex.

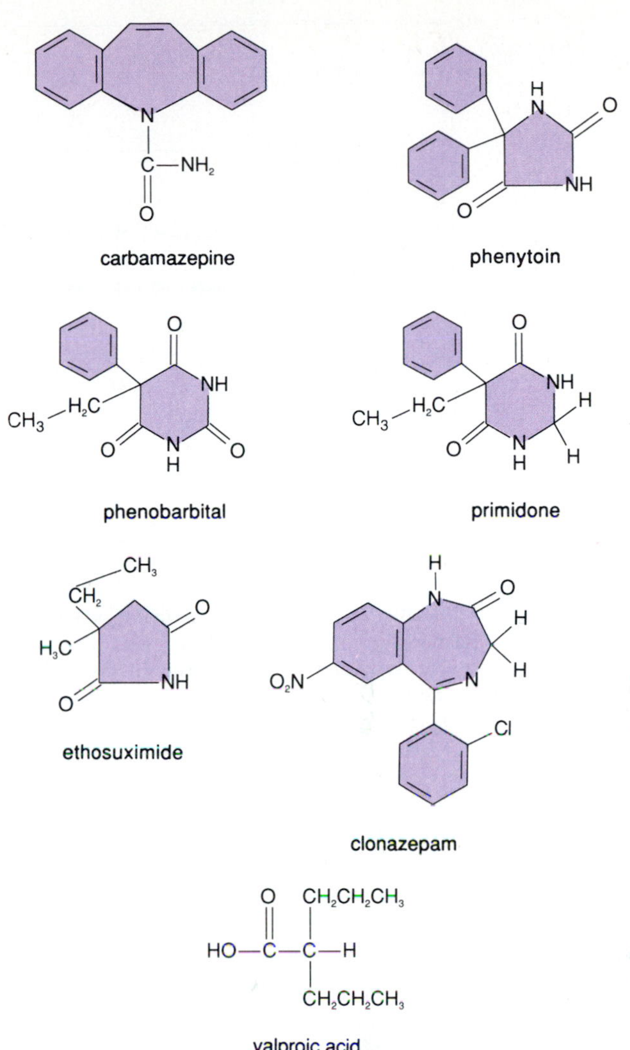

FIGURE 26-2 Structure of major antiepileptic drugs.

years depends on the diagnosis (type of seizure and epileptic syndrome), cause, and response to therapy. With certain epileptic syndromes, antiepileptic drugs may be discontinued, but with others, such as recurrent seizures secondary to a structural lesion, antiepileptic medication should be continued for life.

When seizures recur with increasing frequency such that base-line consciousness is not regained between seizures, **status epilepticus** exists. The patient is considered to be in status epilepticus when seizures last at least 30 minutes. Status epilepticus is a medical emergency with a mortality of 15% or less. Status epilepticus leads to systemic hypoxia, acidemia, hyperpyrexia, cardiovascular collapse, and renal shutdown.

MECHANISMS OF ACTION

Seizure Mechanisms

The pathophysiology of epilepsy is not fully understood for any of the seizure types described. However, multiple mechanisms are known to be involved. Some mechanisms operate in one seizure type and do not operate in others. However, no single seizure type is explained by a single mechanism. Currently, the pathophysiology of focal seizures is better understood than that of general seizures. A focal seizure (Figure 26-1, *A*) arises when pathological alterations in a restricted region of the brain initiate a seizure. Additional features serve to synchronize neurons into epileptic discharges and to propagate the discharges to areas surrounding the focus (Figure 26-1, *B* and *C*).

Available Drugs

The structures of the main-line antiepilepsy drugs available in the United States are shown in Figure 26-2. The drugs include carbamazepine, phenytoin, valproate,

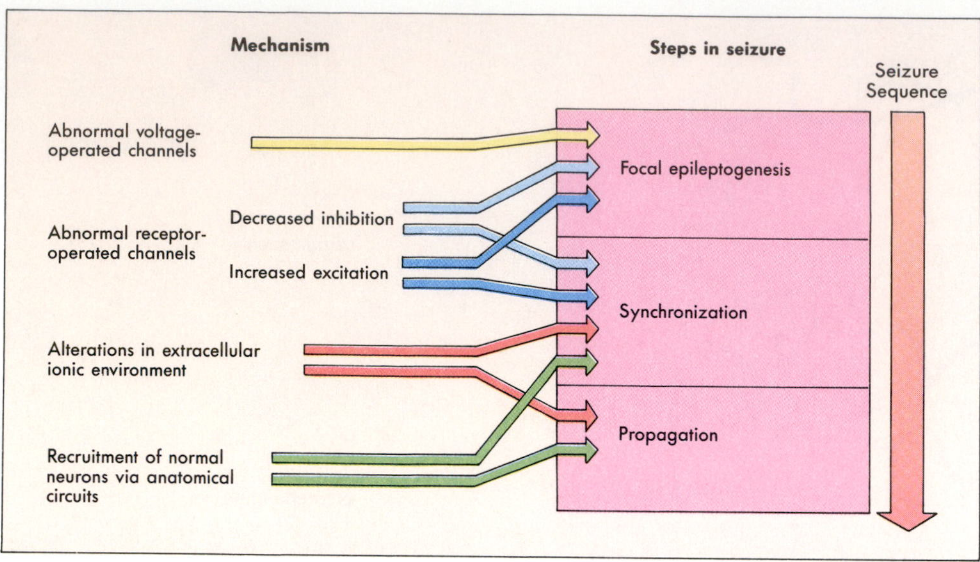

FIGURE 26-3 Cellular and synaptic mechanisms of epileptic seizures. A seizure can be divided into three phases: *(1)* focal epileptogenesis (initiation), *(2)* synchronization of the surrounding neurons, and *(3)* propagation of the seizure discharge to other areas of the brain. Arrows indicate where each of the mechanisms on the left participates in the three phases involved in seizure generation.

ethosuximide, phenobarbital, primidone, and clonazepam. Additional drugs used secondarily in the treatment of epileptic seizures include clorazepate, diazepam, ethotoin, methsuximide, phensuximide, phenacemide, paramethadione, mephenytoin, felbamate, trimethadione, gabapentin, and lamotrigine.

Drug Mechanisms

There are several points in the initiation and spread of seizures at which antiepileptic drugs may act (Figure 26-3). The first is to block abnormal epileptic events within single neurons. The second is to block or slow the synchronization of epileptic discharges among neurons involved in the seizure. A third is to block the propagation of seizure activity. A drug may act by multiple mechanisms and have actions at one or more points.

At least four different mechanisms are involved in the genesis and spread of epileptic discharges, and all are amenable to disruption by drugs. The first includes alterations in neuronal membrane function such as changes in voltage-regulated ion channels in neuronal membranes. These changes lead to excessive depolarization (paroxysmal depolarization shift) or excess action potential firing (loss of inactivation). Examples of useful drugs are carbamazepine and phenytoin, which reduce repetitive firing of neurons by producing a use-dependent blockade of sodium channels (Figure 26-4). By prolonging the inactivated state of the sodium channel and thus the relative refractory period, phenytoin and carbamazepine do not alter the first action potential but rather reduce the likelihood of repetitive action potentials. Neurons retain their ability to generate action potentials at the low frequencies operational in physiological states.

The second broad mechanism of drug-modifiable origin and spread of epileptic discharge is decreased inhibition, which allows excessive neuronal firing to occur. γ-Aminobutyric acid (GABA) is the major inhibitory neurotransmitter in the forebrain. GABA opens receptor-operated chloride channels, hyperpolarizing the neurons and making epileptic firing less likely. In experimental animals, increased GABA-ergic inhibition has antiepileptic activity, whereas administration of agents that diminish GABA-ergic inhibition causes seizures. The GABA receptor/channel complex contains the receptor site for the transmitter GABA (this is a prime target for antiepileptic drug action) and also includes benzodiazepine and barbiturate recognition sites (see Chapter 25). Binding of a benzodiazepine (diazepam, clonazepam, lorazepam) modulates the effectiveness of inhibition by increasing the frequency of chloride-channel opening when GABA combines with its receptor. Barbiturates interact with the GABA receptor at a binding site adjacent to the chloride channel but separate from the benzodiazepine site. Some barbiturates have **GABA-mimetic** (direct action on chloride

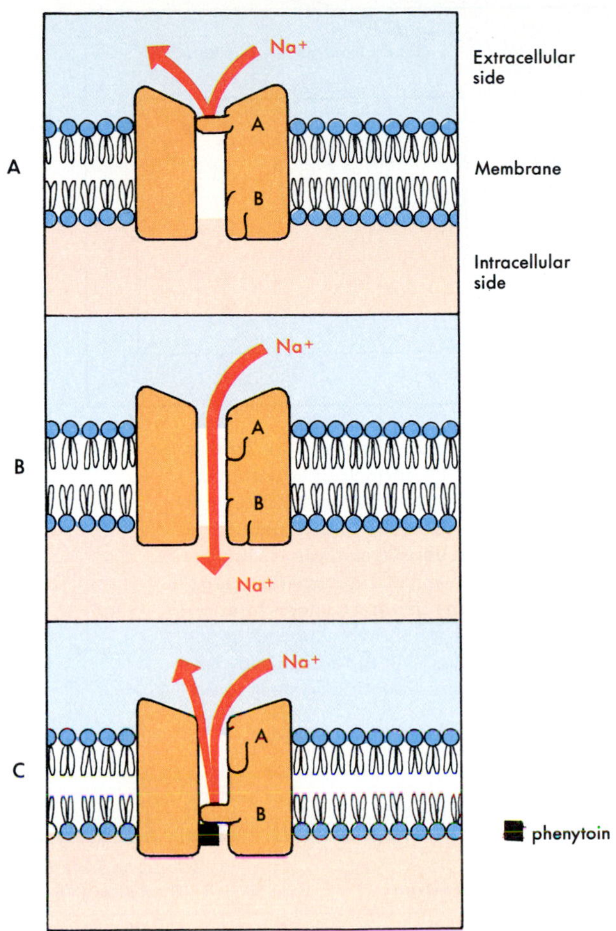

FIGURE 26-4 Action of phenytoin on sodium channel. *A*, Resting state in which sodium-channel activation gate *(A)* is closed. Arrival of an action potential, in *B*, causes depolarization and opening of activation gate *(A)* and Na^+ ions flow into the cell. When depolarization continues, *C*, an inactivation gate *(B)* moves into the channel. Phenytoin prolongs the inactivated state of the sodium channel presumably by preventing reopening of the inactivation gate *(B)*.

channels) and **GABA-potentiating** effects (prolonging the opening of chloride channels achieved by a given amount of GABA) (Chapter 25). Barbiturates that are effective antiepileptic compounds (suppressing seizures with minimal sedation) have strong GABA-potentiation but little or no GABA-mimetic actions. Some barbiturates suppress seizures but are not useful clinically as antiepileptics because of strong sedative effects through GABA-mimetic action. Valproic acid may enhance the GABA-inhibitory system, but this is controversial.

Adenosine, which decreases neurotransmitter release from terminals (presynaptic effect) and binds to adenosine receptors that activate second messengers (postsynaptic effect), is an effective antiepileptic agent in experimental animals. Carbamazepine interacts with the adenosine system, enhancing inhibition and therefore reducing **epileptogenesis** (the initiation of seizure) at all levels, including focal development of epileptic discharges, synchronization of discharges, and seizure propagation throughout the brain.

A third mechanism by which drugs interrupt the origin and spread of epileptic discharges is by reducing excitation. Excitatory neurotransmission is mediated predominantly through glutamate or related compounds. One type of glutamate receptor, the *N*-methyl-D-aspartate (NMDA) receptor, may have a role in epileptogenesis. The NMDA receptor is predominantly involved in high-frequency discharges, such as those occurring with seizures, and is activated only minimally in physiological neuronal activity of the brain. Antagonists of the NMDA receptor are anticonvulsant in animals and in vitro models of epilepsy. A drug that effectively reduces abnormal excitatory transmission by blocking the NMDA receptor could reduce focal epileptogenesis, slow synchronization of the discharge, and slow or block spread of the seizure.

A fourth mechanism involved in drug-interrupted origin and spread of epileptic discharges is an alteration in the extracellular concentrations of potassium and calcium. During seizures, the extracellular concentrations of potassium increases and the concentration of calcium decreases. Both changes cause greater excitability of neurons and may promote seizure initiation and spread. The ability of phenytoin to produce frequency-dependent blockade of action potentials is augmented when extracellular potassium is elevated to concentrations characteristic of seizure activity. This makes phenytoin more effective in epileptic tissue than in normally functioning brain areas.

After seizure initiation, there is excessive synchronization of large numbers of neurons that normally act independently, leading to propagation of the seizure discharge. During a partial seizure the synchronization of neuronal firing may be limited to a portion of the brain or may spread to ultimately involve the entire brain **(secondary generalization).** The exact mechanisms involved in secondary generalization are not known.

For generalized seizures, large areas of the brain are involved at the onset of the seizure. Some clues about the cellular mechanisms of absence seizure initiation are now being elucidated. Absence seizures are characterized by the sudden appearance of spike-wave discharges synchronized throughout the brain, as noted by modified patterns on the electroencephalogram compared to that of generalized tonic-clonic seizures or partial seizures (Figure 26-5). Thalamic neurons may play a role in the generation of thalamocortical rhythms, including the paroxysmal discharges of absence seizures.

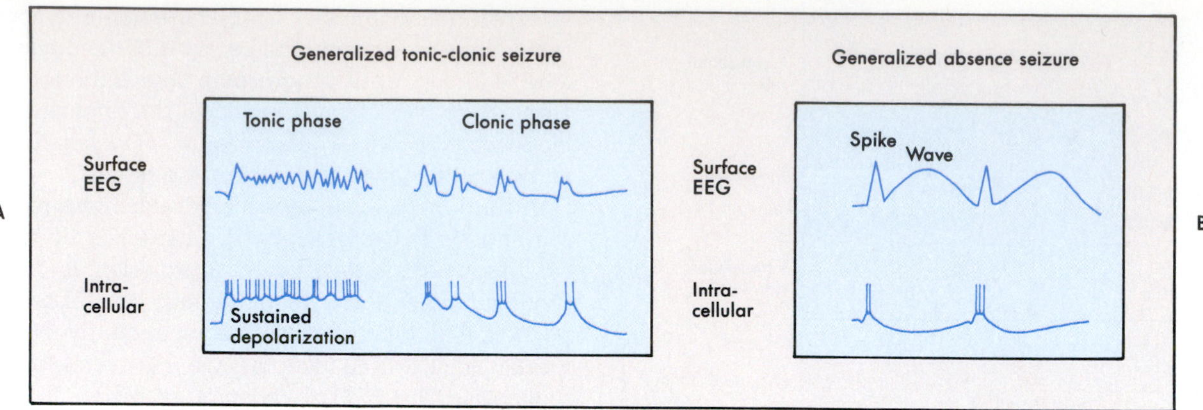

FIGURE 26-5 Neuronal correlates of paroxysmal discharges. *A,* A tonic-clonic seizure begins with a tonic phase of rhythmic high-frequency discharges (recorded by surface EEG) with cortical neurons undergoing sustained depolarization with generation of protracted trains of action potentials (recorded intracellularly). Subsequently, the seizure converts to a clonic phase characterized by groups of spikes on the EEG and periodic neuronal depolarizations with clusters of action potentials. *B,* Absence seizures are distinguished by the spike and wave discharge that is recorded on the surface EEG. During the spike phase, neurons generate short-duration depolarization and a burst of action potentials but, unlike in *A,* neither show sustained depolarization nor produce sustained repetitive firing of action potentials. This difference may explain why drugs that are effective against sustained firing in vitro are effective against tonic-clonic seizures in humans, but not absence seizures.

Table 26-2 Pharmacokinetic Parameter Values

Drug	Administered	$t_{1/2}$ (hour)*	Disposition	Bound to Plasma Proteins (%)
carbamazepine	Oral	10-15	M (60%),† R (40%)	75
phenytoin	Oral	12-36	M (95%), R (5%)	90
phenobarbital	Oral	48-144	M (75%), R (25%)	50
primidone	Oral	6-15	M (60%),† R (40%)	10
ethosuximide	Oral	24-60	M (80%), R (20%)	10
valproic acid	Oral	6-15	M (>95%)	90
clonazepam	Oral	24-36	M (>95%)	>50

M, metabolized (in liver); *R,* eliminated unchanged by renal mechanisms.
*Age dependent.
†Produces an active (antiepileptic) metabolite.

The thalamic neurons generate depolarizations based on calcium currents that may be a crucial cellular mechanism in the generation of normal and abnormal thalamocortical rhythms. Recent results indicate that certain antiepileptic drugs (ethosuximide) may block absence seizures by reducing calcium currents in these thalamic neurons.

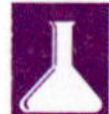

PHARMACOKINETICS

Pharmacokinetic parameters are summarized in Table 26-2 for antiepileptic drugs. Because antiepileptic drugs are used to treat a chronic medical condition, they must be absorbed orally and cross the blood-brain barrier. All the antiepileptic drugs are metabolized to a significant extent, and all bind to plasma proteins, many to a high degree. This is important clinically because the usual determinations of blood concentrations indicate total drug (bound plus free) in the serum. Concentrations of the free fraction of antiepileptic drugs can be measured, but the tests are expensive and time consuming. In addition, there is less experience with what constitutes a therapeutic range for free drug concentrations than for total drug concentration. Therefore the determination of free drug concentrations is reserved for special circumstances.

The metabolism of phenytoin is characterized by saturation, or zero-order kinetics (see Chapter 4) that arise because the liver enzymes that catalyze phenytoin metabolism become saturated and operate at maximum velocity when serum concentrations rise above a certain value. At lower doses there is a linear relationship between the dose of phenytoin and the serum concentration of the drug. At higher doses a much greater rise in serum concentration develops for a given increase in dose (nonlinear). The dose at which this transition occurs varies from patient to patient but is usually in the range of 400 to 600 mg/day. As a result of this kinetic pattern, doses of phenytoin must be individualized.

Phenobarbital causes induction of liver microsomal enzyme systems. Thus phenobarbital typically accelerates its own metabolism and that of other drugs taken concurrently. Primidone is metabolized in the liver to phenobarbital and to phenylethylmalonamide, which also has some antiepileptic action. Carbamazepine is metabolized in the liver to produce a 10,11-epoxide, which is relatively stable and accumulates in the blood. This metabolite has antiepileptic properties, and some believe that the epoxide is a contributor to the neurotoxicity that often develops in patients taking carbamazepine. Carbamazepine also induces its own metabolism, with the rate of metabolism of carbamazepine increasing during the first 4 to 6 weeks so that larger doses become necessary to maintain constant serum concentrations. Ethosuximide has a long half-life, which allows for once-a-day dosing. However, the gastrointestinal side effects are frequently intolerable with once-a-day dosing and are reduced with divided dosing. The half-life of antiepileptic agents varies with the age of the patient and exposure to other drugs.

Many antiepileptic drugs are available as brand name and generic products, but differences in formulation result in a wide range of bioavailability among the several preparations of a given drug. This can lead to problems in seizure control when formulations are changed and should be considered in prescribing antiepileptic drugs.

Table 26-3 Treatment of Epilepsies

Seizure Disorder	Drug Therapy	Therapeutic Serum Concentration ($\mu g/ml$)
PRIMARY GENERALIZED TONIC-CLONIC (GRAND MAL)		
Drugs of choice	carbamazepine	6-12
	phenytoin	10-20
	valproate†	50-100
Alternatives	phenobarbital	15-35
	primidone	6-12
PARTIAL, INCLUDING SECONDARILY GENERALIZED		
Drugs of choice	carbamazepine	6-12
	phenytoin	10-20
Alternatives	phenobarbital	15-35
	primidone	6-12
GENERAL ABSENCE (PETIT MAL)		
Drugs of choice	ethosuximide	40-100
	valproate*	50-100
Alternative	clonazepam	0.013-0.072
ATYPICAL ABSENCE, MYOCLONIC, ATONIC		
Drug of choice	valproate†	50-100
Alternative	clonazepam	0.013-0.072

*First choice if primary generalized tonic-clonic seizure is also present.
†Not approved unless absence seizure is involved.

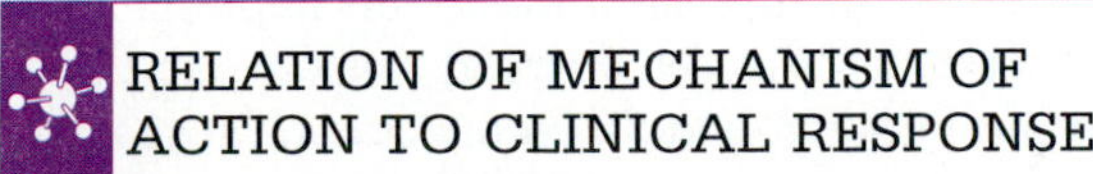

RELATION OF MECHANISM OF ACTION TO CLINICAL RESPONSE

Treatment of Epilepsies

The first line and alternative drugs for different types of seizures are listed in Table 26-3, including the "therapeutic" serum concentration ranges. However, these therapeutic ranges are determined empirically from general clinical experience in diverse and heterogeneous populations of epileptic patients and should not be taken as absolute recommendations for individual patients.

Antiepileptic Drugs During Pregnancy

Because antiepileptic agents are taken for many years or a lifetime, the issue of taking these drugs during pregnancy must be addressed. During pregnancy, seizures increase in 25% of epileptic women, do not change in frequency in 50%, and decrease in frequency in 25%. The possibility of seizures, or even status epilepticus, with hypoxia and other metabolic changes places the epileptic mother and her child at risk. However, the teratogenic properties of antiepileptic drugs are also a concern. The epileptic mother is at heightened risk for obstetrical complications and her child at increased risk for perinatal difficulties. Children of mothers who have epilepsy have an increased risk of malformations even if antiepileptic drugs are not used during pregnancy. No antiepileptic drug has been shown unequivocally to cause birth defects, but none has been proved absolutely safe either. Profound changes in the distribution and metabolism of antiepileptic drugs occur in pregnant women, resulting in a decrease of serum total drug concentrations, and monitoring of serum

Table 26-4 Treatment of Status Epilepticus in Adults

	Drugs of Choice	Initial Dose	Rate (mg/min)	Repeat Dose
INITIAL	diazepam, IV	5-10 mg	1-2	5-10 mg every 20-30 min
	lorazepam, IV	2-6 mg	1	2-6 mg every 20-30 min
FOLLOW-UP	phenytoin, IV	15-20 mg/kg	30-50	100-150 mg every 30 min
	phenobarbital, IV	10-20 mg/kg	25-50	120-240 mg every 20 min

drug concentrations at regular intervals before, during, and after pregnancy is advised.

Whenever possible, prepregnancy counseling should be undertaken. If discontinuation of antiepileptic medication is not an option, monodrug therapy and the smallest dose of the antiepileptic agent should be used. Studies show that the highest incidence of birth defects occurs with multiple drug use. Some drugs, including phenytoin and carbamazepine, are linked to particular fetal malformations, including cardiac defects, cleft lip and palate, and craniofacial anomalies, but not all clinicians agree that these are specific effects rather than examples of a more general syndrome. There is evidence that trimethadione is teratogenic, and this drug should be avoided. Valproic acid is cited as causing neural tube effects in 1% to 2% of offspring of mothers with epilepsy.

The newborn infants of mothers who have received phenobarbital, primidone, or phenytoin during pregnancy may develop a deficiency of vitamin K–dependent clotting factors, which can result in serious hemorrhage during the first 24 hours of life. This hemorrhaging can be prevented by administration of vitamin K to the newborn shortly after birth.

Treatment of Status Epilepticus

The general strategy for treating status epilepticus involves support of cardiovascular and respiratory systems and treatment of seizure activity (Table 26-4). Initially a rapidly acting antiepileptic such as IV diazepam or lorazepam (longer duration) is given to stop the seizures. Because the effect wears off rapidly, long-term antiepileptic therapy with IV phenytoin or phenobarbital is also instituted. Phenobarbital is more sedating and, when the effects are added to the CNS depression produced by the benzodiazepine, can lead to respiratory compromise. Therefore IV phenytoin is more frequently, used as the second drug. It, however, has the potential side effect of producing hypotension or cardiac arrhythmias if administered too rapidly. If status epilepticus develops during withdrawal of a particular drug (e.g., phenobarbital or a benzodiazepine), consideration should be given to reinstating that compound.

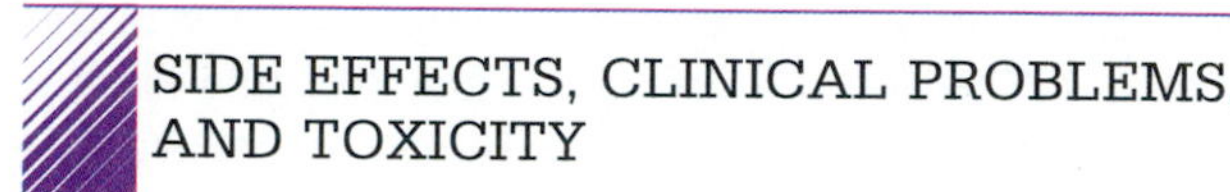

SIDE EFFECTS, CLINICAL PROBLEMS, AND TOXICITY

Side Effects and Toxicity

Antiepileptic drugs cross the blood-brain barrier and thus have potential for systemic and neurologic toxicity (see box). These side effects may be dose related or idiosyncratic. Dose-related side effects are more common at higher serum concentrations and can be reduced by lowering of the drug dose. Idiosyncratic reactions are unique to a particular patient and drug combination, may pose a serious risk to the patient, and often necessitate stopping the drug.

In several studies, side effects of antiepileptic drugs are reported in 30% to 50% of patients. However, these are frequently tolerable and require only monitoring. In other cases, the side effects can be reduced or eliminated by changing the dose or administration schedule. In 5% to 15% of patients another antiepileptic drug must be prescribed because of toxicity. Except for phenobarbital and phenytoin, which can be introduced at maintenance dosage, most antiepileptic drugs should be introduced slowly to minimize side effects.

With carbamazepine, patients often initially experience nausea and visual disturbances, which can be minimized by slow introduction of the drug. Carbamazepine may have hematological effects, particularly leukopenia or sometimes thrombocytopenia. These may disappear with continued use or may persist as a dose-dependent side effect. The most problematic hematological effect with carbamazepine is depression of granulocytes in the blood. If good seizure control is achieved and other serious side effects are absent, an absolute granulocyte count of ≥1000 is acceptable. An aplastic anemia syndrome is associated with carbamazepine, but it is very infrequent (<1 per 50,000) and appears to be idiosyncratic. Other idiosyncratic reactions with carbamazepine include rash in 5% of cases and rare hepatitis. Dose-related side effects for carbamazepine include nausea, dizziness, visual symptoms, and, infrequently, inappropriate antidiuretic hormone secretion. Use of serum concentrations of carbamazepine to assess

CLINICAL PROBLEMS

CARBAMAZEPINE

autoinduction of metabolism
nausea and visual disturbances (dose related)
granulocyte suppression
aplastic anemia (idiosyncratic)

PHENYTOIN

ataxia and nystagmus (dose related)
cognitive impairment
hirsutism, coarsening of facial features, gingival hyperplasia
saturation metabolism kinetics

PHENOBARBITAL

sedation, cognitive impairment
behavioral changes
induction of liver enzymes

PRIMIDONE

see phenobarbital

VALPROIC ACID

tremor
nausea and vomiting
elevated liver enzymes
weight gain

ETHOSUXIMIDE

stomachaches and vomiting
hiccups

CLONAZEPAM

sedation and lethargy
ataxia
tolerance to antiepileptic effects

toxicity can be problematic because the 10,11-epoxide metabolite may also cause toxicity.

The common idiosyncratic reaction with phenytoin is a rash (5% of cases); less common reactions are hepatitis, a lupus-like connective tissue disease, lymphadenopathy, and pseudolymphoma. Dose-related side effects are more common and include ataxia and nystagmus, commonly detected with total serum concentrations <20 μg/ml, and slight dulling of cognitive performance, especially at high doses. Other side effects with chronic phenytoin therapy are hirsutism, coarsening of facial features, and gingival hyperplasia. These should be considered when prescribing phenytoin for children.

Valproic acid may produce nausea, vomiting, and lethargy, particularly early in therapy. The availability of enteric-coated tablets of valproic acid has significantly decreased the gastrointestinal side effects. Elevation of liver enzymes and blood ammonia in patients receiving valproic acid is common. This is important because fatal hepatitis may occur in patients taking valproic acid; overall the risk is small (approximately 1 per 40,000) but heightened considerably for patients less than 2 years of age treated with multiple antiepileptic drugs. Two uncommon dose-related side effects of valproic acid are thrombocytopenia and changes in coagulation parameters, secondary to depletion of fibrinogen. These changes usually are not serious clinically, though they may be associated with bruising and can often be reduced by lowering of the drug dosage. Other side effects of valproic acid are weight gain, alopecia, and tremor.

Phenobarbital frequently produces depression of CNS function, resulting in sedation and depression. This may occur during initiation of phenobarbital therapy or as a dose-dependent phenomenon later in the treatment. Idiosyncratic reactions with phenobarbital are rare but include rash (3%) and bone marrow suppression. Common side effects in children include motor hyperactivity, irritability, decreased attention, or mental slowing. The side effects of primidone are similar to those for phenobarbital.

Dose-related side effects of ethosuximide include gastrointestinal problems (stomachaches and vomiting) and hiccups. Tolerance develops to these effects. Ethosuximide may also lead to bone marrow suppression. The side effects of clonazepam relate to its depressive action on the CNS, causing sedation and lethargy, or ataxia.

Drug Interactions

Antiepileptic drugs may interact with each other in two ways (Table 26-5): (1) one compound alters the metabolism of another by inducing hepatic enzymes or by competing for reactive sites on those enzymes, or (2) one drug changes the binding of another to plasma proteins. For example, valproic acid may increase the toxicity of phenobarbital or phenytoin by decreasing the hepatic metabolism of phenobarbital or by displacing phenytoin from plasma binding sites.

Antiepileptic drugs can also interact with nonantiepileptic drugs; for example, antibiotics (isoniazid, chloramphenicol, erythromycin) have a propensity to elevate serum concentrations of phenytoin, phenobarbital, or carbamazepine. Cimetidine frequently displaces benzodiazepines from plasma proteins and may do the same with phenytoin and valproic acid. Salicylates also compete for plasma protein binding sites, especially with phenytoin. Some antiepileptic drugs decrease the con-

Table 26-5 Antiepileptic Drug Interactions

Drug	Interaction Mechanism
ANTIEPILEPTIC DRUGS	
carbamazepine, with:	
phenobarbital	Increased metabolism to epoxide
phenytoin	Decreased carbamazepine effect (increased metabolism)
phenytoin, with:	
primidone	Increased conversion of primidone to phenobarbital
valproic acid, with:	
clonazepam	May precipitate nonconvulsive status epilepticus
phenobarbital	Increased phenobarbital toxicity (decreased metabolism)
phenytoin	Increased phenytoin toxicity (displacement from binding)
OTHER DRUGS	
antibiotics	Elevates serum concentrations of phenytoin, phenobarbital, or carbamazepine
anticoagulants	Some antiepileptic drugs (particularly phenytoin and phenobarbital) augment metabolism of coumadin anticoagulants
cimetidine	Displaces benzodiazepines (and possibly phenytoin and valproic acid) from plasma proteins
isoniazid	Increased toxicity of phenytoin (inhibits metabolism)
oral contraceptives	Antiepileptics increase metabolism
salicylates	Compete for plasma protein binding sites, especially with phenytoin and valproic acid
theophylline	Carbamazepine and phenytoin may decrease effects of theophylline

centration of coumadin-like anticoagulants by augmenting their metabolism. Antiepileptics also hasten the metabolism of oral contraceptives, resulting in a contraceptive failure rate threefold above normal.

A few specific interactions needing emphasis include the combination of valproic acid and benzodiazepines, which may precipitate absence status epilepticus in some unusual cases and the exacerbation of absence seizures by carbamazepine, phenytoin, and phenobarbital.

NEW DIRECTIONS

The development of new anticonvulsant drugs has entered an era of evaluation based on putative physiological epileptogenic mechanisms. A drug could be a GABA agonist (muscimol), a prodrug for GABA (progabide), or an inhibitor of GABA metabolism. Gabapentin is an antiepileptic drug that was designed as a structural analogue of GABA. Whereas GABA does not cross the blood-brain barrier, the new molecule is more lipophilic and can cross membranes. However, the activity of gabapentin against seizures appears to be distinct from any GABA-related actions. Present clinical evaluation has shown that gabapentin has some efficacy in patients with partial seizures resistant to conventional treatment.

Because of the crucial role of extracellular calcium in the regulation of seizure initiation and propagation, agents that interfere with the entry of calcium might be considered as potential antiepileptic agents. Most of the calcium-channel blockers do not appear to cross the blood-brain barrier, but some, including nimodipine and flunarizine, appear to be centrally active.

In addition, antagonists of the NMDA subclass of excitatory amino acid receptors are being investigated for their antiepileptic activity. So far, the use of the NMDA antagonists has been limited by side effects. There are many more agents under study; for some, a mechanism

TRADE NAMES

In addition to generic and fixed-combination preparations, the following trade-named materials are available in the United States.

PRIMARY ANTIEPILEPTIC DRUGS

Klonopin, clonazepam
Depakene, Depakote, valproic acid
Dilantin, phenytoin
Luminal and others, phenobarbital
Mysoline, primidone
Tegretol, carbamazepine
Zarontin, ethosuximide

SECONDARY ANTIEPILEPTIC DRUGS, INCLUDING ADJUNCTS

Celontin, methsuximide
Diamox, acetazolamide
Felbatol, felbamate
Lamictal, lamotrigine
Mebaral, mephobarbital
Mesantoin, mephenytoin
Milontin, phensuximide
Neurontin, gabapentin
Paradione, paramethadione
Peganone, ethotoin
Phenurone, phenacemide
Tranxene, chlorazepate
Tridione, trimethadione

DRUGS FOR THE TREATMENT OF STATUS EPILEPTICUS

Ativan, lorazepam
Valium, diazepam

of action has been postulated, some are related structurally to the currently available drugs, and for others the mechanism of action is speculative.

In addition to pharmacological therapy, it has become more apparent in the last decade that there are some patients with seizures who could benefit from modern surgical treatment. One goal of surgical therapy is the removal of identifiable lesions such as arteriovenous malformations, brain tumors, abscesses, and hematomas. The overall results of this surgery have been gratifying. Another goal of epilepsy surgery has been the treatment of the patient who is refractory to medical therapy. The seizures must originate in a well-circumscribed region of the brain that can be removed without risk of producing a major neurological handicap. Epilepsy surgery is usually undertaken at a specialized comprehensive epilepsy center and involves a team effort.

REFERENCES

Consensus statement on febrile seizures. In Nelson KB, Ellenberg JH, editors: *Febrile seizures,* New York, 1991, Raven Press.

Drugs for epilepsy, *Med Lett Drugs Ther* 31:1-4, 1989.

Dreifuss FE: Classification of epileptic seizures and the epilepsies, *Pediatr Clin North Am* 36:265-279, 1989.

Lüders, H.O.: *Epilepsy surgery,* New York, 1992, Raven Press.

Regor SR, Kutt H: The medical treatment of epilepsy, New York, 1992, Marcel Dekker.

Scheuer ML, Pedley TA: The evaluation and treatment of seizures, *N Engl J Med* 323:1468-1474, 1990.

Treatment of convulsive status epilepticus: recommendations of the Epilepsy Foundation of America's working group on status epilepticus, *JAMA* 270:854-859, 1993.

SELF-ASSESSMENT QUESTIONS

1. Which of the following is a true statement?
   a. GABA is an excitatory neurotransmitter in the CNS.
   b. Barbiturates and benzodiazepines interact with the GABA receptor/channel complex.
   c. Augmentation of GABA promotes seizure initiation.
   d. During seizures extracellular potassium falls.
   e. Spike-wave discharges recorded on the EEG are associated with tonic-clonic seizures.
2. The drug of choice for absence seizures is:
   a. phenytoin.
   b. clonazepam.
   c. primidone.
   d. carbamazepine.
   e. ethosuximide.
3. All of the following statements about the metabolism of the antiepileptic drugs is true *except* that:
   a. Primidone is metabolized to compounds with antiepileptic properties.
   b. Phenobarbital induces liver microsomal enzymes.
   c. Phenytoin dosing must be individualized because of its linear elimination kinetics.
   d. Carbamazepine is metabolized to a metabolite with antiepileptic activity.
   e. One antiepileptic drug may effect the metabolism of another.
4. Which of the following statements about phenytoin is false?
   a. It commonly causes hiccups, stomachache, and vomiting.
   b. It causes dose-related ataxia and nystagmus.
   c. It is associated with hirsutism and gingival hyperplasia.
   d. It is used to treat generalized tonic-clonic seizures.
   e. It has saturation (nonlinear) kinetics.
5. Which of the following statements is true?
   a. The use of two antiepileptic agents together never exacerbates seizures.
   b. Carbamazepine causes autoinduction of its own metabolism.
   c. Antiepileptic drugs should always be stopped during pregnancy.
   d. The antiepileptic drugs are mainly excreted unchanged by the kidney.
   e. Ethosuximide is the drug of choice for partial seizures with secondary generalization.
6. Which of the following statements about the treatment of status epilepticus is false?
   a. IV carbamazepine is the most commonly used drug for the treatment of status epilepticus.
   b. General strategy includes support of cardiovascular and respiratory systems.
   c. Phenytoin can be given IV but may cause hypotension if given too rapidly.
   d. The use of phenobarbital may lead to respiratory compromise.
   e. Rapidly acting benzodiazepines, such as diazepam or lorazepam, are used initially to control seizure activity.
7. Seizures can be caused by all of the following *except:*
   a. hyponatremia.
   b. alkalosis.
   c. brain tumor.
   d. mental retardation.
   e. drug withdrawal.
8. An epileptic syndrome consists in all of the following *except:*
   a. etiology of the seizures.
   b. family history.
   c. obsessive-compulsive personality.
   d. prognosis.
   e. age of onset.

CHAPTER 27 Drugs for the Treatment of Movement Disorders

JAMES P. BENNETT, JR.

MAJOR DRUGS

L-dopa
dopamine agonists
selegiline
anticholinergic drugs
benzodiazepines
baclofen

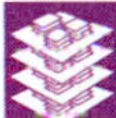

THERAPEUTIC OVERVIEW

Movement disorders involve abnormalities of voluntary and involuntary movement, which usually arise spontaneously. Sometimes movement disorders occur after insults to the nervous system, such as stroke, head trauma, brain infection, or demyelinating lesions of multiple sclerosis. It is useful to divide movement disorders into two categories: those characterized by a paucity of normal movement (the "hypokinetic-rigid" disorders) and those characterized by an excess of movements (the "hyperkinetic-choreic" disorders).

The hypokinetic-rigid disorders are associated with slowing of voluntary movement **(bradykinesia)** and also an increased resistance to muscle stretch **(rigidity).** The most frequently occurring hypokinetic-rigid disorder is idiopathic Parkinson's disease, which is the second most prevalent neurodegenerative disorder of adults (after Alzheimer's disease). All patients with Parkinson's disease will, at some time during their illness, have a 4 to 6 Hz resting tremor of one or more body parts, usually beginning in a hand or arm. This tremor can lessen or disappear in the later stages of the disease, when bradykinesia and rigidity become more dominant. For most Parkinson's patients loss of postural reflexes is ultimately the most disabling symptom and increases the tendency to fall, usually backwards.

ABBREVIATIONS

COMT	catechol-*O*-methyl transferase
GABA	γ-aminobutyric acid
L-dopa	L-dihydroxyphenylalanine
MAO	monoamine oxidase
MPTP	*N*-methyl-4-phenyltetrahydropyridine

Degeneration of certain neuronal systems will mimic Parkinson's disease but will usually have additional signs and symptoms at presentation. Occurrence of one or more of the symptoms of Parkinson's disease is referred to as **parkinsonism.**

Conditions in which parkinsonism is observed include (1) loss of voluntary vertical ocular gaze in progressive supranuclear palsy, (2) disturbances of autonomic nerve function (orthostatic hypotension, impotence, bladder/bowel incontinence) in Shy-Drager syndrome, (3) ataxia and bulbar cranial nerve deficits in olivopontocerebellar atrophy, (4) limb apraxia (loss of complex coordinated motor function) and upper motor neuron defects in corticonigral degeneration, and (5) progressive bradykinesia with minimal or no rigidity and no tremor in striatonigral degeneration.

The distinctions between idiopathic Parkinson's disease and parkinsonism secondary to systems degeneration can be difficult to detect but is of great therapeutic importance. Whereas the signs and symptoms of Parkinson's disease usually respond to the therapeutic agents discussed below, parkinsonism caused by systems degeneration is much less responsive to these drugs. Drug-induced parkinsonism is a common side effect of treatment with neuroleptic drugs but also can be seen in older patients given metoclopramide. Drug-induced parkinsonism is also refractory to drug therapy.

Several hyperkinetic syndromes are named according to the characteristics of the abnormal movements.

Myoclonus refers to brief contractions of one or more muscles. Severe generalized myoclonus can resemble seizures. Distinguishing between the two conditions is important, since they require different therapeutic approaches. Most myoclonus is attributable to drug toxicity or metabolic derangements, particularly renal failure, and effective treatment requires correction of the underlying abnormality.

Tics mimic focal myoclonus and are often benign disorders of childhood and adolescence. **Tourette's syndrome,** possibly an inherited disorder, is characterized by appearance of tics before 12 years of age. The tics commonly become more complex through adolescence and may include vocalizations and complex gestures, sometimes obscene. Apart from Parkinson's disease, **tremor** can result from metabolic disturbances (i.e., hyperthyroidism) or be a side effect of different drugs, such as lithium carbonate, valproic acid, and caffeine. The most common spontaneously occurring tremor, known as **familial,** or **essential, tremor** is not usually seen at rest but occurs with use of the limb (or voice).

Dystonias are abnormal muscle contractions, usually with simultaneous activation of opposing agonist and antagonist groups, that intrude into normal movement, produce abnormal postures, and can be painful. Dystonias can be generalized or focal.

Chorea and **athetosis** refer to more complex semipurposeful involuntary movements. Athetotic movements are usually slower and "serpentine" in quality, whereas choreic movements are more rapid. The two types commonly occur together ("choreoathetotic") and may be attributable to different conditions. A rare but dramatic inherited choreoathetotic disorder appears in the natural course of the neurodegenerative illness **Huntington's disease.** Other causes include metabolic disorders; pregnancy or oral contraceptive use; and complications of rheumatic fever, systemic lupus erythematosus, or hyperthyroidism; or side effects of drug therapy (psychosis, Parkinson's disease) or drug abuse (cocaine, amphetamine).

Spasticity has elements of both hypokinetic and hyperkinetic disorders and arises whenever lower motor neurons are chronically separated from upper motor neuron innervation. Spasticity can follow stroke, spinal cord injury or lesions, prenatal or neonatal insults, or multiple sclerosis.

Parkinson's disease responds well to drugs that facilitate dopaminergic neurotransmission at degenerating brain synapses, whereas parkinsonism associated with systems degeneration is more difficult to treat. Drug therapy of these conditions is empirical and generally unsatisfactory. Treatment of hyperkinetic disorders are also primarily empirical and current strategies are summarized in the box.

THERAPEUTIC OVERVIEW

HYPOKINETIC MOVEMENT DISORDERS

Idiopathic Parkinson's disease
- Primary agents—carbidopa/L-dopa; bromocriptine; pergolide
- Secondary agents—trihexyphenidyl; benztropine; amantidine

Olivopontocerebellar atrophy
- 5-HTP (5-hydroxytryptophan) (for ataxia)

Progressive supranuclear palsy
- bromocriptine; pergolide (for parkinsonism); amitriptyline (for ocular gaze)

Shy-Drager syndrome
- mineralocorticoid; ephedrine

HYPERKINETIC MOVEMENT DISORDERS

Tics
- neuroleptics

Myoclonus
- carbidopa/5-HTP (for anoxic myoclonus); benzodiazepines; baclofen

Essential tremor
- propranolol; primidone, benzodiazepine

Dystonias
- anticholinergics; *Clostridium botulinum toxin*

Chorea

Huntington's disease
- neuroleptic drugs

Tardive dyskinesia
- clozapine; reserpine; L-dopa; clonidine

SPASTICITY

Benzodiazepine; baclofen

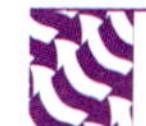

MECHANISMS OF ACTION

L-Dopa

Parkinson's disease is a forebrain dopamine-deficiency state arising from the loss of more than 75% of midbrain (substantia nigra) dopamine-manufacturing neurons. Partial forebrain dopamine replacement occurs after administration of L-dihydroxyphenylalanine (L-dopa), the amino acid precursor of dopamine. L-Dopa crosses tissue barriers (intestine-blood, blood-brain) and enters nerve cells by carrier-mediated diffusion. The large neutral amino acid carrier that transports L-dopa is driven by sodium-ion gradients across cell membranes and also transports dietary amino acids such as tyrosine and leucine. L-Dopa is catabolized in the periphery by decarboxylation to dopamine or methylation

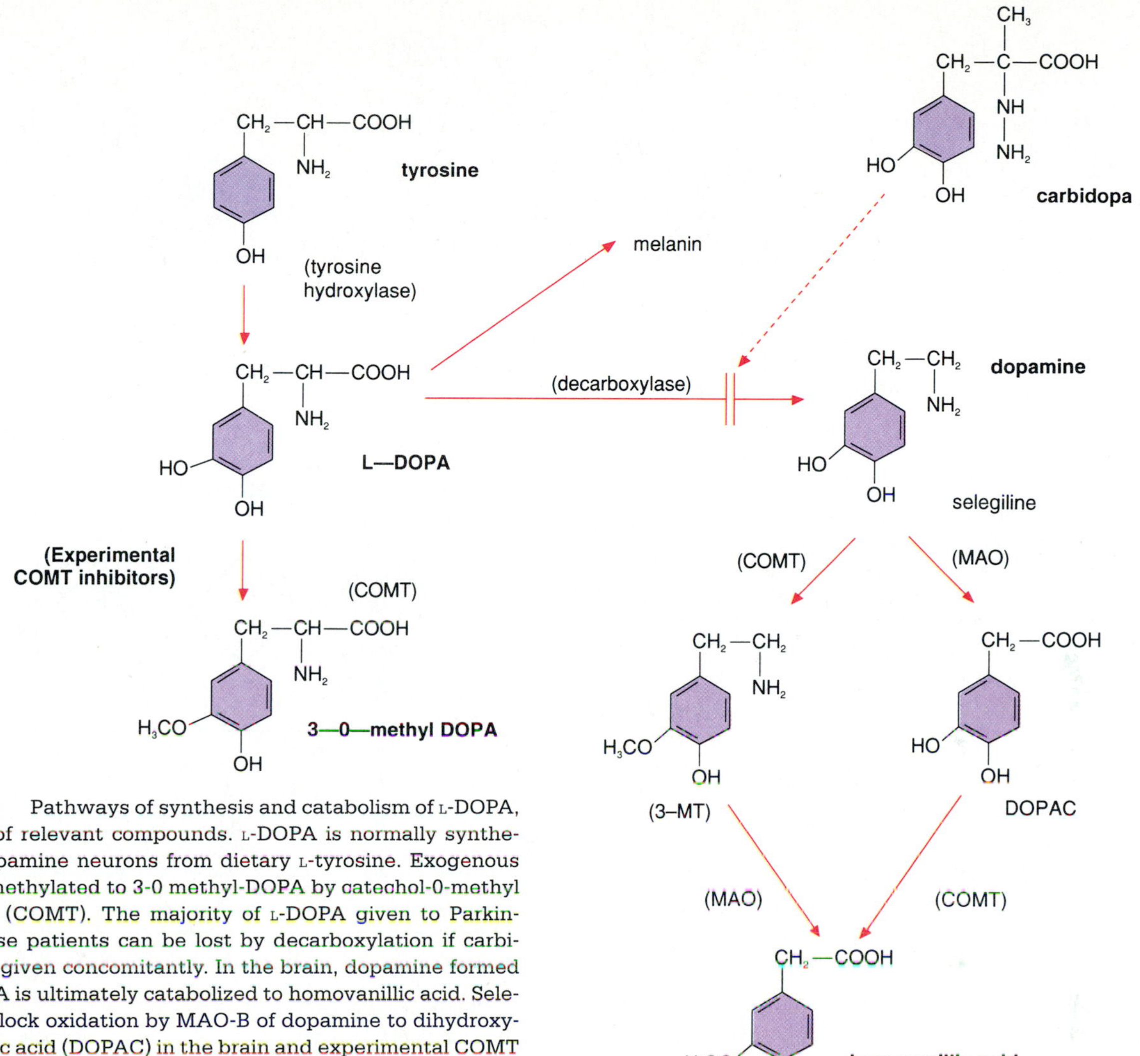

FIGURE 27-1 Pathways of synthesis and catabolism of L-DOPA, structures of relevant compounds. L-DOPA is normally synthesized in dopamine neurons from dietary L-tyrosine. Exogenous L-DOPA is methylated to 3-0 methyl-DOPA by catechol-0-methyl transferase (COMT). The majority of L-DOPA given to Parkinson's disease patients can be lost by decarboxylation if carbidopa is not given concomitantly. In the brain, dopamine formed from L-DOPA is ultimately catabolized to homovanillic acid. Selegiline can block oxidation by MAO-B of dopamine to dihydroxyphenylacetic acid (DOPAC) in the brain and experimental COMT inhibitors that block peripheral conversion of L-DOPA to 3-0-methyl DOPA are presently in clinical trials.

by catechol-*O*-methyl transferase (COMT) to 3-*O*-methyldopa (Figure 27-1). The decarboxylating enzyme (dopa decarboxylase, L-aromatic amino acid decarboxylase) is found in many tissues and is inhibited by carbidopa. Coadministration of carbidopa lessens L-dopa decarboxylation in the periphery, reduces peripheral side effects of L-dopa, and increases L-dopa bioavailability in the brain.

L-Dopa crosses the blood-brain barrier and is converted to dopamine, the endogenous agonist, in neurons and glia, but is retained mainly by catecholamine neurons. Other drugs also exert direct agonist actions at dopamine receptors. Apomorphine is the oldest of the known agonists but has limited effect orally and is administered parenterally in experimental studies. Two orally active, direct dopamine agonists, bromocriptine and pergolide, have recently been introduced (Figure 27-2). These drugs alleviate symptoms of Parkinson's disease by binding to and activating dopamine receptors in the basal ganglia. There are presently five subtypes of brain dopamine receptors known (D_1-D_5; see Table 27-1, but D_1 and D_2 subtypes predominate in the basal ganglia (Figure 27-3). The other subtypes (D_3 to D_5) are found primarily in the limbic forebrain, where they may contribute to some of the CNS side effects of L-dopa and dopamine agonists.

D_1-dopamine receptors activate adenylate cyclase through a stimulatory guanine nucleotide binding protein (G protein). Activation of D_1-receptors increases several ionic currents and can either excite or inhibit neuronal firing. D_2-receptors inhibit adenylate cyclase through an inhibitory G protein and can also inhibit phospholipase C, reducing conversion of phosphatidyl inositol to inositol trisphosphate and diacylglycerol (Figure 27-4). D_2-receptor activation increases potassium influx, which can hyperpolarize neurons and inhibit firing.

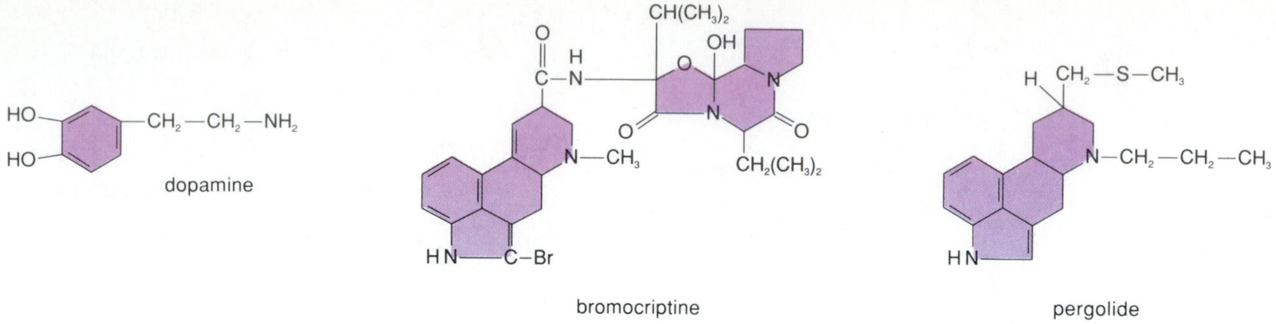

FIGURE 27-2 Structures of the dopamine agonists bromocriptine and pergolide. Notice that both of these agonists contain the basic structure of dopamine.

Table 27-1 Characteristics of the Dopamine-Receptor Families

Subtype	Amino Acids	Coupling
D_1 FAMILY		
D_{1A}	446	↑AC
D_{1B}	475	↑AC
D_{1C} (D_5)	477	↑AC
D_2 FAMILY		
D_{2S}	415	↓AC ↑K^+
D_{2L}	444	↓AC ↑K^+
D_3	400-446	?
D_4	387	?

Most abundant subtypes in brain are D_{1A} and D_2 (D_{2L} >> D_{2S}). Classic neuroleptics interact more strongly with members of the D_2 family compared with the D_1 family. D_4-receptors are located mainly in the limbic system and have an unusually high affinity for the atypical neuroleptic clozapine. *AC*, Adenylate cyclase.

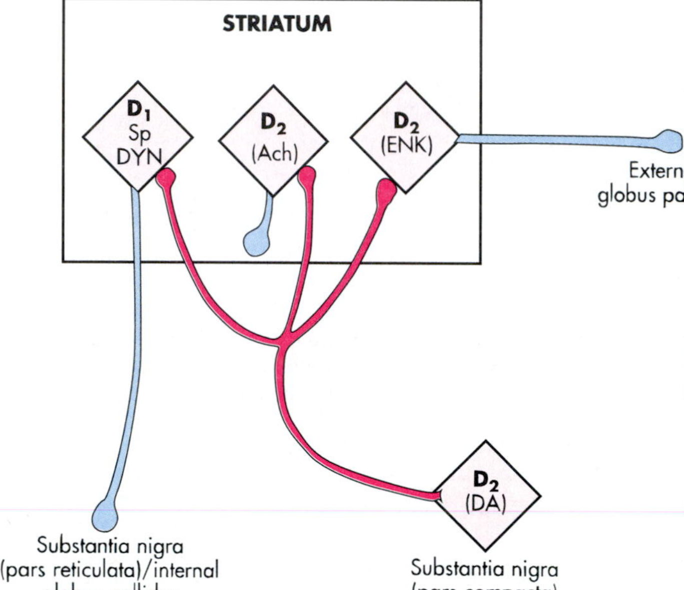

FIGURE 27-3 Location of dopamine subtype–bearing neurons in basal ganglia. D_1-receptors are found on medium spiny neurons that project to substantia nigra (pars reticulata) and internal globus pallidus. D_2-receptors are found on medium spiny neurons that project to external globus pallidus. Localized neuropeptides include substance P *(SP)*, dynorphin *(DYN)*, and enkephalin *(ENK)*. D_2-receptors are also found on large aspiny interneurons, which manufacture acetylcholine *(Ach)*, and on the cell bodies and terminals of substantia nigra neurons, which manufacture dopamine *(DA)*.

All dopamine-receptor subtypes share similar primary structures and belong to a "superfamily" of receptors that signal through G proteins. The major structural differences between D_1- and D_2-receptors are in the third cytoplasmic loop and the length of the cytoplasmic carboxyl terminus. In addition, D_2-receptors exist in both "short" and "long" isoforms, differing by 29 amino acids in the third cytoplasmic loop. Because this structure is believed to be important in G-protein activation, these structural differences may account for the different effects of D_1- and D_2-receptors (Figure 27-5). There is as yet no evidence for functional differences between the short and long isoforms of D_2-receptors.

Anticholinergic Drugs and Amantadine

Before the development of L-dopa, antagonists of muscarinic cholinergic receptors had been used for decades as the only effective therapy for Parkinson's disease. Several anticholinergic drugs are still used for treating early Parkinson's symptoms, particularly tremor. They are generally less effective in treating rigidity and bradykinesia. These drugs differ primarily in potency and cause many peripheral (dry mouth, mydriasis, bladder weakness, constipation) and central (memory loss, confusion) side effects.

Another drug used in treatment of Parkinson's disease symptoms is amantadine. Amantadine appears to

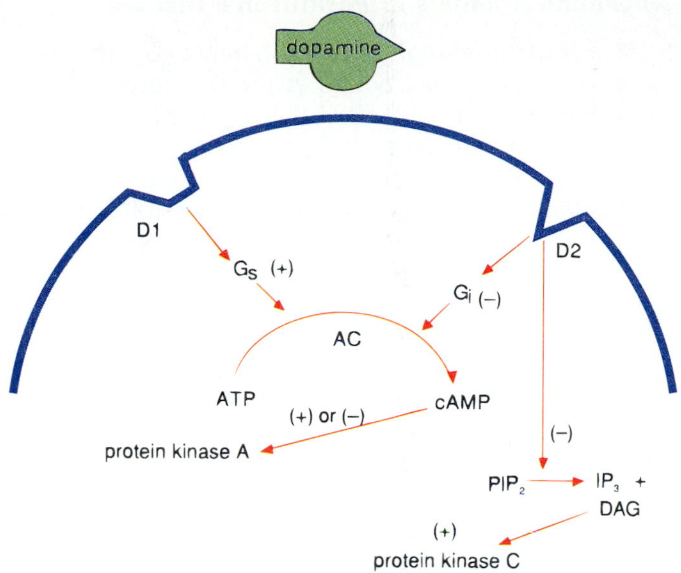

FIGURE 27-4 Second messengers involved in the mechanisms of action at D_1 and D_2 dopamine receptors. D_1-receptors couple to adenylate cyclase *(AC)* through a stimulatory G protein *(G_s)* to increase the intracellular production of cyclic adenosine monophosphate *(cAMP)* from adenosine triphosphate. cAMP stimulates phosphorylation of a variety of cellular proteins by protein kinase A. D_2-receptors couple to AC through an inhibitor G protein *(G_i)* to decrease cAMP production. D_2-receptors also reduce the rate of conversion of phosphatidyl inositol 4,5 bisphosphate *(PIP_2)* to inositol trisphosphate *(IP_3)* and diacylglylcerol *(DAG)*. DAG stimulates protein phosphorylation by protein kinase C.

increase dopamine release from nerve terminals and is thus effective mainly in early Parkinson's patients in whom neuronal degeneration is still minimal. It is usually well tolerated but occasionally causes confusion in elderly patients.

Monoamine Oxidase Inhibitors

Dopamine is degraded in the brain by both the A and B subtypes of monoamine oxidase (MAO). Because the problems of nonselective MAO inhibitors, such as the "tyramine" effect (see Chapter 10), derive from inhibition of intestinal MAO-A, treatment with selective MAO-B inhibitors is usually well tolerated and safe. Selegiline, a selective MAO-B inhibitor, is available for concurrent use with L-dopa therapy in Parkinson's patients who are experiencing declining therapeutic responses. Selegiline also improves symptoms and slows the rate of clinical progression of early Parkinson's disease, thereby delaying the time before dopamine replacement therapy is needed. This latter property indicates that selegiline may be "neuroprotective" and slow the rate of death of dopamine neurons, but its known symptomatic properties complicate this interpretation.

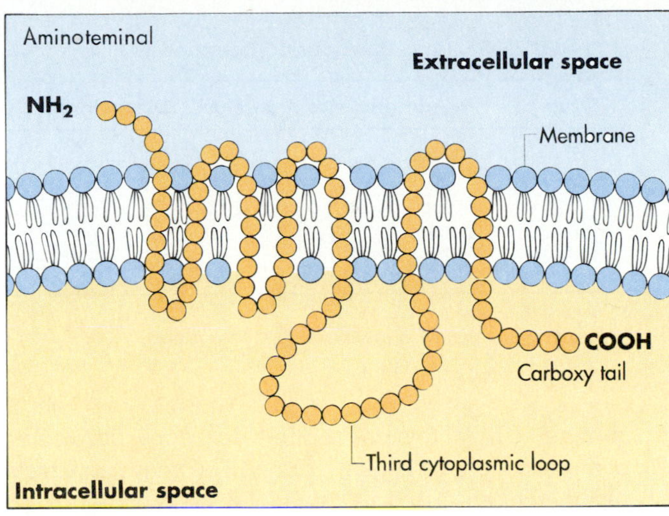

FIGURE 27-5 Basic structures of G protein–coupled receptors. Dopamine receptors possess unique structures in their third cytoplasmic loop (where interactions with G proteins are believed to take place) and in the carboxy tail.

Drugs to Treat Spasticity

Drug treatment of spasticity involves agents that bind to γ-aminobutyric acid (GABA) receptors. Baclofen is an agonist at the GABA-B receptor subtype, located on both neurons and nerve endings in the brain and spinal cord. Presynaptic GABA-B receptors are abundant on dorsal root afferent fibers in the spinal cord and brainstem, they are not restricted to GABA neurons, and their activation inhibits release of several neurotransmitters. Benzodiazepines bind to a subunit of the GABA-A neuronal receptor complex and potentiate the ability of GABA to open chloride-ion channels (See Chapter 25).

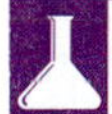

PHARMACOKINETICS

The serum half-life of L-dopa is short, usually about 1 to 2 hours, and therefore L-dopa/carbidopa effectiveness can be prolonged by timed-release formulations. 3-*O*-Methyldopa (Figure 27-1) accumulates with administration of higher L-dopa/carbidopa doses, primarily because of its longer serum half-life (about 20 hr). Because 3-*O*-methyldopa can compete with L-dopa for entry into the brain, reduction of its blood concentrations may improve clinical responses to L-dopa. Trials of COMT inhibitors are being performed to address this hypothesis.

Despite the short serum half-life of oral L-dopa, most patients with early Parkinson's disease achieve good symptom control with two or three doses of L-dopa/carbidopa per day. The duration of L-dopa action in these patients likely derives from the ability of surviving do-

Table 27-2 Pharmacokinetic Parameters

Drug	Administered	t½ (hr)	Disposition
L-dopa	Oral	1-2	M (main)
baclofen	Oral	—	R (main)
	Intrathecal	4-5 in CSF	
bromocriptine	Oral	4-6	M (main)
pergolide	Oral	—*	M (about 100%)

M, Metabolism; *R,* renal.
*No parent drug detected in plasma after oral administration.

pamine neurons to store and release L-dopa–derived dopamine in a physiological manner. The pharmacokinetic parameters are listed in Table 27-2.

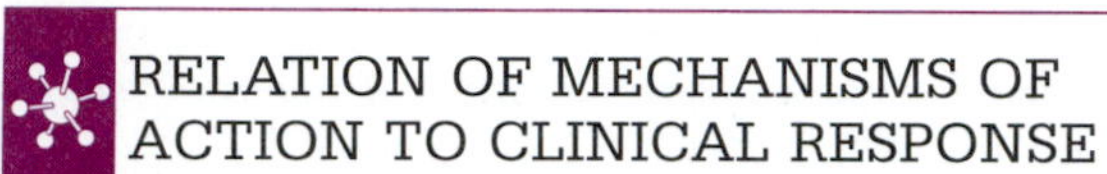

RELATION OF MECHANISMS OF ACTION TO CLINICAL RESPONSE

L-Dopa in Parkinson's Disease

Studies in animal models of parkinsonism demonstrate that L-dopa must be decarboxylated to dopamine for improvements in motor function to be apparent. A close temporal association between increased motor activity and elevation in brain extracellular dopamine after L-dopa treatment can also be demonstrated in animal models, an indication that the primary therapeutic effects are attributable to formation of dopamine.

Dopamine activates both D_1 and D_2 dopamine receptors in basal ganglia (and also the D_3 to D_5 subtypes in the limbic system). In general, D_1 and D_2 subtypes are located on different neuronal populations in the basal ganglia, though there is some overlap in their distribution. Normally, D_1- and D_2-receptors appear to be functionally "coupled" through unknown mechanisms, such that D_1 - and D_2-receptor agonists do not act independently of each other. This "coupling" may occur because both receptors are co-localized on some neurons or involve interactive networks of neurons with different receptor types. When dopamine innervation degenerates, as occurs in Parkinson's disease, D_1- and D_2-receptors "uncouple" from each other and become functionally independent. However, simultaneous activation of both D_1 and D_2 subtypes is still necessary for maximum motor improvement in parkinsonism, probably because separate striatal outflow pathways must be stimulated to restore function. Since dopamine activates both subtypes, L-dopa is the most appropriate agent for treatment of Parkinson's disease, though its efficacy in advanced stages of the disease is less than satisfactory.

Dopamine Agonists in Parkinson's Disease

Bromocriptine and pergolide both bind to D_1- and D_2-receptors but are more potent at the D_2 subtype. Bromocriptine acts as a full agonist at D_2-receptors and a mixed agonist-antagonist at D_1-receptors. Pergolide is also a full agonist at D_2-receptors, but is about 10 times more potent than bromocriptine and has less D_1 antagonist activity. In experimental parkinsonism, selective D_2 agonists are effective in relieving signs and symptoms of parkinsonism, whereas selective D_1 agonists are generally ineffective. However, the combination of D_1 and D_2 agonist activity provides optimum improvement. Thus, D_2 agonists are rarely used alone to treat parkinsonism, except at the early stages of the disease when some endogenous dopamine is still present. In later stages, directly acting agonists are combined with L-dopa/carbidopa for maximum benefit.

Anticholinergic Drugs in Parkinson's Disease

Cholinergic neurons in the basal ganglia possess D_2-receptors, which, when activated, inhibit their firing. With progressive loss of dopamine in Parkinson's disease, this disinhibition results in increased synthesis and release of acetylcholine. Anticholinergic drugs block the effects of elevated acetylcholine, though they do not alleviate other effects of dopamine deficiency. The two most commonly used anticholinergic drugs, benztropine and trihexyphenidyl, have the additional therapeutically desirable action of blocking dopamine reuptake into nerve terminals. This may provide additional improvement in patients with early disease, who have not completely lost their dopaminergic innervation.

Monoamine Oxidase (MAO) Inhibitors in Parkinson's Disease

In most experimental animals (rodents) MAO-A is chiefly responsible for degradation of dopamine in the brain. In humans, however, MAO-B is present in higher levels in substantia nigra and may assume a greater role in dopamine catabolism. Selegiline, a selective MAO-B inhibitor, decreases catabolism of dopamine derived from L-dopa and increases dopamine concentrations in brain extracellular space. This may be an explanation for its ability to potentiate the effects of L-dopa in Parkinson's patients.

Some evidence has indicated that daily treatment with an MAO-B inhibitor may protect dopaminergic neurons and lessen the rate of progression of symptoms (Figure 27-6). If selegiline treatment is neuroprotective in early Parkinson's disease, two mechanisms might ap-

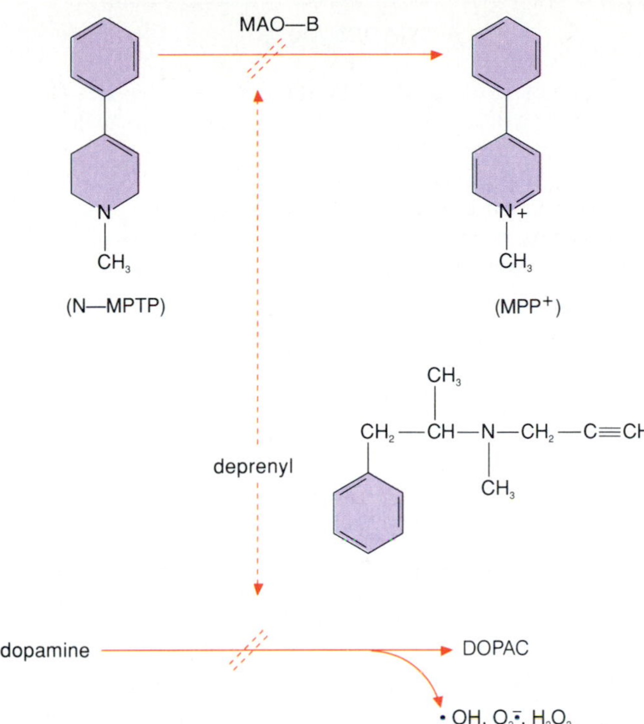

FIGURE 27-6 Potential mechanisms of protective action of selegiline in Parkinson's disease. Selegiline blocks the oxidation by MAO-B of the dopamine neuron protoxin *N*-methyl-4-phenyltetrahydropyridine *(N-MPTP)* to the toxic derivative *N*-methylpyridinium ion *(MPP+)*. Deprenyl also blocks the normal intraneuronal oxidation of dopamine to dihydroxyphenylacetate *(DOPAC)*, during which free radicals (hydroxyl, OH; superoxide, $O_2^=$ and peroxide, H_2O_2) can be formed.

ply. By the reduction of oxidative deamination of dopamine, decreased concentrations of toxic free radicals would be produced. Selegiline can prevent development of parkinsonism after treatment of primates with the substituted pyridine *N*-methyl-4-phenyl tetrahydropyridine (MPTP). This compound was responsible for human parkinsonism in opiate addicts who ingested MPTP-contaminated street drugs. MPTP is oxidized by MAO-B to methylpyridinium ion, which is taken up into dopamine nerve terminals where it poisons mitochondrial respiratory complex I. Selegiline treatment might prevent the neurotoxic effects of environmental pyridines on dopaminergic neurons.

Selegiline is metabolized to methamphetamine and then to amphetamine, which can release dopamine. It also increases brain concentrations of phenylethylamine, which activates dopamine receptors. All these effects may contribute to the ability of selegiline to provide mild improvement of Parkinson's symptoms. It is not yet clear whether selegiline's ability to slow Parkinson's disease progression is attributable to relief of symptoms or to "neuroprotective" actions.

Therapy of Other Hypokinetic-Rigid Disorders

Parkinsonism associated with systems degeneration is usually poorly responsive to dopamine replacement therapy. Large doses of dopamine agonists can sometimes be helpful in progressive supranuclear palsy. Ocular gaze palsies may respond to tricyclic antidepressants through mechanisms that are unclear. Orthostatic hypotension in Shy-Drager syndrome responds to liberalization of salt intake, mineralocorticoid, and α-adrenergic agonist administration (i.e., ephedrine, pseudoephedrine). Ataxia in olivopontocerebellar atrophy may respond to 5-hydroxytryptophan, the amino acid precursor of serotonin, but this is controversial.

Therapy of Hyperkinetic Disorders

Myoclonus Myoclonus arising from a toxic or metabolic disturbance is treated by removal of the primary etiological factor. 5-Hydroxytryptophan (with carbidopa) has been found to be effective in suppressing myoclonus after hypoxic brain injury.

Tics Neuroleptic drugs are helpful in suppressing simple and complex tics in Tourette's syndrome. The risk of tardive dyskinesia with long-term use of neuroleptics must be balanced against the emotional and social consequences of tics. A commonly used strategy is to administer the drug on week days but not on weekends.

Tremor Essential tremor is often reduced by low doses of β-adrenergic receptor antagonists such as propranolol. Structure-activity studies indicate that β-adrenergic receptor antagonism may not be responsible for their efficacy and that they may exert their primary actions outside the CNS. Other effective therapies for tremor include primidone or benzodiazepines with a likely common site of action being the GABA-A receptor. Small doses of alcohol can be used for tremor suppression in social situations, though the risk of alcoholism in susceptible individuals must be kept in mind.

Dystonia Torsion dystonia may be partially alleviated by high doses of muscarinic cholinergic receptor antagonists, which are tolerated well by younger patients. Some focal dystonias may respond transiently to anticholinergic drugs, benzodiazepines, or baclofen but most ultimately require more specific therapy. A recent advance in treatment of focal dystonias is the local intramuscular injection of purified type A toxin ("botox") from *Clostridium botulinum*. Botox treatments involve a small fraction of the toxin dose that would produce clinibaclofen

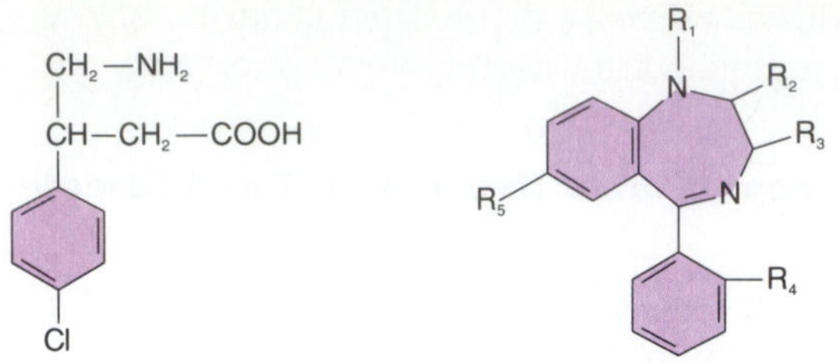

benzodiazepines
(R groups vary)

FIGURE 27-7 Structure of baclofen (β-*para*-chlorophenyl GABA) and benzodiazepines.

CLINICAL PROBLEMS

L-DOPA (FOR PARKINSON'S DISEASE)

Fluctuations in response; confusion and hallucinations; tardive dyskinesia; problems with L-dopa uptake (by food)

BACLOFEN (FOR SPASTICITY)

Major side effect is sedation

SELEGILINE

Protective doses have very few side effects

cal botulism. The toxin is injected into symptomatic muscles and is rapidly taken up into cholinergic nerve endings, where it inhibits acetylcholine release. This leads to temporary denervation and atrophy of associated muscle fibers. Botox injections can be helpful in relieving pain and muscle contraction in focal dystonias but are not curative and are commonly repeated at intervals of 3 to 6 months.

Chorea and Athetosis Use of neuroleptics to block dopamine neurotransmission in basal ganglia will reduce the intensity of choreoathetosis in both Huntington's disease and tardive dyskinesia. Unfortunately, the improvement is usually not long lasting in either condition. Neuroleptic therapy in Huntington's disease can also lead to superimposed tardive dyskinesia. Reserpine in high doses can reduce movements in both disorders but carries a high risk of depression. The appearance of tardive dyskinesia must always prompt reevaluation of the necessity for continued neuroleptic therapy. The atypical neuroleptic clozapine may provide an alternative because it appears to have no risk of causing tardive dyskinesia and is capable of suppressing the abnormal movements in preexisting tardive dyskinesia. It is not known whether clozapine will influence chorea in Huntington's disease.

TRADENAMES

In addition to generic and fixed-combination preparations, the following trade-named materials are available in the United States.

Artane, trihexyphenidyl
Cogentin, benztropine
Lioresal, baclofen
Mysoline, primidone
Parlodel, bromocriptine
Permax, pergolide
Sinemet, carbidopa/L-dopa
Symmetrel, amantadine

Therapy of movement disorders in Wilson's disease is directed at removal of the copper deposition in brain and liver. Dietary copper restriction and copper-chelating agents such as penicillamine prevent further accumulation and accelerate removal of excessive stores.

Spasticity Relief of spasticity by baclofen and benzodiazepines is caused by reduction of excessive afferent input to ventral motor neurons, subsequently reducing the increased outflow to muscles. Sedation is the dose-limiting side effect for most patients and can be reduced by continuous intrathecal (directly into the spinal subarachnoid space) baclofen administration. Baclofen is an agonist at GABA type B receptors. This is primarily a presynaptic receptor in the brainstem and spinal cord that is localized to terminals of dorsal root afferent fibers. Activation of GABA type B receptors inhibits neurotransmitter release, probably by inhibition of inward calcium current. The structure of baclofen is shown in Figure 27-7 (see Chapter 25 for discussion and structures of benzodiazepines).

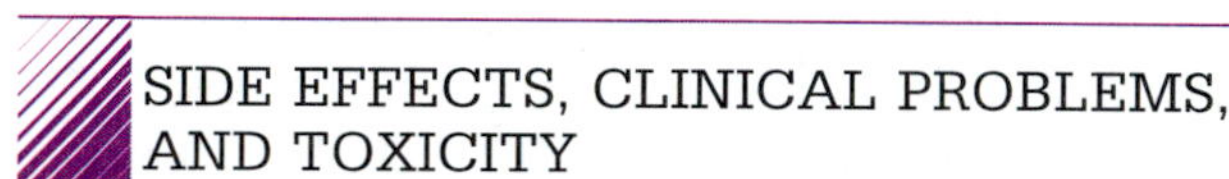

SIDE EFFECTS, CLINICAL PROBLEMS, AND TOXICITY

The major challenges in treating Parkinson's disease are to discover more effective means to slow progression of the disease and to provide long-term control of signs and symptoms as the disease does progress. Initial experience using selegiline demonstrates that MAO-B activity is not exclusively responsible for disease progression. Symptomatic treatment with L-dopa is limited by the tendency toward fluctuating responses after 3 to 5 years of treatment. Patients experience declining efficacy at the end of each dose interval ("wearing off"), which can often be managed when doses are taken more frequently or a directly acting dopamine agonist is added. As therapy continues, dyskinesias, similar to the spontaneous movements of Huntington's disease, appear and become more intense. Still later, unpredictable swings of signs and symptoms not related to drug dosing (random "on-off") appear. In patients with unstable L-dopa responses, peripheral pharmacokinetics of L-dopa are unchanged. Variations in central pharmacodynamics are much more pronounced, with fluctuating patients having much greater sensitivity to small changes in L-dopa blood concentrations.

Fluctuations in response and dyskinesias can be reduced by continuous intravenous L-dopa administration, but such therapy is obviously not practical for outpatient use. Some patients have nearly as good improvement with continuous jejunal L-dopa infusion, which can be undertaken on an outpatient basis. Dyskinesias can be suppressed by addition of the neuroleptic drug clozapine, which can be given to Parkinson's patients. There are some indications that continuous parenteral administration of directly acting dopamine agonists may be effective in managing treatment fluctuations.

L-Dopa and dopamine agonists can cause psychiatric disturbances, commonly visual hallucinations or paranoid psychosis. These side effects can appear in demented persons consuming small drug doses or nondemented persons consuming larger doses. Clozapine is effective in suppressing these effects. Lastly, a severe akinetic-rigid syndrome resembling neuroleptic malignant syndrome can appear if L-dopa or dopamine agonist therapy is abruptly withdrawn from a Parkinson's patient.

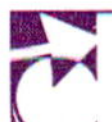

NEW DIRECTIONS

Future directions in Parkinson's therapy include the testing of additional MAO inhibitors without symptomatic actions and newer free-radical scavenging agents as potential neuroprotective agents. Improvements in delivery of potent dopamine agonists, such as transdermal patches and subcutaneous infusion, will alter treatment at all disease stages. Parkinson's disease may derive fundamentally from a defect in mitochondrial oxidative function, particularly that of complex I, in which case restorative therapy may be possible. Brain grafting of both normal fetal brain cells and genetically modified carrier cells has shown preliminary success and will be further refined.

Tardive dyskinesia may be eliminated if atypical neuroleptics such as clozapine can replace traditional drugs for long-term use. Movements of Huntington's disease may improve with grafting of genetically engineered cells that produce the missing neurotransmitters.

REFERENCES

Lang, AE, Weiner WE, editors: Drug-induced movement disorders. Mount Kisco, NY, 1992, Futura.

Stern MB, Koller WC, editors: Parkinsonian syndromes. Marcel Dekker, NY, 1993.

Weiner WJ, Lang AE: Movement disorders: a comprehensive survey, Mount Kisco, NY, 1989, Futura.

SELF-ASSESSMENT QUESTIONS

1. Carbidopa administration:
   a. increases the half-life of L-dopa in plasma.
   b. increases the half-life of dopamine in brain.
   c. reduces decarboxylation of L-dopa in plasma.
   d. reduces decarboxylation of L-dopa in brain.
   e. reduces signs and symptoms of Parkinson's disease.
2. Which of the following directly activate D_2 dopamine receptors?
   a. baclofen
   b. selegiline
   c. L-dopa
   d. bromocriptine
   e. clozapine
3. Spasticity can often be alleviated with:
   a. baclofen.
   b. clozapine.
   c. selegiline.
   d. all of the above.
   e. none of the above.
4. Myoclonus:
   a. usually represents underlying brain damage and is untreatable.
   b. commonly accompanies drug therapy of Parkinson's disease.
   c. has multiple causes, usually related to underlying metabolic derrangement or drug toxicity.
   d. usually has the same therapy as seizures, which it can clinically mimic.
5. The tremor of Parkinson's disease:
   a. occurs at rest and is helped by beta adrenergic antagonists or neuroleptics.
   b. occurs at rest and is worsened by bromocriptine.
   c. occurs mainly with intention or use and is increased by L-dopa.
   d. occurs at rest and is reduced by benztropine or amantadine.

CHAPTER 28

Pain Control with Opioid Analgesics

WILLIAM L. DEWEY
DAVID BRASE
SANDRA P. WELCH

MAJOR DRUGS

opioid analgesics
opioid antagonists

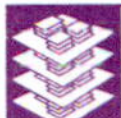

THERAPEUTIC OVERVIEW

Several groups of compounds are used to relieve pain, depending on the severity and duration and on the nature of the painful stimulus. These drugs are classified in several ways. Drugs used to relieve pain without causing unconsciousness are called **analgesics** and are subdivided into three groups according to their ability to relieve mild, moderate, or severe pain. Mild analgesics are termed **nonnarcotic** and include such agents as aspirin (Chapter 29). This chapter primarily covers the narcotic (opioid) analgesics used to control moderate to severe pain, of which morphine is the prototype. Included in this chapter is a discussion of opioid antagonists, partial agonists, and mixed agonists/antagonists.

The Sensation of Pain

The specific anatomical pathways that transmit pain impulses within the CNS are summarized in Figure 28-1. Two different types of nociceptive (noxious) stimuli are intense enough to be perceived as pain and can be alleviated by opioid drugs. One type, sometimes called **somatic pain,** appears as an intense, localized sharp or stinging sensation. This is mediated by fast-conducting lightly myelinated A-delta (Aδ) fibers, which have a high threshold (i.e., require a strong mechanical stimulus) and enter into the spinal cord through the dorsal horn where they terminate mostly in lamina I of the cord.

ABBREVIATION

P_{CO_2}	partial pressure of carbon dioxide

The second type of pain, sometimes called **visceral pain,** is characterized as a diffuse, dull, aching, or burning sensation. This type is mediated by largely unmyelinated, slower conducting C fibers, which are polymodal (i.e., mediate mechanical, thermal, and chemical stimuli). These C fibers also enter the spinal cord through the dorsal horn, where they ascend by the paleospinothalamic and the neospinothalamic tracts and terminate mostly in the outer layer of lamina II.

Endogenous pain control systems descend the spinal cord through the dorsolateral funiculus to the spinal dorsal horn where they inhibit neurons that are activated by nociceptive stimuli. The higher centers connected to these descending systems include the periaqueductal gray region and various subregions of the medulla (e.g., the *nucleus raphe magnus, nucleus reticularis magnocellularis,* and *nucleus reticularis paragigantocellularis lateralis).* These regions contain opioid receptors, and the ability of morphine to inhibit the perception of nociceptive stimuli may involve the activation of these descending pathways.

Although much remains to be learned about the neurotransmitters involved in both the afferent nociceptive and descending antinociceptive pathways, prime candidates for the afferent pathways include peptidergic neurotransmitters (e.g., substance P, somatostatin, vasoactive intestinal polypeptide, cholecystokinin, and calcitonin gene-related peptide). The descending antinociceptive pathways appear to involve norepinephrine and serotonin as neurotransmitters, as well as endogenous opioid peptides. The spinal cord also contains opioid receptors, which are mainly localized within laminae I to III of the dorsal horn and within the tract of

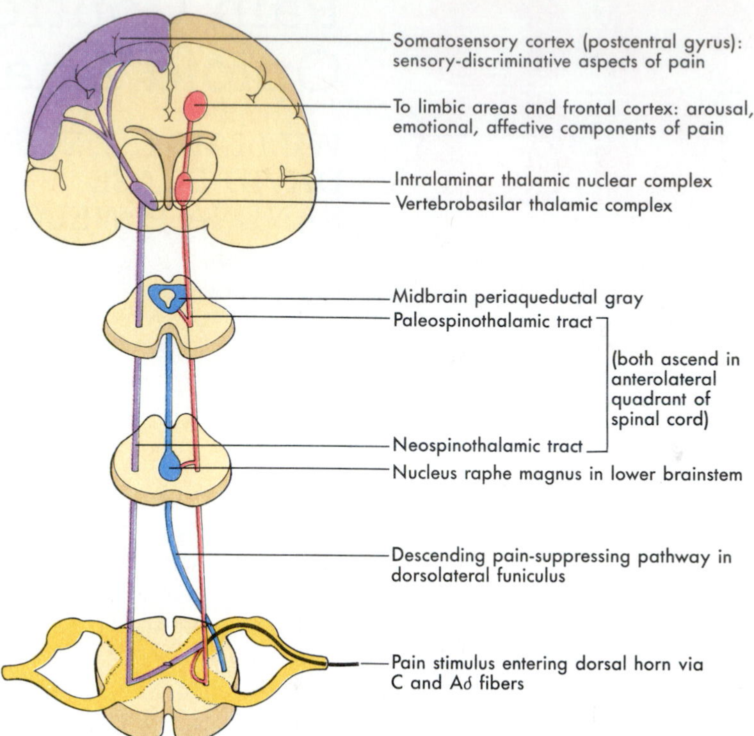

FIGURE 28-1 Schema of the paleospinothalamic and neospinothalamic pain-transmission pathways and the descending pain-suppression pathway.

THERAPEUTIC OVERVIEW

DESIRED EFFECT IS TO RETAIN CONSCIOUSNESS

Relief of moderate-to-severe pain
- Narcotic analgesics
- Morphine and related opioid receptor agonists

Overdose reversal, addiction treatment
- Opioid receptor antagonists

Antidiarrheal action

Antitussive

Lissauer. The highest density of opioid receptors is localized in the inner segment of lamina II.

Since pain is both a sensation (objective feeling) and an emotion (subjective feeling), it is not surprising that opioid drugs affect these components differently. A continuous, dull pain is more effectively relieved by opioid drugs than is sharp, intermittent pain. At usual therapeutic doses, opioid drugs greatly increase the ability to tolerate pain, whereas the capacity to perceive it may be little affected. Higher doses, however, also interfere with pain perception.

The therapeutic uses of narcotic agonists and antagonists are summarized in the box.

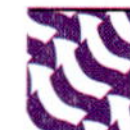

MECHANISMS OF ACTION

Morphine is the prototype opioid. The structures of morphine and related compounds are shown in Figure 28-2. Although sap from unripe seed pods of the opium poppy plant, which contains morphine, was being used medicinally as early as 400 to 300 BC, not until the early 1800s was morphine isolated; in the 1900s its chemical structure was determined. By the mid-1900s, it was determined that only a small fraction of a dose of morphine crosses the blood-brain barrier into the central nervous system to produce analgesia. The presence of binding sites in CNS membranes was used to show that the analgesic *levo*-isomer of an opioid bound with high affinity, but the inactive *dextro*-isomer did not. Specific opioid antagonists were also shown to bind to these sites with high affinity, which provided a mechanism to explain why antagonists can block the analgesic, as well as other agonist effects of morphine and related opioid agonists.

Opioid Receptors and Endogenous Opioid Peptides

Multiple types of opioid receptors in the CNS are classified as μ, κ, and δ, with evidence for additional classes or subclasses. μ-Receptor activation in the brain is presumed to be responsible for the analgesic effect of morphine-like drugs. κ-Receptors, which exist in the brain and spinal cord, also appear capable of producing analgesia, particularly at the spinal level. The majority of the psychotomimetic effects of opioid drugs (e.g., dysphoria and hallucinations) are apparently mediated by σ-receptors. However, it is doubtful that σ-receptors are strictly "opioid" in character because they appear also to be activated by such nonopioid compounds as phencyclidine. The δ-receptor is believed to be the primary receptor for endogenous opioid pentapeptides known as **enkephalins.** These receptors are found not only in the brain and spinal cord, but also in some peripheral tissues.

The opioid analgesics have pharmacological effects similar to those of the endogenous opioid peptides. The first endogenous opioid peptides to be identified were methionine-enkephalin and leucine-enkephalin. Eventually three different classes of endogenous opioid peptides emerged. Each of these is derived from a different gene. One gene encodes the precursor peptide pro-opiomelanocortin, which is cleaved to produce the opioid peptide β-endorphin. A second gene encodes pro-enkephalin A, which gives rise to methionine-enkephalin, and a third encodes prodynorphin, which gives rise to the dynorphin family of opioid peptides. Both pro-enkephalin A and prodynorphin also contain the pentapeptide sequence of leucine-enkephalin. The structures of these three types of endogenous peptides and the pathways for their production are shown in Figures 28-3 to 28-5.

The pharmacological profiles of the several families of opioid peptides are described on p. 376. Dynorphin A is an agonist at κ-receptors. β-endorphin binds to both μ- and δ-receptors, in addition to the ϵ-receptor.

β-Endorphin and dynorphin are located in the pituitary gland and in the CNS proper. The three types of peptides have a distinct distribution throughout the CNS, indicating separate enkephalinergic (δ-receptor) neurons, endorphinergic (μ- and δ-receptor) neurons, and dynorphinergic (κ-receptor) neurons. Small amounts of the peptides appear in human cerebrospinal fluid (CSF). CSF also contains appreciable amounts of incompletely processed opioid peptides with the leu-enkephalin-Arg^6 - and met-enkephalin-Lys^6-amino acid sequences. The endogenous opioid peptides are involved with modulation of nociception and may be important in other physiological processes as well. Endogenous opioid peptides regulate respiration; respiratory depression is therefore a very significant side effect of the opioid analgesic drugs. Finally, some endogenous opioid peptides exist in tissues and organs other than the brain, including the gastrointestinal tract, a principal site of opioid action.

The interaction of opioid agonists with opioid receptors on neuronal membranes generally leads to decreased firing rates or reduced excitability. μ, δ and κ-Receptors are coupled to potassium channels. Agonists promote K^+ efflux and neuronal hyperpolarization. κ-Receptors are negatively coupled to Ca^{++} channels. This mechanism is believed to be responsible for the presynaptic inhibitory effect of κ-receptor agonists. Agonists of μ- and δ-receptors decrease neuronal cAMP synthesis by inhibiting adenylate cyclase coupled to the inhibitory G protein, G_i (see Chapter 2). The mechanism of action of μ-receptor agonists is shown in Figure 28-6. The effect of morphine on pain perception is different from the effect of a local anesthetic. Local anesthetics (Chapter 30) interfere with pain perception by decreasing conduction along the axon. Opioids have very lim-

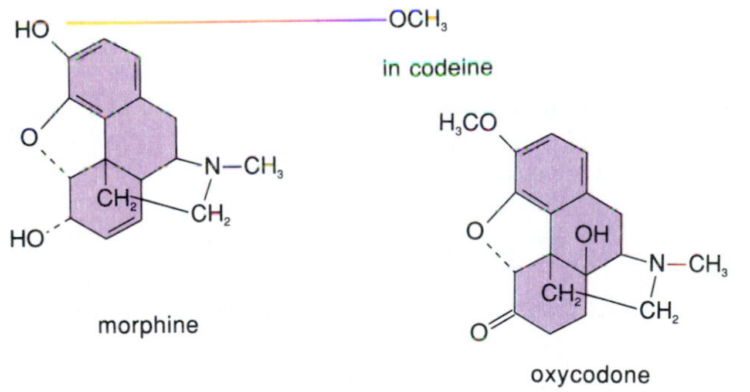

FIGURE 28-2 Chemical structures of morphine and related compounds. Codeine results when the —OH of morphine is replaced by —OCH_3.

Primary Gene Product:

H_2N—| SIGNAL / —— / γMSH / —— / ACTH / —— / β-MSH / β-endorphin |—COOH

β-endorphin: Tyr—Gly—Gly—Phe—Met—Thr—Ser—Glu—Lys—Ser—Gln—Thr—Pro—Leu—Val—Thr—Leu—Phe—Lys—Asn—Ala—Ile—Ile—Lys—Asn—Ala—Tyr—Lys—Lys—Gly—Leu

FIGURE 28-3 Order of compounds encoded by the pro-opiomelanocortin peptide gene and amino acid sequence of β-endorphin. The same gene also encodes adrenocorticotrophic hormone (ACTH) and a family of melanocyte-stimulating hormones (MSH), as well as for other peptides.

Primary Gene Product:

H_2N— | SIGNAL / — / ME / ME / — / MERGL / — / Peptide E / — / MERP | —COOH

Peptide—E: Try—Gly—Gly—Phe—Met—Arg—Arg—Val—Gly—Arg—Pro—Trp—Trp—Met—Asp—Tyr—Gln—Lys—Arg—Tyr—Gly—Gly—Phe—Leu

ME: Tyr—Gly—Gly—Phe—Met (δ>μ>κ)

LE: Tyr—Gly—Gly—Phe—Leu (δ>μ>κ)

MERP: Tyr—Gly—Gly—Phe—Met—Arg—Phe (δ>μ>κ)

MERGL: Tyr—Gly—Gly—Phe—Met—Arg—Gly—Leu (δ>μ>κ)

FIGURE 28-4 Order of opioid peptide sequence encoded by the pro–enkephalin A gene and the amino acid sequences. The order of preference in binding to brain membrane receptor types is shown in parentheses (either δ, μ, or κ). Notice that ME differs from LE by the substitution of leucine for methionine at the C terminus. MERP is met-enkephalin enlarged by arginine *(R)* and phenylalanine *(P)* at the C terminus. MERGL is met-enkephalin enlarged by arginine (*R*), glycine *(G)*, and leucine *(L)* at the C terminus. E begins with the met-enkephalin *(ME)* sequence and ends with the leu-enkephalin *(LE)* sequence.

Primary Gene Product:

| SIGNAL /—— /α –Neoendorphin / —— / Dynorphin-A / Dynorphin–B / | —COOH

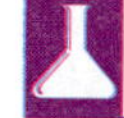

dynorphin—A: Tyr—Gly—Gly—Phe—Leu—Arg—Arg—Ileu—Arg—Pro—Lys—Leu—Lys—Trp—Asp—Asn—Gln (κ>μ>δ)

dynorphin—B: Tyr—Gly—Gly—Phe—Leu—Arg—Arg—Gln—Phe—Lys—Val—Val—Thr (κ>μ>δ)

α–neo–endorphin: Try—Gly—Gly—Phe—Leu—Arg—Lys—Tyr—Pro—Lys (κ>δ>μ)

leu—enkephalin: Tyr—Gly—Gly—Phe—Leu (δ>μ>κ)

FIGURE 28-5 Order of opioid peptide sequence encoded by prodynorphin gene and the amino acid sequences. The order of preference in binding to brain membrane receptor types is shown in parentheses (either δ, μ, or κ). Notice that all the opioid products of this gene begin with the leu-enkephalin sequence.

ited activity on neuronal conduction. Unlike aspirin and the nonnarcotic analgesics, opioid drugs do not have antiinflammatory activity. Because of the ability of many opioid drugs to release histamine, their intracutaneous injection can lead to a mild inflammatory reaction.

Opioid Drug Types

Opioid analgesic drugs can be grouped into categories according to the opioid receptor subtype they activate and whether the compounds act as agonists or antagonists.

The drugs that act primarily at μ-receptors as agonists are listed in the box. The chemical structures of some of these drugs are shown in Figure 28-7.

Additional drugs that act as partial agonists at μ-receptors, including buprenorphine, are shown in Figure 28-8. Structures of the antagonists naloxone and naltrexone also are shown in Figure 28-8.

PHARMACOKINETICS

The pharmacokinetic parameters for the opioid analgesic drugs are summarized in Table 28-1.

Morphine is usually administered IM. Varied bioavailability limits oral administration to low-dose preparations of opium (e.g., paregoric) for treating diarrhea. Despite poor absorption, oral preparations are also used in some terminally ill cancer patients to limit the discomfort of frequent injections. Slow-release oral preparations are becoming more common. The bitter taste of morphine limits its sublingual use.

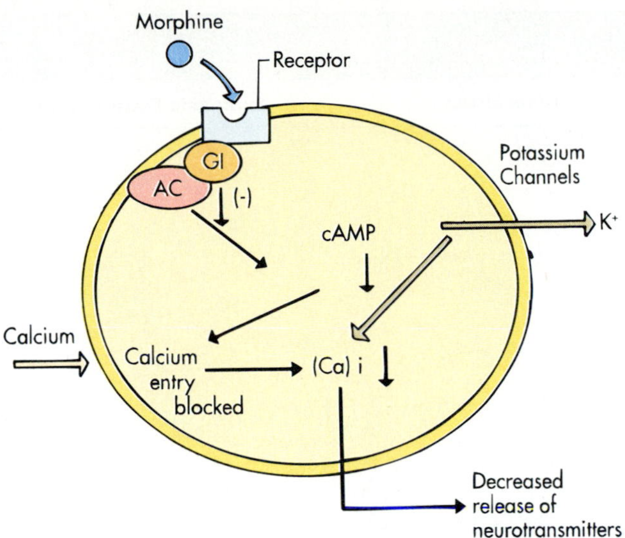

FIGURE 28-6 Mechanism of action of morphine. Binding of morphine to the μ-receptor results in modulation of a G protein (G_i) and a decrease in the activity of adenylate cyclase, resulting in a decrease in the production of cyclic adenosine monophosphate (cAMP). In addition, activation of the μ-receptor results in K^+ efflux and cellular hyperpolarization. Both the decrease in cAMP and the enhanced K^+ efflux lead to decreased Ca^{++} entry and lower free intracellular levels of Ca^{++} ($[Ca]_i$).

OPIOIDS ACTING ON μ-RECEPTORS	
morphine	diphenoxylate
codeine	loperamide
hydromorphine	fentanyl
oxymorphine	alfentanil
levorphanol	sufentanil
oxycodone	methadone
meperidine	1-α-acetylmethadol
alphaprodine	propoxyphene

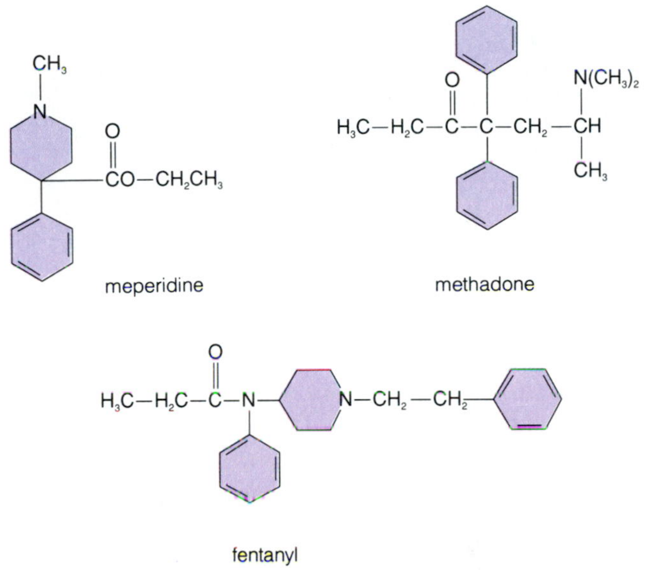

meperidine

methadone

fentanyl

FIGURE 28-7 Chemical structures of additional opioid analgesics as they act as agonists at μ-receptors (in addition to those in Figure 28-2).

Partial μ agonist

buprenorphine

Agonist-antagonist

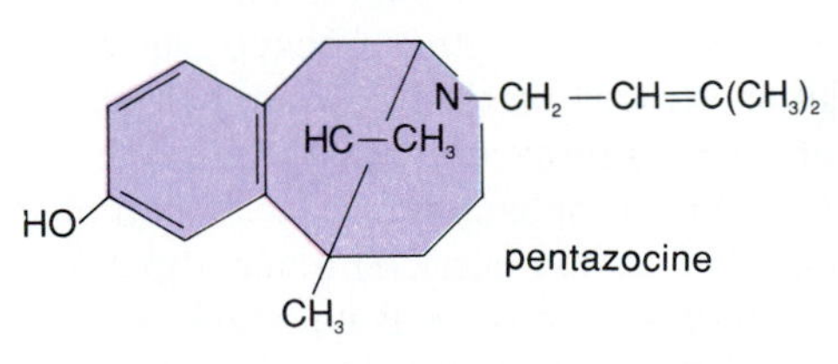

Antagonist

naloxone

in naltrexone

FIGURE 28-8 Several partial μ- or κ-receptor agonists and antagonists.

Table 28-1 Pharmacokinetic Parameters

Drug	Administration	Elimination $t_{1/2}$ (hr)	Disposition	Analgesia Duration (hr)
alfentanil	IV	1.6	—	<0.5
alphaprodine	IV, SC	2.2	—	1-2
buprenorphine	IM, IV, SC	5	—	5-9
butorphanol	IM, IV, nasal spray	2.7	—	3-4
codeine	Oral, SC, IV	3	M† (converted to morphine)	4-6
fentanyl	IV, Transdermal, oral	3.7	M	0.5
hydromorphone	Oral, SC	2.6	M	4-5
levorphanol	SC, oral	11	M	4-5
meperidine	IM, oral	3.2	M†	2-4
meptazinol		1.6	M	1-2
methadone	Oral, SC	25	M	3-5
morphine	IM, IV, SC, oral	2.9	M*	4-5
nalbuphine	IM, SC, IV	5.1	—	4-5
naloxone	IV	1.2	M*	1-4‡
naltrexone	Oral	9.7	M†	10-24‡
oxycodone	Oral	?	M	4-5
oxymorphone	IM, IV, SC	?	M	4-5
pentazocine	Oral, IM	2.9	—	3-4
propoxyphene	Oral	6-12	M†	1-3
sufentanil	IV	2.6	—	0.5

M, Metabolized
*Indicates primary route of disposition; large first-pass effect.
†Active metabolite.
‡Duration of antagonistic action.

Levorphanol, fentanyl, and methadone, with longer half-lives than durations of action, may accumulate in plasma and tissue. The duration of action of methadone can increase from 4 to 12 hours with repeated dosing, making it difficult to titrate individual patients. After IV administration of a single dose, fentanyl, alfentanil, and sufentanil have rapid onsets of action. Their short durations relative to their plasma half-lives is caused by redistribution from brain to peripheral tissues. Fentanyl is 80% to 85% bound to plasma protein, whereas alfentanil and sufentanil are 90% to 95% bound. Morphine is only minimally bound (30%) to plasma proteins. Many opioid analgesics undergo extensive "first-pass" metabolism after oral administration. For example, studies of the oral use of morphine in cancer patients have indicated bioavailabilities ranging from 15% to 49%. The decreased bioavailability of orally administered morphine compared with morphine given parenterally is largely attributable to first-pass hepatic metabolism; the major urinary metabolite of morphine is morphine-3-glucuronide. This same 3-OH position of morphine is derivatized with a methyl group in oxycodone and codeine, both of which have greater oral bioavailability (50% to 65%). The major urinary metabolite of codeine is codeine-6-glucuronide. Methadone and levorphanol also have reasonably good oral bioavailability (approximately 50%).

Morphine is now known to have an active metabolite, morphine-6-glucuronide. Other opioid drugs also have active metabolites. For example, meperidine is metabolized in part to normeperidine, which has about one half the analgesic potency of meperidine but with greater excitatory effects than meperidine. Administration of high doses of meperidine at frequent intervals, particularly in patients with decreased renal function, can lead to an accumulation of normeperidine and result in excitatory signs and symptoms, including seizures. Repeated dosing with propoxyphene leads to its accumulation as well as to the accumulation of an active metabolite, norpropoxyphene. This results in an increased half-life of propoxyphene (3 to 12 hours) and norpropoxyphene (6 to 40 hours). The major unconjugated-metabolite of naltrexone, 6-β-naltrexol, can achieve higher plasma concentrations than naltrexone itself and has a half-life of approximately 11 hours. Although 6-β-naltrexol possesses opioid antagonist activity, it is considerably less potent than naltrexone.

RELATION OF MECHANISMS OF ACTION TO CLINICAL RESPONSE

Major Effects of Opioid Analgesics

Clinical use of opioid analgesics consists primarily in balancing the analgesia against adverse side effects. Morphine and most other opioid analgesics elicit a mixture of stimulatory and inhibitory effects, with the major sites of action being the brain and the gastrointestinal tract. Areas of the brain receiving input from the ascending spinal pain-transmitting pathways are rich in opioid receptors, with a major effect of opioid analgesics being a depression of neuronal activity. This increases the pain threshold, sedation, and is often accompanied by euphoria. Although morphine and other opioids produce drowsiness and promote sleep, this clearly is distinct from and not the cause of the analgesia. Depressant and stimulant effects of morphine are summarized in the box.

An important specific CNS effect of opioids is their ability to depress the cough reflex (antitussive). Most commonly used opioids, except meperidine, possess antitussive activity, with the prototype antitussive drug being codeine. Although the *levo*-isomers of opioids are analgesic, both *dextro*- and *levo*-isomers possess antitussive activity. Several of the dextro-isomeric compounds (e.g., dextromethorphan) have been developed as antitussives and are found in a variety of nonprescription cough remedies. The advantages of *dextro*-isomers, (e.g., dextromethorphan), which are active orally, is that they do not produce physical dependence. The dependence liability of opioid drugs, like the analgesia, resides in the levo-isomer. Great care should therefore be observed in using levo-isomers as antitussives in patients who show a high propensity for dependence liability or a pattern of drug abuse.

Opioid analgesics depress respiratory function at the same doses that produce analgesia. This effect is from depression of respiratory centers in the brainstem and from depression of respiratory reflexes. This can lead to respiratory failure from overdose and is also one of the most limiting side effects of these drugs.

Although CNS depression is usually the overriding effect, certain excitatory effects are sometimes observed. These include restlessness, delirium, mania, and strychnine-like stimulation of the spinal cord. They do not occur in all individuals and are more prevalent with specific opioids (e.g., meperidine).

A stimulatory effect observed with most opioids is constriction of the pupils (miosis). Increased neuronal activity in the Edinger-Westphal nucleus of the oculomotor (third cranial) nerve leads to increased parasympathetic tone. The pupillary constriction aids in clinical identification of heroin addicts. Ophthalmic application of parasympatholytic agents (e.g., scopolamine) blocks opioid-induced miosis.

Opioid drugs sometimes cause nausea and vomiting, especially in ambulatory patients. Nausea and vomiting are induced by stimulation of the chemoreceptor trigger zone in the area postrema of the medulla. This stimulatory action is tempered by an inhibitory effect of opioid drugs on the vomiting (emetic) center in the lateral reticular formation of the medulla.

A second major site of action of opioid drugs is the gastrointestinal tract. Actions on the gastrointestinal tract can be either therapeutically useful or produce strong side effects, especially in patients requiring opioids for prolonged periods of time. Since opioid drugs produce constipation, they are effectively used in treating diarrhea. Clinically significant tolerance does not develop to this effect.

SUMMARY OF DEPRESSANT AND STIMULANT EFFECTS OF MORPHINE

DEPRESSANT EFFECTS

- Suppression of pain, analgesia
- Drowsiness and decreased mental alertness, sedation
- Decreased respiration, increased intracranial pressure
- Decreased myocardial oxygen demand
- Suppression of cough, antitussive
- Decreased peristalsis
- Inhibition of fluid and electrolyte accumulation in intestinal luman
- Decreased gastric acid secretion
- Inhibition of emetic center
- Slight decrease in body temperature
- Decreased release of gonadotropin luteinizing hormone (LH) and follicle-stimulating hormone (FSH)

STIMULANT EFFECTS

- Euphoria
- Constriction of pupils, miosis
- Stimulation of chemoreceptor trigger zone
- Increased tone of intestinal smooth muscle
- Increased tone of sphincter of Oddi, increased biliary pressure
- Increased tone of detrusor muscle
- Increased tone of vesical sphincter
- Increased release of prolactin and antidiuretic hormone
- Proconvulsant in overdose

The mechanisms by which opioids produce constipation involve (1) prolongation of gastric emptying time, (2) decreased propulsive contractions of the small intestine and increased tone of the large intestine to slow transit, and (3) increased tone of the anal sphincter and inattention to normal sensory stimuli for defecation. In addition, the antidiarrheal actions of opioids may also involve blockade of ion and water flow into the intestinal lumen caused by certain bacterial toxins (e.g., cholera toxin) (see also Chapter 60).

Other effects of morphine-like opioids on smooth muscle include increased bile duct pressure with increased sphincter tone, leading to difficulty in micturition. Morphine therefore is contraindicated in treatment of biliary colic. Atropine is used to decrease this effect of morphine without interfering with analgesia. Agonist-antagonist drugs, discussed later, usually cause little if any increase in biliary pressure. The morphine-induced increase in the tone of the urethral sphincter may be tempered by a reduced volume of urine production. On the other hand, agonists of κ-receptors can be used to produce a water diuresis.

Morphine and opioid drugs at therapeutic doses have limited effects on the cardiovascular system, especially in supine patients. However, depressant effects including orthostatic hypotension may be observed at higher doses. Morphine is useful to treat the pain and apprehension in myocardial infarction: It is also useful in treating acute pulmonary edema associated with left ventricular failure, where it reduces the left ventricular work by peripheral pooling of blood. In contrast, some agonist-antagonist opioids (e.g., pentazocine and butorphanol) increase ventricular afterload and myocardial oxygen requirement. Such deleterious hemodynamic effects can result in infarct extension. Pentazocine and butorphanol are therefore not recommended for use in patients with acute myocardial infarction.

A major therapeutic use of opioids is as preanesthetic agents before surgery to produce analgesia, sedation, reduced anxiety, and decreased need for general anesthetic agents. Nonopioid benzodiazepines (e.g., diazepam) are also often used as preanesthetic agents; however, they do not produce analgesia. Some opioids (e.g., morphine or fentanyl) are used as the major agent in balanced anesthesia, especially for cardiac surgery.

Opioid Analgesics that Interact Primarily with μ-Receptors

Morphine Morphine, widely used to relieve severe pain, does not affect other sensory modalities, including touch, taste, smell, or hearing. The IV and spinal uses of morphine are limited to patients whose respiratory function is carefully monitored for potential respiratory depression. Respiratory depression from morphine administered intrathecally is avoided by elevation of the upper part of the body to prevent the rostral flow of morphine in cerebrospinal fluid. Spinal administration of morphine has the advantages of increased potency and duration, reduced incidence of side effects, and temporary relief from tolerance that develops in patients who require long-term analgesia, such as patients with terminal cancer. However, severe itching, not relieved by antihistamines, or urinary retention, especially in elderly men, may prevent spinal use. In general, the therapeutic ratio (see Chapter 1) of morphine is quite good.

Heroin Heroin, diacetyl morphine, is used orally for pain relief in European countries and has been tested in the United States. Because of its great propensity for intravenous abuse, it has no legal medical use in the United States. Heroin is two or three times as potent as morphine but is not more effective than morphine in treating acute pain. Its use in chronic pain is controversial, and some have proposed that heroin should be legalized for treating patients with terminal cancer.

Heroin must first be deacetylated to 6-acetylmorphine and then to morphine to produce analgesia. The 3-acetyl group is removed by plasma and tissue esterases. The 6-acetylmorphine produced, as well as heroin itself, penetrates the blood-brain barrier more readily than morphine. Heroin and 6-acetylmorphine enter the brain by passive diffusion and undergo enzymatic deacetylation to produce morphine. Since heroin itself does not have a high affinity for opioid receptors, its analgesic effects are likely mediated by morphine and 6-acetylmorphine.

Codeine Codeine, the most commonly used opioid analgesic, is often combined with acetaminophen and with aspirin. Codeine is less efficacious than morphine, but it is nevertheless useful in the relief of mild to moderate pain. Orally administered codeine has more predictable bioavailability than morphine and is thus the prototype antitussive agent, with less addiction potential than morphine has. Codeine does not have a high affinity for opioid receptors, but since it is partially metabolized to morphine, a part of its analgesic activity is morphine related.

Other Morphine Congeners Other morphine-like analgesics include hydromorphone, oxymorphone, levorphanol, and oxycodone (see Figure 28-2). Compared with an analgesic dose of morphine, hydromorphone is about 8 times as potent, oxymorphone 10 times, and levorphanol 5 times, and oxycodone is equipotent. They are as effective as morphine for moderate-to-severe pain and have similar durations of action. Except for hydromorphone, these have greater oral bioavailability than morphine, retaining about half of their analgesic potencies compared to parenteral administration. All have addiction potentials similar to morphine.

Meperidine and Other Phenylpiperidine Derivatives Meperidine is widely used to treat moderate to severe pain. Being a piperidine derivative, it does not have a morphine-like chemical structure. Meperidine has a faster onset of action than morphine, with analgesic effects 10 minutes after SC or IM injection and 15 minutes after oral administration. However, it has a shorter duration than morphine because of its more rapid metabolism. Its effects last 2 to 4 hours compared with 4 to 5 hours for morphine. The shorter duration may account, at least in part, for the decreased constipation and decreased potential for biliary spasm. Its slightly lower addiction potential is still considerable, however, as indicated by its history of extensive abuse, particularly by physicians and other health professionals. Meperidine and other phenylpiperidine derivatives do not have useful antitussive activity.

Diphenoxylate and loperamide are used only as antidiarrheal agents with use limited to oral administration. Although doses of diphenoxylate higher than those required for antidiarrheal activity can produce morphine-like euphoria, analgesia, and physical dependence, chronic abuse potential is limited by the addition of atropine to diphenoxylate preparations. Atropine causes undesirable parasympatholytic side effects when taken in high doses. The relative insolubility of diphenoxylate in aqueous solutions also prevents intravenous abuse. Loperamide, which also has low aqueous solubility, binds to intestinal tissue. Most of what is absorbed undergoes efficient enterohepatic circulation, leading to low blood concentrations and poor distribution to the brain. Both antidiarrheal agents are considered to have low abuse potential, with that of loperamide being less than that of diphenoxylate. Loperamide has recently been made available as a nonprescription preparation. Opioid antidiarrheal agents are contraindicated in diarrheal diseases accompanied by high fever or blood in the stool.

Fentanyl and Derivatives Fentanyl, alfentanil, and sufentanil are extremely potent opioid drugs of the piperidine series. Fentanyl is about 100 times as potent as morphine, with a much shorter duration of action (about 30 minutes) after a single IV injection, a result of redistribution from brain to peripheral tissues. Alfentanil is about one fourth as potent as fentanyl, and sufentanil is 5 to 10 times as potent as fentanyl. Both have shorter durations of action than fentanyl. Given IV, these opioids are used primarily as components of balanced anesthesia for surgical procedures, and their use generally requires mechanical ventilation. The muscle rigidity that high doses of these agents sometimes produce can interfere with artificial ventilation. Administration of a muscle relaxant may be necessary.

With fentanyl and related compounds, cases of a delayed respiratory depression have been reported.

Lofentanil is 6000 times as potent as morphine and has a significantly longer duration of action. It binds so tightly to opioid receptors that its effects cannot be antagonized by narcotic antagonists. These characteristics increase the possibility of death from overdose of fentanyl derivatives. Also, some deaths among heroin addicts have occurred from illicit production and use of 3-methylfentanyl (China White), which has nearly 1000 times the potency of heroin.

Methadone and Its Congeners Methadone is a synthetic opioid analgesic not structurally related to morphine. Its potency is equal to or slightly greater than that of morphine, with a similar duration of action after a single dose. Orally administered methadone has greater bioavailability than morphine. These properties, in addition to its longer half-life, have led to its widespread use as a heroin substitute in treatment programs for opioid addiction.

A methadone congener, 1-α-acetylmethadol, has been approved as an alternative to methadone in treatment of addiction because of its ability to suppress appearance of withdrawal signs (i.e., to maintain physical dependence) for as long as 72 hours after a single oral dose. The long duration of action is probably related to formation of long-acting metabolites.

Propoxyphene is chemically similar to methadone but is much less potent and less effective. Its use is limited to oral administration and, compared with orally administered codeine, is about one half to two thirds as potent. Propoxyphene is not effective for treating severe pain and in mild-to-moderate pain it is about as effective as aspirin. With less abuse liability than codeine, propoxyphene use has declined recently after reports of poisoning and death from overdose, particularly when taken with alcohol, tranquilizers, or other CNS depressants. Many deaths occurred from deliberate overuse, abuse, or suicide attempts. Propoxyphene toxicity is characterized by respiratory and CNS depression. However, seizures, cardiotoxic effects, and pulmonary edema can also occur. Some effects are antagonized by naloxone.

Opioid Analgesics That Are Partial μ-Receptor Agonists

Buprenorphine, an opioid agonist of μ-receptors, displays some properties not typical of most morphine-like drugs. In the therapeutic range, doses of buprenorphine equianalgesic with morphine also depress respiration to a similar extent but with a delayed onset. Once developed, the respiratory depression caused by buprenorphine is only partially reversible by the narcotic antagonist naloxone. Buprenorphine can itself antagonize the greater respiratory-depressant effects of higher doses of morphine or fentanyl used during cardiac surgery and still provide postoperative analgesia. Buprenorphine also causes less euphoria than morphine, and physically dependent subjects on buprenorphine experience a milder but more prolonged morphine-like abstinence syndrome that cannot be precipitated by naloxone. These features are characteristic of a compound that is only a partial agonist of μ-receptors and that dissociates very slowly from these receptors. It also appears to be a κ-receptor antagonist. Buprenorphine has somewhat less abuse liability than morphine.

Opioid Analgesics That Are Mixed Agonist/Antagonists

Nalorphine, Levallorphan, and Cyclazocine Analgesic properties of nalorphine are equivalent to those of morphine, but it produces dysphoria rather than the euphoria observed with morphine. Nalorphine has significantly less addiction liability than morphine. Other synthetic opioids, levallorphan and cyclazocine, have similar properties to nalorphine. Unfortunately, the dysphoric side effects at analgesic doses have discouraged the development of these drugs as opioid analgesics. None are in clinical use today. Nalorphine and levallorphan enjoyed wide use as opioid antagonists to treat opioid overdose until the development of more specific antagonists such as naloxone.

Pentazocine Pentazocine was the first in the series of agonist-antagonist analgesics used clinically. Pentazocine, less potent than morphine, appears to be less efficacious, particularly for an anxiolytic effect. When pentazocine is given IM, three to four times as much is required to be equianalgesic to morphine when morphine is given IM. Pentazocine is also active orally in somewhat higher doses than morphine. Unlike morphine, as the dose of pentazocine is increased above the therapeutic range, the respiratory depression caused by pentazocine does not increase to the point of causing death. Thus, there appears to be a ceiling to the respiratory-depressant effect of pentazocine and other related opioid agonist/antagonists. However, increasing the dose of pentazocine above the therapeutic range results in progressively higher incidence of psychotomimetic side effects, including the inability to suppress unpleasant thoughts, dysphoria, and hallucinations.

Butorphanol Unlike pentazocine, butorphanol is given parenterally because of its low oral bioavailability (about 17%). A comparison of butorphanol with other drugs given IM for the relief of postoperative pain indicates that butorphanol is up to seven times as potent as morphine, 40 times that of meperidine, and 20 times that of pentazocine. Butorphanol has antitussive activity but is not used for this purpose. The incidence of psychotomimetic side effects is less than that with pentazocine. Butorphanol tartrate has become available as a nasal spray, providing a convenient route of administration. Intranasal butorphanol appears effective versus both postoperative and migraine-induced pain.

Nalbuphine Nalbuphine is given only parenterally. Its analgesic potency is approximately the same as that of morphine and three to four times that of pentazocine. It may have a slightly longer duration of action than pentazocine, but its peak analgesic effect is decreased, with incidence of psychotomimetic side effects being less than with pentazocine.

Most opiate analgesic drugs can interact with multiple opioid receptors, though the dosage required to activate the different receptors varies. The possibility that pentazocine, butorphanol, and nalbuphine can produce analgesia, at least in part, by acting as partial agonists on μ-receptors has not been ruled out. However, the agonist activity of these drugs is predominantly by κ-receptors. Like the partial μ-receptor agonist buprenorphine, these agonist-antagonist drugs can precipitate a withdrawal syndrome in persons who are highly physically dependent on morphine-like drugs. Nalbuphine has greater antagonistic activity at analgesic doses than the other agonist-antagonist analgesics have. Pentazocine, nalbuphine, and butorphanol generally have much less excitatory effect than morphine on smooth muscles, and so constipation and exacerbation of biliary colic are rarely encountered. The most common side effect of these agonist-antagonist opioids is sedation. The diuretic effects of these drugs have not been reported in humans, though butorphanol has a limited diuretic effect in animal studies, which has led to the postulate that it may be a partial agonist of κ-receptors.

Opioids Used Solely as Antagonists

Naloxone Naloxone was the first relatively pure antagonist available for treating opioid overdose and has now largely replaced nalorphine and levallorphan for this use. A major caution with naloxone is that the patient must be carefully monitored for possible recurrence of respiratory depression after a single bolus dose. The reason is that the duration of action of naloxone is short relative to the duration of the depressant effects of most opioid agonists. This short duration is circumvented by use of multiple injections of naloxone until the patient is stable. The great utility of naloxone, administered IV, is that a physically dependent patient can be titrated

Table 28-2 Summary of Clinical Responses Produced by Opioid Analgesics

Drug	Analgesia	Antitussive	Constipation	Respiratory Depression	Abuse Liability
buprenorphine	++/+++	±	+	++/+++	±
butorphanol	++/+++	−	±	++/+++	±
codeine	+	++	++	+	±
heroin	+++	++	+++	+++	++++
hydromorphone	+++	++	++	+++	+++
levorphanol	+++	++	++	+++	+++
meperidine	++/+++	−	±	+++	++
methadone	+++	++	++	+++	++
morphine	+++	++	+++	+++	+++
nalbuphine	++/+++	−	±	++/+++	±
oxycodone	++	++	++	++	+++
oxymorphone	+++	+	++	+++	+++
pentazocine	++/+++	−	±	++/+++	+
propoxyphene	+	−	±	+	+

++++, Strongest effect; +, weak effect; ±, weakest effect

very carefully to reverse the respiratory depression without precipitating a severe withdrawal syndrome. Naloxone has a higher affinity for μ-receptors than for κ-receptors. This might explain why a higher dose of naloxone is required to reverse the respiratory depression caused by pentazocine-like drugs than that caused by morphine-like drugs. Naloxone produces a significant increase in blood pressure in various forms of shock (e.g., from acute spinal cord injury or septicemia), indicating its possible use to counteract the deleterious hemodynamic effects of endogenous opioids that are apparently released during shock.

Naltrexone Naltrexone, another opioid antagonist, is about three times more potent than naloxone. It has a much longer duration of action and a relatively good oral bioavailability. The long duration of action and oral effectiveness has led to its experimental use as an "extinction" therapy in the treatment of opioid addiction. Chronic oral use of naltrexone has been associated with a low but significantly increased incidence of headache and other pain and an accompanying elevation of serum transaminase concentration that returns to normal upon discontinuation of the drug.

Very recently, naltrexone has been used experimentally to treat apneic disorders associated with elevated concentrations of β-endorphin–like immunoreactivity in the cerebrospinal fluid. These include the infant apnea syndrome, which may be involved in some cases of sudden infant death syndrome; Rett syndrome, observed only in girls and involving several neurological problems in addition to respiratory disturbances; and several disorders in which naltrexone blocks apnea and enhances seizure control by antiepileptic drugs. Naltrexone does not appear to be useful for the treatment of apnea in premature infants; theophylline is the drug treatment of choice.

Summary of Clinical Responses

The major effects of the opioid analgesics are summarized in Table 28-2.

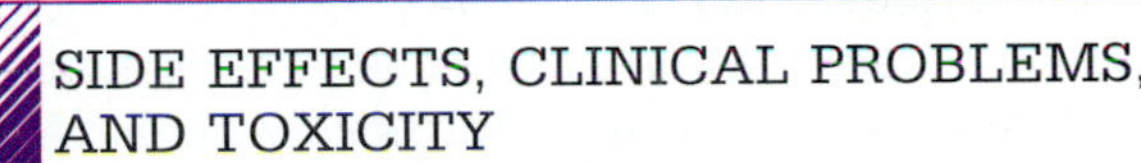

SIDE EFFECTS, CLINICAL PROBLEMS, AND TOXICITY

Respiratory depression, constipation, opioid abuse and addiction, development of tolerance, and development of physical dependence are the most troublesome side effects and problems associated with the use of opioid analgesics.

Respiratory Depression

Except for the investigational drug meptazinol, all the strong analgesics produce a comparable degree of respiratory depression at equianalgesic doses, regardless of whether they act predominantly at μ- or κ-opioid receptors. Although the respiratory depression produced by therapeutic doses of these agents is generally not deleterious to patients with normal respiratory and cardiovascular function, great caution should be exercised when administering these agents to patients with compromised respiratory function (e.g., those with sleep apnea, asthma, or emphysema). Opioid drugs are contraindicated during an asthmatic attack and in patients with head injury that may have caused brain trauma. The respiratory depression produced by therapeutic doses increases the partial pressure of carbon dioxide (P_{CO_2}), which in turn causes cerebral vasodilatation with increased intracranial pressure, which can worsen brain trauma. Mechanical ventilation to prevent increase in P_{CO_2} can be used to prevent increased intracranial pressure.

Since respiratory depression occurs at therapeutic doses, it often is a limiting factor in the use of opioid analgesics in obstetrics. If an opioid analgesic is administered to the mother, it can cross the placenta and cause respiratory depression in the newborn. Obviously women who abuse opioids also place their offspring in jeopardy.

Tolerance and Physical Dependence

Tolerance, best described as the need for an increased dose of drug to produce the same pharmacological effect, is associated with continuous use of opioid analgesics. Rate and degree of tolerance development are related to the frequency, dose, and duration of drug use. Although the molecular mechanism for opioid tolerance is unknown, studies with animals and cultured neurons have indicated that tolerance may involve multiple types of adaptation by neuronal cells that possess cell membrane opioid receptors. Mechanisms include decreased affinity of receptors for agonists, decreased numbers of cell-membrane opioid receptors, or decreased efficiency of coupling between agonist-occupied receptor and control of second messengers such as cAMP, or all three mechanisms. Alternative hypotheses for tolerance include a compensatory increase (or decrease) in excitability of target neurons or tissues innervated by neurons that possess the opioid receptors or recruitment of redundant pathways to bypass the inhibited functional pathway.

Whatever the mechanism, tolerance does not develop uniformly to all actions of the opioid drugs. For example, with chronic morphine administration, as the morphine is increased to achieve the desired level of analgesia, less tolerance develops to the constipating and miotic effects than to the analgesic effect.

Another related characteristic of tolerance is cross-tolerance. Although it is generally accepted that tolerance to one opioid confers cross-tolerance to other opioids, recent animal studies indicate that not all opioids are completely cross-tolerant of each other. A lack of total cross-tolerance could be attributable to differences in intrinsic activity (the efficiency with which the drug couples to receptor-mediated second messengers). One drug may produce a response by occupying only 10% of the receptors that mediate its response, whereas the same response observed with another drug may require the 50% occupation of those receptors. As tolerance develops (and receptor number decreases), the intrinsic activity of drugs that require occupancy of a large fraction of receptors may fall off faster than the activity of drugs that require occupancy of a smaller fraction of receptors. Thus, it is theoretically possible to circumvent partially or delay the tolerance by appropriate switching of drug therapies. However, this has not been exploited clinically. Switching from chronic administration of a μ-receptor agonist to a κ- or partial μ-receptor agonist could also result in precipitation of a withdrawal syndrome, unless there is an opioid-free period between the administration of the two drugs. For patients requiring chronic opioid administration to relieve pain, addition of a nonnarcotic analgesic to the therapeutic regimen often provides beneficial additive effects.

Another major adverse effect of opioid analgesics is their propensity for producing both psychic and physical dependence (see also Chapter 32). Psychic dependence is best characterized by the continued desire or craving for a substance. Physical dependence is observed when the cessation of administration of a substance (abstinence) causes physical signs of withdrawal. The distinction between psychic and physical dependence becomes less clear when one considers that both emotional and vegetative body functions are modulated by neurotransmitters and hormones acting on receptors and that many drugs alter such systems. Opioid drugs clearly produce both psychic and physical dependence.

Although physical dependence can develop with relatively low doses of morphine-like drugs, seldom does a patient become dependent with short-term therapy. Opioid physical dependence is probably closely related to the development of tolerance because the physical signs of withdrawal generally represent physiological actions opposite to acute actions of opioid drugs. For example, if an acute opioid effect is constipation, the corresponding physical withdrawal sign is diarrhea. The typical features and time course of withdrawal from morphine are summarized in Table 28-3. The intensity of a given abstinence sign is not always proportional to the degree of physical dependence. The reason is that physical dependence and tolerance are dynamic phenomena that undergo constant adjustments according to the concentration of agonist present at the receptors. If an agonist has a long half-life (e.g., methadone), agonist withdrawal results in a milder though more prolonged withdrawal than that which occurs if agonist activity is suddenly blocked by the injection of the antagonist naloxone. Generally the overall intensity of naloxone-precipitated withdrawal is directly related to the degree of physical dependence. The extent to which endogenous opioid peptides may function to modify the withdrawal syndrome is unknown. Single-dose physical dependence in ex-addicts has been demonstrated in both clinical and animal studies, indicating that one cycle of physical dependence and withdrawal apparently causes long-lasting changes, which increase the liability for initiating another cycle of dependence (recidivism).

Table 28-3 Symptoms and Their Course after Withdrawal of Morphine and Heroin

Time After Withdrawal	Symptoms
6-12 hr	Drug-seeking behavior; restlessness, lacrimation, rhinorrhea, sweating, yawning
12-24 hr	Restless sleep for several hours and feeling more miserable than previously after awakening; irritability, tremor, dilated pupils, anorexia, gooseflesh
24-72 hr	Increased intensity of above signs plus weakness, depression, nausea, vomiting, intestinal cramps, diarrhea, alternating chills and flushes, various aches and pains, increased heart rate and blood pressure, involuntary movements of arms and legs, dehydration, and possible electrolyte imbalances
Later	Above symptoms of autonomic hyperactivity alternate with brief periods of restless sleep and gradually decrease in intensity until addict feels better in 7 to 10 days but may still exhibit strong craving for the drug. In addition, some mild signs may be detectable for up to 6 months. Delayed growth and development of infants born to addicted mothers may be detected for up to 1 year

Abuse Liability

The capacity of an opioid drug to produce physical dependence requiring continued drug use to suppress unpleasant withdrawal symptoms is only one of the factors that contribute to the abuse liability of an opioid (see also Chapter 32). Other factors include the drug's ability to produce euphoria, the occurrence of toxic side effects when the dose is increased beyond the usual therapeutic range, and the ability to suppress abstinence symptoms caused by withdrawal of other agents in this class. Of these factors, the degree to which a drug induces euphoria or positively reinforcing effects is a major one in determining abuse liability and drug-seeking behavior. The intensity of the euphoric effect depends to some extent on the physical characteristics of the drug. A high degree of lipid solubility, which allows the drug to penetrate the blood-brain barrier rapidly after IV administration, leads to a shorter latency and more intense euphoria. On the other hand, the drug must be sufficiently soluble in water so that it can be injected IV. Heroin has both of these characteristics.

It is generally considered that analgesics acting through κ-receptors (e.g., pentazocine) produce less euphoria and have less overall abuse liability than the morphine-like drugs have. In 1977, however, some addicts discovered that the combination of the antihistamine tripelennamine with pentazocine was as euphoric as heroin, and the IV abuse of this mixture became widespread. This led to more control over the distribution of pentazocine, and since 1983 one oral form of this drug has included a small amount of naloxone hydrochloride to discourage IV abuse by dependent individuals. Because of extensive first-pass metabolism by the liver when administered orally, this amount of naloxone does not antagonize the analgesic effect of pentazocine, but, if administered IV, naloxone blocks the euphoric effect of pentazocine.

Pharmacological Treatment of Opioid Addiction

The most widely used treatment of addiction is the substitution method in which methadone is administered in place of the opioid drug being abused. As with cross-tolerance to morphine-like drugs, there is also cross-dependence among the members of this class, which allows the orally active methadone to substitute for the opioid drug. The methadone, supplied free by licensed clinics, one hopes would reduce the engagement of addicts in criminal activities to meet illicit drug costs. Since methadone is orally active, this also removes the possibility of infection from the sharing of needles and syringes. This is particularly important because of the increased incidence of acquired immunodeficiency syndrome among intravenous drug abusers (Chapters 32 and 54).

The original theory of methadone treatment of addiction is based on first maintaining a high degree of tolerance, so that no euphoric "high" is experienced with heroin and then gradually decreasing the methadone. The rationale for this theory is that the addicts will not undergo as severe a withdrawal as they do with the abrupt withdrawal of opioid drugs with a shorter half-life than that of methadone. One of the problems has been that withdrawal from methadone, at least in some patients, has been equal to or worse than withdrawal from injected opioid drugs, particularly with respect to withdrawal duration. However, methadone maintenance is effective and is widely used to treat opioid addiction.

A second method for treating opioid addiction involves oral use of an opioid antagonist such as naltrexone. Although not widely used clinically, it is being tested in patients who appear particularly motivated to become drug free. The patient is taken off all opioid drugs, undergoes withdrawal, and then is treated with a long-acting antagonist. The theory behind opioid an-

CLINICAL PROBLEMS

RESPIRATORY DEPRESSION

Caused by all potent narcotic analgesics

PHYSICAL AND PSYCHIC DEPENDENCE

Withdrawal problems and abuse potential

TOLERANCE

Degree varies with site of action and drug; cross-tolerance among various opioids

CONSTIPATION

Prolongs gastric emptying and decreases propulsive intestinal movement; basis for use as antidiarrheal agents

DRUG INTERACTIONS

Analgesic dose should be reduced when used with other CNS drugs (e.g., sedatives, anxiolytics)

SMOOTH MUSCLE STIMULATION

Increase in bile duct pressure and urethral sphincter tone; contraindicated in biliary colic

CNS STIMULATION

Nausea and vomiting caused by stimulation of area postrema in medulla

ROUTE OF ADMINISTRATION

Some analgesics have poor oral bioavailability

TRADE NAMES

In addition to generic and fixed-combination preparations, the following trade-named materials are available in the United States.

Alfenta, alfentanil
Astromorph, morphine sulfite injection
Buprenex, buprenorphine
Darvon, Propoxyphene
Demerol, meperidine
Dilaudid, hydromorphone
Dolophine, methadone
Levo-Dromoran, levorphanol tartrate
MS Contin, morphine sulfate tablets
Narcan, naloxone
Nubain, nalbuphine
Numorphan, oxymorphone
Pantopon, opium alkaloids mixture
Roxanol; MSIR; morphine sulfate solution or tablets
Roxicodone, oxycodone
Stadol, butorphanol
Sublimaze, fentanyl
Synalgos-DC, dihydrocodeine
Talwin, pentazocine
Trexan, naltrexone

tagonist therapy is that if subsequent injections of an opioid are received, the antagonist will block the euphoric effects, thereby discouraging further opioid use. During withdrawal, some clinics use the α_2-adrenergic agonist clonidine to suppress withdrawal signs that result from excessive autonomic nervous system activity. Clonidine does not alleviate the dysphoria or drug craving that occurs during withdrawal.

The major difference between these two types of treatment is that in one methadone is substituted for another opioid drug and the patient does not go into withdrawal, whereas in the other (antagonist) approach the patient must first go through complete withdrawal and be completely devoid of opioid drugs before treatment with an opioid antagonist begins. Otherwise, the antagonist could precipitate an immediate and severe withdrawal syndrome.

A major problem with both of these types of treatment is the high frequency of drug administration. Methadone or naltrexone must be taken at least once a day, but thus far the longer acting 1-α-acetylmethadol has not gained widespread clinical acceptance. The shorter acting drugs necessitate more frequent appearance of the addict or postaddiction patient at the treatment center, providing an opportunity for psychological support, an important component of treatment. Buprenorphine, a mixed agonist/antagonist, has been proposed as a possible opioid alternative to methadone for maintenance therapy in opiate addiction treatment. In preliminary studies, it blocks self-administration of opiates in addicts while showing low abuse liability. However, it does produce mild physical dependence. The sublingual preparation (available only in Europe) produces dependence and has significant abuse potential.

The clinical problems with the opioid analgesics are summarized in the box.

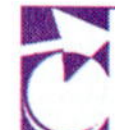

NEW DIRECTIONS

After nearly a decade of attempts, opioid receptors have finally been cloned. The first opioid receptor cloned was the δ-receptor, followed by the μ-receptor and the κ-receptor. All these receptors are G-protein coupled, an indication that they belong to a family of receptors regulated by GTP binding. The molecular characterization of these receptors indicates significant homology of sequence. In addition, the sequences show homology to the somatostatin receptor and that of certain neuromodulators called **tachykinins.** The determination of the molecular biology of these receptors could lead to the design of drugs with increased specificity for the respective receptors. In addition, the interaction of the drugs with their receptors in the modulation of second messengers can be clarified. Since modulation of second messengers by the opioids leads to analgesia and has been implicated in tolerance and physical dependence, drug interventions in such modulation of second messengers may become possible in the future. The ability to design drugs that can be coadministered with the opiates leading to less dependence on the opiate may also be possible in the future. In addition, the knowledge of the molecular sequence of the receptors may lead to development of "antisense," or complementary, sequences of the receptor, which may prove clinically useful in regulating events mediated by the receptors.

Meptazinol is an investigational drug in the United States that is used in the United Kingdom. Unlike other opioid analgesics, meptazinol does not produce as much respiratory depression in therapeutic doses as morphine does. It also produces less miosis, and does not have antidiarrheal properties. However, it may produce a higher incidence of nausea and vomiting than morphine does. It has poor oral bioavailability (<10%) and a shorter duration of action (2 hours) than morphine has. Although not recognized as an opioid by experienced addicts and although no physical dependence has been noted with chronic administration, meptazinol possesses antagonist activity and thus can precipitate withdrawal symptoms in subjects dependent on other opioid drugs. Its analgesic effects can be blocked by naloxone. Meptazinol may be a selective agonist of a postulated subtype of μ-receptor, denoted as the μ_1 opioid receptor.

The development of ketorolac (Toradol), an indol derivative and nonopioid used for the alleviation of pain, has opened a new area of research. Ketorolac, now widely used, is the first parenteral NSAID to be marketed in the United States. Currently it is used extensively for relief of moderate to severe pain in postoperative patients. When administered intramuscularly, 30 mg of ketorolac appears to be equivalent in analgesic effectiveness to 10 mg of morphine or 100 mg of meperidine. Two obvious advantages of ketorolac use are that tolerance does not develop and that drug dependence does not occur. It has no effect on respiration. A disadvantage of its use in patients after surgical procedures is a prolongation of bleeding time by blockade of prostaglandin biosynthesis and resultant inhibition of platelet aggregation. Ketorolac must be used with caution in elderly patients and in those with compromised renal function.

REFERENCES

Basbaum AI, Fields HL: Endogenous pain control systems: brainstem spinal pathways and endorphin circuitry, *Ann Rev Neurosci* 7:309, 1984.

Bobill JG, Sebel PS, Stanley TH: Opioid analgesics in anesthesia: with special reference to their use in cardiovascular anesthesia, *Anesthesiology* 61:731, 1984.

Foley KM, Inturrisi CE: Analgesic drug therapy in cancer pain: principles and practice, *Med Clin North Am* 71(2):207, 1987.

Millan MJ: Multiple opioid systems and pain, *Pain* 27:303, 1986.

Yaksh TL: Opioid receptor systems and the endorphins: a review of their spinal organization, *J Neurosurg* 67:157, 1987.

SELF-ASSESSMENT QUESTIONS

1. Which of the following is a *true* statement?
   a. There is very good oral absorption of morphine (between 90% and 95%).
   b. Extensive first-pass metabolism of codeine enhances the drugs effectiveness.
   c. The half-life of morphine is 24 hours, with 90% of the dose being excreted in 5 days.
   d. The duration of action of methadone analgesia is 25% longer than that of morphine.
   e. None of the above are true statements.
2. All the following statements concerning pentazocine (Talwin) are true *except* that:
   a. it produces pharmacological actions similar to butorphanol (Stadol).
   b. it produces analgesia, sedation, and respiratory depression.
   c. it will not precipitate opioid withdrawal symptoms.
   d. its use is intended to produce a nonaddicting analgesia.
   e. All of the above are false statements.
3. Which one of the following opioids is *inactive* after oral administration?
   a. naloxone (Narcan)
   b. pentazocine (Talwin)
   c. hydromorphone (Dilaudid)
   d. codeine (Tylenol)
   e. meperidine (Demerol)
4. All the following statements concerning opioid drugs are true *except* that:
   a. meperidine (Demerol) is an extremely effective antitussive and antidiarrheal agent.
   b. pentazocine (Talwin NX) is a special formulation with limited intravenous abuse potential.
   c. naltrexone (Trexan) is an orally active antagonist for maintenance of a drug-free state.
   d. heroin-withdrawal syndrome includes anxiety, muscle pain, mydriasis, and sweating.

e. All of the above statements are false.

5. Tolerance develops to all the following actions of morphine *except:*
   a. analgesia.
   b. lethality, or the lethal dose.
   c. euphoria.
   d. constipation.
   e. respiratory depression.
6. All the following statements concerning opioid drugs are true *except* that:
   a. morphine is a strong (potent) agonist.
   b. simple alteration of morphine's chemical structure does not affect pharmacological activity.
   c. changing an —OH group in morphine's structure to an $—OCH_3$ can produce a mild agonist.
   d. addition of a $—CHCH_2$ group to morphine's structure can produce an antagonist.
   e. All of the above statements are false.
7. There are three generally recognized groups of opioid peptides. Which of the following are opioid peptides?
   a. enkephalins
   b. endorphins
   c. dynorphins
   d. All of the above are opioid peptides.
   e. None of the above are opioid peptides.
8. Which of the following is a correct statement?
   a. Pentazocine is a mixed opioid agonist-antagonist.
   b. Methadone is an analgesic that is more potent than morphine as an analgesic.
   c. Opiates produce analgesia by decreasing the release of β-endorphin.
   d. Naloxone is orally active as an opioid antagonist.
   e. None of the above.
9. Which of the following statements is true?
   a. The kappa opioid receptor mediates the dysphoric effects of the opioids.
   b. The mu opioid receptor mediates analgesia, physical dependence, and respiratory depression.
   c. The delta opioid receptor mediates effects such as miosis and diuresis.
   d. The endogenous ligand for the epsilon receptor is dynorphin.
   e. The endogenous ligand for the delta receptor is dynorphin.
10. Which of the following statements are true?
    a. Methadone is a long-acting opioid that is useful in the treatment of addiction because of its long duration of action and oral efficacy.
    b. Opioids such as codeine are often formulated in combination with aspirin or acetaminophen in order to provide maximal pain relief with the least amount of opioid.
    c. Fentanyl is at least eighty-fold more potent than morphine as an analgesic.
    d. All of the statements are true.
    e. None of the statements are true.
11. Side effects of morphine include:
    a. diarrhea.
    b. respiratory depression.
    c. blockade of histamine release.
    d. hypertension.
    e. none of the above.
12. Which of the following are signs of heroin overdose?
    a. miosis (pinpoint pupil size), respiratory depression, hypotension
    b. mydriasis, hypertension, coma
    c. cardiac arrhythmias, convulsions, hypertension
    d. hypothermia, mydriasis, hypotension
    e. none of the above.
13. Which of the following are true statements?
    a. Fentanyl is useful in anesthesia because it has a long duration of action.
    b. Oxycodone and methadone are equal to morphine in analgesic potency.
    c. Propoxyphene is useful in treating severe pain.
    d. Pentazocine is similar to morphine in that it does not alter heart rate or blood pressure when taken in analgesic doses.
    e. Nalorphine is a pure opiate agonist.

CHAPTER 29

Pain and Inflammation Control with Nonsteroidal Antiinflammatory Drugs

THEODORE M. BRODY

MAJOR DRUGS
NSAIDS
acetaminophen

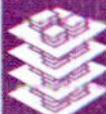

THERAPEUTIC OVERVIEW

Nonsteroidal antiinflammatory drugs (NSAIDs) are used to treat (1) mild pain or elevated body temperature, (2) arthritis and other inflammatory disorders, and (3) gout and hyperuricemia. These disorders may be acute or chronic and affect large segments of the population. Although symptoms may be extremely undesirable and often disabling, these disorders generally are not life threatening. The mild-to-moderate pain of headache, myalgia, neuralgia, and arthralgia that generally arises from integumental structures, and certain kinds of postoperative pain and dysmenorrhea can usually be treated with analgesics such as aspirin and acetaminophen or with other NSAIDs. These drugs at low doses are analgesic and antipyretic, and aspirin, because of its ability to inhibit platelet aggregation, is also useful in the prophylaxis of myocardial infarction. These drugs are excellent examples of rational therapeutic use of drugs based on an understanding of their mechanisms of action.

The arthritic disorders include rheumatoid arthritis, juvenile arthritis, ankylosing spondylitis, psoriatic arthritis, Reiter's syndrome, and osteoarthritis. They are characterized by inflammation and subsequent tissue damage. Although immunological factors play an important role in the causes of these diseases, the precise pathogenesis is largely unknown.

Gout, a disorder characterized by the deposition of uric acid crystals in joints, is accompanied by an increase in blood urates **(hyperuricemia).** This condition may also be present secondary to other diseases or can result from other drug treatments. Therapies for acute or chronic arthritis conditions and underlying hyperuricemia can be successfully carried out with the drugs described in this chapter.

ABBREVIATION	
NSAID	nonsteroidal antiinflammatory drug

MECHANISMS OF ACTION

Drugs Used to Treat Pain and Fever

Drugs used to reduce mild to moderate pain and fever include acetylsalicylic acid (aspirin), diflunisal, salsalate, acetaminophen, ibuprofen, naproxen, and fenoprofen (see boxes).

The mechanism by which these drugs act to reduce mild to moderate pain is based on the relationship between drugs such as aspirin and prostaglandin synthesis. Studies in humans have shown that IV administration of certain prostaglandins elicits headache and pain and produces hyperalgesia, sensitizing the individual to stimuli that normally would not produce pain. Aspirin and related compounds inhibit the enzyme cyclooxygenase and prevent the formation of prostaglandin endoperoxides, PGG_2 and PGH_2, which are normally formed from arachidonic acid (Figure 29-1). The details are described

Therapeutic Overview

PROBLEMS TO BE CONSIDERED

- Mild-to-moderate pain
  - headache
  - myalgia
  - neuralgia
  - postoperational pain
  - dysmenorrhea
- Elevated temperature
- Arthritis
  - rheumatoid
  - juvenile
  - ankylosing spondylitis
  - osteoarthritis
  - immunological factors
- Hyperuricemia
  - acute gout
  - chronic gout

Drugs Used in the Treatment of Mild-to-Moderate Pain

acetylsalicylic acid (aspirin)
diflunisal
salsalate
acetaminophen
ibuprofen
naproxen
fenoprofen
Several of these are also appropriate combined with narcotic analgesics for this purpose and include aspirin (650 mg) plus codeine (32 or 65 mg); acetaminophen (650 mg) plus codeine (32 or 65 mg).

in Chapter 18. The production of all prostaglandins derived from these endoperoxides therefore is blocked. Prostaglandins are not stored within cells, and so their release depends on their biosynthesis. Practically all mammalian cells synthesize prostaglandins; however, the efficacy of inhibitory drugs varies with the tissue. Thus drug selection is based on pain location. In contrast to the effects of the opioids, cyclooxygenase inhibitors act locally to block pain rather than to influence its recognition in the brain.

The chemical structures of some of the analgesic and antipyretic compounds are shown in Figure 29-2.

The ability of aspirin-like drugs to reduce fever depends on their inhibition of prostaglandin E_2 biosynthesis within the preoptic hypothalamic region, which regulates body temperature. Fever usually is caused by

NSAIDs Used for the Treatment of Arthritic Disorders

CARBOXYLIC ACIDS

aspirin
diflunisal
salsalate
choline magnesium trisalicylate
sodium salicylate

PROPIONIC ACIDS

ibuprofen
naproxen
fenoprofen
ketoprofen
flurbiprofen

FENAMATES

meclofenamate
mefenamic acid

ACETIC ACIDS

indomethacin
sulindac
tolmetin
diclofenac
etodolac

PYRAZOLONES

phenylbutazone
oxyphenbutazone

OXICANS

piroxican

NONACID COMPOUNDS

nabumetone

Drugs Used for the Treatment of Gout

colchicine
indomethacin
allopurinol
probenecid
sulfinpyrazone
Several of the drugs used to treat mild-to-moderate pain are also used (see text and box at left).

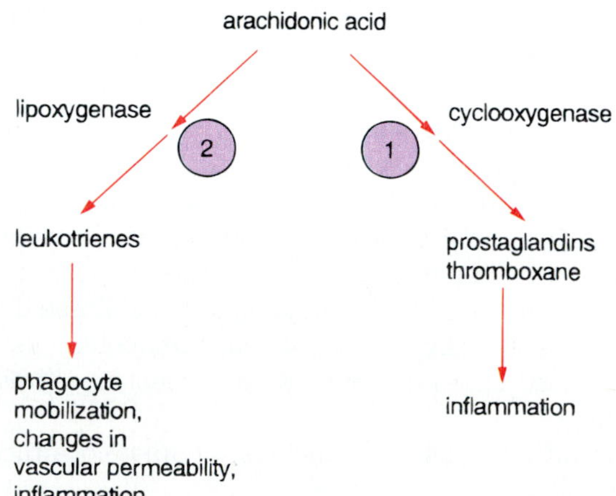

FIGURE 29-1 Proposed mechanisms of action of nonnarcotic analgesics. Most nonnarcotic analgesics act at *(1)* to block prostaglandin and thromboxane formation, and several antiinflammatory agents may also act at *(2)* to block leukotriene formation. (See Chapter 18 for more details.)

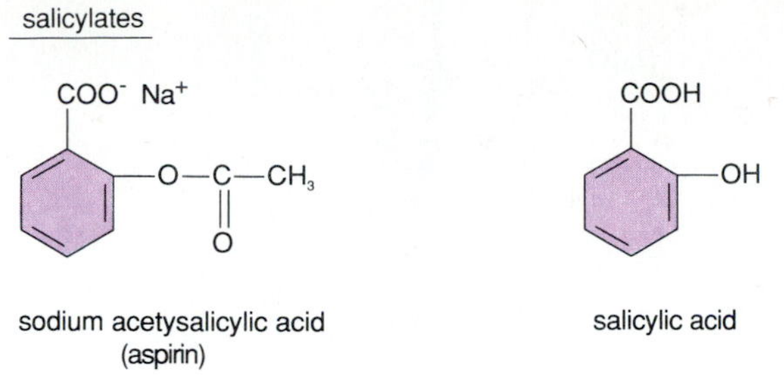

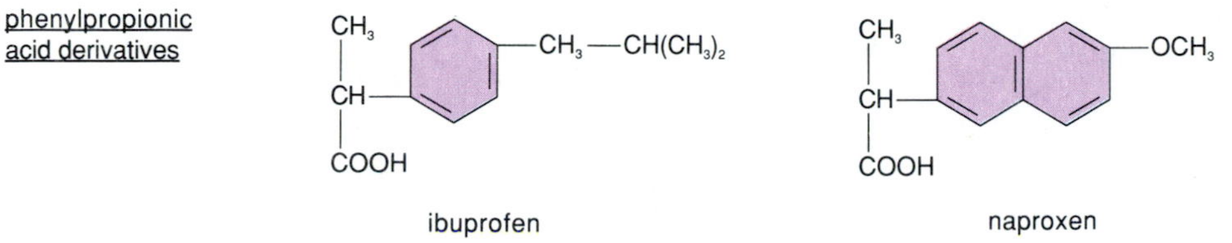

salicylates

$COO^- Na^+$ — $O—C—CH_3$ (=O)

sodium acetysalicylic acid (aspirin)

COOH — OH

salicylic acid

phenylpropionic acid derivatives

CH_3—CH—COOH — $CH_2—CH(CH_3)_2$

ibuprofen

CH_3—CH—COOH — OCH_3

naproxen

FIGURE 29-2 Structures of salicylates and phenylpropionic acid derivatives used as analgesics, antipyretics (some), or antiinflammatory drugs.

viral or bacterial infections. Certain cell wall products of pyrogenic microorganisms stimulate the synthesis and release of a pyrogen that enters the central nervous system and promotes prostaglandin release in the hypothalamus. The cyclooxygenase inhibitors lower elevated body temperature by blocking prostaglandin synthesis.

Antiinflammatory Effect

The inflammatory response is mediated by a host of endogenous compounds, including immunological and chemotactic factors, proteins of the complement system, histamine, serotonin, bradykinin, leukotrienes, and prostaglandins. Both leukotrienes and prostaglandins are major contributors to the symptoms of inflammation. Prostaglandins E_2 and I_2 promote edema and leukocyte infiltration and enhance the pain-producing properties of bradykinin. The leukotrienes increase vascular permeability and further increase the mobilization of endogenous mediators of inflammation. As already noted, by blocking cyclooxygenase activity, the salicylates and related nonsteroidal antiinflammatory drugs prevent the formation of endoperoxides and subsequent prostaglandin metabolites. The lipoxygenase pathway, which converts arachidonic acid to leukotrienes (Figure 29-1 and Chapter 18), is inhibited by diclofenac and indomethacin but not by salicylates. Piroxicam inhibits superoxide anion generation, and indomethacin, piroxicam, ibuprofen, and salicylates inhibit neutrophil function. NSAIDs may unmask T-cell suppressor activity to inhibit the production of rheumatoid factor. Such effects have been attributed to the mechanism by which gold or penicillamine modify the inflammatory response. Other processes unrelated to the inhibition of prostaglandin biosynthesis and postulated to result from high NSAID doses include effects on phospholipase C, chondrocyte proteoglycan synthesis, ion flux, and cell-cell binding.

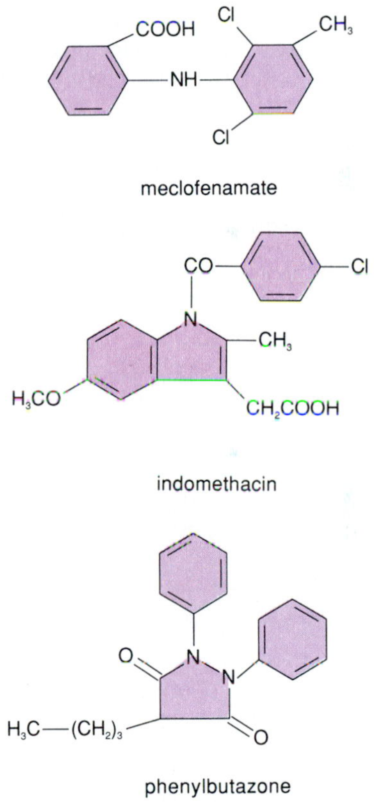

COOH — NH — Cl — CH_3 — Cl

meclofenamate

CO — Cl — N — CH_3 — H_3CO — CH_2COOH

indomethacin

O — N — N — $H_3C—(CH_2)_3$ — O

phenylbutazone

FIGURE 29-3 Structures of drugs used in treatment of arthritis and other inflammatory disorders (see also Figure 29-2).

When rheumatoid arthritis does not respond to conventional drug therapy, remission-inducing drugs are sometimes added to the treatment regimen. These include the gold salts, antimalarials, penicillamine, corticosteroids, and immunosuppressants such as methotrexate (see also antimalarials, Chapter 56; penicillamine, Chapter 47; azathioprine and methotrexate, Chapter 43; and prednisone and prednisolone, Chapter 35).

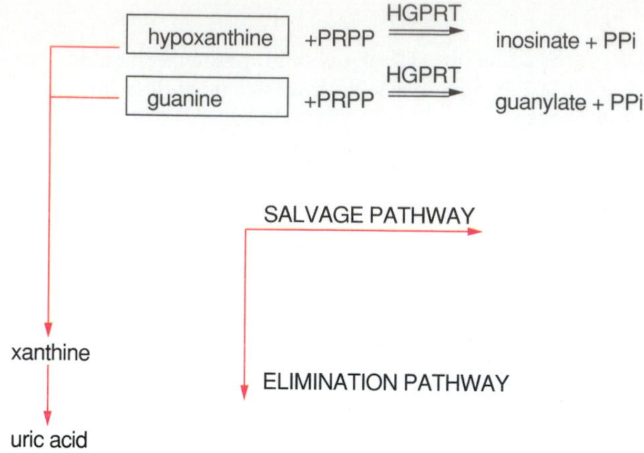

FIGURE 29-4 Salvage pathway for recycling of purine bases to form nucleotides, inosinate, and guanylate. A decrease in the salvage pathway activity can lead to an increase in uric acid formation. *HGPRT,* Hypoxanthine-guanine phosphoribosyltransferase; *PPi,* pyrophosphate; *PRPP,* 5-phosphoribosyl-1-pyrophosphate.

colchicine

probenecid

allopurinol

sulfinpyrazone

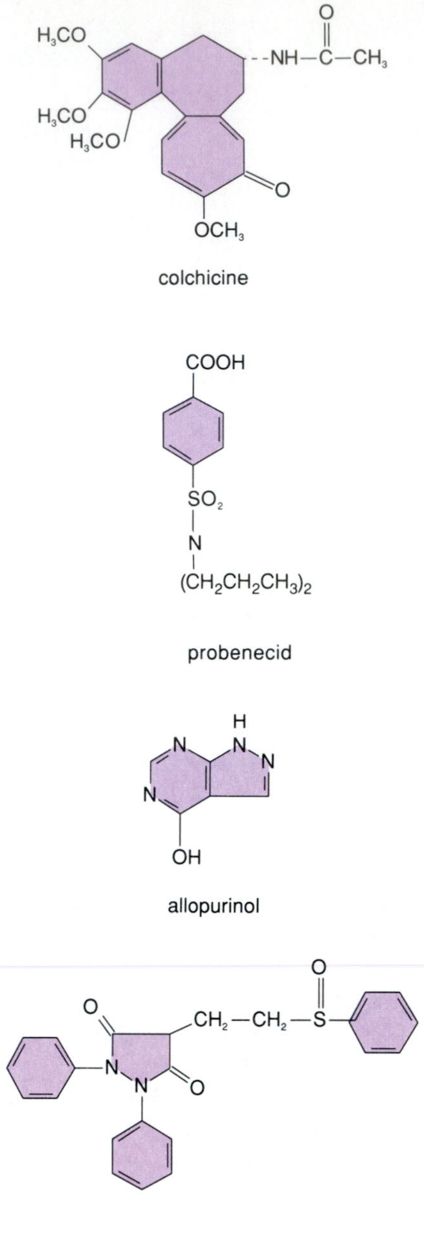

FIGURE 29-5 Some of the drugs used to treat gout.

Drugs Used to Treat Gout and Hyperuricemia

Overproduction of uric acid and decreased uric acid secretion in primary hyperuricemia usually are classified as an inborn error of metabolism. Overproduction can be caused by a deficiency of hypoxanthine-guanine phosphoribosyltransferase activity or by increased phosphoribosyl pyrophosphate synthetase. Both enzymes can produce increased concentrations of 5-phosphoribosyl-1-pyrophosphate (PRPP), a key intermediate in the salvage pathway for purines and uric acid formation (Figure 29-4).

Drugs frequently used to treat acute gouty arthritis are colchicine and indomethacin. Adrenal steroids are also sometimes used, and phenylbutazone, though extremely toxic, can be effective in refractory patients. Several newer antiinflammatory nonsteroidal agents (sulindac, ibuprofen, naproxen, fenoprofen) are also clinically effective in acute gout. Probenecid, sulfinpyrazone, and allopurinol are effective in chronic gout and other conditions where it is essential to decrease plasma uric acid concentrations. (See Figure 29-5 for chemical structures.)

In gout, body fluids become supersaturated with urate and needlelike crystals of urate precipitate in tissues. The inflammation is largely caused by the migration of leukocytes to the joint in an attempt to phagocytize the urate crystals, with the concomitant release of inflammatory mediators. Colchicine acts by binding to a cellular microtubular protein, tubulin, causing the microtubules to disintegrate. Intact microtubules are necessary to maintain leukocyte cell structure and movement. By effecting microtubule disaggregation, colchicine prevents the local infiltration of leukocytes to joint tissue. By blocking phagocytosis, colchicine also prevents the release of lactic acid–rich granulocyte contents into the joint. Lowering pH would tend to further precipitate urate crystals.

Allopurinol is an analog of hypoxanthine but is a better substrate for xanthine oxidase and, when oxidized, forms oxypurinol (alloxanthine). The latter compound is an irreversible, i.e., "suicide," inhibitor that binds very

Table 29-1 Pharmacokinetic Parameters

Drug	Administration	$t_{1/2}$ (hr)	Disposition	Plasma Protein Binding (%)
CARBOXYLIC ACIDS				
acetylsalicylate	Oral	0.25	M (100%)	50-80
sodium salicylate	Oral	2-12	M (main), R	50-80
diflunisal	Oral	8-12	M (main), R	—
PROPIONIC ACIDS				
naproxen	Oral	12-14	M (main), R	99
ibuprofen	Oral	2-4	M (main)	99
fenoprofen	Oral	2-3	M (main), R	High
ketoprofen	Oral	2-3	M (main), R	99
flurbiprofen	Oral	3-5	M (main)	High
ACETIC ACIDS				
diclofenac	Oral	1-2	M (main)	High
indomethacin	Oral	3-5	M, R	90
sulindac	Oral	15-17	M†, R (small)	High
tolmetin	Oral	1-7	M, R (50%)	99
etodolac	Oral	5-7	M (main), R	99
OTHERS				
acetaminophen	Oral	1-3	M (main)	20-50
meclofenamate	Oral	2-3	M, R	99
piroxicam	Oral	40-58	M, R (small)	99
nabumetone	Oral	20-30	M † R	99

M, Metabolized; *R,* renal elimination as unchanged drug.
†Active metabolite.

tightly to the catalytic site of xanthine oxidase. Inhibition of xanthine oxidase results in decreased blood urate concentrations and increased excretion rates of the more water-soluble xanthine and hypoxanthine (Figure 29-6).

In some patients reduced excretion of uric acid results from decreased renal tubular secretion or increased tubular reabsorption, or both. Thus, agents that promote the excretion of urate are also useful in the treatment of hyperuricemia and related conditions. Such uricosuric agents include probenecid and sulfinpyrazone, which increase urate excretion by competing for the renal tubular acid transporter so that less urate is reabsorbed. Normally, about 90% of filtered urate is reabsorbed, with only 10% excreted.

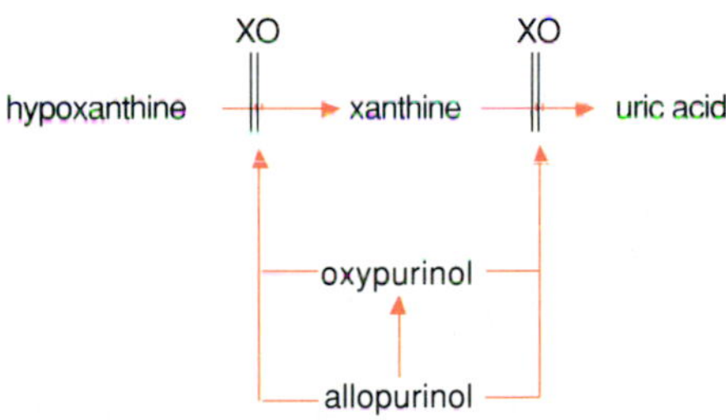

FIGURE 29-6 Blockade of uric acid synthesis by allopurinol and its oxidation agent, oxypurinol. *XO,* xanthine oxidase. See text for details.

PHARMACOKINETICS

Pharmacokinetic parameters are summarized in Table 29-1.

Salicylates

Oral absorption of salicylates occurs rapidly from the stomach but to an even greater extent from the lower gastrointestinal tract by passive diffusion. The pH of the stomach favors absorption because salicylates are weak acids and have a low pK_a. These drugs are found in plasma within 30 minutes, and peak plasma concentrations are achieved 1 to 2 hours after oral administration.

Highly buffered effervescent solutions of *aspirin* are less irritating to the stomach and are more rapidly absorbed. Enteric-coated preparations are also available, but the absorption rate varies among different products. Rectal suppositories are of limited use because of the variable absorption.

Salicylates are distributed across membranes primarily by passive diffusion and can be detected in most body tissues and fluids. However, because plasma sa-

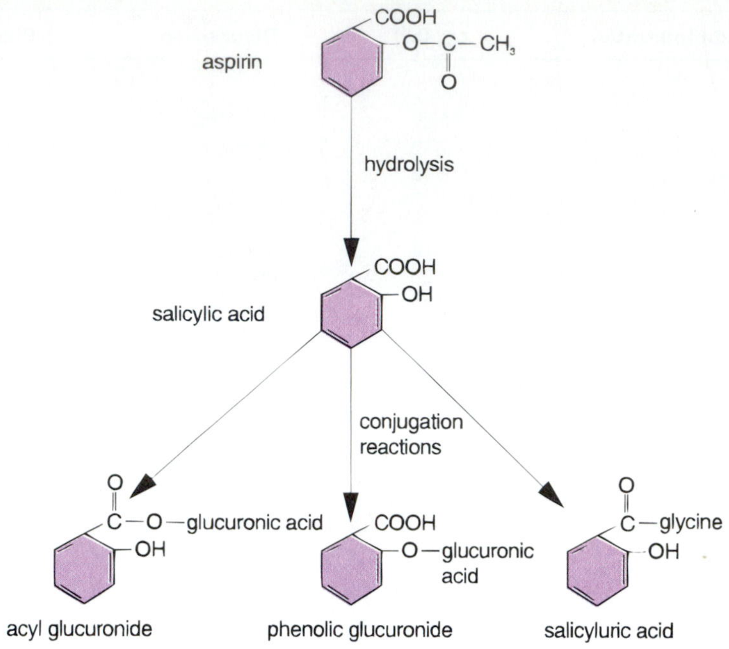

FIGURE 29-7 Metabolism of aspirin.

licylate is largely ionized, only a small amount of salicylate crosses the blood-brain barrier. Aspirin and salicylic acid are bound to plasma proteins (50% to 80%).

Aspirin has a plasma half-life of 15 minutes, undergoing rapid hydrolysis to salicylate, though both acetylsalicylate (aspirin) and salicylate readily enter body tissues and fluids, as already stated. The half-life of salicylate varies from 2 to 3 hours for analgesic doses, up to 12 hours for antiinflammatory doses, and up to 20 hours at toxic doses. The primary metabolites of aspirin and salicylate are shown in Figure 29-7 (see also Chapter 5). The conjugates are inactive pharmacologically and are excreted. The percentage of each metabolite (Chapter 5) depends on the metabolic pool of glucuronic acid or glycine. Although salicylate is secreted by the proximal tubule, the extent of renal excretion as salicylate also can vary, since salicylate can undergo passive backdiffusion. Thus the net renal elimination of salicylate depends on urine pH in the tubular lumen. At alkaline pH, more free salicylate is cleared from the body. Discussed in Chapter 5, alkalinization of the urine by administration of sodium bicarbonate is used to lower toxic concentrations of salicylate. Since the conjugation of salicylate is enzyme catalyzed, the reactions can become saturated (zero order) (see Chapter 5). The limited availability of glycine and glucuronide for conjugation of salicylic acid results in the elimination of salicylate according to first-order kinetics at lower doses and zero-order kinetics at higher doses. This is reflected in the plasma half-lives, which increase with dose.

The pharmacokinetics of *diflunisal* are similar to those of aspirin. Diflunisal is rapidly absorbed with peak plasma concentrations achieved in 2 to 3 hours. The drug is extensively conjugated to water-soluble glucuronides and excreted in the urine. Like salicylate, diflunisal exhibits zero-order elimination kinetics at high doses.

Other NSAIDs

Pharmacokinetic parameters for the NSAIDs are presented in Table 29-1. Most are well absorbed from the gastrointestinal tract, have little first-pass metabolism, are bound to plasma proteins, and have small apparent volumes of distribution. The differences between responders and nonresponders to NSAID antirheumatic effects are unrelated to the pharmacokinetics of the particular drug. Only with some of the NSAIDs is there a linear relationship between the blood concentration and the antirheumatic or toxic effects.

The NSAIDs are metabolized to inactive or active compounds by several mechanisms. Some drugs are demethylated (naproxen, indomethacin) before conjugation and excretion of the conjugated product. *Piroxicam* and *fenoprofen* are hydroxylated, whereas *ibuprofen* and *meclofenamate* are both hydroxylated and carboxylated before conjugation with glucuronic acid and excretion. Sulindac is metabolized to an active sulfide and undergoes extensive enterohepatic cycling, accounting for its longer half-life. *Nabumetone,* a newer agent, is itself a weak cyclooxygenase inhibitor but is converted to the 6-methoxy-2-naphthylacetic acid, a potent inhibitor of the enzyme.

Half of the currently used NSAIDs are cleared rapidly (half-life less than 6 hours), whereas others have elimination half-lives greater than 10 hours. Several of the longer-acting agents are prodrugs (sulindac, nabumetone). Sustained-release preparations of some of the shorter-acting NSAIDs (ketoprofen, indomethacin) have been developed.

With some NSAIDs renal excretion plays a prominent role in drug clearance (Table 29-1). Clearance of these drugs may be slightly decreased in patients with renal failure. Some propionic acid derivatives are converted to acyl glucuronides and recycled and should therefore be used with caution in these patients.

Most NSAIDs are extensively bound to plasma proteins. With ibuprofen and naproxen, binding is saturable and free drug concentrations rise at higher doses, particularly in elderly patients.

Acetaminophen, which is not an anti-inflammatory, is a very weak acid with a pK_a of 9.5, is rapidly absorbed from the gastrointestinal tract. Peak plasma concentrations are achieved within 1 hour. Distribution is relatively uniform throughout all body tissues. The parent compound is almost completely biotransformed to inactive metabolites by the liver, forming conjugates with glucuronic acid, sulfate, and cysteine, which are excreted in the urine. Overdose with acetaminophen results in the formation of a reactive intermediate catalyzed by the cytochrome P-450 pathway. The intermediate is normally conjugated with glutathione and excreted. When glutathione concentrations are depressed in the liver, toxic intermediates form adducts with hepatic proteins resulting in necrosis and resultant hepatitis.

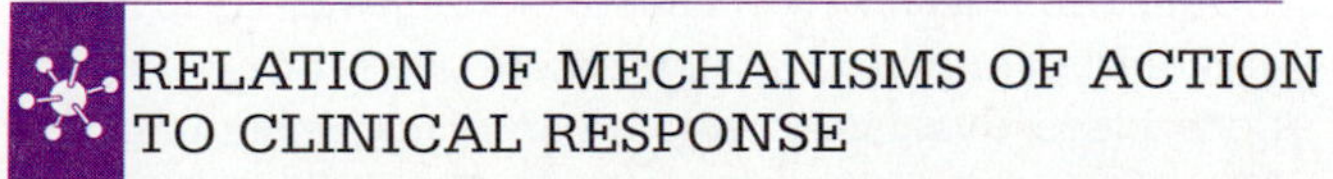

RELATION OF MECHANISMS OF ACTION TO CLINICAL RESPONSE

Drugs commonly used to treat mild pain, arthritis or inflammatory disorders, and gout are listed in the boxes.

Salicylates

Aspirin remains one of the most commonly used and effective agents for analgesia and antipyresis. Salicylates are used to treat headache and joint, muscle, and nerve pain of mild-to-moderate intensity. However, they are not effective in treatment of deep visceral pain, where the opioids are used.

Several analogs of aspirin also are used clinically, including *sodium salicylate, diflunisal, salsalate, salicylic acid,* and *methyl salicylate.* The latter two compounds are used only externally. Salicylic acid is applied topically as a keratolytic agent, and methyl salicylate is used as a counterirritant.

Aspirin shows no tolerance development to its analgesic effects, no psychological or physical dependency, or addiction liability as seen with the opioids. Nor do salicylates produce central nervous system depression. Although aspirin is extremely effective in reducing elevated body temperature, its use for this purpose has diminished because of epidemiological data that indicate a relationship between aspirin use (especially in the treatment of chickenpox or influenza infections) and the occurrence of Reye's syndrome. Alternative therapy is advised, generally with acetaminophen. There is a dose-dependent distinction between the analgesic and antirheumatic actions of the salicylates. At low doses, only the analgesic effect is observed, whereas at much larger doses and over extended periods an antirheumatic effect is obtained. For relief of mild-to-moderate pain, 650 mg of aspirin is as effective as 50 mg of pentazocine, 65 mg of propoxyphene, or 650 mg of acetaminophen.

Aspirin has a long and successful history in treating rheumatic disorders. Because of side effects, this agent is sometimes not well tolerated, and patient compliance is frequently a problem in long-term use. As a result several nonacetylated derivatives of aspirin are now available, but for patients who experience no side effects, aspirin is still the drug of choice.

Buffered aspirin is of some use in reducing gastrointestinal effects, though the antacid content of these preparations is quite small. A disadvantage of the buffered preparations is the large amount of sodium present, which may be undesirable for some patients. Enteric-coated tablets are also available to minimize gastric distress.

Among the nonacetylated derivatives, *diflunisal* is an effective cyclooxygenase inhibitor used for analgesic and antiinflammatory activities but has only weak antipyretic action. Sodium salicylate, choline salicylate, magnesium salicylate, choline magnesium trisalicylate, and salsalate are other nonacetylated compounds with similar pharmacologic effects. These agents are as effective as aspirin in treating inflammatory disorders such as osteoarthritis and rheumatoid arthritis.

Acetylsalicylate is more effective than sodium salicylate as an analgesic, antipyretic, or antiinflammatory agent. Although the reason for this difference is not clear, it may result from the ability of aspirin to acetylate an active site on cyclooxygenase. Although sodium salicylate has no acetylating capacity, it does reduce prostaglandin biosynthesis in vivo. Since acetylsalicylate is metabolized to salicylate, it appears that both compounds possess similar but not equivalent pharmacological activities. Some but not all of the salicylates are effective inhibitors of platelet aggregation, which is related to aspirin's ability to irreversibly acetylate platelet cyclooxygenase (see Chapter 18) (regeneration of platelet cyclooxygenase has a half-life of 7 to 10 days). Because of this activity, aspirin is effective for prophylaxis of myocardial infarction and also has been used in certain thromboembolic diseases. Diflunisal is a weak, reversible inhibitor of platelet aggregation.

Acetaminophen

Because of its lower incidence of side effects, lower potential for toxicity in the event of overdose, and better tolerance by many patients, acetaminophen is an effective alternative to aspirin for the treatment of headache, mild-to-moderate pain, and fever. **It has essentially no antiinflammatory activity.** Other members of this group, such as phenacetin and acetanilid, are no longer used in the United States because of their toxic effects. Acetaminophen is a major metabolite of both these agents. The lack of antiinflammatory action of these agents is not well understood. Acetaminophen is a weak inhibitor of prostaglandin biosynthesis, yet it is an effective analgesic/antipyretic. This may result from greater inhibition of cyclooxygenase in the CNS compared to peripheral tissues. No association is known between acetaminophen and Reye's syndrome, and acetaminophen produces no methemoglobinemia, like acetanilid or phenacetin. Acetaminophen (unlike aspirin) fails to inhibit platelet aggregation. It does not cause CNS depression, nor does it produce tolerance or dependence.

Phenylpropionic Acids

Among the other NSAIDs, several of the phenylpropionic acid derivatives are used to treat mild-to-moderate pain. These include ibuprofen, naproxen, and fenoprofen. All have a lower potential for adverse side effects than aspirin has and also are effective antipyretic and antiinflammatory agents. All of these agents are potent inhibitors of cyclooxygenase and have similar ranges of pharmacological activity. Clinically, 200 mg of ibuprofen or fenoprofen are equivalent in analgesic effectiveness to 650 mg of aspirin or acetaminophen. *Ibuprofen* is somewhat more effective than aspirin in the treatment of dysmenorrhea.

Naproxen is analgesic, antipyretic, and antiinflammatory. It is used to treat most rheumatoid disorders and acute gout. Its pharmacological properties, toxicity, and therapeutic indications are similar to those for the other nonsteroidal antiinflammatory drugs.

Fenoprofen is similar in action to ibuprofen. It is analgesic, antipyretic, antiinflammatory, and equipotent with ibuprofen. It is an effective alternative to aspirin in the treatment of rheumatoid arthritis and osteoarthritis.

Ketoprofen also has good analgesic/antipyretic and antiinflammatory activity and is used to treat rheumatoid arthritis and osteoarthritis. It inhibits both cyclooxygenase and lipoxygenase and stabilizes lysosomal membranes. *Florbiprofen,* another similar derivative, is used to treat rheumatoid arthritis, osteoarthritis, and ankylosing spondylitis.

Acetic Acid Derivatives

This group includes indomethacin, sulindac, and tolmetin. *Indomethacin,* introduced in the 1960s as an antiinflammatory drug, has limited clinical use as an analgesic/antipyretic because of toxicity. It is still widely used to treat acute gouty arthritis, ankylosing spondylitis, osteoarthritis in Reiter's syndrome, and psoriatic arthritis. One of the most potent inhibitors of prostaglandin biosynthesis, like colchicine, it also interferes with the migration of leukocytes, contributing to its utility in the treatment of gout. Neonates who suffer from cardiac failure as a result of incomplete closure of the ductus arteriosus may be helped by treatment with indomethacin. Closure of the ductus is accomplished in 70% of patients.

Sulindac is a prodrug that undergoes hepatic conversion to the sulfide to produce analgesic, antipyretic, and antiinflammatory actions. It is used in adults with rheumatoid arthritis, osteoarthritis, and ankylosing spondylitis.

Tolmetin is a suitable substitute in indomethacin intolerant patients and is one of the few drugs suitable for treatment of juvenile arthritis, rheumatoid arthritis, osteoarthritis, and ankylosing spondylitis.

Pyrazolone Derivatives

Phenylbutazone is an effective analgesic, antipyretic, and antiinflammatory agent, but its use is limited by serious blood dyscrasias which can occur, including leukopenia, agranulocytosis, and aplastic anemia. It should be used only after all other therapeutic regimens have failed and the risk-benefit ratio carefully evaluated. It is also an effective alternative to colchicine for treatment of acute gout and acute episodes of rheumatoid arthritis, but long-term therapy is not recommended. Oxyphenbutazone is an active metabolite of phenylbutazone with a range of pharmacological activity and toxicity similar to that of the parent drug.

A new pyrazolone derivative, *apazone,* is a prostaglandin synthesis inhibitor related to phenylbutazone but has a lower incidence of blood dyscrasias. It is used to treat rheumatoid arthritis, osteoarthritis, psoriatic arthritis, and gout and also serves as an effective uricosuric agent.

Other Antiarthritis Drugs

Meclofenamate, mefenamic acid, and *diclofenac* have analgesic/antipyretic and antiinflammatory action, with the antiinflammatory action of mefenamic acid weaker than the others and more toxic. Piroxicam has similar analgesic/antipyretic and antiinflammatory actions. It inhibits cyclooxygenase and is reported to inhibit neutrophil aggregation and lysosomal enzyme release. It is used to treat rheumatoid arthritis, osteoarthritis, ankylosing spondylitis, and gout.

Elemental gold compounds such as *aurothioglucose, gold sodium thiomalate,* and *auranofin* are used to suppress immune responsiveness and thereby arrest the progress of active adult and juvenile arthritis. Penicillamine has immunosuppressive actions similar to gold, but the high incidence of adverse reactions with this agent limits its use.

Several other immunosuppressive agents used to treat rheumatic disorders include *azathioprine, methotrexate,* and *cyclophosphamide* (Chapter 45). Bone marrow depression and other toxicities limit their use to situations where all other therapies have failed.

The pharmacology of the corticoids is considered in Chapter 35. Prednisone and prednisolone are effective when given orally, and long-acting corticoids (e.g., triamcinolone) are also available for intraarticular administration. The effects of these drugs may last from weeks to months. The corticoids are not regarded as remission-inducing drugs.

Some of the antimalarials such as *chloroquine* and *hydroxychloroquine* also produce remission in arthritic disorders, including juvenile arthritis and systemic lupus erythematosus. They also may produce functional improvement rather than remission.

Drugs for the Treatment of Gout

Colchicine is effective in the treatment of acute gouty arthritis and appears to be relatively specific for this disease. It relieves both pain and inflammation and is frequently the first-line drug for an initial attack. These effects of colchicine are secondary to its action in blocking the mobilization of leukocytes and macrophage release of inflammatory mediators into the joint. Indomethacin and phenylbutazone are also used to treat acute urate crystal–induced gout, apparently through inhibition of urate crystal phagocytosis. The new antiinflammatory drugs fenoprofen, ibuprofen, naproxen, and sulindac also are effective in large doses and serve as alternatives to colchicine for prophylactic therapy. Adrenal glucocorticoids may be effective in severe attacks that do not respond favorably to other antiinflammatory agents. The intraarticular injection of a corticosteroid can relieve pain if a single joint is involved.

Allopurinol is recommended for the therapy of chronic tophaceous gout and other hyperuricemias. Plasma and urine concentrations of uric acid are reduced because of the ability of allopurinol to inhibit xanthine oxidase and de novo purine biosynthesis. Excretion of urates is reduced, lowering the potential incidence of renal injury. Reduction in symptoms and in serum urate concentrations usually occurs in several days to 2 weeks.

In chronic gout, *probenecid* and *sulfinpyrazone* reduce plasma uric acid concentrations and prevent or reduce joint inflammation in chronic gout in patients with adequate renal function. Because acute attacks may occur, early treatment with these uricosuric agents, colchicine, or other antiinflammatory agents may be given concurrently. Other acids (e.g., salicylate) should not be given concomitantly because they compete with uric acid for the same renal transport system.

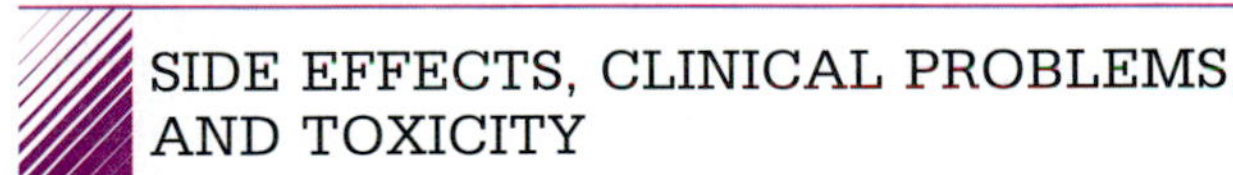

SIDE EFFECTS, CLINICAL PROBLEMS, AND TOXICITY

Salicylates

The most frequent problem with the salicylates is a propensity to cause gastrointestinal distress. With larger doses used to treat rheumatoid diseases, gastrointestinal problems occur in about 20% of patients. Occult bleeding is quite common though blood loss is minimal. The nonacetylated derivatives (other than salicyclic acid) cause fewer gastrointestinal problems. Special preparations, such as buffered or enteric-coated aspirin tablets, afford some further protection. Long-term use of salicylates is believed to contribute to the incidence of peptic ulcers, and salicylates should be avoided, if possible, in patients with active ulcers. Gastritis can be reduced if the patient takes aspirin with meals and with an adequate amount of water to ensure tablet dissolution.

With large doses of salicylate, CNS effects are prominent. So-called **salicylism** is characterized by tinnitus, hearing loss, and vertigo, reversible on reducing drug intake. These are not reliable signs of a maximally tolerated dose in elderly patients or in children, whose early signs of toxicity may vary. Slightly larger doses may stimulate the respiratory center and cause respiratory alkalosis. At moderate toxicity, a metabolic acidosis is observed, which is apparently the consequence of impaired carbohydrate and lipid metabolism from salicylate's effect to uncouple oxidative phosphorylation.

A small number of patients are hypersensitive to aspirin and may develop a rash or an anaphylactoid reaction. They frequently have nasal polyps. Such individuals may also be sensitive to other nonsteroidal antiinflammatory drugs that inhibit prostaglandin biosynthesis. Because aspirin inhibits platelet aggregation, it should be avoided in patients who are taking coumarin or other anticoagulants. Very large doses of aspirin can produce liver injury, and this drug is not recommended in patients with chronic liver disease. Aspirin and related drugs can cause retention of salt and water and can reduce renal function in susceptible patients. Salicylates, when used alone, are not generally associated with renal toxicity; however, combination therapy with other nonnarcotic analgesics has been reported to cause papillary necrosis and interstitial nephritis. There is no indication of a potential hazard in pregnant women taking occasional moderate doses of aspirin.

Acute intoxication from accidental overdose of aspirin is common in children and may have a fatal outcome. Metabolic acidosis, nausea, vomiting, stupor, and coma may develop. Hyperthermia is frequently observed. Extent of intoxication can be estimated from blood salicylate concentrations, with 50 mg/dl considered mildly toxic and 100 to 150 mg/dl potentially lethal. Treatment depends on the severity of the intoxication. Gastric lavage, activated charcoal, and alkalinization of the urine are used to reduce the body burden of salicylate. Dehydration, acidosis, and hypoglycemia, if they occur, should be corrected.

Other NSAIDs

The spectrum of adverse reactions with NSAIDs is broad. Gastrointestinal problems are most common, followed by adverse renal effects. Hepatic problems have been most frequently reported with the pyrazolone, propionic acid, and acetic acid classes of agents. Other adverse effects include skin and central nervous system reactions. Blood dyscrasias are rare. NSAIDs have been long known for their deleterious effects on gastrointestinal function. They produce gastric erosion, peptic ulcer formation and perforation, and inflammation of the duodenum and large intestine. There is little evidence at present that one NSAID is less prone than others with respect to risk of gastrointestinal side effects. The histamine H_2-histamine receptor blockers, and also omeprazole and misoprostol have been used to reduce or prevent the ulcerogenic effect of NSAIDs (Chapter 59).

The kidney is also adversely affected with long-term use of NSAIDs. This is not surprising, since the prostaglandins have a prominent role in normal renal blood flow, glomerular filtration, and salt and water metabolism. Fluid retention is the most common renal complication. Clinically detectable edema, however, occurs in less than 5% of patients and is reversible on discontinuation of the drug. In patients with a preexisting reduced blood flow, NSAIDs can produce renal failure. This results from inhibition by NSAIDs of the biosynthesis of the vasodilator prostaglandins, which are needed to maintain renal perfusion. Other rarer adverse reactions are hyperkalemia, nephrotic syndrome with interstitial nephritis and papillary necrosis. Although the overall risk of renal failure with NSAID use is low, because of the extremely wide use of the NSAIDs in the general population, the number of at-risk patients may be significant.

NSAIDs have been reported to reduce the antihypertensive effects of diuretics, β-adrenergic receptor antagonists and angiotensin-converting enzyme inhibitors. This effect, if it occurs, appears to be quite small. Interpatient variability however may be considerable. The rationale is apparent, since some prostaglandins play a key role in modulating vascular tone.

The adverse effects of the NSAIDs on the central nervous system are less well documented and less frequent than those occurring in other organs. NSAIDs are reported to be responsible for the aseptic meningitis described in patients with systemic lupus erythematosus. Serious psychotic episodes have been observed with sulindac and indomethacin use. Other more subtle effects such as cognitive dysfunction and depression have also been identified in patients on NSAIDs, particularly the elderly.

Clinical Problems

Gastrointestinal disturbances
Renal dysfunction
Bleeding disorders
Hypersensitivity, dermatologic problems
Hematologic reaction (rare)
CNS effects

TRADE NAMES

In addition to generic and fixed-combination preparations the following trade-named materials are available in the United States.

Ansaid, flurbiprofen
Anturane, sulfinpyrazone
Benemid, probenecid
Butazolid, phenylbutazone
Clinoril, sulindac
Cuprimine, penicillamine
Disalcid, salsalate, salicylsalicylate
Dolobid, diflunisal
Feldene, piroxicam
Indocin, indomethacin
Lodine, etodolac
Meclomen, meclofenamate
Motrin, Advil, Nuprin, Rufen, ibuprofen
Myochrysine, gold sodium thiomalate
Nalfon, fenoprofen
Naprosyn, naproxen
Orudis, ketoprofen
Plaquenil, hydroxycloroquine
Relafen, nabumetone
Ridaura, auranofin
Solgangal, aurothioglucose
Tanderil, oxyphenbutazone
Tolectin, tolmetin
Trisilate, choline magnesium trisalicylate
Voltaren, diclofenac
Zyloprim, allopurinol

Acetaminophen

At usual therapeutic doses, acetaminophen is remarkably safe. However, normally a small quantity of the parent compound is converted by the cytochrome P-450 mixed-function oxidase system to a highly reactive toxic intermediate, which is detoxified by conjugation with glutathione. When an overdose of acetaminophen occurs, the conjugation process is overwhelmed and the toxic intermediate becomes covalently bound to hepatic macromolecules, resulting in hepatic necrosis and hepatitis, which can be fatal. Factors that decrease glutathione concentrations enhance toxicity. Treatment of the toxicity involves reducing the body burden of acetaminophen and the administration of *N*-acetylcysteine as a specific antidote.

The major clinical problems are summarized in the box.

NEW DIRECTIONS

Academic and industrial researchers in this field are attempting to develop a new generation of antiinflammatory drugs as effective as the current NSAIDs yet devoid of the undesirable gastrointestinal actions. This research has been stimulated by a recent observation that two different enzymes may be involved subserving separate functions. One is the regulation of prostaglandin-induced inflammation (cyclooxygenase II, or COX II), and the second (cyclooxygenase I, or COX I) is inhibition of gastric acid secretion. The classical concept is that a single enzyme, cyclooxygenase, controlled prostaglandin production and therefore inflammation and inhibition of gastric acid production. Currently available drugs block both COX I and COX II and are therefore ulcerogenic and antiinflammatory. Although COX I and COX II both catalyze the conversion of arachidonic acid into prostaglandins G_2 and H_2, the enzymes have different tissue distributions. COX I is ubiquitous, whereas COX II activity is confined to monocytes and macrophages, which have important roles in inflammation.

Thus the thrust is to find COX II–specific antiinflammatory candidates. Several groups are also attempting to uncover cell lines that are specific for gene expression of COX I or COX II, with the purpose of using such cell lines to screen for potential antiinflammatory agents.

REFERENCES

Brooks PM, Day RO: Nonsteroidal antiinflammatory drugs—differences and similarities, *N Engl J Med* 322:1716, 1991.

Hart FD, Huskisson EC: Non-steroidal anti-inflammatory drugs: current status and rational therapeutic use, *Drugs* 27:232, 1988.

Hess EV, Tangnijkul Y: A rational approach to NSAID therapy, *Ration Drug Ther* 20:1, 1986.

Rumack BH: Mechanisms of acetaminophen toxicity. In Haddad LM, Winchester J, editors: Clinical management of poisoning and drug overdose, Philadelphia, 1983, Saunders.

Whelton A, Hamilton CW: Nonsteroidal anti-inflammatory drugs: effects on kidney function, *J Clin Pharmacol* 31:588, 1991.

SELF-ASSESSMENT QUESTIONS

1. Which of the following is not true of aspirin?
   a. It is deacetylated to salicylic acid.
   b. It irreversibly inhibits platelet cyclooxygenase.
   c. It is converted to inactive glucuronides.
   d. It inhibits lipooxygenase.
   e. It has a $t_{1/2}$ of 15 to 30 minutes.

2. Which of the following is not true of acetaminophen?
   a. It is metabolized to a reactive intermediate, which can be hepatotoxic.
   b. It possesses analgesic, antipyretic and antiinflammatory properties.
   c. It can be used in children with Reye's syndrome.
   d. It is a weak acid with a pK_a of 9.5.
   e. It fails to inhibit platelet aggregation.
3. Colchicine is effective in the treatment of acute gout because it
   a. inhibits xanthine oxidase.
   b. blocks de novo synthesis of urate.
   c. acts to promote excretion of urate.
   d. inhibits cyclooxygenase and lipooxygenase.
   e. prevents mobilization of leukocytes.
4. Which of the following NSAIDs has the shortest pharmacological $t_{1/2}$?
   a. naproxen
   b. nabumetone
   c. piroxicam
   d. sulindac
   e. ketoprofen
5. The most common adverse side effect of the NSAIDs is
   a. immunologic.
   b. gastrointestinal.
   c. on the central nervous system.
   d. hepatic.
   e. renal.
6. Which of the following is a prodrug and must be metabolically transformed to an active compound?
   a. aspirin
   b. indomethacin
   c. ibuprofen
   d. sulindac
   e. acetaminophen
7. Which of the following is not true of the NSAIDs?
   a. They are rapidly absorbed from the GI tract
   b. There is little to no first-pass metabolism
   c. They are extensively bound to plasma protein
   d. They show are linear relationship between blood concentration and antirheumatic effect
   e. They are inhibitors of cyclooxygenase

CHAPTER 30 Pain Control with General and Local Anesthetics

This chapter is divided into two sections. The first considers general anesthetic agents, administered either by inhalation or IV injection. The second section describes local anesthetic agents, which produce their effects at discrete anatomical sites.

General Anesthetics

YUNG-FONG SUNG
STEPHEN G. HOLTZMAN

MAJOR INHALATIONAL ANESTHETICS

nitrous oxide
desflurane
sevoflurane
enflurane
isoflurane
halothane
methoxyflurane

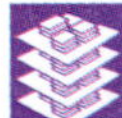

THERAPEUTIC OVERVIEW

Modern surgical procedures would not be possible without anesthetic agents to block the traumatic pain, emotional and physical, that would otherwise be experienced by the patient. Such agents have been available since the 1840s, when diethyl ether was first used successfully to anesthetize patients undergoing surgery.

General anesthesia can be viewed as a controlled reversible state of loss of sensation. From a clinical perspective, the ideal general anesthetic state should comprise analgesia, amnesia, loss of consciousness (absence of awareness), relaxation of skeletal muscles, suppression of somatic, autonomic and endocrine reflexes, and hemodynamic stability. Although most objectives of general anesthesia can be achieved with diethyl ether, this inhalation agent has become obsolete largely because of its flammability and explosiveness. Nevertheless, a range of general anesthetic agents remains available. These typically are subdivided on the basis of their mode of administration: by inhalation or by intravenous injection.

Intravenous administration of an anesthetic agent produces a more rapid and smoother induction of anesthesia that is more pleasant for the patient than induction with an inhalational anesthetic agent is with its slower onset, vapors that may be unpleasant, and facemask delivery. Hypnotic and opioid drugs are often administered intravenously for anesthesia management. In general balanced anesthesia, a combination of various anesthetic agents is used, each in small dosage, to reduce the chance of significant side effects. Combining inhalational and intravenous anesthetic drugs to

ABBREVIATIONS

GABA	γ-aminobutyric acid
MAC	minimum alveolar concentration
N_2O	nitrous oxide
Pco_2	carbon dioxide tension (partial pressure)

THERAPEUTIC CONSIDERATIONS FOR GENERAL ANESTHETIC AGENTS

INHALATIONAL

- Chemical stability
- Irritation upon inhaling
- Speed of onset (time to loss of consciousness)
- Ability to produce analgesia, amnesia, and muscle relaxation
- Side effects, especially cardiovascular and respiratory depression and toxicity to the liver
- Speed and safety of emergence
- Extent of metabolism

INTRAVENOUS

- Chemical stability
- Pain at injection site (water soluble?)
- Speed of onset
- Side effects
- Ability to produce analgesia, amnesia, and muscle relaxation
- Speed and safety of emergence
- Rate of metabolism or redistribution

Structure	Agent
N_2O	nitrous oxide
$CF_3-CHBrCl$	halothane
$CF_3-CHCl-O-CHF_2$	isoflurane
$CHFCl-CF_2-O-CHF_2$	enflurane
$CHCl_2-CF_2-O-CH_3$	methoxyflurane
$CHF_2-O-CHF-CF_3$	desflurane
$CH_2F-O-CH(CF_3)_2$	sevoflurane
$CH_3-CH_2-O-CH_2-CH_3$	diethyl ether

FIGURE 30-1 Structures of principal inhalational general anesthetic agents.

achieve balanced anesthesia is now a common practice.

The safe and effective use of general anesthetic agents is a dynamic process that must be individualized for each patient and surgical situation. The needs of both the surgical team and the patient change during the course of a surgical procedure and may alter anesthetic requirements. For example, at different times there may be a need to (1) blunt the tachycardia and hypertension that result from an intense sympathetic nervous system stimulus, (2) produce greater relaxation of skeletal muscle, or (3) provide additional analgesia. All anesthetic interventions must be reversible, and tissue hypoxia must be prevented.

The primary therapeutic considerations in the use of general anesthetic agents are summarized in the box.

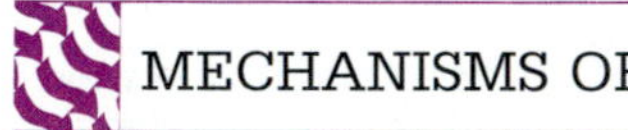

MECHANISMS OF ACTION

Inhalational Anesthetics

The molecular basis for the anesthetic action of inhalational agents is poorly understood. The absence of any obvious structure-activity relationship (Figure 30-1) indicates that, unlike most other therapeutic agents that act on the central nervous system, anesthetic drugs may not exert their effects by interacting with specific cell-surface receptors. More than 90 years ago, Meyer and Overton observed that the potency of anesthetic agents correlates highly with their lipid solubility, as measured by the oil:gas partition coefficient (Table 30-1 and Figure 30-2). Indeed, the relationship between lipid solubility and anesthetic potency holds not only for agents that are in clinical use, but also for inert gases, such as xenon and argon, which are not used clinically. This correlation has given rise to several theories of anesthetic action, none of which has been substantiated.

According to the volume-expansion theory, molecules of an anesthetic agent dissolve in the phospholipid bilayer of the neuronal membrane, causing the membrane to expand. This, in turn, impedes the opening of membrane ion channels necessary for the generation and propagation of action potentials. That anesthesia in laboratory animals can be reversed by increasing the atmospheric pressure provides some support for this theory. Another hypothesis is that anesthetic molecules bind to specific hydrophobic regions of lipoproteins in the neuronal membrane that either are part of or are close to an ion channel. The resulting conformational changes in the protein prevent effective function of the ion channel. Anesthetic agents also might affect the fluidity of membrane lipids. This action could prevent or limit increases in ion conductances.

It also is possible that the seemingly "nonspecific" membrane effects of anesthetic agents may occur at specific cell-surface receptors for neurotransmitters or neuromodulators. For example, in synaptosomal preparations from rat cerebral cortex, volatile anesthetic agents stimulated Cl^- uptake through Cl^- channels gated by receptors for γ-aminobutyric acid (GABA). Clinically relevant concentrations of halothane, enflu-

Table 30-1 Characteristics of Inhalational Anesthetic Agents

Anesthetic Agent	Minimum Alveolar Concentration (MAC—% of 1 atmosphere)	Oil:Gas Partition Coefficient	Blood:Gas Partition Coefficient	Approximate Anesthetic Dose Metabolized (%)
nitrous oxide	105*	1.4	0.47	nil
desflurane	7.0	19	0.42	0.5
sevoflurane	2.0	53	0.63	3
diethyl ether	1.9	65	12	—
enflurane	1.7	98	1.9	3
isoflurane	1.2	98	1.4	0.5
halothane	0.75	225	2.3	15
methoxyflurane	0.16	825	13	60

*Possible only in a hyperbaric chamber.

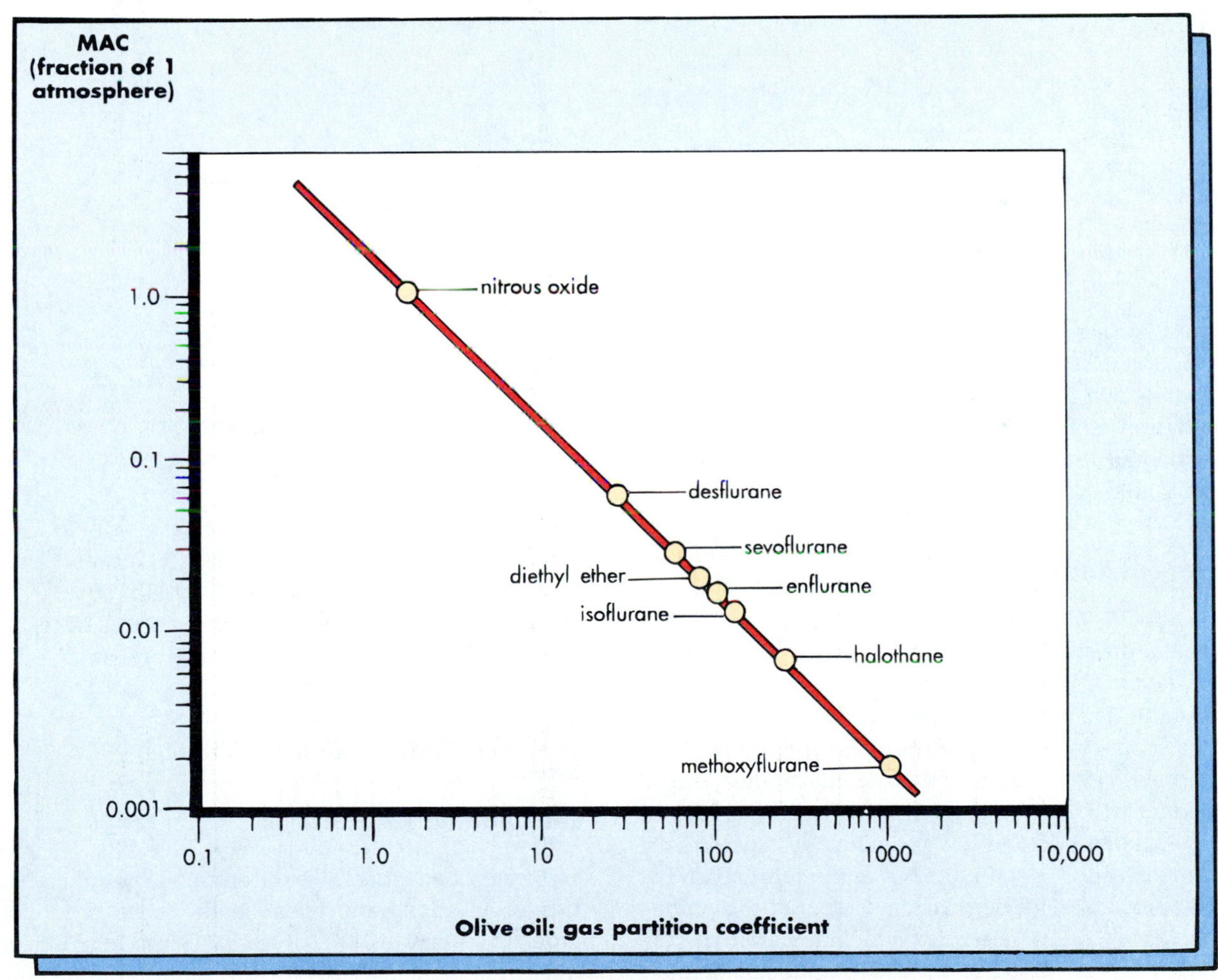

FIGURE 30-2 The potency of an inhalational anesthetic agent is determined by its lipid solubility, as measured by its oil:gas partition coefficient. Methoxyflurane is the most potent, and nitrous oxide (N_2O) is the least potent of the agents considered above.

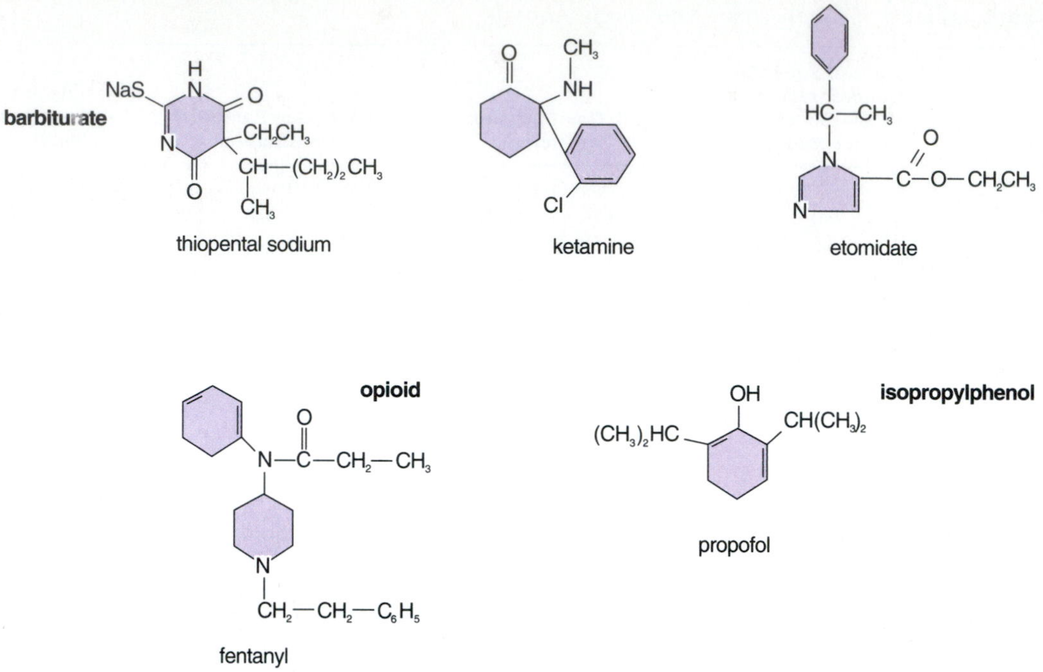

barbiturate

thiopental sodium

ketamine

etomidate

opioid

fentanyl

isopropylphenol

propofol

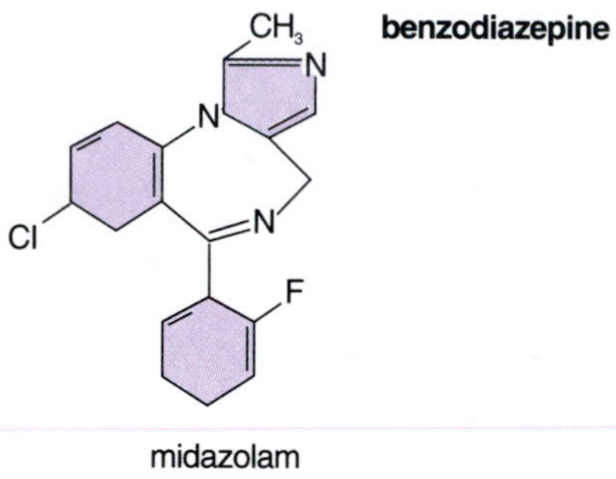

benzodiazepine

midazolam

FIGURE 30-3 Structures of representative IV general anesthetic drugs.

rane, and isoflurane greatly increased the Cl^- conductance induced by GABA in neurons of the rat dorsal root ganglion. Because GABA is the principal inhibitory neurotransmitter in the brain, activation or enhancement of GABA-mediated Cl^- conductance would serve to inhibit neuronal activity in the central nervous system.

Intravenous Anesthetics

In contrast to the uncertainty surrounding the mechanism of anesthetic action of inhalational agents, most intravenous anesthetic drugs (Figure 30-3) have well-documented effects at specific cell-surface receptors that account for much of their therapeutic activity. For example, barbiturates and benzodiazepines act at two distinct recognition sites on the $GABA_A$ receptor/chloride channel molecular complex to potentiate GABA-mediated Cl^- conductance and neuronal inhibition (Chapter 25). The depressant effects of morphine-like opioids on neuronal activity are mediated by the μ-opioid receptor, those of agonist-antagonist opioids by the μ- and κ-opioid receptors (Chapter 28). Ketamine appears to act not by enhancing neuronal inhibition but by blocking neuronal excitation. Ketamine binds to the phencyclidine receptor, a site located within the cation channel that is gated by the *N*-methyl-D-aspartate type of glutamate receptor. Binding to this receptor blocks cation conductance through the channel, thereby blocking the actions of glutamic acid, the principal excitatory neurotransmitter in the brain. The mechanisms of action of etomidate and propofol remain obscure at this time, though a facilitatory effect on the $GABA_A$ receptor/chloride ionophore complex is promising.

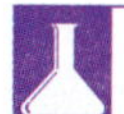

PHARMACOKINETICS

Inhalational Anesthetics

Depth of anesthesia is determined by the concentration of an anesthetic agent in the brain. Therefore, in order to induce a level of anesthesia adequate for surgery, it is necessary to transfer an appropriate amount of general anesthetic agent from the anesthetic machine to the brain of the patient. Unlike most of the other therapeutic agents covered in this textbook, inhalational anesthetic agents are administered as gases or vapors. Therefore a different set of physical principles applies.

In a mixture of gases, the partial pressure of an anesthetic agent is directly proportional to its concentration in the mixture. Thus, in a mixture of 5% halothane, 70% nitrous oxide, and 25% oxygen, used during induction of anesthesia, the partial pressures of the component gases in millimeters of mercury (mm Hg) are 38, 532, and 190, respectively, at 1 atmosphere (760 mm Hg) of pressure. This relationship is illustrated in Figure 30-4.

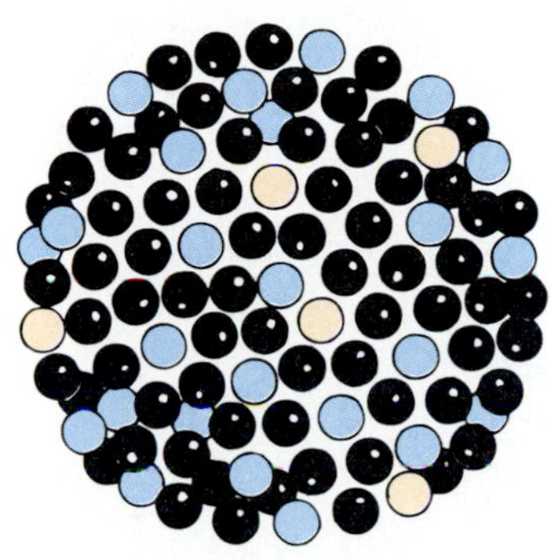

	Concentration %		Partial pressure (mm Hg)
Nitrous oxide	70	(x 760 =)	532
Oxygen	25	(x 760 =)	190
Halothane	5	(x 760 =)	38
	100%	(=)	760 mm Hg (1 atmosphere)

FIGURE 30-4 The partial pressure of any one gas in a mixture of gases is directly proportional to its concentration.

When a gas is dissolved in blood or other body tissues, *its partial pressure is directly proportional to its concentration but inversely proportional to its solubility in that tissue.* The concept of partial pressure is of central importance because the partial pressure of a gas is the driving force that moves the gas from one phase to the next, from anesthetic machine to lung, from lung to blood, from blood to brain. At theoretical equilibrium, the partial pressures will be equal in all body tissues, in alveoli, and in the inspired gas mixture. However, because solubility varies from tissue to tissue, the concentration of the anesthetic agent must also vary from tissue to tissue if partial pressures are equal throughout the body. For example, if halothane was administered in a concentration of 1%, at theoretical equilibrium its concentration would be 0.39 millimolar in alveoli, 0.9 millimolar in blood, and 3.2 millimolar in brain while its partial pressure in each of these locations would be a uniform 7.6 mm Hg.

Figure 30-5 is a schema of the path followed by an inhalational anesthetic agent during induction of and emergence from anesthesia. Induction of anesthesia is

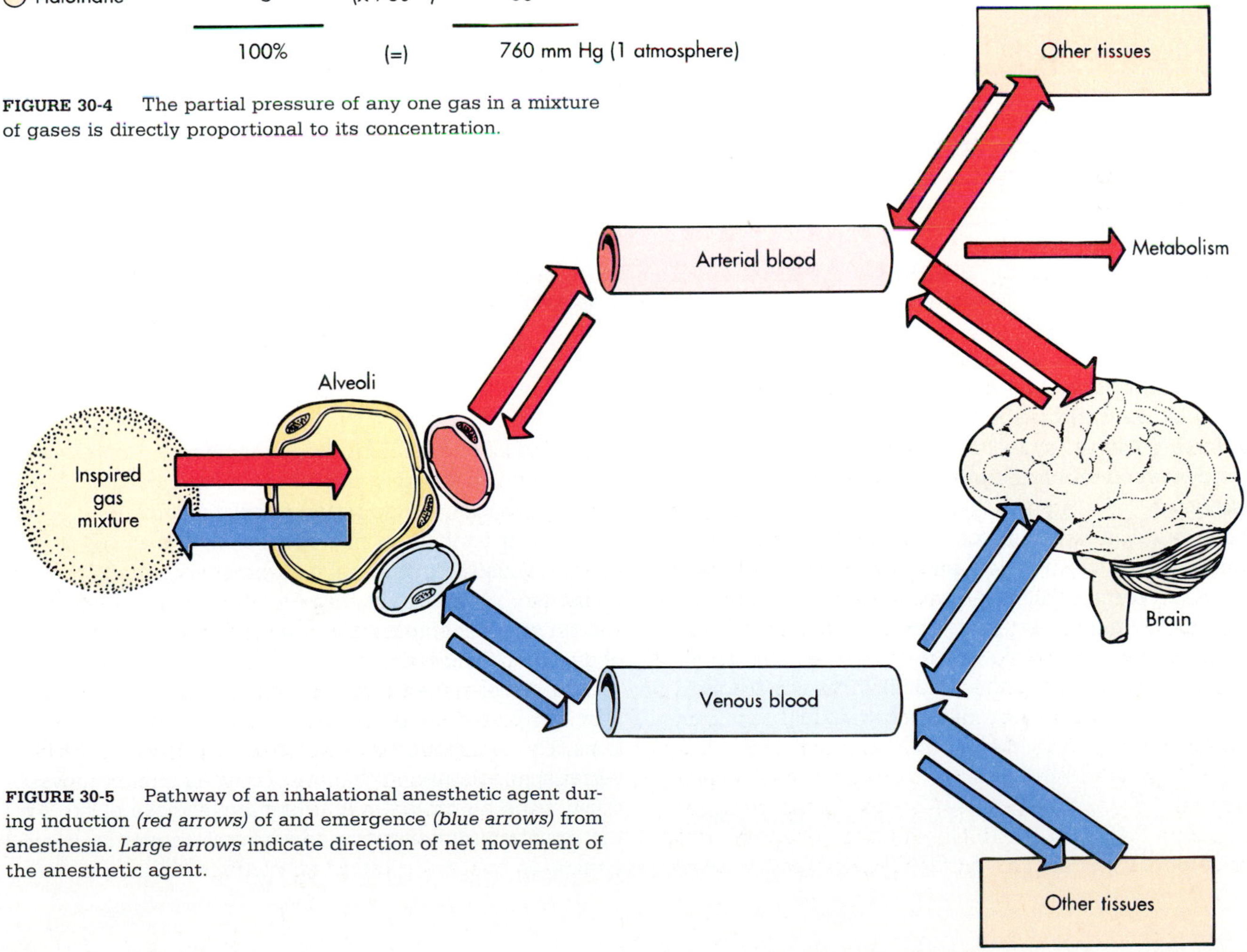

FIGURE 30-5 Pathway of an inhalational anesthetic agent during induction *(red arrows)* of and emergence *(blue arrows)* from anesthesia. *Large arrows* indicate direction of net movement of the anesthetic agent.

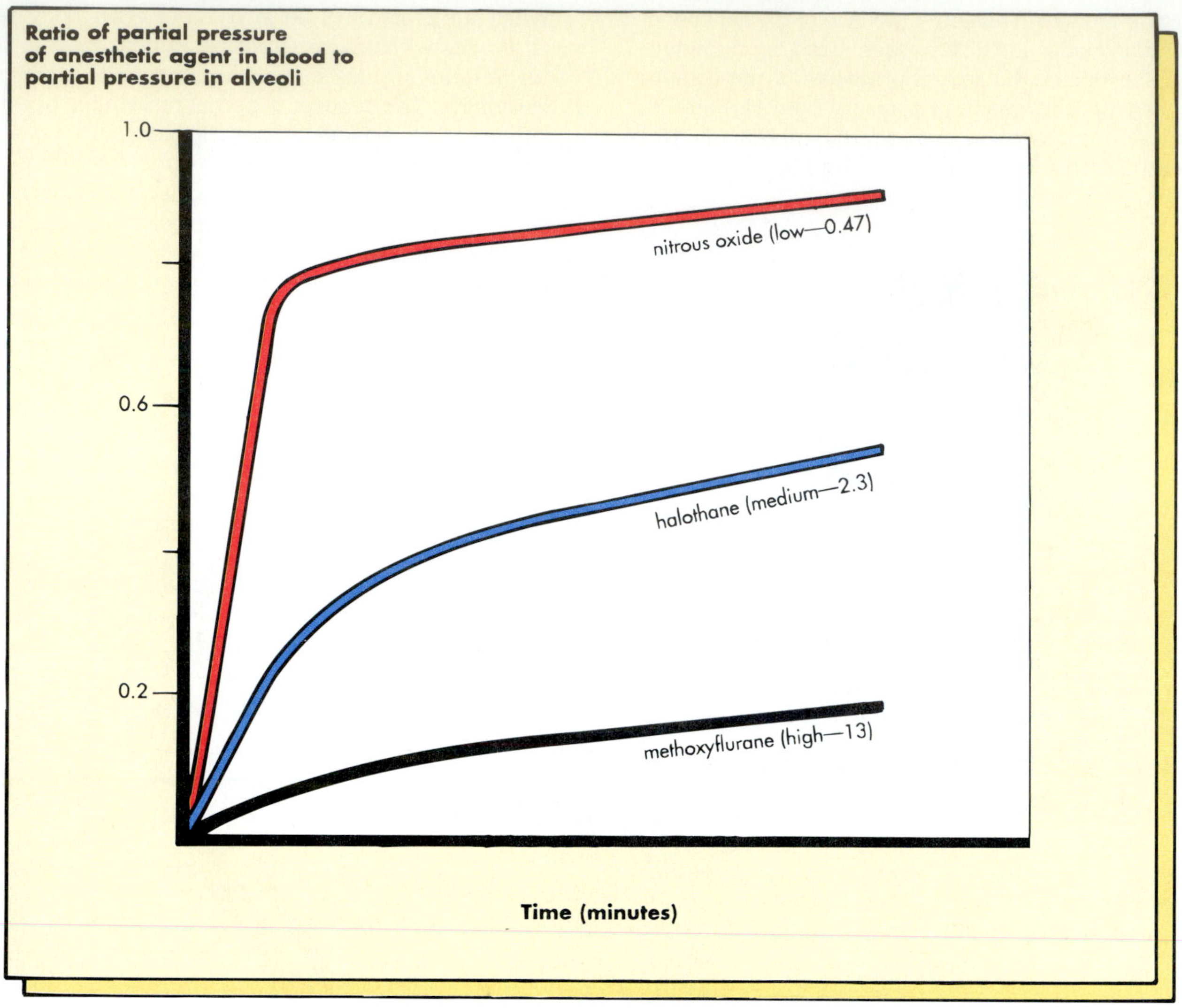

FIGURE 30-6 The rate of rise of partial pressure of an inhalational anesthetic agent in arterial blood is determined by its solubility in blood (blood: gas partition coefficient).

facilitated by factors that maintain a high partial pressure of the anesthetic agent in the inspired gas mixture, in the alveolar space, and in arterial blood, in order to deliver as much of the gas as quickly as possible to the brain.

The partial pressure (or concentration) of the anesthetic agent in the inspired gas mixture is the factor most easily controlled by the anesthesiologist. This is accomplished simply by adjustment of the anesthetic machine to optimize partial pressures during induction.

Alveolar ventilation is the product of rate of respiration and tidal volume less pulmonary dead space, as shown:

$$\text{Alveolar ventilation} = \text{Respiratory rate} \times (\text{Tidal volume} - \text{Dead space})$$

The rate of induction is decreased by factors that reduce alveolar ventilation. For example, preoperative treatment of the patient with respiratory depressant drugs, such as a barbiturate or an opioid analgesic, decreases the rate of respiration or tidal volume, decreasing alveolar ventilation in the absence of assisted ventilation. Alveolar dead space is great in patients with pulmonary disorders, such as emphysema or atelectasis, which also decrease alveolar ventilation and the rate of anesthetic induction.

The alveolar membrane poses no barrier to gases, permitting unhindered diffusion of a gas in both directions. Therefore, once the anesthetic gas reaches the alveolar space, following the law of mass action, it moves down its partial-pressure gradient into alveolar blood. At the initiation of anesthetic administration, partial pres-

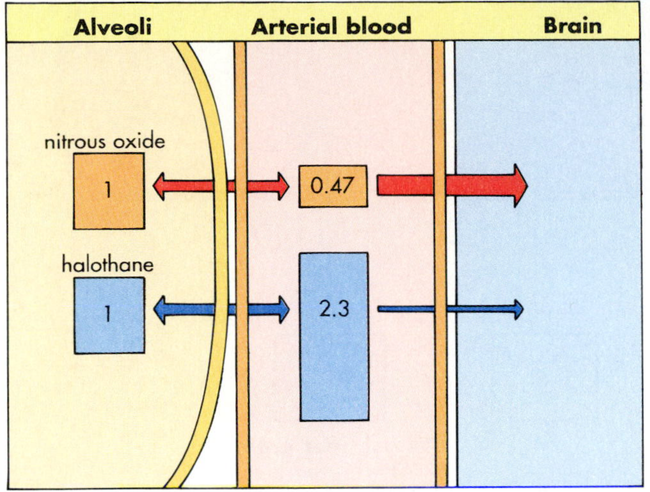

FIGURE 30-7 The solubility of an inhalational anesthetic agent in blood determines how rapidly its partial pressure will rise in blood and brain with a change in its partial pressure in the inspired gas mixture. If the alveolar space and blood were a closed system and nitrous oxide (N_2O) and halothane were allowed to equilibrate between the two, there would be 0.47 parts of N_2O in blood for every 1 part in the alveoli; there would be 2.3 parts of halothane in blood for every 1 part in the alveoli. An increase in the partial pressure of N_2O in the inspired-gas mixture would result in almost a fivefold larger increase in its partial pressure in blood than a similar increase would in the partial pressure of halothane in the inspired-gas mixture, driving N_2O into the brain more rapidly.

sure of the anesthetic agent in the alveolar space is much higher than that in blood. Therefore the partial-pressure gradient between alveolar space and arteriolar blood is high, and initially the anesthetic gas moves rapidly into blood. As the partial pressure of the anesthetic agent in blood increases, the gradient between alveolar space and blood becomes smaller, and the rate of uptake slows. This relationship is illustrated in Figure 30-6.

Another important factor in the rate of rise of the arterial partial pressure of an inhalational anesthetic agent is the solubility of the gas in blood. This relationship is expressed as a blood:gas partition coefficient. The higher the solubility of an anesthetic agent in blood, the more must be dissolved in blood to produce a change in partial pressure (as partial pressure is inversely proportional to solubility). This relationship is illustrated in Figure 30-7 for nitrous oxide and halothane.

Nitrous oxide (N_2O) has a blood:gas partition coefficient of 0.47, and so relatively little needs to be dissolved in blood for its partial pressure in blood to rise. In contrast, blood serves as a larger reservoir for halothane, retaining at equilibrium 2.3 parts for every 1 part in the alveolar space. Induction depends *not* on dissolving the anesthetic agent in blood but on raising arterial partial pressure to drive the gas from the blood to the brain. Therefore, the rate of rise of arterial partial pressure and speed of induction are fastest for those gases least soluble in blood. This relationship also can be seen in Figure 30-6. The blood:gas partition coefficients of inhalational anesthetics are shown in Table 30-1.

Cardiac output determines the rate of pulmonary blood flow. Intuitively, it would seem that an increase in cardiac output and hence an increase in pulmonary blood flow would increase the speed of induction of anesthesia. However, the opposite is true; the rate of anesthetic induction decreases with increasing cardiac output for two reasons. First, with all other factors being constant, an increased pulmonary blood flow means that the same volume of gas from the alveoli diffuses into a larger volume of blood per unit time. The initial consequence is a reduced concentration of anesthetic agent in blood. Because partial pressure is directly proportional to concentration, partial pressure in arterial blood will increase more slowly. Second, the brain normally receives an optimal percentage of cardiac output. Therefore, any increase in cardiac output usually will benefit tissues other than brain, such as muscle, thereby increasing the apparent volume of distribution of anesthetic agent. In a patient with heart failure, blood loss, or other conditions that result in decreased cardiac output, the volume of distribution of anesthetic agent will be reduced and the rate of induction will be increased.

Transfer of anesthetic agent from arterial blood to brain depends on factors analogous to those involved in the movement of gas from alveoli to arterial blood. These include the partial-pressure gradient between blood and brain, the solubility of anesthetic agent in brain, and cerebral blood flow. The brain is part of the vessel-rich group of tissues that compose 9% of body mass but receive 75% of cardiac output. When the anesthetic uptake curve levels off (Figure 30-6), this leveling reflects the attainment of equilibrium of the vessel-rich group of tissues. By contrast, the muscle group represents 50% of the mass of the body but receives only 18% of the cardiac output. Fat represents, on the average, 19% of body mass and receives 5% of cardiac output, whereas the vessel-poor group, bone and tendon, account for 22% of body mass yet receive less than 2% of cardiac output. Thus approximately 41% of total body mass receives a mere 7% of cardiac output. As a consequence, in most surgical procedures poorly perfused tissues do not contribute meaningfully to the apparent volume of distribution of the inhalational anesthetic, and true total equilibration does not occur. The importance of tissue perfusion as a factor determining the uptake of an anesthetic drug is illustrated for halothane in Figure 30-8.

The major factors that affect the rate of induction of

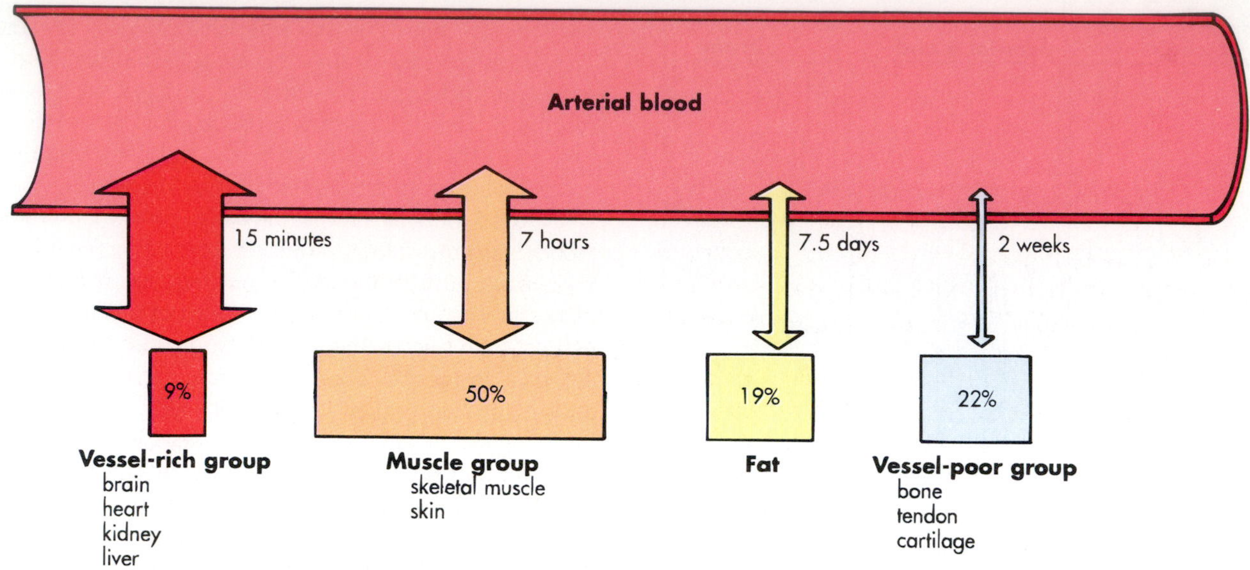

FIGURE 30-8 The rate at which an inhalational anesthetic agent is taken up by a tissue depends on the fraction of the cardiac output that the tissue receives. The approximate time for halothane to equilibrate between blood and tissues is indicated next to the arrows; the percentage of body mass that the tissue represents is shown in the boxes.

Table 30-2 Factors Affecting the Rate of Induction with an Inhalational Anesthetic Agent

Condition	Rate of Induction
↑Concentration of anesthetic in inspired-gas mixture	↑
↑Alveolar ventilation	↑
↑Solubility of anesthetic in blood (blood:gas partition coefficient)	↓
↑Cardiac output	↓

anesthesia with an inhalational agent are summarized in Table 30-2.

When administration of the anesthetic agent is terminated, the anesthetic gas flows from venous blood to the alveolar space (Figure 30-5). The factors that affect the rate of elimination of an inhalational anesthetic agent are analogous to those that determine the rate of uptake. Therefore the rate of loss of an anesthetic gas during emergence from anesthesia is directly proportional to its rate of uptake, and emergence from anesthesia is thus a mirror image of induction.

Although inhaled anesthetics are cleared from the body via the lung, most undergo some degree of metabolism, primarily in the liver. Although metabolism of inhalational anesthetics is not primarily responsible for the termination of drug action, their metabolites have been implicated in organ toxicity associated with some of these agents. Extensive metabolism of methoxyflurane, 50% to 60% of an administered dose, results in the release of fluoride ions, which can reach nephrotoxic concentrations during long surgical procedures. This is the principal reason for the rapid decline in methoxyflurane use. The extent of biotransformation of the other inhalational anesthetic agents ranges from approximately 15% for halothane to negligible amounts for nitrous oxide (see Table 30-1). Fewer toxic effects are generally observed with agents that are minimally metabolized.

Intravenous Anesthetics

Intravenous anesthetic drugs are administered directly into the bloodstream. Thereafter, movement of the drug molecule from blood to brain determines the time to its onset of action. The most rapid induction of anesthesia is produced by the short-acting barbiturates propofol and etomidate; 30 to 50 seconds from injection to loss of the eyelash reflex during one arm-to-brain circulation. A similar degree of reflex obtundation may require several minutes after the administration of a benzodiazepine.

A good intravenous anesthetic drug should have effects within one arm-to-brain blood circulation. Blood flow to the brain is also an important factor. The onset of drug effect may be delayed in a patient with extremely low cardiac output and therefore relatively low blood flow to the brain.

The duration of effect of a single induction dose of an intravenous anesthetic is determined by the rate of redistribution or metabolism of the drug. Redistribution of the drug from the brain into less well-perfused tissues (i.e., abdominal viscera, skeletal muscle, and fat) is the predominant mechanism responsible for termination of the effect. This mechanism can be so efficient that within minutes of induction of anesthesia with a single dose of anesthetic, reflex activity and then consciousness return. The several intravenous induction agents have different speeds of onset, durations of action, and rates of redistribution. The pharmacokinetic and physicochemical characteristics of the ideal intravenous anesthetic are listed in the box.

Thiopental has been used extensively for intravenous induction because of its rapid smooth onset and short duration of action. It is highly lipid soluble, rapidly crosses the blood-brain barrier, and is rapidly redistributed from the brain to other tissues. These pharmacokinetic characteristics of thiopental preclude its use as a maintenance agent for lengthy procedures. Because of its long terminal elimination half-life (Table 30-3), thiopental will accumulate in the body upon repeated dosing. With repeated administration its duration of action increases, and patients may remain unconscious after the operation is finished. Thiopental is primarily metabolized in the liver. Its metabolites are water soluble and are excreted in the urine. The pharmacokinetic properties of other barbiturates available for use as intravenous anesthetic agents, such as methohexital, are generally similar to those of thiopental.

Induction of anesthesia with diazepam is relatively slow, often taking several minutes. Diazepam has a long redistribution half-life of from 30 to 60 minutes, a long duration of action, and a long terminal elimination half-life (Table 30-3). It is metabolized by microsomal enzymes in liver, but the majority of its metabolites are pharmacologically active and, like the parent compound, have long half-lives. Midazolam, on the other hand, is a water-soluble benzodiazepine twice as potent as diazepam. For intravenous induction, midazolam has an onset time (2 to 3 minutes) more rapid than that of diazepam, but slower than that of thiopental.

Propofol is twice as potent as thiopental. After induction, loss of consciousness will occur within one arm-to-brain circulation time. The induction dosage is much lower in the elderly patient and slightly higher in younger children. Propofol can be used as both an induction and a maintenance anesthetic agent. Duration of sleep after a single propofol injection is 5 to 10 minutes. To achieve a more sustained effect after induction, the patient either should be given another bolus dose within 5 minutes or should receive continuous infusion. The latter is preferred for smooth maintenance and constant plasma concentrations. The redistribution half-life is 5 to 10 minutes. A long terminal-elimination half-life indicates that propofol may accumulate in the body after prolonged use.

The duration of action of ketamine is 11 to 16 min-

CHARACTERISTICS OF IDEAL INTRAVENOUS ANESTHETIC DRUG

PHYSICOCHEMICAL

water soluble
stable on shelf and to light exposure
lipophilic
small injection volume

PHARMACOKINETIC

rapid onset of action
short duration of action
nontoxic metabolites

PHARMACODYNAMIC

wide margin of safety
no interpatient variability in effects
nonallergenic
nontoxic to tissues

Table 30-3 Comparison of Intravenous Anesthetic Induction Agents in Healthy Adults

Drug	Water Soluble	Induction Dosage (mg/kg)	Termination $t_{1/2}$ (hours)	Active Metabolites
thiopental	Yes	3.0-6.0	10-12	None
diazepam	No	0.3-0.6	50	Several
midazolam	Yes	0.2-0.4	2-6	One
propofol	No	2.0-4.0	3-6	None
ketamine	Yes	1.0-3.0	2-3	None
etomidate	No	0.2-0.4	2-5	None
methohexital	Yes	1.0-1.5	3-5	None

utes. In addition to its use for induction of anesthesia, ketamine is used for sedation and analgesia at IV doses of 0.5 to 1.0 mg/kg.

Morphine, the prototypical opioid, is given in doses of 8 to 15 mg subcutaneously or intramuscularly to allay anxiety and ease pain before, during, and after surgery, and intravenously in substantially higher doses combined with an inhalational or intravenous agent for induction and maintenance of anesthesia. Because of low lipophilicity, morphine crosses the blood-brain barrier slowly, and plasma concentrations of the drug may not accurately reflect those in the brain. It is metabolized in the liver primarily by conjugation with glucuronic acid; morphine-6-glucuronide retains considerable morphine-like activity but has limited access to the CNS.

The other opioids commonly used in anesthesia differ from morphine in potency and in rate of onset and duration of action but are generally similar to morphine in their basic profiles of pharmacological activity. Meperidine is ⅕ to ⅒ as potent as morphine and has a slightly shorter duration of action. An intermediary metabolite of meperidine has been implicated in drug interactions that cause convulsions. Fentanyl is 100 to 200 times more potent than morphine. Its high lipophilicity is responsible for its rapid onset of action and short duration. The drug is redistributed from the brain to other tissues in a manner similar to thiopental. Sufentanil is 5 to 10 times more potent than fentanyl, alfentanil is ⅓ to ⅕ as potent; both have a shorter duration of action than fentanyl has.

The physicochemical properties of some intravenous anesthetic drugs render them insoluble in water at physiological pH, necessitating the use of solvents (Table 30-3), which can lead to clinical problems. The alkaline pH of a 2.5% solution of thiopental makes it unsuitable for mixing with acidic drugs, especially opioid analgesics and muscle relaxants. In addition, thiopental solutions will cause tissue damage if injected intra-arterially or extravascularly. Acidic etomidate solution can cause pain and thrombophlebitis after intravascular injection. All alcohol-based solvents and buffers are venous irritants, causing pain when injected IV. For this reason, diazepam solution is sometimes mixed with a solution of lidocaine for a less painful IV injection. Midazolam, in contrast, is water soluble and poses no special problems for IV administration.

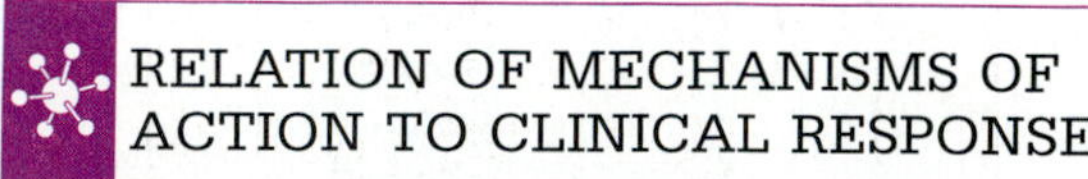

RELATION OF MECHANISMS OF ACTION TO CLINICAL RESPONSE

Inhalational Anesthetics

The potency of an inhalational anesthetic agent is expressed in terms of the minimum alveolar concentration (MAC) that prevents 50% of patients from responding to a painful stimulus, such as a skin incision. MAC is analogous to the median effective dose (ED_{50}), which is used to express the relative potency of nongaseous drugs. Clearly, one should administer an inhalational anesthetic agent at a concentration higher than 1.0 MAC to achieve an acceptable level of surgical anesthesia in which there is no movement in the patient. The dose-effect curve of inhalational anesthetic agents is steep: 1.0 MAC defines the ED_{50}, 1.1 MAC is approximately an ED_{84}, and 1.2 MAC an ED_{97}. A level of anesthesia satisfactory for most surgical procedures is achieved at an alveolar gas concentration of 1.3 MAC.

Doses of inhalational anesthetic agents are additive, and so 0.5 MAC of one can be combined with 0.5 MAC of another to give an inspired-gas mixture that has MAC value of 1.0. For example, 1 MAC of halothane is 0.75% (5.7 mm Hg, or 5.7 torr at 1.0 atmosphere of pressure), and 1 MAC of isoflurane is 1.15% (8.7 torr). Therefore an inspired gas mixture containing 0.375% halothane and 0.507% isoflurane will have a MAC of 1.0.

Except for nitrous oxide, all inhalational anesthetic agents in clinical use are sufficiently potent (i.e., have a low enough MAC) to produce surgical levels of anesthesia when administered in a gaseous mixture containing at least 25% oxygen (see Table 30-1). Therefore, MAC is not an important factor in determining inhalational anesthetic agent selection. Nevertheless, it provides a convenient point of reference for comparing properties of anesthetic agents. For example, it can be useful to compare the amount of hypotension or relaxation of skeletal muscles produced by two different anesthetic agents when each is administered at 1.0 MAC.

The MAC of an inhalational anesthetic is independent of the duration of the surgical procedure, remaining unchanged over time, and is unaffected by gender. It also is relatively independent of the type of noxious stimulus applied (e.g., pressure versus heat). Indeed, increasing the intensity of the noxious stimulus, within limits, has little affect on MAC, though some traumatic surgical manipulations require higher anesthetic concentrations. MAC is unaffected by the acid-base status of the patient and is independent of the size of the patient's body mass. However, at a fixed alveolar concentration, it will take longer to anesthetize a larger patient than it will to anesthetize a smaller patient because of differences in the apparent volume of distribution. Although the MAC of an anesthetic agent is relatively independent of many patient and surgical parameters, it is affected by other factors. One is the age of the patient. The anesthetic requirement (i.e., MAC) is higher for infants and lower for geriatric patients. The general health of the patient also determines the anesthetic requirement. Not surprisingly, MAC is lower in a debilitated patient than in an otherwise healthy one. Another determinant of MAC is the presence of other drugs. In general, the MAC of an inhalational anesthetic agent is reduced in patients who have received CNS depressants. In the surgical patient, these drugs are commonly opioid analgesics, antianxiety agents, sedative drugs, and intravenous anesthetic agents used for induction. Indeed, CNS depressants frequently are administered preoperatively or intraoperatively for the purpose of lowering the MAC of an inhalational anesthetic agent. Nitrous oxide, which cannot be used safely by itself to produce surgical levels of anesthesia, is a common component of anesthetic-gas mixtures. A concentration of 70% nitrous oxide in an inspired gas mixture lowers the MAC of the halogenated agent by one half to two thirds. On the other hand, alcoholic patients who have developed a tolerance to the CNS-depressant effects of ethanol often have an increased anesthetic requirement, as do patients who have developed tolerance to barbiturates and benzodiazepines. CNS stimulants also increase MAC. Although a stimulant drug is unlikely to be administered to a hospitalized patient, because of the widespread abuse of stimulant drugs, it is possible to encounter a patient undergoing emergency surgery who has appreciable tissue concentrations of cocaine or amphetamine.

Intravenous Anesthetics

One monitors the onset of induction of anesthesia with intravenous agents by administering a single dose and following the loss of lash or cough reflex, etc. Factors that alter the apparent volume of distribution of intravenous agents, including protein binding and dilutional effects, can change the amount of agent required to obtund body reflexes. Administration of an insufficient dosage of a single intravenous agent may lead to transient excitation. For example, methohexital may produce hiccups, etomidate myoclonic twitches, and thiopental and propofol unpurposeful movements. Thiopental may also cause laryngeal spasm in an asthmatic patient, especially where dosage is insufficient or the patient is inadequately premedicated.

The majority of intravenous anesthetic agents (hypnotics, opioids) do not have muscle relaxant effects. Most hypnotics except ketamine have no analgesic effects. In fact, thiopental has antianalgesic effects, as mentioned previously.

Ketamine may produce both hypnotic (dissociative) and analgesic effects. However, it often causes "bad dreams" if not combined with a small dosage of a benzodiazepine.

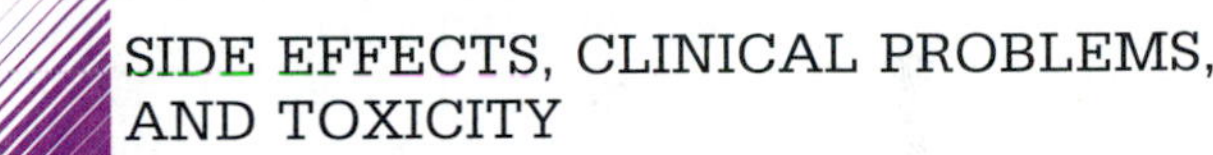

SIDE EFFECTS, CLINICAL PROBLEMS, AND TOXICITY

Inhalational Anesthetics

All inhalational anesthetic agents reduce spontaneous respiration in a concentration-dependent manner by depressing medullary centers in the brainstem. General anesthetic drugs decrease the responsiveness of chemoreceptors in respiratory centers to elevations in carbon dioxide tension (P_{CO_2}) in blood and cerebrospinal fluid. The P_{CO_2} normally serves as a potent stimulus for increasing minute ventilation. Inhalation anesthetic agents flatten the P_{CO_2} ventilation-response curve and shift it to the right (Figure 30-9). Thus the ventilatory response to hypercapnia is attenuated. Opioid analgesics also reduce the responsiveness of brainstem chemoreceptors to elevations in carbon dioxide tension. By themselves, opioid analgesics shift the P_{CO_2} ventilation-response curve in a manner similar to that of general anesthetics. When an opioid analgesic is given concurrently with an inhalational anesthetic drug, the effects of the two on respiration are at least additive and often synergistic, as shown in Figure 30-9. Carbon dioxide exerts a local effect on the cerebrovasculature by dilating small vessels. The increase in intracranial pressure that results is a cause for concern in patients with head trauma.

Although all inhalational anesthetic agents will depress myocardial contractility in a concentration-dependent manner in isolated heart preparations, in patients the effects on myocardial function vary, depending on the agent and the concentration needed for surgical anesthesia and the drug's effects on the sympathetic nervous system. N_2O has minimal effects on cardiovascular function, whereas halothane signifi-

CLINICAL PROBLEMS

INHALATIONAL AGENTS

Depression of respiratory drive because of lower response to CO_2 or to hypoxia
Depressed cardiovascular drive
Gaseous space enlargement by nitrous oxide
Fluoride-ion toxicity from methoxyflurane
Malignant hyperthermia

INTRAVENOUS AGENTS

Depression of respiratory drive because of lower response to CO_2 or to hypoxia
Depressed cardiovascular drive
Muscular rigidity (opioids, ketamine)
Ketamine hallucinations and emergence delirium
Etomidate steroidogenesis inhibition
Thiopental reduces pain threshold

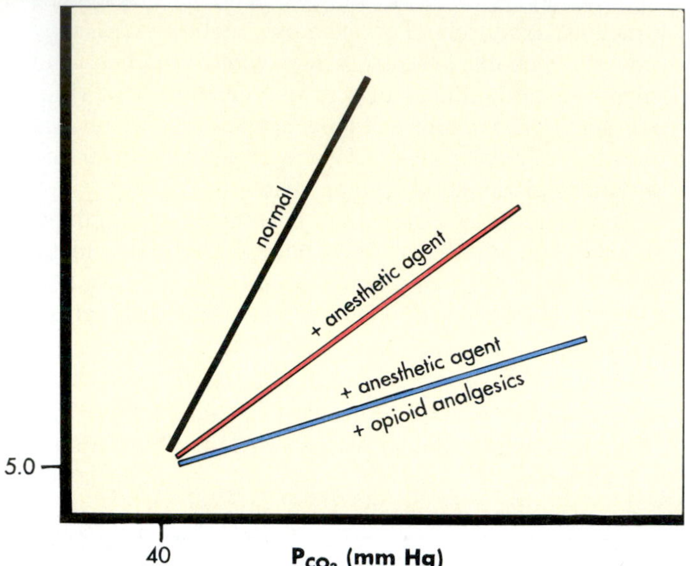

FIGURE 30-9 Anesthetic agents reduce the ventilatory response to increases in carbon dioxide tension (P_{CO_2}) in blood and cerebrospinal fluid. This effect is exacerbated by opioid analgesics.

cantly depresses most cardiovascular parameters. The other anesthetic agents fall between N_2O and halothane with respect to effects on the cardiovascular system. In addition to directly depressing myocardial contractility and reducing cardiac output, halothane depresses the central outflow of the sympathetic nervous system, depresses the baroreceptor reflex, and relaxes peripheral vascular smooth muscle. The last effect is attributable both to a direct action of halothane on vascular smooth muscle and the secondary consequence of elevated blood concentrations of carbon dioxide from depression of brainstem respiratory centers. The overall effect is hypotension and decreased general organ perfusion. Halothane also sensitizes the conducting tissue of the myocardium to arrhythmias induced by catecholamines. This action is shared with methoxyflurane and, to a lesser extent, with enflurane. Therefore, caution must be exercised when one is administering pressor drugs to counteract the hypotension induced by these anesthetic agents.

The liver and the kidney are the most prominent targets of undesirable effects of anesthetic agents. Generally, metabolites of the anesthetic drugs rather than the parent drugs have been implicated in organ toxicity. "Halothane hepatitis" occurs in 1 of 10,000 to 20,000 cases, with fatal hepatic necrosis occurring in about half of these instances. A metabolite of halothane is postulated to form a hapten that triggers an immunological response. However, it is difficult to determine which toxic effects are attributable to the anesthetic agent itself or to its metabolites. Some adverse effects are probably secondary to the anesthetic-induced decrease in cardiac output and blood flow to the liver or may result from blood transfusions administered during surgery. Liver function tests commonly show abnormalities for 1 or more days after administration of inhalational anesthetics. Although halothane has been administered safely countless times, the specter of hepatic toxicity has reduced its use, particularly in the United States, in favor of newer (and more expensive) halogenated agents.

Renal blood flow and glomerular filtration rate are decreased during general anesthesia, resulting in decreased urine formation. Methoxyflurane undergoes extensive metabolism in the liver and releases free fluoride ions, which can be nephrotoxic during lengthy surgical procedures, particularly if the concentration of methoxyflurane is maintained close to the MAC. Impaired renal function is manifested by a high output of urine, similar to that in diabetes insipidus, followed by renal failure. The possibility of nephrotoxicity has rendered methoxyflurane largely obsolete. Free fluoride ions also are released during the metabolism of enflurane and sevoflurane. However, with these agents, free fluoride ions do not reach concentrations toxic to the kidney. Nevertheless, enflurane should be avoided in patients with impaired renal function. Halothane, though metabolized to an appreciable extent (Table 30-1), does not release significant amounts of free fluoride ions.

Halogenated inhalational anesthetic agents, and halothane in particular, can precipitate malignant hyperthermia in genetically susceptible patients. Drugs that relax skeletal muscle by depolarization, notably succinylcholine, can also trigger this event, which is manifest as a sustained contraction of the musculature with a dramatic increase in oxygen consumption. Body temperature can rise by 0.2° C per minute. The syndrome apparently results from a failure of sarcoplasmic reticulum to resequester Ca^{++}, preventing dissociation of actin and myosin filaments of muscle. The resultant hyperthermia is an emergency requiring prompt treatment, including rapid cooling and administering dantrolene to counteract the excessive release of Ca^{++} from the sarcoplasmic reticulum, thus ensuring adequate oxygenation. The overall incidence of malignant hyperthermia is 1 of 15,000 to 50,000 cases. Its highest incidence occurs when halothane and succinylcholine are used together, and it is lowest when a halogenated anesthetic agent other than halothane is used with another muscle relaxant.

Nitrous oxide, the only gaseous anesthetic agent currently in use, lacks sufficient potency to produce surgical levels of anesthesia safely by itself and does not relax skeletal muscles. Nevertheless, now in its second century of clinical use, it remains the most widely used inhalational anesthetic agent in technologically advanced countries. It can produce analgesia comparable to that of a therapeutic dose of morphine and induces amnesia as well. However, between these latter two effects, it can induce a state of disinhibited behavior and raucousness in patients not receiving other drugs concurrently (Table 30-4). It is this action of N_2O that gives rise to the term "laughing gas." Most often, N_2O is administered in combination with a halogenated anesthetic agent to lower the anesthetic requirement for the latter, as well as to promote rapid induction (see Figure 30-6). The minimal effect of N_2O on cardiovascular function is another advantage of its use.

Nitrous oxide diffuses into enclosed air-filled cavities in the body where it becomes exchanged with nitrogen. Because of a difference in the blood:gas partition coefficients of these two gases, blood can carry much more nitrous oxide than it can nitrogen. N_2O diffuses out of blood and into air-filled cavities about 35 times faster than nitrogen leaves these cavities and enters the blood. The result is an increase in pressure and distention of enclosed air-filled nitrogen-containing spaces. This unwanted situation might be encountered where there is occlusion of the middle ear, pneumothorax, obstructed intestine, air emboli in the bloodstream, or after a pneumoencephalogram. These conditions, if not absolute contraindications to the use of N_2O, are at least signals for caution.

Nitrous oxide oxidizes components of vitamin B_{12}, which decreases the availability of this vitamin and inhibits the activity of methionine synthetase, a vitamin B_{12}–dependent enzyme. This results in a decrease in protein and nucleic acid synthesis, megaloblastic anemia, and other signs of vitamin B_{12} deficiency. Inhalation of N_2O for as little as 2 hours can result in a detectable decrease in methionine synthetase activity, and megaloblastic anemia has been observed in severely ill patients several days after exposure. Generally, clinical sequelae do not occur unless exposure time is lengthened from hours to days. However, chronic exposure to low concentrations of N_2O, as might occur in personnel working in settings where N_2O is used without adequate safeguards to avoid contamination of room air, has been linked to neuropathies stemming from vitamin B_{12} deficiency. There is also some evidence that chronic occupational exposure to N_2O reduces fertility in women.

Enflurane initially replaced halothane in popularity before being replaced itself by isoflurane. In general, effects on the cardiovascular system are similar to those of halothane, though cardiac arrhythmias occur less frequently; analgesia and skeletal muscle relaxation are superior to that which can be achieved with halothane.

Table 30-4 Concentration-Related Effects of Nitrous Oxide

% Nitrous Oxide	Effect
20	Analgesia
40	Behavioral disinhibition
60	Amnesia
80	Unconsciousness

Concentrations of enflurane above its MAC, especially during hypocapnia, can cause a characteristic pattern of seizure activity seen on the electroencephalogram, coupled with increased motor activity in the nonmedicated patient. This excitatory effect of enflurane has minimal or no adverse consequences to the patient, who, upon awakening, has no recall of the event. Nevertheless, this action of enflurane may be a consideration in patients with known seizure disorders.

Isoflurane, a structural isomer of enflurane, does not evoke seizures. In fact, isoflurane suppresses electrical activity of the brain and can, in combination with thiopental, provide some protection to the brain against injury from hypoxia.

Desflurane and sevoflurane are the would-be successors to isoflurane. Desflurane was recently approved for clinical use in the United States and sevoflurane is presently in late stages of clinical trials . Their effects on respiration and cardiovascular function appear to be similar to those of isoflurane. Sevoflurane has the disadvantages of undergoing metabolism, with release of fluoride ions, and of interacting with the soda lime in the rebreathing circuit of anesthesia systems. The high vapor pressure of desflurane requires using special vaporizers for administration.

Intravenous Anesthetics

Thiopental, like all barbiturates, is contraindicated in the patient who may be allergic to barbiturates or have a familial history of acute intermittent porphyria. Because it depresses respiration, it should not be used in situations where instrumentation for supporting respiration is not available. Thiopental is contraindicated in cases of cardiovascular instability, such as patients in shock, because it decreases myocardial contractility and also dilates peripheral vessels. Because thiopental decreases the pain threshold, exerting an antianalgesic effect, it must be combined with an analgesic drug before surgery. Thiopental causes less nausea and vomiting postoperatively than inhalational anesthetic agents do, but causes more than propofol.

Because diazepam is a respiratory depressant, its use as a sole induction agent is contraindicated in ultrashort procedures, in chronic obstructive airway disease, or where no facilities exist for airway and respiratory management. Midazolam depresses cardiovascular function equally to thiopental when equivalent doses for induction are compared. However, a smaller dose of midazolam given incrementally will not cause myocardial depression and, because of its prominent amnestic effect, can result in a pleasant induction in patients with severe hypovolemia.

The availability of a selective $GABA_A$ receptor antagonist, flumazenil, is an important advantage to the use of benzodiazepines. Flumazenil acts competitively at the benzodiazepine recognition site of the $GABA_A$ receptor complex to reverse residual sedative effects of benzodiazepine agonists (Chapter 25). Because of its receptor selectivity, flumazenil will not antagonize depressant effects of drugs other than benzodiazepines.

Flumazenil does not reverse the respiratory-depressant effects of benzodiazepines. Therefore, equipment for airway management and resuscitation must be available. Although flumazenil acts rapidly, within one arm-to-brain circulation time, its duration is short, approximately 60 minutes. Therefore, resedation may occur after reversal (so-called residual sedation), especially in patients receiving a large dose of a long-acting benzodiazepine, requiring additional doses of flumazenil. Flumazenil can precipitate a withdrawal syndrome in the benzodiazepine-dependent individual.

A single induction dosage of etomidate can suppress steroid synthesis in the adrenal cortex for at least 4 to 8 hours, suppressing also release of corticosteroids in response to stress. Therefore, etomidate is not suitable for IV infusion for maintenance of anesthesia. It can cause pain on injection and myoclonus and thrombophlebitis at the injection site. The incidence of postoperative nausea and vomiting limits its use in an outpatient setting. Etomidate causes hypertension, cardiac arrhythmias, hypoventilation, hyperventilation, laryngospasm, and sometimes hiccups. Etomidate can replace thiopental in the patient with decreased myocardial function and cardiac output. Etomidate has no analgesic activity and is contraindicated in patients with known hypersensitivity or a history of porphyria.

The use of propofol is contraindicated in any individual with hypersensitivity to the drug. Respiratory and cardiovascular support systems must be available while one is using propofol because it is a respiratory and cardiovascular depressant, especially when injected rapidly and in large doses. Use in obstetrical procedures should be avoided until there is adequate data on the safety of propofol to the fetus.

Ketamine is related structurally to phencyclidine and the two drugs have many actions in common. Although ketamine produces analgesia and amnesia, skeletal muscle tone is maintained. At appropriate dosages the patient may appear to be awake but is unresponsive to or dissociated from the environment (hence the term "dissociative anesthesia"). Although ketamine is indicated for use as a general anesthetic drug, its practical usefulness for maintenance of anesthesia is limited by its cardiovascular stimulant actions and, in particular, by the high incidence of unpleasant dreaming and other dysphoric episodes during emergence from anesthesia. For these reasons, ketamine is used primarily as an induction agent in patients in hypovolemic shock and for brief painful procedures, such as changing burn dressings, where its analgesic and amnestic effects are advantageous. A benzodiazepine is often administered with ketamine to minimize postoperative psychotomimetic reactions.

Because opioids are potent respiratory depressants, they should be used only where equipment is available to provide assisted ventilation. Postoperative nausea and vomiting are common side effects of all μ-opioid receptor agonists. Rapid IV administration of morphine can evoke the release of histamine from mast cells, which in turn causes arterial and venous dilatation and hypotension. This effect can be prevented by pretreatment with H_1- and H_2-histamine receptor blockers, such as diphenhydramine and cimetidine respectively. Rigidity of respiratory muscles is produced by all μ-agonist opioid drugs, notably with fentanyl and its derivatives, often necessitating the use of muscle-relaxing drugs so that assisted ventilation can be provided.

The specific opioid antagonist naloxone can be given postoperatively to reverse any depression of respiration produced by opioid analgesics and to arouse the patient. However, because naloxone will reverse all effects of opioid analgesics, including analgesia, it should not be used routinely for this purpose. The duration of action of naloxone is short. Therefore, when antagonist administration is indicated, dosing should be repeated periodically. Since it is exquisitely selective, naloxone will not reverse effects of drugs other than opioids.

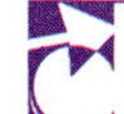

NEW DIRECTIONS

Efforts to reduce the rising cost of health care in the United States may result in as many as 70% to 75% of all surgical procedures being performed in ambulatory surgical facilities. Surgery in hospitals will be reserved for those patients requiring the most intensive medical care. This trend in surgery has important implications for drug development. Because the majority of surgical patients are discharged within hours of their surgery, the effects of anesthetic drugs will have to be dissipated rapidly and completely, so that the patient has a clear

TRADE NAMES

In addition to generic and fixed-combination preparations the following trade-named materials are available in the United States. Drugs available only in generic preparations are not listed.

INHALATIONAL ANESTHETICS

Ethrane, enflurane
Fluothane, halothane
Forane, isoflurane
Penthrane, methoxyflurane
Suprane, desflurane

INTRAVENOUS ANESTHETICS

Alfenta, alfentanil
Amidate, etomidate
Brevital, methohexital
Demerol, meperidine
Diprivan, propofol
Inapsine, droperidol
Innovar, fentanyl and droperidol
Ketalar, ketamine
Pentothal, thiopental
Sublimaze, fentanyl
Sufenta, sufentanil
Valium, diazepam
Versed, midazolam

ANTAGONIST DRUGS

Romazicon, flumazenil
Narcan, naloxone

sensorium, with no residual postoperative hangover, nausea, or impairment of motor function, judgment, or memory. The pharmacokinetics of inhalational anesthetic agents makes it unlikely that suitable drugs can be developed from this class. Therefore, general anesthesia will come to rely more heavily on intravenous drugs that are rapidly inactivated by simple mechanisms (such as plasma cholinesterase activity), so that drug effects will disappear within moments of ending drug administration. New drugs should possess the characteristics of the ideal agent listed in the box on page 409.

Inhalational agents will still be widely used. They have good potency, low solubility in blood for rapid onset and offset of effects, and should undergo minimal biotransformation, since the metabolites of inhalational anesthetics are responsible for some of the undesirable side effects.

SELF-ASSESSMENT QUESTIONS

1. Cardiac output and blood pressure are reduced the most by:
   a. nitrous oxide.
   b. halothane.
   c. ketamine.
   d. isoflurane.
   e. fentanyl.
2. The ventilatory response to carbon dioxide is blunted during anesthesia with:
   a. halothane.
   b. morphine.
   c. enflurane.
   d. isoflurane.
   e. all of the above.
3. The minimum alveolar concentration (MAC) of an inhalational anesthetic agent is higher:
   a. in an obese patient than in a patient of average body weight.
   b. during a long surgical procedure than during a short surgical procedure.
   c. in an infant than in an elderly patient.
   d. in a patient pretreated with morphine than in an otherwise drug-free patient.
   e. in males than in females.
4. Competitive receptor antagonists are available for reversing undesirable postoperative effects of:
   a. thiopental.
   b. halothane.
   c. propofol.
   d. midazolam.
   e. isoflurane.

REFERENCES

Davis PJ, Cook DR, editors: Clinical pharmacokinetics of the newer intravenous anaesthetic agents, *Clin Pharm* 11:18, 1986.

Domino EF, editor: *PCP (phencyclidine): historical and current perspectives,* Ann Arbor, Mich, 1981, NPP Books.

Eger EI, editor: *Anesthetic uptake and action,* Baltimore, 1974, Williams & Wilkins.

Eger EI, editor: *Nitrous oxide,* New York, 1985, Elsevier.

Katz R, editor: Propofol: clinical update and implications. In *Seminars in Anesthesia,* vol 3, no 1, suppl 1, New York, 1988, Grune & Stratton.

Miller RD, editor: *Anesthesia,* New York, 1981, Churchill Livingstone.

Olsen RW, editor: Drug interactions at the GABA receptor-ionophore, *Annu Rev Pharmacol Toxicol* 22:245, 1982.

Roth SH, Miller KW, editors: Molecular and cellular mechanisms of anesthetics, New York, 1986, Plenum Press.

5. Potential advantages of fentanyl over morphine for induction or maintenance of anesthesia include:
   a. superior relaxation of skeletal muscles.
   b. absence of postoperative nausea and vomiting.
   c. lack of depressant effect on spontaneous respiration.
   d. all of the above.
   e. none of the above.
6. Nitrous oxide does all of the following *except:*
   a. relax skeletal muscles.
   b. produce analgesia.
   c. produce amnesia.
   d. increase the pressure in enclosed air-filled cavities in the body.
   e. reduce the anesthetic requirement for a concurrently administered halogenated inhalational agent.
7. Activation of the electroencephalogram sometimes occurs with:
   a. halothane.
   b. enflurane.
   c. isoflurane.
   d. thiopental.
   e. diazepam.

Local Anesthetics

KENNETH P. MINNEMAN
THEODORE M. BRODY

MAJOR LOCAL ANESTHETICS

bupivacaine
chloroprocaine
etidocaine
lidocaine
mepivacaine
procaine
tetracaine

Therapeutic Considerations

Speed of onset
Duration of effect
Side effects
- seizures
- cardiovascular depression

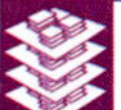

THERAPEUTIC OVERVIEW

Local anesthetics cause a reversible blockade of action potential generation or conduction in neurons. They have many uses in medicine to make a specific section of the body impervious to the perception of painful stimuli. These uses range from dentistry to obstetrics and include procedures as simple as local infiltration for removal of a superficial skin lesion, to a regional anesthetic used entirely for a hip replacement, including management of postoperative pain. Therapeutic considerations are indicated in the box.

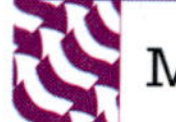

MECHANISMS OF ACTION

Local anesthetics act directly on nerve cells to block their ability to transmit impulses down their axons. By blocking action potential propagation in sensory neurons, they eliminate sensations of pain. Local anesthetics are not specific to any nerve cell type and act on all sensory, motor, and autonomic neurons and all neurons in the central nervous system. However, by local administration the actions of these compounds can be restricted. Also, certain practical pharmacokinetic considerations make them particularly useful in blocking sensory transmission of pain impulses. The greatest advantage of local anesthetics is their reversibility. When the drug is eliminated by metabolism or excretion, its action is terminated and the nerve resumes completely

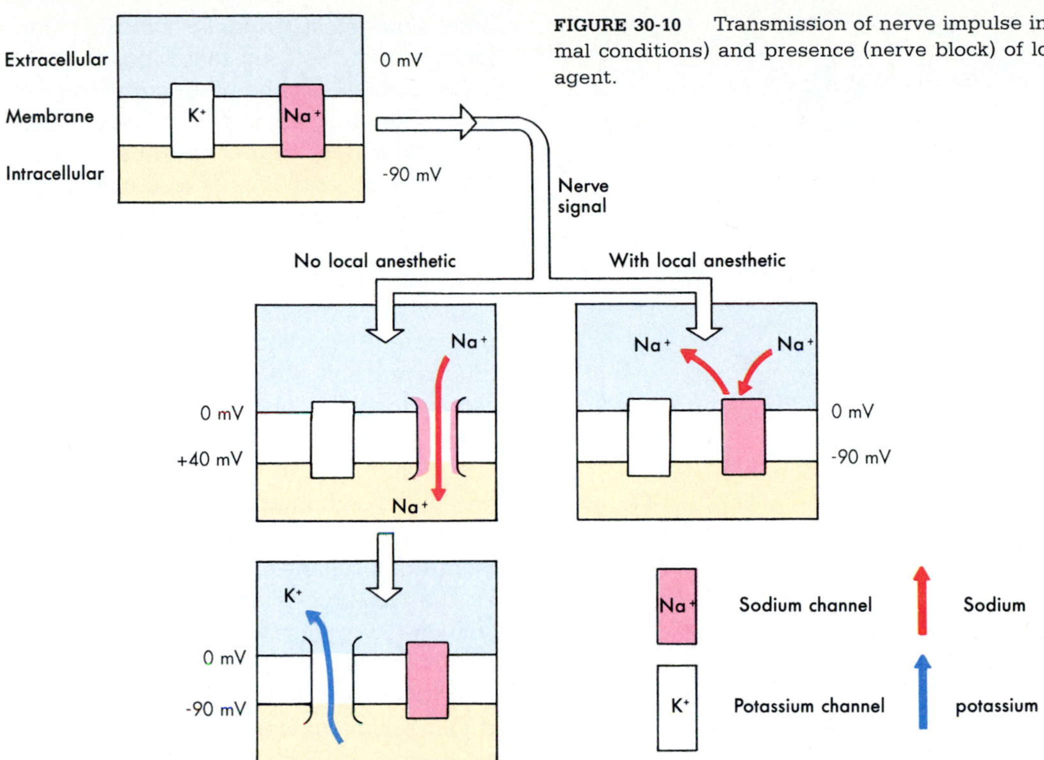

FIGURE 30-10 Transmission of nerve impulse in absence (normal conditions) and presence (nerve block) of local anesthetic agent.

normal function. There are generally no long-term consequences of local anesthetic use. Thus these drugs are highly effective in providing regional, localized, and reversible pain relief.

The molecular targets for local anesthetic action are the voltage-dependent sodium channels, which occur in all neurons. As reviewed in Chapter 22, these channels are responsible for the regenerative action potentials that occur along neuronal axons to carry messages from cell bodies to nerve terminals. Voltage-dependent sodium channels are usually closed at normal resting membrane potentials, preventing the high concentration of sodium in the extracellular fluid from entering the cell. When membranes are depolarized, these channels open and allow sodium to flow into the cell down its concentration gradient. This influx of positive charge depolarizes the cell further, opening more channels, and causes a self-regenerating action potential as discussed in Chapter 22. Sustained depolarization causes an automatic inactivation of the voltage-dependent sodium channels, shutting off sodium influx, and a concurrent opening of voltage-dependent potassium channels. The resultant potassium efflux returns the membrane potential to its normal resting value.

The mechanism by which local anesthetics block conduction of nerve impulses is well understood. These drugs bind selectively to the intracellular surface of sodium channels and block the entry of sodium into the cell (Fig. 30-10). By blocking sodium influx, these drugs eliminate the depolarization necessary for action potential propagation and, at sufficient concentrations, block impulse conduction. Since the binding of local anesthetics to sodium channels is completely reversible, when drug administration is stopped the drug diffuses away and is metabolized and nerve function is completely restored. The ability of local anesthetic drugs to block sodium channels is highly dependent on the conformation (or state) of the channel. As discussed in Chapter 22, sodium channels exist in three major states. In the resting state the channels do not allow sodium influx and are highly sensitive to depolarization-induced opening; in the open state they allow sodium influx; and in the refractory state they do not allow sodium influx and are not opened by depolarization (see Fig. 22-5).

Local anesthetics have different potencies in binding to the several states of sodium channels. Local anesthetics are much more likely to block sodium channels that are open or refractory and bind to resting channels with a much lower potency. This phenomenon is called "state dependence" and has great practical importance. Because local anesthetics will preferentially block nerves in which sodium channels are open or are refractory, they are more potent in rapidly firing nerves than in nerves in which action potentials are less frequent. Since sensory neurons often fire at substantially greater frequencies than motor fibers do, sensory neurons are

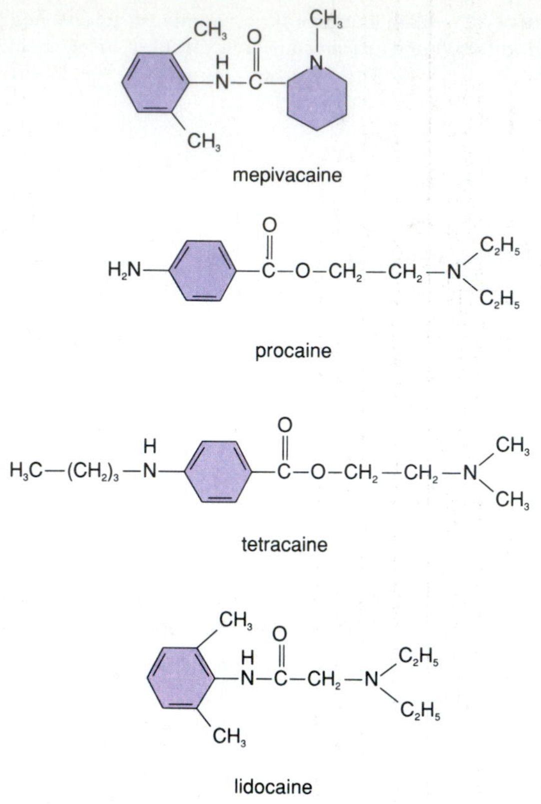

mepivacaine

procaine

tetracaine

lidocaine

FIGURE 30-11 Structures of local anesthetic agents shown as free base forms.

often preferentially blocked by a given concentration of local anesthetic.

The structures of local anesthetic drugs have several interesting aspects that have a direct bearing on their therapeutic actions (Fig. 30-11). All these drugs contain a hydrophobic group (almost always an aromatic moiety) linked through an alkyl chain of intermediate length to a hydrophilic group (usually a tertiary amine). The presence of both hydrophilic and hydrophobic groups reflects the dual requirements for local anesthetic drug action. The drug must be partially water soluble to be able to diffuse to the nerves to be blocked after local injection; however it must also be sufficiently lipid soluble to be able to penetrate the cell membrane and reach its binding site on the inner surface of the voltage-dependent sodium channels. Thus the hydrophilic tertiary amine facilitates diffusion to the cells of interest, and the hydrophobic aromatic group allows the drug to enter the cell and reach its actual site of action.

Another relevant aspect of the chemistry of these drugs is the effect of pH. Local anesthetic drugs are weak bases, with pK_a values usually in the range of 8 to 9. This means that most of the drugs will be in the charged cationic form at normal body pH. This is fortunate, since most evidence indicates that it is the cationic form of the drug that binds to and blocks the sodium channel. On the other hand, the cationic-charged form of the drug is much less likely to penetrate the cell membrane (despite the presence of the hydrophilic aromatic group) and thus is less able to reach its site of action. The constant equilibrium between cationic and unprotonated drug explains this dichotomy. As a weak base, although most drug will be protonated at physiological pH, a certain proportion (1% to 10%) will be nonprotonated. This minor nonprotonated fraction of the drug is probably the primary species that permeates the cell membranes and accumulates in the cytoplasm. Once across the membrane, equilibrium is reestablished, and most of the drug will again be protonated, facilitating sodium-channel blockade.

The type of bond linking the aromatic and amine groups in local anesthetic drugs has major implications for the duration of action and toxicity of these compounds. Two types of linkages are found in the alkyl chains connecting the hydrophobic and hydrophilic regions of local anesthetic molecules. An ester linkage, as is found in procaine, allows the drug to be inactivated by esterases, which are widely distributed throughout the body. Because hydrolysis of the ester bond eliminates the biological activity of the drug, the presence of an ester bond usually, though not always, results in a drug with a relatively short duration of action. In contrast, an amide linkage, as is found in lidocaine, cannot be hydrolyzed by esterases and usually results in drugs that are longer acting. Finally, since hydrolysis of the ester type of local anesthetic drugs results in metabolites that resemble *para*-aminobenzoic acid derivatives, the ester type of local anesthetic drugs are more likely to provoke hypersensitivity reactions than the amide type of local anesthetic drugs would (although these actually are relatively infrequent with either drug class). This is discussed in more detail later.

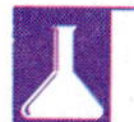

PHARMACOKINETICS

Local anesthetics are generally administered by injection close to the nerves to be blocked. Since the point where local anesthetics act is the inner surface of the nerve membrane, agents must diffuse through tissues from the injection site to reach the appropriate nerve fibers. Several factors influence rate of onset of anesthesia. Because local anesthetics are weak bases (forming salts by combining with acids) and have pK_a values between 8 and 9, they exist as the nonprotonated form in an alkaline or less acidic environment. The nonprotonated form more readily traverses tissue membranes to reach the site of action than the charged, or protonated,

Table 30-5 Pharmacokinetic Parameter Values for Local Anesthetics

Drugs	Administration	Elimination ($t_{1/2}$, hr)	Disposition	Plasma Protein Bound (%)	Onset Time (min)
mepivacaine	PN	1.9-3/2 (adults)	R, B, M, (main)	75	3-20
		2.7-9/0 (neonates)	—	—	—
bupivacaine	PN	2.7 (adults)	—	—	—
		8.1 (neonates)	M	95	2-10
lidocaine	PN, IV	1.5-2	M* (95%), R	70	—
procaine	PN, IV	<60 sec	M	—	—
etidocaine	PN	2.5	M, R	95	3-5

B, Biliary; *M*, metabolism; *PN*, perineural (around the nerve); *R*, renal.
*Large first-pass effect.

form does. Inside the nerve membrane, it is the latter species that interacts with sodium-channel proteins and is responsible for the pharmacological effect.

Other determinants of rate of onset of local anesthesia include drug concentration and potency, drug binding to plasma protein, rate of metabolic biotransformation, and vascularity at the site of drug injection. The last is of primary importance in that any diffusion into blood vessels will reduce the regional drug concentration at the nerve fibers to be blocked. Vasoconstrictors, such as epinephrine, are frequently used to diminish local blood flow and reduce systemic absorption. Although vasoconstrictor drugs tend to extend the duration of action of local anesthetics, they are apparently more effective in prolonging the actions of the less lipid-soluble agents (lidocaine, chloroprocaine, mevipacaine) than those of the more lipid-soluble etidocaine and bupivacaine. Some local anesthetics are marketed in combination with fixed concentrations of vasoconstrictor drugs.

Local anesthetics vary considerably in the rates at which they are converted to inactive metabolites by body tissues. Since all local anesthetics diffuse into the systemic circulation to some extent, metabolic fate becomes a prominent factor in the potential of these agents to produce undesirable side effects or overt toxicity. In addition to drug biotransformation, plasma protein binding to α_1-acid glycoprotein will also reduce the concentration of free drug in the systemic circulation.

Several local anesthetics (procaine, chloroprocaine, tetracaine) are esters (see Figure 30-11) and are rapidly metabolically transformed to inactive products by hydrolysis by plasma cholinesterase and liver esterases. These agents generally have a relatively short half-life in the body (Table 30-5). In the absence of esterase activity, such as in spinal fluid, the duration of spinal anesthesia with the esters is considerably extended. The amide type of local anesthetics are metabolized by microsomes of the liver endoplasmic reticulum. This involves an initial N-dealkylation followed by hydrolysis. Relative rates of biotransformation of amide-linked local anesthetics are lidocaine (fastest) followed by mepivacaine and bupivacaine (slowest; see Table 30-5). Some products of lidocaine metabolism possess local anesthetic activity.

The amides are also extensively bound to plasma proteins, and nonspecific tissue binding also occurs near the injection site. Preexisting liver disease is more likely to result in toxicity with these agents as a result of both reduced drug biotransformation and a lower plasma protein concentration, since plasma proteins are synthesized in the liver.

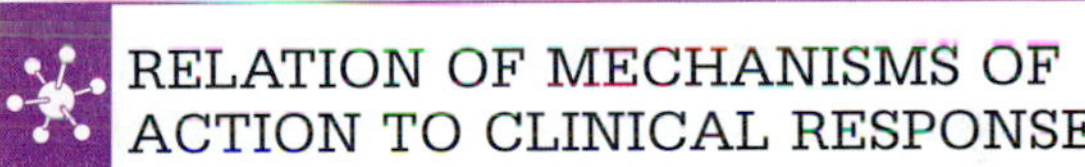

RELATION OF MECHANISMS OF ACTION TO CLINICAL RESPONSE

Anatomical, physiological, and chemical factors all play an important role in determining the susceptibility of nerve fibers to block by local anesthetics. The rate of onset, intensity, and duration of nerve block are dramatically affected by the size, myelination, firing rate, and anatomical location of the nerves. Chemical considerations such as pH also have important practical effects on the clinical response to these drugs. Because the same types of sodium channels are present in most types of neurons, local anesthetics block impulse conduction in all types of nerve cells, including sensory, motor, autonomic, and CNS neurons. Sodium channels also play an important role in electrically excitable muscle cells, and local anesthetics can also have prominent actions on muscle. The result of actions on cardiac sodium channels is the basis for some of their therapeutic uses in the treatment of cardiac arrhythmias (see Chapter 14), and actions on smooth and cardiac muscle allow one to explain some of their toxicity (see below). However, local anesthetics are not equally potent and effective in all cells in which sodium channels are found. In

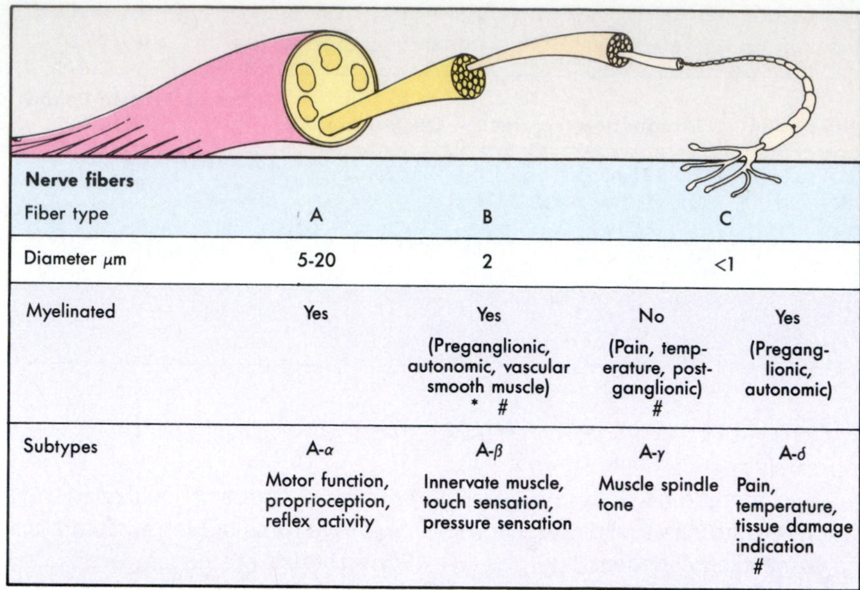

Nerve fibers				
Fiber type	A	B	C	
Diameter μm	5-20	2	<1	
Myelinated	Yes	Yes (Preganglionic, autonomic, vascular smooth muscle) * #	No (Pain, temp-erature, post-ganglionic) #	Yes (Pregang-lionic, autonomic)
Subtypes	A-α Motor function, proprioception, reflex activity	A-β Innervate muscle, touch sensation, pressure sensation	A-γ Muscle spindle tone	A-δ Pain, temperature, tissue damage indication #

* Spinal and peridural anesthesia
\# Pain transmission fibers

FIGURE 30-12 Summary of anatomical types of nerve fibers, including those over which pain signals are conducted.

fact, these drugs show remarkable selectivity between different types of neurons and muscle cells. This selectivity is based primarily on pharmacokinetic considerations of penetration, physiological aspects concerning firing rate, and anatomical considerations of nerve size and degree of myelination.

Neurons differ from each other substantially based on diameter, frequency of firing, and degree of myelination. Most pain impulses in humans are carried on two types of primary afferent fibers, Aδ and C (Figure 30-12). Aδ fibers are distributed primarily in skin and mucous membranes, are small and finely myelinated, and are associated with sensations of sharp pricking pain. C fibers are widely distributed, are small and unmyelinated, and are associated with long-lasting, burning pain. Some pain impulses are also carried by myelinated B fibers.

Because the binding of local anesthetics to sodium channels is state dependent, rapidly firing neurons such as those carrying pain impulses are generally blocked at lower concentrations than are more slowly firing neurons (discussed above). It is also clear that small nerve fibers are generally more sensitive than large nerve fibers are and that myelinated nerves are more sensitive than unmyelinated nerves. Size (diameter of the axon) is important because it relates to the critical length along the axon that must be affected to block transmission. Small fibers generally have shorter critical lengths than large fibers have. Myelination is important because of the different types of current spread in unmyelinated and myelinated axons (see Fig. 22-8). Spread of current along myelinated fibers is generally discontinuous, involving only the small unmyelinated areas at the nodes of Ranvier. Since this involves much less surface membrane to be blocked, local anesthetics usually block myelinated fibers more effectively than unmyelinated fibers of the same size.

The situation is complicated further when one considers the anatomical localization of the different nerve types. Nerve cells in the outer portion of nerve trunks will generally be exposed to higher drug concentrations than will nerve cells located in the center of nerve trunks, where diffusion of drug will be restricted. Although these general principles can explain the differential sensitivity of nerve fibers to undergo blockade by local anesthetics, it is clearly difficult to predict precisely what will happen in a given situation. There is, however, a general order in which sensory modalities are usually lost: pain first, then cold, warmth, touch, and finally deep pressure. Motor functions are often more resistant to local anesthetics, probably because of considerations of size, firing rate, and anatomical localization discussed above.

Local anesthetic drugs are generally found to be less effective in infected tissues than in normal tissues. The reason is that infection usually results in a local metabolic acidosis, lowering the pH. As discussed above, the ability of local anesthetic drugs to penetrate cell membranes depends on the acid-base equilibrium, since the small proportion of the nonprotonated form is better able to permeate cell membranes. Infection-induced acidosis alters this equilibrium, greatly reducing the proportion of the drug in the nonprotonated form. Consequently, the ability of the drug to cross the cell membrane to its site of action is greatly reduced. Since local anesthetics are often used to treat pain associated with inflammation or infection, this reduced efficacy has substantial clinical relevance.

Local anesthetic drugs are widely used to provide temporary pain relief in localized regions of the body. By varying the drug, its concentration, its dose, and the method by which it is administered, one can obtain a wide range of effects. A very localized intensely numb area of skin can be achieved for a short time by infiltration of the area with a short-acting drug. On the other hand, a mostly sensory block can be achieved by administration of a dilute solution of a long-acting local anesthetic drug through an indwelling catheter to the epidural space, providing complete anesthesia while preserving motor function and a mother's ability to deliver an infant. Anesthetics can be used to provide analgesia (relief of pain) and muscle relaxation at the same time, by administration of a potent compound to the central neuraxis (spinal or epidural) or a major peripheral nerve complex (e.g., the brachial plexus). Dilute solutions of local anesthetics mixed with narcotics are increasingly used in postoperative pain to provide excellent analgesia with a lower total narcotic drug dose than would be required with conventional therapies. Finally, local anesthetics are used in the management of more complicated acute and chronic pain states as both diagnostic and therapeutic tools. There are many different drugs available that differ primarily in their duration of action, side effects, and toxicity.

SIDE EFFECTS, CLINICAL PROBLEMS, AND TOXICITY

Because the termination of local anesthetic action ultimately depends on movement of drug into the systemic circulation, side effects and toxicity can result from blockade of impulse propagation in excitable organs and tissues perfused by blood. The central, peripheral, and autonomic nervous systems and all muscle are potential targets.

CNS effects may be manifest as depression or stimulation, or both, depending on the nervous pathways affected by the local anesthetic. Depression of cortical inhibitory neurons, without the balancing depression of excitatory nerves, may result in tremor and restlessness and culminate in overt clonic convulsions, coma, and respiratory failure (see box). However, a variety of symptoms, including general depression and drowsiness, are common clinical consequences. Seizures can be treated or prevented by injection of diazepam intravenously, and oxygen can protect against hypoxemia in the convulsing patient. An overdose of local anesthetics results in reduced transmission of impulses at the neuromuscular junction and at ganglionic synapses, producing weakness or muscle paralysis. Support of respiration is an important component of treatment. Smooth muscle appears to be only minimally affected by local anesthetics.

Local anesthetics do have potential deleterious actions upon pacemaker activity, electrical excitability, conduction times, and contractile force of the heart. Arrhythmias are also possible; however, cardiac toxicity is infrequently observed, apparently only when high blood concentrations of anesthetic agent are attained. Cardiovascular failure has also been reported to occur, however, from small doses used in infiltration anesthesia.

Lidocaine is also used therapeutically to depress abnormal pacemaker activity in certain arrhythmogenic states (Chapter 14). Cocaine, a potent local anesthetic that had wide clinical use several decades ago, also has prominent side effects upon the heart and the CNS (Chapter 32). Among the local anesthetics in current use, bupivacaine is considered to be more cardiotoxic than other agents are.

Local hypersensitivity reactions can result from the use of some ester type local anesthetics, particularly

CLINICAL PROBLEMS WITH LOCAL ANESTHETICS

CNS seizures and convulsions at high agent concentrations

Cardiac sodium-channel blockade (also used therapeutically for antiarrhythmic effects) (see Chapter 14)

TRADE NAMES

In addition to generic and fixed-combination preparations, the following trade-named preparations are available in the United States.

LOCAL ANESTHETICS

Carbocaine, mepivacaine HCl
Duranest, etidocaine HCl
Marcaine, Sensorcaine, bupivacaine HCl
Nesacaine, chloroprocaine HCl
Novocaine, procaine HCl
Pontacaine, tetracaine HCl
Xylocaine, lidocaine HCl

procaine and related compounds. These can be ameliorated by the systemic administration of antihistaminics.

REFERENCES

Butterworth JF, Strichartz GR: Molecular mechanisms of local anesthesia, *Anesthesiology* 72:711-734, 1990.

Catterall WA: Common modes of action on Na+ channels: Local anesthetics, antiarrythmics and anticonvulsants. *Trends Pharmacol Sci*, 8:57-65, 1987.

Ritchie JM: An overview of the mechanisms of local anesthetic action; past, present and future. In Roth SH, Miller KW, editors: *Molecular and cellular mechanisms of anesthetics*, New York, 1984, Plenum.

Saverese JJ, Covino BG: Basic and clinical pharmacology of local anesthetic drugs. In Miller RD, editor: *Anesthesia*, ed 2, New York, 1986, Churchill, Livingstone.

SELF-ASSESSMENT QUESTIONS

1. Which of the following is *not* true of local anesthetics?
   a. Their molecular sites of action are voltage-dependent sodium channels.
   b. Local anesthetics bind selectively to the intracellular surface and block entry of sodium into the cell.
   c. The binding of local anesthetics to sodium channels is completely reversible.
   d. The ability to block the sodium channel depends on the conformational state of the channel.
   e. All of the above are correct.
2. Which of the following is correct about local anesthetics?
   a. They are weak acids.
   b. They are largely in the charged cationic form at normal body pH.
   c. The charged form of the drug readily penetrates the cell membrane because of the presence of a hydrophilic group.
   d. The protonated form of the drug blocks the sodium channel.
   e. b and d are correct.
3. All of the following are correct *except:*
   a. Local anesthetics form salts by combining with acids.
   b. They possess both hydrophilic and hydrophobic groups.
   c. Anesthetics with amide linkages have longer durations of action than those with ester linkages.
   d. Vascularity of the tissue reduces the effectiveness of the local anesthetic action.
   e. All of the above are correct.
4. Toxic effects of local anesthetics include the following *except:*
   a. cardiac arrhythmias.
   b. seizures.
   c. hypersensitivity.
   d. CNS depression.
   e. All of the above are correct.

CHAPTER 31

Alcohol

RICHARD A. DEITRICH
JOHN D. PALMER

Ethanol is a prime example of a chemical with limited medicinal use that is nevertheless widely used for nonmedical purposes. In cultures in which ethanol use is accepted, the substance is misused and abused by some fraction of the population. Such use is associated with serious social, medical, and economic problems, including the potential for life-threatening damage to most major organ systems and the development of psychological and physical dependence in individuals who use the drug excessively. In the United States, its use causes almost insurmountable problems. It is estimated that 65% to 70% of the population uses alcohol (i.e., ethanol) and that more than 10 million are alcohol dependent. An additional 10 million are subject to negative consequences of alcohol abuse such as arrests, automobile accidents, violence, occupational injuries, and deleterious effects upon job performance and health. About 50% of all traffic deaths are estimated to be alcohol related. The annual cost of alcohol-related problems in the United States is over 100 billion dollars. Since individuals who abuse alcohol probably overuse the health care system, alcoholics constitute a substantial fraction of many medical practices: therefore a medical history designed to elicit information on alcohol use is an essential feature of a modern medical work-up. Clearly, alcohol abuse is a significant public health problem. This chapter covers these behavioral and toxicological problems associated with the use of ethanol as a recreational drug or drug of abuse and reviews the deleterious effects of other alcohols.

ABBREVIATIONS

ADH	alcohol dehydrogenase
ALDH	aldehyde dehydrogenase
BAC	blood alcohol concentration
ETS	electron transport system
GABA	γ-aminobutryic acid
LDH	lactic dehydrogenase
NAD^+	nicotinamide adenine dinucleotide
NADH	nicotinamide adenine dinucleotide, reduced
NADPH	nicotinamide adenine dinucleotide phosphate, reduced

USES OF ETHANOL

Ethanol is used primarily as a social drug, with only limited application as a therapeutic agent (see the box). Ethanol is used topically to lower elevated body temperature by promoting evaporation, as a rub to prevent pressure sores in bedridden patients, and sometimes by injection to produce irreversible nerve block or tumor destruction. It is also effective in the treatment of methanol and ethylene glycol poisonings, where it acts competitively to prevent the conversion of these alcohols to toxic intermediates until the unmetabolized parent compounds are removed from the body (see below for details). Ethanol is only rarely prescribed for its antianxiety and sedative properties and as an appetite stimulant. Ethanol mist has been used to reduce the frothing in acute pulmonary edema resulting from left ventricular failure.

MOLECULAR MECHANISMS OF ACTION

For many years alcohol and the general anesthetic agents were assumed to share a common mechanism of action in that both (1) require millimolar concentrations to produce their effects and (2) show excellent correlation between the oil/water partition coefficients (see Chapter 30) of these agents and their ability to depress the CNS. Before the advent of ether, ethanol was used as the "anesthetic" agent before surgical intervention.

Pharmacological and genetic evidence now indicate

THERAPEUTIC OVERVIEW

Ethanol is used:
- Topically to reduce body temperature and as an antiseptic
- By injection to produce irreversible nerve block by protein denaturation
- By inhalation to reduce foaming in pulmonary edema
- Orally for sedative effect
- Orally to increase appetite
- In treatment of methanol and ethylene glycol poisoning

that ethanol, like general anesthetics, "fluidizes," or "disorders," the physical structure of cell membranes, particularly those low in cholesterol. In studies with animals previously exposed to ethanol or that exhibit pharmacological tolerance to ethanol intoxication or in species genetically resistant to the effects of ethanol, the neuronal cell membrane is not readily disordered by ethanol. Also, cell membranes from animals selectively bred for sensitivity to ethanol are more easily fluidized than those obtained from animals genetically resistant to alcohol.

At the molecular level ethanol may interfere with the packing of molecules in the phospholipid bilayer of the cell membrane, thus increasing membrane fluidity. However, this fluidizing effect of ethanol is small and probably is not responsible for ethanol's CNS depressant effects. However, this fluidizing effect may be relevant to lipid structures in discrete areas of the brain, such as those surrounding important neurotransmitter receptors or ion channels, and thereby generating greater CNS disruption. Current experimental techniques do not permit measurements in small enough areas of the cell membrane to explore this theory; however, at some concentration, ethanol affects most ion channels and receptors. Table 31-1 lists some of the ion channels influenced by ethanol. Ethanol may also act by binding directly to receptor or enzyme proteins, whether or not they are in a lipid milieu. Although the significance of these findings has not been established, ethanol appears to have both inhibitory and facilitatory effects, depending on the channel. In each case, the effect is depression of the CNS. Because both barbiturates and benzodiazepines exhibit additive CNS depression and cross tolerance to ethanol, all three agents may share a common mechanism, perhaps through the γ-aminobutyric acid $GABA_A$-benzodiazepine-chloride channel complex (see Chapter 25).

Recent studies in animals demonstrate a selective effect of low concentrations of ethanol on guanine nucleotide binding proteins (G proteins). Ethanol apparently promotes the activation of G_s (see Chapter 2), thus enhancing adenylate cyclase activity. Whether this event plays an important role in the mechanism of action of ethanol in humans is not determined. It has been suggested that the adenylate cyclase system may provide a biochemical marker of genetic predisposition to alcoholism.

OBSERVED EFFECTS OF ETHANOL ON THE CENTRAL NERVOUS SYSTEM

Like the general anesthetic agents, ethanol depresses all areas and functions of the brain. As with most CNS depressants, an excitement stage is observed initially as depression of higher inhibitory centers releases the normal control mechanisms responsible for social and behavioral restraints. Thus, ethanol is described as a disinhibitor or euphoriant. The higher integrative areas of the brain are affected first, with thought processes, fine discrimination, judgment, and motor function sequentially impaired. These effects may be observed with blood ethanol concentrations of 0.05% (50 mg/dl) or lower. Specific behavioral changes are difficult to predict and depend to a large extent upon the environment and the personality of the individual. As blood ethanol concentration increases to 0.1%, errors in judgment are frequent, motor systems are impaired, and responses to complex auditory and visual stimuli are altered. Patterns of involuntary motor action are affected. Ataxia is noticeable, with walking becoming difficult, and staggering common as the blood alcohol concentration approaches 0.15% to 0.2%. Reaction times are increased and the individual may become extremely loud, incoherent, and emotionally unstable. Violent behavior may occur at these concentrations. These effects are the result of depression of the excitatory areas throughout the brain. At blood ethanol concentrations from 0.2% to 0.3%, intoxicated individuals frequently experience periods of amnesia or "blackout," with failure to recall events occurring at that time.

With increased blood ethanol concentrations to 0.25% to 0.30%, anesthesia ensues. Ethanol, although sharing many properties with the general anesthetics, is less safe as an anesthetic because of its low margin of safety (ratio of anesthetic to lethal concentration). It is also a poor analgesic. Coma in humans occurs with blood alcohol concentrations above 0.3%. The lethal range for ethanol, in the absence of other CNS depressants, is between 0.4% and 0.5%, though individuals with much higher blood concentrations have survived. Death from

Table 31-1 Some Ion Channels That Are Functionally Altered by Ethanol

Channel	Effect	Ethanol Concentration
Sodium (voltage-gated)	Inhibited	100 mM and higher*
Potassium (voltage-gated)	Facilitated	50-100 mM
Calcium (voltage-gated)	Inhibited	50 mM and higher
Calcium (glutamate-activated)	Inhibited	20-50 mM
Chloride (GABA-gated)	Facilitated	10-50 mM

*100 mM ethanol is 460 mg/dl.

acute ethanol overdose is relatively rare compared to death resulting from the combination of alcohol with other CNS depressants such as barbiturates and benzodiazepines. Death occurs as a result of a depressant effect on the medulla, resulting in respiratory failure (Table 31-2).

Table 31-2 Physiological or Behavioral State as a Function of Blood Alcohol Concentrations

Blood Concentrations (mg/dl)	Reaction
0-50	Loss of inhibitions, excitement, incoordination, impaired judgment, slurred speech, body sway
50-100	Impaired reaction time, further impaired judgment, impaired driving ability, ataxia
100-200	Staggering gait, inability to operate a motor vehicle
200-300	Respiratory depression; danger of death in presence of other CNS depressants; blackouts
>300	Unconsciousness, severe respiratory and cardiovascular depression, death
>1200	Highest known blood concentration with survival in a chronic alcoholic

Tolerance and Dependence

Both acute and chronic tolerance occurs with ethanol use. Acute tolerance can occur within a matter of hours and can rapidly dissipate. Acute tolerance may develop in minutes in in vitro experiments in which ethanol is applied directly to nerve cells. If alcohol is ingested daily for periods of weeks to months, chronic tolerance ensues with high chronic tolerances developing in some individuals. Approximately a doubling of blood alcohol concentrations is required to produce effects in tolerant compared to nontolerant individuals. This is much less, however, than is observed with opiate drugs where a tolerance of 10- to 30-fold can be seen. With alcohol, tolerance development has greater implications than tolerance with other agents has, because other organ systems are now exposed to much higher concentrations with deleterious consequences, particularly to the liver. Although tolerance develops to some of the CNS effects with ethanol, there is only a very minor increase in the concentration of drug that produces death. In late-stage alcoholism with serious liver damage, the metabolism of ethanol may be impaired.

Both psychological and physical dependence are characteristics of chronic alcohol use. The clinical manifestations of ethanol withdrawal are divided into early and late effects. The early symptoms occur between a few hours and up to 48 hours after cessation of drinking, with peak effects around 24 to 36 hours. Tremor, agitation, anxiety, anorexia, and insomnia are some of the usual symptoms. Seizures can also occur during the early phase of withdrawal. Late withdrawal symptoms or delirium tremens are relatively rare but can be life threatening. They consist of confusion, disorientation, auditory or visual hallucinations, disturbed sensory perception, and hyperthermia. Coma and death can occur if these are untreated. Complicating factors in alcohol withdrawal are trauma from falls or accidents, bacterial infections, and problems associated with other organ systems, such as liver and heart. The withdrawal syndrome after ethanol consumption is much more severe than that with opioids and depends largely on the blood alcohol concentration before withdrawal and the duration of the consumption. Management is aimed at preventing severe complications that may lead to a fatal outcome and includes prevention or treatment of seizures, delirium, and cardiac arrhythmias. Intravenous benzodiazepines, particularly those not converted to active metabolites, are the drugs of choice. Phenobarbital can also be used. Other barbiturates and phenothiazines should be avoided. Phenytoin should not be used unless there is preexisting epilepsy.

Table 31-3 Pharmacokinetic Parameters of Ethanol

Administered	Topically, orally, sometimes by inhalation, or by injection into nerve trunks
Absorption	Slight topically, complete from stomach and intestine by passive diffusion, rapid via lungs
Elimination	>90% metabolized to CO_2 and H_2O by liver and other tissues, excreted in air, urine, milk, sweat.
Rate of metabolism	Normally about 100 mg/kg/hr of total body burden, or 0.015%/hr; higher or lower in liver enzyme induction or in liver disease; zero-order kinetics
Distribution	Total body water; therefore the volume of distribution is 68% of body weight in men and 55% in women; varies widely

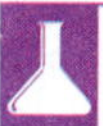

PHARMACOKINETICS

Absorption and Distribution

The pharmacokinetic parameters for ethanol are summarized in Table 31-3. Alcohol taken orally is absorbed throughout the gastrointestinal tract. Absorption depends on passive diffusion and is governed by the concentration gradient and the area available for absorption. Several factors influence absorption, the most important being the presence of food in the stomach. This tends to dilute the alcohol, delay emptying time, and retard absorption from the small intestine (where absorption is favored because of the large surface area). There is significant first-pass metabolism in both the stomach and liver. The slower absorption caused by the presence of food in the stomach will prolong the time for metabolism of the ethanol in the stomach and liver. Higher ethanol concentrations in the gastrointestinal tract cause a greater concentration gradient and therefore hasten the rate of absorption. The absorption process continues until the alcohol concentration in the blood and that in the gastrointestinal tract are at equilibrium. Since ethanol is rapidly metabolized and removed from the blood, eventually all the alcohol is absorbed from the gastrointestinal tract. Ethanol vapor is also rapidly absorbed from the lung.

Once ethanol reaches the systemic circulation it is immediately distributed to other body compartments at a rate proportional to the blood flow to that area and is eventually distributed equally to total body water. Because the brain receives a rapid blood flow, high concentrations in the brain are achieved rapidly.

Metabolism and Elimination

The major pathway for the disappearance of ethanol from the body is metabolism by the liver and to a minor extent by other organs (however, see below), with metabolism accounting for about 90% of the total eliminated. Expired air contains ethanol in proportion to the vapor pressure of ethanol at body temperature. The ratio of ethanol concentrations between exhaled air and blood alcohol, 1/2100, forms the basis for the "breathalyzer" test, in which blood alcohol concentration is determined by extrapolation from analysis of the alcohol content of the expired air.

Blood alcohol determination varies with hematocrit; people living at higher altitudes have a higher hematocrit and therefore a lower water content in blood. Urine is also available for determining ethanol concentration, and spinal or ocular fluid is generally used for postmortem analyses.

Blood concentrations of ethanol can be estimated from the weight and sex of the individual and the amount of ethanol consumed orally. These estimates are somewhat higher than actual blood concentrations unless the ethanol is given IV because there is rapid first-pass metabolism after oral administration. After consuming comparable amounts of ethanol, women have higher blood ethanol concentrations than men, even after correcting for differences in weight. Women also are more susceptible to alcoholic liver disease. Much of the first-pass metabolism of ethanol occurs in gastric tissue. The first-pass metabolism of ethanol is about 50% less in women than in men because of lower alcohol dehydrogenase activity in the female gastric mucosa. This occurs in nonalcoholic and alcoholic women and explains the increased vulnerability of women to the effects of acute and chronic alcoholism. It had been assumed earlier that the higher ethanol concentrations in women were entirely dependent on a difference in the apparent volumes of distribution between men and women. Body water content is 55% of body weight for women and 68% for men (Widmark factors), but these differences do not account entirely for the higher ethanol concentrations in women.

Calculation of Blood Alcohol Concentration from the Amount Ingested

Physicians are frequently called on as expert witnesses in cases involving alcohol intoxication. Moreover, in the course of taking a medical history it is valuable to be able to estimate the blood alcohol concentration and the subsequent effects of the alcohol from the amount ingested. In the calculation of the amount of ethanol ingested, the percentage of alcohol in the beverage (usually indicated on a volume/volume percent-

	Drinks in one hour 1	2	3	4	5
Body weight (pounds) 100	30	60	90	120	150
120	25	50	75	100	125
140	22	44	66	88	110
160	19	39	58	78	97
180	17	34	52	69	86
200	16	31	47	62	78

Blood alcohol concentration (BAC) mg/dl

FIGURE 31-1 Approximate percentages of ethanol in blood (BAC) in male subjects of different body weights, calculated as percent, weight/volume (w/v), after indicated number of drinks. One drink is 12 oz of beer, 5 oz of wine, or 1 oz of 80 proof distilled spirits. Individuals with BAC of 0.10% (100 mg/dl) or higher) are considered intoxicated in most states; those with BAC of 0.05% to 0.09% (50 to 99 mg/dl) are considered impaired. *Light pink area,* impaired; *dark pink area,* legally intoxicated. BAC can be 20% to 30% higher in female subjects. Notice the small number of drinks that can result in a state of intoxication.

age, with 100 proof equivalent to 50% ethanol by volume) and the density of 0.8 g for each ml of ethanol must be known. Blood alcohol concentrations (BAC) are calculated as milligrams of alcohol per liter of blood. The legal limit for operating a motor vehicle in most states is 1000 mg/L, 100 mg/dl, or 0.1%. An example of a typical calculation for a 70 kg person ingesting 1.0 oz, or 30 ml, of 80 proof distilled spirits is as follows:

$$\left(\frac{80}{2} \text{ proof} = 40\%\right) (30 \text{ ml}) = 12 \text{ ml } 100\% \text{ EtOH (by volume)}$$

$$(12 \text{ ml})(0.8 \text{ g/ml}) = 9.6 \text{ g EtOH (by weight)}$$

If absorbed immediately and distributed in total body water (assuming blood is 80% water):

$$\text{BAC (male)} = \frac{9.6\text{g}}{(70\text{kg})(0.68)} \times 0.8 = 0.16 \text{ g/L, } 16 \text{ mg/dl, } .016\%$$

$$\text{BAC (female)} = \frac{9.6\text{g}}{(70 \text{ kg})(0.55)} \times 0.8 = 0.2 \text{ g/L, } 20 \text{ mg/dl, } 0.02\%$$

An average rate for metabolism of ethanol by nontolerant individuals is 100 mg/kg of body weight/hr or 7 g/hr in a 70 kg individual. Chronic alcoholics metabolize ethanol at a higher rate, because of stimulation of the microsomal ethanol metabolizing system, or cytochrome P-450 system (see below). In the calcuation below, left, the man with a body burden of 9.6 g of ethanol would totally metabolize the alcohol in less than 2 hours.

Figure 31-1 provides an approximation of the maximum blood alcohol concentrations (BACs) in men ingesting 1 to 5 drinks in 1 hour for individuals of different body weights if one assumes rapid absorption. This figure emphasizes how little consumption can produce impaired motor skills and inability to drive an automobile safely, as indicated by the legal limit of 0.10% ethanol in most states and 0.08% in some states.

Enzyme Systems that Metabolize Ethanol

Most of the metabolism of ethanol takes place in the liver parenchyma catalyzed by alcohol dehydrogenase (ADH). The metabolic disposition is shown in Figure 31-2. Ethanol is metabolized to acetaldehyde by ADH, which in turn is oxidized to acetate by aldehyde dehydrogenases (ALDH). Acetate is then oxidized to CO_2 and H_2O, primarily in peripheral tissues. Both ADH and ALDH are dependent on nicotinamide adenine nucleotide (NAD^+) with the oxidation of 1 mole of ethanol to acetate producing 2 moles of nicotinamide adenine dinucleotide, reduced (NADH). Thus, for continuation of ethanol oxidation, mechanisms must exist both for acetaldehyde removal and for recycling of NAD^+ from

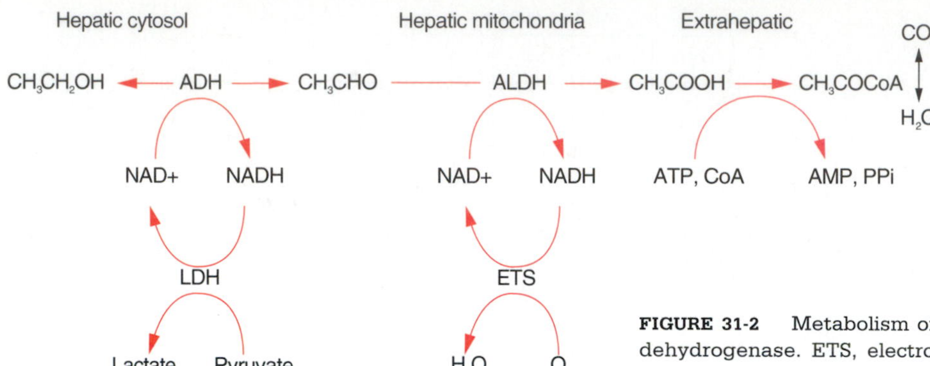

FIGURE 31-2 Metabolism of ethanol by alcohol and aldehyde dehydrogenase. ETS, electron transport system; LDH, lactate dehydrogenase.

NADH. Liver mitochondria contain a particularly efficient form of ALDH with a very low K_m that removes the acetaldehyde. The NADH is reoxidized to NAD^+ by several mechanisms including the mitochondrial electron transport system and the conversion of pyruvate to lactate by lactate dehydrogenase. During ethanol oxidation the concentration of NADH rises substantially, and NADH product inhibition can become rate-limiting. The K_m for various isozymes of human liver ADH varies from 0.05 to 30 mM (0.23 mg/dl to 138 mg/dl). Depending on the mix of these isozymes in an individual, alcohol disappearance kinetics will vary with the concentration of blood alcohol, especially at low blood alcohol concentrations. During fasting, ethanol metabolism decreases, an effect that can be accounted for by the decrease in liver ADH. Because of these factors, the metabolism of ethanol is limited and exhibits zero-order kinetics (Figure 31-3).

Another system for metabolizing ethanol in the liver is that catalyzed by cytochrome P-450. This system has also been called the *microsomal ethanol metabolizing system* and converts ethanol to acetaldehyde. The K_m for the system is relatively high (~30 mM) and normally would not be responsible for a significant fraction of ethanol metabolism. This enzyme system, however, is induced by prolonged ethanol exposure and can be important in chronic alcoholism. During the oxidation of ethanol with this system, one molecule of nicotinamide adenine dinucleotide phosphate reduced (NADPH) is utilized for every molecule of ethanol oxidized to acetaldehyde. Therefore the $NADH/NAD^+$ ratio does not increase. Since this enzyme system also metabolizes other exogenous compounds, when ethanol is present, their metabolism may be inhibited in chronic alcoholics, or stimulated if the cytochrome P-450 system is induced (see Chapter 5). A third system capable of metabolizing ethanol is the peroxidative reaction of catalase, a system limited by the amount of hydrogen peroxide available, which is normally low. There is disagreement in the literature as to the relative contributions from the cytochrome P-450 and catalase systems. Small amounts of ethanol are also metabolized by formation of phosphatidylethanol and ethyl esters of fatty acids.

Table 31-4 ADH Genetic Model*

Gene	Allele	Subunit
ADH_1	ADH_1	α
ADH_2	ADH_2^1	β_1
	ADH_2^2	β_2
	ADH_2^3	β_3
ADH_3	ADH_3^1	γ_1
	ADH_3^2	γ_2

*From Schuckit MA: *Ann Emerg Med* 15:991, 1986.

Table 31-5 Frequency of ADH_2, ADH_3, and $ALDH_2$ Alleles in Racial Populations

	ADH_2^1	ADH_2^2	ADH_2^3	ADH_3^1	ADH_3^2	$ALDH_2^1$
White Americans	>95%	<5%	<5%	50%	50%	100
White Europeans	85	15	<5	60	40	100
Asians	15	85	<5	95	5	50
African-Americans	85	<5	15	85	15	100

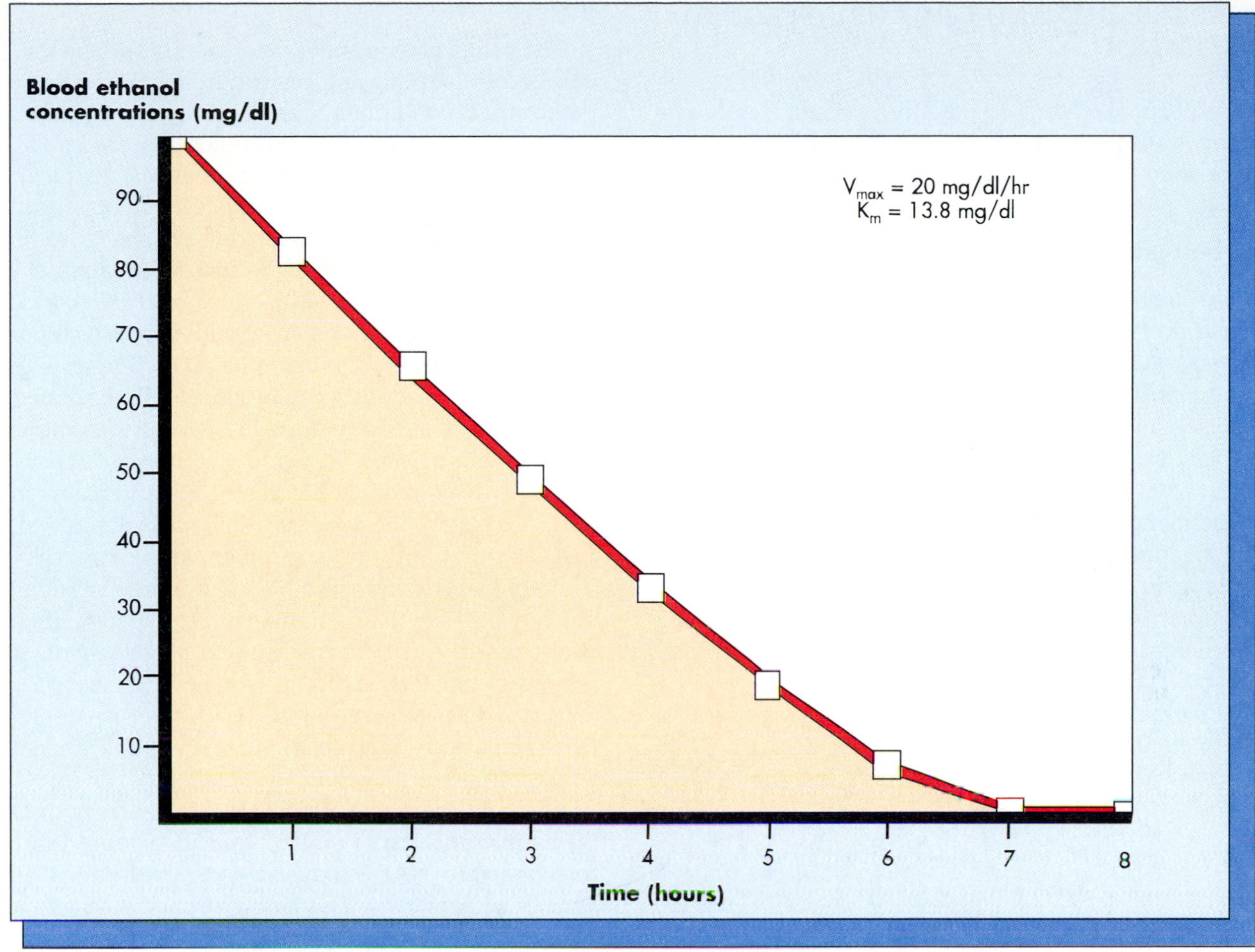

FIGURE 31-3 Disappearance of ethanol after oral ingestion follows zero-order kinetics.

Genetics of Ethanol-Metabolizing Enzymes

Human ADH is a cytosolic zinc-containing dimeric enzyme made up of six separate subunits, α, β_1, β_2, and β_3 and γ_1 and γ_2 (see Table 31-4). These subunits are encoded by three genes, ADH_1, ADH_2, and ADH_3, and their respective alleles. Because homodimers and heterodimers exist, many combinations of isozymes are possible. Whites, Asians, and blacks have different percentages of isozymes, which contribute to differences in the metabolism of ethanol among the races (Table 31-5). The several isozymes also have different K_m values.

The second enzyme in ethanol metabolism is aldehyde dehydrogenase. This mitochondrial enzyme has a K_m of about 1 μM, and so the very large amounts of aldehyde generated are handled efficiently. (There are also cytosolic and microsomal aldehyde dehydrogenases with higher K_m values.) This is fortunate because acetaldehyde is very reactive and potentially toxic. With this enzyme there are significant genetic differences that influence the responses to ethanol. Some Asians have a different mitochondrial ALDH than Caucasians have. About 50% of Asians have an inactive ALDH, caused by a single base change in the gene that encodes for the enzyme. This renders some Asians incapable of oxidizing acetaldehyde efficiently. High concentrations of acetaldehyde bring about a flushing reaction and other unpleasant effects, and so individuals with this genetic condition become only rarely alcoholic. Advantage is made of the strongly undesirable response to acetaldehyde accumulation in the aversive treatment of chronic alcoholism by the use of disulfiram (Antabuse). Disulfiram inhibits ALDH and in the presence of ethanol brings about flushing, headache, nausea and vomiting, sweating, and hypotension, shortly after alcohol ingestion.

Other agents such as metronidazole, the sulfonylureas, griseofulvin, some cephalosporins, and chloramphenicol may also provoke the acetaldehyde effect. Disulfiram also inhibits dopamine β-hydroxylase.

OTHER TISSUES AND ORGANS AFFECTED BY ETHANOL

The effects of ethanol on other organs and tissues are also important in the assessment of the hazards of ethanol ingestion.

Gastrointestinal Tract

It has been known for many years that tissues other than the liver have the capacity to metabolize ethanol. The metabolism of alcohol by the stomach and small intestine contributes to first-pass metabolism (discussed previously) and the greater susceptibility of women to ethanol. The oral mucosa, esophagus, stomach, and small intestine are also exposed to higher concentrations of ethanol than other tissues of the body. Thus they are susceptible to direct toxicity from ethanol. The alcohol dehydrogenase in the gastrointestinal tract is different from that in the liver and has a particularly high K_m. These tissues are also capable of metabolizing ethanol by the cytochrome P-450 system.

Acute gastritis resulting in nausea and vomiting is a result of ethanol abuse. Bleeding, ulcers, and cancer of the upper gastrointestinal tract are possible consequences.

Liver

The consequences of ethanol metabolism by the liver can be devastating and contribute significantly to the pathological conditions seen in this organ. The metabolism of ethanol causes a large increase in the NADH/NAD^+ ratio, which produces serious biochemical disruption in liver metabolism. The cell attempts to maintain NAD^+ concentrations in the cytosol by reducing pyruvate to lactate, leading to increased lactic acid in the liver and blood. Lactate is excreted by the kidney and competes with urate for elimination, which can increase blood urate. The excretion of lactate also apparently leads to a deficiency of zinc and magnesium. A more direct effect of increased NADH concentrations in the liver is increased fatty acid synthesis, since NADH is a necessary cofactor. Since NADH participates in the citric acid cycle, the oxidation of lipids is depressed, further contributing to fat accumulation in liver cells.

Acetaldehyde may also play a prominent role in liver damage. If there is an initial insult to the liver, the concentration of ALDH decreases and acetaldehyde is not removed efficiently and can react with many cell constituents. Possible consequences to the liver of chronic alcoholism and other deleterious effects of ethanol are listed in the boxes, below.

The increase in the NADH/NAD^+ ratio brought about by the metabolism of ethanol and inability of the body to regenerate NAD^+ may cause hypoglycemia and a state of ketoacidosis. The former occurs in the drinking, noneating user of alcohol when hepatic glycogen stores are exhausted (72 hours) and gluconeogenesis is inhibited by the increased NADH/NAD^+ ratio. The metabolic acidosis observed in nondiabetic alcoholics is an anion-gap acidosis with an increase in plasma concentration of β-hydroxybutyrate and lactate.

Effects of Ethanol on the Liver

- Increased NADH/NAD^+ ratio
- Increased acetaldehyde concentration
- Increased lipid content
- Increased protein accumulation
- Decreased protein export
- Increased water content
- Increased oxygen uptake
- Inhibition of gluconeogenesis
- Centrilobular hypoxia
- Proliferation of endoplasmic reticulum
- Increased cytochrome P-450 content
- Increased or decreased drug metabolism
- Increased production of free radicals and lipoperoxidation products
- Decreased production of coagulation factors
- Increased collagen deposition
- Hepatitis
- Scarring
- Cirrhosis with portal hypertension
- Hepatocellular death

Other Consequences of Ethanol

- Gastritis
- Increased incidence of peptic ulcer
- Gastrointestinal bleeding
- Pancreatitis
- Cardiomyopathy
- Cardiac dysrhythmias
- Feminization in males
- Cancers of upper gastrointestinal tract, liver
- Fetal alcohol syndrome
- Wernicke-Korsakoff syndrome

Pancreas

Ethanol is a known cause of acute pancreatitis. Repeated use can lead to pancreatic insufficiency with decreased pancreatic enzyme secretion and diabetes mellitus as possible consequences.

Endocrine System

Large amounts of ethanol decrease testosterone concentrations in men and cause loss of secondary sex characteristics and feminization. Premenopausal women who abuse alcohol may have a disruption of ovarian function seen as oligomenorrhea, hypomenorrhea, or amenorrhea. Ethanol also stimulates the release of adrenocortical hormones by increasing the secretion of adrenocorticotropic hormone.

Heart

Alcoholic cardiac myopathy is also a consequence of ethanol consumption. Other cardiovascular effects include mild increases in blood pressure and heart rate and cardiac arrhythmias. Cardiovascular complications as a result of liver cirrhosis and decreased venous return also occur. Epidemiological data indicate, however, that daily moderate use of alcohol may decrease the incidence of cardiovascular disease by elevating concentrations of high-density lipoprotein.

Kidney

As is well known, ethanol has a diuretic effect unrelated to fluid intake. This is caused by inhibition of secretion of antidiuretic hormone, which decreases the renal reabsorption of water. The inhibition of oxytocin release was formerly used to prevent premature labor.

Brain

There are several well-documented neurological conditions resulting from excessive ethanol intake with concomitant nutritional deficiencies. These include Wernicke-Korsakoff syndrome, cerebellar atrophy, central pontine myelinosis and demyelinization of the corpus callosum, and mammillary body destruction are other effects of ethanol upon the brain.

Fetal Alcohol Syndrome

Although fetal alcohol syndrome has been recognized from early times, it was rediscovered in the 1970s and the general public is well aware of the hazards of drinking by pregnant women on the health of the fetus. Consequences of maternal ingestion of alcohol can include miscarriage, stillbirth, low birth weight, slow postnatal growth, microcephaly, mental retardation, and many other organic and structural abnormalities. The incidence of fetal alcohol syndrome in some parts of the United States is estimated to be as high as 1 in 300 births. It is the most common cause of birth defects that are entirely preventable.

Other Effects

Alcoholics are frequently immunologically compromised, are subject to infectious diseases, and have excess mortality to cancers of the upper gastrointestinal tract as well as the liver. Although the mechanism of this latter effect is not known, alcohol consumption is a risk factor for the development of cancer and may be related to vitamin A metabolism.

Ethanol relaxes blood vessels, and in severe intoxication, hypothermia resulting from heat loss from vasodilatation may occur. Several types of anemias have been described in alcoholic patients.

DIAGNOSIS OF CHRONIC ALCOHOLISM: GENETIC FACTORS

The diagnosis of chronic alcoholism in a patient is a difficult problem for the practicing physician. Success depends on a reliable history from the patient or from a member of the patients' family. If a diagnosis can be made, it is frequently difficult to manage the problem because treatment is initiated when the disorder is well advanced.

Over the past 10 to 15 years the role of genetic factors in the development of chronic alcoholism has been identified with the hope that early intervention may be more successful. Studies involving family members and twins support a predisposition and an increased risk of alcoholism among close relatives. This conclusion that primary alcoholism is genetically influenced is based upon several interesting findings.

Studies among families indicate a threefold to fourfold higher risk for alcoholism primarily in sons but some in daughters of alcoholic parents. Comparisons of the risk of alcoholism in identical twins versus fraternal twins should determine whether alcoholism is related to the childhood environment. Since both types of twins have similar childhood backgrounds, if alcoholism is related to the childhood environment, both identical and fraternal twins should have the same rates of development of the alcoholic disorder. Most results show that in identical twins, which share 100% of their genes, there is a twofold higher concordance for alcoholism compared to fraternal twins. In another study, alcoholic

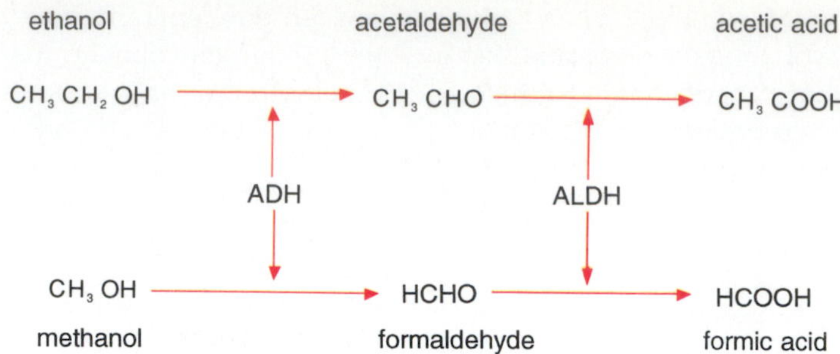

FIGURE 31-4 Ethanol has a greater affinity for alcohol dehydrogenase than methanol does, thereby reducing the conversion of methanol to its metabolic products.

risk was assessed in male children of alcoholics who were raised by adoptive parents (other than their biological parents) who were nonalcoholics. In these males there was a threefold to fourfold higher risk for alcoholism. Being raised by alcoholic adoptive parents did not increase the risk for alcoholism. In some studies there was a protective effect, in fact.

Other studies have categorized alcoholics into several subgroups. One is the alcoholism most frequently seen in men and associated with criminality, and the second is a subtype observed in both sexes and influenced by the environment. Genetic predisposition, however, is merely one of several factors leading to the development of alcoholism. Studies in progress are attempting to seek out possible biological markers with which to identify potential alcoholics (e.g., specific differences in blood proteins, enzymes involved in ethanol degradation, and enzymes concerned with brain neurotransmitters and signaling system components, including G proteins) to encourage such individuals to seek assistance sooner.

TREATMENT OF ALCOHOLISM

Acute Intoxication

Emergency treatment of acute alcohol intoxication includes the maintenance of an adequate airway and support of respiration and blood pressure. In addition to its depressant actions on the CNS, other organs including the heart may be affected. It is also important to assess the level of consciousness relative to blood alcohol concentration, since other drugs may influence the apparent degree of intoxication. As a precaution a short-acting narcotic antagonist is generally administered. Hypoglycemia, ketoacidosis, and dehydration may require the administration of glucose. The loss of body fluids may also necessitate IV fluids containing potassium, magnesium, and phosphate. Thiamine and other vitamins such as folic acid and pyridoxine are administered usually with IV glucose to prevent the neurological deficits that may occur. Extreme caution is needed when one is modifying sodium concentrations, since overcorrection has been associated with central pontine myelinolysis.

Chronic Alcoholism

The effective management of chronic alcoholism includes the social and environmental as well as the medical aspects and also involves the family of the individual undergoing treatment. Several types of treatment are available, including group psychotherapy (e.g., Alcoholics Anonymous), and private and public clinics outside of a hospital setting. Hypnotherapy, psychoanalysis, and aversive therapy with *disulfiram* also have been used. Management regimens have had variable success rates, with many being no more effective over the long term than 10% to 15% of the participants.

OTHER ALCOHOLS

Methanol Intoxication

Alcoholics or others may accidentally or intentionally ingest methanol, which has a toxicological profile quite different from that of ethanol. The two major characteristics of methanol intoxication are optic nerve damage, which can lead to blindness, and severe acidosis. Methanol is metabolized by alcohol dehydrogenase and aldehyde dehydrogenase systems in a manner similar to ethanol but at a much slower rate. The products of methanol metabolism are formaldehyde and formic acid, which are apparently responsible for visual damage and acidosis. Management requires maintenance of an airway and ventilation as with any intoxication, attempts to remove residual methanol, the treatment of the acidosis, and the administration of IV ethanol in order to reduce the formation of the toxic metabolic products. Ethanol is effective since it can compete successfully with methanol for alcohol dehydrogenase and essentially saturate the enzyme (Figure 31-4). This reduces the likelihood of subsequent effects of methanol metabolites and provides the time necessary for removal of methanol from the body by dialysis, which is the treatment of choice.

Ethylene Glycol Intoxication

The dihydric alcohol ethylene glycol is found in antifreeze products and may also be ingested accidentally and cause severe CNS depression and renal damage. Ethylene glycol is also metabolized by alcohol dehydrogenase to glycolic and oxalic acids. Glycolic acid can cause metabolic acidosis, as with methanol intoxication, whereas oxalate appears to be responsible for the renal toxicity. Management is similar to that for methanol intoxication.

Isopropanol Intoxication

Isopropyl alcohol, or rubbing alcohol, is sometimes accidentally ingested and may be used by chronic alcoholics when ethanol may be unavailable. It is a CNS depressant and more toxic to the CNS than ethanol. Signs and symptoms of intoxication are also similar to ethanol. Toxicity is limited, however, because isopropanol produces severe gastritis with accompanying pain, nausea, and vomiting. Isopropanol is metabolized by alcohol dehydrogenase to acetone but at a much slower rate than that of ethanol. In severe intoxication, hemodialysis is used to remove isopropanol from the body.

NEW DIRECTIONS

New drugs have been proposed for treatment of alcohol craving and prevention of relapse. Data from animal studies and from limited clinical trials have pointed to the possibility of serotonin uptake blockers as useful agents. Studies also implicate dopamine in the reward pathway as a target for a variety of drugs of abuse. These observations may lead to useful drugs acting on dopamine receptors. Also clinical trials of opiate antagonists have yielded some promising results in preventing relapse.

REFERENCES

Abel EL: *Fetal alcohol syndrome and fetal alcohol effects.* New York, 1984, Plenum Press.

Deitrich RA, Dunwiddie TV, Harris RA, et al.: Mechanism of action of ethanol: initial central nervous system actions, *Pharmacol Rev* 41:489, 1990.

Frezza M, Di Padova C, Pozzato G, et al.: High blood alcohol levels in women, *N Engl J Med* 322:95, 1990.

Goldstein DB: *Pharmacology of alcohol,* Oxford, 1983, Oxford Press.

Hoffman PL, Tabakoff B: Ethanol and guanine nucleotide binding proteins: selective interaction, *FASEB J* 4:2612, 1990.

Schuckit, MA, Low level of response to alcohol as a predictor of future alcoholism, *Am J Psychiatry* 151:184, 1994.

Schuckit MA: Genetic aspects of alcoholism, *Ann Emerg Med* 15:991, 1986.

SELF-ASSESSMENT QUESTIONS

1. An adequate medical history from a patient should include information concerning alcohol usage because alcohol may be implicated in:
   a. cardiovascular disease.
   b. liver malfunction.
   c. cancer of the larynx and pharynx.
   d. mental retardation of children.
   e. all of the above.
2. Ascites resulting from excessive alcohol intake is most likely caused by:
   a. obstructed venous return.
   b. increased osmolality of the blood.
   c. increased blood uric acid concentrations.
   d. increased magnesium excretion.
   e. increased blood lactate concentrations.
3. Current evidence indicates that genetic risk for developing alcoholism:
   a. is due to a single gene.
   b. is greater for men than for women.
   c. is caused by inheritance of altered genes for liver alcohol dehydrogenase.
   d. is caused by high concentrations of acetaldehyde.
   e. is caused by inheritance of genes coding for increased dopamine concentrations in the reward pathways of the brain.
4. Women's risk for disorders induced by alcohol is greater than that for men in which organ:
   a. pancreas
   b. stomach
   c. larynx
   d. liver
   e. heart

5. Flushing reactions in response to ethanol in Asians resembles the response to ethanol in individual who have taken:
   a. benzodiazepines.
   b. barbiturates.
   c. antihistamines.
   d. disulfiram.
   e. chloral hydrate.

6. As a consequence of the metabolism of ethanol by the cytochrome P-450 system and also its induction by ethanol the following may occur:
   a. Increased rate of metabolism of other drugs.
   b. When ethanol is present, a decreased rate of metabolism of some drugs.
   c. Increased production of carcinogenic compounds from procarcinogens.
   d. Increased clearance of ethanol.
   e. All of the above.

CHAPTER 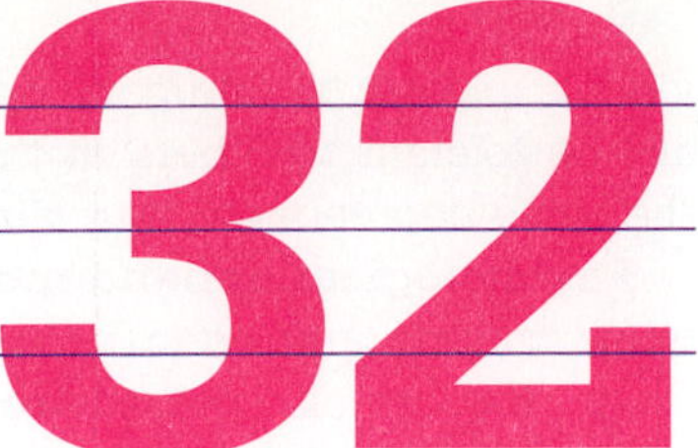

Drug Abuse

ROBERT L. BALSTER

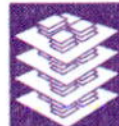

THERAPEUTIC OVERVIEW

Medical problems related to drug abuse have become an important concern of practicing physicians. Many physicians are involved in the treatment of acute overdoses, withdrawal, and the medical sequelae of drug abuse. Although long-term treatment of drug abuse has increasingly become the province of specialized, multidisciplinary treatment programs, the primary care physician plays a key role in diagnosis, referral, and sometimes treatment.

The main types of abused substances are listed in the box, p. 436. Abused substances are defined as drugs or other materials (e.g., solvents) administered repeatedly in a pattern and amount that interferes with the health or normal social and occupational functioning of the individual. This definition does not require the development of tolerance or dependence, though these often accompany substance abuse. **Tolerance** (Chapter 3) is characterized by a reduced drug effect with repeated use and a requirement of higher doses to produce the same effect. Since tolerance does not occur to the same extent for all effects, drug abusers who take increasing amounts of drugs risk exposure to those effects to which tolerance does not develop.

Dependence is characterized by physiological or behavioral changes after discontinuation of drug use referred to as withdrawal. During drug withdrawal, these changes are reversible on resumption of drug administration. **Physical (or physiological) dependence** is evidenced by a characteristic syndrome of signs and symptoms during withdrawal. **The withdrawal syndrome** for drugs within a pharmacological class is similar but differs among various drug classes. The course of the withdrawal syndrome varies according to the rate of elimination of individual drugs or their active metabolites. Withdrawal from long-acting drugs has a delayed onset, is relatively mild, and may occur over many days or weeks (Figure 32-1, *A*), whereas that from more rapidly metabolized or eliminated drugs is more intense but of shorter duration (Figure 32-1, *B*). If an antagonist is administered, withdrawal signs are even more intense and of shorter duration (Figure 32-1, *C*). Physical dependence usually occurs only when substances are used over extended times, with significant blood and brain concentrations achieved for days, weeks, or months. Initially, dependence can be either slight or severe, but with repeated drug use the severity becomes increasingly greater. Occasional drug use does not usually result in a clinically significant physical dependence.

Withdrawal can occur spontaneously or can be precipitated by antagonists (Figure 32-1). **Spontaneous withdrawal** can occur without an antagonist when drug use is discontinued. An example of **precipitated withdrawal** occurs when opiate-dependent individuals given the antagonists naloxone or naltrexone experience an immediate, intense withdrawal syndrome. Similarly, precipitated withdrawal from benzodiazepines can be produced by the benzodiazepine antagonist flumazenil. The duration of the precipitated withdrawal syndrome is determined by the duration of action of the antagonist.

Different drugs within a pharmacological class can generally support physical dependence produced by other drugs in the same class. This phenomenon is

ABBREVIATIONS	
HIV	human immunodeficiency virus
LAAM	*l*-α-acetylmethadol
LSD	D-lysergic acid diethylamide
PCP	phencyclidine
THC	tetrahydrocannabinol
MDMA	methylenedioxymethamphetamine
NMDA	*N*-methyl-D-aspartate

termed **cross-dependence.** Thus, heroin withdrawal can be prevented by administration of other opioids. This is the rationale for the use of methadone in the pharmacotherapy of heroin or morphine dependence. Alcohol, barbiturates, and benzodiazepines also show cross-dependence with each other but not with opioids. **Cross-tolerance** is similar to cross-dependence. Individuals tolerant to a drug in one chemical class will usually be tolerant to others in the same class but not to the same degree as to drugs in other classes.

Psychological dependence is characterized by intense craving and compulsive drug-seeking behavior. Drugs of abuse also possess **reinforcing effects** often accompanied by intense euphoria and feelings of well-being, which contribute to their continued abuse. This is especially true of stimulants such as cocaine and the amphetamines.

Several strategies are used in drug abuse treatment. **Maintenance therapy** utilizes a drug such as methadone to continue opioid dependence while psychological, social, and vocational therapies are used to support the user during abstinence. **Detoxification** is the process of treating physical dependence by reducing drug administration and can be performed abruptly or gradually.

SUBSTANCES OF ABUSE

OPIATES AND OPIOIDS

morphine, codeine, heroin, meperidine, hydromorphone, and other opioid agonists

SYMPATHOMIMETIC STIMULANTS

cocaine, amphetamines, methylphenidate, and other related stimulants

DEPRESSANTS

barbiturates, nonbarbiturate sedatives, benzodiazepines, and ethanol

HALLUCINOGENS

D-lysergic acid diethylamide (LSD), mescaline, methylenedioxymethamphetamine (MDMA), and others

OTHERS

phencyclidine, marihuana, inhalants, nicotine, caffeine

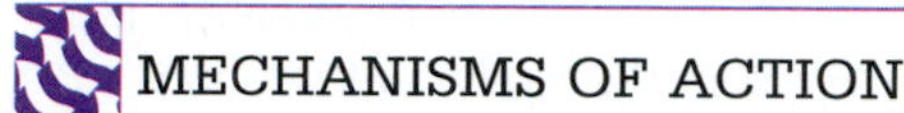

MECHANISMS OF ACTION

Opiates

Opium is the concentrated resinous material obtained from the opium poppy. The two principal naturally occurring opiates are morphine and codeine. Synthetic opioids are also widely available and abused. The most commonly abused opioid is heroin, or diacetyl morphine. Although heroin is about three times more po-

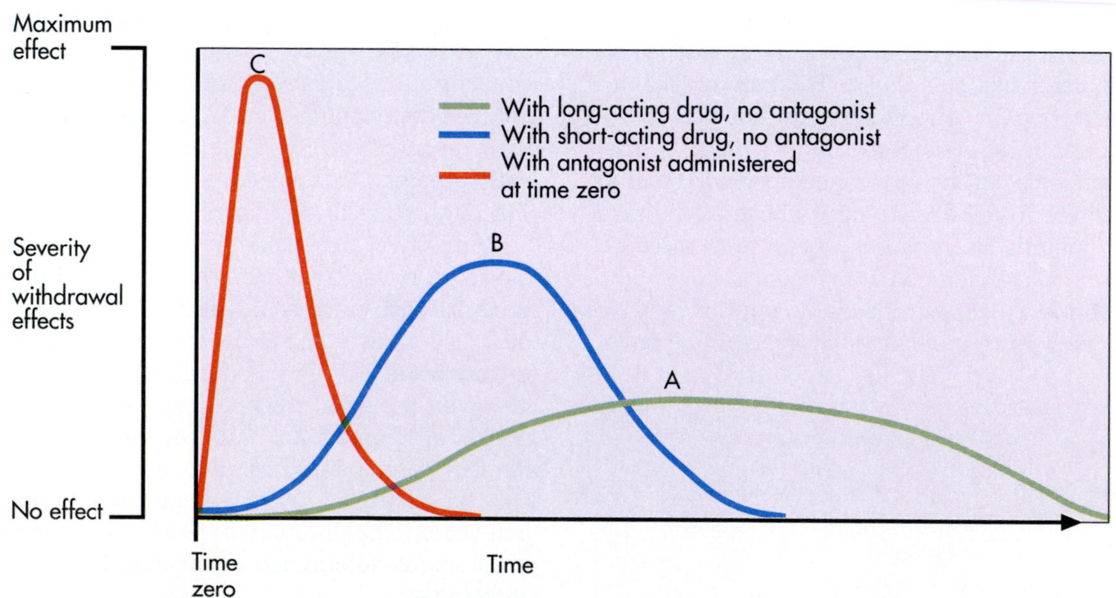

FIGURE 32-1 Schema showing the course of severity of withdrawal effects with dependence on drugs with long *(A)* and short *(B)* durations of action, or after administration of an antagonist *(C)*.

tent than morphine, the two drugs have very similar effects, and even experienced abusers have difficulty distinguishing between them.

Most of the effects of abused opiates, including their reinforcing effects, are mediated by μ opiate receptors (Chapter 28). On the other hand, the biological basis of opiate physical dependence is poorly understood. No biochemical marker has yet been found for opiate dependence. Animal studies have not found consistent changes in μ opiate receptor number or affinity with repeated opioid exposure, nor have changes been found in endogenous opiate peptides. The most consistent correlate of opiate dependence is the increased sensitivity to withdrawal precipitated by opiate antagonists. This sensitivity may begin with the first opiate dose, since under laboratory conditions high doses of an antagonist can precipitate a withdrawal syndrome within a few hours after a single dose of morphine or methadone.

Sympathomimetic Stimulants

The most commonly abused drugs in this class are cocaine and the amphetamines, though other stimulants also have abuse potential. These drugs all act in the CNS to enhance catecholaminergic neurotransmission as discussed in Chapter 10.

The structure of cocaine is shown in Figure 32-7. Cocaine is the principal psychoactive alkaloid present in the coca bush, cultivated principally in South America, where the chewing of coca leaves is a common practice. Cocaine is extracted from the plant and used as either the free base or as the water-soluble hydrochloride salt.

The amphetamines include dextroamphetamine and its *N*-methyl analog, methamphetamine. The amphetamines are synthetic compounds related structurally to the catecholamine neurotransmitters and to substituted phenethylamine hallucinogens (Figure 32-2). Nonamphetamine sympathomimetic stimulants such as methylphenidate and phenmetrazine are also abused. Other such weight-control medications have varying degrees of central stimulant actions and propensity for abuse. The anorectics with potent serotoninergic actions, such as mazindol and fenfluramine, may produce adverse effects at higher doses, which limit their abuse potential.

The reinforcing effects of cocaine and amphetamines arise from enhanced catecholamine neurotransmission at dopamine synapses in the ascending mesolimbic and mesocortical pathways (Figure 32-3). By binding to a specific site on the transporter protein, cocaine blocks the reuptake of dopamine, thus enhancing dopamine action. Amphetamines also have prominent actions on

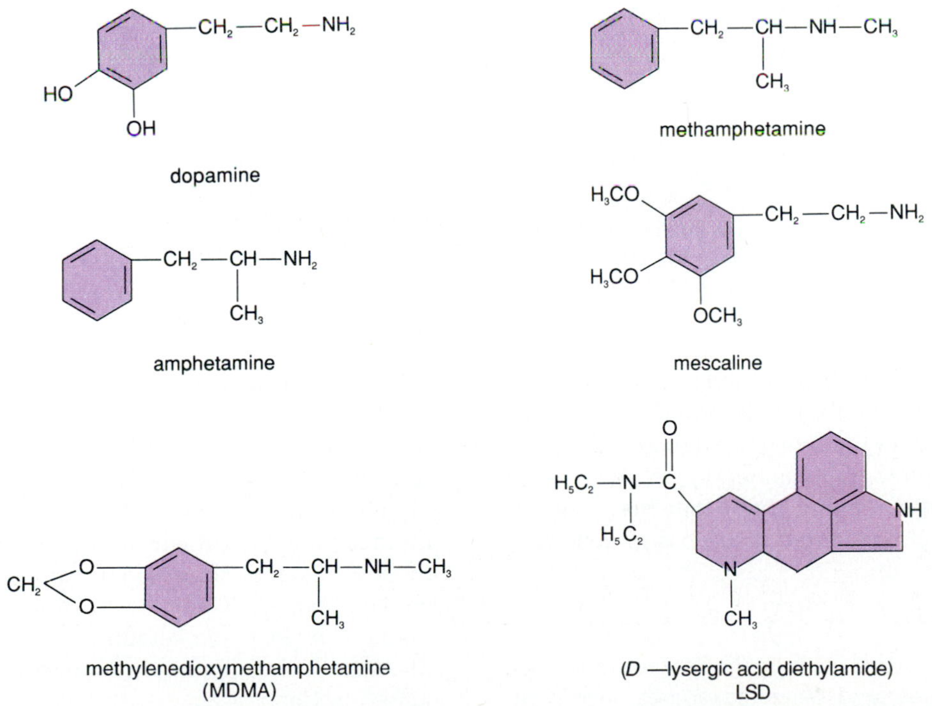

dopamine

methamphetamine

amphetamine

mescaline

methylenedioxymethamphetamine (MDMA)

(*D* —lysergic acid diethylamide) LSD

FIGURE 32-2 Structures of amphetamines, substituted-amphetamine hallucinogens (mescaline and MDMA), and the indolamine hallucinogen LSD. Note structural similarity of amphetamines to dopamine.

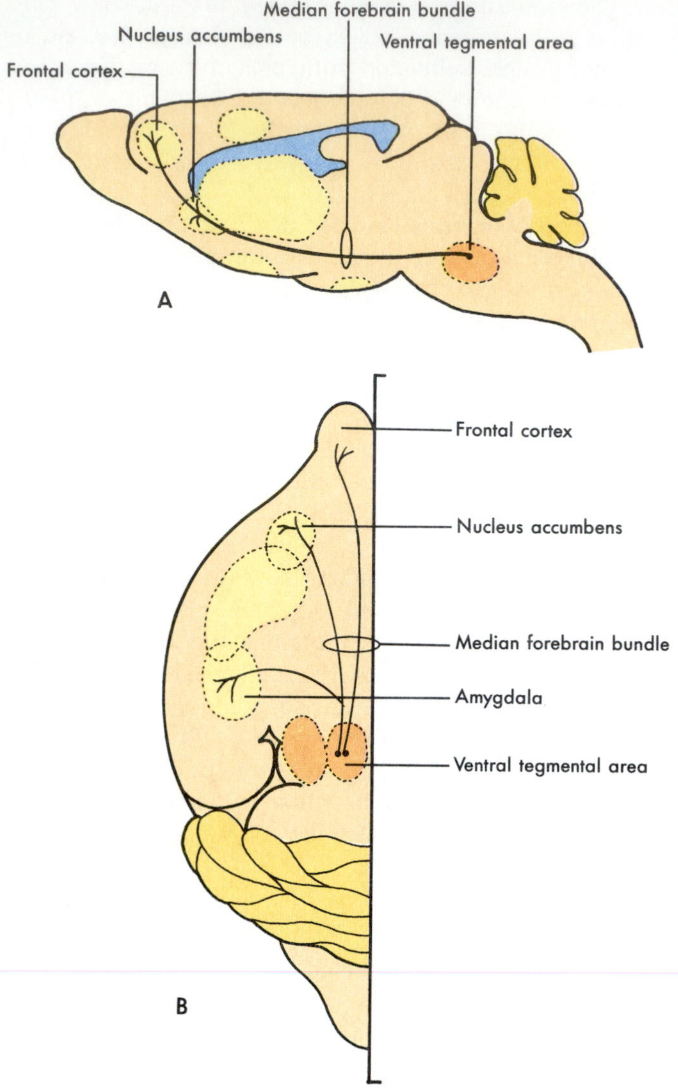

FIGURE 32-3 Schema of ascending dopaminergic pathways in rat brain believed to mediate the reinforcing effects of cocaine and the amphetamines. **A,** Sagittal, or side view. **B,** Coronal, or top view.

dopaminergic neurons in these regions, enhancing neurotransmitter release, inhibiting destruction by monoamine oxidase, blocking reuptake, or directly activating postsynaptic receptors. Dopaminergic pathways activated by stimulant drugs are those that may have an important role in reinforcement processes in general.

CNS Depressants

CNS depressant drugs such as the barbiturates, nonbarbiturate sedatives, and benzodiazepines have pharmacological actions that are fundamentally similar to those of alcohol (Chapters 25, 26, and 31), and this similarity is important to understanding the abuse of these compounds. Like their other pharmacological effects, the reinforcing effects of these drugs appear to be mediated by enhancement of γ-aminobutyric acid neurotransmission. As with opiates, the biochemical and neural basis for physical dependence on depressant drugs is not well understood.

Hallucinogens

Abused hallucinogenic compounds fall into two chemical classes, the substituted phenethylamines and the indolamines. Mescaline is the prototypic substituted phenethylamine hallucinogen (see Figure 32-2). Ring-substituted amphetamines are also commonly abused and include such compounds as methylenedioxymethamphetamine (MDMA), a compound recently referred to as "ecstacy" or "XTC" (see Figure 32-2). D-Lysergic acid diethylamide (LSD) (see Figure 32-2) is the prototypic indolamine hallucinogen; others include psilocybin (from mushrooms) and dimethyltryptamine. The hallucinogens have no recognized medical use. Because of the large number of chemical modifications that can be made without losing psychoactivity, so-called designer drugs have appeared and are abused before they become subject to drug abuse control provisions. Examples of designer drugs in other classes are the potent heroin-like fentanyl derivatives (e.g., "China White") and various phencyclidine analogs.

The sympathomimetic effects of hallucinogens probably result from enhanced catecholaminergic neurotransmission. However, for most hallucinogens the most prominent effects relate to an individual's subjective experiences. These unique psychological effects of hallucinogens are believed to result from modulation of serotoninergic neurotransmission, with recent evidence implicating the activation of the 5-HT_2 (serotonin) receptor subtype.

Others

Phencyclidine Phencyclidine, or PCP, was originally developed as an injectable anesthetic (Figure 32-4). Ketamine, a close structural analog of PCP, is currently used clinically (Chapter 30). PCP was withdrawn from human testing because of the severity of emergence delirium in patients. Until recently, PCP was used as a veterinary anesthetic and used in capture guns to tranquilize wild animals. The type of "dissociative" anesthesia produced by PCP and ketamine does not occur with the inhalational and barbiturate anesthetics and is discussed in Chapter 30.

A unique binding site for PCP has been discovered in mammalian brain. The PCP site may comprise a portion of an ion channel regulated by the excitatory amino

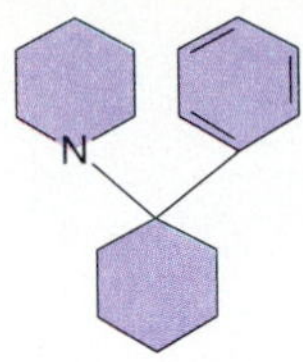

FIGURE 32-4 Structure of phencyclidine (PCP).

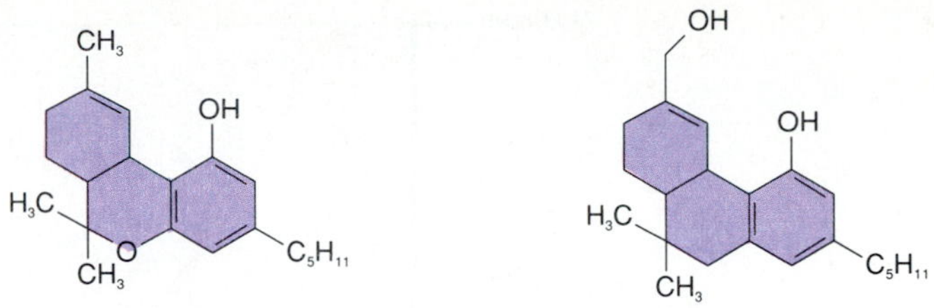

Δ^9 tetrahydrocannabinol (THC)

11-OH- Δ^9-THC

FIGURE 32-5. Structure of Δ^9-tetrahydrocannabinol (THC) and its active metabolite 11-OH-Δ^9-tetrahydrocannabinol

acid neurotransmitter glutamate. PCP antagonizes glutamate action and, in animals, offers some protection against excitotoxicity resulting from overstimulation of the *N*-methyl-D-aspartate (NMDA) subtype of glutamate receptor (see Chapter 2). Evidence is accumulating that glutamate antagonism is the basis for the effects of PCP relevant to its abuse. Interest is developing in studying certain NMDA antagonists as possible anticonvulsants or as neuroprotective agents in ischemic or concussive brain injury where glutamate may play a role.

Cannabis *Cannabis sativa* is the common hemp plant; however, plant varieties suitable for making rope often have little psychoactivity. The leaves and resin from *Cannabis sativa* cultivated for smoking contain chemicals referred to as cannabinoids; $(-)\Delta^9$-tetrahydrocannabinol (or THC) (Figure 32-5) is the major cannabinoid with psychoactivity. THC is metabolically converted to another active compound, 11-OH-Δ^9-THC. Other plant cannabinoids include cannabinol, which has weak biological activity, and cannabidiol, which is inactive. Marihuana is the dried leaf material from the plant and generally contains 1% to 3% THC. Hashish is the dried resinous material exuded by mature plants and generally contains about 10 times greater concentrations of THC than the corresponding leaf material.

A cannabinoid receptor has now been cloned and its amino acid sequence determined. The good correlation between affinity for this receptor and the psychoactivity of THC and various THC analogs indicates strongly that it serves as the molecular target for these drugs and may be involved in the neural basis for *Cannabis* abuse.

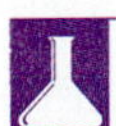

PHARMACOKINETICS

The biodisposition of opiates is discussed in Chapter 28. Since heroin and morphine have poor oral availability, abusers of these drugs usually resort to administration by injection or inhalation.

When cocaine free base is volatilized and inhaled, absorption into the blood is rapid, leading to an onset of action similar to that for IV administration (Figure 32-6). Intranasal and oral administration result in slower onset. The intoxication after IV administration or inhalation of cocaine generally lasts only about 30 minutes, and redosing is frequently employed in an attempt to maintain intoxication. Cocaine is rapidly metabolized by blood and liver esterases (Figure 32-7) to a common final product with metabolites found in urine for up to a week after use. *N*-demethylation in the liver to norcocaine is a minor metabolic pathway with corresponding deesterified norcocaine metabolites also found in the urine. Assay for cocaine metabolites in urine is an important basis for establishing recent cocaine use.

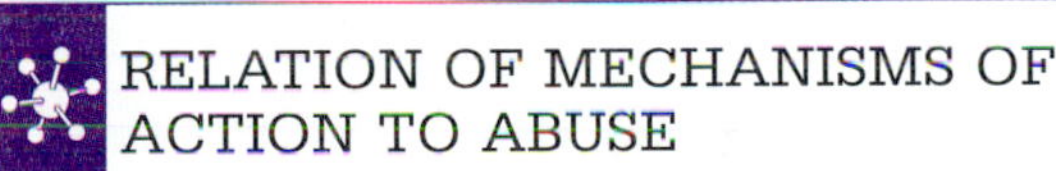

RELATION OF MECHANISMS OF ACTION TO ABUSE

Opiates

Routes of Administration Heroin abusers often begin by smoking or SC injection of the drug; most eventually administer the compound by IV injection. The IV route of administration leads to many medical problems (see box on page 441). A particularly dangerous practice is the sharing of needles and other injection paraphernalia, since *the incidence of blood-borne infection, including human immunodeficiency virus (HIV), in opiate abusers is extraordinarily high.*

Initial Effects The "rush" that accompanies an IV heroin injection is quite intense. When the abuser is in withdrawal, the positive reinforcing effects of the rush are amplified by the instant alleviation of withdrawal sickness. Many physically dependent abusers are tolerant to the positive reinforcing effects, and continued drug use provides only relief from withdrawal.

After a few minutes the IV administration rush subsides, and effects resemble those after oral dosing with opioids. The user feels relaxed and carefree, somewhat dreamy, but able to carry on many normal activities. Un-

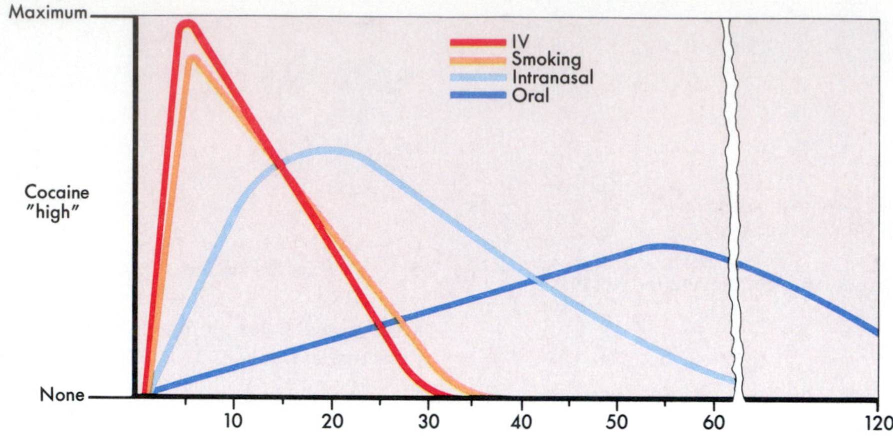

FIGURE 32-6 The intensity and course (in minutes) of cocaine intoxication at equivalent doses by different routes of administration.

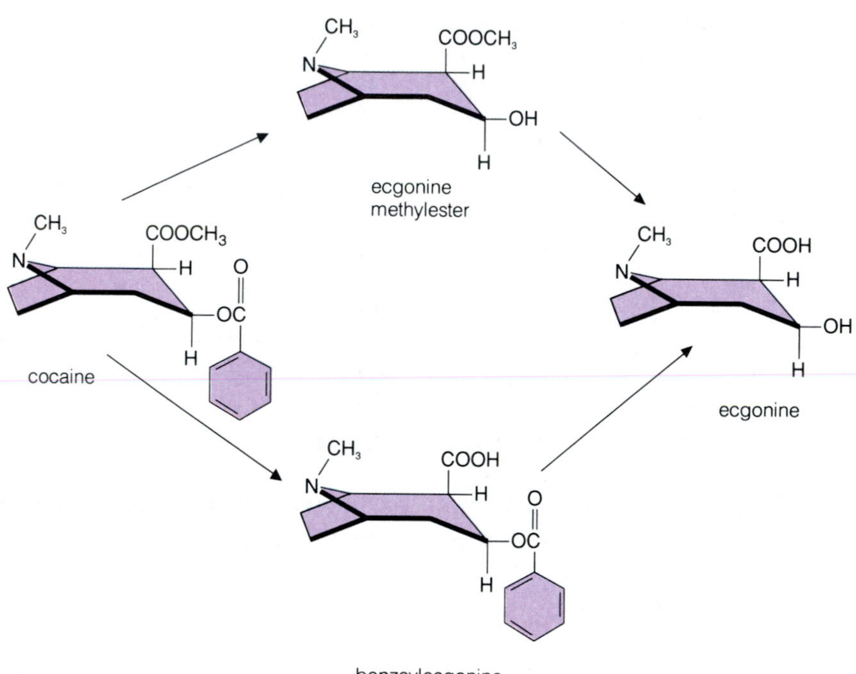

FIGURE 32-7 Deesterification pathways for cocaine metabolism by serum and liver esterases.

like an individual intoxicated with alcohol or another CNS depressant, the opiate abuser is difficult to detect solely on the basis of observable behavioral effects.

The effects of injected heroin persist about 4 to 6 hours, depending on the dose. Users who are not physically dependent recover readily from its effects. Most heroin abusers do not immediately develop a dependence-producing pattern of use. Some may take opiates for many years at intervals that are insufficient to produce physical dependence. It is important to distinguish physically dependent from nondependent abusers, since treatment strategies differ considerably. Unfortunately, most treatment programs are for hard-core dependent abusers. Strategies for preventing escalation from occasional use would be highly desirable, but such users often do not come to the attention of health professionals.

Overdosage leads to unconsciousness, respiratory depression, and extreme miosis, though the last is not always apparent, since severe asphyxia can dilate pu-

Medical Sequelae of Opiate Abuse

Overdosage
Abscesses at site of injection, thrombophlebitis
Pregnancy complications and babies born dependent
Possibilities for subsequent infections:
- HIV and AIDS (see Chapter 51)
- Bacterial endocarditis
- Hepatitis and hepatic dysfunction
- Tuberculosis
- Pneumonia
- Septic pulmonary embolism
- Tetanus

pils. An opiate antagonist such as naloxone can immediately reverse all these effects and cause rapid patient recovery. It is important not to administer too large a dose, since severe withdrawal can be precipitated in a physically dependent patient. The duration of action of naloxone is shorter than that of opioid agonists, and one should be cautious that severe intoxication does not reemerge. Naltrexone has a longer duration of action than naloxone but is not currently available in an injectable form for use in treating overdosage.

Dependence The progression to physical dependence occurs gradually for most opiate abusers. Experimental users are generally confident that they can control their use and initially are only dimly aware that they are becoming dependent. Taking multiple daily doses of heroin or other opioids usually results in clinically significant dependence in a few weeks. Opiate withdrawal rarely constitutes a medical emergency and is considerably less dangerous than withdrawal from alcohol and barbiturates (see box above right).

The significance of physical dependence is the inexorable appearance of the withdrawal syndrome about 6 or more hours after the last heroin injection. Many of the signs and symptoms of withdrawal (see box) are opposite to the effects of acute opiate administration. Unmedicated, the syndrome reaches peak severity in about 24 hours and is terminated in 7 to 10 days. Opiates cross the placental barrier, and in an opioid-dependent mother the newborn will undergo withdrawal beginning 6 to 12 hours after birth. Although the long-term consequences of prenatal opioid dependence are poorly understood, it may be appropriate to maintain the mother on methadone and treat the dependent infant with paregoric or methadone rather than to withdraw the mother before parturition. Otherwise, the mother may leave treatment and resume opiate abuse without adequate prenatal care.

Comparison of Opiate and Depressant Withdrawal

OPIATE WITHDRAWAL	DEPRESSANT* WITHDRAWAL
Anxiety and dysphoria	Anxiety and dysphoria
Craving and drug-seeking	Craving and drug-seeking
Sleep disturbance	Sleep disturbance
Nausea and vomiting	Nausea and vomiting
Lacrimation	Tremors
Rhinorrhea	Hyperreflexia
Yawning	Hyperpyrexia
Piloerection and gooseflesh	Confusion and delirium
Sweating	Convulsions
Diarrhea	Possible death
Mydriasis	
Abdominal cramping	
Hyperpyrexia	
Tachycardia and hypertension	

*Alcohol, barbiturates, or benzodiazepines.

In opiate-dependent individuals, opiate antagonists produce precipitated withdrawal, which has an immediate onset and can be much more severe than spontaneous withdrawal. Its duration is determined by the duration of action of the antagonist (e.g., naloxone-precipitated withdrawal is shorter than naltrexone-precipitated withdrawal). In most other respects, precipitated withdrawal closely resembles spontaneous withdrawal.

Cross-dependence Cross-dependence occurs among all full opioid agonists. For a heroin addict, opioids such as hydromorphone, meperidine, oxycodone, and others can reverse opioid withdrawal signs and at appropriate doses can produce a heroin-like intoxication. Even less efficacious opioid agonists such as codeine and dextropropoxyphene show cross-dependence with heroin. A major problem for prescribing physicians is that heroin abusers often convincingly exhibit symptoms that require potent analgesics, which are used for treatment of their withdrawal symptoms.

Mixed opioid agonist/antagonists and partial opioid agonists such as pentazocine, butorphanol, nalbuphine, and buprenorphine are less abused than full agonists, though each offers a slightly different profile of abuse potential (Chapter 28). Except for buprenorphine, these drugs show little cross-dependence with heroin and can exacerbate withdrawal; thus they offer little attraction for the heroin addict.

On the other hand, pentazocine and related mixed

agonist/antagonists have some positive reinforcing effects and may be abused. Pentazocine abuse has been reduced by reformulation in combination with naloxone. Naloxone is intended to block the positive reinforcing effects of pentazocine after IV injection.

Sympathomimetic Stimulants

Routes of Administration Cocaine hydrochloride is a bitter-tasting, white, crystalline material that is generally inhaled nasally (insufflation) or injected IV. Cocaine salts are often diluted ("cut") with local anesthetics, which are similar in appearance and taste. The abuse of "free-base" cocaine, known as "crack," has recently become common. Crack is volatile at a lower temperature than the salt and can be inhaled after heating. It is usually sold as small hard pieces, or "rocks," and is readily available and relatively inexpensive. Abuse of cocaine by nasal insufflation may lead to irritation of the nasal mucosa, sinusitis, and perforated septum. Needle-sharing among IV cocaine abusers and high-risk sexual behaviors associated with cocaine abuse are important avenues for HIV transmission.

The amphetamines and amphetamine-like stimulants are more commonly abused by oral administration, though insufflation and IV use also occur. Inhaled methamphetamine ("ice"), used in a manner similar to crack cocaine, is a problem in some areas.

Initial Effects The IV or inhalational use of cocaine (see Figure 32-6) produces a rapid onset rush with intense positive reinforcing effects. Cocaine and other stimulants produce increased alertness, feelings of elation and well-being, increased energy, feelings of competence, and increased sexuality. Enhancement of athletic performance has been reported, particularly in sports requiring sustained attention and endurance. Although these effects are small, they provide a significant advantage in competitive sports. Thus all sympathomimetic drugs, including over-the-counter medications such as pseudoephedrine and phenylpropanolamine, are banned by most athletic associations.

Stimulant overdose results in excessive activation of the sympathetic nervous system. The resulting tachycardia and hypertension may result in myocardial infarction and cerebrovascular hemorrhage in susceptible individuals. Cocaine can cause coronary vasospasm and cardiac arrhythmias. CNS symptoms of cocaine users include anxiety, feelings of paranoia and impending doom, and restlessness. Patients exhibit unpredictable behavior and sometimes become violent. Catecholamine receptor blockers alleviate some of these symptoms, though many patients do not require medication.

An important component of stimulant intoxication is the "crash" that occurs as the drug effects subside. Dysphoria, tiredness, irritability, and mild depression often occur within hours after a stimulant intoxication experience.

Abuse Patterns, Dependence and Psychosis A dangerous pattern of stimulant abuse is the extended, uninterrupted sequences referred to as "runs." Runs result from attempts to maintain a continuous state of intoxication, to extend the pleasurable feeling, and to postpone the postintoxication crash. Acute tolerance can occur, particularly with IV use, resulting in a need for increasingly larger doses. This spiral of tolerance and dosage increases is often continued until drug supplies are depleted or the individual collapses from exhaustion. During runs, drug-taking and drug-seeking behavior take on a compulsive character making intervention difficult.

Another typical abuse pattern begins with self-medication. Stimulants are used in certain occupations to achieve sustained attention (e.g., by long-distance truckers or students) or to make tasks appear easier (e.g., housework). These patterns lead to increased dosage and frequency of use, producing tolerance, and further dosage escalation. Alcohol or depressant drugs are frequently used to counteract the resultant anxiety and insomnia, establishing a cycle of "uppers and downers."

In animals, repeated cocaine or amphetamine administration does not produce physical dependence as seen with opiate and depressant drugs in man, but rather results in extended periods of uninterrupted high-dose self-administration. Thus, dependence on stimulants is characterized principally by uncontrolled compulsive episodes of use, a phenomenon referred to as psychological dependence. In stimulant abusers, various sequences of mood and behavior change have been described after cessation of use. Perhaps the most notable aspects of this withdrawal syndrome are fatigue and depression, since they often result in drug-craving and relapse. Sleep disturbances, hyperphagia, and electroencephalographic abnormalities have also been noted during stimulant withdrawal. The psychological sequelae of stimulant withdrawal are important in continued abuse and are important targets of treatment interventions.

Personality changes commonly occur in stimulant abusers and include persecutory delusions, preoccupation with self, hostility, and suspiciousness. With severe abuse, a toxic psychosis can result. Often difficult to diagnose differentially from paranoid schizophrenia, amphetamine and cocaine psychoses require psychiatric management. Antipsychotic medication may be used with some success (see Chapter 23).

Cocaine use during pregnancy may be associated with complications that include abruptio placentae, lower gestational age at birth, lower birth weight, and neurobehavioral impairment of the newborn.

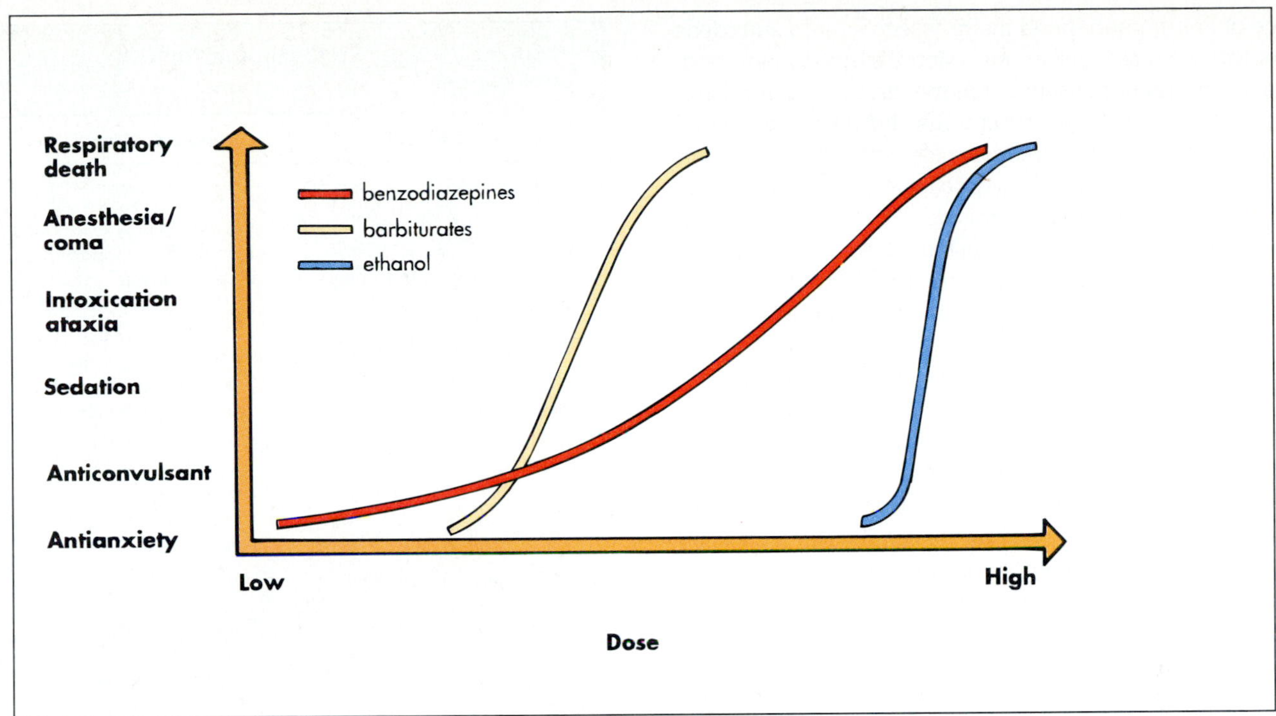

FIGURE 32-8 Comparison of the dose-effect relationships for the acute effects of ethanol, barbiturates, and benzodiazepines.

CNS Depressants

Initial Effects The dose-response curves for abused CNS depressant drugs are essentially the same as for ethanol except for more shallow slopes (Figure 32-8). If one considers that blood ethanol concentrations of 0.1% are only one fourth the lethal level (see Chapter 31), the therapeutic index for alcohol would be among the poorest of any prescription medication. In contrast, gram quantities of benzodiazepines may not be lethal, resulting in over a 500-fold difference between therapeutic and potentially lethal doses. Like ethanol, barbiturates and nonbarbiturate sedatives have dose-effect curves with slopes that are much steeper than those for benzodiazepines.

Barbiturates and nonbarbiturate sedatives such as meprobamate can produce an ethanol-like intoxication and are sometimes abused for this purpose. The rapidly acting barbiturates such as secobarbital and pentobarbital are more widely abused than depressants with a slower onset, such as phenobarbital and the benzodiazepines.

After overdosage with depressant drugs, pupils are sluggish and miotic, respiration is shallow and slow, deep tendon reflexes are absent or attenuated, and patients are unresponsive. There are no known antagonists for barbiturates or nonbarbiturate sedatives, whereas the competitive benzodiazepine antagonist, flumazenil, will completely reverse benzodiazepine intoxication. Although benzodiazepines are rarely lethal when taken alone, they enhance the effects of other depressants that may have been taken concurrently, including alcohol.

Dependence Repeated use of depressant drugs produces physical dependence, and cross-dependence occurs among barbiturates, nonbarbiturate sedatives, benzodiazepines, and alcohol. Signs and symptoms of depressant withdrawal (see box on p. 441) are often opposite to the acute pharmacological effects of these drugs. The occasional appearance of convulsions and delirium make depressant withdrawal a medical emergency. Long-acting benzodiazepines or phenobarbital can be used to treat alcohol and barbiturate withdrawal.

Hallucinogenic Compounds

Initial Effects Nearly all hallucinogens produce varying degrees of sympathomimetic effects such as tachycardia and increased blood pressure. Psychomotor stimulation or euphoria may also be evident. For substituted amphetamines such as MDMA, these effects may predominate, particularly at higher doses. The unique psychological effects of hallucinogens include (1) lability of mood, (2) altered thought processes, (3) altered visual, auditory or somatesthetic perception, (4) experience of having enhanced insights into events and ideas, and (5) impaired judgment. Mood swings can range from profound euphoria to anxiety and even terror. Panic states ("bad trips") are symptoms that most commonly lead abusers to seek medical assistance. Bad trips generally are not the result of overdoses, though larger doses are more likely to produce this result; rather, they result from the propensity of the hallucinogenic drug experience to undergo rapid transformation. For this reason, the nature of hallucinogenic drug intoxication is highly dependent upon the context in which the drugs are ingested. Unexpected or frightening events can transform the experience dramatically. Bad trips usually respond to calm reassurance and removal from the threatening environment until the drug effect wears off. Medication is rarely needed, though excessive stimulation may indicate that treatment with antipsychotics is necessary.

Although acute overdose is not a common problem with hallucinogenic compounds, some other hazards are present. The most significant is the risk of injury from impaired judgment. In addition, psychiatric illness may be precipitated by even an occasional encounter with hallucinogenic compounds in predisposed subjects. With repeated use, this problem is exacerbated. Another potential danger, suggested by animal experiments, is neurotoxicity from the severe depletion of dopamine or serotonin, accompanied by neuronal degeneration. This has been most clearly shown in animal studies with certain substituted-phenethylamine hallucinogens (e.g., MDMA). Whether this occurs in humans is presently unknown. Finally, the effects on fetal development are poorly understood, with conflicting evidence from in vitro and animal studies.

Another poorly understood aspect of hallucinogen abuse are flashbacks, in which users reexperience aspects of hallucinogen intoxication while being drug free. Flashbacks also may occur with marihuana or PCP use. They may be no more than a *déjà vu* experience, or they may be a frightening episode that reflects an emerging psychopathological condition.

Adulterations and Misrepresentations In addition to the classical hallucinogens discussed above, other classes of psychoactive drugs dramatically alter consciousness and perceptual processes. Some of these drugs are sought out for this use, but they also are used as adulterants or substitutes in "street drugs" and frequently are misrepresented as LSD and other drugs.

The most notable class of nonclassical hallucinogens are the antimuscarinics (Chapter 9). Atropine and scopolamine are present in readily available North American plants and mushrooms. Certain groups of native American Indians and Central Americans practice ritual use of these plants because of their ability to produce profound alterations in consciousness. These and other anticholinergic drugs can also be diverted from medical sources. Antimuscarinic intoxication can be accompanied by signs of anticholinergic poisoning. Appropriate treatment is the acetylcholinesterase inhibitor physostigmine.

Table 32-1 Signs and Symptoms of PCP Intoxication

Anticipated Effects	Untoward Effects
LOW DOSE	
Dreamy, carefree state Mood elevation Heightened or altered perception	Impaired judgment Mood swings, panic Partial amnesia
MODERATE DOSE	
Inebriation Dissociation, depersonalization Perceptual distortions Diminished pain sensitivity	Ataxia, motor impairment Confusion, disorientation Preoccupation with abnormal body sensations Amnesia Exaggerated mood swings Panic
HIGH DOSE	
All of the above, hallucinations	Catatonia, "blank stare," delirium, drooling, severe motor impairment, psychotic behavior, hypertensive crisis, meditatio mortis, amnesia

Others

Phencyclidine Phencyclidine (PCP) abuse began in the late 1960s with oral use. A major epidemic of PCP abuse began when smoking and insufflation became common routes for PCP administration, since these routes allowed easier titration of dose. PCP is often referred to as "angel dust," or "dust," and is generally mixed with plant material (e.g., dried parsley or marihuana) and smoked. Although PCP is the major drug abused, many other analogs of PCP produce similar effects. The dissociative anesthetic ketamine also has PCP-like abuse potential.

PCP produces a unique profile of effects, yet it also combines aspects of the actions of sympathomimetic stimulants, barbiturate-like depressants, and hallucinogens. The subjective experience of PCP intoxication is unlike that of classical hallucinogens (see Table 32-1). The perceptual effects are not as profound and relate more to somesthesis. Distortions of body image are common, and one of the motivations for PCP abuse is to enhance sexual experience. PCP users have impaired judgment and may behave unpredictably, sometimes in bizarre and violent ways. PCP intoxication often includes motor incoordination, and at high doses cataleptic behavior may be exhibited accompanied by nystagmus and a blank stare. After smoking, PCP intoxication typically lasts 4 to 6 hours. There is some evidence that combined use of PCP and depressant drugs or alcohol may result in enhanced disruption of behavior. Major dangers with PCP abuse are production of risk-taking behavior and development of progressive personality changes that culminate in a toxic psychosis. PCP overdosage is rarely lethal but may require careful management because of the severe incapacitation of the subject. There is no PCP antagonist available. The use of antipsychotic medications in mild PCP intoxication is controversial, but benzodiazepines may be used to help calm anxiety. PCP is a weak base (pK_a of 8.5), the elimination of which can be increased somewhat by aggressive acidification of the urine (pH less than 5.5).

Although some tolerance can develop during long-term PCP abuse, dramatic dosage escalation is uncommon. The dependence produced by PCP has not been well characterized, but it clearly does not have the physical dependence potential of opioids and depressants.

Heavy use of PCP can result in a toxic psychosis. Schizophrenic patients or individuals with schizophrenic tendencies are particularly at risk for PCP psychosis. PCP psychosis shares many features of schizophrenia and may respond to antipsychotic medication.

Cannabis Marihuana is generally inhaled by smoking. The onset of peak intoxication is delayed 15 to 30 minutes after smoking, making dosage titration more difficult than that with some other drugs. The effects generally last 4 to 6 hours.

Except with very high doses, marihuana intoxication is considerably less intense than intoxication with hallucinogens or PCP. Users exhibit mood lability including euphoria, anxiety, fear, and even panic attacks. They identify heightened sensitivity to music, movies, sexual behavior, and other activities as strong motivation for their usage. Thought processes, judgment, and time estimation are altered. Marihuana has little direct effect on psychomotor coordination, though altered perception and judgment can impair task performance, including driving. Marihuana often produces drowsiness, particularly 1 to 2 hours after smoking. Physiological effects include tachycardia and reddening of conjunctival vessels.

Major dangers of marihuana abuse include the harmful effects of impaired performance, overuse to exclusion of other activities, and development of personality changes and psychopathology. Death from acute overdosage is extremely rare. Bad trips generally respond well to reassurance and removal of patients from threatening environments. Because of the prevalence of marihuana use, accidents and injury during intoxication are important concerns. Cannabinoids can be detected in urine many days after marihuana use.

Inhalants Many volatile chemicals and gases produce CNS effects and are subject to abuse. These chemicals are in the following groups: (1) gases such as nitrous oxide (2) volatile liquids, and (3) aliphatic nitrites.

Nitrous oxide, a clinically used general anesthetic agent (Chapter 30), produces a short-lived mild intoxication that is characteristic of the early onset of anesthesia. Some of the more frequently abused and easily available volatile liquids are (1) toluene-containing paint thinners, correction fluids, and plastic adhesives, (2) other alkylbenzene solvents and cleaners, (3) chlorinated hydrocarbon cleaners and degreasers such as 1,1,1-trichloroethane (methylchloroform) and methylene chloride, and (4) ethyl chloride and chlorofluorocarbon-containing aerosols. Particularly dangerous are products containing chlorofluorocarbons, ketones, organic metals, and *n*-hexane. The chlorofluorocarbons are cardiotoxic, *n*-hexane and methyl *n*-butyl ketone produce well-defined axonopathies, and others may produce hepatotoxicity.

The intoxication produced by inhaling solvent vapors is poorly understood. In animals, toluene, 1,1,1-trichloroethane, and halothane produce alcohol-like behavioral effects. Abusers seem to seek an alcohol-like intoxication with these agents. Motor performance deficits similar to those produced by alcohol and depressant drugs occur with solvent abuse.

Aliphatic nitrites are volatile liquids. Amyl nitrite, supplied in ampules that are crushed and the contents inhaled, are used medically and are subject to abuse. Other organic nitrites have been made available in specialty stores as room "odorizers." Since these nitrites are vasodilators, dizziness and euphoria probably result from hypotension and cerebral hypoxia secondary to peripheral venous pooling. Nitrites are often abused in conjunction with sexual activity and are popular among homosexual males for their claimed ability to enhance orgasms, probably the result of penile vasodilatation. Nitrites use can result in accidents related to syncope.

Nicotine Nicotine self-administration is an important basis of tobacco use and it is clear that nicotine is the component in tobacco that causes dependence. Although the psychological effects of inhaled nicotine are fairly subtle, they occur reliably and include mood changes, stress reduction, and some performance enhancement.

Nicotine withdrawal emerges soon after smoking cessation, peaks in 24 to 48 hours, and may last for 10 days or more, with tobacco craving continuing in many individuals for years after terminating tobacco use. The major symptoms are dysphoria, irritability, anxiety, difficulty in concentrating, fatigue, and sleep disturbances. Observable signs include decreased heart rate and weight gain. Nicotine-containing gum or transdermal patches may be used to treat the withdrawal syndrome while patients are participating in a smoking cessation program. Relapses are common and should be viewed as a normal aspect of nicotine dependence treatment.

Caffeine As with other methylxanthine stimulants, caffeine is found in beverages made from coffee beans or tea leaves and is present in many soft drinks. A typical cup of brewed coffee contains 85 to 150 mg caffeine and mugs of strong coffee can have as much as 200 mg per cup. Caffeine is also present in various over-the-counter medications, including analgesic preparations, stimulants, and weight-control products, with 100 to 200 mg caffeine per tablet typical. Excessive consumption of any of these products or combined consumption can result in an intake of more than 1 g of caffeine per day. Patients receiving theophylline for bronchodilatation may be especially sensitive to caffeine because of the similar pharmacological effects of theophylline.

An effective oral dose of caffeine in nontolerant individuals is 85 to 150 mg. Effects are increased alertness, loss of fatigue, and an apparent greater capacity for activities requiring sustained attention. Higher doses (>200 mg) can produce nervousness, restlessness, and tremors, and very high doses can result in convulsions. Caffeine consumption late in the day can result in insomnia. Anxiety and nervousness associated with caffeine consumption can be misdiagnosed as an anxiety disorder.

Two neurochemical actions of methylxanthines are relevant to their acute effects on the CNS. (1) Caffeine inhibits nucleotide phosphodiesterase resulting in increased concentrations of cAMP. (2) Methylxanthines are also adenosine antagonists at both the adenosine A_1 and A_2 receptors. Both these actions result in enhanced neurotransmission by amplifying the cyclic neucleotide second messenger cascade.

The nature of methylxanthine dependence is becoming clearer from recent research. Regular coffee drinkers who omit their morning coffee report headache, irritability, inability to work effectively, nervousness, restlessness, and lethargy. This syndrome has an onset of 12 to 24 hours, peaks at 20 to 48 hours, and has a duration of about 1 week. These withdrawal effects can be reversed by resumption of caffeine intake.

PHARMACOTHERAPIES FOR OPIATE AND STIMULANT ABUSE

Opiates

Detoxification of patients receiving opioids for pain relief is accomplished by tapering of the dose of prescribed opioid or by substitution of methadone or another longer-acting medication. Only rarely does such iatrogenic dependence lead to illicit opioid use. Medications play an important role in treatment of opiate abuse, but they are only adjuncts to psychosocial and educational interventions.

In the case of dependent heroin abusers, simple detoxification by itself is rarely sufficient to prevent relapse. Most opiate abusers undergo detoxification numerous times, either medically or as a result of interrupted drug supply or incarceration. Nondrug detoxification can be used or, alternatively, dependent heroin abusers can be stabilized on a long-acting oral medication such as methadone. The daily dose is gradually decreased over a period of about 30 days (inpatient) or 180 days (outpatient). Withdrawal signs are mild, though the patient will be uncomfortable for most of the withdrawal period. Another approach is to terminate the opioids abruptly and treat the signs and symptoms of withdrawal, many of which reflect stress and sympathetic nervous system activation. Medications such as clonidine have been used successfully, particularly in mildly dependent subjects. Antianxiety agents may also be useful in alleviating the stress of withdrawal.

Maintenance therapies are based on cross-dependence. Methadone is the drug of choice because of its good oral bioavailability and long duration of action. Methadone maintenance patients receive single, daily oral doses chosen to prevent withdrawal signs but not large enough to produce significant intoxication. Urinalysis for continued illicit drug use is an important feature of most maintenance programs. Although methadone maintenance of opiate abusers is somewhat controversial, it has many proven benefits and has been shown to be effective. It breaks the destructive pattern of continued IV drug abuse and crime. It is attractive to many abusers who would not otherwise seek treatment, provides the opportunity for other therapeutic interventions, and has dependence-producing properties that help ensure continued patient participation in counseling. Take-home medications and other clinic privileges can be used to reinforce positive changes in behavior.

In theory, opiate antagonists could also be used for treatment of opiate abuse. After a sufficient oral dose of naltrexone, positive reinforcement from opiates can be

TRADE NAMES

In addition to generic and fixed-combination preparations, the following trade-named materials are available in the United States.

Habitrol, nicotine patch
Mazicon, flumazenil
Narcan, naloxone
Nicoderm, nicotine patch
Nicorette, nicotine polacrilex gum
Nicotrol, nicotine patch
PROSTEP, nicotine patch
Revia, naltrexone
Talwin Nx, pentazocine with naloxone

prevented for up to 24 hours. Patients given naltrexone must first be detoxified or else precipitated withdrawal will occur. Naltrexone does not produce dependence; thus patient compliance is less assured. On the other hand, the patient must plan ahead to obtain opiates, making a spontaneous relapse less likely.

Stimulants

Antipsychotic medications are useful in treating stimulant overdoses and in management of toxic psychoses. No standard pharmacotherapy is yet available to treat chronic cocaine or amphetamine abuse.

NEW DIRECTIONS

Improvements are continuing in the treatment of drug abuse. One area of interest is the development of improved medications. For opiate abuse, clinical trials have established the utility of a long-acting methadone analog, *l*-α-acetylmethadol (LAAM), which will prevent the appearance of withdrawal symptoms by up to 72 hours. This reduces the necessity of daily clinic visits and may provide some advantages for certain patients. Buprenorphine can also prevent opioid withdrawal and has been evaluated for detoxification and pharmacotherapy of opiate dependence. When buprenorphine is substituted in dependent heroin abusers, the eventual discontinuation of buprenorphine is not accompanied by significant withdrawal signs, perhaps because of its very slow rate of dissociation from the opiate receptor. There is also interest in developing longer-acting opiate antagonists. Research is underway with various depot formulations of naltrexone that, when administered to an opiate-abstinent patient, would prevent opiate reinforcement for many days.

There is also an active search for medications that would be useful for treatment of stimulant abuse. Because of the presumed long-term alterations in dopaminergic regulation resulting from cocaine abuse which may be a factor in relapse, research is focused on the possible use of dopaminergic agonists such as amantadine or bromocriptine and of antidepressants such as desipramine, which may ameliorate abstinence depression and reduce craving. However, further research is needed to establish their effectiveness.

It is clear that drug abuse is a complex biopsychosocial problem that does not lend itself to simple solutions and that no medications are likely to be effective outside of a standard comprehensive treatment milieu. In this context, improvements are also being made in behavioral interventions for drug abusers. One area of considerable interest is the study of classically conditioned drug effects. Patients may experience withdrawal signs and drug craving in certain situations where they had abused drugs in the past. Methods are being developed to teach patients about those conditioning effects that contribute to relapse and to provide them with effective behavioral strategies. New psychosocial treatments are also being developed for stimulant abuse. In the long run, the best solutions are prevention and early intervention.

REFERENCES

Bock GR, Whelan J, editors: *Cocaine: scientific and social dimensions,* CIBA Foundation Symposium 166, Chichester, 1992, John Wiley & Sons.

Galanter M, Kleber HD, editors: *Textbook of substance abuse treatment,* Washington, 1994, American Psychiatric Press.

Goldberg SR, Stolerman IP, editors: *Behavioral analysis of drug dependence,* Orlando, 1986, Academic Press.

Goldstein A: *Addiction: from biology to drug policy,* New York, 1994, W.H. Freeman

Gorelick DA, Balster RL: Phencyclidine (PCP). In Bloom FE, Kupfer DJ, editors: *Psychopharmacology: the fourth generation of progress,* New York, 1995, Raven Press.

Hollister LE: Health aspects of cannabis, *Pharmacol Rev* 38:1, 1986.

Hughes JR, Oliveto AH, Helzer JE, et al: Should caffeine abuse, dependence, or withdrawal be added to DSM-IV and ICS-10? *Am J Psychiatry* 149:33, 1992.

US Department of Health and Human Services: *The health consequences of smoking: nicotine addiction. A report of the surgeon general,* DHHS (CDC) Publication No 88-8406, Washington, DC, 1988, US Government Printing Office.

SELF-ASSESSMENT QUESTIONS

1. An individual who has been taking one drug chronically and experiences a withdrawal syndrome upon discontinuing it finds relief from these symptoms by taking a second drug. This is an example of:
   a. craving.
   b. psychological dependence.
   c. cross-dependence.
   d. tolerance.
   e. drug addiction.
2. Which of the following drugs most likely results in a life-threatening withdrawal?
   a. cocaine
   b. secobarbital
   c. heroin
   d. lysergic acid diethylamide (LSD)
   e. methamphetamine
3. Relative to barbiturates, the dose-effect curves for benzodiazepines are:
   a. steep.
   b. shallow.
   c. parallel.
   d. biphasic.
   e. inverted.
4. Which of the following is *not* a common symptom of opiate withdrawal?
   a. convulsions
   b. lacrimation and rhinorrhea
   c. nausea and vomiting
   d. abdominal cramps
   e. all of the above are symptoms of opiate withdrawal
5. The drug methadone:
   a. can become a substance of abuse.
   b. is orally effective.
   c. is used in heroin detoxification.
   d. should not be used for maintenance in nondependent opiate abusers.
   e. is all of the above.
6. The problems of cocaine abuse are most similar to those of:
   a. heroin abuse.
   b. marihuana abuse.
   c. amphetamine abuse.
   d. alcoholism.
7. Barbiturate withdrawal symptoms are similar to the withdrawal symptoms from:
   a. heroin.
   b. alcohol.
   c. phenothiazines.
   d. benzodiazepines.
   e. more than one of the above.
8. "Crack" cocaine:
   a. is a closely-related chemical analog of cocaine.
   b. is the free base form of cocaine.
   c. volatilizes at a higher temperature than cocaine salts.
   d. is usually self-injected intravenously.
   e. is more than one of the above.
9. Which of the following is the least characteristic of cocaine abuse?
   a. a run (repeated intravenous injections over the course of days or weeks)
   b. significant physical dependence
   c. weight loss and insomnia
   d. hallucinations and delusions
   e. depression and fatigue when the drug is discontinued, followed by prolonged sleep
10. Caffeine:
    a. blocks adenosine receptors.
    b. catalyzes phosphodiesterase.
    c. blocks the accumulation of cyclic AMP.
    d. is an agonist at GABA receptors.
    e. is more than one of the above.
11. Which of the following effectively relieves opiate withdrawal signs and symptoms?
    a. naloxone
    b. naltrexone
    c. both
    d. neither
12. Which of the following has no specific antagonists?
    a. barbiturates
    b. opiates
    c. both
    d. neither
13. On prolonged use, which of the following may produce a paranoid psychosis that may be indistinguishable from schizophrenia?
    a. barbiturates
    b. heroin
    c. amphetamines
    d. marihuana
    e. alcohol
14. Phencyclidine (PCP):
    a. is a weak acid.
    b. has effects that are more similar to those of anesthetic ketamine than those of the hallucinogen LSD.
    c. acts upon brain GABA receptors.
    d. is available for medical use.
    e. is more than one of the above.
15. Detoxification refers to:
    a. methadone maintenance.
    b. the use of opiate antagonists.
    c. the use of disulfiram.
    d. treating physical dependence.
    e. treating opiate overdose.

CHAPTER 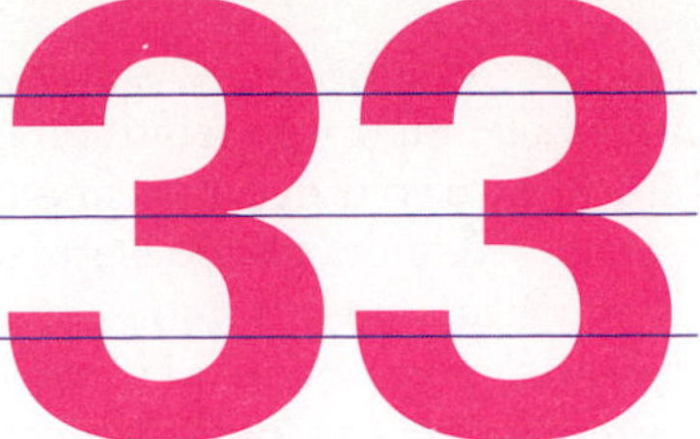

Drugs for Sleep Disorders

EDWARD F. DOMINO

MAJOR DRUGS

Benzodiazepines
Barbiturates
CNS stimulants

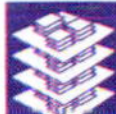

THERAPEUTIC OVERVIEW

Disorders of sleep are a frequent patient complaint. In the United States about one third of all adults have difficulty sleeping. About 6% complain of excessive daytime sleepiness. Medication to treat symptomatic sleep disorders is both widely used and abused by patients and frequently extensively prescribed by physicians.

A classification that is useful in the diagnosis and treatment of sleep disorders consists of four major categories: (1) the **insomnias,** disorders of initiating and maintaining sleep, (2) the **hypersomnias,** disorders of excessive sleep or sleepiness, (3) disturbances in the awake-sleep schedule, circadian rhythm alterations caused by shift-work changes or jet lag, and (4) **parasomnias,** dysfunctions associated with sleep, its various stages, or partial arousals. The use of pharmacological agents to treat categories 1 and 2 are discussed in this chapter. Category 3 symptoms usually are transitory and are alleviated in a few days without the use of medications once a new sleep schedule is established. Category 4 is a group of miscellaneous disorders without specific drug therapies.

Insomnia and daytime sleepiness are symptoms and not specific diseases. Many diseases have symptoms of insomnia. Treating insomnia with drugs provides symptomatic therapy only. If given for an extended period, drugs dramatically alter the normal sleep cycle and may lead to pharmacologically induced sleep disturbances. Hence, **hypnotics** (drugs that promote sleep) should be prescribed temporarily (days to weeks); how long the medication should continue is not completely agreed upon. Clearly, sleep medication for insomnia should not be used indiscriminately without determining what goal is to be accomplished. Before initiation of drug therapy, management of insomnia should be focused on behavior modification, exercise, reduction of caffeine intake, sleep hygiene, and other sleep-promoting modalities.

Sleep-promoting drugs act as central nervous system (CNS) depressants and include the benzodiazepines, barbiturates, and diverse other compounds. Pharmaceutical companies are exploring new chemical entities that will probably alter the types of sleep promoting agents we now have, since our present medications have significant limitations. For the opposite effect, namely, treatment of excessive sleepiness, CNS stimulants are used primarily. These have abuse potential (Chapter 32).

The therapeutic aspects of sleep-related drugs are summarized in the box on page 450.

ABBREVIATIONS

EEG	Electroencephalogram
GABA	γ-aminobutyric acid
NREM	Non–rapid eye movement
REM	Rapid eye movement

MECHANISMS OF ACTION

Sleep Cycle

Sleep is an essential, normal, readily reversible physiological state, distinguished by relative quiescence andl unconsciousness, decreased responsiveness to sensory stimuli, characteristic posture, and reduced activity of most voluntary muscles. It occurs approximately every

24 hours and varies in duration depending on age, normal physiology, and presence of a pathological condition. The average normal adult sleeps about 8 hours, though there are considerable individual differences. Infants and older normal adults tend to have a significant amount of fragmented sleep.

The two major forms of sleep are characterized by distinct behaviors, dreams and their recall, and polygraphic (brainwave, electromyograph, eye movement), metabolic, and temperature changes. These two forms are REM (rapid eye movement) and NREM (non–rapid eye movement) sleep. Both states differ behaviorally from wakefulness in terms of sensation and perception, thought progression, and movement control. There are several subcategories of the state of drowsiness as observed in the electroencephalogram (EEG).

Sleep in humans can be subdivided into five stages, of which stages I to IV characterize NREM sleep and the fifth stage is REM sleep. Different stages of sleep result in different wave patterns in the EEG (Figure 33-1). Of all the stages of sleep, it is most difficult to arouse individuals from REM sleep. The term "deep sleep" is imprecise, can also refer to stages III and IV or stage REM, and should not be used.

The normal sleep cycle of adults shifts dramatically minute to minute between the different stages of sleep, with REM episodes occurring approximately every 90 to 100 minutes and lasting longer later in the sleep period. In a normal adult about 4 to 5 short sleep cycles of NREM (average 95 minutes each) are interspersed with periods of REM to give 6 to 8 hours of total sleep. Vivid, illogical, and bizarre dream recall occurs when an individual is aroused from REM sleep. If unpleasant, these are called *nightmares*. Night terrors (present especially in children) and sleep walking occur during NREM sleep and are not recalled by the individual. Some dreams are remembered after NREM sleep but lack detail and vividness.

As patient age increases, stages III and IV (NREM) become less prominent; geriatric patients spend much less time in these stages. Patients with dementia and serious mental diseases such as schizophrenia and depression have pronounced sleep disturbances, especially in stages III and IV (NREM), with an earlier onset of REM sleep than normal subjects do.

THERAPEUTIC OVERVIEW

SLEEP DISORDERS

INSOMNIAS: Failure to initiate or maintain sleep

Treatment:

Nondrug
- eliminate underlying cause, counseling
- promote sleep hygiene, etc.

Drug
- CNS depressants such as:
- benzodiazepines (flurazepam, triazolam, temazepam, quazapam, lorazepam)
- barbiturates (pentobarbital, secobarbital, amobarbital)
- antihistaminics (doxylamine, pyrilamine)
- others (chloral hydrate, paraldehyde)

HYPERSOMNIAS: excess sleep, narcolepsy

Drug
- CNS stimulants
- *d*-amphetamine
- pemoline
- methylphenidate

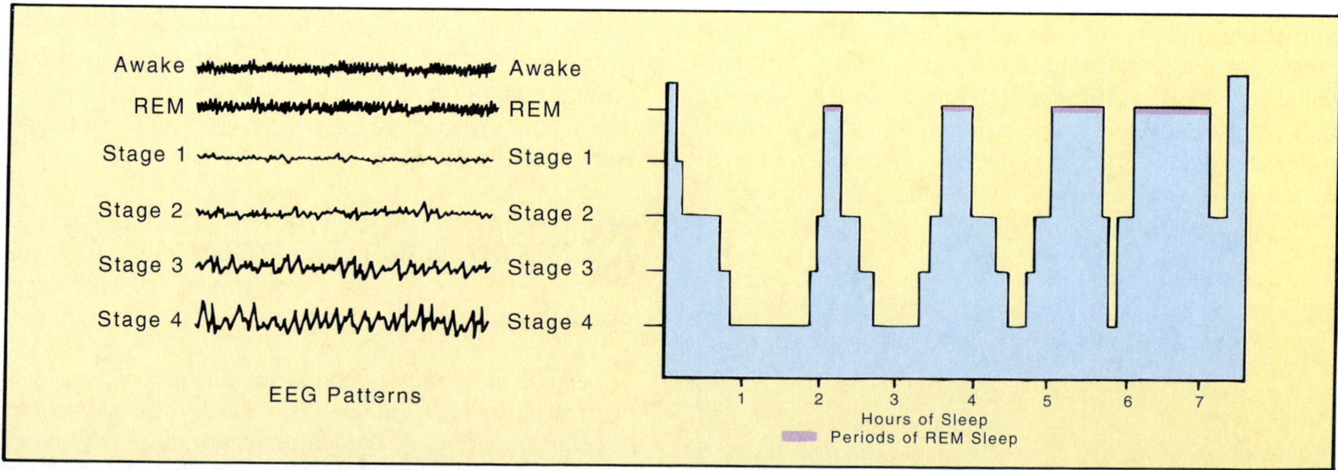

FIGURE 33-1 Characteristic electroencephalographic patterns for different stages of human sleep. The EEG pattern for stage-REM sleep resembles that for the awake state (see text). Also shown are average times spent in each sleep state for a young adult during an 8-hr period.

Sleep-Wakefulness: Neurotransmitters

The neurochemistry of sleep and wakefulness is not well understood. It is not known whether two or more separate systems exist in the brain for these behavioral states. Wakefulness is mediated by the arousal or activating system located in the brainstem reticular formation and hypothalamus. Neurons from these structures innervate wide areas of the neocortex (via the diffuse thalamic projection system) and the paleocortex, or limbic system (via the hypothalamus). The neurotransmitters implicated in wakefulness are acetylcholine, catecholamines (including dopamine and norepinephrine), histamine, and glutamic acid. Acetylcholine and norepinephrine apparently play important roles in REM sleep. Both REM and NREM sleep involve grossly similar brain regions. Serotonin and γ-aminobutyric acid (GABA) are the most important neurotransmitters in NREM sleep. Peptides are also involved in NREM, but, like many of the other chemicals in the brain, their precise role has not been established. An important research area involves sleep-promoting peptides.

Because such a large variety of neurotransmitters are involved in sleep, many drugs acting on these diverse neurotransmitters affect wakefulness as well as the different stages of sleep. From a practical therapeutic point of view, the most widely used sleep-promoting medications at this time are certain benzodiazepines and, much less frequently, barbiturates, both acting on $GABA_A$ receptors in the brain but at somewhat different sites. The benzodiazepines and barbiturates enhance the inhibitory presynaptic or postsynaptic actions of GABA by acting allosterically on $GABA_A$ receptors. Their mechanism of action is well described in Chapters 2 and 25.

Specific Drugs

The primary sleep-promoting drugs are benzodiazepines and barbiturates and a miscellaneous group of diverse chemicals that are not widely used. The chemical structures of some of these compounds are shown in Figure 33-2.

Although the barbiturates and the benzodiazepines act upon the same GABA receptor system, most benzodiazepines produce relatively shallow dose-response curves, whereas the barbiturates have steeper dose-effect properties (see Chapter 32). Clinically, this is very important because if taken in overdosage, most benzodiazepines are much safer compared with barbiturates and other sleep-promoting agents. The molecular mechanisms of action of chloral hydrate and paraldehyde apparently resemble those of ethanol (Chapter 31). The detailed molecular mechanisms of action of other hypnotics such as ethinamate and ethchlorvynol, are

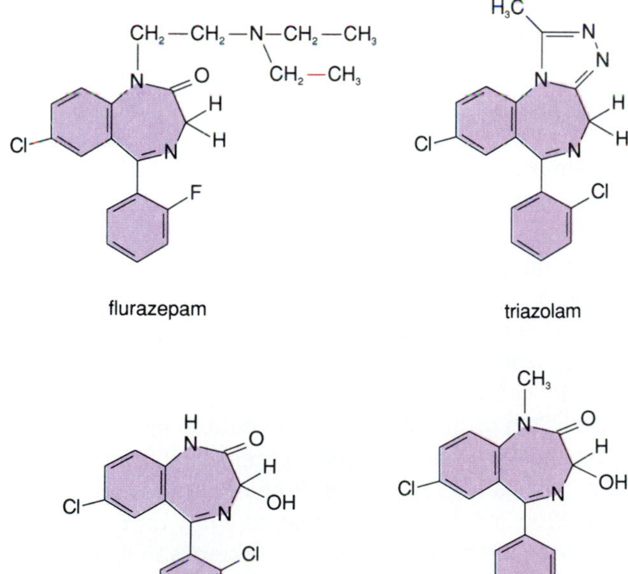

FIGURE 33-2 Chemical structures of frequently used drugs for promotion of sleep. See text for further information.

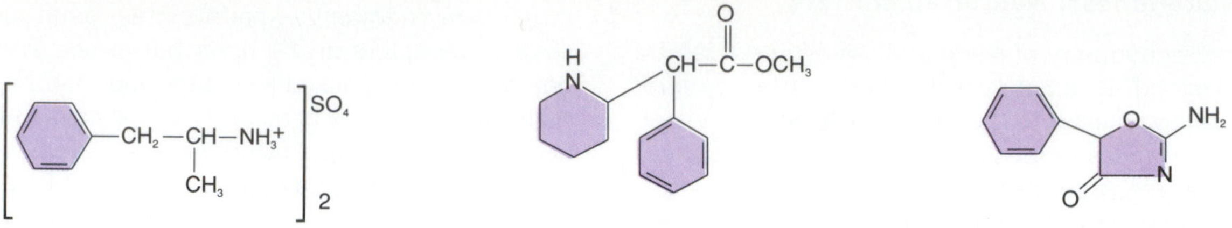

dextroamphetamine sulfate (dextro isomer) methylphenidate pemoline

FIGURE 33-3 Chemical structures of some stimulants used to reduce excessive sleep. See text for further information.

not well studied but may involve actions on other sites or the $GABA_A$ receptors.

Other sleep-promoting medications include muscarinic cholinergic antagonists such as scopolamine, now used chiefly as a preanesthetic agent to promote sleep and reduce secretions before surgery. Over-the-counter nonprescription preparations often contain a sedative H_1 antihistaminic, of which diphenhydramine and doxylamine are frequently used. Diphenhydramine also has muscarinic anticholinergic properties. In view of the role of serotonin in sleep, one of its precursors, L-tryptophan, has been used to promote sleep but was withdrawn from use for a period because of contaminant toxicity (Chapter 61). Many antipsychotic drugs and especially antidepressants promote sleep when given at bedtime, but these drugs are used primarily to treat the specific mental diseases causing the disturbance of sleep (see Chapters 23 and 24).

CNS stimulants used to treat excessive sleep include the amphetamines (Chapters 10 and 32) methylphenidate and pemoline. The structures of these compounds are shown in Figure 33-3.

PHARMACOKINETICS

The pharmacokinetic parameter values for many of these drugs are listed in Table 33-1.

Table 33-1 Pharmacokinetic Parameters

Drugs	Administered	$t_{1/2}$ (hr)	Disposition
BENZODIAZEPINES			
lorazepam	Oral	8-25	M (main)
flurazepam	Oral	50-98	M (main)*
temazepam	Oral	9.5-12.4	M (main)
triazolam	Oral	1.5-5.5	M (main)
quazepam	Oral	40	M*
BARBITURATES			
amobarbital	Oral	16-40	M (main)
pentobarbital	Oral	15-50	M (main)
secobarbital	Oral	15-40	M (main)
MISCELLANEOUS			
chloral hydrate	Oral	4-9.5	M (main)*
paraldehyde	Oral	3.4-9.8	M (main)
NONPRESCRIPTION ANTIHISTAMINICS			
diphenhydramine	Oral	3.7-4.5	—
doxylamine	Oral	4-12	—

M, Metabolized.
*Active metabolites.

Benzodiazepines

All the benzodiazepine hypnotics now in clinical use are reasonably well absorbed after oral administration and reach peak blood and brain concentrations within 1 to 2 hours. Their duration of action varies considerably, and the formation of active metabolites further contributes to their effects. Flurazepam is a long-acting drug that undergoes conversion to desalkylflurazepam, a long-acting active metabolite. Relatively little flurazepam and desalkylflurazepam are excreted unchanged in the urine and undergo further biotransformation in the liver. Hence, their elimination half-life in young adults is long (Table 33-1) and increases even further in older patients and in patients with liver disease.

Temazepam has an intermediate elimination $t_{1/2}$, whereas triazolam has the shortest. Triazolam is an especially potent benzodiazepine that produces significant amnesia. Jet travelers have been known to take triazolam, go to sleep, wake up, and act normally but have no memory of that part of their trip. After nighttime triazolam use, some patients report rebound anxiety and confusion the next day, especially with large doses. This drug should be used cautiously, particularly in the elderly. There has been a great deal of controversy with triazolam in particular. It seems to have a steeper dose-effect relationship compared with other benzodiazepines. Even younger adults taking small, approved amounts may have unwanted side effects.

Lorazepam is used as a hypnotic and antianxiety drug (see Chapter 25). Quazepam, which also is converted to an active metabolite, is almost exclusively used for its sleep-producing effects.

Barbiturates

Barbiturates are weak acids. Those listed in Table 33-1 are well absorbed. The barbiturates undergo biotransformation in the liver, where they are metabolized by the cytochrome P-450 microsomal enzyme oxidative system and conjugated with glucuronic acid for excretion by the kidneys. Tolerance rapidly develops to the sleep-promoting effects of these barbiturates, and so the period of treatment recommended is a maximum of 2 weeks. Their duration of action is about 4 to 6 hours, but their elimination $t_{1/2}$ is much longer. Phenobarbital is not considered here; earlier it had wide use as a sedative-hypnotic but is now used almost exclusively as an anticonvulsant. The ultra–short acting barbiturates are used as IV anesthetic agents and are discussed in Chapter 30.

Miscellaneous Prescription Drugs

Chloral hydrate is an irritating liquid also available as a less irritating sodium salt of the phosphate ester. It is converted to its active metabolite, trichloroethanol, in the liver. Trichloroethanol is conjugated with glucuronic acid and excreted in the urine. The $t_{1/2}$ of trichloroethanol is 4 to 12 hours. The effects of chloral hydrate on the sleep cycle are similar to those of barbiturates, but in low dosage, REM sleep is suppressed less.

Paraldehyde is a cyclic trimer of acetaldehyde. It is a liquid with a rather strong odor and disagreeable taste that alcoholics like because it reminds them of a poor martini. Oral paraldehyde is rapidly absorbed and facilitates sleep within 15 minutes. It is biotransformed in the liver to acetaldehyde and subsequently oxidized by aldehyde dehydrogenase to acetic acid and then to carbon dioxide and water. It is seldom used as a hypnotic but has for over a century been used as a sedative in a variety of psychiatric and medical situations.

Several other hypnotics are available for use. These vary in duration of action and elimination $t_{1/2}$. All are biotransformed in the liver to less active metabolites. Most alter the sleep cycle in a fashion similar to the benzodiazepines and barbiturates with minor differences and offer no advantages over the benzodiazepines.

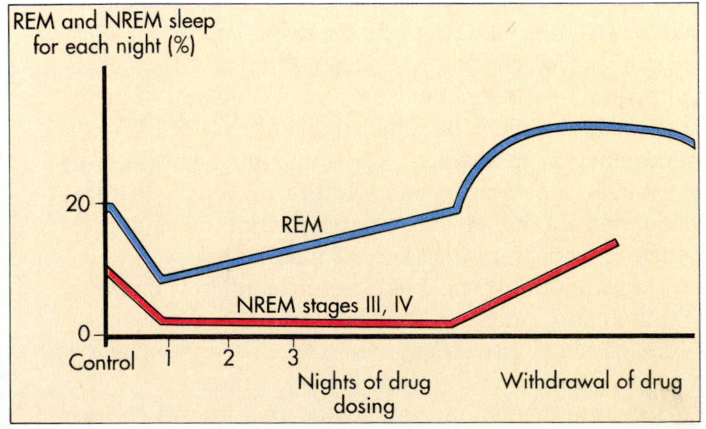

FIGURE 33-4 Typical REM and NREM effects; tolerance and excessive rebound to barbiturate hypnotics. Benzodiazepines produce similar but less pronounced effects (see text).

Nonprescription Drugs

The two drugs widely used as over-the-counter hypnotics are the sedative H_1 antihistamines diphenhydramine and doxylamine. Diphenhydramine has a shorter $t_{1/2}$ than doxylamine (Table 33-1). Tolerance rapidly develops to the sedative effects of both. Good systematic sleep cycle studies with these agents, especially in the small doses approved, are lacking, despite their widespread use in nonprescription preparations.

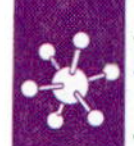

RELATION OF MECHANISMS OF ACTION TO CLINICAL RESPONSE

Drugs that reduce the activity of the brain and spinal cord are termed CNS depressants. Those used clinically to promote sleep are termed *hypnotics,* or less commonly, *soporifics.* The term *hypnotics* for sleep promotion should not be confused with hypnosis, which is a mental state induced in a susceptible individual in response to suggestion. Although sensory perception, mood, memory, and motor performance appear to be altered in the hypnotized state and hypnotic suggestion usually involves statements that the person is "very tired and sleepy," the hypnotic state is quite different from true sleep.

All the drugs used to alter the sleep cycle act on normal as well as ailing subjects. REM sleep, which at one time was considered the most important type of sleep, is suppressed by drugs such as barbiturates and scopolamine. In addition, stages III and IV of NREM sleep are also reduced by the barbiturates. Tolerance to REM suppression occurs, but REM rebound with intense dream recall and nightmares on drug withdrawal is especially characteristic (Figure 33-4). Benzodiazepines also suppress REM sleep to various degrees, as well as stages III and IV of NREM sleep. The latter effect is useful in treating patients with night terrors, which are related to those stages.

All hypnotics alter the normal sleep cycle to suppress REM sleep, decrease stages III and IV of NREM sleep, and produce tolerance on continued use. They may or may not cause REM rebound on withdrawal. Thus the key issue is whether temporarily some sleep with side effects is better than no sleep (insomnia). For short periods (days to a few weeks) some sleep is clearly better than none; however, over a period of a few weeks, months, and especially years, patients with insomnia who take sleep medications nightly develop pronounced drug-induced abnormalities of their sleep cycle. Hence, hypnotics must be prescribed for short-term use only. Unfortunately, in patients with severe insomnia most nondrug treatments are not very successful. Such patients frequently pressure their physicians to continue prescribing medication indefinitely. This situation ultimately greatly alters the patient's sleep cycle detrimentally. Such patients must be weaned from all sleep medications and their primary problems treated in some other fashion, preferably without drugs.

Anesthesia should not be confused with sleep. General anesthesia involves a loss of consciousness. It persists as long as the anesthetic agent is present at sufficient concentrations in the brain (Chapter 30).

The disorders associated with excessive sleep or hypersomnias can be divided into several categories, of which the most common is narcolepsy. **Narcolepsy** is characterized by excessive daytime sleepiness, disturbed nocturnal sleep, and especially pathological REM sleep. This syndrome is characterized by early onset REM periods and other REM patterns that cause cataplexy (extreme muscle weakness induced by emotional activity) and sleep paralysis, both day and night. Although the cause of narcolepsy has not been established, there is a link between DR2, the class II antigen of the major histocompatibility complex, and narcolepsy. The majority of narcolepsy patients are DR2 positive, an indication of an association with or an involvement of the immune system.

The drugs used to treat the symptoms of excessive daytime sleep are CNS stimulants, of which amphetamines, methylphenidate, and pemoline are most frequently used. Dextroamphetamine is the most efficacious but also produces more side effects such as irritability, tachycardia, tolerance, and drug dependence. Methylphenidate is effective, though exhibiting fewer side effects. Pemoline has a longer duration of action than the other two agents. Some tricyclic antidepressants like protriptylene are also used as adjunctive therapy and control certain symptoms of the disorder. The abuse potential and other side effects of the CNS stimulants are described in Chapter 32.

SIDE EFFECTS, CLINICAL PROBLEMS, AND TOXICITY

The therapeutic goal in using hypnotic agents is to promote sleep. Their use in treating insomnia is only symptomatic. All the drugs used alter the normal sleep cycle and should be administered for only days or weeks and almost never for months or years. The rate of tolerance development varies with the chemical class, individual compound, and dosage. With the barbiturates two types of tolerance occur, pharmacokinetic and cellular. In the first type, barbiturates have the well-known property of stimulating their own metabolism by induction of the cytochrome P-450 system enzymes (see Chapter 5). In cellular tolerance, their effect upon the CNS is decreased. Daytime residual sleepiness or hangover may be a problem with some of the longer acting compounds. Rebound anxiety and rebound REM sleep also occur with some of the compounds.

Both psychological and physical dependence are very common with most classes of hypnotics. Physical withdrawal signs and symptoms resemble alcohol withdrawal and may include convulsions misdiagnosed as epilepsy. All substances may produce allergic and idiosyncratic reactions in addition to the side effects that are extensions of their normal pharmacological action. Major side effects of the hypnotics include excessive sedation, dizziness, and an additive or in some cases potentiating action with alcohol, coma, and respiratory depression, which may be fatal. The lethal effects are especially prominent with barbiturates and have led to considerable reduction in their use, concomitant with an increase in the use of benzodiazepines. Benzodiazepines are less toxic but can produce serious toxicity in combination with ethanol. Abuse of hypnotic agents is possible in susceptible individuals and can lead to substance dependence and withdrawal problems similar to that of ethanol. Cross tolerance and cross dependence to alcohol are the rule for most hypnotics.

These agents are capable of crossing the placenta and therefore can cause CNS depression in the neonate. Withdrawal symptoms can occur in the newborn if the mother is dependent on any of these drugs.

Barbiturates are contraindicated in intermittent porphyria, since they can induce the enzymes responsible for porphyrin synthesis.

The clinical problems with sleep drugs are summarized in the box above.

CLINICAL PROBLEMS OF SLEEP DRUGS

PROMOTE SLEEP (TREAT INSOMNIAS)

Greater toxicity problems with barbiturates, thus limitation of treatment cycles to days to a few weeks
Drugs used for symptomatic treatment only

DEPRESS SLEEP (TREAT HYPERSOMNIAS)

CNS stimulants
Produce irritability, tachycardia, tolerance, and drug dependence; have significant abuse potential

TRADE NAMES

In addition to generic and fixed-combination preparations, the following trade-named materials are available in the United States.

BENZODIAZEPINES

Ativan, lorazepam
Dalmane, flurazepam
Dormalin, quazepam
Halcion, triazolam
Restoril, temazepam

BARBITURATES

Amytal, amobarbital
Nembutal, pentobarbital
Seconal, secobarbital

MISCELLANEOUS

Doriden, glutethimide
Noludar, methyprylon
Placidyl, ethchlorvynol
Valmid, ethinamate

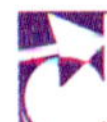

NEW DIRECTIONS

The 1990s are the "decade of the brain." As we learn more about the brain, expect sleep research to take some new directions and provide new therapeutic agents to treat sleep disorders. Sleep-promoting peptides are of special interest. Unfortunately currently identified sleep-promoting peptides do not cross the blood-brain barrier. Analogs that might do so are being actively sought. New sleep-promoting substances promise to be more selective in promoting natural sleep without disturbing the normal sleep cycle.

REFERENCES

Borbey A, Valtax JL, editors: Sleep mechanisms, *Experimental Brain Research* (Suppl 8), Berlin, 1984, Springer-Verlag.

Gillin JC, Byerley WF: The diagnosis and management of insomnia, *N Engl J Med* 322:239, 1990.

Hartman EL: Sleep. In Kaplan HI, Freedman AM, Sadock BJ, editors: *Comprehensive textbook of psychiatry/III*, vol 1, ed 3, Baltimore, 1980, Williams & Wilkins.

Kelly DD: Sleep and dreaming. In Kandel ER, Schwartz JH editors: *Principles of neurosciences,* ed 2, New York, 1985, Elsevier.

Kelly DD: Disorders of sleep and consciousness. In Kandel ER, Schwartz JH, editors: *Principles of neurosciences,* ed 2, New York, 1985, Elsevier.

Kryger MH, Roth T, Dement WC, editors: *Principles and practices of sleep medicine*, Philadelphia, 1989, WB Saunders Co.

Williams RL, Karacan I, editors: *Pharmacology of sleep*, New York, 1976, Wiley & Sons.

SELF-ASSESSMENT QUESTIONS

1. Which one of the following benzodiazepines has the shortest elimination half-life?
   a. flurazepam
   b. diazepam
   c. triazolam
   d. temazepam
2. Which one of the following has no significant active metabolite?
   a. flurazepam
   b. diazepam
   c. chlordiazepoxide
   d. lorazepam
3. Which of the following is considered the mechanism of action of benzodiazepines?
   a. They facilitate the action of GABA at $GABA_A$ receptors.
   b. They facilitate the action of GABA at $GABA_B$ receptors.
   c. They facilitate the actions of serotonin at $5\text{-}HT_{1A}$ receptors.
   d. They inhibit the excitatory effects of glutamic acid at NMDA receptors.
4. Which of the following has the greatest abuse potential?
   a. triazolam
   b. chloral hydrate
   c. pentobarbital
   d. diazepam
5. Which would you *not* prescribe as primary treatment for a patient with narcolepsy?
   a. dextroamphetamine
   b. methylphenidate
   c. pemoline
   d. amitriptyline

ENDOCRINE SYSTEMS: HORMONES AND RELATED COMPOUNDS

PART V

The endocrine system can be defined classically as a diverse group of glands that secretes on demand chemical substances called *hormones* directly into the bloodstream. The secreted hormones are transported in the bloodstream to organs or cells where they regulate organ and cellular activities. The hypothalamus-pituitary, thyroid, parathyroid, pancreas, adrenals, ovary, testes, and sometimes placenta and intestinal mucosa are considered to be the main endocrine glands producing hormones.

The endocrine hormones affect the activities of most organs and many types of cells. These actions occur by extremely intricate pathways, including positive- and negative-feedback control loops and sequences involving hormones from endocrine glands that act to control hormonal secretions from other glands. A given hormone typically exerts multiple actions, and a given function typically is influenced by several different hormones. After synthesis, an endocrine hormone is packaged in the endocrine gland and stored for later release as needed. Special releasing hormones often bring about the secretion of the stored, packaged hormone.

The endocrine hormones can be divided into two chemical structural types: (1) the peptides and amino acid derivatives and (2) the cholesterol-based steroid compounds. The typical plasma concentrations for endocrine hormones range from 10^{-7} to 10^{-9} M for steroids and usually range much lower (10^{-9} to 10^{-11} M) for peptide hormones. The half-lives of many endocrine hormones are quite short (5 to 30 minutes). The steroid hormones can be grouped into six classes: glucocorticoids, mineralocorticoids, estrogens, progestins, androgens, and vitamin D.

Pharmacological intervention in the treatment of endocrine malfunction or disease state generally takes one of three approaches: (1) replacement or supplementation of the natural hormone, (2) use of the hormone to obtain a specific response, or (3) use of drugs to modify the concentration or action of a specific hormone.

A list of the major endocrine hormones and the glands most responsible for their synthesis and secretion is given in Table V-1 on the following page. The chapter in which each hormone is discussed is also indicated but only for those hormones that are involved in pharmacological intervention. Endocrine hormones that are not utilized in therapeutics are not discussed, since their pharmacological roles remain to be established. Most of the diagnostic uses of endocrine hormones also are not included, unless the results are utilized in some way to formulate a pharmacological therapeutic approach.

The endocrine hormones act at target organs and cells through specific receptors. The receptor mechanisms are the same in many respects to the mechanisms of the central or peripheral neurotransmitter systems, already discussed in Chapter 2 and developed further in the peripheral autonomic and central nervous system sections (Chapters 8 to 10 and 22). Because receptors play a key role in the mechanisms of action of endocrine hormone systems, the next chapter contains a summary of the key receptor concepts pertinent to endocrine systems, with special emphasis on the unique features for the endocrine receptors.

Table V-1 Major Endocrine Hormones

Hormone	Secreted by	Chapter
PEPTIDE OR AMINO ACID DERIVATIVE		
insulin	pancreas	39
glucagon	pancreas	39
somatostatin	pancreas	39
pancreatic polypeptide	pancreas	39
thyroid hormones	thyroid	38
antidiuretic hormone (ADH)	pituitary	41
oxytocin	pituitary	41
adrenocorticotropic hormone (ACTH)	pituitary	41
thyroid-stimulating hormone (TSH)	pituitary	41
luteinizing hormone (LH)	pituitary	41
follicle-stimulating hormone (FSH)	pituitary	41
growth hormone (GH)	pituitary	41
prolactin	pituitary	41
gonadotropin-releasing hormone (GnRH) or	pituitary	41
luteinizing-hormone releasing hormone (LHRH)	pituitary	41
thyrotropin-releasing hormone (TRH)	pituitary	41
prolactin-inhibiting factor (PIF)	pituitary	41
parathyroid hormone	parathyroid	42
calcitonin	thyroid	38
catecholamines	adrenals	8,10
STEROID		
estradiol	ovary, adrenals	36
progesterone	ovary, testes, adrenals	36
testosterone	testes, ovary, adrenals	37
cortisol (glucocorticoid)	adrenals	35
corticosterone (glucocorticoid)	adrenals	35
aldosterone (mineralocorticoid)	adrenals	35

CHAPTER 34

Hormone Receptors and Signaling Mechanisms

STEVEN J. JACOBS

HORMONE RECEPTORS: AN OVERVIEW

Complex multicellular organisms require mechanisms for intercellular communication to coordinate independent components. The endocrine and nervous systems have as primary functions long-range communication within the body. Neural transmission is rapid and discrete, sometimes delivering a specific signal to an individual cell, whereas endocrine transmission is relatively slow and diffuse. The reason is that neural transmission is mediated by propagation of an action potential over long distances followed by release of a chemical signal (neurotransmitter) in proximity to its target. Endocrine transmission of information is mediated by chemical signals (hormones) released into the blood and carried to distant target organs.

ABBREVIATIONS	
β-ark	β-adrenergic receptor kinase
cAMP	cyclic adenosine monophosphate
cGMP	cyclic guanosine monophosphate
CURL	compartment of uncoupling of receptor and ligand
EGF	epidermal growth factor
GAP	*ras*-guanosine triphosphatase activator
GDP	guanosine diphosphate
GMP	guanosine monophosphate
GRB-2	one of the SH2-containing proteins
GTP	guanosine triphosphate
HRE	hormone response element
IGF-1	insulin-like growth factor 1
MAP	mitogen-activated protein kinase
PDGF	platelet-derived growth factor
PI3 kinase	phosphoinositol phosphate 3-kinase
SH2, SH3	*src* homology 2 or 3 domain
Sos	one of the cytosolic proteins
T_3	triiodothyronine
TGF	transferring growth factor

In addition to long-range communication by endocrine and nervous systems, virtually all cells in the body release chemical signals that diffuse locally through the extracellular fluid and influence their neighbors (paracrine regulation). Sometimes cells respond to chemical signals that they themselves release into the extracellular fluid (autocrine regulation). Endocrine, paracrine, and autocrine regulation are schematically outlined in Figure 34-1.

Frequently the same or similar chemical mediators and receptor systems are involved in endocrine, paracrine, autocrine, and neural transfer of information. For example, glucagon, secreted by pancreatic islet alpha cells, can be carried by the circulation to the liver to affect glycogen breakdown or act locally on islet beta cells to stimulate insulin secretion. Thyroid releasing hormone is itself both a hormone and a neurotransmitter. In response to growth hormone, insulin-like growth factor I (IGF-I) is secreted by the liver into the blood acting in an endocrine fashion on epiphyseal cartilage. But IGF-I is also produced by chondrocytes and acts in an autocrine fashion.

The same or similar biochemical and cellular mechanisms are involved in hormonal, paracrine, and autocrine signaling. In this chapter, the term *hormone* is therefore used loosely, and the mechanisms by which hormone-like substances trigger a response in their target cells are described.

The initial step by which hormones trigger a response involves their interaction with specific receptors. Receptors have two major functions. First, they recognize the presence of a particular hormone. Second, they trigger a biological response. Usually, several amplification steps intervene between the initial process

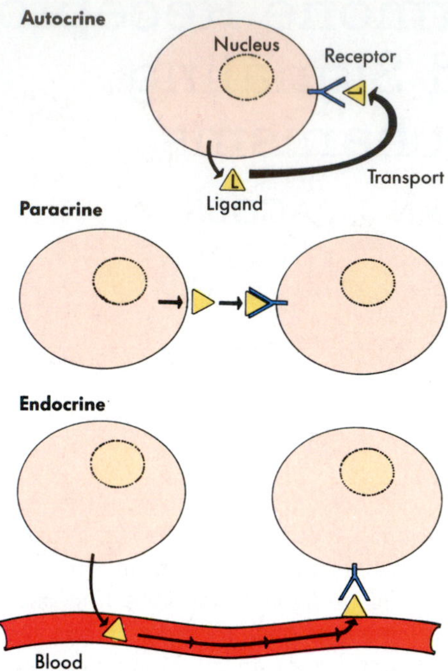

FIGURE 34-1 Three types of cellular regulation: autocrine, paracrine, and endocrine. Secretion of ligand *(L)* is followed by transport and then binding of ligand to a receptor (shown in the shape of Y).

MEMBRANE RECEPTORS
G PROTEIN COUPLED—receptors for biogenic amines, peptides, glycoproteins Activate adenylate cyclase Inhibit adenylate cyclase Activate phospholipase C Regulate ion channels TYROSINE KINASES—receptors for peptide growth factors GUANYLATE CYCLASES—receptors for atrial natriuretic peptide, *Escherichia coli* heat-stable enterotoxin SERINE/THREONINE KINASES—receptors for activin, inhibin, TGF-β, Müllerian inhibiting substance GROWTH HORMONE PROLACTIN AND CYTOKINE RECEPTORS—receptors that associate with tyrosine kinases, receptors for cytokines, growth hormone, prolactin THE STEROID RECEPTOR SUPERFAMILY—transcriptional regulators, receptors for steroids, sterols, T_3, retinoic acid, and vitamin D

activated by the receptor and the classically recognized physiological response.

In addition, most if not all receptors can and do modulate their responses to hormonal stimulation appropriate to the past history of the cell. These modulations include downregulation, desensitization, upregulation, and receptor cross-talk. (see Chapter 2).

Although the precise mechanisms by which different receptors accomplish these functions is diverse, the receptors for most hormones can be classified into a few large families. Six such families are shown in the box. Receptors within a family share structural and functional similarities and most probably have a common evolutionary origin. Usually, receptors within a family interact with structurally similar hormones and trigger common signaling pathways. Much of this chapter is devoted to discussion of these receptor families. However, first some general principles of receptor action that are common among receptors are discussed.

Receptor Recognition

A fundamental principle of receptor action is that hormone-receptor recognition occurs through noncovalent binding with high affinity and specificity. Since hormones are usually present at very low concentrations (nanomolar or less), the affinity of binding must be appropriately high. (A receptor with an affinity constant of 10^9 M^{-1} would be 50% saturated when the hormone concentration was 1 nM.) Since target cells are bathed in a sea of biological molecules, some very closely related to the hormone, binding must also be highly specific so that other molecules do not interfere with hormone binding or inappropriately trigger a response.

High affinity is achieved by multiple interactions between the hormone and receptor working in concert. The individual interactions involved neither have very high affinity nor are very specific. They have the same electrostatic, polar, hydrogen bonding, and hydrophobic interactions involved in all macromolecular interactions. High specificity is achieved by the complementarity between the surface of the hormone and its receptor, dependent on their particular three-dimensional configurations. For many hormone-receptor pairs, a large surface on the hormone reacts with a large surface of the receptor to provide these multiple interactions.

Specificity, though high, may not be absolute. At sufficiently high concentration, molecules that do not normally bind to a receptor will indeed do so. This is particularly true for closely related hormones. For example, insulin and IGF-I are related polypeptide hormones with approximately 40% of their amino acids identical. Although each has its own receptor to which it binds with high affinity, each also will bind to the other's receptor but with about a 100-fold lower affinity. Normally this cross-reactivity is not significant, since physiological

Table 34-1 Second Messengers Involved in Hormone-Receptor Signaling Pathways

second messenger	Pathway
cAMP	G protein–coupled receptors, cAMP-dependent protein kinase
cGMP	cGMP-dependent protein kinase
diacylglycerol	C-kinase
inositol trisphosphate	Ca^{++} release from endoplasmic reticulum and cell entry
calcium ions	Ca^{++}-calmodulin–dependent protein kinase
nitric oxide	Guanylate cyclase

concentrations of the hormones are not sufficiently high. However, in certain pathological conditions or when very high pharmacological concentrations of the hormone are used or when synthetic analogs of the hormone are administered, cross-reactivity can be a problem.

Signaling and Receptor Aggregation

For a hormone to be active, receptor binding alone is not sufficient. Binding must trigger a signal. Signaling may result from the intrinsic catalytic activity of the receptor or by the receptor interacting with other proteins and regulating their catalytic activity. The molecular mechanisms by which hormone binding induces an active receptor conformation are not fully understood; however, for many receptors, dimerization or aggregation plays a role. Upon hormone binding, receptors of the steroid receptor superfamily and many tyrosine kinase receptors self-associate to form homodimers. Receptors may also associate with closely related receptor family members to form heterodimers. These typically have slightly different hormone binding and signaling properties from those of receptor homodimers.

Retinoic acid and triiodothyronine (T_3) receptors are examples of receptors that associate to form heterodimers. Sometimes the hormone itself is also a dimer, and this determines the nature of the receptor dimer that forms. For example, platelet-derived growth factor (PDGF) hormone, itself a heterodimer, induces the formation of PDGF receptor heterodimers. Cytokine receptors also form heterodimers after hormone binding. Receptor association with guanosine nucleotide regulatory proteins (G proteins) provide another type of interaction, discussed in Chapter 2 (also see box, p. 460).

Not only is receptor dimerization or aggregation important in signaling, but it can also quantitatively affect hormone binding. In Chapter 2, the equilibrium binding properties of hormone-receptor interactions that followed simple biomolecular reactions were derived. More complex reactions require different equations. For example, a hormone (H) such as growth hormone that causes its receptor (R) to dimerize has the stoichiometric binding equation

$$H + 2R \gtreqless HR_2$$

This would follow the equilibrium binding equation

$$K_e = [HR_2]/[H][R^2]$$

and would result in nonlinear Scatchard plots.

Signal Relay Pathways

Several steps intervene between the initial activation of a hormone receptor and most physiological responses such as secretion, motility, substrate transport, gene expression, or cell-cycle control. These allow for (1) amplification of the initial signal, (2) branching or diffusion of the signal so that a single receptor can effect multiple responses, (3) feedback control, and (4) integration with other cellular signaling systems.

Three types of mechanisms are frequently utilized in the signaling relay pathways: second messengers, protein phosphorylation-dephosphorylation, and protein-protein interactions. All three mechanisms may be involved in a single signaling pathway.

The second messengers involved in hormone receptor signaling pathways triggered by receptor activation include cyclic adenosine monophosphate (cAMP), cyclic guanosine monophosphate (cGMP), diacylglycerol, and inositol trisphosphate (Table 34-1). *Calcium ions released from the endoplasmic reticulum by inositol trisphosphate,* or entering the cytoplasmic compartment through membrane channels, also serve as second or tertiary messengers.

Three families of serine/threonine protein kinases are targets for these second messengers: cAMP-dependent protein kinases, protein kinase C isoforms (diacylglycerol/calcium sensitive), and calcium-calmodulin–dependent protein kinases. These protein kinases have broad substrate specificity and cause wide branching of the signaling pathways. Other more specific protein kinases with restricted substrate specificity are also involved in signaling. These may be members of a chain or cascade of protein kinases that are activated by hormone binding.

Although the importance of second messengers and protein phosphorylation in signaling pathways has been appreciated since the work of Sutherland and Rall and their collaborators on cAMP, it has only more recently been appreciated that direct protein-protein interactions are important in some signaling systems. Members of the steroid receptor superfamily regulate gene expression by forming protein-protein interactions with the transcription complex. Tyrosine phosphorylation serves as a signal for direct protein-protein interactions. Receptors or proteins with phosphorylated tyrosines associate with other proteins containing src homology in 2 or 3 domains (SH2 or SH3) and thus form complexes with downstream elements of signaling pathways (signaling complexes).

Regulation of Hormonal Responsiveness

The responsiveness of a cell to a hormone is tightly regulated and varies with cell state. For example, when a cell is exposed to a hormone, it may become desensitized. Not only can a hormone affect the way a cell responds to itself (homologous effects), but it can also affect the way a cell responds to other hormones (heterologous effects). For example, exposure to estrogen is required to sensitize many cells to the effects of progesterone. Modulation of responsiveness occurs at the level of both the receptor and the downstream signaling pathways.

Changes in receptor affinity and signaling efficiency occur rapidly. Changes in receptor number attributable to internalization or degradation have an intermediate course. A change in the rate of receptor synthesis occurs even more slowly. Receptor phosphorylation on serine or threonine residues is a common mechanism of regulating responsiveness. Phosphorylation can rapidly change receptor affinity or signaling efficiency. It can also target a receptor for internalization and degradation.

Homologous and heterologous receptor desensitization of the β-adrenergic receptor have been studied extensively (Fig. 34-2). Receptor phosphorylation on serine/threonine by three different protein kinases plays a role. These include β-adrenergic receptor kinase (β-ark), cAMP-dependent protein kinase, and protein kinase C. Phosphorylation of the β-receptor inhibits its ability to interact with G proteins and subsequently leads to its sequestration or internalization to a compartment where it cannot interact with extracellular hormone. The enzyme β-ark is particularly important in homologous desensitization. This kinase is capable only of phosphorylating the active agonist bound form of the receptor. It is this property that makes it so specific for homologous desensitization.

Other protein kinases, for example, cAMP-dependent protein kinase, may also prefer the agonist-bound form of the receptor but not to the same extent as β-ark. Although β-ark was originally described as a kinase specific for the β-adrenergic receptor, probably β-ark or

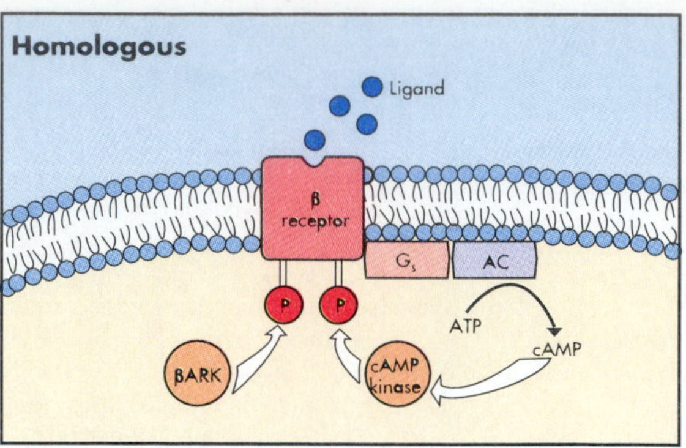

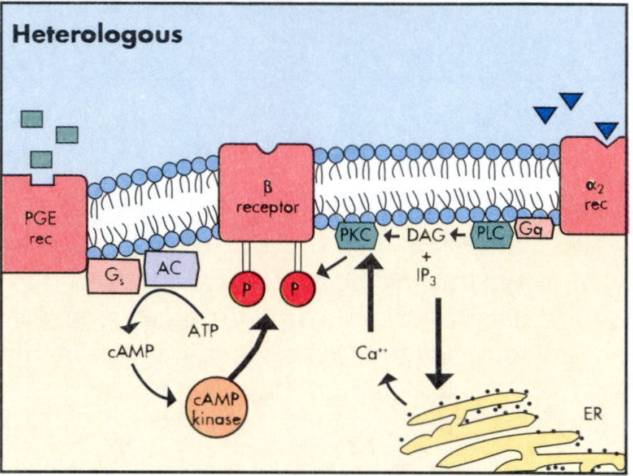

FIGURE 34-2 Phosphorylation is important in receptor desensitization. Pathways of stimulation of β-adrenergic receptor kinase (*β-ARK*), cAMP-dependent protein kinase in homologous desensitization, and cAMP-dependent protein kinase and protein kinase C *(PKC)*, in heterologous desensitization by α-adrenergic receptor *(α rec)* and prostaglandin PGE receptor *(PGE rec)*. *AC*, adenylate cyclase; *DAG*, diacylglycerol; *ER*, endoplasmic reticulum; *GP*, G protein; IP_3, inositol trisphosphate; *P*, phosphorylated state; *PLC*, phospholipase C.

closely related protein kinases can phosphorylate several receptors in this family when they are in an agonist-bound, active state. This aspect indicates that this kinase may have an extensive role in homologous desensitization of G protein–coupled receptors.

Modular Design and Combinatorial Shuffling in Receptor Signaling

Various elements in hormone-responsive signaling pathways including receptors, coupling proteins, and downstream regulators belong to families of closely related proteins, undoubtedly a consequence of evolution as already mentioned. Important functional consequences can ensue. One family member can be substituted for another to create a functionally unique pathway. Such shuffling can create enormous biological diversity with a minimum of individual elements. By independently regulating individual components, the cell

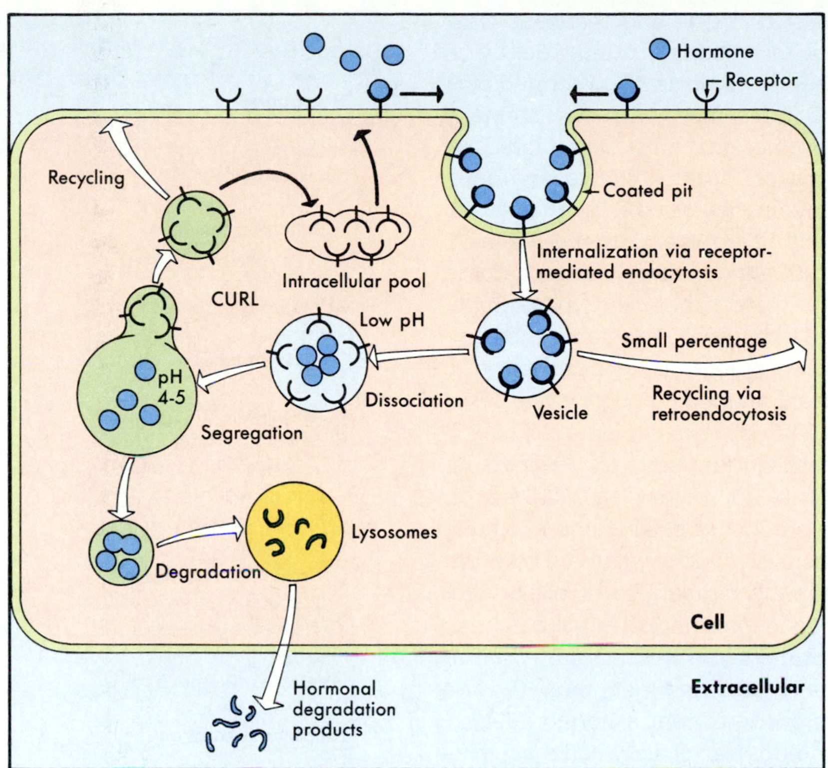

FIGURE 34-3 Pathways of receptor internalization and recycling. *CURL,* Compartment of uncoupling of receptor and ligand.

can dramatically alter the way it responds to the same hormonal stimulus. For example, there are at least 11 different isotypes of protein kinase C expressed in different amounts in different tissues. All but two are stimulated by diacylglycerol but vary with respect to sensitivity to calcium ions, the degree of downregulation by prolonged stimulation, and to some extent their substrate specificity. Thus, some effects of protein kinase C persist after prolonged stimulation, whereas others do not. Furthermore, sustained and transient activation of protein kinase C can produce quantitatively different behavior varying in different tissues.

Internalization and Recycling of Membrane Receptors

Most known protein and peptide hormone receptors are transmembrane proteins. Intracellular receptors bind the lipid-soluble hormones (including steroids, retinoic acid, vitamin D and thyroid hormones), which readily pass through the cell membrane. The transmembrane receptor proteins are amphipathic in nature; that is, they characteristically have both extracellular and cytoplasmic domains with polar residues located on their surfaces, membrane-spanning α-helical domains composed of 19 to 24 nonpolar hydrophobic amino acids, which interact with hydrophobic membrane lipids. This amphipathic nature of receptors prevents them from moving into and out of the membrane lipid bilayer or from changing orientation by flip-flopping across the membrane. However, membrane receptors freely diffuse laterally in the plane of the membrane. This lateral mobility allows membrane receptors to associate with other membrane components and with themselves. As already discussed, these interactions in some cases are required for triggering a response.

In the absence of hormone, most receptors are not localized to particular regions of the cell membrane. When hormone binds, receptors rapidly migrate to coated pits. These are specialized invaginations of the membrane that are surrounded by an electron-dense cage formed by the protein clathrin. At these sites receptor mediated endocytosis occurs. Segments of membranes within coated pits rapidly pinch off to form intracellular vesicles, which are rich in receptor-ligand complexes (Fig. 34-3). These vesicles then fuse with tubular-reticular structures called compartment of uncoupling of receptor and ligand (CURL). The internal pH of CURL is maintained at about 4.5 to 5 by an adenosine triphosphate–dependent proton pump. The low pH favors the dissociation of hormone and receptor, making it possible for them to be sorted independently. In most cases, dissociated hormone is incorporated into vesicles that fuse with lysosomes, with the hormone then degraded by lysosomal enzymes. Dissociated receptor recirculates to the cell surface. However, a fraction of internalized hormone may also be recirculated to the cell surface along with receptor and then is released. This process is called *retroendocytosis*. Free receptor in CURL may recirculate to the cell surface or may temporarily be sequestered in an intracellular membrane compartment. Alternatively, receptor may be transported to lysosmes where it is also degraded. The latter two cases result in a net decrease in cell receptor number.

There are several possible functions for receptor internalization and redistribution. It is clearly an important way by which the number of cell surface receptors and thereby hormone sensitivity is regulated. Hormonal surface receptors frequently regulate intracellular processes (e.g., nuclear gene expression). Thus it has been postulated that receptor-mediated hormone internalization may bring hormone or activated receptor to the site where these processes occur, or that a hormone or receptor fragment generated intracellularly could serve as a second messenger. Currently, no conclusive experimental evidence supports such hypothetical roles.

Table 34-2 G Protein–Coupled Receptors

Hormone	Action
Glucagon	stimulate AC
Somatostatin	inhibit AC, activate K^+ channels
Antidiuretic hormone	stimulate AC, stimulate PLC
Oxytocin	stimulate AC
Adrenocorticotrophic hormone	stimulate AC
Thyroid-stimulating hormone	stimulate AC
Luteinizing hormone	stimulate AC
Follicle-stimulating hormone/human chorionic gonadotropin	stimulate AC
Growth hormone–releasing hormone	stimulate PLC, stimulate AC
Corticotrophin-releasing hormone	stimulate AC
Thyrotrophin-releasing hormone	stimulate AC, stimulate PLC
Luteinizing hormone releasing hormone	stimulate PLC
Parathyroid hormone	stimulate AC
Calcitonin	stimulate AC

AC, Adenylate cyclase; *PLC,* phospholipase C.

G PROTEIN–COUPLED RECEPTORS

Many hormone receptors interact with G proteins (see box, p. 460). These activate or inhibit adenylate cyclase, activate phospholipase C, or regulate ion channels. Characteristically, these receptors have seven transmembrane domains. They have been discussed in Chapter 2 and briefly in earlier sections of this chapter. A partial list of hormones that bind to receptors in this family and their actions is given in Table 34-2. Some hormones have more than one action. These may be mediated by the hormonally activated distinct but closely related receptor subtypes. For example, antidiuretic hormone stimulates adenylate cyclase through the V_2-receptor, and phospholipase C through the V_1-receptor. Receptor subtypes have different structure activity relationships, and synthetic agonists or antagonists can be highly specific for each subtype.

TYROSINE-SPECIFIC PROTEIN KINASE RECEPTORS

The tyrosine-specific protein kinase receptors (Fig. 34-4) are hormonally regulated protein kinases. They differ from the usual protein kinases in that they phosphorylate proteins exclusively on tyrosine hydroxyl residues. They include receptors for insulin and several growth factors. They also include proteins, which because of their structures appear to be transmembrane tyrosine kinase receptors for yet-to-be-identified hormones. The biological effects resulting from activation of the tyrosine kinase receptors have as a general theme, stimulation of anabolic processes, growth, and differentiation. Because of the important role these receptors play in regulating growth and differentiation, somatic mutations of these receptors may result in tumor formation. Abnormal forms of these receptors have been identified as oncogenes.

Tyrosine Kinase Receptor Structure

Receptors in this family have a single membrane spanning the α-helix, which divides the receptor into an extracellular hormone binding aminoterminal domain and a cytoplasmic carboxy-terminal domain that contains a tyrosine kinase (see Figure 34-4). Receptors for insulin and IGF-I vary slightly from this arrangement. Although their genes code for a protein with these characteristics, early in its biosynthesis this protein forms a disulfide linked homodimer that is subsequently cleaved proteolytically to produce a disulfide-linked tetramer.

The extracellular portions of receptors in the tyrosine

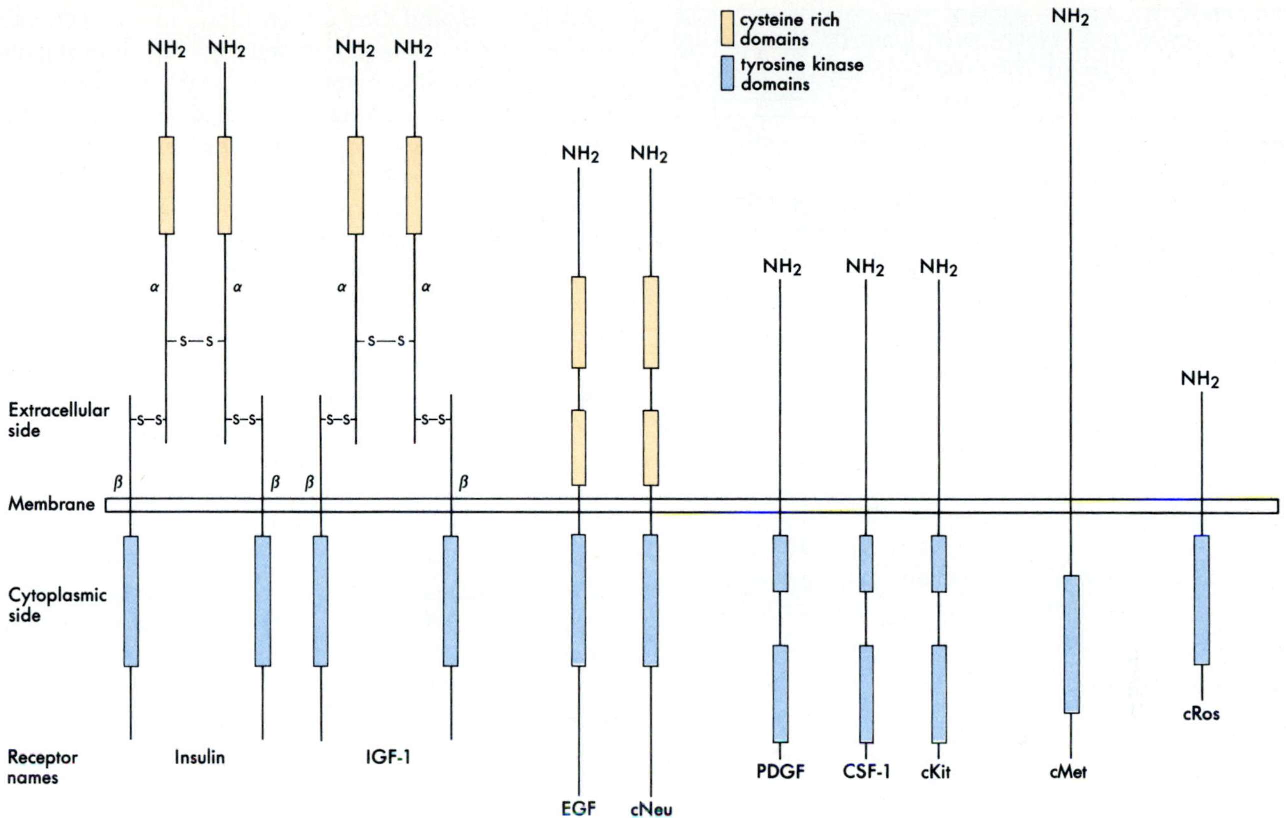

FIGURE 34-4 Comparative structures of several tyrosine kinase receptors shown as linear amino acid sequences and illustrating cysteine-rich domains and tyrosine kinase domains. Many of these receptors belong to three subfamilies. Note that the tyrosine kinase domain may be present as one segment or as two divided segments. *cNeu, cKit, cRos, cMet,* protoncogenes.

kinase family vary widely though within subfamilies high degrees of similarity exist. Some receptors have cysteine-rich sequences, which are imperfectly repeated several times.

The tyrosine kinase domain is the most highly conserved region particularly between members of different subfamilies. There is a well defined adenosine triphosphate binding site near the amino terminus of the domain. The variable regions that flank or in some receptors (PDGF receptor family, fibroblast growth factor [FGF] receptor family) interrupt the tyrosine kinase domain may have a role in substrate binding, thereby accounting for the differing substrate specificity of different members of this family.

Tyrosine Kinase Signal Transduction and Signaling Pathways

Only a small group of proteins become tyrosine phosphorylated in response to tyrosine kinase receptor activation. These include the receptors themselves (autophosphorylation) and other proteins with important regulatory functions. Tyrosine phosphorylation can effect the function of a protein in two ways.

First, tyrosine phosphorylation can directly alter the activity of a phosphorylated substrate. The receptors themselves are examples of this. Autophosphorylation directly increases their tyrosine kinase activity.

Second, tyrosine phosphorylation targets a protein for association with SH2 domains of other cellular proteins. These domains, named because they are conserved in the nonreceptor *src* family of tyrosine kinases, recognize phosphotyrosine in the context of adjacent peptide sequences. The activities of SH2-containing proteins can be altered by this association. For example, phosphatidylinositol phosphate 3-kinase (PI3 kinase) is activated by association with tyrosine phosphorylated proteins or peptides. SH2 domain proteins can associate with autophosphorylation sites on the receptors themselves. For example, PI3 kinase and phospholipase C-γ both react with separate autophosphorylation sites on the PDGF receptor. Alternatively, SH2 domain proteins

PROXIMAL ELEMENTS IN TYROSINE KINASE SIGNALING PATHWAYS

IRS-1

Major substrate of insulin and IGF-1 receptor kinase.
Contains multiple tyrosine phosphorylation sites capable of binding several SH2-containing proteins.

grb-2

Contains a single SH2 and SH3 domain. An adapter protein that functions in the activation of *ras* by insulin, PDGF, and EGF.
Binds to autophosphorylated EGF and PDGF receptors and tyrosine phosphorylated IRS-1.

PI3-KINASE

Contains two SH2 domains. Activated by insulin and PDGF as a consequence of binding to autophosphorylated PDGF receptor and tyrosine phosphorylated IRS-1.

PHOSPHOLIPASE C-γ

Contains two SH2 domains. Activated by EGF and PDGF as a result of binding to their autophosphorylated receptors. Not activated by insulin.

ras-GAP

Contains two SH2 domains. Associates with autophosphorylated EGF and PDGF receptor. This may result in functional inhibition of its activity to stimulate the GTPase activity of *ras* resulting in *ras* inactivation as a signal transducer.

can react with phosphorylated tyrosines on receptor substrates. For example, PI3 kinase reacts with tyrosine phosphorylated IRS-1, a major substrate of insulin and IGF-1 receptor kinases (see box).

Ras plays a central role in linking tyrosine kinase receptors to downstream signaling pathways. Like the G proteins, which couple seven transmembrane receptors to their effectors, *ras* tightly binds guanosine triphosphate (GTP) and hydrolyses it to guanosine diphosphate (GDP), which remains tightly bound. *Ras* is able only to activate downstream pathways in the GTP-associated state. In a fashion analogous to the activation of G proteins by the seven transmembrane receptors, tyrosine kinase receptors activate *ras* by dissociating bound GDP allowing fresh GTP to bind. However, tyrosine kinase receptors do this indirectly with the help of two intervening cytosolic proteins, *Grb*-2 and *sos*. *Grb*-2 is an SH2-containing protein that binds to autophosphorylated tyrosine kinase receptors or their tyrosine phosphorylated substrates. Bound *Grb*-2 then binds to *sos*, activating *sos* as a GDP-dissociation factor for *ras*. The signaling pathway downstream of *ras* consists in a cascade of serine-threonine kinases that include *raf*, MAP kinase kinase, MAP kinase, and a ribosomal protein S6 kinase. MAP kinase phosphorylates c-*jun*, providing a link between tyrosine kinase receptors and a transcription factor involved in regulating the cell cycle.

The signaling pathways activated by tyrosine kinase receptors are complex (Fig. 34-5). They branch diffusely, are redundant, and have extensive positive- and negative-feedback loops. Although *ras* plays a central role, other effectors are directly involved as well. For example, phospholipase C-γ, and PI3 kinase are activated by many tyrosine kinase receptors. Different tyrosine kinase receptors trigger different physiological responses. This is largely because they have different cellular distributions. However, even when present on the same cells, they activate different but overlapping physiological responses. This reflects their overlapping but distinct range of substrates and signaling pathways. For example, the PDGF receptor binds to and phosphorylates the *ras*-GTPase activator (GAP) and phospholipase C-γ and activates PI3 kinase; the EGF receptor binds to and phosphorylates GAP and phospholipase C-γ but does not (or weakly) activates PI3 kinase; and the insulin receptor activates PI3 kinase but does not bind to or phosphorylate GAP or phospholipase C.

GUANYLATE CYCLASE RECEPTORS

This family (see box, p. 460), which includes both cell membrane receptors (atrial natriuretic factor receptor) and cytosolic receptors (nitric oxide receptors), catalyses the hormone-dependent formation of cyclic guanosine monophosphate (cGMP) from guanosine triphosphate. The cGMP formed then activates a serine threonine protein kinase. The pathway activated by cGMP to cause smooth muscle relaxation is best understood (see Chapter 17). cGMP-dependent protein kinase phosphorylates myosin light-chain kinase, decreasing its activity and thereby decreasing the phosphorylation of the light chains of smooth muscle myosin. Unlike receptors coupled to adenylate cyclase, which have seven membrane-spanning regions and are coupled to adenylate cyclase by guanosine triphosphate binding proteins, receptors linked to cGMP either lack or have single membrane-spanning domains and have both ligand binding and catalytic activity in a single molecule. The catalytic domain, which is homologous in all family members, shares lesser homology with regions of adenylate cyclase. Cytosolic guanylate cyclase has an attached iron heme moiety, which is nitrosylated by nitric oxide and regulates cyclase activity. Aside from this, its functional significance is unknown.

Soluble guanylate cyclase is a heterodimer composed of homologous alpha-beta subunits. The atrial natriuretic factor receptor is a disulfide-linked tetramer of guanylate cyclase A receptors. Guanylate cyclase C is activated by heat-stable enterotoxins. It is not clear if guanylate cyclase B and C have their own unique endogenous ligands.

SERINE-THREONINE KINASE RECEPTORS

The TGF-β (transferring growth factor-beta) (see box, p. 460) family of polypeptide hormones that regulate growth (inhibitory and stimulatory), morphogenesis, differentiation, and secretion are homodimers or heterodimers consisting of closely related family members. Extensive diversity results from shuffling combinations of subunits within subfamilies. For example, inhibin A and B are heterodimers of a common α-chain with a β_A- or a β_B-chain. The β-chains can also dimerize to form activin A, B, or AB species.

The gene for the TGF-β receptor and two distinct genes that give rise to activin receptor subtypes have been identified. They have a short cysteine-rich extracellular portion, a single membrane-spanning domain, and an intracellular portion that is almost entirely a serine kinase domain. Currently, nothing is known about their substrates or early signaling pathways. It is likely but not yet proved that other members of this hormone family will have serine kinase receptors.

TGF-β has several other high-affinity cell surface-binding sites in addition to this transmembrane serine kinase. Currently, it is not clear what these have to do with TGF-β signaling. However, they may somehow cooperate with the TGF-β serine kinase.

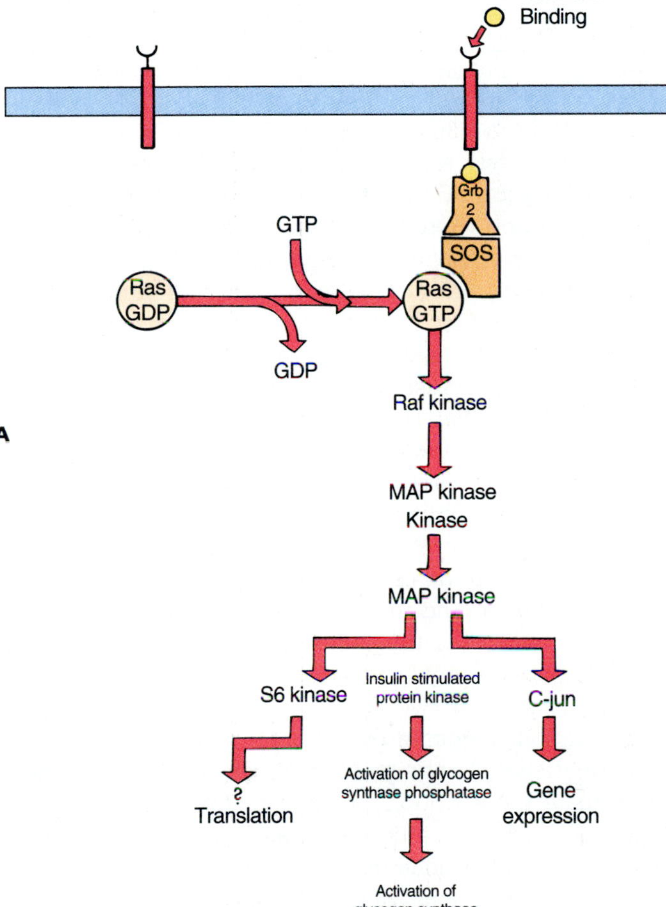

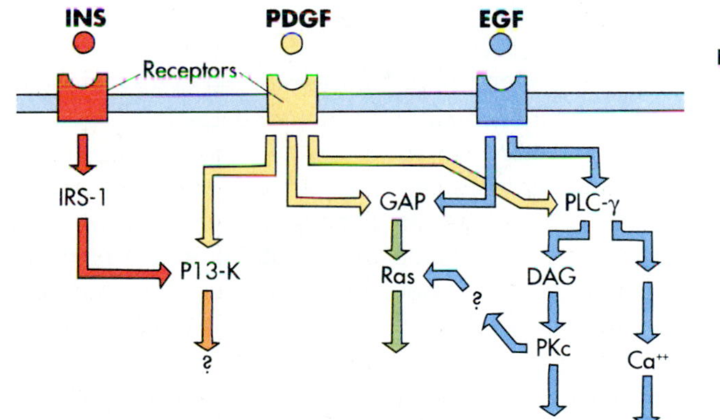

FIGURE 34-5 *A,* Binding of a hormone such as insulin leads to autophosphorylation and activation of receptor tyrosine kinase. This in turn leads to phosphorylation on tyrosine of upstream binding proteins on SH2 domains including Grb2 and *sos,* activating *ras. ras* in turn hydrolyzes GTP to GDP and becomes inactive. *sos* enhances GDP dissociation from *ras* promoting its activation by rebinding GTP. *ras* in turn activates *raf,* a serine threonine protein kinase. *raf* phosphorylates and activates *Map* kinase kinase, a bifunctional tyrosine and threonine/serine protein kinase. *Map* kinase kinase activates *Map* kinase by phosphorylation on both tyrosine and threonine. *Map* kinase itself phosphorylates and activates S6 kinase, which activates microsomal polypeptide translation. In addition, glycogen synthase is activated by phosphorylation and activation of glycogen synthase phosphoprotein phosphatase. In addition, nuclear gene expression is also activated by phosphorylation. Thus three anabolic pathways are stimulated by insulin, *B,* Signaling mechanisms initiated by insulin, PDGF, and EGF. Insulin activates IRS-I and PI3 kinase. PDGF also activates PI3 kinase but also the *ras-gap* sequence and phospholipase C-γ (PLC-γ). EGF also activates the *ras-gap* sequence and PLC γ. Thus cross-talk is present in these signaling pathways as well as separate actions.

GROWTH HORMONE, PROLACTIN, AND CYTOKINE RECEPTORS

Receptors in the diverse family of growth hormone prolactin, and cytokine receptors are transmembrane proteins with single membrane-spanning domains (see box, p. 460). The greatest homology within the family is in their extracellular portions. These consist of two closely spaced β-sandwich immunoglobulin-like domains. X-ray crystallography of the growth hormone–receptor complex indicates that the N-terminal immunoglobulin-like domain is involved in hormone binding and the juxtamembrane immunoglobulin-like domain is involved in receptor dimer formation. Their intracellular domains vary considerably in sequence and length, though there is greater similarity within subfamilies.

Growth hormone receptors and several of the cytokine receptors form dimers when they bind hormone. The nature of the dimer varies for different family members. The growth hormone receptor is an homodimer. Interleukin-3, interleukin-5, and interleukin-6, and granulocyte macrophage–colony stimulating factor form high-affinity heterodimers consisting of a low-affinity α-subunit and a β-subunit, which does not bind the cytokine on its own. IL-3, IL-5, and granulocyte macrophage–colony stimulating factor share a single common β-subunit but have unique specificity-determining α-subunits. The IL-2 receptor dimer is different. An intermediate-affinity β-subunit associates with a low-affinity α-subunit, not a member of the cytokine family, to produce a high-affinity ternary complex.

The mechanisms for cytokine receptor transmembrane signaling are becoming known. Many of these receptors are tyrosine phosphorylated or are associated with tyrosine phosphorylated proteins in the presence of hormone. This association indicates that they may activate nonreceptor tyrosine kinases. Signaling occurs by tyrosine phosphorylatin of a cluster of cell membrane bound proteins which are activated and rapidly enter the nucleus to control gene expression.

Alternative splicing of growth hormone receptor messenger ribonucleic acid results in a receptor form truncated just proximally to the membrane-spanning domain. This results in the secretion of a growth hormone–binding protein that circulates in the serum. The physiological significance of this circulating receptor is unknown, but it is useful to monitor receptor status in various genetic receptor disorders.

THE STEROID RECEPTOR SUPERFAMILY

Several hormones including steroids, retinoic acid, vitamin D, and thyroid hormone exert their effects by binding to intracellular receptors (Table 34-3). They belong to a closely related family that controls specific gene expression by the hormone-dependent regulation of transcription. Regulation can be either positive or negative as exemplified by T_3 stimulation of growth hormone expression and repression of thyroid-stimulating hormone expression. Hormones activating these receptors are, as previously discussed, hydrophobic, and therefore freely diffuse through the cell membrane to reach the receptor. However, cell membrane-binding sites have also been described, and may play a role in their transport into the cell.

Table 34-3 The Steroid Receptor Superfamily and Their DNA-Binding Sequences

Receptor	Hormone Response Element
Glucocorticoid receptor	GGTACA N3 TGTTCT
Mineralocorticoid receptor	GGTACA N3 TGTTCT
Progesterone receptor	GGTACA N3 TGTTCT
Androgen receptor	GGTACA N3 TGTTCT
Thyroid Hormone receptor-α	AGGTCA TGACCT
Thyroid Hormone receptor-β	GATCA N6 TGACC
Retinoic acid receptor (α, β, γ)	GATCA N6 TGACC
Vitamin D receptor	GACTCA TGAACG

N represents any nucleotide.

Activated receptors bind to specific regions of DNA called the *hormone response element* (HRE) and regulate the transcription of adjacent genes. Closely related family members bind to the same or similar HREs. Receptors that bind to the same HRE have different biological functions largely because of their different tissue distributions.

Activation, triggered by hormone binding, include a conformational change making the receptor competent to regulate transcription. Some receptors, for example, glucocorticoid receptors, are located in the cytosol in the absence of hormone. Activation includes their translocation to the nucleus. However, other receptors, for example, T_3 and retinoic acid receptors, are tightly associated with the nucleus even in the basal state. Furthermore, some receptors are associated with heat-shock proteins, which act as inhibitory subunits, under basal conditions. Receptor activation results in their dissociation.

Steroid superfamily receptors bind to DNA as dimers (Fig. 34-6), and the DNA sites recognized (HREs) have specific short consensus sequences which are imperfectly repeated in a palindromic (complemented and inverted) fashion (Table 34-3). Each subunit of the dimer binds to one of the repeated elements. Homodimers or heterodimers composed of closely related family members are observed. For example, two different T_3 receptor genes code for different receptor subtypes. Each

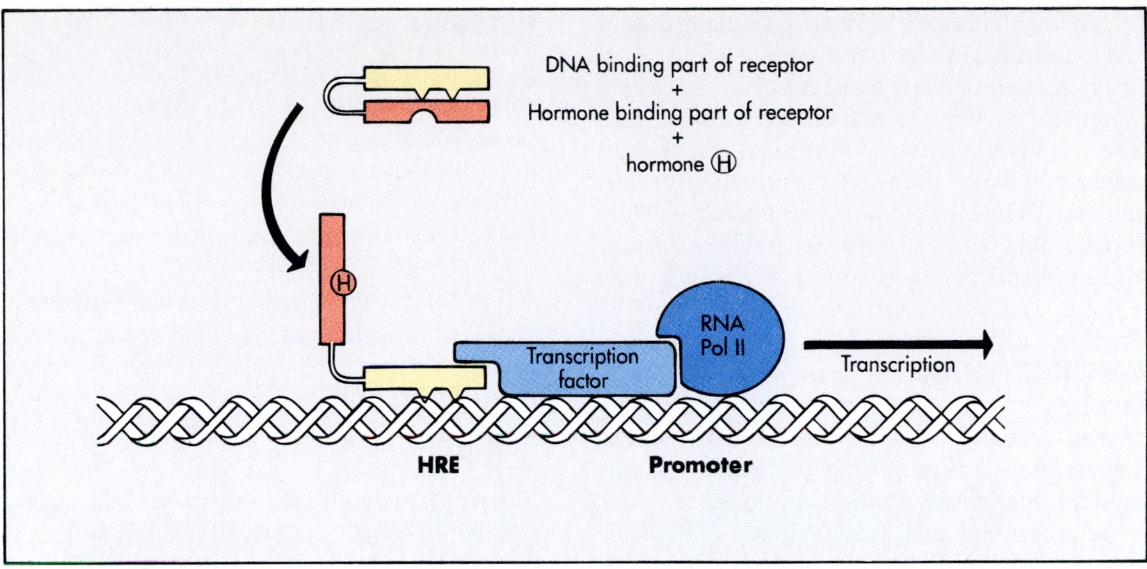

FIGURE 34-6 Nuclear receptors bind to DNA at the hormone response element (HRE) and facilitate (or inhibit) formation of an "active transcription complex" at the promotor. *RNA Pol II,* RNA polymerase II.

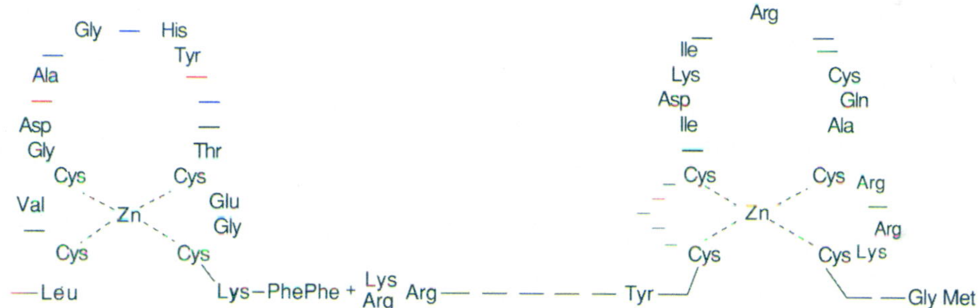

FIGURE 34-7 Hypothetical "zinc fingers" in the DNA binding domain of nuclear receptors. Amino acid residues, for which a strong consensus exists, are indicated. If no consensus exists, residues are indicated by a dash.

gene gives rise to additional receptor subtypes by differential RNA splicing. Three different genes code for closely related retinoic acid receptor subtypes. These form a very large variety of heterodimers having different properties. Through the formation of heterodimers a single defective receptor may adversely affect the function of other receptors with which it associates. This may explain how some forms of thyroid hormone resistance that map to a T_3 receptor gene can have an autosomal dominant inheritance.

HREs are generally located upstream of the promoters of target genes. Binding of activated receptor to the HRE either stabilizes (positive regulation) or interferes with (repression) the binding of accessary transcription factors. These are necessary for RNA polymerase II to tightly bind to the promoter and initiate transcription. Whether and how a specific gene will respond to one of these hormones depends on the presence of an HRE, on other neighboring regulatory elements to which accessory transcription factors bind, and on the specific promoter. Different promoters have different requirements for accessary factors. There is usually considerable flexibility in the position and in some instances the orientation of the HRE with respect to the promoter.

Receptors in this family have a similar overall architecture. They are single polypeptide chains that contain two particularly highly conserved regions. The most highly conserved is the DNA-binding region. It is rich in cysteines and contains two zinc-binding fingers (Fig. 34-7) also identified in several other DNA-binding proteins. Mutating these zinc fingers alters a receptor's HRE specificity. The carboxy-terminal portion of the receptor contains the hormone binding and dimerization domains. Within this domain is the second highly conserved region. It is particularly well conserved in closely related receptors, for example, those for steroid hormones. The hypervariable amino-terminal region and the hinge region between the two conserved regions are not essential for DNA binding but may modify it. They contain regions that interact with transcription factors and target the receptors to the nucleus.

NEW DIRECTIONS

Despite the huge amount that has been learned about receptors and their signaling pathways, the application of this information to therapeutics is only beginning. The realization that most receptors have isotypes indicates the possibility of developing receptor agonists and antagonists that are far more specific than believed possible a few years ago. The ability to express a single well-defined isotype using recombinant DNA techniques has greatly facilitated the identification of such specific ligands. Molecular modeling of hormone-receptor interactions will facilitate their design. The accuracy of modeling increases dramatically if the structure of a close family member is known. The structure of the growth hormone–receptor complex is the first to be determined by crystallography. Others will follow rapidly.

Aside from the G protein–coupled receptors, it has been very difficult to design antagonists for polypeptide hormone receptors. Antireceptor antibodies may be a useful general approach. There has been considerable progress in using recombinant techniques to "humanize" murine antibodies and minimize their immunogenicity. Anti-HER-2 antibodies and anti–epidermal growth factor receptor antibodies are being evaluated for use in cancer.

The discovery of "orphan receptors" (receptor-like molecules with no known ligands) has lead to the subsequent discovery of potentially useful hormones and growth factors. For example, the C-*kit* ligand was found to be a pleuripotential hematopoietic growth factor. A large number of orphan receptors, particularly in the nuclear receptor family, remain to have their ligands and biological functions determined.

In addition to targeting hormone receptor interactions, pharmacologists are beginning to target newly discovered signaling pathways. For example, tyrosine kinase inhibitors are being evaluated as cancer therapies, and protein kinase C inhibitors are being evaluated in inflammatory diseases, cancer, and psoriasis.

REFERENCES

Cantley LC, Auger KR, Carpenter C, et al: Oncogenes and signal transduction, *Cell* 64:281-302, 1991.

De Vos AM, Ultsch M, Kossiakoff AA: Human growth hormone and extracellular domain of its receptor: crystal structure of the complex, *Science* 255:306-312, 1992.

Evans RM: The steroid and thyroid hormone receptor superfamily, *Science* 240:889-895, 1989.

Jacobs S, Moxham C: Hybrid receptors, *New Biol* 3:110, 1991.

Larner AC, David M, Feldman GM, et al: Tyrosincphosphorylation of DNA binding proteins by multiple cytokines, *Science* 261:1730-1733, 1993.

Massague J: Receptors for the TGF-β family, *Cell* 60:1067-1070, 1992.

Nicola NA, Metcalf D: Subunit promiscuity among hemopoietic growth factor receptors, *Cell* 67:1-4, 1991.

Rhee SG, Choi KD: Regulation of inositol phospholipid-specific phospholipase C isozymes, *J Biol Chem* 267:12393-12396, 1992.

Sibley DR, Benovic JL, Caron MG, et al: Regulation of transmembrane signaling by receptor phosphorylation, *Cell* 48:913-922, 1987.

Ullrich A, Schlessinger J: Signal transduction by receptors with tyrosine kinase activity, *Cell* 61:203-212, 1990.

SELF-ASSESSMENT QUESTIONS

1. Hormone receptors are characterized by:
   a. high affinity.
   b. high specificity.
   c. being amphipathic in nature.
   d. ability to move laterally in the cell membrane.
   e. all are correct.
2. Receptors are downregulated by:
   a. phosphorylation on serine/threonine.
   b. internalization by coated pits.
   c. phosphorylation on tyrosine.
   d. association with G proteins.
   e. a and b are correct.
3. Hormone signaling can occur by:
   a. tyrosine phosphorylation.
   b. receptor association with G proteins.
   c. formation of second messengers such as cAMP.
   d. mobilization of Ca^{++} from endoplasmic reticulum.
   e. all are correct.

4. Which is *not* a second messenger involved in hormone action?
   a. nitrous oxide
   b. Ca^{++}
   c. cGMP
   d. triglyceride
   e. inositol trisphosphate
   f. a, b, c, e are correct.
5. G-protein–coupled receptors include:
   a. steroid hormone.
   b. thyroid hormone.
   c. ACTH.
   d. oxytocin.
   e. d and e are correct.
6. Guanylate cyclase receptors include:
   a. nitric oxide receptors.
   b. atrial natriuretic factor receptors.
   c. *Escherichia coli* heat stable enterotoxin.
   d. glucagon.
   e. insulin.
   f. d, b, c are correct.
7. Examples of nuclear receptors include:
   a. insulin.
   b. IGF I.
   c. steroids.
   d. retinoic acid.
   e. c and d are correct.

CHAPTER 35

Glucocorticoids and Mineralocorticoids

ANDREW N. MARGIORIS
ACHILLE GRAVANIS
GEORGE P. CHROUSOS

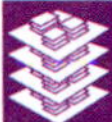

THERAPEUTIC OVERVIEW

Cortisol (also called *hydrocortisone*, or *compound F*) is the main endogenous glucocorticoid in humans. It is synthesized in the adrenal cortex. Cortisol exerts a wide range of physiological effects including regulation of intermediate metabolism, the stress response, some aspects of central nervous system function, and particularly immunity. Thus cortisol is necessary for the maintenance of life, and because of its pivotal biological significance, its synthesis and secretion are tightly regulated. The hypothalamic-pituitary-adrenal axis is very sensitive to negative feedback by circulating cortisol or synthetic glucocorticoids. High plasma concentrations of glucocorticoids suppress the hypothalamic-pituitary-adrenal activity, resulting in decreased cortisol biosynthesis, thus, lower concentrations of circulating cortisol. This suppression of hypothalamic-pituitary-adrenal axis persists for prolonged periods of time. Thus an abrupt cessation of a chronically administered synthetic glucocorticoid may cause the simultaneous lack of both exogenous and endogenous glucocorticoids, resulting in serious morbidity and even mortality. Gradual reduction of the exogenously administered glucocorticoids may require extended periods, since the hypothalamic-pituitary-adrenal system needs up to a year to recover (i.e., to secrete cortisol at a normal rate).

Aldosterone is the major mineralocorticoid in humans synthesized in the adrenal cortex. Aldosterone is the primary regulator of sodium and potassium in the extracellular fluid.

The main therapeutic uses of glucocorticoids are (1) as a replacement of cortisol in cases of adrenal insufficiency (i.e., inadequate endogenous production of cortisol), (2) as an antiinflammatory-immunosuppressant agent, and (3) as an adjuvant in the treatment of myeloproliferative diseases and other malignancies. The major therapeutic use of mineralocorticoids is as a replacement of aldosterone in cases of primary adrenal insufficiency or isolated aldosterone deficiency.

ABBREVIATION	
ACTH	corticotropin

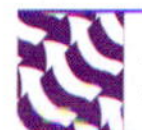

MECHANISMS OF ACTION

Glucocorticoids

Cholesterol is the main precursor of cortisol and aldosterone synthesis. It is taken up from the circulation rather than synthesized de novo in the adrenal cortex, though the cortex is capable of de novo cholesterol biosynthesis. Plasma cholesterol is carried by both low-density and high-density lipoproteins; the adrenal cortex has receptors for these lipoproteins. In humans, low-density lipoproteins are the major source of adrenal cholesterol. The uptake of circulating cholesterol and the de novo synthesis of cholesterol by the adrenals are interchangeable sources, and so blockade of one or the other causes no significant decrease in cortisol or aldosterone biosynthesis.

Adrenocortical cholesterol is esterified and stored inside cytoplasmic lipid droplets. Esterified cholesterol is hydrolyzed by cytoplasmic cholesterol ester hydrolase and transported into the mitochondria by a sterol carrier protein where it is converted to **pregnenolone.** This conversion requires nicotinamide adenine dinucleotide phosphate (reduced), oxygen and the cytochrome P-450 mixed-function oxidase system and involves (1) the removal of a portion of the side chain of cholesterol (which is attached to its seventeenth carbon) and (2) the addition of a double-bonded oxygen at carbon position 20. The synthesis of the major glucocorticoids and mineralocorticoids is shown in Figures 35-1 and 35-2.

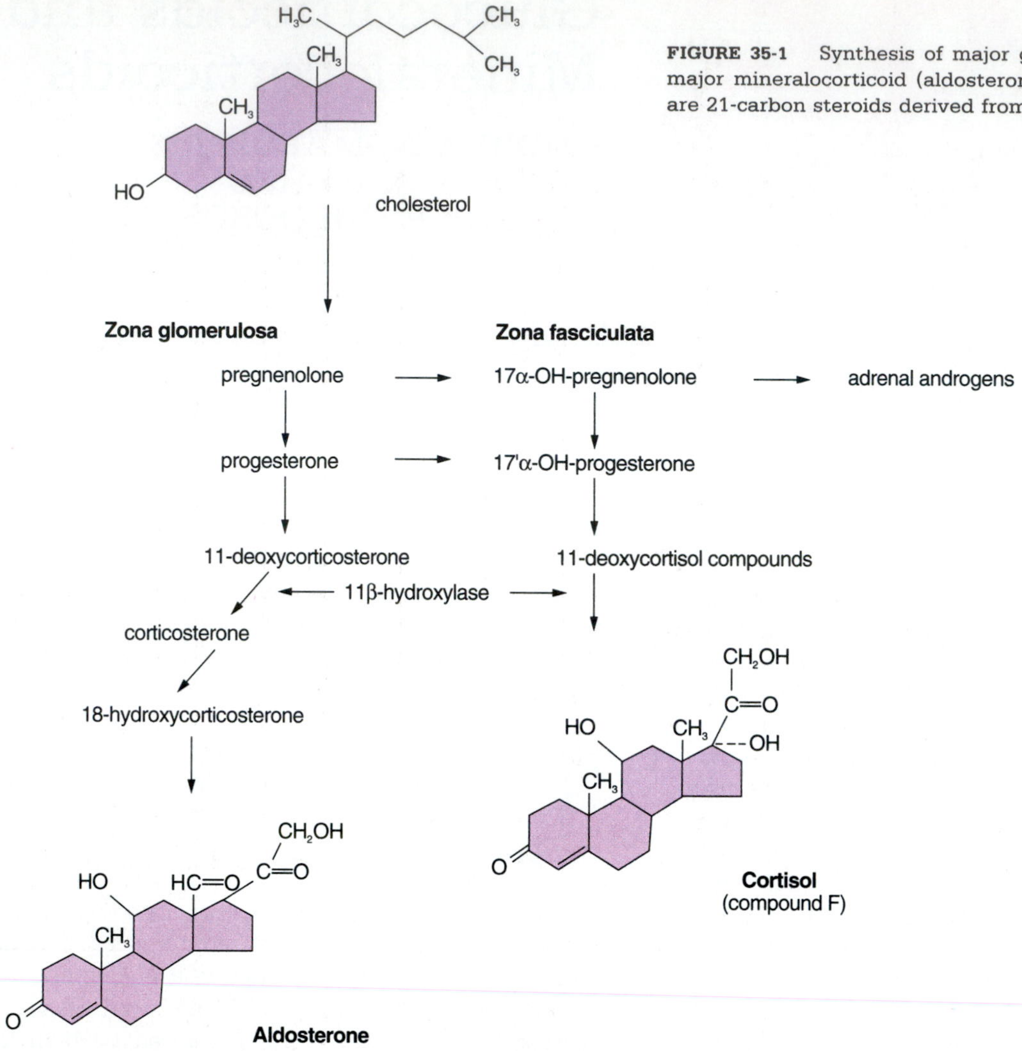

FIGURE 35-1 Synthesis of major glucocorticoid (cortisol) and major mineralocorticoid (aldosterone) by adrenal cortex. Both are 21-carbon steroids derived from cholesterol.

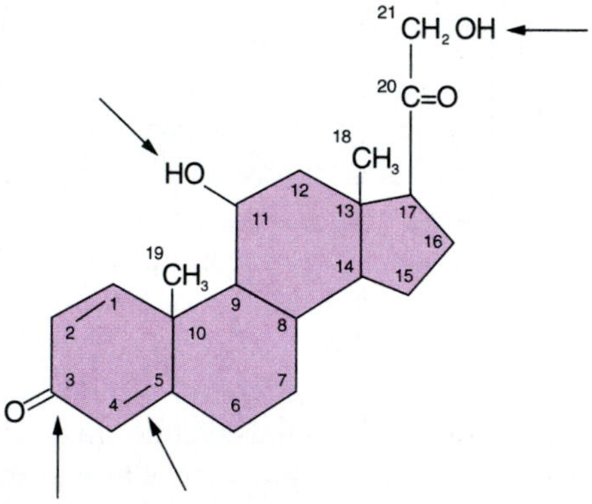

FIGURE 35-2 Corticoid structure indicating sites for bioactivation and biotransformation to inactive products.

THERAPEUTIC OVERVIEW

GLUCOCORTICOIDS

Replacement therapy in adrenal insufficiencies
Antiinflammatory and immunosuppressive action
Myeloproliferative diseases
Drugs used:
hydrocortisone, cortisone, prednisone, prednisolone, fludrocortisone, methylprednisolone, betamethasone, triamcinolone, dexamethasone

MINERALOCORTICOIDS

Replacement therapy in adrenal insufficiencies
Hypoalderosteronism
Drugs used: fludrocortisone

STEROID SYNTHESIS INHIBITORS

Adrenocortical hyperfunction
Drugs used: metyrapone, ketoconazole aminoglutethimide, trifostane

Pregnenolone is transferred from the mitochondria to the smooth endoplasmic reticulum where most of it is hydroxylated by the 17α-hydroxylase enzyme into **17α-hydroxypregnenolone,** which in turn is converted to **17α-hydroxyprogesterone** through replacement of a 5,6 double bond by a 4,5 double bond. The latter reaction is catalysed by the 3β-hydroxysteroid dehydrogenase/Δ5-isomerase enzyme complex. A small percentage of pregnenolone is first converted by this enzyme complex to **progesterone** and then hydroxylated at the 17 position to 17α-hydroxyprogesterone. 17α-Hydroxyprogesterone is a strategically located steroid. In the zona fasciculata, this compound undergoes two successive hydroxylations. First, it is hydroxylated at position 21 by the 21-hydroxylase enzyme (located in the endoplasmic reticulum) resulting in **11-deoxycortisol** (also called *compound S*). Compound S is then hydroxylated at position 11 by the 11β-hydroxylase enzyme (located inside the mitochondria) to cortisol (also called *compound F*). In the zona glomerulosa there is no 17α-hydroxylase enzyme present, and thus all available pregnenolone is transformed to progesterone, which in turn follows the pathway for the synthesis of the mineralocorticoid aldosterone.

Cortisol synthesis and secretion is regulated by the pituitary hormone corticotropin (ACTH). ACTH is synthesized and secreted by the corticotrophs of the adenohypophysis, as discussed in Chapter 41. Pituitary ACTH is secreted in the peripheral circulation and reaches the ACTH receptors located on the surface of the adrenocortical cells. ACTH interacts with these receptors and initiates a cyclic adenosine monophosphate (cAMP)–dependent increase of the transcription of almost all enzymes involved in cortisol biosynthesis, which results in increased cortisol production and secretion. In addition, ACTH acts as a growth factor for the adrenal cortex, and so a lowering of plasma ACTH results not only in a decrease of cortisol synthesis and secretion, but also in the gradual atrophy of the adrenal cortex. Pituitary production of ACTH is very sensitive to suppression by exogenous glucocorticoids. Manipulations of this system for therapeutic purposes should be approached with the utmost care, since chronic administration of exogenous glucocorticoids results in adrenocortical atrophy and thus impaired glucocorticoid biosynthesis.

Most ACTH is released as a series of secretory episodes followed by an equal number of bursts of cortisol secretion in plasma. These secretory episodes of ACTH and cortisol are characterized by a sharp rise of their plasma concentration followed by a slower decline. In a 24-hour period approximately 8 to 10 such ACTH and cortisol peaks are detected (Fig. 35-3). A circadian periodicity in the frequency and the magnitude of these secretory episodes is present, with generally greatest frequency and magnitude in early morning and less frequency and magnitude in late afternoon.

The Glucocorticoid Receptor All natural and synthetic glucocorticoids act by binding to a specific cytoplasmic glucocorticoid receptor. This receptor is a protein of about 800 amino acids and can be divided into three domains (see Chapter 34). The glucocorticoid-binding domain is located at the carboxy-terminus of the molecule and is the area where the hormone binds. The deoxyribonucleic acid (DNA)–binding domain is located in the middle of the protein and contains nine cysteine residues. This region folds into a "two-finger" structure stabilized by zinc ions connected to cysteines to form two tetrahedrons. This part of the molecule binds to specific sites of DNA, called *glucocorticoid-responsive elements,* which regulate glucocorticoid action on glucocorticoid-regulated genes. The zinc fingers represent the basic structure by which the DNA-binding domain recognizes specific nucleic acid sequences. The amino-terminal domain of the receptor is highly antigenic. Its exact function is not known, but there is evi-

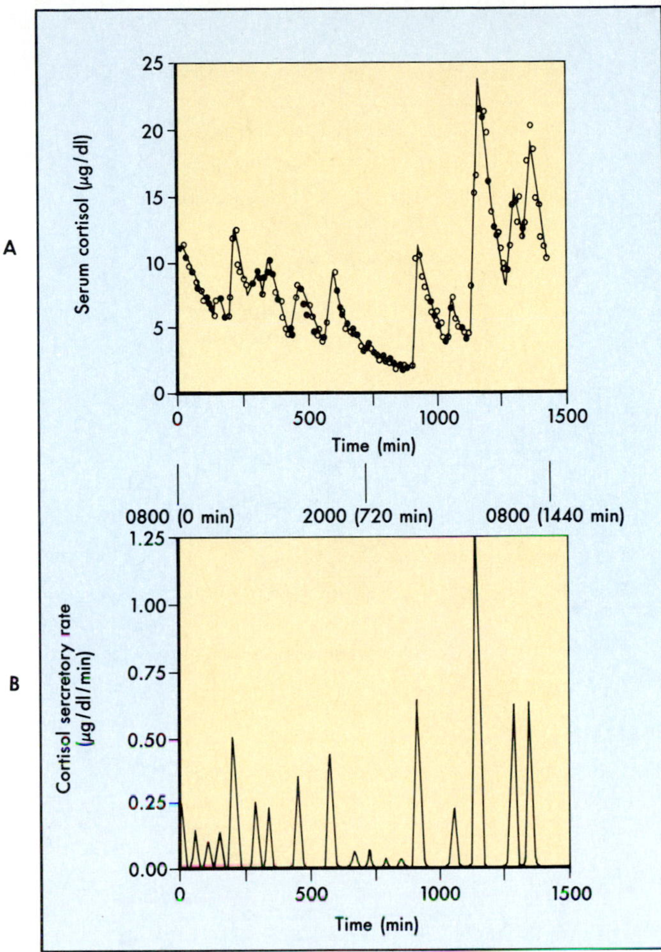

FIGURE 35-3 Serum cortisol concentrations in a healthy man. Serial blood samples collected at 10-minute intervals were assayed for serum cortisol concentrations. **A,** Concentrations plotted, with continuous line calculated using a special multiple parameter model of combined secretion and clearance of cortisol. **B,** Calculated rates of cortisol secretion as a function of time. Zero minutes = 0800 = start of experimental period. (Modified from Veldhuis JD, Iranmanesh A, Lizarralde G, Johnson ML: *Am J Physiol* 257:E6, 1989.)

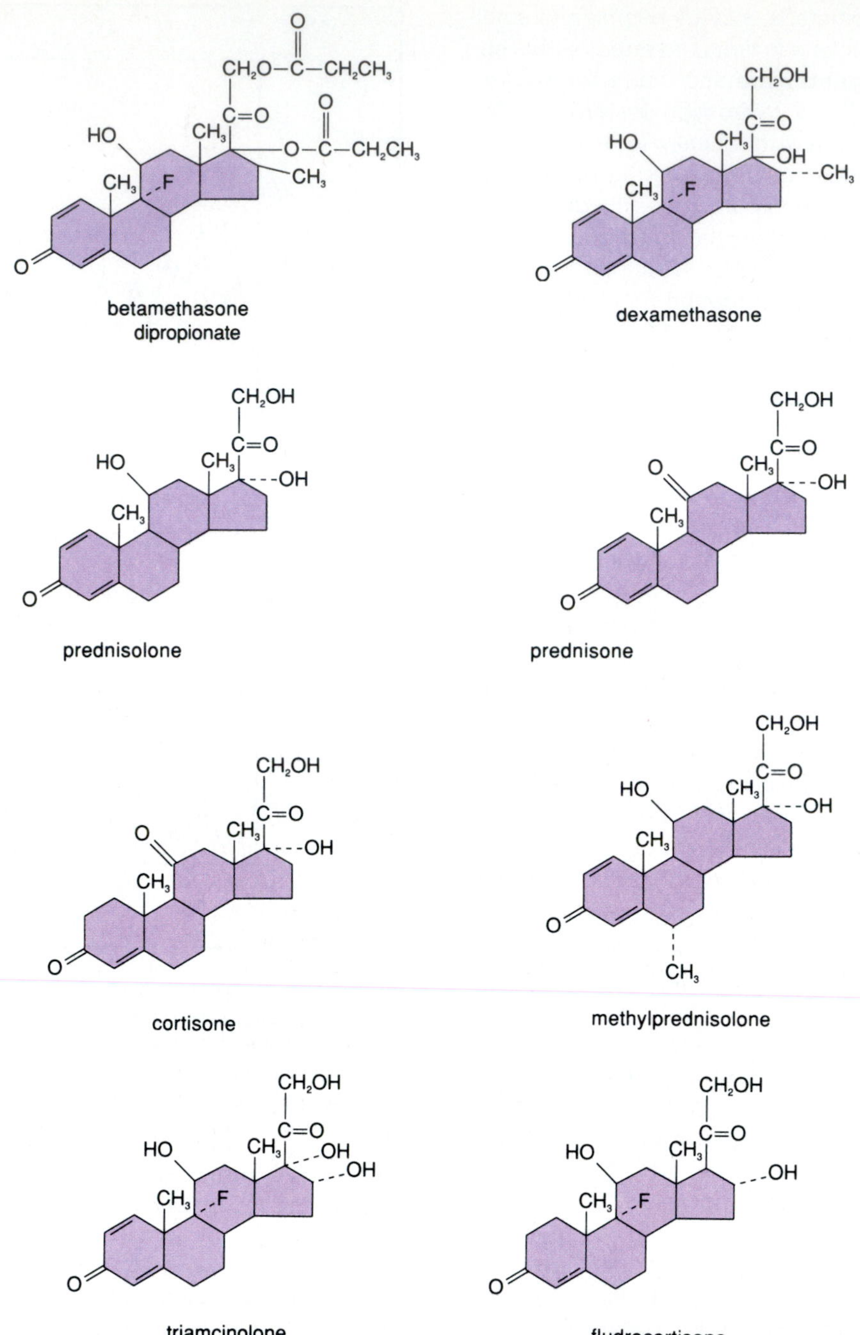

FIGURE 35-4 Principal clinically used glucocorticoids and mineralocorticoids (see also Figure 35-1).

dence that it is involved in the translocation of the receptor into the nucleus and its subsequent interaction with chromatin.

The inactive form of the glucocorticoid receptor is located in the cytoplasm as a heteromer associated with other proteins, one of which is heat shock protein 90. This heteromer is unable to exert any effect. Binding of a glucocorticoid to its receptor results in the dissociation of the hormone-receptor complex from the heat-shock protein 90, thus freeing the DNA-binding domain of the receptor, which now is available for its interaction with DNA. This sequence of events is generally called *glucocorticoid receptor activation.* The activated glucocorticoid-receptor complex then enters the nucleus (translocation). Inside the nucleus, two molecules of activated receptor are associated to form a

Table 35-1 Pharmacokinetic Parameters

Drugs	Administration	$t_{1/2}$	Disposition
GLUCOCORTICOIDS			
cortisol*	IM, IV, oral†	Short	M
cortisone	Oral, IM, IV	Short	M
prednisone	Oral	Intermediate	M
prednisolone	IM, IV	Intermediate	M
methylprednisolone	IM, IV, oral†	Intermediate	M
dexamethasone	IM, oral,† topical, IV	Long	M
betamethasone	Oral, topical, inhaled	Long	M
triamcinolone	Intraarticular, topical, inhaled	Long	M
MINERALOCORTICOIDS			
fludrocortisone	Oral	Intermediate	M
aldosterone (for reference)	—	Short	M
desoxycorticosterone acetate	IM	Long	M

Short, 10-90 minutes; *intermediate,* several hours; *long,* 5 hours or more; *M,* metabolism.
*Same as hydrocortisone.
†Intralesional, intraarticular, nasal, and inhaled. Collectively, they are called "compartmentalized" administration.

homodimer that binds to glucocorticoid response elements, located near the promoter region of specific genes, resulting in altered transcription rates (see Chapter 34).

Mineralocorticoids

Aldosterone is the major mineralocorticoid produced by the adrenal cortex. Aldosterone acts mainly at the distal portion of the convoluted renal tubule, where it promotes the reabsorption of sodium and the excretion of potassium. (See Chapter 19 for extensive discussion.) The adrenal secretion of aldosterone is controlled by the renin-angiotensin system and the concentration of potassium. ACTH plays a secondary role in the regulation of aldosterone secretion.

Receptors for mineralocorticoids are found in appropriate target tissues as well as in other tissues. They have the same affinity for glucocorticoids as for mineralocorticoids.

The structures of the principal clinically used glucocorticoids and mineralocorticoids are shown in Figures 35-1 and 35-4.

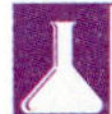

PHARMACOKINETICS

The pharmacokinetic parameters for the clinically used glucocorticoids and mineralocorticoids are summarized in Table 35-1.

Most glucocorticoids are rapidly and readily absorbed from the gastrointestinal tract, as a result of their lipophilic character. Glucocorticoids are also absorbed from the synovial and the conjunctival spaces. The absorption of glucocorticoids through the skin is very slow. Chronic use of steroids by nasal spray for control of seasonal rhinitis can lead to nasal and pulmonary epithelial atrophy. Consequently, topical administration of glucocorticoids is used only briefly for local action. Excessive and prolonged local application may result in enough absorption to cause systemic effects. The presence of a hydroxyl group at carbon position 11 confers glucocorticoid activity on both cortisol and prednisolone. Cortisone and prednisone with a keto group at the 11 position must be hydroxylated by the 11β-hydroxylase to become active (Figure 35-2). This hydroxylation takes place mainly in the liver. Consequently, the administration of 11-keto corticoids to patients with abnormal liver function should be avoided. For the same reason, topical application on the skin of the 11-ketocorticoids is ineffective.

Most circulating cortisol is bound to plasma proteins: 80% to 90% is bound (with high affinity) to cortisol-binding globulin, also called *transcortin* and 5% to 10% loosely bound to albumin. The free (bioactive) fraction is approximately 3% to 10%. The cortisol-binding globulin can also bind synthetic glucocorticoids, such as prednisone and prednisolone. However dexamethasone does not bind cortisol-binding globulin, and, consequently, almost 100% of its plasma concentration is in the free (bioactive) form. Estrogens increase the biosynthesis of cortisol-binding globulin from the liver. Thus, in conditions in which estrogens are elevated, such as exogenous estrogen administration (contraception) or during pregnancy, the cortisol-binding globulin is elevated, resulting in increased concentrations of total plasma cortisol.

The introduction of a fluorine atom in carbon position 9 and a CH3 group on carbon 16 enhances glucocorticoid receptor activation and prolongs its half-life (Figure 35-2).

The liver and kidney are the major sites of glucocorticoid inactivation. Pathways leading to inactivation of glucocorticoids include (1) reduction of the double bond at positions 4 to 5, (2) reduction of the keto group at carbon position 3, and (3) hydroxylation of carbon atom 6. About 30% of the inactivated cortisol is metabolized to tetrahydrocortisol-glucuronide and tetrahydrodeoxycortisol-glucuronide and excreted in the urine. An important cortisol inactivation pathway mentioned previously, takes place in the kidneys and results in its conversion to cortisone by the 11β-dehydroxysteroid dehydrogenase enzyme. Cortisone does not bind to the kidney mineralocorticoid receptor and thus does not exert a salt-retaining effect. A rare clinical syndrome has been observed in which this enzyme complex does not function efficiently, resulting in salt retention, hypokalemia, and hypertension.

Established inducers of hepatic drug metabolism, such as rifampicin, phenobarbital, and phenytoin may accelerate liver biotransformation of glucocorticoids. Thus the administration of these medications may increase the required dose of glucocorticoids. Hypothyroidism may decrease the metabolism of glucocorticoids.

Aldosterone does not bind specifically to a plasma protein. It binds only weakly to several plasma proteins, from which it dissociates very rapidly. The half-life of aldosterone is very short.

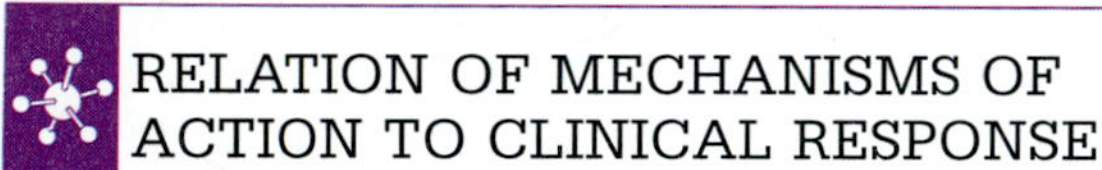

RELATION OF MECHANISMS OF ACTION TO CLINICAL RESPONSE

Glucocorticoids

Glucocorticoids have actions on glucose, protein, and bone metabolism and possess antiinflammatory and immunosuppressant actions. Glucocorticoids affect the immune system at multiple levels: (1) leukocyte movement, (2) antigen processing, (3) eosinophil cells, and (4) lymphatic tissues. (See box.)

Within hours after the administration of glucocorticoids the number of circulating neutrophils increases as a result of alterations of their trafficking dynamics. The neutrophilia may result from glucocorticoid-induced decrease of neutrophil adherence to vascular endothelium and the inability of neutrophils to egress toward bone marrow or inflammatory sites. In addition, glucocorticoids inhibit antigen processing by the macrophages, suppress T-cell helper function, inhibit synthesis of cellular mediators of the inflammatory response (i.e., interleukins, other cytokines, and prostanoids), and also inhibit phagocytosis. In addition, glucocorticoids induce eosinopenia and lymphopenia. The latter may be attributable to modification of cell production, or distribution, or cell lysis and are more profound on T than on the B lymphocytes. This feature may explain the beneficial effect of glucocorticoids in the treatment of certain leukemias, such as the acute lymphoblastic leukemia of childhood.

Therapeutically, the most important effect of glucocorticoids is the inhibition of the accumulation of neutrophils and monocytes at the site of inflammation and the suppression of their phagocytic, bactericidal, and antigen-processing activity. However, these effects compromise the immune system and thus predispose the patient to several common or uncommon pathogens and saprophytic sepsis. This condition represents the single most dangerous complication of chronic glucocorticoid treatment.

EFFECTS OF GLUCOCORTICOIDS

METABOLIC

Increased glycogenolysis and gluconeogenesis
Increased protein catabolism and decreased protein synthesis
Decreased osteoblast formation and activity
Decreased calcium absorption from the gastrointestinal tract
Decreased thyroid-stimulating hormone secretion

ANTIINFLAMMATORY

Local and systemic effects including:
- Decreased production of prostaglandins, cytokines, and interleukins
- Decreased proliferation and migration of lymphocytes and macrophages

Mineralocorticoids

The endogenous mineralocorticoid aldosterone is not used therapeutically because the duration of its biological action is very short. The synthetic mineralocorticoid fludrocortisone (9α-fluorohydrocortisone) is indicated for the treatment in the following: (1) primary adrenocortical insufficiency, (2) isolated aldosterone insufficiency, (3) salt-losing congenital adrenal hyperplasia, and (4) idiopathic orthostatic hypotension.

Selection of Drugs

Cortisol and cortisone are used only for replacement in patients with adrenal insufficiency (i.e., diminished production of endogenous glucocorticoids). They have no role in any antiinflammatory therapeutic regimen because of their high mineralocorticoid activity relative to the antiinflammatory activity.

Prednisone, prednisolone, and methylprednisolone, on the other hand, have considerable antiinflammatory activity, intermediate plasma half-lives, and relatively low mineralocorticoid activity. These characteristics make them first-choice drugs for chronic antiinflammatory and immunosuppressant therapeutic regimens. Indeed, prednisone and its derivatives are the most commonly used glucocorticoids for the treatment of several autoimmune diseases such as (1) collagen diseases (systemic lupus erythematosus and polymyositis-dermatomyositis), (2) vasculitis syndromes (polyarteritis nodosa, giant cell arteritis, Wegener's granulomatosis), (3) gastrointestinal inflammatory diseases (Crohn's disease and ulcerative colitis), and (4) renal autoimmune diseases (glomerulonephritis and the nephrotic syndromes). Intermediate-action glucocorticoids are also used for the treatment of bronchial asthma and chronic obstructive pulmonary disease.

Dexamethasone and betamethasone exhibit minimal mineralocorticoid activity, maximal antiinflammatory activity, and have prolonged plasma half-lives and pronounced growth-suppressing properties. They represent the best choice in cases in which a maximum antiinflammatory therapy is needed acutely (e.g., in cases of septic shock or brain edema). Because of their prolonged action, growth suppression, and bone demineralization properties, dexamethasone and betamethasone are not considered as first-choice drugs for chronic antiinflammatory treatment.

During the last few years, a new mode of glucocorticoid administration in which glucocorticoids are given every other day instead of daily has also been used. This "alternate-day" glucocorticoid administration presents both advantages and problems. The antiinflammatory effect of the glucocorticoids with intermediate duration of action persists longer than their suppressive effect on the hypothalamic-pituitary axis and bone growth rate. Therefore, by administering prednisone or prednisolone every other day, suppression of the hypothalamus and anterior pituitary can be lessened and bone growth suppression can be avoided, while a beneficial antiinflammatory effect can be achieved. However, there are two potential problems. First, in some patients the antiinflammatory effect of an alternate-day glucocorticoid therapeutic regimen may be not sufficient to control inflammation. Second, an abrupt switch from a daily dose of glucocorticoids to an alternate day regimen may cause symptoms and signs of clinical hypocortisolism (i.e., sense of being tired, nausea, vomiting, hypotension) on the days between the doses.

CLINICAL PROBLEMS

Side effects caused mainly by high (pharmacological as compared to physiological) concentrations and for long times

Most common side effects:

- Development of cushingoid habitus (trunkal obesity, moon facies, buffalo hump), salt retention, and hypertension (i.e., iatrogenic Cushing's syndrome)
- Suppression of the immune system (rendering the patient vulnerable to common and opportunistic infections)
- Osteoporosis (rendering the patient vulnerable to fractures)
- Peptic ulcers (resulting in gastric hemorrhages or intestinal perforation)
- Suppression of growth in children
- Behavioral problems
- Reproductive problems
- Prolonged suppression of the hypothalamic-pituitary-adrenal axis after drug discontinuation

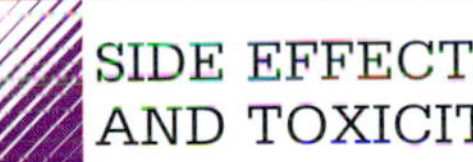

SIDE EFFECTS, CLINICAL PROBLEMS, AND TOXICITY

The primary clinical problems in the therapeutic use of glucocorticoids and mineralocorticoids are listed in the box.

Glucocorticoids and the Hypothalamic-Pituitary-Adrenal Axis

Suppression of the hypothalamic-pituitary-adrenal axis is the most common side effect of chronic glucocorticoid therapy. The suppressive effect of glucocorticoids on the hypothalamic-pituitary-adrenal axis appears within days after glucocorticoid treatment is started. Patients who receive glucocorticoids in doses equivalent to 5 mg or more of prednisone daily for more than 2 weeks should be considered as having suppressed hypothalamic-pituitary-adrenal axis. The time needed for the axis to recover depends on the type of glucocorticoid given, dose and frequency of administration (i.e., daily versus alternate days), and length of treatment. In cases of prolonged glucocorticoid administration, recovery may take up to a year or even longer. Assessment of recovery of the axis is based on the short ACTH test, in which ACTH or an analog is given IV and plasma cortisol concentrations are measured at 30 and 60 minutes.

Glucocorticoids and Bone

A major side effect of glucocorticoids, especially if given in pharmacological doses and for prolonged periods, is their detrimental action on bone. Patients with the highest risk in developing glucocorticoid-induced osteoporosis are children and postmenopausal women. This osteoporosis involves bone trabeculae, the most metabolically active site. Glucocorticoids cause osteoporosis by disrupting the regulation of calcium metabolism at several levels (1) by decreasing intestinal absorption and renal reabsorption of calcium, (2) by a direct antianabolic and catabolic action on bone and (3) by blockading the protective effect of calcitonin.

Glucocorticoids increase the 1α-hydroxylation of 25-hydroxyvitamin D to the 1,25-dihydroxyvitamin D, the active form of the vitamin (which facilitates intestinal absorption of calcium). However, it appears that glucocorticoids block the biological effect of the active form of vitamin D, so that despite high concentrations of circulating 1,25-dihydroxyvitamin D, the absorption rate of calcium is decreased. The parathyroid gland responds to the resulting hypocalcemia by increasing the secretion of parathyroid hormone, which catabolizes bone in an attempt to increase calcium concentrations in the extracellular fluid.

Glucocorticoids also affect bone directly by inhibiting osteoblastic activity as documented by the low concentrations of osteocalcin, a protein produced by osteoblasts. Furthermore, glucocorticoids may stimulate osteolysis by increasing the number of osteoclasts (i.e., they increase the transformation of precursor cells to osteoclasts). This results in increased bone resorption, as documented by the increased concentrations of urine hydroxyproline (an index of increased bone collagen catabolism). Finally, glucocorticoids block the bone-sparing effect of calcitonin, a 32-amino acid peptide synthesized by the parafollicular cells of the thyroid gland that inhibits osteoclastic bone resorption (see Chapter 42).

Glucocorticoids and Glucose

Glucocorticoids obtained their name from their role in glucose metabolism. Glucocorticoids increase plasma glucose by (1) increasing gluconeogenesis and glucose secretion by liver, (2) increasing the sensitivity of liver to the gluconeogenic action of glucagon and catecholamines, (3) decreasing glucose uptake and utilization by peripheral tissues, and (4) increasing the substrate for gluconeogenesis (increasing proteolysis and inhibiting protein synthesis in muscles). As a consequence, chronic administration of glucocorticoids may cause hyperglycemia and the development of diabetes mellitus in susceptible individuals.

TRADE NAMES

In addition to generic and fixed-combination preparations, the following trade-named materials are available in the United States.

Aristocort, Kenalog, triamcinolone

Carmol HC, Cortogen, Hydrocortone, Cortril, Cortef, Hydrocort, hydrocortisone and cortisol and related esters

Decadron, Hexadrol, dexamethasone

Deltasone, prednisone

Fluorinef, fludrocortisone

Maxivate, Celestone, Diprolene, Betatrex, betamethasone

Methapred, Depo-Medrol, methylprednisolone and esters

Other Side Effects

Chronic administration of glucocorticoids increases the incidence of peptic ulcers. It has been proposed that glucocorticoids (1) increase gastric acid output and (2) inhibit synthesis of mucopolysaccharides, which protect gastric mucosa from acid. Since even short (less than 1 month) treatment with glucocorticoids may cause gastric irritation or ulcers, some physicians prescribe antacids or H_2-blockers with glucocorticoids (see Chapter 59 and 60).

The main acute effect of glucocorticoids in the central nervous system is the promotion of arousal and general euphoria. However, prolonged treatment with glucocorticoids may cause depression, sleep disturbances, and, in some cases, true psychotic ideation.

Glucocorticoids can suppress the synthesis and secretion of gonadotropins and their effect on gonads. In men, chronic glucocorticoid treatment may cause hypogonadism associated with decreased plasma testosterone. In women, they can cause anovulation, oligomenorrhea, or dysfunctional uterine bleeding.

Most children on chronic glucocorticoid therapy have their linear growth rate impaired. Although chronic glucocorticoid administration decreases the secretion of growth hormone from the anterior pituitary, it is now believed that this adverse effect of glucocorticoids on growth is attributable to inhibition of the biological effects of insulin-like growth factor-I (formerly somatomedin C).

NEW DIRECTIONS

In the last decade efforts were undertaken to find agents that might reduce excessive cortisol production. Thus, several glucocorticoid antagonists were tested, the most promising being mepristine. Mepristine is a synthetic steroid that binds with high affinity to glucocorticoid receptors. This compound is a partial glucocorticoid antagonist, exerting also mild glucocorticoid agonistic effects. Mepristine was recently tested as antiglucocorticoid in patients with hypercortisolemia (Cushing's syndrome), reversing most of the associated symptoms. Furthermore, since RU 486 exhibits a proinflammatory action in experimental animals, it can be used as an immunopotentiating agent in patients with compromized immune systems.

REFERENCES

Axelrod L: Corticosteroid therapy. In Becker K.L., Bilezikian J.P., Bremner W.J., editor: *Principles and practice in endocrinology and metabolism,* Philadelphia, 1990, Lippincott.

Boumpas DT, Chrousos GP, Wilder RL, et al: Glucocorticoid therapy for immune-mediated diseases: basic and clinical correlates, *Ann Intern Med* 119(12):1198-1208, 1993.

Chrousos GP, Detera-Wadleigh SD, Karl M: Syndromes of glucocorticoid resistance, *Ann Intern Med* 119(11):1113-1124, 1993.

Arai K, Chrousos GP: Syndromes of glucocorticoid and mineralocorticoid resistance, Steroids 60(1):173-179, 1995.

Edwards CRW, Stewart PM, Bent D, et al: Localization of 11β-hydroxysteroid dehydrogenase-tissue specific protein of the mineralocorticoid receptor, *Lancet* 2:986-919, 1988.

Evans RM: The steroid and thyroid hormone receptor superfamily, *Science* 240:889, 1988.

SELF-ASSESSMENT QUESTIONS

1. Which is considered the most suitable glucocorticoid in the treatment of septic shock?
   a. cortisol
   b. prednisone
   c. dexamethasone
   d. methylprednisolone
   e. prednisolone
2. Which is the best test to assess the recovery of the hypothalamus-pituitary-adrenal axis in patients withdrawing from exogenous glucocorticoids?
   a. morning serum cortisol
   b. evening serum cortisol
   c. morning plasma ACTH
   d. insulin-tolerance test
   e. ACTH stimulation test
3. Which moiety confers glucocorticoid activity to the corticoid molecule?
   a. the hydroxyl group at carbon 17
   b. the hydroxyl group at carbon 11
   c. the keto group at carbon 3
   d. the keto group at carbon 11
   e. the hydroxyl group at carbon 20
4. All the following are the advantages of the alternate-day glucocorticoid therapy *except* which one?
   a. minimizes the clinical manifestations of hypercortisolism (Cushing's syndrome)
   b. facilitates the recovery of the hypothalamus-pituitary-adrenal axis
   c. beneficial in the treatment of adrenocortical insufficiency
   d. lessens growth suppression in children
   e. does not compromise the antiinflammatory effects of glucocorticoids
5. Each of the following is an indication for mineralocorticoid treatment *except:*
   a. primary adrenocortical insufficiency (Addison's disease).
   b. diabetic hyporenin-hypoaldosteronism.
   c. autoimmune glomerulonephritis.
   d. salt-losing congenital adrenal hyperplasia.
   e. idiopathic orthostatic hypotension.

CHAPTER 36 Estrogens, Progestins, and Oral Contraceptives

MICHAEL K. FRITSCH
FERN E. MURDOCH

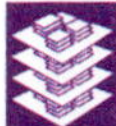

THERAPEUTIC OVERVIEW

The two major classes of female sex hormones are the estrogens and the progestins. Together they serve important functions in the development of female secondary sex characteristics, the control of pregnancy, the control of the ovulatory/menstrual cycle, and the modulation of many metabolic processes.

Estrogens

There are three natural human estrogens: 17β-estradiol, the principal ovarian estrogen; estriol, the principal placental estrogen;, and estrone, a metabolite of 17β-estradiol and a major ovarian and postmenopausal estrogen.

Estrogens coordinate the systemic responses during the ovulatory cycle, including regulation of the reproductive tract, pituitary, breasts, and other tissues. They also play a role in progression of some tumors. The target organs for hormone action are shown in Figure 36-1, *B*. The hypothalamic-pituitary-ovarian organs are shown in Figure 36-1, *A*.

Estrogens are also responsible for the development of secondary sex characteristics when a female enters puberty, including the progressive development of the fallopian tubes, uterus, vagina, and external genitalia. With estrogen stimulation, fat deposition increases in the breast, buttocks, and thighs, leading to the characteristic female habitus. Estrogens also (1) initiate breast development by increasing ductal and stromal growth, (2) contribute to accelerated growth at puberty, (3) stimulate closure of the epiphyses in the shafts of the long bones, (4) stimulate synthesis and secretion of prolactin from pituitary lactotrophs, (5) produce increased cellular proliferation of uterine endometrium and stroma, in the absence of progesterone as occurs in the follicular phase of the menstrual cycle, (6) induce ribonucleic acid (RNA) and protein synthesis in cells, (7) generate thickening of vaginal mucosa and thinning of cervical mucus, (8) aid in maintaining bone mass, as evidenced by substantial but preventable (with estrogen replacement therapy) bone loss in postmenopausal women, (9) stimulate hepatic production of sex hormone–binding globulin, thyroid-binding globulin, blood-clotting factors (VII to X), plasminogen, and high-density lipoprotein (HDL) but inhibit antithrombin III and low-density lipoprotein (LDL) formation. Estrogens also increase retention of sodium and water, occasionally causing edema. Estrogens can decrease bowel motility as well.

Estrogens may play a direct role in the progression of some endometrial tumors, and estrogen or antiestrogen therapy is used in the treatment of breast cancer and some prostate tumors. Continuous exposure of the uterus to unopposed estrogen results in abnormal endometrial hyperplasia with episodes of breakthrough bleeding and an increased incidence of endometrial cancer.

ABBREVIATIONS	
GnRH	gonadotropin-releasing hormone
FSH	follicle-stimulating hormone
HDL	high-density lipoprotein
LDL	low-density lipoprotein
LH	luteinizing hormone

Progestins

The important natural progestin is progesterone, but 17α-, 20α-, and 20β-hydroxyprogesterones have weak progestational activities. Progesterone is partially responsible for mammary glandular development and may play a role in ductal growth. Progesterone concentrations rise rapidly in the luteal phase of the menstrual cycle, resulting in modulation of estrogen's action on the uterus. Under the influence of progesterone, the estrogen-primed uterus initiates secretory changes in preparation for embryo implantation. Without estrogen, progesterone receptor concentrations are low and estrogen priming is necessary for progesterone receptor induction in almost all progesterone-responsive tissues, including the uterus. Progesterone is responsible for increased basal body temperature observed in the luteal phase. In the absence of pregnancy, plasma progesterone concentrations fall, resulting in sloughing of the endometrial lining. A variety of disorders of the menstrual cycle are treated with estrogens, progestins, or a combination of both.

Progesterone also (1) aids in the maintenance of pregnancy, (2) inhibits uterine contraction, (3) can alter carbohydrate metabolism, (4) may lead to decreased HDL and increased LDL concentrations, and (5) increases sodium and water elimination through competition with aldosterone for binding to mineralocorticoid receptors.

Combined Effects

There are several other ways these hormones act together. Progesterone and estrogen coordinate events associated with the luteal phase of the ovulatory cycle and pregnancy. In primary hypogonadism, estrogens and progestins are administered to optimize normal development of secondary sex characteristics. An important pharmacological use of estrogens and progestins is as oral contraceptives. Estrogens and progestins act predominantly to decrease the production of the gonadotropins, follicle-stimulating hormone (FSH), and luteinizing hormone (LH) at the pituitary-hypothalamic axis. This inhibits the midcycle LH surge and thereby prevents ovulation. Interestingly, antiestrogens have been developed that aid in the treatment of infertility by inducing an increase in circulating FSH, which leads to ovulation.

A summary of the major therapeutic uses of steroid hormones, antihormones, and steroidogenesis inhibitors is shown in the box.

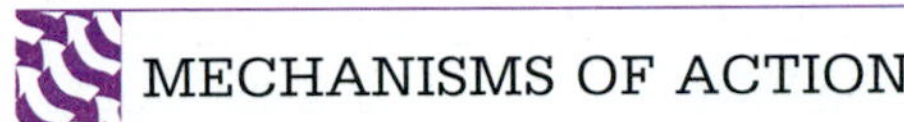

MECHANISMS OF ACTION

Ligand Structure

Estrogens can be classified structurally as either steroidal or nonsteroidal, with steroidal estrogens further divided into natural and synthetic compounds. The

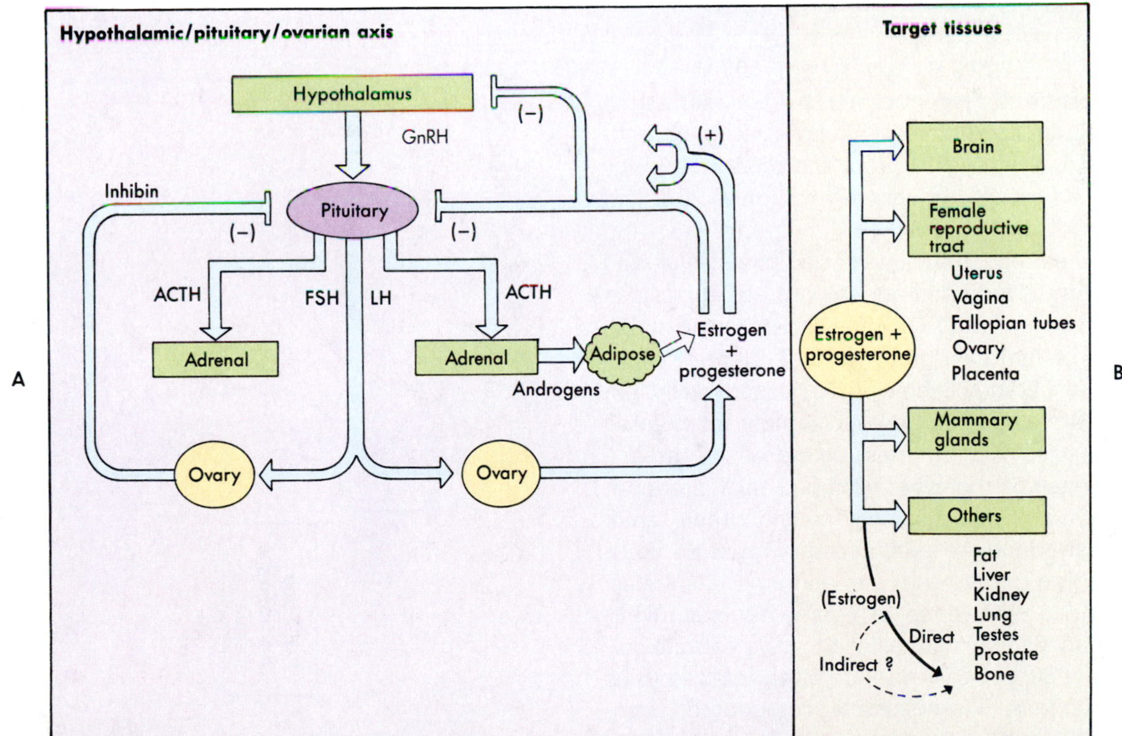

FIGURE 36-1 Feedback loops and target tissues. **A,** Schema demonstrates negative and positive feedback action of estrogens and progesterone on the hypothalamic-pituitary-ovarian axis. **B,** Other target tissues for these steroid hormones. *GnRH,* Gonadotropin-releasing hormone.

THERAPEUTIC OVERVIEW

FERTILITY CONTROL

Combination oral contraception (estrogens, progestins)
Progestin-only contraception (progestins)
Postcoital contraception (estrogens, progestins)
Contragestation (antiprogestins)

HORMONE REPLACEMENT THERAPY

Menopause (estrogens, progestins [?])
Osteoporosis (estrogens, progestins [?])
Ovarian failure (estrogens, progestins)
Dysfunctional uterine bleeding (progestins, estrogens)
Luteal phase dysfunction (progestins)

OVULATION INDUCTION

Infertility (clomiphene citrate)

CANCER CHEMOTHERAPY

Breast cancer (estrogens, progestins, antiestrogens, steroidogenesis inhibitors)
Endometrial cancer (progestins, antiestrogens [?])
Prostate cancer (estrogens)

OTHERS

Endometriosis (danazol, progestins, gonadotropin-releasing hormone)
Diagnostic use (progestins)

natural estrogens and progestins are steroids with structures derived from cholesterol. The most common natural human estrogens and some of the most frequently used synthetic ligands are shown in Figures 36-2 and 36-3.

The natural estrogens include estradiol, estrone, and estriol. They have 18 carbon atoms with an aromatic A ring, a methyl group at C13, a phenolic hydroxyl at C3, and a ketone or hydroxyl group at C17. Natural estrogens have low potency when administered orally because they are poorly absorbed and rapidly inactivated by the liver. Estradiol is the most potent of the three.

The conjugated estrogens are coupled at C3 predominantly to sulfate but occasionally to glucuronic acid. Conjugated estrogens are prepared directly from pregnant mare's urine to give estrogen and equilin sulfates. Equilin is an estrogen found in horses but not in humans. They can also be synthesized to give estrone sulfate contents of 80% to 85% and are often referred to as *esterified estrogens*. Water-soluble conjugated estrogens have virtually no estrogenic activity and must be activated (hydrolyzed at C3) to be able to bind to the estrogen receptor.

The synthetic steroidal estrogens include orally active ethinyl estradiol and mestranol, used predominantly

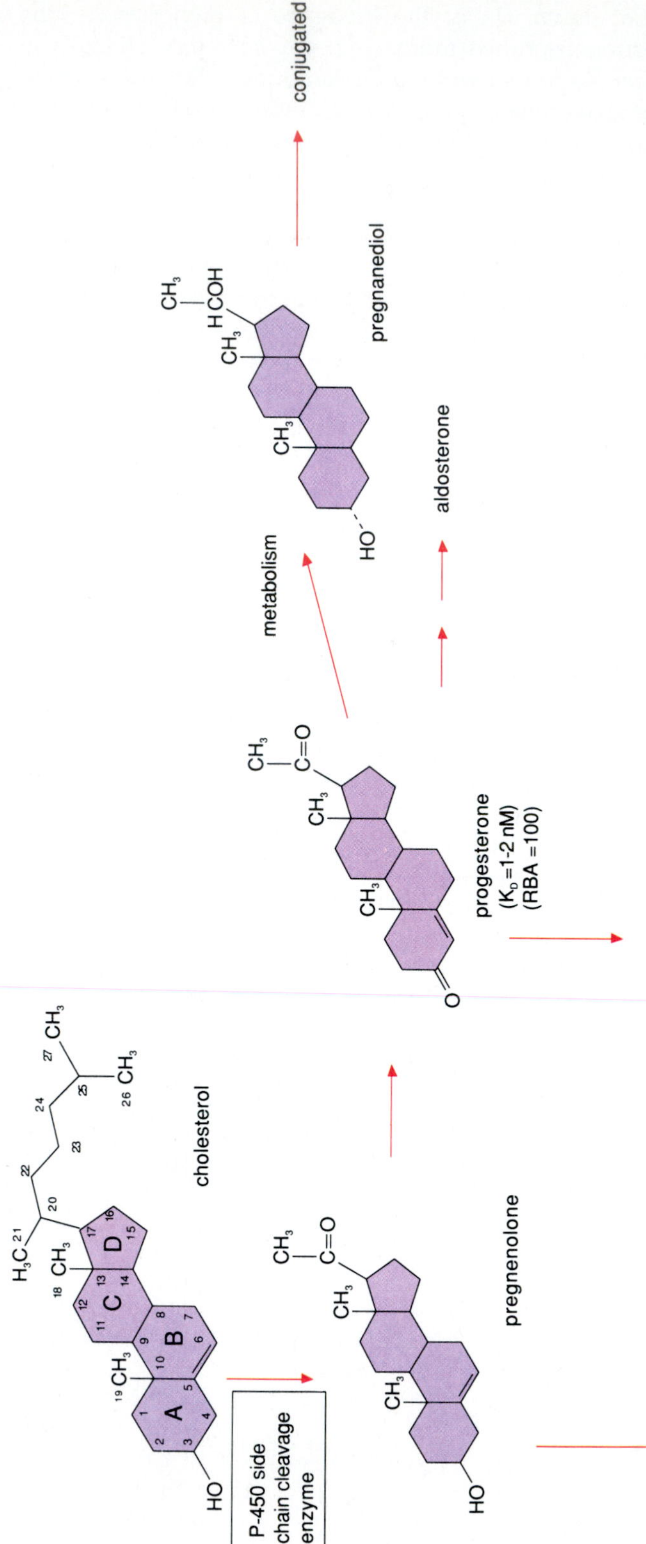

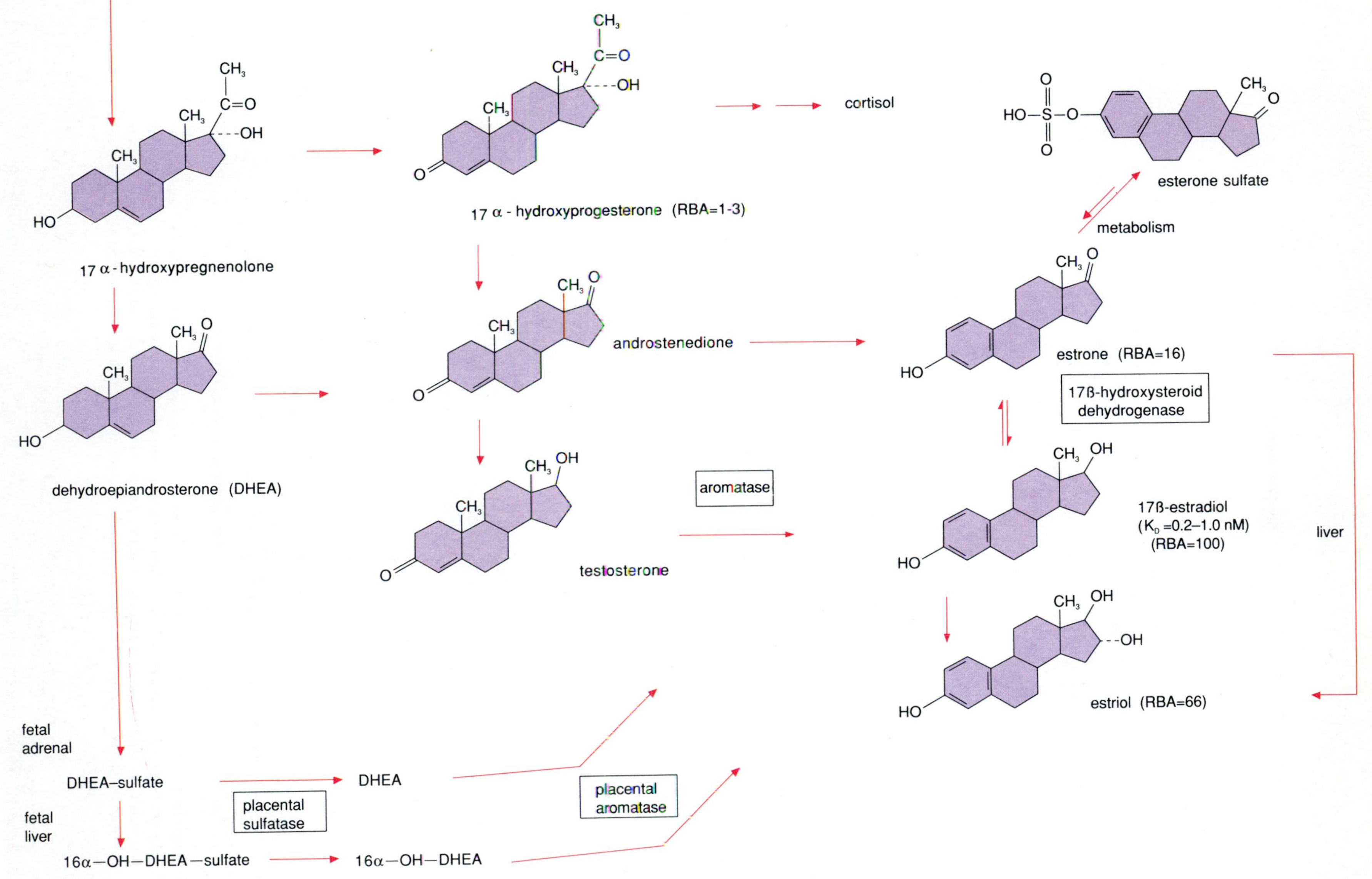

FIGURE 36-2 Steroidogenesis. Biosynthetic pathways of progesterone and the natural estrogens are illustrated. Included are the absolute binding affinities of progesterone and estradiol for their respective receptors and the relative-binding affinities (RBA) of estrone and estriol when that of estradiol is set at 100%. Also shown are important metabolites of progesterone and the estrogens. *Boxed area,* Pathway of estrogen production in the fetal-placental unit.

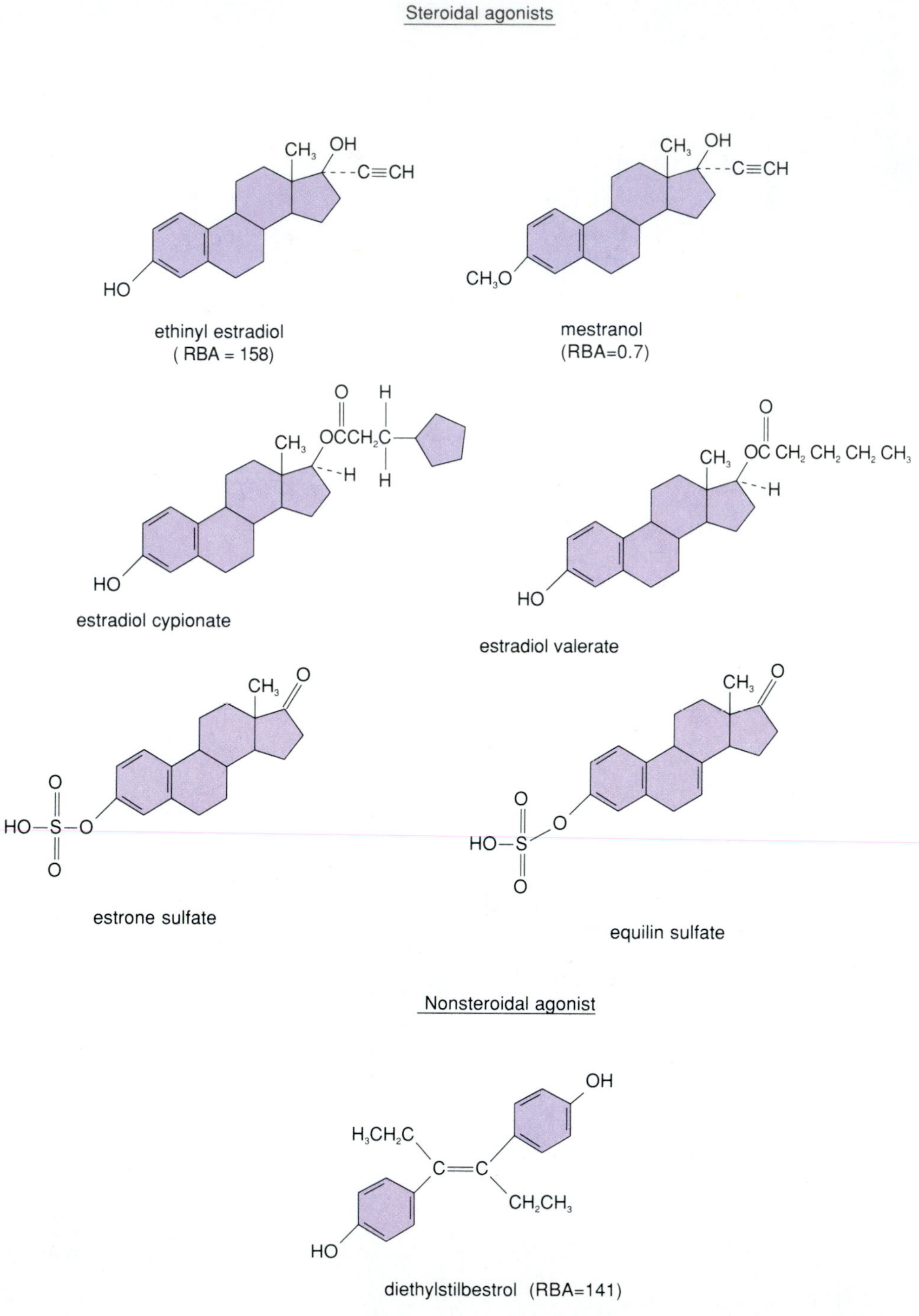
Steroidal agonists
CH3 OH
C≡CH
HO
ethinyl estradiol
(RBA = 158)
CH3 OH
C≡CH
CH3O
mestranol
(RBA=0.7)
O H
CH3 OCCH2C
H H
HO
estradiol cypionate
O
CH3 OC CH2 CH2 CH2 CH3
H
HO
estradiol valerate
CH3 O
O
HO—S—O
O
estrone sulfate
CH3 O
O
HO—S O
O
equilin sulfate
Nonsteroidal agonist
OH
H3CH2C
C=C
CH2CH3
HO
diethylstilbestrol (RBA=141)

FIGURE 36-3 Commonly used estrogens and antiestrogens. Structures for several ligands for the estrogen receptor are shown. Relative binding affinity *(RBA)* for the ligand to the estrogen receptor, as compared to estradiol, is also shown (RBA for estradiol, 100%). Mestranol is converted to ethinylestradiol. Esterified estrogens are hydrolyzed and converted to active species.

Antagonists

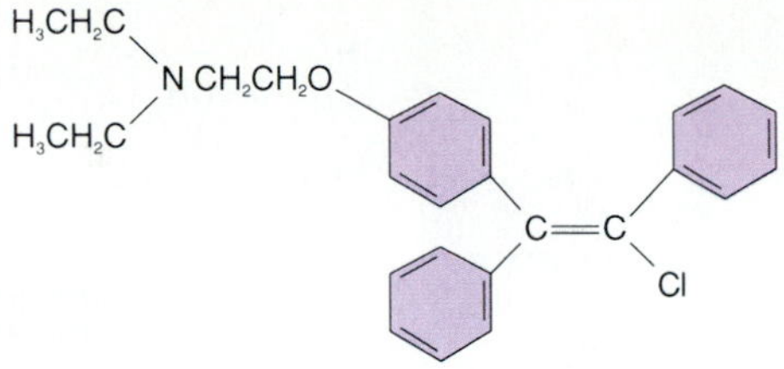

enclomiphene
(RBA=8)

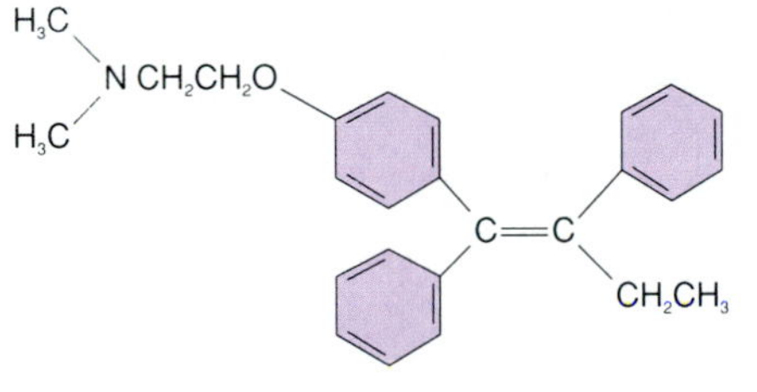

tamoxifen
(RBA=3–5)

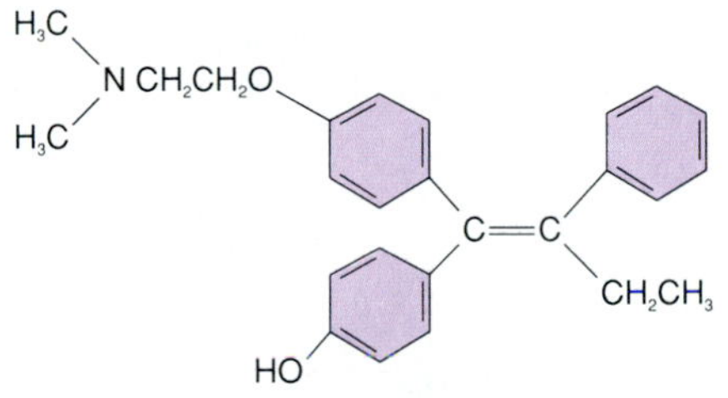

monohydroxy tamoxifen
(RBA=100–290)

FIGURE 36-3, cont'd. For legend see opposite page.

C_{21} Agonists

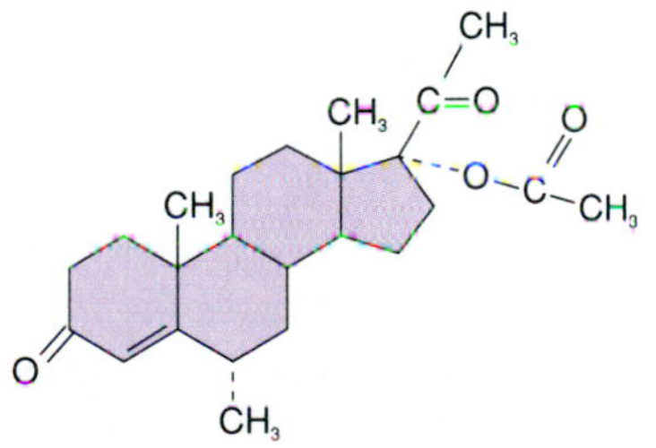

medroxyprogesterone acetate
(RBA=78)

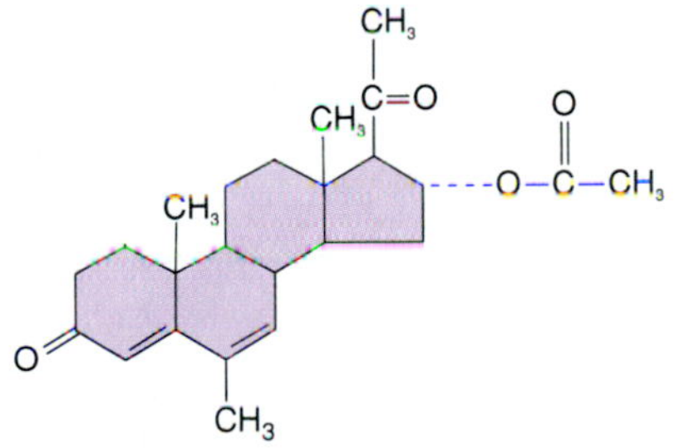

megestrol acetate

Antagonist

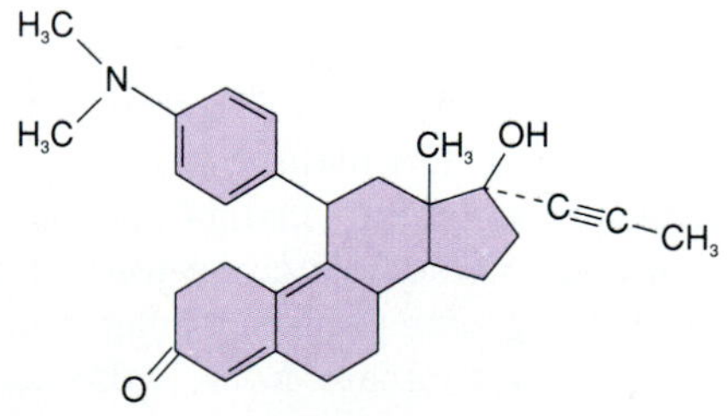

mifepristone (RU 486)
(RBA=530)

FIGURE 36-4 Commonly used progestins and antiprogestin. Structures for several ligands for the progesterone receptor are shown. Relative binding affinity *(RBA)* for the ligand to the progesterone receptor, as compared to progesterone, is also shown (RBA for progesterone, 100%). *Continued.*

in combination oral contraceptives. Ethinyl estradiol and mestranol have an ethinyl group at C17, which protects against inactivation by the liver. Mestranol is inactive until converted to ethinyl estradiol in the liver. Other orally active synthetic steroids include estropipate and quinestrol.

The parenterally administered synthetic steroids include estradiol cypionate, estradiol valerate, and polyestradiol phosphate. The synthetic, nonsteroidal estrogens include diethylstilbestrol, chlorotrianisene, and dienestrol.

The antiestrogens used clinically include tamoxifen and enclomiphene citrate (see Figure 36-3). Clomiphene citrate is a racemic mixture of two stereoisomers and has both estrogenic and antiestrogenic properties. Tamoxifen is a nonsteroidal triphenylethylene derivative structurally similar to clomiphene. The *trans* isomer of

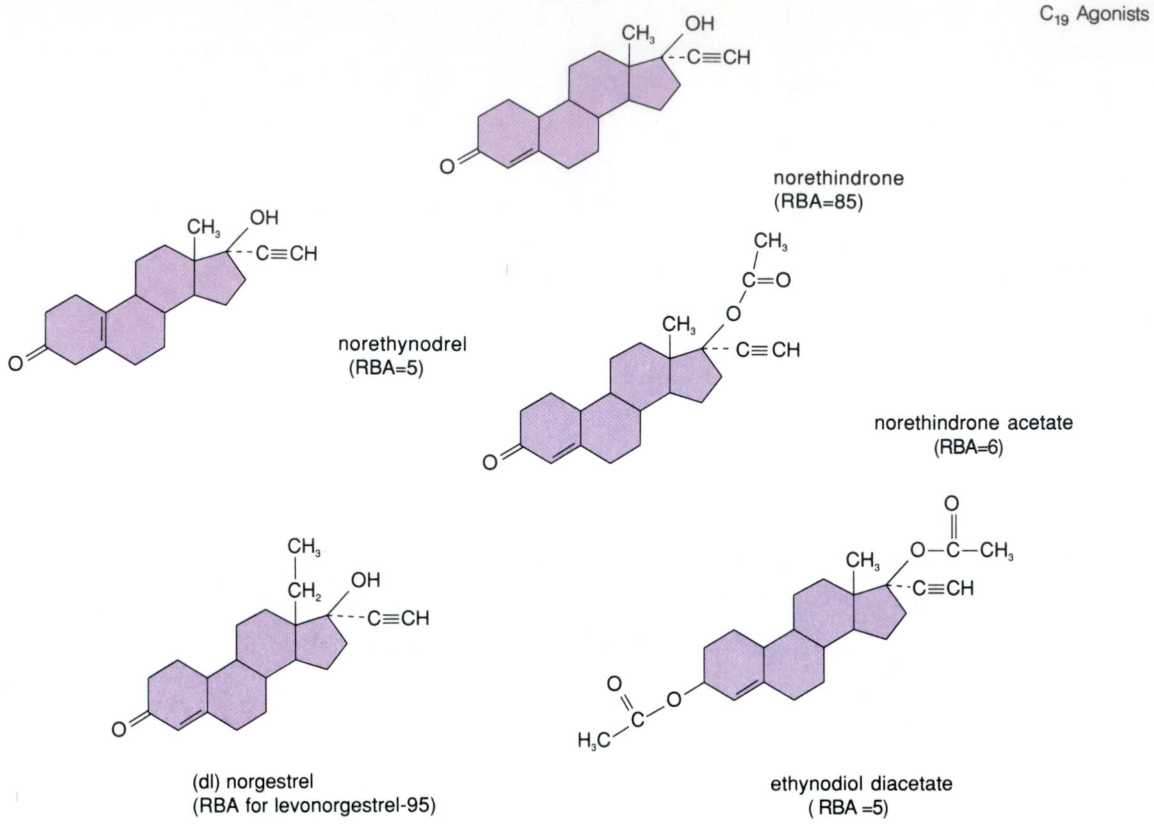

C$_{19}$ Agonists

norethindrone
(RBA=85)

norethynodrel
(RBA=5)

norethindrone acetate
(RBA=6)

(dl) norgestrel
(RBA for levonorgestrel-95)

ethynodiol diacetate
(RBA =5)

FIGURE 36-4, cont'd. For legend see previous page.

tamoxifen is believed to produce the antiestrogenic properties.

The most common naturally occurring progestins in humans and several important synthetic progestins are shown in Figures 36-2 and 36-4. Progestin derivatives can be classified based on positions C21 or C19 (19-nortestosterone).

The C21 derivatives include the natural progestins, progesterone, and 17α-hydroxyprogesterone, which utilize the same carbon backbone as pregnenolone, from which they are derived. The other C21 compounds are derivatives of 17α-hydroxyprogesterone and include medroxyprogesterone acetate, megestrol acetate (6,7 double bond to medroxyprogesterone), and hydroxyprogesterone caproate (6-methyl deleted and 17-acetate replaced by 17-caproate from hydroxyprogesterone acetate). The presence of an acetate ester in medroxyprogesterone acetate and megestrol acetate helps protect these compounds from inactivation in the liver and allows their oral use.

The 19-nortestosterone derivatives are similar to testosterone but lack the C19 methyl group. They include synthetic levonorgestrel and norgestrel, a racemic mixture of active levonorgestrel and the inactive stereoisomer. Therefore, on a weight basis, levonorgestrel is twice as potent as norgestrel.

The other synthetic progestins include norethindrone, norethindrone acetate, norethynodrel (norethindrone with C—H instead of C—CH at C17), and ethynodiol diacetate. Norethindrone acetate and norethynodrel are metabolized to the active progestin norethindrone. These synthetic compounds are orally active with an ethinyl group present at C17 to slow inactivation in the liver.

In general synthetic progestins are more potent than C21 derivatives when administered orally. Norgestrel is 5 to 10 times more potent than the same dose of norethindrone. Synthetic progestins can also display some estrogenic and androgenic activity, with progesterone and C21 derivatives showing less androgenic and no estrogenic properties.

Biosynthesis of Estrogens and Progestins

Estrogens and progestins are produced by steroidogenesis in various tissues. In nonpregnant premenopausal women, the ovary is the predominant source. During pregnancy the fetal-placental unit produces large amounts of both steroids. A significant amount of estrogen is also produced by skeletal muscle, liver, and adipose tissue by conversion of circulating androgens to estrone. Certain brain areas in males and females may produce estrogens by conversion of circulating androgens. Small amounts of estradiol are produced in the male testes.

In the biosynthesis of natural estrogens and progestins (see Figure 36-2), the rate-limiting step in ovarian production of steroid hormones is the conversion of cholesterol to pregnenolone by cytochrome P-450 side-chain cleavage enzymes. Most cholesterol derives from the blood LDL form, but it can also be synthesized in the cell from acetyl CoA. Pregnenolone can then be directly converted to progesterone or 17α-hydroxypregnenolone. Two pathways lead to androgenic steroids, androstenedione and testosterone. These androgens can then be converted to estrone and 17β-estradiol, respectively, by the aromatase enzyme. The aromatase in the ovary and peripheral tissues is responsible for aromatization of the A ring and loss of the C19 methyl group, producing a molecule with estrogenic properties.

Estriol can be produced in the liver as an oxidation product derived mainly from estrone; some estriol is also made from estradiol. During pregnancy, estriol can be synthesized in the fetal-placental unit.

Although progesterone is readily made in the placenta, direct placental conversion of cholesterol to estrogen cannot occur. Maternal cholesterol is converted to dehydroepiandrosterone sulfate in fetal adrenals and then hydroxylated to the 16α-hydroxy derivative in fetal liver. In the placenta, which is rich in sulfatase and aromatase enzymes, the 16α-hydroxy derivative is converted to estriol, whereas dehydroepiandrosterone sulfate is converted to estrone.

The quantities of the various steroids produced in the adrenals, testes, ovaries, and placenta are probably regulated by the enzymic activity at each step of steroidogenesis in particular cell types.

During the menstrual cycle estrogen and progesterone are synthesized and released from the ovary under regulation of pituitary gonadotropins FSH and LH. Pulsatile release of hypothalamic gonadotropin-releasing hormone regulates FSH and LH synthesis and release. Gonadotropin-releasing hormone concentrations are regulated through negative and positive feedback by the steroid hormones. Estrogens and progestins also act directly on the pituitary gonadotrophs to decrease FSH and LH concentrations. In addition, an ovarian protein, inhibin, negatively affects FSH synthesis. A schema of the pathways for integrated control of hormone concentrations is shown in Figure 36-1.

A normal ovulatory/menstrual cycle lasts 25 to 35 days. The steps in the ovarian and endometrial cycles are shown in Figure 36-5. The ovarian cycle is divided into the follicular (preovulatory) phase, which is predominantly concerned with the maturing follicle, and the luteal (postovulatory) phase, which is controlled by the corpus luteum. The follicle is the basic reproductive unit of the ovary and consists of the oocyte surrounded by granulosa cells, which are separated by a basement membrane from the theca cells. During follicular development both the cell layers and a follicular cavity containing fluid (the antrum) enlarge. After ovulation the remnants of the antral fluid, granulosa, and theca cells make up the corpus luteum.

At the beginning of a menstrual cycle, several follicles increase their rates of maturation under FSH stimulation. FSH binds to its cell surface receptor on granulosa cells, leading to increased enzymatic activity to aromatize androgens to estradiol. One follicle becomes dominant while the others undergo atresia. By days 8 to 10, FSH concentrations are falling, but the dominant follicle has an increased number of FSH receptors and thereby becomes more sensitive to circulating gonadotropin concentrations. LH concentrations rise slightly during this time.

In the late follicular phase blood estrogen concentration rises rapidly and peaks at 0.3 to 0.7 ng/ml, initiating the midcycle LH surge (16 to 24 hours before ovulation) through positive feedback to the hypothalamic-pituitary axis. The LH surge leads to follicular production of progesterone, prostaglandin $F_{2\alpha}$, and proteolytic enzymes and to follicular rupture and ovulation.

The length of the follicular phase can vary, but the luteal phase is consistently about 14 days. The corpus luteum produces predominantly progesterone, which rises through the first half of the luteal phase (peak concentrations of 10 to 20 ng/ml). The estrogen concentrations reach 0.2 ng/ml. These high steroid concentrations feedback negatively to the hypothalamic-pituitary axis to keep the concentrations of FSH and LH low. Unless pregnancy occurs, the progesterone and estrogen concentrations fall and luteolysis occurs, leading to menses (steroid withdrawal bleeding) and the beginning of a new cycle. The negative-feedback effect of high concentrations of estrogens and progestins is exploited by oral contraceptives to inhibit the FSH and LH peaks and thereby prevent follicular maturation and ovulation.

In the event of pregnancy, the placenta secretes chorionic gonadotropin into the maternal circulation. The chorionic gonadotropin concentration rises rapidly after implantation and peaks about 6 to 8 weeks into pregnancy. Chorionic gonadotropin maintains the corpus luteum and stimulates progesterone production, which helps maintain pregnancy. The feto-placental unit eventually becomes the major source of circulating progesterone and estrogens, especially estriol, sometime after the fifth week of pregnancy.

As women age, the number of follicles present in the ovaries diminishes, predominantly because of atresia. Eventually, no follicles remain and the normal menstrual cycles cease (menopause). The lack of follicles means estradiol and progesterone can no longer be made in the ovary. Without these two steroid hormones to feed back on the hypothalamic-pituitary axis, FSH and LH rise to very high concentrations. Adrenal androgens, predominantly androstenedione, are still produced and can be converted by aromatase to estrone in peripheral tissues. However, because these concentrations are low, women experience some symptoms related to the absence of estrogens during this time.

Transport of Hormones in the Blood

Before estrogen or progesterone can lead to a response it must be secreted into the blood and transported to a target tissue. The steroid hormones are transported in the blood complexed with proteins. Estrogens are bound by sex hormone–binding globulin and progesterone by corticosteroid-binding globulin. These are relatively high-affinity, low-capacity interactions compared to those of albumin. Clearly the concentration of these binding globulins in relation to hormone determines the concentration of free hormone available to target tissues. The free concentration of hormone (not bound to serum proteins) represents the true hormone concentration available to elicit a response. The concentrations of these proteins are hormonally regulated. Estrogen administration leads to increased production of both binding globulins. Serum albumin also can bind estrogens and progesterone, but the amount of albumin in the blood is unaffected by these hormones. These are low-affinity, high-capacity interactions. Synthetic ligands show variable affinities for the serum proteins.

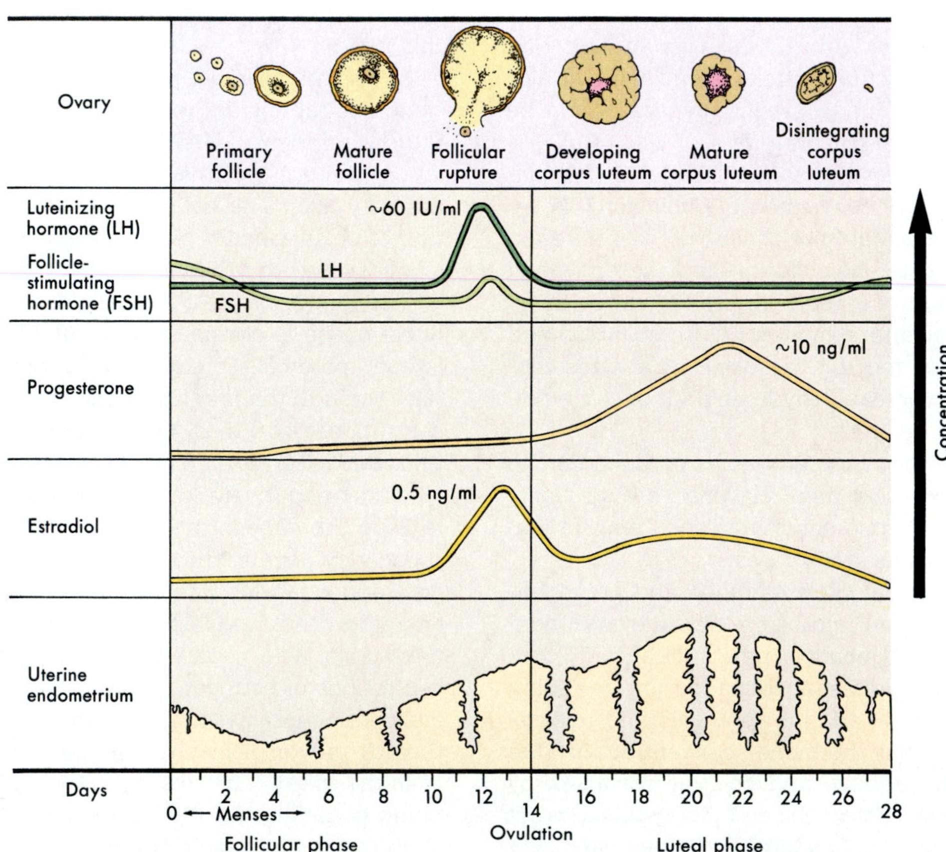

FIGURE 36-5 Ovulatory and menstrual cycle. Schema of ovarian and uterine changes that occur with the cyclical hormonal changes during the normal human menstrual cycle. Note the increase in LH, FSH, and estradiol concentration before ovulation during the follicular phase. Progesterone rises and peaks in the midluteal phase, concomitant with reductions in LH, FSH, and estradiol.

Receptor Mechanisms

All steroid hormones appear to act by a similar mechanism. After delivery to the target tissue, free hormone passively diffuses into the cell and through the cytoplasm and binds to a specific receptor protein in the nucleus in the case of estrogen and progesterone receptors. If a particular receptor molecule is present, the target tissue produces a response to the hormone. Different tissues can respond differently to the same hormone, though probably only one estrogen receptor protein species exists in target tissues. Therefore factors other than the receptor alone must determine the type and magnitude of response by a target tissue. The binding of estrogen or progesterone to its particular receptor in the nucleus is a high-affinity interaction. Each binds tightly to its own receptor but weakly to the other receptor. However, progesterone cross-reacts with glucocorticoid and androgen receptors. Although progesterone binds with higher affinity to its own receptor, this cross-reactivity may have mechanistic importance, since some progestins can elicit androgenic responses.

Cellular receptor concentrations are strongly influenced by hormonal environment. Progesterone receptors are expressed in direct response to estrogen exposure of the target tissue. High concentrations of progesterone decrease estrogen receptor concentrations, which in turn lead to decreased progesterone receptor concentrations. Furthermore, each hormone can directly regulate its own receptor concentration (down or up) in some circumstances.

The ultimate response to estrogen in the uterus and breast is increased cellular proliferation, whereas the response to progesterone in these same estrogen-primed tissues is decreased cellular growth and increased cellular differentiation. The events that occur between a hormone binding to its receptor and the final expression of cellular responses remain unclear. One step by which steroid hormones promote metabolic changes in target tissues is by increasing the rate of target gene transcription. These metabolic changes eventually lead to increased DNA synthesis and cell division. The hormone-receptor complex may also elicit cellular responses by repression of gene transcription or stabilization of mRNA.

Binding of ligand to its receptor induces a conformational change in the protein, allowing the receptor to modify the expression of specific genes and probably involves interaction between the steroid-receptor complex and specific DNA sequences or other nuclear proteins involved in regulating transcription. This specific DNA sequence is termed a *hormone response element* and is often found upstream from the target gene (see Chapter 34 for further discussion).

Regulation of the tissue's ability to respond in a particular way to a specific hormone occurs at a minimum of three levels. First, the cell must express the appropriate receptor. Second, the gene must have a hormone response element to be a target for the hormone. Third, the target gene must have an appropriate array of chromatin proteins and transcription factors for transcription to be regulated in that tissue.

The receptor-steroid complex turnover is not completely understood. The half-life for the estrogen receptor is 2 to 4 hours, with or without bound ligand. Possibly the receptor is processed by proteolysis, though dissociation of estradiol from the receptor may also occur.

The molecular basis for hormone action, including estrogen and progesterone, is summarized in Chapter 34. Considerable progress has been made in understanding molecular mechanisms of steroid hormone action; active research continues on the role of hormones in receptor function, the variable response of target genes, the mechanism by which receptors modulate gene transcription and mRNA stabilization, and the role of the steroid hormones in fetal development.

Antihormone action is produced by competitive binding of ligands to hormone receptors, directly blocking binding of the hormone. Antiestrogens such as clomiphene or tamoxifen bind to the estrogen receptor with relatively high affinity, preventing estrogen access to the binding site. The antiestrogen-receptor complex may still bind to the hormone response element but does not initiate increased transcription of the target gene. Other genes may be directly activated by the antiestrogen-receptor complex. Interestingly, some antiestrogens have partial agonist (estrogen-like) properties in some tissues while displaying antagonist activities in other tissues.

PHARMACOKINETICS

Pharmacokinetic parameter values for these agents are summarized in Table 36-1.

Estrogens

Estrogens are rapidly absorbed from the gastrointestinal tract, skin, and mucous membranes and after parenteral injection. The unconjugated, natural estrogens are rapidly inactivated in the gastrointestinal tract and liver if taken orally; therefore other modes of delivery (transdermal, vaginal, nasal, or intramuscular) are warranted. Micronized estradiols, steroidal estrogens that contain an ethinyl group at C17, the conjugated estrogens, and nonsteroidal estrogens are orally active. Once absorbed, these drugs are rapidly metabolized in the

Table 36-1 Pharmacokinetic Parameters

Drug	Administration	Absorption	$t_{1/2}$	Plasma Protein Binding	Disposition
estradiol	Oral (esters), IM, topical, suppository	Rapid if micronized	30 min	50%-80% SHBG; 18%-48% albumin	M (main)*, R
ethinyl estradiol	Oral	Rapid	~6-20 hr	98% albumin	M (main)*, R
progesterone	IM	Poor	5 min	50% CBG; 48% albumin	M, R
levonorgestrel	Oral	Rapid	11-45 hr	80% SHBG	M
norethindrone	Oral	Rapid	5-14 hr	60%-70% SHBG; 30%-35% albumin	M
clomiphene citrate	Oral	Rapid	4-10 hr *(trans)*, >18 hr *(cis)*	—	M
tamoxifen citrate	Oral	Slow	7 days	Albumin	—
mifepristone (RU 486)	Oral	< 25%	10-24 hr	95% albumin	R (10%)
aminoglutethimide	Oral	Rapid	10-15 hr	20%-35%	R (35%-50%)
danazol	Oral	Rapid	~15 hr	—	M

CBG, Corticosteroid-binding globulin; *M,* metabolism; *R,* renal; *SHBG,* sex hormone-binding globulin.
*Enterohepatic cycling.

liver. Chlorotrianisene and quinestrol have prolonged durations of action because of storage in and slow release from adipose tissue.

Estrogens are distributed to most body tissues with selective uptake by target and adipose tissues. Estradiol is tightly bound to sex hormone–binding globulin and somewhat to albumin, whereas estrone and estriol bind mainly to albumin. The conjugated estrogens bind weakly to albumin only.

Estrogens are excreted primarily as polyhydroxylated forms conjugated at C3 with sulfate or glucuronic acid. Free estrogens are distributed to the bile, reabsorbed in the gastrointestinal tract, and recirculated to the liver (enterohepatic recirculation). About one fifth of the estrogen is excreted in the feces and the remainder in the urine. Estradiol is rapidly cleared from the blood. In the liver estrone is converted to estrone sulfate, which is then excreted or hydrolyzed back to estrone. The serum half-life for estrone sulfate is about 12 hours. The common synthetic steroidal estrogens, ethinyl estradiol and mestranol, are metabolized slower than estradiol because of the ethinyl group at C17. Brain tissue can metabolize 17β-estradiol to form catechol estrogens, structurally similar to catecholamines but of unclear function in the brain. The synthetic nonsteroidal estrogens may be excreted as glucuronide or sulfate conjugates.

Progestins

Oral progesterone is almost completely inactivated in the liver, and so synthetic modification is necessary to produce the orally active progestins listed in Figure 36-4. Progesterone can be given parenterally but has an elimination half-life of only a few minutes. It is converted in the liver to pregnanediol and conjugated with glucuronic acid at C3, and the conjugate is excreted mainly in urine. The 19-nortestosterone derivatives are all orally active. Medroxyprogesterone acetate can be used orally or IM, whereas megestrol acetate is only used orally. The C21 derivatives and the 19-nortestosterone compounds all have longer plasma half-lives than progesterone has. Most of these compounds are metabolized in the liver and conjugated to glucuronides, and the conjugates are excreted in the urine.

Combination Oral Contraceptives

The low doses of estrogens and progestins in current combination oral contraceptives decrease side effects. Further decreases in dosage formulation without altering contraceptive effectiveness are unlikely because of metabolic variability. First-pass losses in the liver limit the bioavailability and rate of metabolism of these steroids. The dosage of estrogens and progestins in oral contraceptives must be high enough to produce biologically active serum concentrations in virtually 100% of users, and so the minimal effective dose to ensure prevention of pregnancy is limited.

Antiestrogens

Clomiphene citrate is orally administered and readily absorbed from the gastrointestinal tract. It may enter the enterohepatic circulation with about 50% excreted in the feces within 5 days, but the serum half-life is shorter than this. Both enclomiphene and zuclomiphene reach peak plasma concentrations within 3 to 6 hours after an oral dose. However, enclomiphene has a shorter plasma elimination half-life (4 to 10 hours) than zuclomiphene (greater than 18 hours).

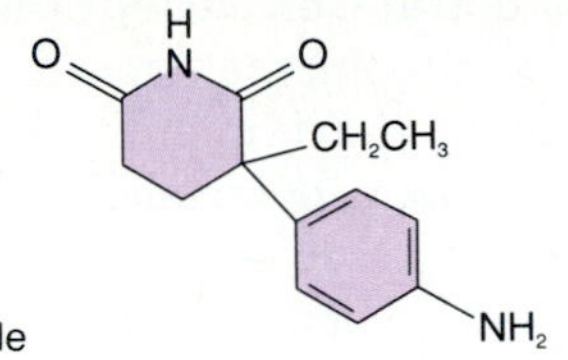

aminoglutethimide

CH_2CH_3 NH_2

danazol
(progesterone receptor RBA=5-20)
(androgen receptor RBA ≅ 40)

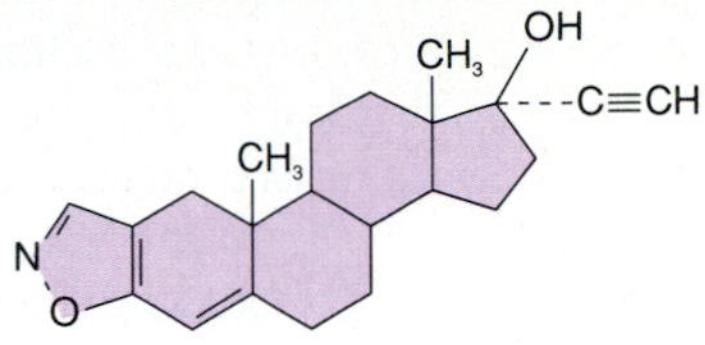

FIGURE 36-6 Structures of aminoglutethimide and danazol. Relative binding affinity *(RBA)* for danazol to the progesterone or androgen receptors, as compared to progesterone (RBA, 100%) or dihydrotestosterone (RBA, 100%), is shown.

Conjugated metabolites after oral tamoxifen are primarily excreted by the biliary route into the feces. Enterohepatic recirculation of the metabolites, binding to serum albumin, and high-affinity binding to tissues all contribute to the long half-life. The major metabolites of tamoxifen include *N*-desmethyltamoxifen, which binds only weakly to the estrogen receptor but is present in greater concentrations than tamoxifen itself, and 4-hydroxytamoxifen, which binds much more tightly to the estrogen receptor than tamoxifen but is present in low concentrations. The antiestrogen action of tamoxifen may be aided by its metabolites.

Steroidogenesis Inhibitors

Aminoglutethimide is rapidly absorbed after oral administration, with maximum circulating concentrations reached in 1.5 hours. From 20% to 35% of the drug is bound to plasma proteins, and 35% to 50% is excreted unchanged in the urine, whereas 4% to 15% is excreted as acetylaminoglutethimide. None of the observed metabolites block adrenal steroidogenesis.

Oral danazol is rapidly absorbed and metabolized but takes 7 to 14 days to reach a steady-state concentration. There are several metabolites excreted in both urine and feces (Figure 36-6).

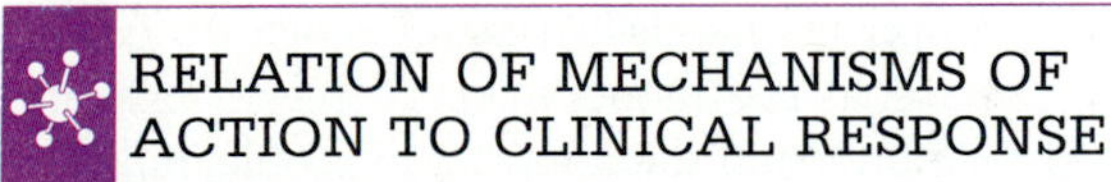

RELATION OF MECHANISMS OF ACTION TO CLINICAL RESPONSE

Fertility Control

Combination Oral Contraception The most common use for administered estrogens and progestins is oral contraception. Oral contraceptives are the most effective reversible method for preventing pregnancy in the United States. The failure rate is less than 0.7 per 100 women-years for users of combination oral contraceptives. The only method of birth control with a lower failure rate is sterilization.

Oral contraceptives available in the United States consist of progestin alone (the so-called minipill) or a combination of one of two synthetic estrogens with one of five synthetic progestins (the combination pill). The estrogen component is either ethinyl estradiol or mestranol, with mestranol being slightly less potent. The progestins include norethindrone, norethindrone acetate, and ethynodiol diacetate, as well as norgestrel and its active isomer, levonorgestrel.

The present low-dose estrogen contraceptives have decreased the incidence of adverse side effects and have still prevented pregnancy at rates equal to earlier higher-dose estrogen formulations. The most commonly used oral contraceptives consist of a combination preparation taken for 21 days followed by 7 days without any steroids to induce withdrawal bleeding, but other dosing regimens also may be used to reduce side effects.

Combination oral contraceptives prevent pregnancy by inhibiting ovulation, presumably as a result of gonadotropin suppression induced by the estrogen and progestin effects on the hypothalamic-pituitary axis. The increased early follicular phase FSH concentrations and midcycle peaks of FSH and LH are not observed in patients taking combination oral contraceptives. The lower concentration of FSH results in decreased ovarian function with minimal follicular development. In addition, lower concentrations of endogenous steroids are secreted during both phases of the menstrual cycle.

Oral contraceptives also act directly on the cervix and uterus. The cervical mucus of oral contraceptive users is usually thick and in lower quantity than that seen in a normal postovulatory phase. This may also aid in preventing pregnancy by inhibiting sperm penetration. Also the endometrium may be inhibited from developing into the appropriate state for implantation. Missing two or more doses during a cycle substantially increases the risk of pregnancy. Therefore a high compliance rate is needed to ensure adequate contraception, especially with low-concentration ethinyl estradiol preparations.

Oral contraceptives provide several well-documented health benefits beyond the control of fertility including a decreased incidence of ovarian and endometrial cancers. Although ovarian malignancy carries a relatively high mortality, long-term oral contraceptive users (more than 5 years) have a relative risk of 0.6 compared to 1.0 for nonusers. This protective effect continues for 10 to 15 years after discontinuance of oral contraceptives. Endometrial cancers have relatively low mortality but occur fairly commonly in women. A causal link between increased incidence of endometrial cancer and use of sequential oral contraceptives led to cessation of their use in 1976 (sequential oral contraceptives consisted of estrogen alone for 14 to 16 days, then 5 to 6 days of estrogen plus progestin, and then 7 days without steroid). Many studies on the association between combination oral contraceptive use and the development of endometrial cancer show a protective effect of the contraceptives. Users have a relative risk of 0.5 compared to 1.0 for nonusers. This effect appears after as little as 1 year of use and lasts 10 to 15 years after discontinuance of the contraceptive. It is postulated that the mechanism is related to the use of daily progestin to oppose the proliferative actions of the synthetic estrogens on the endometrium.

Other benefits of long-term oral contraceptive use include a 50% decrease in fibroadenomatous and fibrocystic breast disease, 10% to 70% reduction of acute pelvic inflammatory disease, and decreases in other less critical problems.

Progestin-only Contraception Progestin-only formulations were developed to avert the adverse side effects of estrogens in oral contraceptives. Major problems with this approach are a slightly higher failure rate of 2 to 3 per 100 woman-years and a much higher incidence of irregular menstrual bleeding, often leading to discontinuation of the medication.

Progestin-only medication suppresses FSH and LH concentrations and ovulation to variable degrees, however, these actions cannot be the only explanation for the observed 97% to 98% success rate. Continuous progestin alone leads to scant, thick cervical mucus, endometrial atrophy (which could prevent implantation), and often quite variable length and duration of bleeding. Several new modalities have been developed and are being used for long-term contraception (see New Directions, p. 499).

Medroxyprogesterone acetate is approved in 80 countries as a contraceptive but, because of an increased incidence of breast tumors in beagle dogs, is not approved in the United States for contraception, but only for use in the treatment of advanced endometrial and renal carcinomas and endometriosis. Its mode of action is similar to other progestin-only contraceptives. Three new progestin oral contraceptives used in Europe (desogestrel, norgestimate, and gestodene) are not available in the United States.

Postcoital Contraception Large doses of estrogens alone or in combination with progestins may prevent pregnancy after unprotected coitus but must be used within 72 hours of coital exposure to prevent pregnancy and are currently recommended only in cases of rape, incest, failure of a barrier method, or unprotected intercourse. The preparations probably act by preventing implantation because the endometrium is made nonreceptive to the blastocyst by high-dose hormone treatment.

Contragestation Mifepristone (RU 486) (see Figure 36-4) is a synthetic potent antiprogestin with 50 times less antiglucocorticoid than antiprogestin activity, which is widely used in Europe. It binds to the progesterone receptor, preventing binding by endogenous progesterone, thereby preventing the usual hormone response. It also binds weakly to the androgen receptor and tightly to the glucocorticoid receptor (affinity greater than dexamethasone).

Replacement Therapy

Menopause Menopause, the natural cessation of menses, results from ovarian failure after the depletion of functional ovarian follicles. This produces decreased estrogen and progesterone production and causes various physiological and psychological changes. Vasomotor symptoms, genitourinary atrophy, osteoporosis, and cardiovascular disease in postmenopausal women can be substantially decreased if estrogen replacement therapy is begun during menopause. Controversy remains, however, regarding patient selection, treatment regimens, addition of progestin, and possible adverse effects.

An additional benefit of estrogen replacement therapy is reduced risk of cardiovascular disease, especially coronary artery disease. Women have a lower incidence of coronary artery disease before menopause than men of the same age, but after menopause the incidence increases with age and eventually parallels that in males. Estrogen replacement therapy provides a 50% to 70% reduction in the risk of arteriosclerotic cardiovascular disease in postmenopausal women. This may be related to changes in the lipoprotein profile, since after menopause HDL concentrations fall and LDL concentrations rise in women. In males these changes have been correlated with increased risk of coronary artery disease. Estrogen replacement therapy increases HDL and lowers LDL concentrations and may thereby provide a protective effect. The presence of estrogen receptors in several large arteries and the direct effects of estrogen on endothelial or smooth muscle cells of coronary arteries may contribute to the protection.

The best time to initiate estrogen therapy to treat menopausal symptoms is as promptly as menopause begins. Estrogen is more effective in preventing osteoporosis, genitourinary atrophy, and cardiovascular disease than in reversing them once they have occurred. The beneficial changes in the lipoprotein profiles can be negated by the addition of progestins to the regimen. Several progestogens, especially the 19-nortestosterone derivatives, create a dose-dependent decrease in HDL and increase in LDL. The C21 progestins such as medroxyprogesterone acetate have less of an effect on lipoproteins. It is important to choose a progestin carefully and to use as low a dosage as possible to minimize the adverse effects on the lipoprotein profile. The use of progestins with estrogen replacement therapy remains controversial.

Other Uses Other clinical problems in which estrogen replacement therapy is useful include osteoporosis, primary hypogonadism, dysfunctional uterine bleeding, and luteal phase deficiency.

Osteoporosis represents reduced bone mass per volume. Bone loss occurs naturally in both males and females with age and accelerates in women in the perimenopausal period. This involves primarily trabecular (spongy) bone, but cortical bone is also lost.

Estrogen replacement therapy can decrease the rate of bone loss as well as the incidence of vertebral, wrist, and hip fractures in postmenopausal women.

Estrogen therapy initiated near the time of puberty may help stimulate normal sexual development and may be used to treat female primary hypogonadism. Concurrent treatment with androgens is discussed in Chapter 37.

Dysfunctional uterine bleeding occurs during irregulare menstrual cycles often characterized by prolonged bleeding. High-dose progestin therapy can be used to stop an episode of prolonged bleeding but should be followed by long-term cyclic therapy with an orally administered progestin to ensure occurrence of regular withdrawal bleeding.

Luteal phase deficiency results from insufficient progesterone. Ovulation is normal, but the corpus luteum functions subnormally with insufficient progesterone production to maintain pregnancy. The most popular method of treatment is natural progesterone supplementation.

Ovulation Induction

About 20% to 30% of infertility may be attributable to an anovulatory condition. Agents that induce ovulation in these patients include gonadotropins, gonadotropin-releasing hormone, and clomiphene citrate. Clomiphene citrate (see Figure 36-3), a partial estrogen agonist, is used to treat ovulatory failure in patients desiring pregnancy whose mates are fertile and potent. This agent may act as an antiestrogen at the hypothalamus and may relieve estrogen-induced negative feedback on gonadotropin-releasing hormone release.

After clomiphene administration, pulse frequency (but not amplitude) of LH release rises significantly possibly because of an increased pulse frequency of gonadotropin-releasing hormone release. Clomiphene functions best in women with normal concentrations of estrogen before therapy and is not useful in patients with primary ovarian or pituitary dysfunction. Bromocriptine is used specifically to treat the underlying anovulation of hyperprolactinemia.

Cancer Chemotherapy

Approximately one third of patients with advanced breast cancer show tumor regression or prolongation of disease-free survival with therapy that decreases estrogen production or action. Early trials with high-dose progestins, androgens, glucocorticoids, and estrogens resulted in 10% to 40% response because of unknown mechanisms but with adverse side effects. More recently the antiestrogen tamoxifen has produced an overall response of 30% to 40% with fewer adverse effects. Tamoxifen is discussed further in Chapter 44.

Reduction of estrogen production in postmenopausal women for prevention of breast cancer is discussed also in Chapter 43 and can be aided by adrenalectomy. To avoid such surgery, adrenal steroidogenesis inhibition may be used. Aminoglutethimide (shown in Figure 36-6) inhibits a cholesterol side-chain cleaving enzyme, which converts cholesterol to pregnenolone, and the aromatase enzyme, which converts adrenal androstenedione to estrone and testosterone to estradiol (see Figure 36-2). Patient supplementation with glucocorticoid replacement therapy is needed mainly to inhibit the compensatory rise in adrenocorticotropic hormone, which can override the action of aminoglutethimide. Hydrocortisone is used because aminoglutethimide stimulates the metabolism of dexamethasone. Aminoglutethimide plus hydrocortisone replacement can also reduce circulating concentrations of estrogens. Aromatase inhibitors are also under investigation.

Endometrial cancer formation is enhanced with long-term unopposed estrogen therapy but can be treated with progestins. Progestational therapy is used as adjunctive and palliative treatment with approximately one third of advanced cases of metastatic endometrial carcinoma showing a favorable response. Medroxyprogesterone acetate often is used and likely acts through the progesterone receptor to downregulate the estrogen receptor and to induce formation of 17β-hydroxysteroid dehydrogenase to increase estradiol metabolism. In addition, it may have direct cellular actions leading to decreased cell division. High progesterone receptor concentrations in the tumor correlate with increased survival.

High doses of estrogens such as diethylstilbestrol are used to treat advanced prostate cancer. Newer therapies decrease the high incidence of cardiovascular deaths, which are predominantly thromboembolic in nature, associated with these high doses of estrogen.

Ovarian cancer may or may not demonstrate hormonal dependence. Some studies indicate that estrogen use may increase the risk of developing ovarian cancer, though some conflicting results indicate the usefulness of determining estrogen and progesterone receptor concentrations in predicting therapeutic response.

Others

Endometriosis results from ectopic endometrial cell implants occurring outside the uterus. These endometrial cells continue to respond to steroid hormones but may show subtle differences to estrogen and progesterone receptor concentrations and function.

The goal of therapy in endometriosis is to induce a hormone-poor environment, especially with low estrogen concentrations, to inhibit the growth of implants and thereby alleviate symptoms. The three main pharmacological agents used in the United States to treat endometriosis are danazol, progestins, and gonadotropin-releasing hormone derivatives. Gestrianone, a slightly androgenic and strongly antiestrogenic synthetic hormone, is also under investigation for treating endometriosis but is not currently available in the United States.

Danazol, shown in Figure 36-6, effectively relieves the symptoms of endometriosis and may act by inhibiting either the LH/FSH surge or the action of several steroidogenic enzymes or both. Danazol can interact with both androgen and progesterone receptors (see Chapter 35) and produces amenorrhea and pain relief without decreasing the basal concentrations of gonadotropins or estrogen. Between 80% and 100% of patients report lessened pain within 3 to 12 months of therapy.

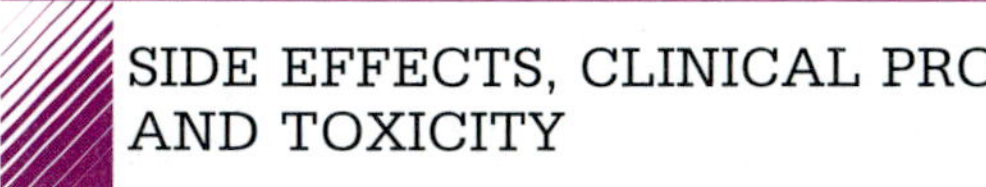

SIDE EFFECTS, CLINICAL PROBLEMS, AND TOXICITY

A brief summary of the potential problems for some of the important drugs is shown in the box.

CLINICAL PROBLEMS

ESTROGENS
- GI disturbances
- Menstrual disorders
- Breast discomfort
- Thromboembolic disorders
- Hypertension
- Endometrial cancer
- Decreased lactation
- Drug interactions
- Adverse effects on fetus (diethylstilbestrol)

PROGESTINS
- GI disturbances
- Menstrual disorders
- Adverse changes in lipoprotein levels
- Abnormal glucose tolerance
- Drug interactions
- Adverse effects on fetus

CLOMIPHENE CITRATE
- GI disturbances
- Vasomotor symptoms
- Ovarian enlargement
- Visual disorders
- Multiple gestations

TAMOXIFEN
- GI disturbances
- Menstrual disorders
- Vasomotor symptoms

MIFEPRISTONE (RU 486) (INVESTIGATIONAL)
- Menstrual disturbances (rare)

AMINOGLUTETHIMIDE (INVESTIGATIONAL)
- GI disturbances
- CNS disturbances

DANAZOL
- Androgenic effects in women
- Antiestrogen-like effects
- Adverse changes in lipoprotein concentrations
- Adverse effects on the fetus

Estrogens

Some less serious adverse effects of high-dose estrogen therapy include nausea, occasional vomiting, abdominal cramps, bloating, diarrhea, appetite changes, fluid retention, dizziness, headache, breast discomfort and enlargement, weight gain, mood changes, ocular changes, allergic rash, and changes in some serum protein concentrations.

More serious side effects occasionally encountered include increased incidences of thromboembolic disorders, high blood pressure, gallbladder disease, and endometrial cancer.

In humans an etiological role for diethylstilbestrol in the development of clear cell adenocarcinoma of the vagina and cervix has been postulated from epidemiological data of the 1950s. Female offspring that received fetal exposure to diethylstilbesterol subsequently developed increased cancers of these types. In children endogenous or exogenous estrogen exposure can lead to precocious puberty.

Progestins

The occasional and less serious side effects of high-dose progestin therapy, as it is used to treat advanced endometrial cancer or in progestin-only oral contraceptives, include breakthrough bleeding, spotting, changes in menstrual flow, amenorrhea, edema, weight changes, nausea, bloating, headache, allergic rash, mood changes, and changes in lipoprotein concentrations (HDL decreases and LDL increases). High-dose progestin results in abnormal glucose-tolerance tests in 4% to 16% of women. Diabetic women or those with a prior history of glucose intolerance should be monitored after oral contraceptive preparations are started. A progestin with as low a dose and potency as possible should be used.

The most common side effects of IM medroxyprogesterone acetate as a contraceptive are menstrual abnormalities, characterized by irregular bleeding early, followed by amenorrhea in 50% to 70% of patients after 2 years of treatment.

Combination Oral Contraceptives

Despite over 30 years of oral contraceptive use, a great deal of controversy remains concerning the risks. Several factors must be considered: (1) many early studies that associated oral contraceptive use with specific side effects were conducted with much higher doses than present formulations; recent studies with low-dose oral contraceptives show fewer adverse effects; (2) several early studies were criticized for study design in that subgroups were not identical; and (3) restricting certain high-risk patient subgroups from oral contraceptive use has decreased the association between cardiovascular side effects and oral contraceptive use.

An overview of epidemiologic studies reveals an association between oral contraceptive use and thromboembolic disease in the absence of other predisposing factors. The association between oral contraceptive use and stroke or myocardial infarction is less consistent. The death rate associated with childbirth exceeds that of oral contraceptive use for all age groups except oral contraceptive users who are more than 40 years of age and who smoke.

The risk of idiopathic venous thrombosis associated with oral contraceptive use ranges from twofold to sixfold over nonusers. These thromboembolic events are directly related to the dose of estrogen. Since the risk of thromboembolic disease rapidly returns to normal (up to about 1 month) after oral contraceptives are discontinued, their use should be stopped at least 2 to 4 weeks before elective surgery and not restarted until at least 2 weeks after surgery.

An infrequent but proved side effect of oral contraceptive use is increased blood pressure over time in 1% to 5% of users. Usually the increase is small, but occasionally a rapid rise in blood pressure is observed, often within the first few months of therapy. The elevated blood pressure almost always resolves when oral contraceptives are discontinued. This increased blood pressure appears to relate to estrogen more than progestin because women on progestin-only oral contraceptives usually do not experience the increase.

Cerebrovascular accidents are not definitively correlated with oral contraceptive use; some studies show an increased incidence of stroke, whereas others do not. A recent large prospective study found no increased risk of stroke in oral contraceptive users. The association between oral contraceptive use and subarachnoid hemorrhage also remains controversial.

Older studies indicated an increased risk of myocardial infarction, but most of the myocardial infarctions occurred in women with other risk factors, especially older age and smoking. Nearly all new epidemiological studies have shown no increased risk of myocardial infarction in former oral contraceptive users. Studies excluding women with other major risk factors for cardiovascular disease have shown no increased incidence of myocardial infarction or cerebrovascular accidents in oral contraceptive users over controls.

Multiple case-control studies and at least five large cohort studies published before 1987 have assessed the risk of breast cancer. The majority of studies have shown no change in the incidence of breast cancer with oral contraceptive use. A few studies showed increased risk of breast cancer with prolonged use (greater than 4 to 8 years) in women who began the medication before 25 years of age. Three epidemiological studies published in 1988 and 1989 showed significantly increased risk of breast cancer in long-term oral contraceptive users under 45 years of age. In two of the studies the increased risk was found only in certain groups of oral contraceptive users, and they were not the same subgroups in both studies. Because these results contradict the large amount of earlier data, the FDA in 1989 recommended further research but maintains that there is no overall increased risk of breast cancer associated with oral contraceptive use.

Studies have indicated increased risk of cervical dysplasia and carcinoma in situ of the cervix in long-term oral contraceptive users; however, controls for these studies were difficult to obtain. Women using oral contraceptives may be at high risk for cervical cancer if they have used these drugs for more than 5 years and should have screening cervical cytology at least once a year.

Combination oral contraceptive formulations diminish the amount of milk produced in women who breastfeed. This effect is caused by the estrogen, even in low-dose formulations. Alternative methods of birth control (e.g., progestin-only contraceptives) should be considered for women wishing to use oral contraceptives and breastfeed.

Oral contraceptives are contraindicated in women with a current or past history of thrombophlebitis or thromboembolic disorders, cerebrovascular or coronary artery disease, known or suspected pregnancy, undiagnosed abnormal genital bleeding, known or suspected carcinoma of the breast, uterus, cervix, vagina or other estrogen-dependent neoplasm, hepatic adenoma or carcinoma, or cholestatic jaundice of pregnancy or jaundice with prior oral contraceptive use. Oral contraceptives should be used with caution in patients with liver or renal disease, asthma, migraine headaches, diabetes, hypertension, and congestive heart failure, and in patients receiving medication that can interfere with its effectiveness. Women who smoke and use oral contraceptives should be advised to use alternative methods of birth control after the 35 years of age.

Oral contraceptives are less effective with increased incidence of breakthrough bleeding when used simultaneously with rifampin, resulting from induction of hepatic microsomal enzymes. Similar interactions may occur with enzyme inducers including griseofulvin, barbiturates, carbamazepine, and phenytoin.

Estrogen Replacement Therapy

Fewer adverse effects are seen with lower physiological-dose estrogen replacement than with oral contraceptive or high-dose estrogen use because the incidence of thromboembolic disorders remains at age-appropriate levels with postmenopausal estrogen replacement therapy. Although women using exogenous estrogen can show altered coagulation profiles (i.e., elevated concentrations of factors VII, VIII, IX, and X and decreased antithrombin III concentrations), this does not lead to a functionally hypercoagulable state. Also, the synthetic estrogens (ethinylestradiol) are more likely to alter these concentrations than estradiol or conjugated estrogens used more generally in estrogen replacement therapy. Similarly, estrogen replacement therapy seems to pose little if any increased risk of hypertension or cholelithiasis.

Estrogen-only replacement therapy can increase risk of endometrial cancer, but not all women receiving unopposed estrogen therapy develop endometrial cancer. An adverse effect of the use of estrogen-progestin combined therapy in postmenopausal women is continued cyclic endometrial withdrawal bleeding that some women find undesirable. The association between breast cancer and postmenopausal estrogen use is less clear. Summarizing the studies up to now, if estrogen replacement therapy increases the risk of developing breast cancer, it is a very small increased risk and progestins may or may not affect this risk.

Antiestrogens

With clomiphene citrate the frequency and severity of adverse effects are dose related and include hot flashes that resemble those in menopausal patients. Visual problems occasionally occur and have been correlated with increasing total dose. Other high-dose side effects include ovarian enlargement or cyst formation, abdominal discomfort, nausea and vomiting, abnormal uterine bleeding, breast tenderness, headache, dizziness, depression, allergic dermatitis, and urinary frequency. Multiple gestations, particularly twins, occur at an incidence of 6% to 12% as compared to about 1% in the general population. Clomiphene citrate is contraindicated in patients with ovarian cysts, during pregnancy, or in patients with a past history of liver disease.

Side effects from tamoxifen therapy are minimal, with the most common being hot flashes, nausea, and vomiting. The possibility of using tamoxifen as long-term adjuvant treatment in some patients with breast cancer has raised questions about osteoporosis, alteration in serum lipoproteins, and increased incidence of cardiovascular disease. Preliminary results show no significant loss of bone in breast cancer patients on tamoxifen therapy for over 2 years versus controls not on tamoxifen. Also, recent studies demonstrate a beneficial effect of tamoxifen on the serum lipoprotein profile, and in one study the treatment group had a lower incidence of fatal myocardial infarction compared to the control group.

Pregnancy should be avoided while one is taking tamoxifen. The teratogenic effects of this drug in humans are unknown, but numerous defects in animal models have been demonstrated.

Other

Mifepristone (RU 486) is well tolerated, with only occasional prolonged uterine bleeding. The most frequent, reversible side effects of aminoglutethimide include drowsiness, skin rash, nausea, anorexia, fever, dizziness, and ataxia, but these usually diminish with continued use.

The use of danazol is fraught with multiple antiestrogen-like and androgenic side effects, including weight gain, muscle cramps, decreased breast size, deepening of the voice, edema, amenorrhea, emotional lability, flushing, sweating, acne, mild hirsutism, oily skin and hair, altered libido, nausea, headache, dizziness, insomnia, rash, increased LDL concentrations, decreased HDL concentrations, and increased hepatic enzymes. Most of these are reversible with cessation of the drug. Also, urogenital abnormalities are possible in offspring if danazol is used during pregnancy or while breastfeeding.

TRADE NAMES

In addition to generic drugs and fixed-combination preparations (other than oral contraceptives), the following trade-named materials are available in the United States.

STEROIDAL ESTROGENS

Depo-Estradiol, depGynogen, Depogen, Dura-Estrin, Estro-Cyp, Estrofem, Estronol-LA; estradiol cypionate
Estinyl, Feminone; ethinylestradiol
Estrace, Estraderm (transdermal); estradiol
Estradurin, polyestradiol phosphate
Estroject, Estronol, Gynogen, Kestrin, Theelin, Ungen, Wehgen, estrone
Estrovis, quinestrol
Ogen, estropipate
Premarin, Estratal, Menest; conjugated estrogen
Valergen, Dioval, Delestrogen; estradiol valerate

NONSTEROIDAL ESTROGENS

DV, dienestrol
Stilphostrol, diethylstilbestrol phosphate
TACE, chlorotrianisene

ANTIESTROGENS

Clomid, Serophene; clomiphene citrate
Nolvadex, tamoxifen

PROGESTINS

Aygestin, Norlutate; norethindrone acetate
Enovid, norethynodrel
Gesterol, Progestaject-50; progesterone
Hyprogest, Pro-Depo, Duralutin, Hylutin, Prodrox; hydroxyprogesterone caproate
Megace, megestrol acetate
Norlutin, norethindrone
Provera, Cycrin, Curretab, Amen; medroxyprogesterone acetate

ANTIPROGESTINS

Mifepristone, RU 486

OTHER

Cytadren, aminoglutethimide
Danocrine, danazol

ORAL CONTRACEPTIVES	*progestin*	*estrogen*
Ovrette, Micronor, Nor-QD		
Progestin only	norgestrel norethindrone	
COMBINATION		
Brevicon, Nelova, Genora, Modicon, Ovcon	norethindrone	ethinyl estradiol
Demulen	ethynodiol diacetate	ethinyl estradiol
Levien	levonorgestrel	ethinyl estradiol
Loestrin, Norlestrin	norethindrone acetate	ethinyl estradiol
Lo/Ovral	norgestral	ethinyl estradiol
Norinyl, Ortho-Novum, Norethin, Nelova	norethindrone	mestranol

NEW DIRECTIONS

To avoid the inconvenience of taking a daily pill and to try to obtain lower continuous doses of steroid as a means to minimize side effects, alternative methods of administration are under investigation. Norplant-2 consists of six Silastic (silicone elastomer) capsules containing levonorgestrel. These capsules are placed subdermally, usually in the arm. The major benefits of this form of contraception are that it is effective for up to 5 years and much lower doses of steroid are released. The problems include irregular uterine bleeding and the necessity of surgical insertion and removal. Norplant has been extensively used in several less developed countries and was recently approved by the Food and Drug Administration for use in the United States.

RU 486 (mifepristone) is currently used in Europe as a potential once-a-month oral contragestational agent. Studies indicate an 82% to 89% success rate of interrupting early pregnancy if given before the fifth week of amenorrhea. After 5 weeks the placenta probably produces enough local progesterone to overcome the antihormone. The mechanism of pregnancy termination by RU 486 is mediated directly at the level of the endometrium. RU 486 blocks progesterone action, leading to endometrial shedding (progesterone withdrawal bleeding) and prostaglandin release within 2 to 4 days. The conceptus is detached from the uterine wall and human chorionic gonadotropin concentrations drop, resulting in luteolysis. RU 486 is effective only after implantation, which can be delayed in some women. The most effective dosage is a single dose of 600 mg given on the day of expected menses. The 15% failure rate needs to be improved if RU 486 is to be competitive with other methods of contraception. The addition of low doses of prostaglandin E_2 to RU 486 is under investigation; data indicate a 96% success rate with this combination. Its use as a contragestational agent has not been approved in the United States.

REFERENCES

Boulieu EE: Contragestation and other clinical applications of RU486, an antiprogesterone at the receptor, *Science* 245:1351-1357, 1989.

Brown KH, Hammond CB: The risks and benefits of oral contraceptives, *Adv Intern Med* 34:385-305, 1989.

Carson-Jurica MA, Schrader WT, O'Malley BW: Steroid receptor family: structure and function, *Endocrine Rev* 11:201-220, 1990.

Institute of Medicine: Oral contraceptives and breast cancer, Washington, DC, 1991, National Academy Press.

Jordan VC, editor: Estrogen/antiestrogen action and breast cancer therapy, Madison, Wisc, 1986, University of Wisconsin Press.

Lindsay R: Prevention of postmenopausal osteoporosis, *Ob Gyn Clin North Am* 14:63-88, 1987.

Metzger DA, Luciano AA: Hormonal therapy of endometriosis, *Ob Gyn Clin North Am* 16:105-122, 1989.

Mishell DR: Contraception, *N Engl J Med* 320:777-787, 1989.

Robinson SP, Jordan VC: Metabolism of steroid modifying anticancer agents, *Pharmacol Ther* 36:41-103, 1988.

Romieu I, Berlin JA, Colditz G: Oral contraceptives and breast cancer: review and meta-analysis, *Cancer* 66:2253-2263, 1990.

Sarrell PM: Estrogen replacement therapy, *Ob Gyn* 72 (suppl):25-55, 1988.

Szarewski A, Guillebaud J: Contraception, *Br Med J* 3023: 1224-1226, 1991.

Wharton C, Blackburn R: Lower-dose pills, *Population Reports* 16:1-31, 1988.

SELF-ASSESSMENT QUESTIONS

1. What enzyme is directly responsible for the conversion of testosterone to 17β-estradiol and is therefore a target for the steroidogenesis inhibitor aminoglutethimide?
   a. cytochrome P-450 side-chain cleavage enzyme
   b. placental sulfatase
   c. aromatase
   d. Megestrol acetate
   e. none of the above
2. Which compound is not an estrogen?
   a. 17β-estradiol
   b. estriol
   c. levonorgestrel
   d. diethylstilbestrol (DES)
   e. estrone
3. Progestins commonly can result in all of the following *except:*
   a. increased DNA synthesis and cellular proliferation in target cells.
   b. maintenance of pregnancy.
   c. altered carbohydrate metabolism.
   d. increased LDL and decreased HDL levels.
   e. increased basal body temperature in the luteal phase.
4. The side effects of progestins include all of the following *except:*
   a. GI disturbances.
   b. abnormal glucose tolerance.
   c. thromboembolic disorders.
   d. adverse effects in lipoprotein profiles.
   e. menstrual disorders.
5. The ethinyl side chain (HC≡C−) at the carbon 17 position is added to several synthetic estrogens and progestins to:
   a. increase metabolism of the compound and decrease its half-life.
   b. alter the receptor binding specificity of the compound.
   c. alter the affinity of the ligand for the receptor.
   d. decrease the metabolism of the compound and prolong its half-life.
   e. alter the molecular weight of the compound.

CHAPTER 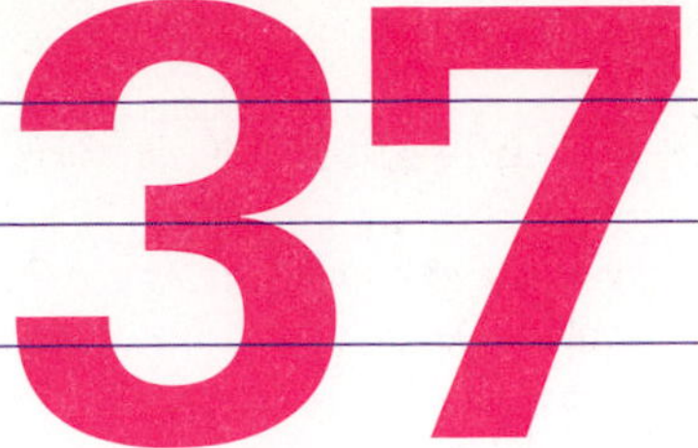

Androgens and Antiandrogens

STEPHEN J. WINTERS

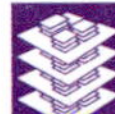 THERAPEUTIC OVERVIEW

Androgens are produced by the testis, ovary, and adrenal glands. Testosterone, the most important androgen in males, is produced by the Leydig cells of the testis (see Chapters 35 and 36). It stimulates virilization and is an important spermatogenic hormone. Within the ovary, testosterone and androstenedione are precursor steroids for estradiol production. In both sexes, androgens stimulate body hair growth, positive nitrogen balance, bone growth, muscle development, and erythropoiesis. The mechanism of action of testosterone at its target organs is similar to that of other steroid hormones. The major use of androgens in clinical medicine is for replacement therapy in men whose production of testosterone is impaired, which is a relatively common condition. Testosterone synthesis inhibitors and antiandrogens are used to limit the effects of androgens in patients with androgen-dependent disorders, such as prostatic cancer, hirsutism, and precocious puberty.

Principal therapeutic considerations with androgens and related pharmacological preparations are summarized in the box.

ABBREVIATIONS

FSH	follicle-stimulating hormone
GnRH	gonadotropin-releasing hormone
hCG	human chorionic gonadotropin
LH	luteinizing hormone
SHBG	sex hormone–binding globulin

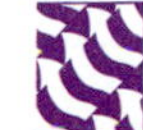 MECHANISMS OF ACTION

Testosterone Synthesis

Testosterone, a 19-carbon steroid hormone is synthesized from cholesterol in the Leydig cells of the testis, the adrenal cortex, and the theca cells of the ovary following the pathways shown in Figure 37-1. In the adult gonads, the principal regulator of testosterone synthesis and secretion is luteinizing hormone (LH), which is produced by the anterior pituitary gland (see Chapter 39). In fetal testis, human chorionic gonadotropin (hCG) promotes androgen formation. The precursor cholesterol is itself synthesized in the Leydig cells from acetate and stored as cholesterol esters in lipid droplets. A cholesterol ester hydrolase mobilizes free cholesterol from the lipid droplets, which in turn is transferred to the inner mitochondrial membrane. Stimulation of this transfer may represent a major action of LH. Mitochondrial oxidation occurs at positions C20 and C22, followed by lyase cleavage of the C—C bond between positions 20 and 22, resulting in the production of pregnenolone (Figure 37-1). These steps are catalyzed by the cytochrome P-450 enzyme system.

Pregnenolone, a 21-carbon steroid with a double bond in the 5-6 position, is converted to a 21-carbon androgen in two steps; 17α-hydroxylation and lyase action at position 17-20, now known to be catalyzed by the same cytochrome P-450 enzyme located in Leydig cell microsomes. Two possible pathways exist for the synthesis of testosterone from pregnenolone, as shown in Figure 37-1. One path is through 17α-hydroxypregnenolone to dehydroepiandrosterone (the Δ^5-pathway), and the second is through progesterone to 17α-hydroxyprogesterone and androstenedione (the Δ^4 pathway). Δ Refers to the position of the double bond in the A or B steroid ring. The A and B rings of pregnenolone or dehydroepiandrosterone are converted to a

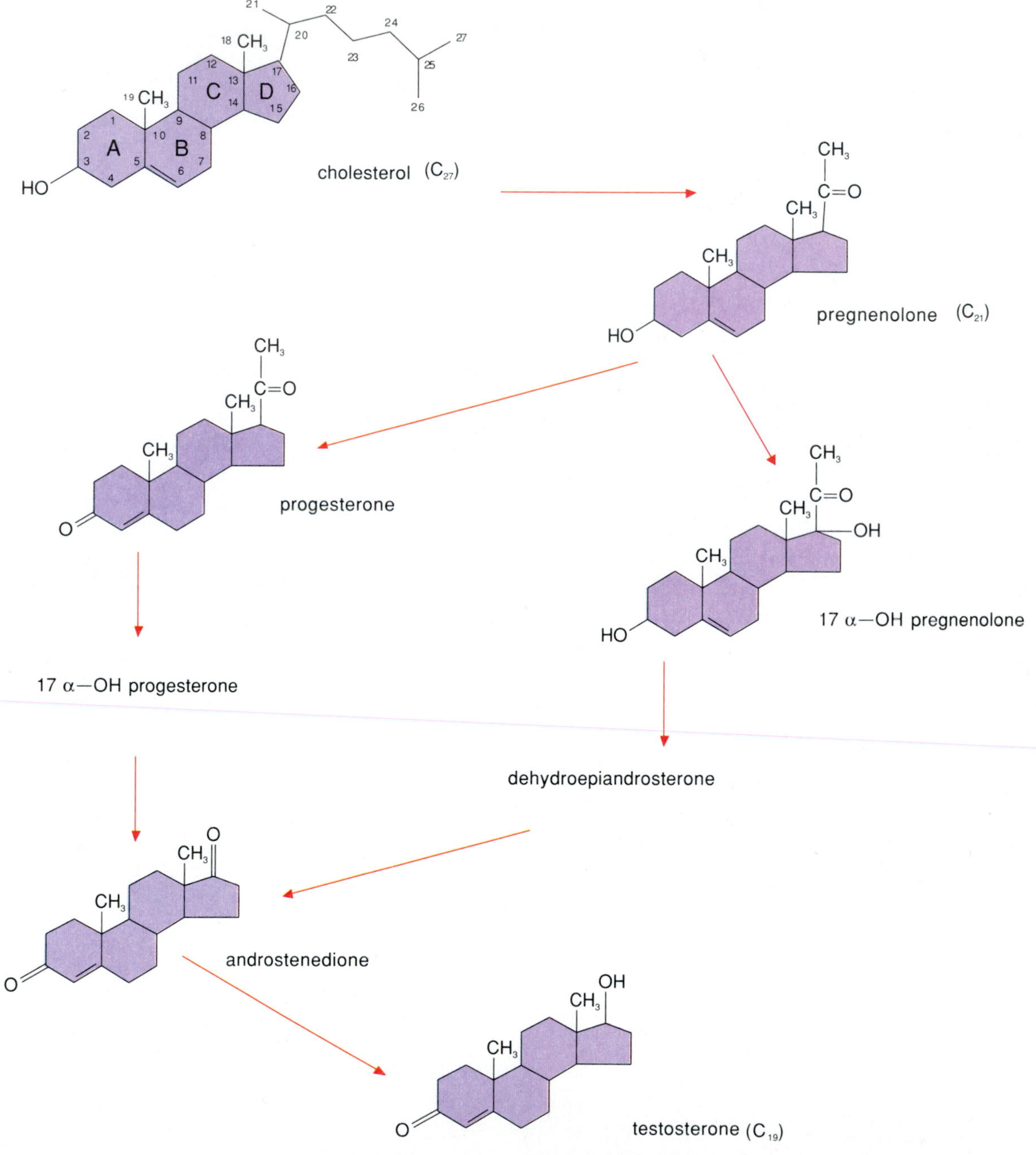

FIGURE 37-1 Pathways of testosterone synthesis in the Leydig cell. Also shown, structures of compounds and numbering system for steroid rings *(A, B, C, D)*.

THERAPEUTIC OVERVIEW

ANDROGENS

Primary testicular insufficiency
Hypogonadotropic hypogonadism
Constitutional delay of growth and adolescence
Osteoporosis, anemia
Testosterone and derivatives used for replacement therapy

ANTIANDROGENS AND ANTAGONISTS

Virilization in women
Precocious puberty in boys
Male contraceptive
Drugs used to decrease androgen synthesis or block androgen action

$\Delta^{4,5}$-keto structure by Δ^5,Δ^4-isomerase coupled to a 3β-hydroxysteroid dehydrogenase, also located within the microsomes. Finally, the microsomal enzyme 17β-hydroxysteroid dehydrogenase catalyzes the conversion of androstenedione to testosterone. Leydig cells also convert a small fraction of the testosterone produced to estradiol.

In contrast to peptide hormones, there is little intracellular storage of steroid hormones before secretion. The content of testosterone in the human testis is approximately 300 ng/g of wet tissue. Since an adult human testis weighs about 15 g, the total testicular content of testosterone in an adult approximates 9 μg. This quantity is about 0.1% of the usual daily production of testosterone in normal adult men (i.e., an average of 5 to 7 mg produced per 24 hours).

Fetal testosterone synthesis begins during the first trimester of pregnancy when the fetal testis is stimulated by hCG of placental origin to produce the testosterone required for male sexual differentiation. Gonadotrophs are not present in the fetal pituitary until the end of the first trimester, with LH and follicle-stimulating hormone (FSH) secretion beginning in the second trimester. The principal stimulus to the fetal gonadotroph, as in the adult, is gonadotropin-releasing hormone (GnRH). Gonadotropin secretion and sex steroid production decline late in fetal life followed by a prominent postnatal surge that lasts 2 to 3 months. By 3 or 4 months of age, little testosterone is secreted. There is presently no explanation for this transient postnatal surge and subsequent attenuation in these secretions.

At puberty, gonadotropin secretion rises and reawakens the Leydig cell to produce testosterone. Gonadotropin secretion exhibits a striking diurnal rhythm in early puberty, with elevated concentrations of luteinizing hormone and testosterone at night. In adult men it is more difficult to demonstrate a diurnal rhythm for LH, though testosterone concentrations are approximately 25% higher in the early morning hours compared to late afternoon. There are also fluctuations in LH secretion in adults that occur every 1 to 2 hours as a result of intermittent stimulation of gonadotrophs by GnRH from the anterior hypothalamus. Gonadotropin-releasing hormone secretory episodes in turn are coupled to the excitatory discharges of an incompletely identified neural oscillator system. Intermittent gonadotropin-releasing hormone secretion is required for the pituitary to function normally, but whether pulsatile gonadotropin secretion is needed for normal testicular function remains to be clarified. However, testosterone is released into the circulation in a pulsatile fashion in response to the pulsatile stimulation of Leydig cells by LH. FSH release is less clearly pulsatile in the circulation. Glycoprotein hormone α subunit secretion is also pulsatile and coupled to gonadotropin-releasing hormone stimulation, whereas free β-gonadotropin subunits do not appear to be released in measurable quantities into the circulation from the normal pituitary.

Androgen Production by the Adrenal Glands and Ovaries

The adrenal glands also secrete dehydroepiandrosterone, androstenedione, and testosterone, as well as some dehydroepiandrosterone sulfate and estrone. Glucocorticoids and mineralocorticoids are the principal products of the adult adrenal gland. The concentrations of dehydroepiandrosterone, dehydroepiandrosterone sulfate, and androstenedione in the circulation rise between 7 and 10 years of age. This process has been termed *adrenarche,* to distinguish it from puberty, or gonadarche, which refers to the onset of adult gonadal function. Since adrenocorticotropin stimulates the adrenal to secrete cortisol as well as sex steroids, some additional mechanisms must be responsible for adrenarche, since there is no concomitant increase in cortisol secretion in children at this age. Adrenal androgen secretion also declines in the elderly and during severe illness.

Control of Testosterone Synthesis and Secretion

The major regulator of testosterone synthesis and secretion is luteinizing hormone. Leydig cells have cell surface receptors for luteinizing hormone, which are coupled to adenylate cylase and to specific guanosine triphosphate–binding proteins. The steroidogenic response also requires intracellular calcium ions and the calcium-binding protein calmodulin. Like other protein hormones, luteinizing hormone action may also involve activation of phospholipase C, which produces diacylglycerol and inositol trisphosphate from membrane phosphoinositides (see Chapter 2). Diacylglycerol can activate protein kinase C, which phosphorylates membrane and intracellular proteins. Other hormones that may influence testosterone synthesis include prolactin, cortisol, insulin, insulin-like growth factors, estradiol, and inhibin. There is a growing awareness that multiple incompletely characterized factors produced within the seminiferous tubules by germ cells and Sertoli cells or peritubular myoid cells can also regulate testosterone synthesis. Together these factors maintain the concentration of testosterone in adult men at 300 to 1000 ng/dl (10 to 30 nM).

Sertoli cells are somatic cells within the seminiferous tubules. Tight junctions between these cells at the base of seminiferous tubules form a blood-testis barrier, which prevents circulating proteins from entering the tubular compartment. Sertoli cells secrete a large number of proteins. Some enter the tubular lumen and are important in spermatogenesis. Other proteins are secreted through the basal end of the cell and enter the circulation. Among these Sertoli cell proteins are androgen-binding protein, transferrin, and inhibin. Follicle-stimulating hormone is the major regulator of Sertoli cell function. The follicle-stimulating hormone receptor is membrane bound and acts through the second messengers cyclic adenosine monophosphate and calcium. Insulin and insulin-like growth factors, testosterone, vitamin A, and β-endorphins also influence Sertoli cell function.

The hormones of the hypothalamus, pituitary, and testes form an internally regulated unit (Figure 37-2), which is discussed further in Chapter 41. Not only are the testes stimulated by pituitary gonadotropins, but also the testes regulate luteinizing and follicle-stimulating hormone secretion through negative-feedback mechanisms (Chapter 41). Testosterone suppresses gonadotropin secretion by slowing the pulsatile release of gonadotropin-releasing hormone. A secondary action of testosterone limits pituitary responsiveness to gonadotropin-releasing hormone. Although estradiol inhibits gonadotropin release at both the hypothalamic and the pituitary levels, its exact mechanism of action depends on gonadal status, dose, and duration of steroid exposure. Inhibin, a heterodimeric glycoprotein produced by the Sertoli cells of the testis, reduces FSH synthesis and secretion and limits both LH and FSH release by antagonizing the action of gonadotropin-releasing hormone.

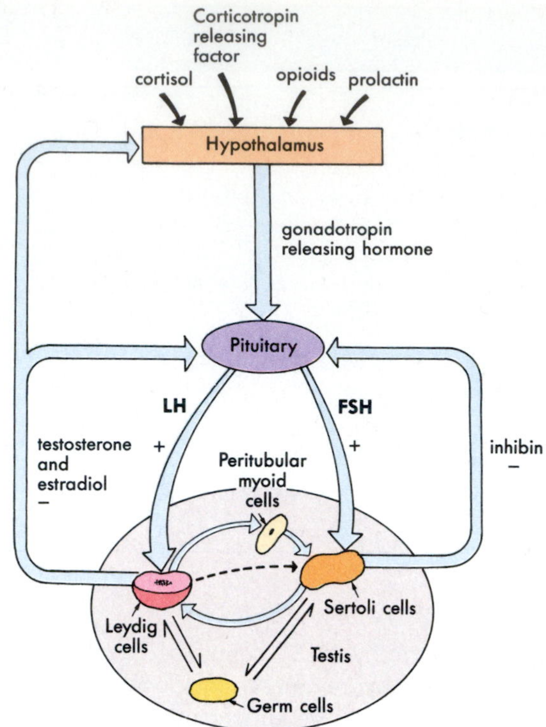

FIGURE 37-2 Hormonal control of testicular function. See the text for further information.

Normal women produce approximately 0.25 mg of testosterone per day, compared to the 5 to 7 mg/day for adult men. The majority of testosterone circulating in women is derived from the peripheral conversion of androstenedione secreted by the ovary as well as the adrenal. Benign and malignant tumors of the adrenal and ovary, congenital steroidogenesis enzyme defects, and disturbances of gonadotropin secretion can be associated with increased androgen production in women.

Androgen Action

Circulating endogenous testosterone or exogenous testosterone derivatives (Figure 37-3) are transported to the target tissues, where testosterone or the exogenous androgen derivatives enter the cells.

Circulating testosterone is bound tightly to a serum glycoprotein of hepatic origin, called sex hormone-binding globulin (SHBG), and weakly to albumin. Less than 1% to 2% of the circulating testosterone is believed to be unbound. However, binding to albumin is of such low affinity that it is functionally equivalent to unbound testosterone. Together the free and weakly bound testosterone, which account for approximately 50% of the testosterone found in adult male serum, can enter target tissues. SHBG is a heterodimer of molecular weight 88,000 daltons, identical in sequence to the androgen-binding protein produced by Sertoli cells; however, the

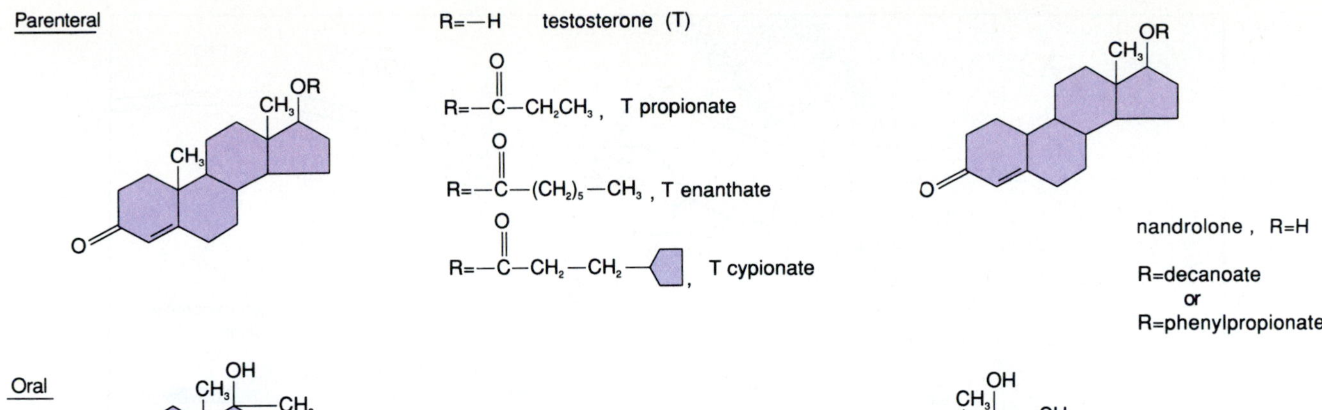

FIGURE 37-3 Structure of major testosterone derivatives in clinical use. See the text for further information.

two androphilic binding proteins differ in carbohydrate content. There is some evidence to indicate that SHBG binds to or enters androgen target cells, and so the transport proteins may also play a role in the action of testosterone. Estrogens and thyroxine increase, and androgens, growth hormone, and insulin decrease SHBG production. So the concentrations of SHBG are twofold to threefold greater in women than in men, and are increased in hyperthyroidism. Perhaps because of hyperinsulinemia, obesity in humans is associated with low concentrations of SHBG.

Once the androgens enter the target tissue cell, they may be enzymatically converted to another compound that shows greater or less androgen activity, or they may interact directly with androgen receptors (Figure 37-4). When testosterone enters certain target tissues such as the prostate gland, it is preferentially metabolized to 5α-dihydrotestosterone, but in other target tissues such as muscle and kidney, testosterone remains unchanged. There is no clear explanation for the presence of testosterone 5α-reductase in only certain androgen target tissues. However, the clinical syndrome of ambiguous genitalia in patients who lack normal testosterone 5α-reductase activity underscores the importance of the latter enzyme in the normal development of the external genitalia in human males. Dihydrotestosterone binds with slightly higher affinity to the androgen receptor than does testosterone. This difference reflects the slower kinetics of dissociation of dihydrotestosterone from the receptor. In this way 5α-reduction appears to amplify the actions of testosterone in target cells. There is now evidence for the presence of at least two isozymes for 5α-steroid reductase in man.

Intracellular receptor binding of androgens and the postreceptor events are similar to those of other steroid hormones. Androgen receptors have been purified and shown to be proteins with molecular weights of approximately 120 kilodaltons with synthesis guided in humans by genes on the X chromosome. The steroid-binding monomer (4.4S) is present in cells bound to receptor-associated protein and to small molecules producing a 9S inactive oligomer. Testosterone or dihydrotestosterone binds to a hormone-binding site near the carboxy terminus of the receptor, thereby activating the receptor complex so it can bind to a nuclear DNA acceptor site, known as the *hormone-response element* (HRE). Receptor activation involves the disaggregation of the

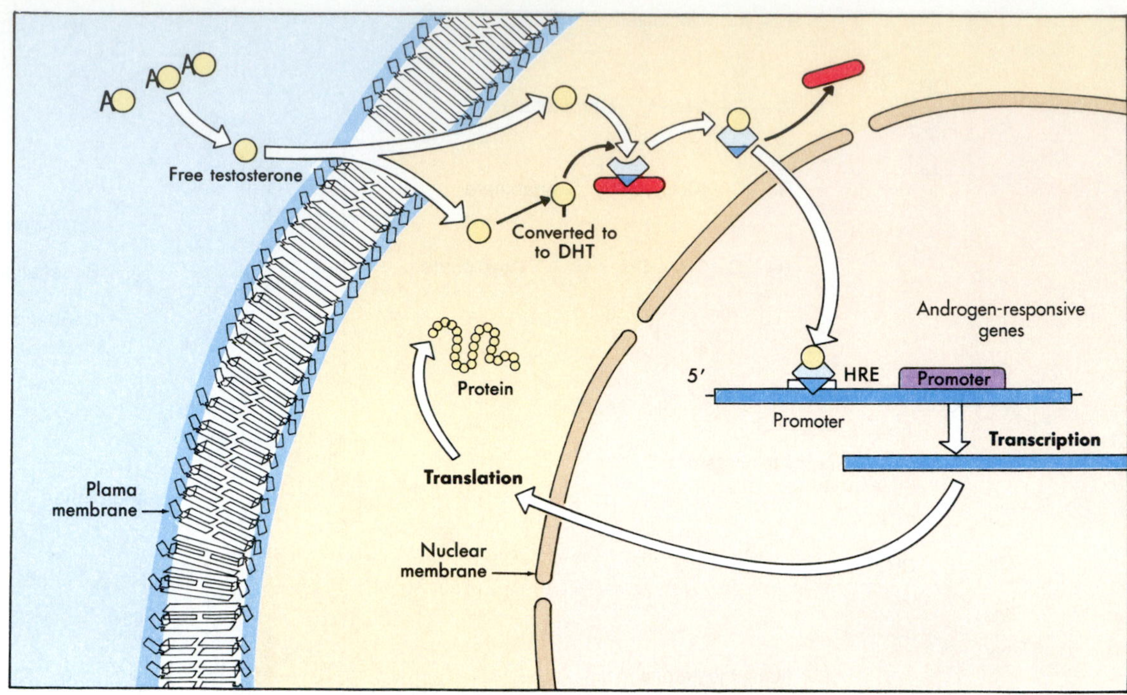

FIGURE 37-4 Schema of androgen action at target cells. See the text for further information.

Key:
- Androgen
- DHT (dihydrotestosterone)
- Androgen bound to plasma/tissue protein
- Receptor / DNA binding site
- Steroid binding monomer
- HRE Hormone response element

macromolecular complex with the release of an accessory protein exposing the DNA binding site on the 4.4S receptor. This region of the protein is rich in cysteines and is highly homologous with suggested DNA-binding domains of other steroid hormone receptors (see Chapter 34). Binding of the receptor to DNA is followed by the transcription of mRNAs for tissue-specific proteins, which constitutes the hormonal response.

Androgen regulation of target tissues may not only be positive, as in the stimulation of androgen-dependent proteins within the prostate, but also negative, as in the inhibition of gonadotropin-releasing hormone release by the hypothalamus. The molecular mechanisms for the inhibitory action of androgens are unknown.

Antiandrogens and Antagonists

The mechanism of action of antiandrogens is to block the synthesis of endogenous testosterone, whereas antagonists bind to the androgen receptor or otherwise block androgen action. Several drugs, including spironolactone and ketoconazole decrease testosterone production by reducing the activity of cytochrome P-450 in testicular microsomes responsible for conversion of progesterone to androstenedione through 17α-hydroxylation and C17-20 lyase cleavage. These drugs are substrate analogs, which compete with the natural substrates for binding to the active site of the enzyme. They are also used in the treatment of several diseases. Their structures are shown in Figure 37-5.

Finasteride, a 5α-reductase inhibitor, blocks the conversion of testosterone to 5α-dihydrotestosterone in tissues containing this enzyme, including the prostate. This drug decreases prostate size and is used to treat benign prostatic hyperplasia (see New Directions, p. 512).

Spironolactone, a synthetic steroid, also acts as an androgen antagonist by binding to the androgen receptor, as do the nonsteroidal compounds flutamide and cimetidine. The latter compound is a relatively weak antiandrogen with limited clinical usefulness, whereas flutamide is used clinically, together with GnRH agonists such as leuprolide acetate, to treat metastatic prostate cancer, and together with estrogens to treat hirsutism in women.

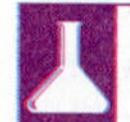

PHARMACOKINETICS

Pharmacokinetic parameter values for clinically used androgens and spironolactone are listed in Table 37-1.

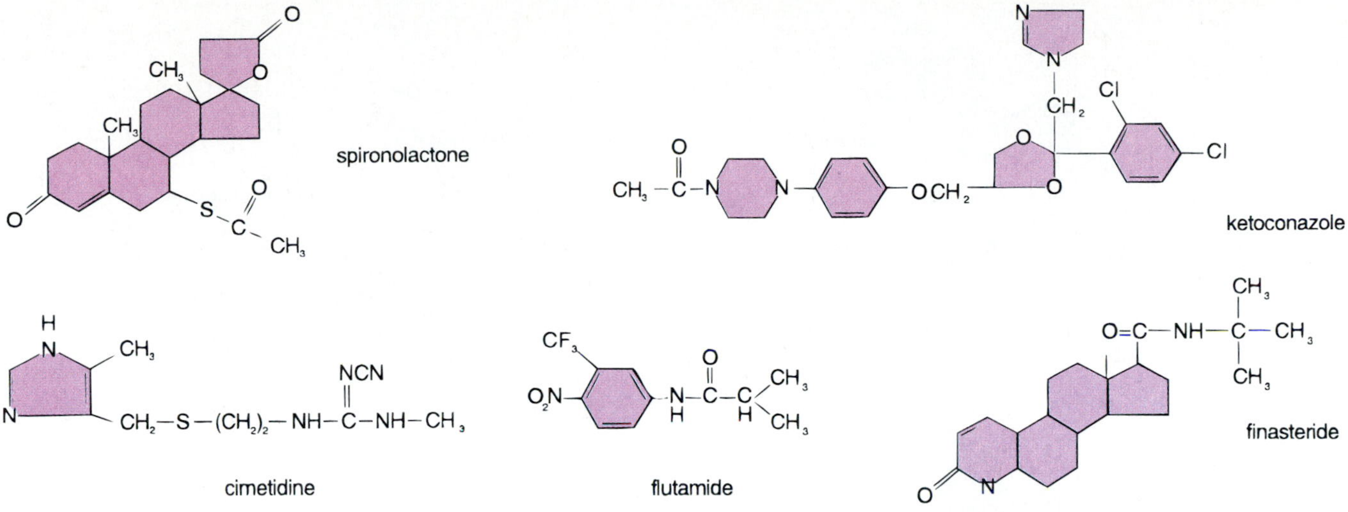

FIGURE 37-5 Structures of antiandrogens and antagonists. See the text for further information.

Table 37-1 Pharmacokinetic Parameters

Drug	Administration	Duration and use	Disposition
methyltestosterone	Oral, buccal	Short acting, daily	M
testosterone propionate	IM	Short acting, q 2-3 days	M
testosterone cypionate	IM	Long acting (depot)	M
testosterone enanthate	IM	Long acting (depot), q 2-3 weeks	M
fluoxymesterone	Oral	Short acting, daily or twice daily	M
danazol	Oral	Short acting, daily	M
nandrolone	IM	Long acting (depot)	M

M, Metabolized.

See Chapter 53 for values for ketoconazole, Chapter 59 for cimetidine, and Chapter 59 for spironolactone pharmacokinetics.

Testosterone Metabolism

The metabolism of testosterone is summarized in Figure 37-6. Metabolism in liver is primarily to the 17-ketosteroids 5α-androsterone and 5β-etiocholanolone. However, these compounds form only a small fraction of the 17-ketosteroids found in urine. The majority of the 17-ketosteroids in urine are the metabolites of androstenedione and dehydroepiandrosterone produced by the adrenal gland. Testosterone is also conjugated to sulfuric and glucuronic acids and excreted in the urine and bile.

The conversion of testosterone to estradiol by the enzyme complex aromatase occurs in the testis, adipose stroma, skin, and brain. A portion of the feedback regulation of gonadotropin secretion at the level of the gonadotropin-releasing hormone pulse generator may involve the pituitary and conversion of testosterone to estradiol. Other physiological actions of estradiol in males remain incompletely defined.

Androgen Preparations

Androgens are available for clinical use in oral and parenteral forms (see Figure 37-3 and Table 37-1). Natural testosterone taken orally or injected IM is rapidly cleared by the liver, rendering these routes ineffective for clinical use. Testosterone esterified at the 17-hydroxyl position is used for IM injection in an oil suspension. Esterification increases the lipid solubility of testosterone and prolongs its action. Testosterone propionate has a relatively short duration of action, 1 to 2 days. The more commonly used enanthate or cypionate esters can be given by deep IM injection every 2 to 3 weeks. The esters are converted to free testosterone in the circulation. Subcutaneous pellets containing testos-

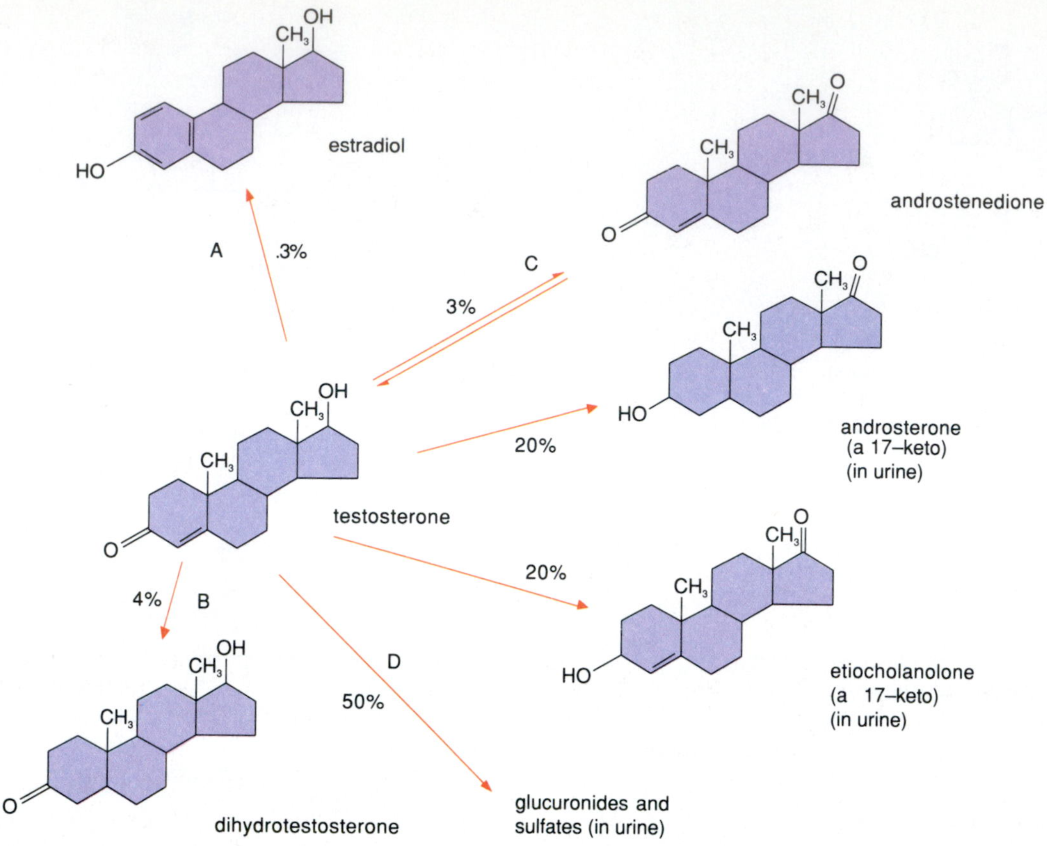

FIGURE 37-6 Metabolism of testosterone. Enzymes are, *A*, aromatase; *B*, 5α-reductase; *C*, 17β-hydroxysteroid dehydrogenase; *D*, hydroxylases and transferases.

terone have been used in Europe and Asia but have achieved little popularity in the United States.

Transdermal delivery of testosterone has been accomplished in an effort to produce stable physiological drug concentrations. A thin, flexible, self-adhering polymer is applied to the scrotal skin, since absorption through this surface is considerably greater than through thicker epidermis elsewhere. Another method for testosterone delivery (being tested) is drug encapsulation in biodegradable microspheres injected IM.

Several testosterone derivatives are available for sublingual or oral use. Alkylation produces androgens that are slowly metabolized by the liver but without testosterone as a metabolite. These derivatives interact directly with the androgen receptor. However, their androgenic potency is difficult to determine, since the end point upon which to base normal androgen action is uncertain. The pharmacokinetics of these compounds are not well established.

Danazol is only weakly androgenic and interacts with progesterone as well as androgen receptors. It inhibits pulsatile release of gonadotropins with a subsequent decline of serum concentrations of estradiol and estrone in women. A half-life of 4.5 hours has been reported.

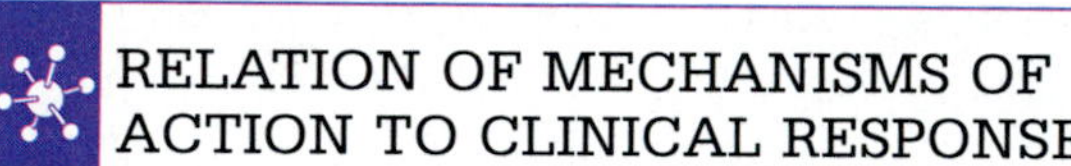

RELATION OF MECHANISMS OF ACTION TO CLINICAL RESPONSE

Replacement Theory

Testosterone is required for the normal development of the internal ducts of the male reproductive tract. Its 5α-reduced product, dihydrotestosterone, is responsible for the development of male external genitalia during the first trimester of fetal life. Therefore, when fetal synthesis of androgen is insufficient (e.g., an inborn enzymatic error), or there is an ineffectiveness of androgen action at its target tissues (e.g., a receptor defect), the genital phenotype may be female or ambiguous.

At puberty in males, an increase in circulating androgens stimulates the expression of adult secondary sex characteristics. The scrotum darkens and become rugated; beard and body hair growth are stimulated; sebaceous glands are stimulated; phallus, prostate, seminal vesicles, and larynx enlarge; and the voice deepens. There is an increase in muscle mass, skeletal development, and linear growth. Finally, androgens affect the brain to stimulate libido. These processes are incomplete if androgen synthesis or actions are impaired.

Testosterone is also an important spermatogenic hormone. Both Sertoli and myoid cells contain intracellular androgen receptors and appear to be androgen target cells. Thus androgen deficiency is associated with hypospermatogenesis, and hypogonadal men are often infertile.

Aging is associated with a decline in testicular function; for example, Leydig cell volume decreases with a fall in serum testosterone concentrations after 60 years of age. Both primary testicular failure and a disturbance in GnRH secretion appear to be responsible.

Several situations can develop where androgen concentrations or synthesis rates are depressed and where replacement therapy is sometimes used. Testosterone deficiency may result from a disorder intrinsic to the testis or from insufficient stimulation of the testes by pituitary gonadotropins. The former condition is termed *primary testicular failure,* and the latter syndrome is termed *hypogonadotropic hypogonadism.* Although testosterone treatment stimulates the expression of secondary sex characteristics in men with primary testicular failure, they remain infertile.

Androgen excess is not a clinical problem in adult men. The production of excess androgens in preadolescents however, causes precocious puberty and in women can lead to infertility, disturbed menstrual rhythms, hirsutism, and, if sufficiently severe, to the development of a male body habitus (virilization). Precocious puberty refers to the onset of sexual development in boys before 9 years of age and in girls before 8 years of age. Approximately 50% of boys with true precocious puberty have a tumor of the hypothalamus.

Androgens are used to treat adult men with testosterone deficiency from primary gonadal failure or hypogonadotropic hypogonadism. The goal of therapy is to stimulate or restore androgenization to normal. Androgens stimulate body and beard hair growth, phallic enlargement, muscle development, voice deepening, and other phenomena. In adult men who have previously established normal sexual development, androgens may increase libido and potency. These latter end points are often difficult to quantitate and are influenced by factors other than sex steroids.

Testosterone is also used to treat congenital microphallus. Most boys with a small phallus will ultimately prove to be hypogonadal as adults. Impaired androgen production in utero or resistance to androgen action presumably explains the failure of the phallus to develop normally. Treatment is usually begun with intermittent small doses of parenteral testosterone and monitored carefully to prevent unwanted virilization.

Androgen replacement to increase the height of short children and short teenagers with constitutional delay of puberty is complex and controversial, since the role of androgens in normal growth and development remains ill-defined. Further, premature closure of the epiphyseal plates with resultant growth arrest and unacceptable virilization may occur. For children with constitutional delay of growth and adolescence, monthly injections of the long-acting testosterone esters can hasten pubertal growth and adolescent development without compromising adult height. Normal puberty in both males and females is accompanied by an acceleration in growth rate known as the *pubertal growth spurt,* presumably related to the increase in sex steroid secretion. Androgens increase the daily production rate and the amplitude of spontaneous growth hormone secretory episodes. Treatment of growth hormone-deficient teenagers with growth hormone together with androgens is more effective in increasing linear height than are androgens alone. In children with normal growth hormone secretion, androgen therapy initially increases growth velocity; however, accelerated epiphyseal closure may reduce ultimate adult height. Androgens may also be used to treat boys of exceptionally tall stature to accelerate epiphyseal closure and limit final height, but this use is equally debatable.

Anabolic Steroids in Normal Men

Androgens known as anabolic steroids are used by athletes to increase muscle mass and physical performance as well as used therapeutically with children to promote linear growth. These drugs are believed to be more anabolic than androgenic. This drug classification is based on in vivo bioassays in immature male rats in which increased levator ani muscle weight was found to occur at lower doses than those that stimulated the growth of the seminal vesicles and prostate. The interpretation of this bioassay has been criticized however, because the levator ani is not a typical skeletal muscle but instead is a sexual dimorphic muscle of the reproductive tract. Whether anabolic steroids differ appreciably from androgens is controversial because the androgen receptor in skeletal muscle is not known to differ from that in seminal vesicles and prostate. However, the latter tissue contains 5α-reductase whereas skeletal muscle does not. This enzyme amplifies the action of testosterone but does not influence the potency of most testosterone derivatives and may reduce the potency of 19-nortestosterone. Thus local metabolism may influence the potency of various androgens differently, and this effect may vary among target tissues.

Drugs commonly used for their anabolic activity include derivatives of 19-nortestosterone, oxandrolone, oxymetholone, and stanazolol.

Miscellaneous Androgen Uses

The erythropoietic effect of androgens is well established. Hemoglobin concentration is 1 to 2 g/dl higher in sexually mature men than in women or children, and mild anemia is common in hypogonadal men. Polycythemia may occur as an unwanted effect of androgen therapy. Androgens have been shown to stimulate erythropoiesis by increasing renal erythropoietin production (Chapter 65). There is also a direct effect of androgens on erythrocyte maturation. Since 5β-androgens (which bind weakly to androgen receptors) are more effective than 5α-androgens, the binding may constitute a novel mechanism to explain the direct effect of androgens on bone marrow cells. Androgens may be used to treat patients with aplastic anemia, and such patients occasionally respond to androgen therapy; however, responses vary. Both parenteral testosterone esters and oral androgens have been used, with the less potent androgens employed in women to limit undesirable virilization. Hypogonadism is common in both men and women with chronic renal failure. There is a mean increase in hematocrit in patients with chronic renal failure treated with androgens. Patients who need frequent transfusions and who have had bilateral nephrectomy may respond more poorly.

Danazol is an androgen derivative used for treatment of endometriosis, fibrocystic disease of the breast, and premenstrual tension syndrome (see Chapter 36). Danazol is also used to prevent attacks of hereditary angioneurotic edema, a disorder characterized by recurrent edema of the skin and mucosa. These patients lack the function of the inhibitor of the activated first component of complement, and androgens increase the serum concentration of this protein. Danazol is used rather than testosterone because it is weakly androgenic.

Other indications for the use of androgens have included inoperable breast cancer, postpartum breast pain and engorgement, and the wasting of chronic diseases and malnutrition in both sexes. The mechanism through which androgens affect the normal breast and modify the growth of breast cancer cells is uncertain. Positive responses of breast cancer, which average 30%, are less than for other hormonal therapies. Potent androgens are unacceptable in women because of virilization. Less potent androgens such as danazol have also been examined, but their efficacy is uncertain. Although androgens produce a positive nitrogen balance, clinical improvement in malnourished patients with chronic disease may reflect improved nutritional status.

Antiandrogens and Antagonists

Blockade of androgen synthesis or action is used as a treatment for female hirsutism, alopecia, acne, precocious puberty in males, benign prostate tumors, and other diseases. In this connection, several gonadotropin suppressants including leuprolide, buserelin, nafarelin, and goseralin which, in turn, inhibit testosterone productions have been approved for use in the United States. Although the role of androgens in the pathogenesis of benign and malignant prostate disease remains uncertain, disseminated prostatic cancer may be treated by decreasing testosterone production and impeding its action because the symptoms of bone pain are improved and survival is prolonged slightly. The limiting of production can be accomplished by orchidectomy or by drugs.

Androgen antagonists exert their effects by competing for binding to the testosterone-dihydrotestosterone binding site on the intracellular androgen receptor. Antiandrogens may be either steroidal or nonsteroidal. Steroidal antiandrogens may also bind to progesterone receptors and act as weak agonists in the absence of testosterone. Nonsteroidal antiandrogens, such as flutamide, though dissimilar from testosterone in planar structure, undergo sufficient folding to allow them to simulate the structure of androgens and bind to the receptor to form an antagonist-receptor complex that fails to undergo activation. Receptor binding to nuclear acceptor sites generally does not occur, and the biological actions of circulating androgens are blocked. This mechanism differs from that of antiestrogens, which bind to one or more classes of receptors and accumulate in target cell nuclei but are inactive biologically.

One of the antiandrogens, spironolactone, is a synthetic steroid primarily used as an aldosterone antagonist in the treatment of primary and secondary hyperaldosteronism, or as an antihypertensive agent. In addition to occupying aldosterone receptors, spironolactone interacts with androgen receptors. Further, spironolactone reduces the concentrations of the cytochrome P-450 17α-hydroxylase C17-to-C20 lyase enzyme complex in testicular microsomes, resulting in a decline in testosterone synthesis. Progesterone concentration increases because its further conversion is inhibited. However, a decrease in serum androgen concentration in men produces an increase in gonadotropin secretion, which may return the serum testosterone concentration to normal. The rise in gonadotropin secretion may increase aromatization to estradiol, leading to impotence and gynecomastia. Because of its action to block testosterone synthesis and to impede androgen action, spironolactone is used in the treatment of hirsute women.

The histamine H_2-receptor antagonist cimetidine, widely used to decrease gastric acid secretion in the treatment of peptic ulcer disease and esophagitis, acts as an antiandrogen. Thus it has been reported to produce gynecomastia when given in large doses like those used in the treatment of patients with Zollinger-Ellison syndrome. Gynecomastia occurs in less than 1% of patients treated with dosages in peptic ulcer disease. Cimetidine interacts with the androgen receptor about 0.01% as effectively as testosterone. Cimetidine also is used to treat hirsutism in women.

Ketoconazole is a broad-spectrum antimycotic agent used in the treatment of systemic fungal infections (see Chapter 52). Ketoconazole inhibits the synthesis of ergosterol in fungi, resulting in altered membrane permeability; inhibits the synthesis of cholesterol; and interferes with the action of cytochrome P-450 enzyme complexes in several mammalian cell types, including Leydig cells. The result is a dose-dependent decline in circulating testosterone concentrations in adult men and a rise in serum 17α-hydroxyprogesterone concentrations, suggestive of an effect on the C17-20 lyase. Serum luteinizing and follicle-stimulating hormone concentrations rise because of the decline in testosterone negative feedback. This action of ketoconazole has prompted its investigational use in the treatment of prostatic cancer and also in gonadotropin-independent precocious puberty in boys. However, the extent of suppression of testosterone synthesis is highly variable among men. Ketoconazole also inhibits cortisol biosynthesis, and has been used as an adjunctive therapy in patients with Cushing's syndrome. Ketoconazole-treated men may develop gynecomastia.

Cyproterone acetate, a synthetic steroid derived from 17α-hydroxyprogesterone, is an antiandrogen that is not available for clinical use in the United States, in part because it has some intrinsic suppressive effects on the corticotropic axis. Cyproterone also binds to the androgen receptor approximately 10% as well as testosterone and is a potent progestin. When given to women, it disrupts cyclic menstrual bleeding. The combination with estrogen suppresses gonadotropin secretion, inhibits ovulation, and reduces circulating testosterone concentrations. The aromatase inhibitor testolactone is also antiandrogenic.

Flutamide is a nonsteroidal antiandrogen recently approved in the United States for clinical use in combination therapy with GnRH analogs for the treatment of metastatic prostatic cancer. It binds weakly to the androgen receptor and requires hydroxylation for metabolic activity in vivo.

SIDE EFFECTS, CLINICAL PROBLEMS, AND TOXICITY

Many side effects of androgens are dose related and occur when target tissues are stimulated excessively. These include priapism (sustained erection), acne, polycythemia, and prostatic enlargement. Androgens should not be used in men with suspected prostatic cancer. Androgens also decrease high-density lipoprotein concentrations (and may be atherogenic). Weight gain and sodium retention may occur with androgen therapy, though the mechanism is unclear. Chronic androgen treatment suppresses gonadotropin secretion, decreases testis size, and depresses spermatogenesis. For this reason testosterone has been evaluated as a male contraceptive. However, azoospermia (zero sperm output) does not always occur, perhaps because of the direct stimulatory effect of testosterone on seminiferous tubules. Occasionally patients treated with testosterone develop gynecomastia. This may be from the bioconversion (aromatization reaction) of administered testosterone to estradiol. Obstructive sleep apnea has been reported to be exacerbated in susceptible men treated with testosterone.

The 17α-methylated androgens may disturb hepatic function, which appears to be an idiosyncratic response. Serum transaminase concentrations may rise, and 1% to 2% of patients develop jaundice because of intrahepatic cholestasis. Peliosis hepatitis and hepatocellular carcinoma have each been reported in a few patients treated with very high doses of alkylated androgens. Accordingly, these compounds are usually reserved for individuals in whom parenteral administration is contraindicated (e.g., bleeding dyscrasias).

Danazol may produce acne, oily skin, decreased breast size, hirsutism, and decreased high-density lipoprotein cholesterol in treated women (as noted in Chapter 36).

Spironolactone and several of its long-acting metabolites are antiandrogenic. As many as 50% of men treated with spironolactone develop gynecomastia. Libido may decline and impotence may occur. Amenorrhea and breast tenderness occur in women.

Professional and amateur athletes often use multiple androgens in dosages that far exceed estimated physiological replacement amounts. These androgens, like testosterone, suppress gonadotropin section and thereby reduce testicular function, including spermatogenesis. Nonaromatizable androgens reduce high-density lipoprotein synthesis and thereby high-density lipoprotein concentrations. This may increase the risk of atherosclerosis in these men. Long-term, high-dose androgen treatment may also increase the risk of benign prostatic hyperplasia and cause prostatic cancer when these men age. Because numerous variables influence athletic performance and because the efficacy of pharmacological androgen treatment of normal men remains controversial and the side-effects are unequivocal, the use of these drugs has been banned by the International Olympic Committee. Legislation is currently planned to

CLINICAL PROBLEMS

Masculinization in women
Priapism in men
Growth disturbances in children
Fetal masculinization during pregnancy
Jaundice
Edema
Acne
Hypertension
Weight gain

limit their availability in the United States.

The clinical problems with these drugs are summarized in the box. See Chapter 53 for ketoconazole, Chapter 59 for cimetidine, and Chapter 19 for spironolactone.

NEW DIRECTIONS

Finasteride is a 4-azasteroid inhibitor of prostatic testosterone 5α-reductase and was introduced recently as a treatment for benign prostatic hyperplasia. This approach to therapy is based upon the reduction in the size of the normal or hyperplastic prostate that occurs after androgen deprivation. Unlike agents that reduce testosterone production or block testosterone action, 5α-reductase inhibitors are more specific to prostate because almost all the testosterone entering the prostate is converted to dihydrotestosterone, and dihydrotestosterone is several times more potent an androgen than testosterone. Finasteride treatment in approved doses reduces prostatic dihydrotestosterone content by 80% but increases prostate testosterone sevenfold. Prostate size is reduced in some patients, and the symptoms of prostatism improve. The urine flow rate also increases when compared to placebo treatment. Because circulating concentrations of dihydrotestosterone are only 10% of testosterone concentrations, the 50% decline in serum dihydrotestosterone that accompanies finasteride treatment appears not to produce unwanted effects. For example, there are negligible changes in serum LH and FSH concentrations, and impotence and gynecomastia seem to occur rarely. The long-term influence of this therapy on the natural history of benign prostatic hyperplasia remains to be established, but the hope is that medical therapy will improve symptoms and reduce the need for surgery.

Current methods of androgen replacement are inadequate. Long-acting testosterone esters, which are currently the preferred therapy, produce high concentrations of not only testosterone but also estradiol in the first few days after intramuscular injection. Normal concentrations are variably sustained from 10 days to 3 weeks. Transdermal delivery produces stable physiological testosterone and estradiol concentrations over 24 hours, but daily treatment is needed. Moreover, to reproduce the testosterone concentrations of normal adult men, testosterone-impregnated membranes were applied to the thin skin of the scrotum from which absorption is high. Unexpectedly, high concentrations of dihydrotestosterone were produced, presumably because of the reduction of testosterone by 5α-reductase in scrotal skin. The long-term consequences of high dihydrotestosterone concentrations are not known. Biodegradable microspheres containing testosterone injected intramuscularly release testosterone for absorption into the circulation over a period of weeks to months. Thus, infrequent treatment is needed. Differences in bioavailability leading to variable hormone concentrations among subjects and pain at the injection site have been observed.

Antiandrogens and testosterone 5α-reductase inhibitors may prove to be useful treatments for benign and malignant disease of the prostate. Androgen-responsive growth factors may be identified, and methods may be developed to prevent the development of these disorders. Acne and male-pattern alopecia may also benefit from androgen deprivation. Use in women is limited by potential teratogenic effects on the developing fetus and will require combining these agents with oral contraceptives. Lack of target tissue specificity also limits the usefulness of antiandrogens in many conditions.

TRADE NAMES

In addition to generic and fixed-combination preparations, the following trade-named materials are available in the United States.

ANDROGENS

Anadrol, oxymetholone
Anavar, oxandrolone
Android, Metandren, Testred, Virilon, methyltestosterone
Danocrine, danazol
Deca-Durabolin, nandrolone decanoate
Delatestryl, testosterone enanthate
DEPO-testosterone, Virilon IM, testosterone cypionate
Durabolin, nandrolone
Halotestin, fluoxymesterone
Testoderm transdermal system, testosterone
Winstrol, stanozolol

ANTIANDROGENS AND ANTAGONISTS

Aldactone, spironolactone
Eulexin, flutamide
Proscar, finasteride

REFERENCES

Nieschlag E, Behre HM, editors: *Testosterone: action, deficiency, substitution*, New York, Springer-Verlag, 1990.

Sciara F, Toscano V, Concolino G, Silverio F: Antiandrogens: clinical applications, *J Steroid Biochem* 37:349-362, 1990.

Sokol RZ, Swerdloff RS: Practical considerations in the use of androgen therapy. In Santen RJ, Swerdloff RS, editors: Male reproductive dysfunction: diagnosis and management of hypogonadism, infertility, and impotence, New York, 1986, Marcel Dekker.

Sonino N: The use of ketoconazole as an inhibitor of steroid production, *N Engl J Med* 317:812, 1987.

Stoner E: The clinical development of a 5α-reductase inhibitor finasteride, *J Steroid Biochem* 37:375-378, 1990.

Wilson JD: Androgen abuse by athletes, *Endocr Rev* 9:181, 1988.

Winters SJ: Clinical disorders of the testis. In DeGroot LJ, editor: *Endocrinology*, Philadelphia, 1995, WB Saunders.

SELF-ASSESSMENT QUESTIONS

1. Gynecomastia may occur during treatment with all of the following *except:*
   a. spironolactone.
   b. testosterone.
   c. finasteride.
   d. cimetidine.
   e. flutamide.
2. Which of the following is not associated with testosterone treatment?
   a. testis growth
   b. polycythemia
   c. acne
   d. pubic hair growth
   e. nitrogen retention
3. All of the following statements about anabolic steroid use are true *except* that:
   a. LH and FSH secretion are suppressed.
   b. spermatogenesis is inhibited.
   c. SHBG concentrations decline.
   d. HDL-cholesterol is increased.
   e. hypertension may occur.
4. All of the following inhibit testosterone biosynthesis *except:*
   a. ketoconazole.
   b. spironolactone.
   c. cimetidine.
   d. estradiol.
   e. leuprolide.
5. An androgen-deficient adult man with a pituitary adenoma should be treated with:
   a. testosterone propionate.
   b. testosterone cypionate.
   c. GnRH.
   d. danazol.
   e. flutamide.
6. All of the following increase LH and FSH secretion *except:*
   a. clomiphene.
   b. GnRH.
   c. spironolactone.
   d. flutamide.
   e. danazol.
7. All of the following statements about dihydrotestosterone are true *except* that:
   a. it is the major androgen in the prostate.
   b. it is the major androgen in the circulation of adult men.
   c. it is secreted by the testis.
   d. it binds to sex hormone–binding globulin.
   e. it is metabolized in the liver.
8. Fluoxymesterone should not be used in patients with:
   a. chronic renal failure.
   b. pituitary adenomas.
   c. gynecomastia.
   d. hepatitis.
   e. congestive heart failure.
9. A biologically active metabolite of testosterone is:
   a. estradiol.
   b. 17-hydroxypregnenolone.
   c. 17α-hydroxyprogesterone.
   d. androsterone.
   e. testosterone glucoronide

CHAPTER 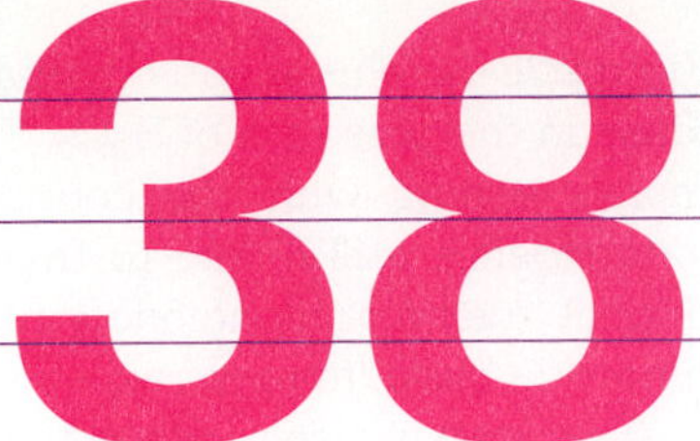

Thyroid and Antithyroid Drugs

ANN D. DUNN
JOHN T. DUNN

MAJOR DRUGS

iodides
thioureylenes
thyroid hormones

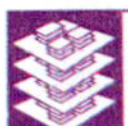

THERAPEUTIC OVERVIEW

The thyroid, like most endocrine glands, can secrete too much or too little hormone, producing hyperthyroidism or hypothyroidism. Hypothyroidism is most commonly caused by the end stages of autoimmune thyroid disease (Hashimoto's thyroiditis), in which autoantibodies have destroyed the thyroid gland. Other causes include familial goiter and surgical removal of the thyroid. Whatever the cause, hypothyroidism can be completely corrected by pharmacological preparations of thyroid hormone, either thyroxine or triiodothyronine.

The treatment of hyperthyroidism is more complex. The most common causes of hyperthyroidism are Graves' disease (another form of autoimmune thyroid disease) and toxic nodular goiter. In Graves' disease, autoantibodies directed to thyroid membrane receptors stimulate the thyroid to overproduce thyroid hormone. The optimal approach to therapy would be to block the immunological stimulation, but such an approach is currently impractical. Instead, antithyroid drugs, radioactive iodine, or surgery are used to block the synthesis or effects of excess thyroid hormone. Radioactive iodine and surgery are ablative approaches that can control the hyperthyroidism definitively when their use is sufficiently aggressive. The treatments of hypothyroidism and hyperthyroidism are summarized in the box, p. 516.

ABBREVIATIONS

ClO_4^-	perchlorate
T_3	triiodothyronine
T_4	thyroxine
TcO_4^-	pertechnetate

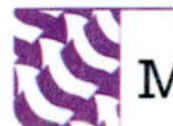

MECHANISMS OF ACTION

Thyroid Hormones

The thyroid hormones 3,5,3′,5′-tetraiodothyronine (thyroxine) (T_4) and 3,5,3′-triiodothyronine (T_3) are iodinated derivatives of tyrosine (see Figure 38-1 for structures). T_3 and T_4 are synthesized in the thyroid gland, or in the treatment of hypothyroidism, are administered to the patient. The chemical structures are the same whether T_3 and T_4 are synthesized in vivo or prepared in vitro.

The in vivo synthesis and storage of T_3 and T_4 occurs as part of the synthesis of the large glycoprotein thyroglobulin. The thyroid gland is unique among endocrine organs in having an extracellular compartment, the follicular lumen, in which hormone is stored. The intrathyroidal processing steps in the synthesis of thyroid hormones are outlined in Figure 38-2.

Circulating iodide is concentrated by thyroid epithelial cells by an active-transport system believed to be located in basal membranes. The system, which operates against an electrochemical gradient, requires energy in the form of oxidative phosphorylation and can be demonstrated only in the intact cell. Although details of the transport mechanism remain unknown, phospholipids may serve as iodide carriers across the cell membrane. Once within the thyroid cell, iodide passes down its electrochemical gradient across the apical cell membrane and into the follicular lumen. Meanwhile the peptide chain of thyroglobulin and part of its carbohydrate moiety are synthesized within the endoplasmic reticulum. Completion of the carbohydrate units occurs as the protein passes through the Golgi apparatus. The as-yet un-iodinated thyroglobulin is then transported in small vesicles to the apical cell membrane where it also is released into the lumen.

Next, iodide is oxidized and then attached to tyrosyl residues in thyroglobulin, forming the thyroid hormone precursors monoiodotyrosine and diiodotyrosine (see Figure 38-1). This step is mediated by a thyroid peroxidase in the presence of H_2O_2. The formation of the hormones occurs with the coupling of an acceptor, diiodotyrosine, still linked to thyroglobulin, and a donor, diiodotyrosine or monoiodotyrosine, which loses its alanine side chain to form respectively T_4 or T_3 (Figure 38-3). This step is also mediated by thyroid peroxidase. Iodination and coupling are believed to occur at the apical cell membrane where both the peroxidase and an H_2O_2-generating source are present. Under normal circumstances, a thyroglobulin molecule contains an average of three to four residues of T_4 and zero or one residue of T_3. At least four major hormonogenic sites exist in the thyroglobulin polypeptide chains.

As thyroid hormone is needed by the body, thyroglobulin is retrieved from the follicular lumen by endocytosis in the form of either small vesicles or large colloid droplets, where proteolytic processing is initiated by cathepsins D, B, and L. The latter two are stimulated by thyroid-stimulating hormone and have their major activities respectively at the N- and C-termini of the thyroglobulin polypeptide chain. The hormone-enriched peptide intermediates are then processed by lysosomal exopeptidases, such as lysosomal dipeptidase-1, to release the iodoamino acids, with T_3 and T_4 being rapidly transferred intact from lysosomes into the bloodstream by unknown mechanisms.

THERAPEUTIC OVERVIEW

HYPOTHYROIDISM

Administer exogenous thyroxine (T_4) or triiodothyronine (T_3)

HYPERTHYROIDISM

Surgery
Radioactive iodine
Drugs
- thioureylenes
- β adrenergic receptor blockers
- corticosteroids
- iodides

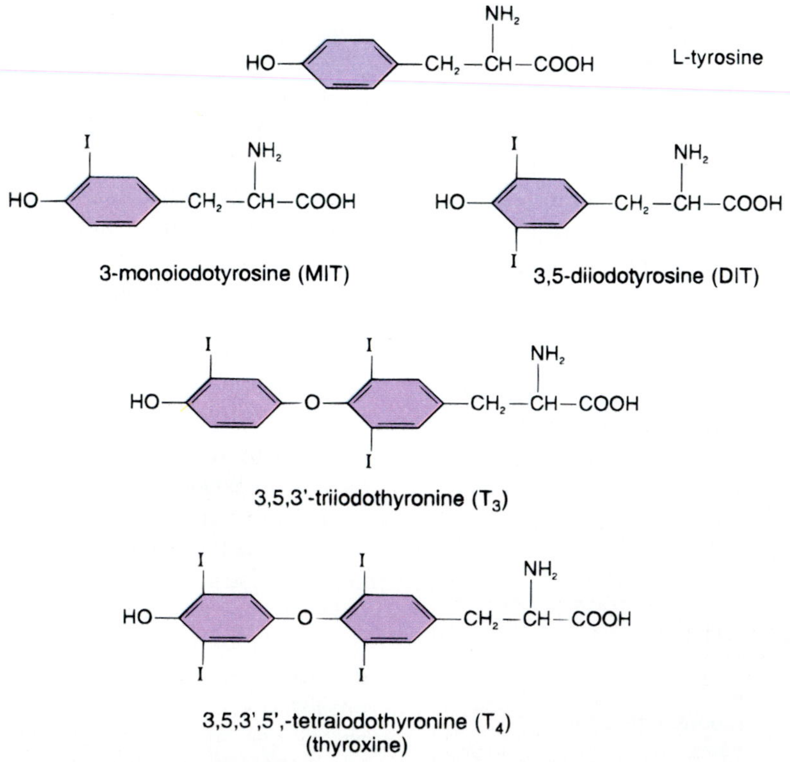

HO–C₆H₄–CH₂–CH(NH₂)–COOH — L-tyrosine

3-monoiodotyrosine (MIT)

3,5-diiodotyrosine (DIT)

3,5,3'-triiodothyronine (T_3)

3,5,3',5',-tetraiodothyronine (T_4)
(thyroxine)

FIGURE 38-1 Structures of thyroid hormones and precursors.

Most of the circulating thyroid hormones are noncovalently bound to plasma transport proteins. In humans this transport is mediated primarily by thyroxine-binding globulin and to a lesser extent by transthyretin (thyroxine-binding prealbumin) and albumin. The affinities of each of these proteins are much greater for T_4 than for T_3. Before entry into the target cell, the hormones are released from plasma proteins. The final processing of T_4 occurs in peripheral tissues, where it is deiodinated to T_3.

The thyroid hormones act through nuclear receptors to alter the expression of specific genes in target tissues. These receptors, identified in all thyroid hormone–responsive tissues, are nonhistone proteins of 47,000 to 57,000 daltons and are structurally related to the glucocorticoid hormone receptors. Unlike the latter, however, the thyroid hormone receptors are tightly bound to DNA even in the absence of hormone. Several isoforms of thyroid hormone receptors exist and are expressed in a specific manner. Each may bind to DNA by itself as either monomer, dimer, or heterodimer with several cell type–specific proteins.

Direct control of gene expression by thyroid hormones has been established in several systems. In some, regulation occurs primarily or exclusively at the transcriptional level. These include the systems coding for two pituitary hormones, growth hormone (positive control) and thyrotropin (negative control). In both cases addition of T_3 to cultured pituitary hormone–producing cells results in rapid changes in concentrations of hor-

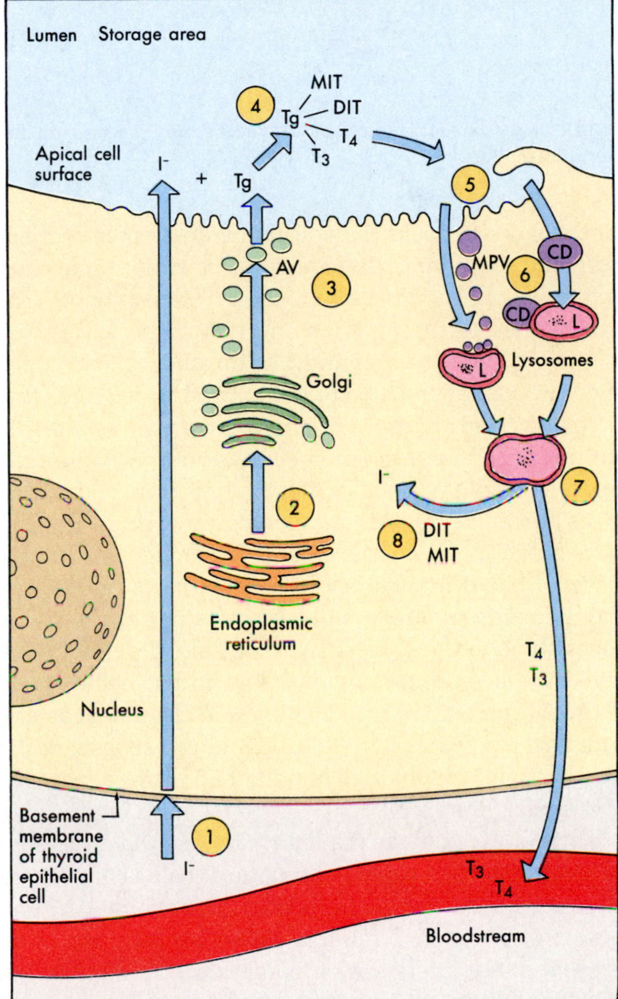

FIGURE 38-2 Intrathyroidal processing during synthesis of T_3 and T_4 hormones. *(1)*, Trapping iodide at the basement cell membrane and passage to the apical cell surface. *(2)*, Synthesis of polypeptide chains of thyroglobulin *(Tg)* including synthesis of carbohydrate units within the rough endoplasmic reticulum *(rER)*, with completion of the carbohydrate units in the Golgi *(G)*. *(3)*, Transport of newly formed Tg to the cell surface in small apical vesicles *(AV)*. *(4)*, Iodination of Tg, coupling of iodotyrosyl precursors to form T_4 and T_3 at the apical cell surface, and storage of iodinated Tg in the lumen. *(5)*, Retrieval of Tg by micropinocytosis into small vesicles *(MPV)* or by massive engulfment of colloid droplets *(CD)*. *(6)*, Fusion of lysosomes *(L)* with CD and MPV, proteolysis of Tg, and release of iodinated amino acids, T_3, and T_4. *(7)*, Entrance of T_4 and T_3 into bloodstream. *(8)*, Deiodination of DIT and MIT with recirculation of iodide.

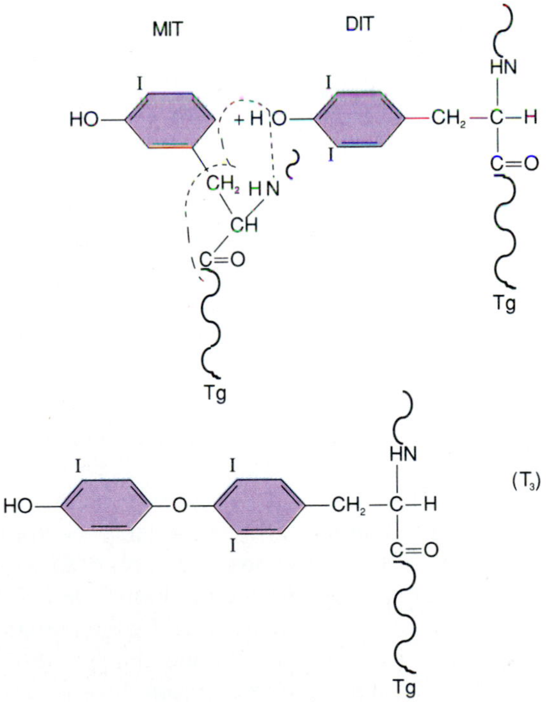

FIGURE 38-3 Formation of 3,5,3′-triiodothyronine (T_3) by coupling of an "acceptor" diiodotyrosine residue with a "donor" monoiodotyrosine residue with loss of the alanine side chain of the latter. T_4 is formed in the same manner by the coupling of two diiodotyrosine residues.

Table 38-1 Antithyroid Compounds

Inhibited Step (see Figure 38-2)	Compounds
Iodide concentration (step 1)	Complex anions: ClO_4^-, SCN^-
Iodination (step 2)	Thioureylenes, SCN^-
Coupling (step 4)	Thioureylenes
Hormone release (step 6)	Iodide, lithium salts, ClO_4^-
Deiodination (step 8)	propylthiouracil
Peripheral action (block deiodination)	Adrenal steroids, β-adrenergic blockers

ClO_4^-, Perchlorates; *SCN^-*, thiocyanides

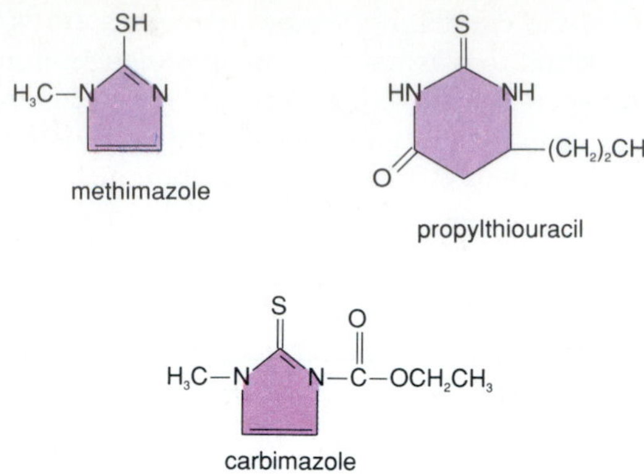

FIGURE 38-4 Structures of thioureylenes. See the text for further information.

mone mRNA that are commensurate with changes in transcription rates.

T_3 control of gene expression may not be directly related to transcription in all systems. An example of this is the hepatic S14 protein. Although the function of this protein is still unknown, it appears to be associated with lipogenesis and may provide information on the role of thyroid hormones in controlling thermogenesis. Administration of T_3 in this and similar systems may act primarily to stabilize a nuclear precursor of mRNA.

Antihyperthyroid Drugs

Drugs can inhibit the synthesis of T_3 and T_4 or the action of these hormones at several steps in the synthesis sequence, as listed in Table 38-1, with reference to Figure 38-2.

Thioureylene Drugs The primary clinical drugs are the thioureylenes, propylthiouracil, methimazole, and carbimazole (not available in the United States), which inhibit the thyroid peroxidase-mediated iodination and coupling steps (see Table 38-1 and Figure 38-2). The structures of these drugs are shown in Figure 38-4. Although carbimazole has potent antithyroid activity in vitro, it probably exerts most of its in vivo effects after metabolic conversion to methimazole.

The thioureylene drugs act in vitro either by reversibly inhibiting iodination or by irreversibly inactivating thyroid peroxidase. The scheme proposed to explain these different actions is outlined in Figure 38-5. Under normal conditions the heme group of thyroid peroxidase is oxidized by H_2O_2 (reaction 1) and then in turn oxidizes iodide to form a complex between the enzyme and the new iodide species, depicted as the iodinium ion I^+ (reaction 2).

In the absence of antithyroid drugs the iodide is transferred to tyrosyl residues in thyroglobulin to form monoiodotyrosine (reaction 3). In the presence of methimazole or propylthiouracil the drug is preferentially iodinated, depriving thyroglobulin of iodide and shutting down the synthesis of T_3 and T_4 (reaction 4). The drug is then further oxidized by thyroid peroxidase-I^+; as the concentration of drug diminishes, more of the thyroid peroxidase-I^+ complex is used to iodinate thyroglobulin, and thyroid hormone formation resumes. In the presence of sufficient concentrations of iodide, the inactivation of thyroglobulin iodination is transient, thyroid peroxidase itself is unaffected, and drug metabolism is extensive. In the absence of sufficient iodide, however, the drug reacts with the oxidized form of thyroid peroxidase, irreversibly inactivating the enzyme (reaction 5). In the case of methimazole, the drug is believed to become covalently linked to the heme group of thyroid peroxidase, and iodination does not resume until new enzyme is synthesized and metabolism of the drug becomes much more limited than under conditions of reversible inhibition.

Thyroid peroxidase–mediated coupling is more sensitive to inhibition than is iodination. This is in part explained by the kinetics of iodothyronine formation and in part by a direct inhibitory effect on coupling independent of the inhibition of iodination. The mechanism for this inhibition of coupling is unknown. One suggestion has been that the thioureylenes, which bind to thyroglobulin, may alter the steric configuration of this protein so that coupling between two iodotyrosine residues can no longer occur.

Propylthiouracil, but not methimazole, affects the processing of T_4 in peripheral tissues. Although the thyroid gland secretes some T_3, about 80% of the T_3 in humans originates from 5′-deiodination of T_4 in extrathyroidal tissues. Since T_3 is 10 times as active as T_4, this conversion step has considerable physiological importance. Although the relative contributions of different organs to circulating T_3 concentrations has not been established, liver and kidney are very active. The enzymes

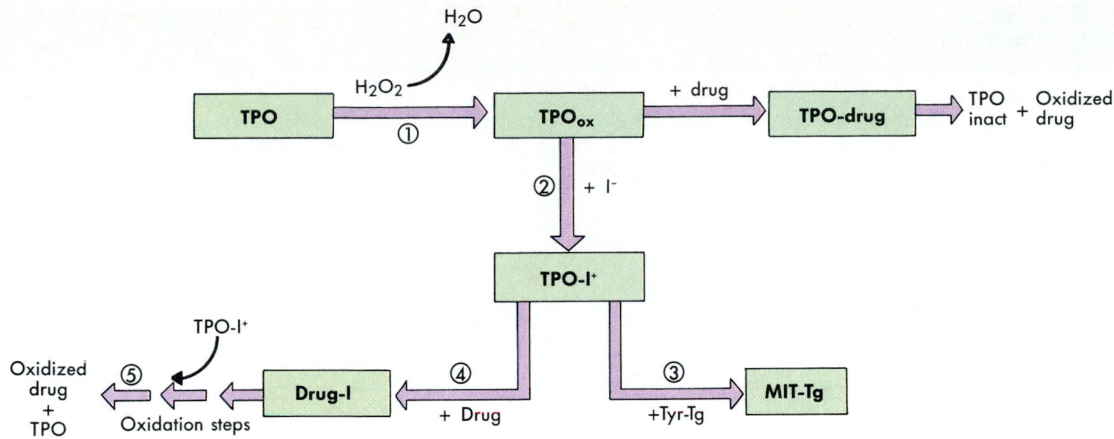

FIGURE 38-5 Inhibition of thyroid peroxidase (TPO)–mediated iodination. I^-, Iodide; I^+, iodinium; *MIT,* monoiodotyrosine; T_g, thyroglobulin; *TPO,* thyroid peroxidase; *Tyr,* tyrosine.

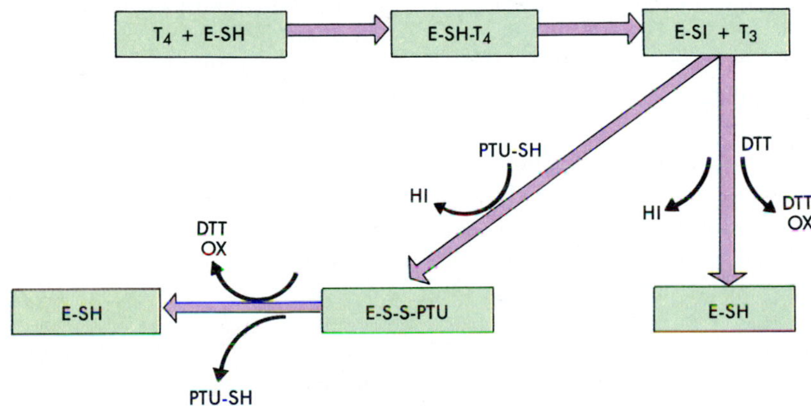

FIGURE 38-6 Pathway for liver-kidney 5′-deiodination of T_4 to produce T_3 and inhibition by propylthiouracil (PTU). DTT is dithiothreitol cofactor: E-SH is an SH group on the enzyme.

involved in 5′-deiodination have not been fully characterized. At least two different T_4-5′-deiodinase systems appear to be involved. The microsomal enzyme in liver and kidney is very sensitive to propylthiouracil inhibition, whereas the microsomal enzyme in pituitary, brain, and brown adipose tissue is insensitive to propylthiouracil inhibition. The latter enzyme may regulate local intracellular rather than circulating T_3 concentrations.

Propylthiouracil inhibits the liver-kidney deiodinase reaction noncompetitively with respect to T_4 and competitively with respect to the needed reduced thiol factor (Figure 38-6). In the first part of the reaction, T_3 and an enzyme-sulfinyl-iodide complex are formed. This step is unaffected by propylthiouracil; however, the drug prevents regeneration of the native enzyme by binding covalently to the enzyme, presumably at an essential SH site, forming a propylthiouracil-enzyme mixed disulfide as shown in Figure 38-6.

Other Antithyroid Drugs

Several monovalent anions block thyroid hormone synthesis by competitively inhibiting the active transport of iodide into the thyroid gland. Both pertechnetate (TcO_4^-) and perchlorate (ClO_4^-) have a higher affinity for the transport system than iodide itself does. Radiolabeled TcO_4^- is used clinically as a test ion to indicate trapping by the thyroid. Perchlorate, in addition to inhibiting iodide uptake, also accelerates the release of iodide. This anion is effective as an antithyroid drug but is rarely used because of a high incidence of side effects, notably aplastic anemia.

Table 38-2 Pharmacokinetic Parameters

Drugs	Administration	Absorption	$t_{1/2}$ (hrs)	Disposition	Plasma Protein Bound (%)
thyroxine (T_4)	Oral, IV	Fair (50%-80%)	5 days	M (to T_3), E	99.97
triiodothyronine (T_3)	Oral	Good	2 days	M (conjugated)	99.70
thioureylenes					
propylthiouracil	Oral	Good	2	M (oxidized and conjugated)	82
methimazole	Oral	Good	13-18	M (oxidized and conjugated)	8
carbimazole*	—	—	—	M (to methimazole)	—

M, Metabolized; *E*, enterohepatic circulation.
*Not available in the United States.

Hormone secretion by the thyroid can be inhibited by excess iodide. Several mechanisms have been proposed, including inhibition of thyroglobulin endocytosis and suppression of lysosomal proteolytic activity.

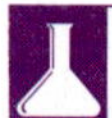

PHARMACOKINETICS

Thyroxine must be converted to T_3 for its clinical effects, providing the body some control in regulation of hormonal effect, which is probably an important benefit. The dose of T_4 varies widely among subjects. Important factors influencing the dose are variability of absorption and of conversion of T_4 to T_3. The half-life of T_4 in the serum is about 5 days; thus several weeks are required for assessment of the effects of dose changes. The optimal dose can be gauged by clinical response and laboratory tests, particularly the concentration of serum thyroid-stimulating hormone, which should be normal when the proper dose is administered to subjects with primary hypothyroidism.

The pharmacokinetic parameter values for thyroid hormone preparations and thioureylenes are listed in Table 38-2. (See Chapter 10 for value for β-blockers and Chapter 35 for values for corticosteroids.)

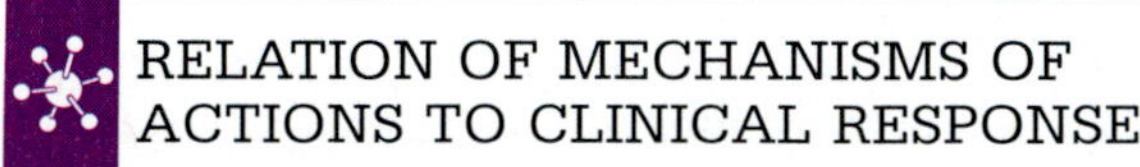

RELATION OF MECHANISMS OF ACTIONS TO CLINICAL RESPONSE

Hyperthyroidism

For patients with hyperthyroidism the usual therapeutic choice is between antithyroid drugs and radioiodine. Subtotal thyroidectomy has largely been replaced by radioiodine, which is simpler, safer, and equally effective. The antithyroid drugs can be expected to be effective in almost all patients. However, if the gland is still hyperplastic when antithyroid drugs are withdrawn, hyperthyroidism will probably recur.

Individuals with autoimmune thyroid diseases, of which Graves' disease is an example, have antibodies that stimulate the thyroid (producing hyperthyroidism) as well as antibodies that destroy the thyroid (producing hypothyroidism). The clinical status of an individual patient depends on the balance between these stimulating and destructive antibodies. Thus the natural course of Graves' disease includes a period of hyperthyroidism that is eventually replaced by euthyroidism and later hypothyroidism. Patients treated with antithyroid drugs during the entire duration of this hyperthyroid phase have no recurrence when the drugs are terminated. However, if the antithyroid drugs are withdrawn too early, clinical hyperthyroidism will reappear. The clinician would like to predict how long this period of intrinsic hyperthyroidism will last and on that basis decide whether a temporary means of treatment like antithyroid drugs is satisfactory, or whether an ablative method like radioiodine is necessary. Many attempts have been made to predict this natural course, but none has been entirely successful. In general, the milder the hyperthyroidism and the smaller the thyroid gland, the shorter is the period of spontaneous hyperthyroidism. Based on these considerations many clinicians choose radioiodine for patients with large thyroids or moderately severe hyperthyroidism and reserve antithyroid drugs for those patients with small glands, mild disease, or an absolute contraindication to radioiodine, such as pregnancy.

β-Adrenergic receptor blocking drugs provide an adjunct to the treatment of hyperthyroidism. In contrast to the other drugs mentioned so far, the β-blockers act peripherally (at the site of thyroid hormone effect) rather than at the thyroid gland. The mechanism of action is not certain but may relate to β-receptor inhibition of deiodination since the major source of T_3 is not that resulting from release from the thyroid but is the T_3 from deiodination of T_4 in the periphery. This action of the β-blockers makes them useful as adjuncts because they do not interfere with the actions of the thioureylenes or radioiodine on the thyroid. Their effect is much more rapid than what can be achieved by blocking thyroid hormone synthesis, as with the thioureylene drugs. Also, the β-blockers are most effective at those tissues, particularly the heart, where emergency treatment for arrhythmias associated with hyperthyroidism is frequently needed.

Corticosteroids are also occasionally useful in the treatment of hyperthyroidism, particularly of Graves' disease. They have no specific effect on the thyroid itself but do have several important peripheral actions. Corticosteroids lower peripheral conversion of T_4 to T_3, have an immunosuppressive effect on thyroid-stimulating antibodies, and are antipyretic. It has not been shown convincingly that patients with severe hyperthyroidism are truly hypoadrenal. However, these steroids are used empirically when patients with severe hyperthyroidism become hypotensive. The introduction of these agents into clinical practice has coincided with improved survival of patients with severe hyperthyroidism.

Most patients show some response to thioureylene drugs within 2 weeks, though months may be needed to obtain a maximal response. For the usual patient the duration of treatment may be a year or more. With a favorable response the gland decreases in size and the patient remains euthyroid as the dose of propylthiouracil is decreased and finally stopped. The success of treatment with antithyroid drugs varies widely with patient selection and probably with iodine content in the diet. In the United States the success rate has usually been well under 50%. However, in patients with mild disease, in those with small glands, and perhaps in those with significant ophthalmopathy with Graves' disease, antithyroid drugs are a reasonable choice. If patients experience no side effects, they may remain taking the drug for several years. However, most patients and physicians find that repeated unsuccessful attempts at withdrawal from antithyroid drugs lead them to choose radioiodine for long term therapy.

Hypothyroidism

Treatment of hypothyroidism usually involves replacement of thyroid hormone adequate to meet the patient's needs. Four types of preparation are available: levothyroxine (T_4), triiodothyronine (T_3), liotrix (a combination of T_4 and T_3), and desiccated thyroid or thyroid extract. Of these, T_4 is preferred and used almost universally. Desiccated thyroid is much less pure, less stable, and less predictable, though still satisfactory for most clinical purposes. Triiodothyronine is more expensive and frequently more difficult to regulate. Its chief use is in patients poor at converting T_4 to T_3, or where an effect of short duration is needed. A mixture of T_4 and T_3 is more expensive and has no clinical advantage over T_4 alone.

CLINICAL PROBLEMS

IODIDE

Angioedema, hemorrhage, sore teeth and gums, salivation, induction of goiter and myxedema

THIOUREYLENES

Agranulocytosis, granulocytopenia, skin rash

THYROID PREPARATIONS (INCLUDING THYROXINE)

Drug interactions with warfarin, bound (T_4, T_3) by cholestyramine in GI tract

TRADE NAMES

In addition to generic and fixed-combination preparations, the following trade-named materials are available in the United States.
Armour thyroid S-P-T; thyroid tablets
Cytomel, liothyronine (T_3)
Euthroid, Thyrolar, liotrix
Levothroid, Synthroid, Levoxine, thyroxine (T_4) (or thyroxine sodium or levothyroxine sodium)

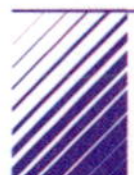

SIDE EFFECTS, CLINICAL PROBLEMS, AND TOXICITY

The treatment of severe, life-threatening hyperthyroidism (thyroid storm) needs special comment. Radioiodine requires several weeks to control the disease—too long for an emergency—thus, the mainstay is drug treatment. In this situation propylthiouracil is given in large doses and iodine (administered as Lugol's solution or potassium iodide) is added because of its more rapid effect on release of stored hormones. The most immediate emergency response, however, is obtained with β adrenergic receptor–blocking drugs, though these must be used cautiously in patients with coexistent heart failure. Corticosteroids are also valuable, particularly in patients with hyperpyrexia or hypotension.

Antithyroid drugs can be used in pregnancy but

should be used at the lowest dose possible because propylthiouracil and methimazole cross the placenta with ease. Fortunately, the immunosuppressive effects of pregnancy allow one to keep antithyroid drug doses to a minimum and frequently to withdraw them.

The clinical problems with these agents are summarized in the box.

NEW DIRECTIONS

The current treatment for hypothyroidism with thyroid hormone provides precisely the substance that the thyroid is unable to produce itself. This treatment is highly satisfactory, and no major changes are likely. Current treatments for Graves' disease, the most common cause of hyperthyroidism, act to prevent the thyroid from synthesizing excess hormone, but do not directly address the immunological cause of the hyperthyroidism. Also, current therapy for hyperthyroidism does not affect other features of Graves' disease, particularly the ophthalmopathy. Immunosuppressive therapy is a more logical approach, but currently available agents produce side effects and are not recommended. However, advances in understanding of the immunology of Graves' disease and development of improved immunosuppressive drugs may alter current treatment practice.

REFERENCES

Cooper DS: Antithyroid drugs, *N Engl J Med* 311:1353, 1984.

Kohrle J, Hesch D, Leonard JL: Intracellular pathways of iodothyronine metabolism. In Braverman LE, Utiger RD, editors: *Werner and Ingbar's the thyroid: a fundamental and clinical text*, 6th ed, Philadelphia, 1991, Lippincott.

Larsen PR, Silva JE, Kaplan MM: Relationships between circulating and intracellular thyroid hormones: physiological and clinical implications, *Endocrine Rev* 2:87, 1981.

Oppenheimer JH, Schwartz JL, Mariash CM, et al: Advances in our understanding of thyroid hormone action at the cellular level, *Endocrine Rev* 8:288, 1987.

Samuels HH, Formanm BM, Horowitz ZD, et al: Regulation of gene expression by thyroid hormone, *J Clin Invest* 81:957, 1988.

Taurog A: Hormone synthesis: thyroid iodine metabolism. In Braverman LE, Utiger RD, editors: *Werner and Ingbar's the thyroid: a fundamental and clinical text*, 6th ed, Philadelphia, 1991, Lippincott.

SELF-ASSESSMENT QUESTIONS

1. In a 60-year-old woman with moderately severe hyperthyroidism and a fairly large thyroid, the best treatment would usually be:
   a. iodides.
   b. radioiodine.
   c. propylthiouracil.
   d. thyroidectomy.
   e. perchlorate.
2. For treating life-threatening hyperthyroidism ("thyroid storm"), which of the following combinations is the best initial approach?
   a. β-blocker and radioiodine
   b. adrenocortical steroids and surgery
   c. β-blocker, adrenocortical steroids, and a thioureylene
   d. β-blocker, adrenocortical steroids, and surgery
   e. surgery followed by radioiodine
3. Which one of the following is the best reason to choose T_4 over T_3 in treating hypothyroid patients?
   a. T_4 acts more rapidly.
   b. T_4, by being converted to T_3 allows the body some control over hormone delivery to tissues.
   c. T_4 is better absorbed.
   d. T_4 has selective actions on the heart and liver that are more effective than T_3.
   e. T_3 causes more allergic reactions than T_4 does.
4. Which of the following statements is *not* true? β-Blockers are useful in treating hyperthyroidism because
   a. they block peripheral conversion of T_4 to T_3.
   b. they do not interfere with radioiodine therapy.
   c. they provide prompt relief of the cardiovascular features of hyperthyroidism.
   d. they do not interfere with thioureylene therapy.
   e. they provide permanent control of hyperthyroidism.
5. Which of the following statements about familial goiter is *not true*?
   a. Most familial goiters can be treated effectively with thyroid hormone, regardless of the level of the biosynthetic defect.
   b. Defective iodide trapping can be overcome, at least theoretically, by treatment with iodine.
   c. Defective iodide organification can be overcome, at least theoretically, by treatment with iodine.
   d. Defective intrathyroidal deiodination can be overcome, at least theoretically, by treatment with iodine.
   e. Iodine treatment should not overcome defective iodotyrosyl coupling.

CHAPTER 39 Insulin and Oral Hypoglycemic Agents

JOHN C. LAWRENCE, JR.

MAJOR DRUGS

insulins
sulfonylureas

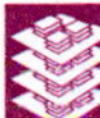

THERAPEUTIC OVERVIEW

The term diabetes mellitus encompasses a group of pancreatic endocrine-based disease states of differing causes and severity.

Diabetes is derived from the Greek word *diabētēs,* meaning 'syphon', to signify the copious urine production in individuals with this affliction. Diabetes has been recognized for at least 2000 years; however, ancient physicians made no distinction between diabetes mellitus and another disease, diabetes insipidus. Both diseases involve the endocrine system and generate increased volumes of urine but are otherwise unrelated. The observation that urine from some types of diabetic patients tasted sweet (a common, if unsavory, diagnostic procedure) whereas that from other types was tasteless led to the first distinction between diabetes mellitus and diabetes insipidus (Figure 39-1).

ABBREVIATIONS

GLUT-4	glucose transporter 4
IDDM	insulin-dependent diabetes mellitus
IGF-1, IGF-2	insulin-like growth factors
IRS-1	insulin receptor substrate 1
MAPK	microtubule-associated protein kinase
NIDDM	non–insulin dependent diabetes mellitus
PP1G	glycogen-bound form of protein phosphatase 1
raf	a protooncogene kinase
UGDP	University Group Diabetes Program

Diabetes insipidus results from a deficiency of antidiuretic hormone (vasopressin), a hormone necessary for the reabsorption of water in the kidney. A person lacking this hormone may produce liters of insipid urine each day. Glucose imparts the sweet taste to the urine in diabetes mellitus (*mellítus* is the Latinized Greek word for 'honeyed'). In untreated disease, blood glucose rises to much higher concentrations than normal, leading to increased concentrations of sugar in the glomerular filtrate. The kidney has an active glucose transport system that normally pumps almost all the sugar out of the urine. However, with glucose concentrations of approximately 200 mg/dl (11 mM), the transport system becomes saturated, and glucose spills into the urine, resulting in osmotic diuresis. Ketone bodies (discussed later) in the urine also can contribute to the diuresis.

In the early 1880s it was discovered that pancreatectomy produced symptoms of diabetes mellitus in dogs, a discovery that indicated that the pancreas produces a substance that prevents the onset of the disease. However, it was not until 1921 that Banting, Best, Collip, and McLeod successfully isolated and used insulin to treat a diabetic human. Before this, the prognosis for a patient with insulin-dependent diabetes mellitus (previously termed *juvenile onset*) was death, usually within a few months. Life could sometimes be extended for a short time by adherence to a diet bordering on starvation. In this setting one can appreciate the immense influence of the discovery of insulin. Insulin was soon isolated in quantities sufficient for treating diabetes.

Diabetes mellitus has been diagnosed in approximately 3% of the general population, probably an underestimate. Although the widespread perception is that the disease is curable with insulin, this is far from true.

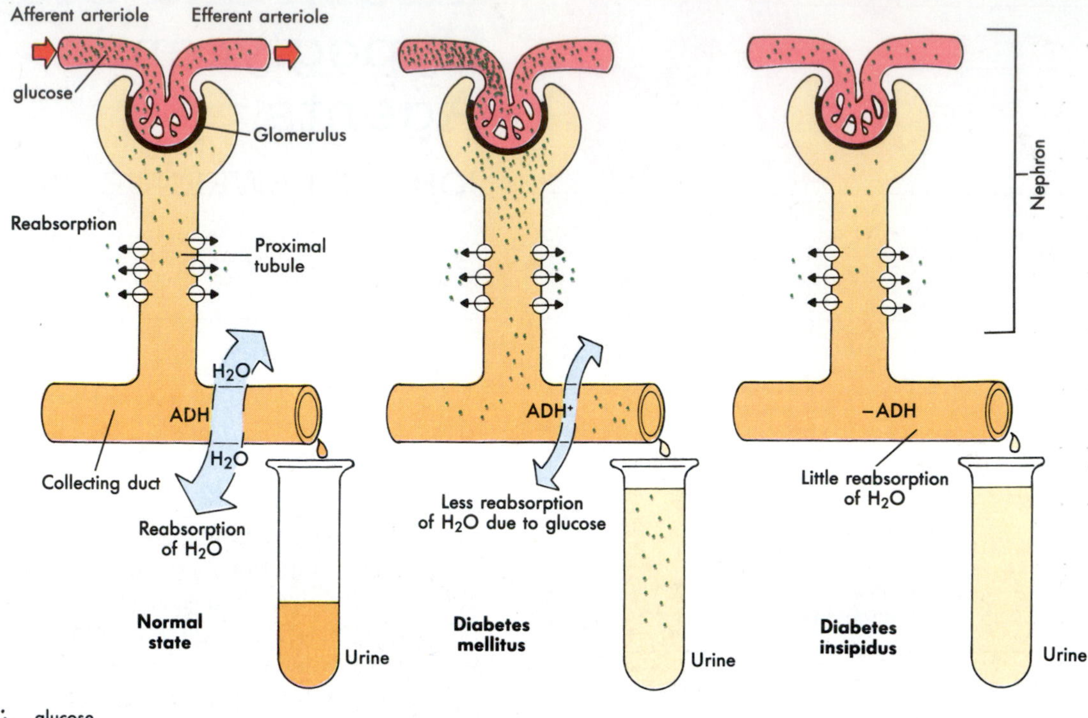

FIGURE 39-1 Schema of renal nephron functionality in the "normal," "diabetes mellitus," and "diabetes insipidus" states. Both types of diabetes produce polyuria. The three diagrams show water and small molecules, such as glucose, passing through the glomerulus into the tubule, where saturable reabsorption of glucose takes place (shown leaving the proximal tubule). In diabetes mellitus the reabsorption process cannot handle all the glucose, and so some glucose is voided in the urine (shown as the test-tube contents). In the normal state, 98% to 99% of the water also is reabsorbed (shown here as water leaving the collecting duct). In diabetes mellitus less water is reabsorbed because of the elevated concentration of glucose in the collecting duct. Diabetes insipidus is characterized by a low concentration of antidiuretic hormone (ADH) necessary for reabsorption of water.

Complications resulting from diabetes mellitus are among the leading causes of blindness, renal failure, cardiovascular disease, and limb amputations.

Types of Diabetes Mellitus

Diabetes mellitus occurs when circulating insulin concentrations decline or when the target cells become resistant to the hormone. Most cases can be divided into two types, which have gone by a variety of names over the past few years (Table 39-1). Juvenile onset and maturity onset were previously used to designate the two types. Either type can occur at either age, and so such terminology is somewhat misleading. The current preferred designations are *insulin-dependent diabetes mellitus* (IDDM) and *noninsulin-dependent diabetes mellitus* (NIDDM).

Table 39-1 Nomenclature and Terminology Used to Differentiate Between the Two Major Types of Diabetes Mellitus

Insulin-dependent Diabetes Mellitus (IDDM)	Non–insulin Dependent Diabetes Mellitus (NIDDM)
TYPE I	TYPE II
ketosis prone	ketosis resistant
juvenile onset	adult onset
growth onset	maturity onset

Insulin-dependent Diabetes Mellitus IDDM results from a degeneration of the pancreatic beta cells, which produce insulin. It is the more serious type and accounts for approximately 15% to 20% of the total cases. There is a genetic link or predisposition, though environmental factors must also be involved, since the incidence of IDDM in homozygous twins is only about 50%.

It is now clear that IDDM results from autoimmune destruction of the β cells. The stimulus that prompts the

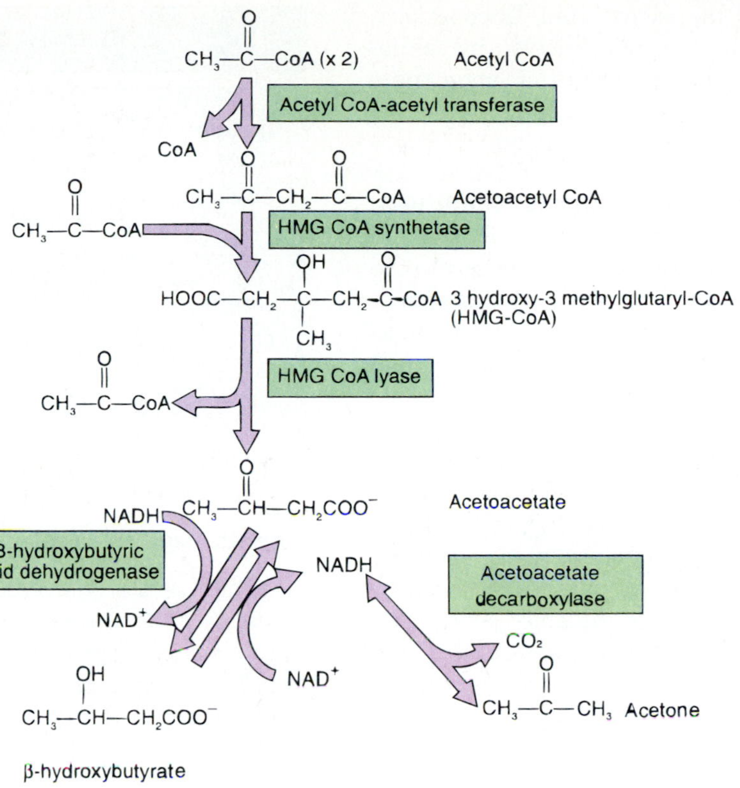

FIGURE 39-2 Progression of IDDM leads to the buildup of acetyl CoA, generated from the sequential β-oxidation of fatty acids. The excess acetyl CoA undergoes conversion to ketone bodies, some of which are acidic, and can lead to a breakdown in the control of blood pH.

immune system to attack the β cells remains a mystery. The disease has an abrupt onset clinically, though evidence now indicates that the process has been occurring slowly over a period of years, usually in childhood or early adulthood, and is associated with the symptomatic triad of polyuria, polydipsia, and polyphagia. The increased urine volume is caused by the osmotic diuresis that results from the increased concentration of glucose (hyperglycemia), and ultimately ketone bodies, in the urine. Thirst and hunger are compensatory responses to the loss of fluid and the inability to utilize nutrients. Weight loss is a hallmark of the untreated disease, as is premature cessation of growth when diabetes develops in childhood.

At the time of onset of IDDM, there may be detectable, though lower than normal, concentrations of serum insulin. However, the concentration of the hormone will decline to negligible values with progression of the disease; and if insulin is not supplied, metabolic acidosis (ketosis) will ensue, followed shortly by diabetic coma and death. Metabolic acidosis results from the production of ketone bodies, which are synthesized from acetyl CoA in the liver. The synthetic pathway is summarized in Figure 39-2. The production of ketone bodies is an ongoing activity of the liver, which releases them into the circulation for transport to the heart, skeletal muscle, and other tissues to be used as an energy source. In the normal fed state, the concentration of ketone bodies is relatively low because insulin stimulates the synthesis of fatty acids, a competing pathway for the use of acetyl CoA. Insulin also inhibits lipolysis, thereby decreasing the supply of fatty acids, which are a major source of acetyl CoA in the liver. Thus, when insulin concentrations are decreased, as occurs in diabetes or fasting, production of ketone bodies is favored. Severe ketosis does not develop in normal individuals because only a small amount of insulin is needed to inhibit lipolysis in adipose tissue.

The use of the term *ketone body* to describe the compounds that produce ketosis is a misnomer because the major ketone body produced during diabetes or fasting in humans, β-hydroxybutyrate, is not a ketone. Except for acetone, all the diabetes ketone bodies are organic acids, explaining why decreased blood pH is associated with their production. Because acetone is volatile, it is excreted to some extent by the lungs, accounting for the "fruity" acetone breath of individuals with severe ketosis.

The later stages of diabetic ketoacidosis are associated with severe fluid depletion, in part because of the osmotic diuresis caused by increased concentrations of glucose and ketone bodies in the urine. Fluid loss also occurs with vomiting, which is one of the ways the body attempts to rid itself of the excess acid. Unconsciousness, referred to as diabetic coma, followed by cardiovascular collapse and death, occurs if appropriate therapy is not instituted. Treatment involves administration of insulin and rehydration with careful monitoring to establish and maintain electrolyte balance.

Non–insulin Dependent Diabetes Mellitus NIDDM usually develops after 35 years of age, and most diabetics of this type are obese. In contrast to the insulin-dependent diabetic, non–insulin dependent diabetics have significant concentrations of the circulating hormone. Indeed, the presence of insulin and the ability of sulfonylureas (discussed later) to evoke release of the hormone are indicative of NIDDM. Because only a small amount of insulin is needed to prevent ketone body formation, the non–insulin dependent diabetic rarely develops ketosis. In some cases of NIDDM the concentrations of insulin are actually higher than normal. The apparent paradox of hyperglycemia despite elevated insulin is explained by the fact that the target cells are relatively insensitive to the hormone. In such resistant cells, a higher concentration of insulin is needed to elicit a response than in normal cells. In some cases of insulin resistance, concentrations of insulin receptors are decreased; in others the problem is distal to the receptor in the pathway of insulin action.

Diabetic coma is rarely seen in non–insulin dependent diabetics, presumably because their endogenous insulin prevents ketosis. However, a related condition, hyperosmolar coma, can occur. It is most often observed in elderly individuals and is usually preceded by an illness or other stressful situation that increases the requirement for insulin. Under these circumstances, the insulin present becomes insufficient to prevent glucosuria. Fluid loss is compounded when vomiting is associated with the precipitating illness. As dehydration becomes severe, urinary output decreases despite the high urinary concentration of glucose. Thus, renal excretion of glucose falls, and blood glucose and serum osmolarity increase to extremely high concentrations, leading to loss of consciousness. Like diabetic coma, hyperosmolar coma is life threatening; it is a particularly grave condition in older diabetics, who may already have compromised cardiovascular function.

Figure 39-3 illustrates the responses of IDDM, early NIDDM, IDDM, and normal subjects to an oral glucose tolerance test. In IDDM patients essentially no insulin is detected, and plasma glucose is elevated. In NIDDM patients plasma glucose is elevated and insulin secretion is delayed. In early IDDM patients plasma glucose is elevated early (30-60 min) and plasma insulin secretion is exaggerated.

THERAPEUTIC OVERVIEW

INSULIN AND HYPOGLYCEMIC AGENTS

IDDM

Insulin
Diet
Exercise

NIDDM

Oral hypoglycemic agents—sulfonylureas
Insulin
Diet
Weight reduction
Exercise

Agents Used in Treatment

Insulin is still the only drug effective in treating IDDM. A class of drugs collectively referred to as *oral hypoglycemic agents* is now used in the therapy of NIDDM. It should be stressed that nonpharmacological methods are of the utmost importance in treating the obese non–insulin dependent diabetic. Weight reduction and a regular program of moderate exercise, when not contraindicated by physical debilitation, should be encouraged in all obese non–insulin dependent diabetics as proved ways of increasing insulin sensitivity. Unfortunately, poor compliance with such programs is the rule rather than the exception, and the majority of the NIDDM diabetics must be treated with insulin or oral agents.

Several classes of oral hypoglycemic agents have been identified, but only one, the sulfonylureas, are currently used in this country. The hypoglycemic action of sulfonylureas was discovered in the early 1940s during clinical trials to investigate the antimicrobial efficacy of sulfonamide derivatives. It was noted that several patients developed hypoglycemia after receiving the sulfonylurea *p*-aminobenzenesulfonamido-isopropylthiadiazole. More than 10 years elapsed before clinical trials established that a related compound, carbutamide, was effective in controlling blood glucose concentrations in selected NIDDM patients.

Two other classes of oral hypoglycemic agents should be mentioned: the biguanides, of which phenformin is the prototype, and the thiazolidinediones, of which ciglitazone is the prototype. Phenformin was previously used in the United States to treat NIDDM; however, it produced serious side effects, notably metabolic acidosis, and is no longer approved for use in this country. A related agent, metformin, has less tendency than phenformin to produce acidosis and is currently used in Europe. Ciglitazone and the related agent piaglita-

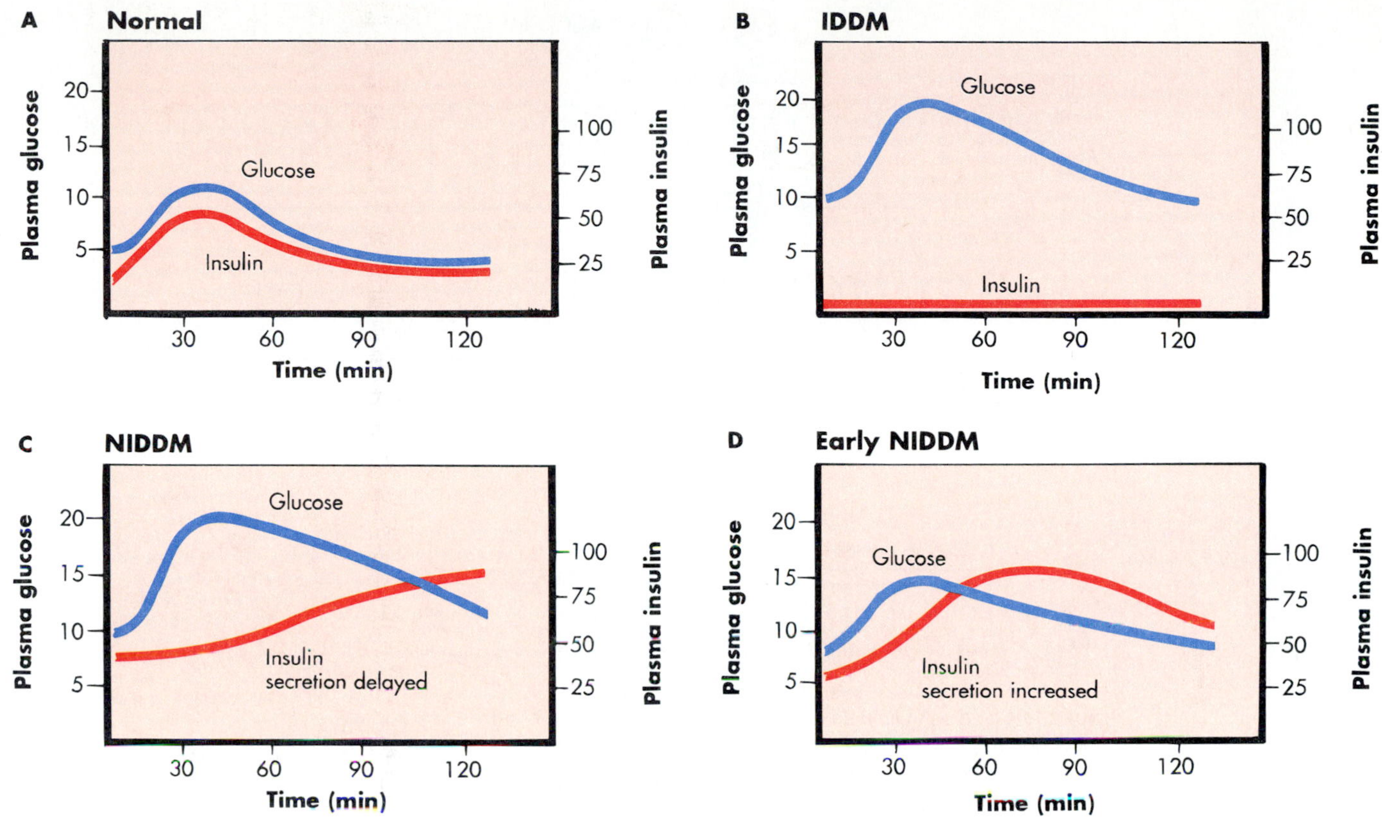

FIGURE 39-3 In normal persons (**A**) plasma glucose rises in an oral glucose tolerance test in 30 minutes and returns to normal in 90 to 120 minutes. Insulin rises and returns to normal during the same time period. In IDDM patients (**B**) plasma glucose is greatly elevated at all time points and plasma insulin is essentially nondetectable. In NIDDM (**C**) patients plasma glucose is elevated at all time points, and plasma insulin response to an oral glucose tolerance test is delayed but prolonged. Total insulin response is normal or increased. In early NIDDM (glucose intolerance) (**D**) plasma glucose is elevated at 30 to 60 minutes but may or may not return to normal at 120 minutes. Plasma insulin is elevated basically, and secretion is exaggerated.

zone are experimental agents that increase insulin sensitivity.

The therapeutic overview is summarized in the box.

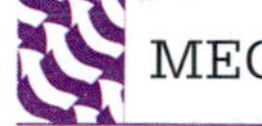

MECHANISMS OF ACTION

Insulin

Insulin is an acidic protein having a molecular weight of approximately 5600 daltons (Figure 39-4). This hormone is composed of two polypeptides, termed the *A* and *B chains,* which are covalently joined by two interchain disulfide bonds. A third intrachain disulfide bridge is present in the A chain. The chains are formed by proteolysis of proinsulin, a larger single-chain precursor, by removal of the intervening sequence of amino acids, referred to as the *C peptide*. The conversion of endogenous proinsulin to insulin occurs in the secretory granule, where most of the insulin undergoes crystallization with Zn^{++}. Approximately equimolar amounts of insulin and C peptide are stored in the granule, along with a much smaller amount of proinsulin. When the β-cell receives the appropriate stimulation, the contents of the granule are released by exocytosis.

The amino acid sequence of insulin is highly conserved across species. Beef insulin differs from human insulin in three amino acids. Pork insulin is more similar to the human type, differing in only a single amino-acid. This explains why pork insulin in less antigenic in humans than beef insulin.

The structure of insulin is similar to those of several other hormones and growth factors, including relaxin and insulin-like growth factors 1 and 2 (IGF-1 and IGF-2). Conservation of the cysteine residues is of particular note, given the role of disulfide bonds in determining the tertiary structure of protein. Not surprisingly, IGF-1 and IGF-2 have some affinity for the insulin receptor; however, both growth factors have their own receptors. In some cases homologies extend to receptor structure and biological action. For example, the receptors and actions of IGF-1 and insulin are similar. In contrast, relaxin

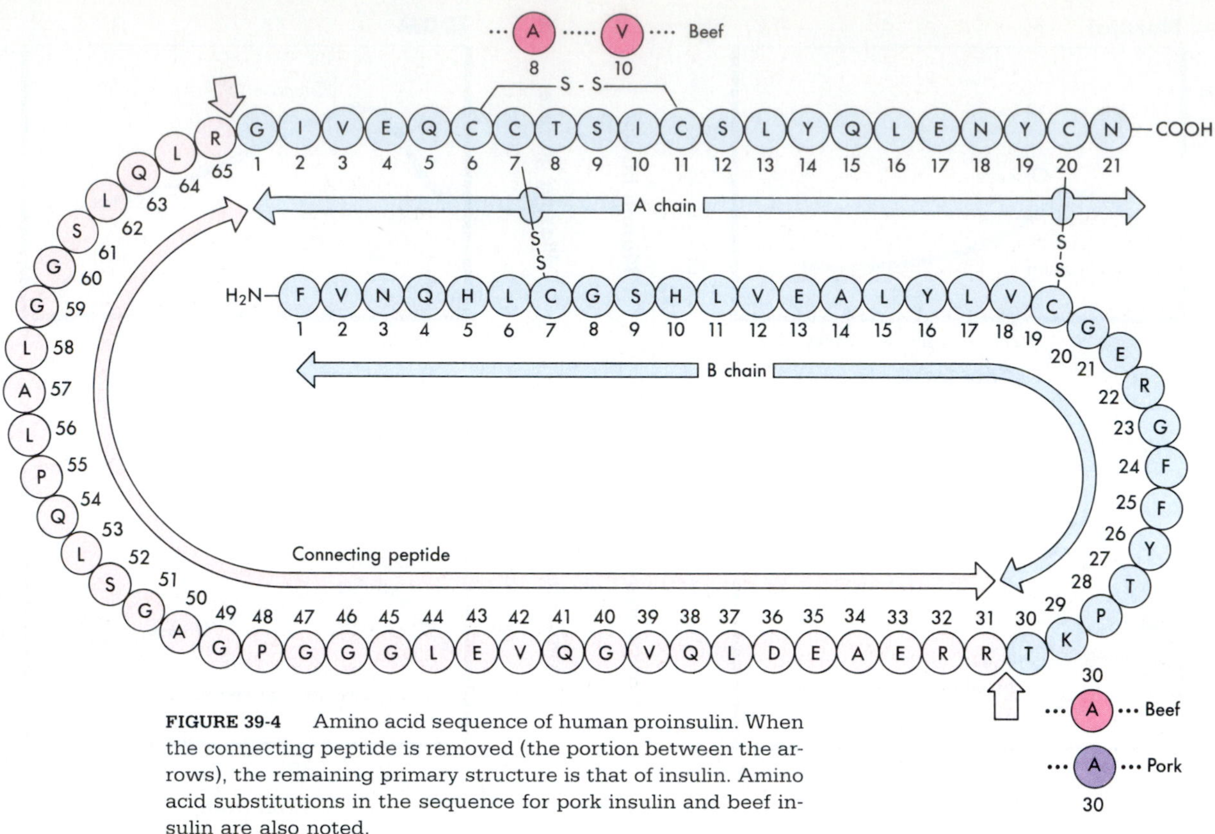

FIGURE 39-4 Amino acid sequence of human proinsulin. When the connecting peptide is removed (the portion between the arrows), the remaining primary structure is that of insulin. Amino acid substitutions in the sequence for pork insulin and beef insulin are also noted.

causes widening of the symphysis pubis immediately before delivery, an effect not produced by insulin.

Insulin stimulates a variety of anabolic processes in muscle, liver, and fat cells. These effects are initiated after insulin binds to a cell-surface receptor (see Chapters 2 and 34). This interaction causes the generation of a signal that is transmitted to the inside of the cell to trigger activation of various anabolic pathways and inhibition of catabolic processes. A brief overview of current knowledge and ideas concerning the signal propagation pathway is provided in the next few paragraphs.

Insulin Receptor The insulin receptor is a tetrameric protein complex composed of two α subunits of approximately 130,000 daltons and two 90,000 dalton β subunits. Subsequent propagation of the signal involves changes in the phosphorylation states of enzymes in several important metabolic pathways. It has been known for many years that insulin promotes dephosphorylation of phosphoserine residues in glycogen synthase, pyruvate dehydrogenase, and hormone-sensitive lipase. Dephosphorylation of glycogen synthase and pyruvate dehydrogenase activates the enzymes, accounting in part for the stimulation of glycogen synthesis and glucose oxidation by insulin. Dephosphorylation inactivates hormone-sensitive lipase, contributing to the antilipolytic action of insulin. Thus, several of the important metabolic actions of insulin are mediated by dephosphorylation of key enzymes. However, as discussed below, the signal transduction pathway leading to dephosphorylation of at least some of these enzymes involves activation of protein kinases and increased protein phosphorylation.

The insulin receptor is a protein tyrosine kinase. Insulin binding to the α subunit activates the kinase, which resides in the β subunit. This is described in greater detail in Chapter 34 and is only summarized here. The resulting autophosphorylation is stimulated by insulin and causes a further increase in receptor protein tyrosine kinase activity. Effects of insulin mediated by the insulin receptor are dependent on the receptor tyrosine kinase. The major substrate for the insulin receptor is insulin-receptor substrate 1 (IRS-1), a protein having an important role in insulin signal transduction. Phosphotyrosine residues in IRS-1 serve as binding sites for proteins having Type 2 src homology (SH-2) domains (see Chapter 34). Thus, when phosphorylated, IRS-1 brings together key elements in various signal transduction pathways. The best defined of these pathways involves the GTP-binding protein ras and leads to cell growth and/or differentiation. The two proteins immediately downstream of IRS-1 in the ras signaling pathway are growth factor receptor binding protein

2 (GRB-2) and mammalian son of sevenless (mSOS), a protein that promotes formation of the GTP-bound(active) form of ras by stimulating the exchange of GDP for GTP. GRB-2 functions to link phosphorylated IRS-1 to mSOS, leading to activation of ras. In a reaction(s) that is still not understood completely, ras activates the protein kinase raf-1. The next steps are well defined and involve a phosphorylation and activation of MAP kinase. MAP kinase phosphorylates several transcription factors, thereby coupling the pathway to the control of gene expression. MAP kinase also phosphorylates and activates ribosomal protein S6 kinase 2 (Rsk-2). This provides a potential link to the control of glycogen synthesis as Rsk-2 phosphorylates and activates PP1G, the protein phosphatase responsible for dephosphorylating glycogen synthase. However, this mechanism can not solely explain the effects of insulin on glycogen synthase because Rsk-2 is activated by a variety of agents that do not activate glycogen synthesis. Additional research will be needed to define fully the mechanism by which insulin stimulates glycogen synthesis.

A different type of mechanism is involved in the stimulation of glucose transport by insulin. Insulin-stimulated glucose transport is most pronounced in skeletal muscle fibers, cardiac myocytes, and adipocytes. These cells express the highest levels of the glucose transporter, GLUT-4. In the absence of insulin, almost all the GLUT-4 is found in intracellular vesicles. Insulin promotes the translocation of GLUT 4 from this intracellular store to the plasma membrane. Thus, glucose transport increases because the number of transporters at the cell surface increases. The signals that cause vesicles containing GLUT-4 to move to the plasma membrane have not been identified but may involve phosphorylation of regulatory elements controlling vesicle trafficking. Insulin also causes translocation of receptors for transferrin and IGF-2 to the plasma membrane, indicating that insulin-stimulated translocation between cellular compartments occurs with other proteins in addition to GLUT-4.

Much remains to be determined regarding the mechanism of action of insulin. For example, it is still not clear how insulin triggers dephosphorylation of pyruvate dehydrogenase, a mitochondrial enzyme. One hypothesis is that insulin activates this enzyme by promoting formation of a soluble low molecular weight substance that appears to be an inositol phosphoglycan formed from glycosylphosphatidylinositol precursors found in the plasma membrane.

Glucagon

Glucagon is a single-chain polypeptide with a molecular weight of about 3500 daltons. It is processed in the alpha cells of the islets of Langerhans of the pancreas by enzymatic cleavage of specific bonds from a large precursor, proglucagon. A related molecule, glycentin (molecular weight about 7000 daltons), containing glucagon within it is formed from proglucagon in the stomach and gastrointestinal tract.

Glucagon acts in the opposite direction from insulin to facilitate the breakdown of macromolecules. As part of its control of catabolism, glucagon acts to decrease anabolic processes in target organs. The major organ where glucagon acts is the liver, but it also produces effects in fat and in the heart. Glucagon, like insulin, interacts with a specific receptor on the outer surface of sensitive cells. The receptor is not yet as well characterized as the insulin receptor but is believed to be a single polypeptide chain of about 60,000 daltons and coupled to at least two intracellular second-messenger systems. These messenger systems are the production of cyclic adenosine monophosphate by activation of adenylate cyclase and the production of IP_3 by activation of phospholipase C. Glucagon secretion is determined by the arterial blood glucose concentration; thus hypoglycemia stimulates and hyperglycemia retards glucagon release. Certain amino acids are reported to be effective secretagogues.

Oral Hypoglycemic Agents

Sulfonylureas Shortly after discovery of the hypoglycemic actions in humans, it was found that these drugs also produced hypoglycemia in normal animals but not in pancreatectomized dogs. This observation led to the suggestion that these drugs decreased blood glucose by releasing insulin from the pancreas. There is no question that the sulfonylureas promote insulin release from beta cells. However, after chronic treatment with sulfonylureas, concentrations of insulin return to the pretreatment values, but the hypoglycemic effect persists. Therefore it is now clear that sulfonylureas also increase insulin sensitivity.

In isolated islet cells, sulfonylureas have little or no effect on insulin release in the absence of glucose, but in the presence of glucose they increase insulin release, sensitizing the beta cells to glucose. The agents act by binding to specific receptors that are coupled to increased entry of Ca^{++} into the beta cells, thus enhancing secretion. The receptor appears to be associated with an ATP-dependent K^+ channel. Binding of sulfonylurea inhibits conductance of the channel. Thus, by decreasing K^+ efflux, sulfonylureas partially depolarize the beta cell membrane. This leads to increased influx of Ca^{++} through voltage-sensitive Ca^{++} channels.

Sulfonylureas enhance the effect of insulin to stimulate glucose uptake into muscle and fat cells. Such ac-carbutamide

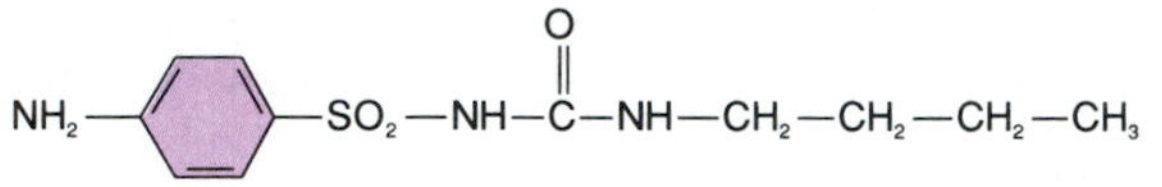

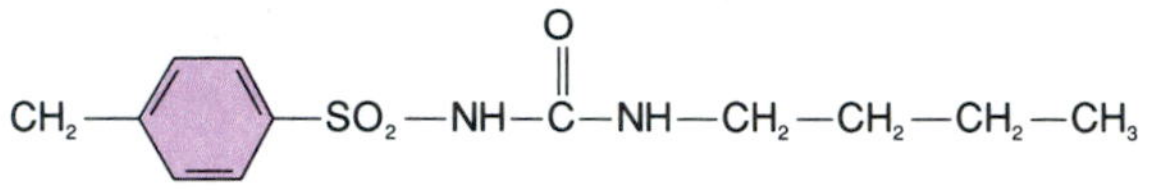

tolbutamide

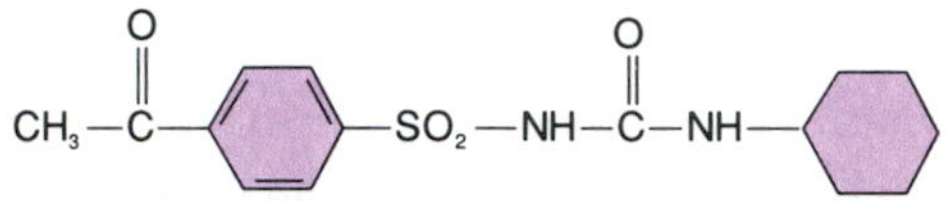

acetohexamide

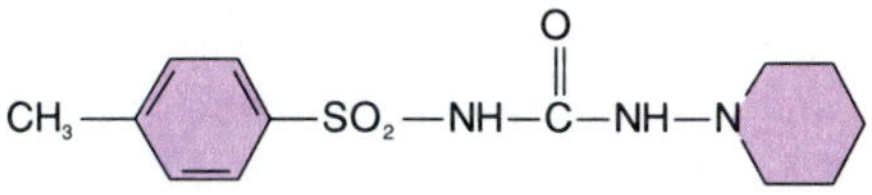

tolazamide

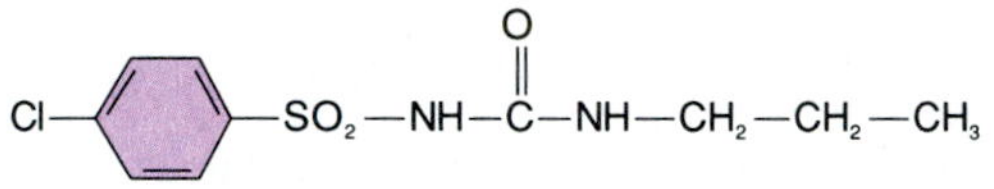

chlorpropamide

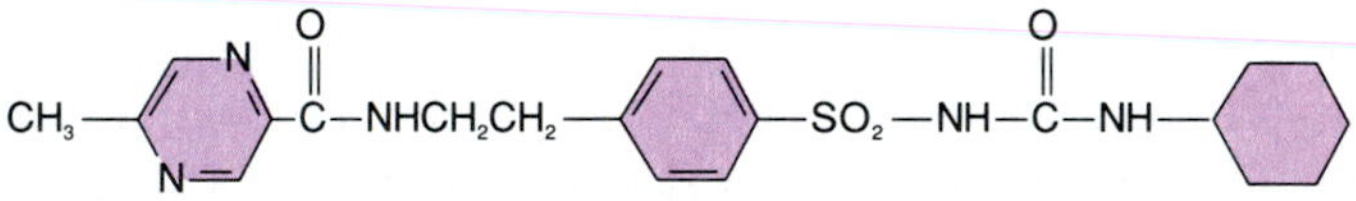

glipizide

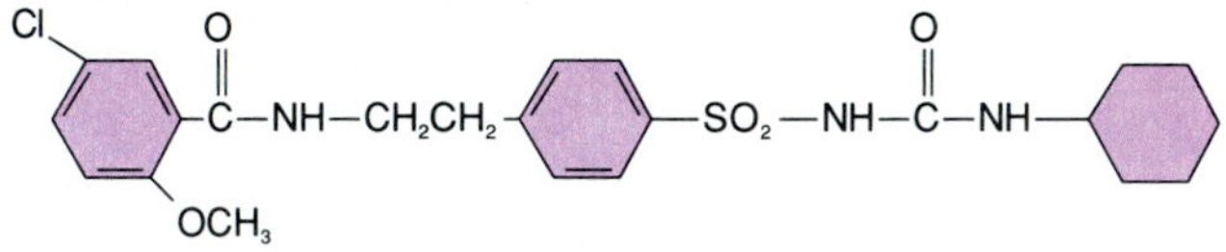

glyburide

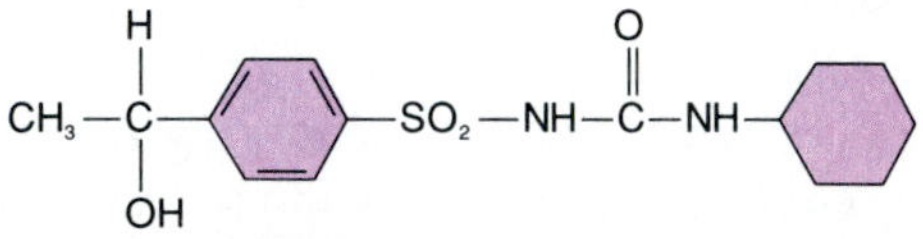

l-hydroxyhexamide (active metabolite of acetohexamide)

FIGURE 39-5 Structures of sulfonylurea hypoglycemic agents. See the text for further information.

Table 39-2 Pharmacokinetic Parameters

Insulin Preparation	Source	Onset (hr)	Duration (hr)
SHORT ACTING			
Crystalline zinc insulin	B, P, H	1	7
Prompt Insulin Zinc Suspension	B, P	1	14
INTERMEDIATE ACTING			
Isophane Insulin Suspension (NPH)	H, B, P	2	24
Insulin Zinc Suspension (Lente)	H, B, P	2	24
LONG ACTING			
Protamine Zinc Insulin Suspension	B, P	4	36
Extended Insulin Zinc Suspension	B, P	4	36

B, Beef; *H,* human; *P,* pork.

tions can be explained, at least in part, by increased sensitivity to insulin.

The first-generation sulfonylureas are tolbutamide, tolazamide, acetohexamide, and chlorpropamide. Glipizide and glyburide are second-generation agents that have been used in Europe for the past 15 years but are now also approved for clinical use in the United States. The structures of the first- and second-generation agents and the common chemical features leading to their classification as sulfonylureas are shown in Figure 39-5. The second-generation drugs are effective at 10 to 100 times lower concentrations, and this difference in potency is a major distinction between the two generations of drugs.

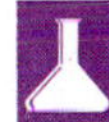

PHARMACOKINETICS

Insulin

Insulin is degraded by proteolytic systems in a variety of tissues, with the liver being the most prominent. In fact, almost half of the insulin released from the pancreas into the portal vein is destroyed by the liver before it can gain access to the general circulation. In humans, the half-life of the circulating hormone is approximately 8 minutes. The effects of insulin on glucose and lipid metabolism occur within minutes of exposing insulin-sensitive cells to the hormone. The onset of action of insulin after IV injections is very rapid, but the duration of action is short. Because of the short half-life, almost all the hormone is cleared within an hour.

All preparations of insulin must be injected. If administered orally, most of the hormone is destroyed by the proteases in the intestinal tract before it can be absorbed. Except in the emergency treatment of diabetic coma, insulin is administered by SC injection. Because of its relatively large size, there is some delay in absorption from the site of injection, and the duration of action is longer than that seen with IV injection. After SC injection, a soluble preparation has an onset of action of approximately 1 hour and a duration of about 6 hours. The original preparations of insulin were soluble, and multiple injections were required to maintain adequate control of blood glucose.

Insulin Preparations The pharmacokinetic parameters for insulin preparations currently available in the United States are summarized in Table 39-2. Crystalline zinc insulin is a clear solution and is the only preparation suitable for IV use. It may be referred to as regular insulin or as crystalline zinc insulin to denote that it was prepared by dissolving crystals of insulin-zinc. The most common use of soluble preparations is in combination with an extended-action insulin to provide a rapid rise in insulin concentrations. Several such longer-acting preparations are now available. A common property of the extended-action preparations is that the insulin is in a precipitated state that can be absorbed only after it has dissolved in the interstitial fluid. Thus the prolonged duration of action is achieved when one creates a depot from which the drug is slowly released, not by increasing the half-life of the circulating drug. *All long-acting preparations of insulin are suspensions, rather than solutions, and should never be injected IV.*

Two extended-action preparations are based on the interaction between insulin and protamine, a basic protein. When insulin is mixed with protamine, a complex of insulin-protamine precipitates. Protamine Zinc Insulin Suspension is a preparation that contains excess protamine so that the insulin dissolves very slowly after injection. Consequently, the preparation has a very long duration of action (approximately 36 hours), too long to achieve good control. Regular insulin cannot be added to achieve a prompt increase in circulating hormone be-

Table 39-3 Pharmacokinetic Properties of Sulfonylureas

Drug	Administered*	$t_{1/2}$ (hr)	Plasma Protein Binding	Duration of Action (hr)	Active Metabolite	Elimination
tolbutamide	Oral	3-5	>90%	6-12	No	95% M, R
acetohexamide	Oral	3-11	>90%	12-18	Strongly active	60% M, R
tolazamide	Oral	7	>90%	12-14	Weakly active	90% M, R
chlorpropamide	Oral	24-48	>90%	60	Yes	90% M, R
glipizide	Oral	3-7	>90%†	24	No	90% M, R
glyburide	Oral	10-16	>90%†	24	No	50% M, R

Half-lives and durations of action vary considerably among individuals, and the values given are approximations.
Metabolite activity refers to the collective hypoglycemic action of the metabolite. *M,* Metabolism; *R,* renal excretion of metabolites.
*All are absorbed from the gastrointestinal tract.
†Not readily displaceable by other ionic-binding drugs.

cause the excess protamine combines with the soluble insulin, converting it to a depot form. To circumvent this problem, a second preparation of insulin that contained low concentrations of uncombined protamine was formulated. This preparation, referred to as either NPH or Isophane Insulin, has a neutral (N) pH, contains protamine (P), and was developed by the Danish scientist Hagedorn (H). Isophane denotes that the preparation contains stoichiometric amounts of insulin and protamine. The onset and duration of action of NPH insulin are shorter than that of Protamine Zinc Insulin Suspension.

The protamine-containing preparations utilized phosphate buffers. If insulin is dissolved in an acetate buffer and excess Zn^{++} is added, the insulin precipitates as either large homogeneous crystals or as small particles. Three preparations of insulin are made from these two precipitated forms. The advantages of these preparations are that they can be mixed in any proportions without impaired activity or stability, and they avoid allergic reactions attributable to protamine while retaining the desired prolonged activity.

Extended Insulin Zinc Suspension is a preparation of the large crystals. These dissolve very slowly at the site of injection so that the onset and duration of action are similar to Protamine Zinc Insulin Suspension. Semilente insulin is a suspension of the small particles. In part because of the large surface area, the crystals dissolve rapidly and the onset and duration of action are similar to crystalline zinc insulin. Insulin Zinc Suspension is a mixture containing 30% semilente and 70% ultralente. The onsets and durations of action are similar to NPH insulin.

Purified insulin has a specific activity of 25 to 30 units/mg. In the United States, the standard insulin preparations contain 100 units/ml, but formulations of 500 units/ml are available for patients with severe insulin resistance.

Insulin is extracted from the pancreases of slaughterhouse animals, mostly cattle and hogs. Although adequate in most cases, there are some problems with these preparations, notably allergic reactions to the animal insulins. Obtaining enough of the hormone to treat all insulin-dependent diabetics worldwide was another problem. These problems have been solved by recombinant DNA technology, which has enabled the large-scale in vitro production of insulin. The recombinant human hormone is now marketed under the tradename Humulin. Another strategy is to prepare human insulin from porcine insulin by converting the alanine in position B-30 to a threonine. Human insulin prepared in this way is marketed as Novolin.

Sulfonylureas

The sulfonylurea drugs share the properties of rapid and complete absorption from the gastrointestinal tract and a high percentage of binding to plasma proteins. Most of the sulfonylurea compounds are converted in the liver to metabolites, which are excreted primarily by the kidney. Hydroxylation reactions are prominent in the metabolism of both first- and second-generation drugs. The hydroxylated products are less lipid soluble and therefore are more rapidly excreted in the urine than their respective parent compounds.

The pharmacokinetic parameters of the sulfonylureas are summarized in Table 39-3. Tolbutamide has the shortest half-life of the agents and is rapidly metabolized in the liver to inactive products. In some cases, the metabolites are active as hypoglycemic agents and thus extend the duration of action of the drug. Tolazamide, the most slowly absorbed, is metabolized to mildly hypoglycemic products, which are rapidly excreted. The metabolism of acetohexamide is notable in that the major metabolite, 1-hydroxyhexamide (see Figure 39-5), is even more active in lowering blood glucose than the parent compound. Although extensively metabolized by the liver, chlorpropamide has the longest half-life and is administered only once daily. The half-lives of glyburide

SOME FACTORS THAT CONTROL THE RELEASE OF ENDOGENOUS INSULIN

STIMULATE	INHIBIT
NUTRIENTS	
Glucose	
Amino acids	
Fatty acids	
Ketone bodies	
HORMONES	
Secretin	Somatostatin
Glucagon	
Pancreozymin	
Gastrin	
Vasoactive intestinal peptide	
Gastric inhibitory polypeptide	
DRUGS	
β-Adrenergic agonists	α-Adrenergic agonists
Cholinergic agonists	
Sulfonylureas	

and glipizide are both approximately 24 hours, and these drugs are metabolized to inactive products by the liver. All of the sulfonylureas bind appreciably to plasma proteins; however, the first-generation drugs are displaceable by other ionic binding drugs, but the second-generation drugs are not readily displaceable.

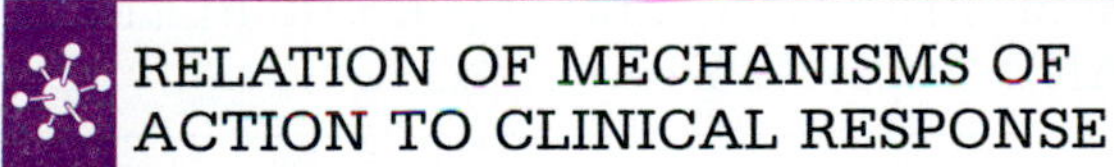

RELATION OF MECHANISMS OF ACTION TO CLINICAL RESPONSE

Insulin

The most important stimulus for release of endogenous insulin is glucose. In keeping with the function of insulin in stimulating storage of nutrients, many of the breakdown products of complex nutrient molecules also stimulate insulin release. These include amino acids, fatty acids, and ketones (see box). In addition, hormones including secretin, pancreozymin, and glucagon stimulate release. These hormones are elaborated from the intestinal tract in response to products of digestion, and their actions on the beta cell explain why insulin concentrations sometimes increase after a meal before glucose concentrations rise.

In fasting humans, approximately 90% of insulin-like activity in serum is not attributable to insulin. This activity became known as nonsuppressible insulin-like activity because it was not suppressed by addition of anti-insulin antibodies to the serum. The substances responsible for nonsuppressible insulin-like activity have been identified as IGF-1 and IGF-2. These growth factors circulate bound to specific carrier proteins. When complexed with these proteins, the IGFs are incapable of interacting with their cellular receptors. Furthermore, unlike concentrations of insulin, IGF concentrations are not controlled by glucose. Consequently, although the actions of IGFs are similar to those of insulin, it is clear that they cannot compensate for the insulin deficit in diabetes mellitus.

ACTIONS OF INSULIN

METABOLISM	ACTION
Carbohydrate metabolism	Increases glucose transport
	Increases glycogen synthesis
	Increases pentose shunt activity
	Increases glucose oxidation
	Decreases gluconeogenesis
Lipid metabolism	Increases fatty acid transport
	Increases triglyceride synthesis (includes fatty acid synthesis and esterification)
	Decreases lipolysis
Protein metabolism	Increases amino acid transport
	Increases protein synthesis (including mRNA transcription and translation)
	Decreases degradation

Carbohydrate Metabolism

The classic action of insulin is to lower blood glucose concentration. Various effects that contribute to the uptake and storage of glucose are summarized in the box.

Insulin stimulates the transport of glucose by facilitated diffusion into muscle and fat cells by promoting translocation of GLUT-4 to the cell surface.

Insulin does not stimulate glucose transport in liver. Glucose transport in hepatocytes is mediated by

GLUT-2. In contrast to the distribution of GLUT-4 in muscle and fat cells, almost all the GLUT-2 is found in the plasma membrane, even in the absence of insulin. However, insulin does act on hepatocytes to inhibit gluconeogenesis, an important action in decreasing blood sugar. Hormonal regulation of glucose production by liver and glucose utilization by muscle, fat, and other tissues is an example of the type of dual control of synthetic and degradative pathways.

Although effects of insulin on gluconeogenesis are restricted to the liver, the hormone affects the activities of a variety of intracellular enzymes involved in energy storage in all the major insulin sensitive tissues. As a result glucose is efficiently converted to glycogen, triglyceride, and protein.

The stimulation of glycogen synthesis by insulin involves dephosphorylation and activation of glycogen synthase, the enzyme catalyzing the rate-limiting step in glycogen synthesis from glucose. This effect was the first clear-cut example of an action of insulin on the activity of an intracellular enzyme.

Lipid Metabolism

Insulin exerts a variety of actions to decrease the concentration of serum lipids (see Box, p. 533). Because of their low water solubility, lipids are transported in blood primarily as particles composed of cholesterol esters complexed with proteins (termed *lipoproteins*). Before the fatty acids can be taken up into cells, the cholesterol esters must be hydrolyzed. The activity of lipoprotein lipase, the enzyme catalyzing this reaction, is stimulated by insulin.

Insulin also stimulates fatty acid synthesis. Dephosphorylation and activation of two key enzymes in the synthetic pathway, pyruvate dehydrogenase and acetyl CoA carboxylase, are involved in this effect of the hormone. Although synthesis is increased, the concentration of free fatty acids is decreased in response to insulin because the hormone decreases lipolysis and increases the rate of fatty acid esterification to form triglyceride. Stimulation of glucose transport into fat cells increases the supply of glycerol phosphate used in esterification. Inhibition of lipolysis involves dephosphorylation and inactivation of triglyceride lipase.

Protein Metabolism

Insulin increases protein synthesis in various cells by stimulation of several steps in the synthetic pathway. Control at the transcriptional level is evident by increases in specific mRNA species. Insulin also stimulates the rate of amino acid transport, increasing the precursors for protein synthesis. It has not been determined whether amino acid transporters are translocated to the membrane in response to insulin. Insulin also increases the rate of translation of mRNA into protein. The finding of increased phosphorylation of ribosomal protein S6 in response to insulin in some cells indicates that phosphorylation of the ribosome may be involved. Finally, insulin decreases the rate of proteolysis, an action that is more sensitive to insulin than the increase in protein synthesis.

Glucagon

Glucagon is used therapeutically to increase blood glucose concentrations in patients with hypoglycemia who are unable to take glucose orally. Its chief use, however, is in radiology. When administered with a radiopaque substance, it relaxes the gastrointestinal smooth muscles, allowing better visualization of tumors and other gastrointestinal disorders.

Glucagon, which has a positive inotropic effect on the heart, can be useful in the treatment of overdosage with β-adrenergic-blocking drugs.

Sulfonylureas

The relative contributions to the hypoglycemic effect of the actions of sulfonylureas on enhancing insulin sensitivity and on promoting insulin release are still being debated. However, both of these actions require the presence of insulin, either circulating or in the beta cells. Thus *sulfonylureas are ineffective in treating IDDM.* Their usefulness is restricted to the therapy of some cases of NIDDM.

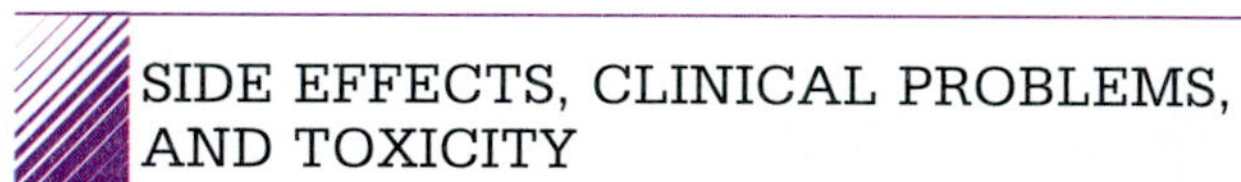

SIDE EFFECTS, CLINICAL PROBLEMS, AND TOXICITY

Problems in Achieving Good Control

The IDDM patient is absolutely dependent on administration of exogenous insulin for normal growth, and to prevent ketosis and death. In contrast, the NIDDM patient may appear to function normally without treatment of any kind. However, the disease has serious complications that are insidious in nature. Seriously impaired function of the renal, nervous, and circulatory systems may develop in both the IDDM and NIDDM patients. In a large multicenter clinical trial it was recently proved that good control of diabetes did prevent, or at least delay, the development of long-term complications.

Maintaining glucose homeostasis with exogenous insulin is complicated by several factors. A major problem is that control of blood glucose cannot be achieved with a fixed concentration of insulin. Blood concentrations of insulin fluctuate dramatically in normal individuals. Figure 39-6 depicts hypothetical changes in blood glucose and insulin concentrations over a 24-hour period. During a period of fasting, as occurs at night in most people, concentrations of insulin and glucose are low. After a meal, the rise in blood glucose is attenuated because insulin concentrations also increase. Without insulin, blood glucose could increase to 500 mg/dl or higher. The pancreatic control system maintains tight control of glucose concentrations by releasing insulin in proportion to need. Thus, serum glucose concentrations are maintained within a relatively narrow range, even though food intake varies greatly. After a light snack, insulin concentrations might double, but after a large meal, the hormone concentration may increase by tenfold or more.

Any of several factors can cause insulin sensitivity to change, foiling even conscientious attempts at control. Exercise or ethanol can greatly increase insulin sensitivity, thus decreasing the hormonal requirement. This is frequently the cause of insulin-induced hypoglycemia. Stress, pregnancy, or drugs including thiazide diuretics and β-adrenergic receptor blockers decrease insulin sensitivity and exacerbate the signs and symptoms of diabetes mellitus.

Insulin

Delivering insulin so that it peaks in a pattern matching that seen in the nondiabetic subject is an objective that is difficult to achieve. If the insulin concentrations do not decrease as blood glucose falls, hypoglycemia ensues. In most cases multiple injections of a short-acting insulin preparation are used to produce the peaks in insulin concentrations, and an extended-action preparation is used to establish a base-line concentration.

Administering insulin with constant infusion pumps provides a means to control more precisely the concentration of circulating insulin, and there is evidence that tighter control of blood glucose is possible with these devices. Unfortunately, there is some reason to believe that simply mimicking the normal circulating insulin concentrations might not be sufficient to prevent diabetic complications. This concern arises from the relationship of the pancreas and liver in the circulatory system. Insulin is released directly into the portal vein and passes through the liver before it reaches the peripheral circulation. More than half the insulin is degraded by a single pass through the liver. Consequently, in normal individuals the hepatic tissues are exposed to insulin concentrations more than twice as high as in the vascular beds of skeletal muscle or adipose tissue. When exogenous insulin is injected in an insulin-dependent diabetic to achieve a normal blood concentration of the hormone, that concentration may be insufficient to initiate appropriate responses in the liver. Pancreas or islet transplantation may ultimately provide a solution to this problem.

Side Effects Insulin has relatively few side effects. The most common are localized fat accumulation or atrophy, allergic reactions, and hypoglycemia.

The insulin concentration is highest at the site of injection. When the hormone is repeatedly administered at the same site, there is a tendency of the adipose tissue to hypertrophy in the surrounding region. This is presumably caused by the action of insulin to promote triglyceride accumulation in fat cells. The problem can be corrected by rotation of sites of injection, a practice now routinely encouraged. Atrophy of adipose tissue at the site of injection has also been a frequent problem in

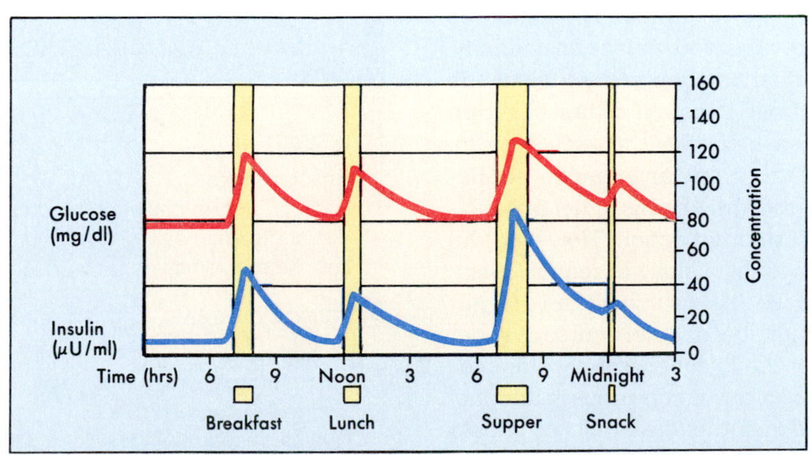

FIGURE 39-6 Typical profile of insulin and glucose concentrations in a normal individual.

the past. This is hard to explain in terms of the defined actions of insulin and is most likely caused by stimulation of lipolysis by contaminants, possibly glucagon, in the insulin preparations. At any rate the incidence of lipoatrophy is lower with the highly purified insulin preparations now available. In fact, injection at the atrophic sites with the new purified insulin preparations has been successful in treating the atrophy.

Allergic reactions occur in a small percentage of individuals, mostly those receiving beef insulin. This occurs because this insulin differs from the human hormone (see Figure 39-4), and is recognized as a foreign substance by the immune system. In some cases, the antibodies are produced in sufficient quantity to increase the concentration of insulin needed therapeutically. Fortunately, the problem associated with allergic reactions can be corrected when one changes from beef insulin to porcine insulin, which is closer to the human hormone, or to recombinant human insulin.

Hypoglycemia is a serious complication and results when circulating insulin concentrations are too high. Among the causes are mistakes in calculating the dosage or in injecting the hormone, changes in eating patterns, or a reduction in insulin requirement. The brain and nervous tissue have an absolute requirement for glucose. When severe, hypoglycemia can cause loss of consciousness, convulsions, brain damage, and death. Therefore the physician and associates of the diabetic patient must be able to recognize the signs and correct the cause of hypoglycemia.

Symptoms of hypoglycemia are generally attributable either to increases in epinephrine or to abnormal functioning of the CNS, or both. When the fall in blood glucose is rapid, epinephrine is released as a compensatory measure to stimulate hepatic glucose production and mobilization of energy reserves. Rapid heart rate, headache, cold sweat, weakness, and trembling are characteristic responses to the catecholamine. The extent to which these symptoms are observed varies considerably, depending on the individual and the rate of fall of the blood glucose concentration. Impaired neural function leads to blurred vision, an incoherent speech pattern, and mental confusion. At this point, an experienced diabetic might be capable of recognizing his or her hypoglycemic state and taking corrective action. However, the mentally disoriented individual is likely to require assistance. The remedy is glucose. If the subject is able, a glucose tablet, candy bar, fruit juice, or other source of sugar may be given. Because of the likelihood of choking, administering food or drink to an unconscious individual should never be attempted. In this case glucose should be administered intravenously by a trained health care professional. Glucagon can also be administered under these circumstances to raise blood glucose.

The unconscious hypoglycemic state induced by overdosage of insulin is referred to as *insulin coma*. Unfortunately, insulin coma is sometimes confused with diabetic coma. The two conditions have opposite causes, and the therapeutic intervention strategies are fundamentally different. Diabetic coma is the result of a chain of events set into motion by an insulin deficit and ultimately involves ketoacidosis, electrolyte imbalance, and dehydration. This condition usually develops over days or weeks, whereas with insulin coma, the patient may be well one minute and seriously debilitated a few minutes later. Thus when the onset is rapid, insulin coma should be suspected, particularly if it is known that the subject has recently received an injection of the hormone.

Even when diabetic coma is suspected, it is good practice to first administer glucose. In the event of a mistaken diagnosis, a hypoglycemic patient will recover as soon as blood glucose concentrations are increased, provided that there is no brain damage. It should be remembered that administering insulin to a patient in insulin coma could easily cause death; giving glucose to a patient in diabetic coma will do no harm, particularly since the subject may actually be hypoglycemic because of the depletion of energy stores. It should also be noted that treatment of diabetic coma involves much more than injections with insulin and should be attempted only in the proper clinical setting where glucose and electrolyte concentrations can be monitored and maintained at proper concentrations.

Sulfonylureas For the past two decades, the use of sulfonylureas in treating non–insulin dependent diabetes mellitus has been controversial. The controversy arose from results of the University Group Diabetes Program (UGDP), a large long-term clinical trial involving 12 university medical centers. The goal of the UGDP

CLINICAL PROBLEMS

INSULIN

Hypoglycemia
Local or systemic allergic reactions
Visual disturbances
Peripheral edema

SULFONYLUREAS

Hypoglycemia
Gastrointestinal disturbances
Hematological disturbances
Flushing especially with concurrent alcohol ingestion
Contraindicated with hepatic or renal insufficiency
Drug interactions

was to determine whether insulin therapy or orally administered hypoglycemic agents were of any benefit in delaying the onset of diabetic complications. Several years into the study, some subjects, notably elderly women, treated with tolbutamide appeared to be dying from cardiovascular disease at a higher rate than individuals in the control groups, and tolbutamide was withdrawn from the trial. Understandably, the UGDP has become best known for its implications concerning the safety of tolbutamide and, by association, the other sulfonylurea hypoglycemic agents.

If sulfonylureas were known to place patients at increased risk of death, their use could not be justified, particularly since insulin affords an effective though less convenient alternative for treating the non–insulin dependent diabetic. Questions that cast serious doubt on the validity of the UGDP's conclusion regarding tolbutamide have been raised. For example, it has been pointed out that only 26% of the patients assigned to the original test groups actually remained in that group throughout the study, and the patients assigned to the tolbutamide group appeared to have had more risk factors (e.g., high blood pressure or elevated serum cholesterol) to begin with. Such problems have prompted the American Diabetes Association to withdraw its support of the UGDP's stance on tolbutamide. Nonetheless, the question of the safety of tolbutamide has not been put to rest.

Side Effects Depending on the sulfonylurea being taken, the incidence of side effects of some type ranges between 3% and 66%. These side effects are usually not serious and the drugs are considered relatively safe, with the possible exception discussed above. The most frequent complication is hypoglycemia, which may be brought on by overdosage, increased insulin sensitivity, change in dietary pattern, or increased energy expenditure. If the hypoglycemic response is mild, it can be corrected by decreasing the dose of the drug. However, severe cases may persist for days after withdrawal of the drug, and require multiple injections of glucose.

Because of the high degree of binding to serum proteins, the potential exists for interactions with other drugs (e.g., phenylbutazone or salicylates) that compete for serum binding sites. This is particularly true for the first-generation drugs tolbutamide, acetohexamide, tolazamide, and chlorpropamide, which bind to serum albumin chiefly by ionic interactions and therefore can be displaced by other drugs. The second generation drugs glipizide and glyburide bind to albumin by nonionic interactions and are less readily displaced by other drugs.

Gastrointestinal disturbances, allergic reactions, dermatological problems, and transient leukopenia can be expected in a small percentage of cases. A disulfiram type of response (i.e., flushing) when taken with alcohol is sometimes a problem, particularly with chlorpropamide. This drug is the only sulfonylurea that causes fluid retention, an effect that appears to be a result of stimulation of the release of antidiuretic hormone.

TRADE NAMES

In addition to generic and fixed combination preparations, the following trade-named materials are available in the United States.

INSULIN

Short acting
- Humulin R, Novolin R, Velosin; human insulin
- Iletin Regular, insulin
- Iletin Semilente, Insulin Zinc Suspension

Intermediate acting
- Humulin L, Novolin L; human insulin zinc suspension (intermediate)
- Humulin N, Novolin N; Isophane Insulin human
- Insulabard NPH, Isophane Human Insulin
- Lente, Insulin Zinc Suspension (intermediate)
- NPH Iletin, Isophane Insulin
- NPH insulin, Isophane Insulin

Long acting
- Protamine Zinc Iletin, Protamine Zinc Insulin Suspension
- Ultralente Iletin, Insulin Zinc Suspension (Extended)

SULFONYLUREAS

Diabinase, chlorpropamide
Dymelor, acetohexamide
Glucotrol, glipizide
Micronase, DiaBeta; glyburide
Orinase, tolbutamide
Tolinase, Ronase, tolazamide

Contraindications

Therapy is contraindicated in individuals not having a proved pancreatic reserve of insulin. Attention to the metabolism and route of excretion of the drugs is required before one begins sulfonylurea therapy in subjects with impaired hepatic or renal function. In these cases, treatment with insulin may be the best choice. Teratogenic effects of sulfonylureas have not been reported, but because of the possibility of such effects and adverse reactions in the newborn, the drugs should not be administered to pregnant or lactating women. Problems are summarized in the box.

Unlike sulfonylureas, biguanides have little hypoglycemic action in nondiabetic subjects, and "antihyperglycemic" might be a more appropriate adjective for describing these agents. Biguanides inhibit the absorption

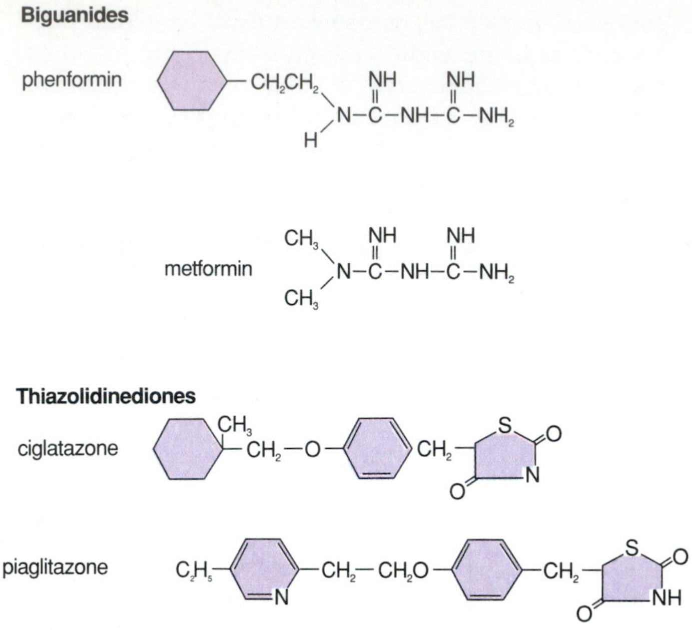

Biguanides

phenformin

metformin

Thiazolidinediones

ciglatazone

piaglitazone

FIGURE 39-7 Structures of biguanide and thiazolidinedione drugs. See the text for further information.

of glucose from the gut, and it is clear that this effect contributes to the lowering of blood glucose. Other effects including decreased hepatic output of glucose and increased glucose uptake by muscle and fat cells have been reported in experimental animals.

Thiazolidinediones do not cause insulin release, and in insulin-resistant animal models they actually increase the insulin content of pancreatic islets. The mechanism of action of the agents is still incompletely understood, but they appear to sensitize the target tissues (muscle, liver, and fat) to insulin by increasing the numbers of glucose transporters and insulin receptors. Since the agents act primarily by increasing insulin sensitivity, rather than insulin release, they show potential for the therapy of NIDDM and perhapsin IDDM when insulin resistance is a problem.

NEW DIRECTIONS

In IDDM, progress is being made in the identification of several candidate autoantigens that may be involved in the pathophysiology of the autoimmune islet beta-cell destruction. Specific mutations in the DQ locus of the histocompatability leukocyte antigens (HLA) have also been implicated. A significant therapeutic advance has been the surgical transplantation of the pancreas and kidney in patients with advanced disease. Trials of antiinflammatory, immunosuppressive interventional therapy in at-risk populations are being designed. A multi center trial with insulin as a possible prophylactic agent for prevention of type I diabetes has begun.

In NIDDM, the insulin resistance has been defined as postreceptor, mainly in muscle, related chiefly (70% to 80%) but not exclusively to nonoxidative glucose disposal and is likely genetic in nature. The beta-cell glucose secretory stimulation defect is under active investigation with a possible relationship to a defect in the glucokinase enzyme under consideration.

A genetic investigation of maturity onset diabetes of youth (MODY) has localized the genetic defect to chromosome 20 with mutations in the glucokinase gene. Mutations in the insulin receptor, glucokinase and the mitochondrial genome have been described in specific families with NIDDM. Chromosome 4 q locus has been associated with insulin resistance in Pima Indians. Thus progress is being made on the genetic heterogeneity of NIDDM.

REFERENCES

Bressler R, Johnson D: New pharmacological approaches to the therapy of NIDDM, *Diabetes Care* 15:792, 1992.

Larner J: Insulin signaling mechanisms, *Diabetes* 37:262, 1988.

Lawrence JC Jr: Signal transduction and protein phosphorylation in the control of cellular metabolism by insulin, *Annu Rev Physiol* 54:177, 1992.

Lebovitz HE: Oral hypoglycemic agents, *J Primary Care* 15:353, 1988.

Saltiel AR, Cuatrecasas P: In search of a second messenger for insulin, *Am J Physiol* 255 (*Cell Physiol* 24):C1, 1988.

Santiago JV: Overview of complications of diabetes. *Clin Chem* 32 (suppl 10):B48, 1986.

Shank WA Jr, Morrison AD: Oral sulfonylureas for the treatment of type II diabetes: an update, *South Med J* 79:337, 1986.

SELF-ASSESSMENT QUESTIONS

All of the following are true except one.

1. Insulin action involves:
   a. stimulation of glycogen synthesis in muscle fiber.
   b. inhibition of lipolysis in the adipocyte.
   c. stimulation of fatty acid synthesis in the hepatocyte.
   d. stimulation of K^+ uptake in muscle fiber.
   e. stimulation of gluconeogenesis in the hepatocyte.
2. All of the following are true except:
   a. regular insulin is frequently used in combination with other preparations.

b. Protamine Zinc Insulin has the longest duration of action of various insulin preparations.
c. Semilente contains protamine-zinc and acetate.
d. NPH insulin has an intermediate duration of action.
e. regular insulin is used to treat acidosis and coma.

3. All of the following are true except:
   a. acetohexamide is metabolized to a compound having more hypoglycemic action than the parent compound.
   b. chlorpropamide causes ADH release.
   c. pioglitazone is a novel agent that acts to sensitize insulin action.
   d. tolbutamide causes hyperpolarization of the beta-cell plasma membrane.
   e. biguanides such as metformin and phenformin have been removed from the approved drugs in the United States because of their metabolic effects to cause acidosis.
4. All of the following are true except:
   a. sulfonylureas are useful in treating IDDM.
   b. sulfonylureas stimulate insulin release from the beta cells of the islets.
   c. sulfonylureas act chronically to sensitize peripheral tissues to insulin.
   d. sulfonylureas can lose their efficacy in a proportion of patients with continued therapy.
   e. sulfonylureas can cause hypoglycemia as a side effect.
5. All of the following are true except:
   a. insulin-stimulated glucose transport involves translocation to the cell membrane and activation of a specific glucose transporter, GLUT-4, in insulin-sensitive tissues such as muscle and fat.
   b. there exists a family of glucose-transporter molecules that is widely distributed in all tissues.
   c. GLUT-4, the insulin-sensitive glucose transporter, is responsible for glucose entry into the CNS.
   d. the insulin receptor contains a tyrosine kinase domain in the β subunit.
   e. there is activated a set of phosphorylation and dephosphorylation events by the initial interaction of insulin with its receptor.
6. The onset and duration of action of NPH insulin are extended because:
   a. protamine decreases the rate at which insulin is absorbed.
   b. protamine blocks insulin metabolism in the liver.
   c. protamine is basic and combines with insulin by charge interactions.
   d. protamine is slowly degraded proteolytically releasing the bound insulin.
   e. protamine is a foreign protein made from animal sources.

CHAPTER 40

Drugs Affecting Uterine Motility

HAROLD E. FOX
THEODORE M. BRODY

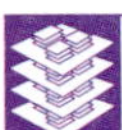

THERAPEUTIC OVERVIEW

Neuroendocrine mechanisms that initiate and control uterine contractility during pregnancy and parturition are complex. Regulation of myometrial (uterine) smooth muscle contraction involves changes in cell membrane function and hormone-receptor interactions.

The initiation and maintenance of uterine contractility involve an alteration in the hormonal milieu. Throughout pregnancy, the effects of high concentrations of progesterone predominate to suppress uterine smooth muscle contractility. Progesterone hyperpolarizes uterine smooth muscle membranes, making the muscle nonexcitable. It also prevents the release of arachidonic acid, the precursor for prostaglandin synthesis. Oxytocin concentrations and the number of oxytocin receptors increase slightly during gestation and may have a permissive role in early labor. However, oxytocin concentration and receptor number do rise significantly during the later stages of labor.

As parturition approaches, the major change in the hormonal environment is an increase in the estrogen-to-progesterone ratio. The increased concentrations of estrogen increase the number of gap junctions that electrically couple myometrial muscle cells. This enhances intercellular communication and raises the resting potential of the cell membrane. In addition, the number of receptors increases greatly for the following contractile agonists: oxytocin, angiotensin, and α-adrenergic receptor agents—heightening the sensitivity of the myometrial cells to contractile stimuli. Increases in fetal estrogen may stimulate prostaglandin biosynthesis, thereby promoting contractions of the myometrium.

Two major classes of drugs affect uterine motility: uterine stimulants and uterine relaxants. Uterine stimulants are used to facilitate parturition, manage postpartum hemorrhage, or stimulate uterine contraction during a therapeutic abortion. Uterine relaxants (tocolytic agents) inhibit uterine contraction and are used primarily to arrest premature labor.

The therapeutic overview is summarized in the box.

ABBREVIATIONS	
cAMP	cyclic adenosine monophosphate
MLCK	myosin light-chain kinase
PGE_2, $PGF_2\alpha$	prostaglandins E_2 and $F_2\alpha$

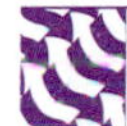

MECHANISMS OF ACTION

Uterine Contraction

The biochemical and molecular events involved in uterine smooth muscle contraction are the same as those that control other smooth muscle tissues (see Chapter 17).

Assuming that the changes previously described in the hormonal environment and in the number of the several hormone receptors on the myometrial cell membrane have taken place before parturition, the uterine

THERAPEUTIC OVERVIEW

UTERINE STIMULATION
Induction of labor
Augmentation of labor
Therapeutic abortion
Postpartum hemorrhage control

UTERINE RELAXATION
Arrest premature labor

DRUGS USED TO PROMOTE UTERINE CONTRACTION OR RELAXATION

ACTION	AGENT
Uterine stimulation	oxytocin prostaglandins
Uterine relaxation tocolysis	β-adrenergic receptor agonists including isoxsuprine, terbutaline, and ritodrine prostaglandin synthesis inhibitors including indomethacin magnesium sulfate calcium-channel blockers diazoxide

smooth muscle is sensitized for contraction to occur. As with other smooth muscles, actin and myosin must interact for uterine contraction to occur, and this depends on phosphorylation of myosin light chains. This phosphorylation in turn is dependent on the activity of myosin light-chain kinase (MLCK), a key enzyme in uterine contraction. MLCK-driven phosphorylation requires cellular Ca^{++} concentrations of 10^{-6} M or more. Additionally the enzyme is active only if associated with calmodulin, and formation of the MLCK-calmodulin complex also is Ca^{++} dependent (see Chapter 17).

Various hormones and drugs interact to enhance the contractile state of the uterus and are used therapeutically to induce or augment uterine contractions. In addition, some drugs may be used in the treatment of postpartum hemorrhage. The types of drugs that promote uterine stimulation are listed in the box. The ergot alkaloids (α-adrenergic receptor agonists) are used in the control of postpartum hemorrhage.

Oxytocin, a nonapeptide (Figure 40-1), is synthesized in the supraoptic and paraventricular nucleus of the hypothalamus and is released from the posterior pituitary. A role for oxytocin in initiation or propagation of normal labor has been postulated for many years, but only small increases in concentrations of oxytocin have been demonstrated before the onset of labor. However, the concentration of oxytocin in maternal serum does increase significantly during the later stages of labor. The number of myometrial oxytocin receptors also increases greatly. The interaction of endogenous or administered oxytocin with myometrial cell membrane receptors pro-

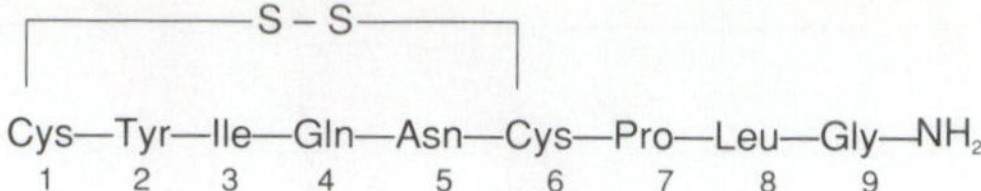

FIGURE 40-1 Structure of oxytocin, a cyclic disulfide-linked nonapeptide that stimulates uterine smooth muscle contraction. See the text for further information.

motes the influx of Ca^{++} from the extracellular fluid and from the sarcoplasmic reticulum into the cell. This increase in cytoplasmic calcium stimulates uterine contraction by activation of myosin light-chain kinase, as discussed previously. In addition, oxytocin acts together with prostaglandins to facilitate uterine smooth muscle contraction.

α-Adrenergic agonists used to stimulate uterine smooth muscle contraction include ergot alkaloids, ergonovine maleate and methylergonovine maleate. The mechanism involves a drug-uterine receptor interaction. The hormone receptor complex facilitates the entry of Ca^{++} into the cell, probably by opening calcium channels through the enzymatic phosphorylation of specific membrane phospholipids. The increase in intracellular cytosolic Ca^{++} facilitates smooth muscle contraction. The sensitivity of the uterus to ergot alkaloids increases steadily during pregnancy, and the number of α-adrenergic receptors increases as the estrogen/progesterone ratio heightens at term.

Prostaglandins are the most recent addition to the list of uterine stimulants. These drugs, discussed in Chapter 18, are formed by action of several enzymes on arachidonic acid. The major prostaglandins important in pregnancy and parturition are E_2 (PGE_2), and $F_{2\alpha}$ ($PGF_{2\alpha}$) (Figure 40-2).

The mechanism by which prostaglandins PGE_2 and $PGF_{2\alpha}$ lead to increased uterine contractility is not well understood but may result from their action on cell surface receptors to moderate cAMP and cAMP-dependent protein kinase activities (see Chapter 17). Decreases in cAMP concentrations may increase myosin light-chain kinase activity and cause contraction. In addition, prostaglandins, in conjunction with oxytocin, may enhance Ca^{++} release into the cytosol.

In summary, the overall mechanisms by which uterine stimulants enhance myometrial smooth muscle contraction are through (1) a receptor-mediated increase in cytosolic (i.e., intracellular) Ca^{++} or (2) an alteration in the production of cAMP. For the effect of these agents to occur, the uterus must be "hormonally primed" so that concentrations of oxytocin, α-adrenergic, and prostadinoprostone (PGE_2)

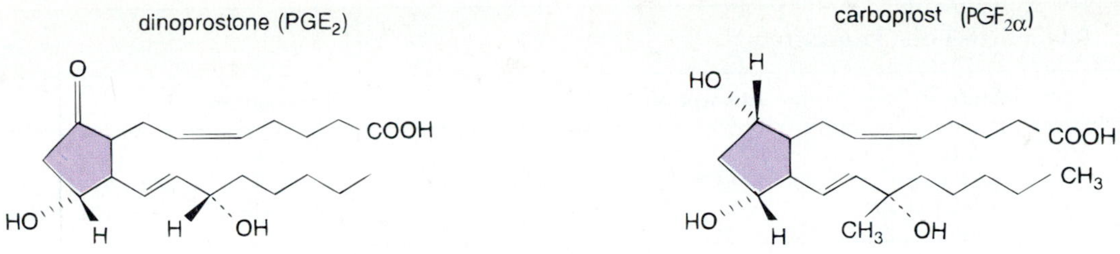

carboprost ($PGF_{2\alpha}$)

FIGURE 40-2 Structures of uterine-stimulant prostaglandins. See the text for further information.

glandin receptors have increased above their early pregnancy values.

Uterine Relaxation

Uterine smooth muscle relaxation is modulated by two distinct regulatory pathways that utilize cAMP. The first mechanism involves inhibition of myosin light-chain kinase through action of a cAMP-mediated protein kinase (see Chapter 17). In addition, cAMP promotes the accumulation of Ca^{++} in the sarcoplasmic reticulum, thus decreasing the concentration of cytosolic calcium. The concentrations of cAMP are determined by two specific enzymatic activities (i.e., synthesis by adenylate cyclase and degradation by cAMP phosphodiesterase). Stimulation of β-adrenergic receptors leads to increased adenylate cyclase activity and subsequent increases in cAMP concentration. These biochemical pathways can be modulated by pharmacological agents to promote relaxation of uterine smooth muscle.

The chief use of uterine relaxants or tocolytic agents is in the arrest of premature labor. Ethanol and inhibitors of prostaglandin synthesis (e.g., indomethacin) act indirectly and prevent the synthesis or release of endogenous uterine stimulants. Magnesium sulfate and β-adrenergic drugs act directly to suppress the contractile response of the myometrial smooth muscle.

Ethanol has been the most widely used tocolytic agent for inhibiting premature labor. Based on the observation that ethanol suppresses antidiuretic hormone release from the posterior pituitary gland, it has been hypothesized that ethanol could suppress oxytocin release and result in uterine relaxation. Analysis of the myometrial dose response to oxytocin before and after administration of ethanol indicates, however, that ethanol not only decreases oxytocin release, but also acts directly on the myometrial cell membrane. Ethanol also may stimulate β-adrenergic receptors, which results in the production of increased concentrations of cAMP. The increased concentrations of cAMP promote relaxation of the uterus.

Prostaglandin synthesis inhibitors (e.g., indomethacin) are theoretically useful for retarding premature labor. This is based on the observation that depletion of prostaglandins prevents stimulation of the uterus by oxytocin agonists; the addition of prostaglandins restores the potency of oxytocin. It is believed that prostaglandin-synthesis inhibitor drugs block spontaneous uterine contractions by reducing the amount of prostaglandins synthesized and released by myometrial cells.

The β-adrenergic receptor agonists are the most recently added class of tocolytic agents. These drugs (i.e., isoxsuprine, terbutaline, ritodrine; structures shown in Chapter 10) are similar in structure to epinephrine. The drugs have a greater effect on β_2-adrenergic receptors (uterus and lung) than β_1-receptors (particularly the heart). These β-adrenergic drugs bind to β_2-adrenergic receptors on the outer surface of the cell membranes of the myometrial cells, activating adenylate cyclase. ATP is converted to cAMP, which activates protein kinases to phosphorylate cellular proteins. The phosphorylated proteins act to sequester intracellular Ca^{++} within the sarcoplasmic reticulum or to inactivate the MLCK. The decrease in intracellular calcium prevents the activation of the actin and myosin elements and therefore inhibits uterine contraction.

There are three other drugs that play a less significant role as uterine relaxants. The calcium-channel blockers (i.e., nifedipine and nicardipine) inhibit the entry of calcium into smooth muscle cells and have been shown to decrease uterine contractility in various animal studies. Up to now these drugs have had only limited use in human pregnancy because potential negative effects on the fetus still need to be clarified. Diazoxide, a potent vasodilator agent known to inhibit uterine activity, is administered to treat hypertensive crises during pregnancy. The mechanism for tocolysis may involve a direct effect on uterine smooth muscle or may involve stimulation of the release of catecholamines. This drug has major side effects that limit its usefulness as a first-line tocolytic agent.

Parenteral administration of magnesium sulfate inhibits uterine contraction. The mechanism of action re-

Table 40-1 Pharmacokinetic Parameters*

Drug	Route	Absorption	$t_{1/2}$	Disposition
Oxytocin	IV, IM	Degraded	1-6 min	Metabolized in liver, kidney
Ergonovine	PO, IM, IV	Fairly well	Several hours	Metabolized in liver, bile
Prostaglandins	IV, IM, IA†, oral	—	—	Metabolized in many tissues, especially lung

0.5 mg, 1 IU for oxytocin.
*Values for uterine stimulants only; values for uterine relaxants are in other chapters (see text).
†Intraamniotic.

sults from ionic magnesium antagonizing the action of Ca^{++} in myometrial cells. The drug may exert its effect by (1) decreasing the frequency of myometrial muscle cell action potentials, (2) uncoupling the excitation and contraction of the uterine smooth muscle cells, or (3) directly relaxing the contractile elements.

PHARMACOKINETICS

Uterine stimulants often are administered by slow IV infusion to maintain control of the response. Oxytocin undergoes hydrolytic cleavage in the gastrointestinal tract if given orally. Ergonovine maleate and its methyl analog both are well absorbed when administered orally. Disposition of oxytocin, ergonovine, and PGE_2 or $PGF_{2\alpha}$ is mainly by metabolism to inactive compounds. The plasma half-life, disposition, and other pharmacokinetic parameters for uterine stimulants are summarized in Table 40-1.

Some of the uterine inhibitors are also discussed in other chapters: indomethacin in Chapter 18; terbutaline and ritodrine in Chapter 10. The disposition, mode of administration, half-life, and other pharmacokinetic factors for these drugs are presented elsewhere. Magnesium sulfate usually is administered IV.

Both the uterine stimulants and uterine inhibitors are titrated to obtain the desired therapeutic response according to the clinical condition of the patient.

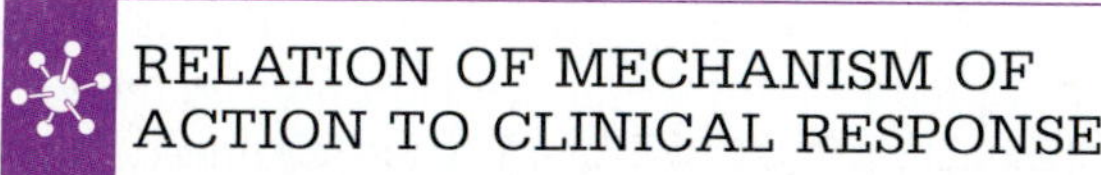

RELATION OF MECHANISM OF ACTION TO CLINICAL RESPONSE

Uterine Stimulants

Induction of Labor Uterine stimulants are used primarily to induce labor and decrease the risk of neonatal morbidity and mortality when a medical or obstetrical problem exists. Common indications for induction include extended pregnancy, early rupture of membranes, or placental insufficiency. Intravenous oxytocin is the preferred agent either to induce labor or to augment a dysfunctional labor, a condition in which contractions are inadequate. Dinoprostone (PGE_2) has recently gained favor for labor induction because the near-term myometrium is exquisitely sensitive to prostaglandins. Drug administered either intravaginally or intracervically show the fewest side effects, since other smooth muscle is less affected when drug is given by these routes. Prostaglandins and oxytocin should never be used concurrently, since the combination may result in uterine rupture. Where tetanic contractions occur with dinoprostone use, the tocolytic agent terbutaline may be administered intravenously. The ergot alkaloids are absolutely contraindicated for the induction of labor.

Other Uses of Uterine Stimulants

Postpartum Bleeding Oxytocin, ergot alkaloids (α-adrenergic receptor agonists), and prostaglandin produce firm contractions in the uterus and thus decrease bleeding after delivery or after an abortion. Oxytocin may be employed intravenously for this purpose. The ergot alkaloids (ergonovine and methylergonovine) can be administered intramuscularly when a longer effect is desired. Because they generate sustained contractions rather than intermittent ones, their use may lead to severe fetal hypoxia. Ergot alkaloids also cause arteriolar constriction further reducing blood loss. The α-adrenergic receptor is coupled to phospholipase C, promoting hydrolysis of phosphatidylinositol bisphosphate with the ultimate activation of protein kinase C leading to an increase in intracellular calcium and contraction (Chapter 8). Prostaglandins (carboprost and dinoprostone) are used to control postpartum hemorrhage when other agents are unsuccessful.

Termination of Pregnancy Prostaglandins are the preferred agents for second-trimester abortion. In contrast to oxytocin, which increases uterine contractions near or at term, prostaglandins stimulate uterine muscle at all times during gestation. Both dinoprostone and carboprost are effective from week 12 through week 20 of gestation. When used for pregnancy termination, prostaglandins increase gastrointestinal smooth muscle as well as uterine contractions.

CLINICAL CONDITIONS OFTEN ASSOCIATED WITH PRETERM LABOR

SITE	CONDITION
Maternal	Acute and chronic severe systemic disease
	Endocrine conditions such as hyperthyroidism or hyperadrenocorticism
	Chronic hypertension
	History of premature birth
	Trauma
	Genital infection
	Age, under 16 or over 40 years
Fetoplacental	Genetic abnormalities
	Fetal death
	Abruptio placentae
	Placenta previa
	Multifetal gestation
	Premature rupture of the amniotic membranes
Uterine	Multiple gestation
	Foreign body
	Infection
	Cervical incompetence or trauma
	Surgery
	Uterine anomalies

Tocolytic Agents

Tocolytics, or agents that relax the uterus, are used to treat premature labor in conditions in which the fetus would benefit significantly from longer intrauterine life. Alcohol infusion, used earlier for this purpose, has been replaced by the β_2-adrenergic receptor agonists. Other agents used in combination with the adrenergic agonists are prostaglandin inhibitors and magnesium sulfate. Nondrug therapies include bed rest, sedation, and hydration. Ritodrine and terbutaline are both widely used where therapeutic intervention is indicated, acting on the β_2-adrenergic receptor to produce relaxation of the uterus. They are effective orally as well as by other routes of administration. The box lists some of the clinical conditions associated with preterm labor.

Magnesium sulfate, which blocks uterine contractions by a competitive action against calcium ion, is administered intravenously and is probably as effective as the β_2-adrenergic agonists. Magnesium sulfate has frequently been used in combination with ritodrine and alone if the cardiovascular side effects of ritodrine are a problem.

Table 40-2 Problems (Stimulants)

Drug	Maternal	Fetal
oxytocin	Uterine hyperactivity	Acidosis
	Uterine rupture	Hypoxia
	Hypotension	Hyperbilirubinemia
	Tachycardia	
	ECG changes	
ergot alkaloids	Hypertension	Hypoxia
	Severe headache	Death
	Nausea and vomiting	
	Blurred vision	
	Convulsions	
	Death	
	Bradycardia	
	Angina	
prostaglandins	Uterine hypertonus	Death
	Nausea and vomiting	
	Diarrhea	
	Tachycardia	
	Headache	
	Flushing	
	Fever	
	Seizures	

Other drugs have been tried experimentally. Because prostaglandins increase uterine contractions, prostaglandin inhibitors have also been examined to arrest premature labor. Although indomethacin has been used with some success, prostaglandin synthesis inhibitors also cause closure of the ductus arteriosus in the fetus, a significant drawback to their use in premature labor. The calcium-channel blocker nifedipine (Chapter 16) has also been studied as a tocolytic agent and has been shown to reduce contractions by blocking calcium entry into uterine cells. Diazoxide, an antihypertensive drug that relaxes smooth muscle directly (Chapter 13), has been used experimentally to retard premature labor.

SIDE EFFECTS, CLINICAL PROBLEMS, AND TOXICITY

The major maternal side effects of the uterine stimulants (Table 40-2) include uterine rupture, cardiovascular effects, and gastrointestinal symptoms. In the fetus, if uterine contractions become too strong, the fetus can experience serious injury, hypoxia, and even death.

The major maternal side effects of the uterine relaxants (Table 40-3) are primarily associated with severe

Table 40-3 Clinical Problems (Tocolytics)

Drug	Maternal	Fetal
β-adrenergic receptor agonists	Tachycardia Hypotension Hyperglycemia Tremors Nausea and vomiting Angina Pulmonary edema	Tachycardia Hypotension
prostaglandin synthesis inhibitors	Anorexia Nausea GI bleeding Headaches Confusion Allergic rashes Bone marrow depression	Premature closure of the ductus arteriosus Pulmonary hypertension Hyperbilirubinemia Coagulopathy
magnesium sulfate	Skin flushing Nausea Headache Palpitations Depressed reflexes Respiratory depression Cardiac conduction problems Cardiac arrest	CNS depression (rare) Muscle relaxation

alterations on the cardiovascular system and changes in the function of the CNS. Fetal toxicities are less common.

NEW DIRECTIONS

Numerous studies since 1988 have dealt with the local application of PGE_2. This agent induces structural changes in the uterine cervix, producing thinning, softening, and dilatation, enhancing ripening. PGE_2 as a gel may be inserted intracervically, intravaginally, or extra-amniotically. The intravaginal insertion, the simplest application, produces a pattern of uterine activity that closely resembles spontaneous labor, in contrast to labor induced by oxytocin and amniotomy. The intravaginal method is favored over intracervical application because of fewer side effects, even though intracervical priming may be more effective.

The role for oxytocin in the initiation and maintenance of labor has led to the development of oxytocin receptor antagonists. Such an antagonist, 1-deamino-2-D-Tyr-(Oet)-4-Thr-8-Orn-oxytocin (RWJ 22164, dTVT), has recently been studied in in vitro and in situ models of uterine contractility to characterize the effects of dTVT on preterm labor. Early data indicate that such drugs may represent a new modality for the treatment of preterm labor.

TRADE NAMES

In addition to generic and fixed-combination preparations, the following trade-name materials are available in the United States.

UTERINE STIMULANTS

Ergotrate, ergonovine maleate
Methergine, methylergonovine maleate
Prostin E_2, PGE_2, dinoprostone
Syntocinon, Pitocin, oxytocin
Hemabate, carboprost, tromethamine

UTERINE RELAXANTS

Brethine, Bricanyl, terbutaline sulfate
Yutopar, ritodrine hydrochloride
Indocin, indomethacin

The antiprogestin, mefipristone (RU 486), prevents uterine implantation by blocking the binding of progesterone to its receptor and thus has wide use in Europe as a contragestational agent (Chapter 36). If implantation has occurred, mefipristone, in combination with a prostaglandin, has been shown to be an effective abortifacient in early pregnancies. It is not available currently in the United States but may be in the future.

A potential area of interest is the possible role for nitric oxide in uterine motility. The uterus contains significant concentrations of nitric oxide synthase. Animal studies have demonstrated that nitric oxide synthase concentrations are reduced at term. Manipulation of this system leaves open the potential for developing agents that may be useful in either arresting premature labor or in inducing labor.

REFERENCES

Andersen LF, Lyndrup J, Akerlund M, Melin P: Oxytocin receptor blockade: a new principle in the treatment of preterm labor? *Am J Perinatol* 6:196-199, 1989.

Besinger RE, Niebyl JR: The safety and efficacy of tocolytic agents for the treatment of preterm labor, *Obstet Gynecol Surv* 45:415-440, 1990.

Cox SM, Sherman ML, Leveno KJ: Randomized investigation of magnesium sulfate for prevention of preterm birth, *Am J Obstet Gynecol* 163:767-772, 1990.

Rayburn WF: Prostaglandin E_2 gel for cervical ripening and induction of labor: a critical analysis, *Am J Obstet Gynecol* 160:529-534, 1989.

Uldbjerg N, Forman A, Petersen LK, et al: Biomechanical and biochemical changes of the uterus and cervix during pregnancy. In Reece EA, et al, editors: *Medicine of the fetus and mother,* Philadelphia, 1992, Lippincott.

Wilkins I, Creasy RK: Preterm labor, *Clin Obstet Gynecol* 33:502-514, 1990.

SELF-ASSESSMENT QUESTIONS

1. Which of the following statements are characteristics of biochemical and molecular processes in uterine smooth muscle contractility?
   a. Adenylate cyclase leads to increases in the concentration of cAMP.
   b. cAMP leads to phosphorylation of myosin light-chain kinase.
   c. Myosin light-chain kinase must form its own active complex with calmodulin.
   d. None of the above.
   e. a, b, c are correct.
2. Magnesium sulfate inhibits uterine contraction by:
   a. decreasing the frequency of myometrial muscle cell action potentials.
   b. uncoupling the excitation and contraction of the uterine smooth muscle cells.
   c. directly relaxing the contractile elements.
   d. all of the above.
   e. none of the above.
3. Indomethacin is used to treat some cases of premature labor because it:
   a. acts directly to suppress the contractile response of the myometrial smooth muscle.
   b. has a greater effect on β_2-adrenergic receptors.
   c. decreases the synthesis of oxytocin.
   d. inhibits prostaglandin synthesis.
   e. all of the above.
4. Which of the following is characteristic of oxytocin?
   a. This drug readily crosses the placenta and can cause deleterious effects to the fetus, including death.
   b. The effects of this drug may persist per several hours.
   c. The plasma half-life is a few minutes.
   d. This drug can be administered orally.
   e. The sensitivity of the uterus to this drug is greater than that to prostaglandins during pregnancy.
5. The maternal side effects associated with β_2-adrenergic receptor agonists include:
   a. hyperglycemia.
   b. headaches.
   c. acidosis.
   d. depressed reflexes.
   e. all of the above.
6. The fetal side effects associated with magnesium sulfate include:
   a. hiccups.
   b. muscle relaxation.
   c. hypotension.
   d. tachycardia.
   e. all of the above.

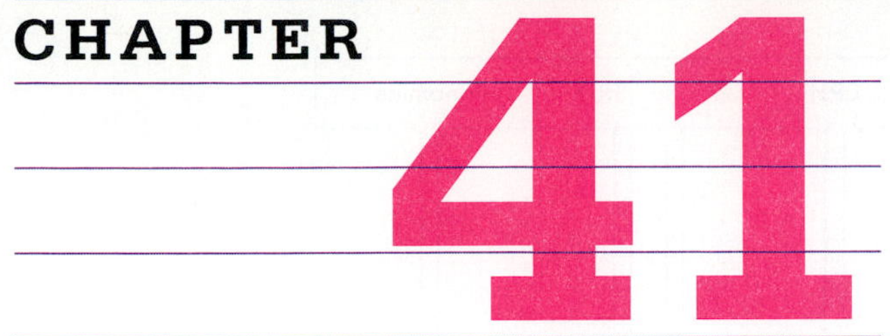

Hypothalamic-Pituitary Hormones

WILLIAM S. EVANS
MICHAEL J. SOLLENBERGER
MARY LEE VANCE

MAJOR DRUGS

hypothalamic hormones and analogs (GnRH, GHRH, bromocriptine, octreotide)
pituitary hormones and analogs (FSH, LH, GH, vasopressin, desmopressin, clomiphene)

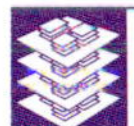 THERAPEUTIC OVERVIEW

The role of the pituitary gland in regulating hormone production by peripheral endocrine organs is well known, but the relationship between the pituitary and the hypothalamic factors that control pituitary function has been defined only recently. Peptides and biogenic amines, synthesized and secreted by specialized neurons within the hypothalamus, are transported by the hypothalamohypophyseal portal circulation to the anterior pituitary where, acting through specific receptors, they stimulate or inhibit hormone secretion (Figure 41-1). Anterior pituitary hormones, in turn, signal the production of hormones by peripheral endocrine organs. Hormones originating from peripheral endocrine organs subserve their own functions and provide feedback at the hypothalamic or pituitary level to modulate the synthesis and release of their particular trophic hormone. Thus hypothalamic gonadotropin-releasing hormone (GnRH) stimulates the secretion of luteinizing hormone (LH) and follicle-stimulating hormone (FSH) by the pituitary, which effect gametogenesis and gonadal hormone production by the testes and ovaries (see Chapter 36 and 37). Thyrotropin-releasing hormone (TRH) stimulates the secretion of thyroid-stimulating hormone (TSH), which in turn controls thyroid function. Corticotropin-releasing hormone (CRH) stimulates the secretion of adrenocorticotropin (ACTH), which promotes the secretion of hormones by the adrenal cortex. Growth hormone–releasing hormone (GHRH) and somatotropin release–inhibiting factor (SRIF) stimulate and inhibit respectively the production of growth hormone (GH), which has numerous effects on growth and metabolism. Hypothalamic dopamine functions to tonically inhibit the secretion of prolactin, the hormone primarily responsible for lactation. The posterior pituitary (or neurohypophysis) secretes arginine vasopressin (AVP) and oxytocin. Unlike the anterior pituitary, which is under hypothalamic control, the neurohypophysis is made up of neurons with cell bodies within the hypothalamus. These cells synthesize and secrete AVP and oxytocin that are transported by carrier proteins (neurophysins) through axons to the posterior pituitary where they are released directly into the systemic circulation.

Except for prolactin, each of the hypothalamic and

ABBREVIATIONS

AVP	arginine vasopressin (or simply vasopressin)
CRH	corticotropin-releasing hormone
DDAVP	desamino-D-arginine vasopressin
FSH	follicle-stimulating hormone
GH	growth hormone
GHRH	growth hormone–releasing hormone
GnRH	gonadotropin-releasing hormone
LH	luteinizing hormone
SRIF	somatotropin release–inhibiting factor (somatostatin)
TRH	thyrotropin-releasing hormone
TSH	thyroid-stimulating hormone
VIP	vasoactive intestinal polypeptide

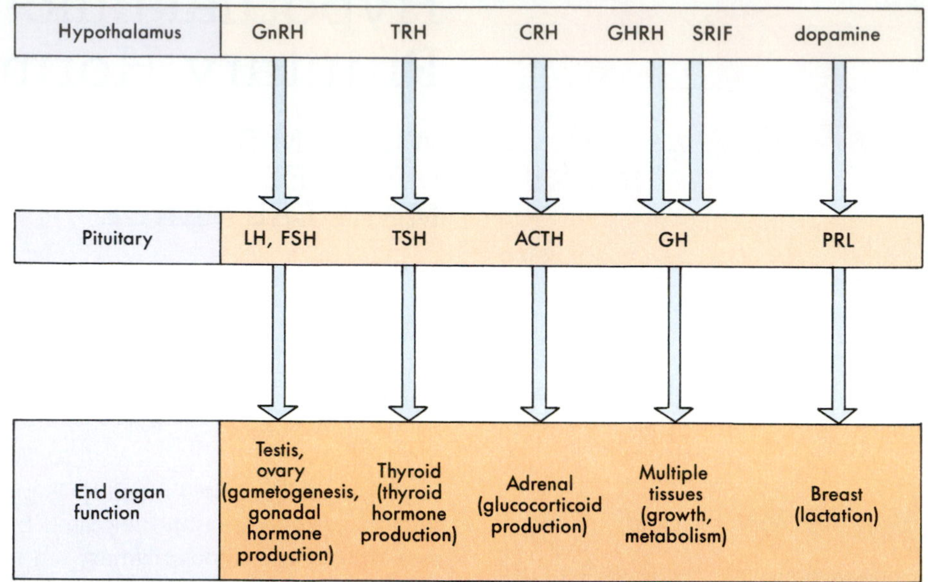

FIGURE 41-1 Relationships among the hypothalamic releasing and inhibiting hormones, the anterior pituitary hormones that the hypothalamic hormones control, and their respective target organs or tissues. *ACTH,* Adrenocorticotropic hormone; *CRH,* corticotropin-releasing hormone; *FSH,* follicle-stimulating hormone; *GH,* growth hormone; *GHRH,* growth hormone-releasing hormone; *GnRH,* Gonadotropin-releasing hormone; *LH,* luteinizing hormone; *PRL,* prolactin; *SRIF,* somatotropin release-inhibiting factor (somatostatin); *TRH,* thyrotropin-releasing hormone; *TSH,* thyroid-stimulating hormone.

pituitary hormones mentioned are used for diagnostic or therapeutic purposes. Because the major roles of TRH, CRH, TSH, and ACTH are diagnostic, these hormones are not discussed further. The hypothalamic hormones (or their analogs and agonists): GnRH, GHRH, dopamine, and somatostatin; the anterior pituitary hormones GH and LH/FSH; and the posterior pituitary hormone AVP are used therapeutically or have therapeutic potential and are discussed in this chapter. The pharmacology of oxytocin is discussed in Chapter 40. A therapeutic overview of hypothalamic and pituitary hormones is listed in the box.

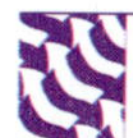

MECHANISMS OF ACTION

Hypothalamic Hormones

The majority of GnRH-positive neurons in humans are located in the medial basal hypothalamus between the third ventricle and the median eminence. Projections from these neurons terminate in the median eminence, in contact with the capillary plexus of the hypothalamic-hypophyseal portal circulation. These capillaries allow GnRH to be delivered into the circulation without passing through a blood-brain barrier. GnRH is formed by processing of a larger prohormone, pre-pro-GnRH, and transported in secretory granules to nerve terminals for storage, degradation, or release into the pituitary portal blood vessels.

At the target, GnRH binds to receptors and initiates the secretion of LH and FSH. The molecular weight of the GnRH receptor is estimated to be 136,000 daltons. Microaggregation also stimulates upregulation of the GnRH receptor and is followed by endocytosis-mediated internalization of the hormone receptor complex (see Chapter 34). Receptor activation results in the influx of extracellular Ca^{++} through the opening of ligand-gated calcium channels and the hydrolysis of phosphatidylinositol 4,5-bisphosphate (see Chapter 34).

GnRH is released in a pulsatile manner by a "hypothalamic pulse generator." This release pattern is essential for normal function. Continuous administration results in an attenuated response mediated by receptor downregulation and postreceptor mechanisms. To achieve the same effect as continuous administration but in a more practical manner, analog agonists with increased half-life and greater receptor binding and competitive antagonists have been synthesized by selective amino acid substitutions in the molecule (Figure 41-2).

Major modulators of gonadotropin secretion are inhibin (a peptide hormone synthesized by ovarian granu-

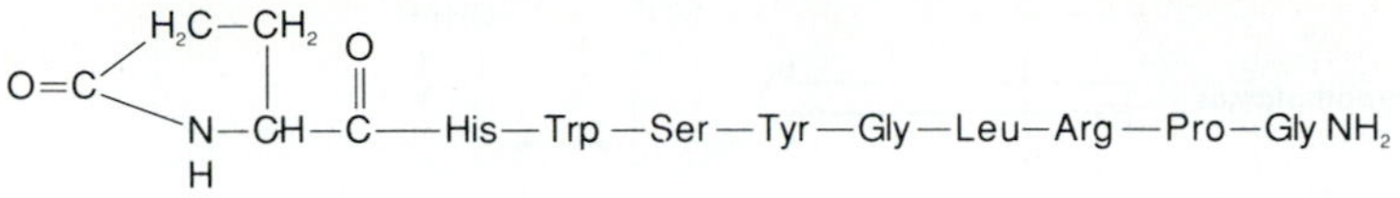

$O{=}C\langle H_2C{-}CH_2 \rangle N(H){-}CH{-}C(=O){-}$His—Trp—Ser—Tyr—Gly—Leu—Arg—Pro—Gly NH_2

FIGURE 41-2 Structure of gonadotropin-releasing hormone (GnRH). See the text for further information.

THERAPEUTIC OVERVIEW

HYPOTHALAMIC HORMONES

GnRH

Replacement therapy
- central amenorrhea
- idiopathic hypogonadotropic hypogonadism

GnRH Analogs

Prostate cancer
Idiopathic precocious puberty
Endometriosis
Contraception

GHRH

Short stature

Dopamine Agonists (Bromocriptine)

Physiological hyperprolactinemia
Pathophysiological hyperprolactinemia
Acromegaly
Parkinson's disease

Somatostatin and Analogs

Carcinoid tumor
VIP secreting tumor

PITUITARY HORMONES

LH and FSH

Infertility in women
Infertility in men with hypogonadotropic hypergonadism

GH

Short stature

AVP

Diabetes insipidus

losa and testicular Sertoli cells) and opioid peptides. In normally ovulating women, estradiol also exerts positive feedback at the pituitary, which may be responsible in part for the preovulatory LH surge.

GHRH Growth hormone's secretion is regulated by two opposing hypothalamic hormones: GHRH and SRIF (see Figure 41-3 for regulation).

Dopamine Agonists Bromocriptine is an inhibitor of prolactin secretion (see Figure 41-4 for structure). It suppresses prolactin release by directly stimulating dopamine receptors on prolactin-secreting lactotropes in the anterior pituitary. Ample evidence implicates hypothalamically derived dopamine as the physiologically significant prolactin-inhibiting factor (see Chapter 22 for dopamine-receptor mechanisms).

Somatostatin and Analogs Somatostatin (SRIF) is a cyclic peptide containing 14 amino acids (somatostatin 14). Recently a family of somatostatin-related peptides, including an amino-terminal extended peptide (somatostatin 28), was discovered. In addition to its presence in the hypothalamus, somatostatin is widely distributed throughout the nervous system, the gut, and various endocrine and exocrine glands. It has several functions depending on its source, acting as a neurohormone to inhibit pituitary GH release, a neurotransmitter in the nervous system, and as an autocrine and paracrine factor outside of the nervous system.

Somatostatin 14 and somatostatin 28 have different functions, as exemplified by the greater suppressive effect of somatostatin 28 than that of somatostatin 14 on insulin secretion. Somatostatin acts through specific receptors that are present in pituitary cells, pituitary plasma membranes, brain synaptosome membranes, and pancreatic islet cells. It appears to act to decrease cytosolic Ca^{++}.

Somatostatin has a fiftyfold greater suppressive effect on glucagon than that on insulin release. Its predominant effect on pancreatic islets is inhibition of glucagon-secreting cells. Somatostatin inhibits gut hormone secretion (e.g., gastrin, vasoactive intestinal polypeptide [VIP], motilin, secretin); exocrine secretion (e.g., gastric acid, pepsin, pancreatic bicarbonate, pancreatic enzymes); and gastric emptying, gallbladder contraction, and intestinal motility. Somatostatin also decreases GI absorption and mesenteric blood flow. In the central nervous system (CNS), somatostatin has both excitatory and inhibitory influences on neurons and on neurotransmitter and neurohormone release. Its predominant role in the CNS is not established.

Pituitary Hormones

LH and FSH LH and FSH are structurally similar glycoproteins, each consisting of two polypeptide chains linked by hydrogen bonds and with internal cross-

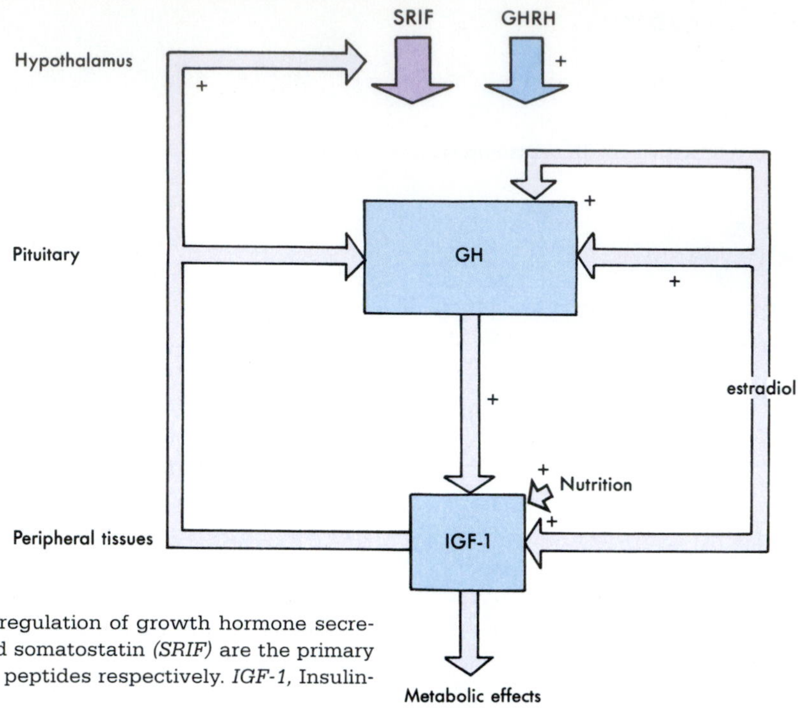

FIGURE 41-3 Schema of regulation of growth hormone secretion in humans. GHRH and somatostatin *(SRIF)* are the primary stimulatory and inhibitory peptides respectively. *IGF-1,* Insulin-like growth factor 1.

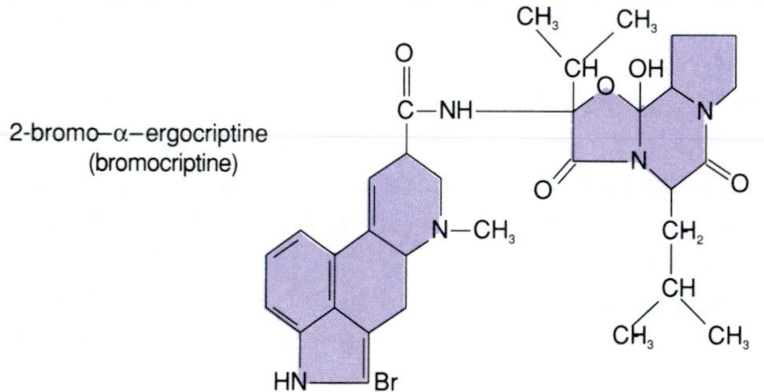

FIGURE 41-4 Structure of the prototypical dopamine agonist 2-bromo-α-ergocriptine (bromocriptine). See the text for further information.

linking by disulfide bonds. LH and FSH are composed of an identical 89 amino acid α chain and a 115 amino acid β chain unique to each hormone and responsible for specific hormonal activity. Two complex carbohydrate side chains are attached to specific locations on the α subunit, two to the FSH-β subunit, and one to the LH-β subunit. A terminal sialic acid is found on approximately 5% and 1% of FSH and LH carbohydrate molecules respectively. Sialic acid prolongs metabolic clearance of glycoproteins and results in a longer half-life for FSH as compared with LH. There is no evidence that other molecular forms of LH and FSH such as prohormones and fragments circulate in the plasma.

The gonadotrope secretes LH and FSH. The α and β chains are synthesized separately and appear to combine before carbohydrate addition.

Gonadotropins bind to high-affinity membrane receptors in the testes and ovary, activating adenylate cyclase. The production of cyclic adenosine monophosphate signals the activation of its protein kinase and, subsequently, the phosphorylation of proteins necessary for steroidogenesis. The LH receptor has a molecular weight of approximately 180,000 daltons and binds one LH. The FSH receptor has not been characterized.

In addition to regulating estrogen production, the gonadotropins have multiple effects on ovarian follicles. FSH directly stimulates follicular growth and maturation and enhances granulosa cell responsiveness to LH. LH is essential for the breakdown of the follicular wall, resulting in ovulation, and for the subsequent resumption of meiotic division of the oocyte.

By contrast, testicular steroidogenesis requires only LH. The Leydig cells, which constitute about 10% of testicular volume, are stimulated to produce testosterone by binding of LH to surface receptors. FSH binds to Sertoli cells and, with testosterone, is essential for cellular maturation and for spermatid differentiation, the first step of spermatogenesis. The Sertoli cell is necessary for maintenance of seminiferous tubule function and germ cell development.

Growth Hormone Growth hormone is a 191 amino acid polypeptide that has 84% identity with placental chorionic somatomammotropin and strong structural homology with prolactin. Growth hormone is synthesized by somatotropes of the anterior pituitary; the major product is a 22,000-dalton peptide. The majority of circulating GH is the 22,000-dalton isoform, with 5% to 10% a 20,000-dalton isoform. GH dimers and tetramers also have been detected.

The precise signaling mechanism by which GH exerts its intracellular effects likely involves interaction with a specific plasma membrane receptor (or receptors) (see Chapter 34). Additionally, GH binds to proteins in both cytosol and plasma. The specificity of the circulating binding protein is similar to the suggested GH receptor.

Numerous direct effects of GH on specific tissues include stimulation of RNA, protein, and insulin-like growth factor 1 synthesis by liver; stimulation of amino acid transport and incorporation into muscle protein; and stimulation of amino acid incorporation into protein and lipolysis in adipose tissue. Additionally, GH exerts a positive influence on hematopoietic tissue.

Vasopressin AVP is a nonapeptide that functions as the primary antidiuretic hormone in humans (Figure 41-5). Synthesized primarily in the magnocellular neuronal systems of the supraoptic and paraventricular nuclei of the hypothalamus, the AVP precursor molecule contains a signal peptide, a neurophysin, and a glycosylated moiety in addition to the AVP sequence. This precursor molecule travels through neuronal axons to the posterior pituitary where granules containing cleaved and uncleaved hormone are stored. Such granules are released in response to a signal that effects Ca^{++} influx into the cell. The mechanisms that prompt the exocytosis of AVP primarily consist of osmotic signals (detected by osmoreceptors in the anterior hypothalamus) and pressure signals (detected by baroreceptors in the heart and large blood vessels). Nausea, emesis, and hypoglycemia may also stimulate the release of AVP.

Of particular clinical relevance is that certain agonists (such as the desamino analog desmopressin) (see Figure 41-5 for the amino acid sequence) possess pronounced antidiuretic effects with minimal pressor effects (see Chapters 12 and 19 for discussion of actions of AVP).

AVP thus has reasonably well defined effects on water balance and on the cardiovascular system. Each of these actions of AVP, including its effect on the production of antihemophilic factor (factor VIII) through as yet poorly understood mechanisms, has been used therapeutically.

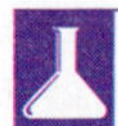

PHARMACOKINETICS

Pharmacokinetic parameters for these hypothalamic and pituitary hormones and analogs are summarized in Table 41-1.

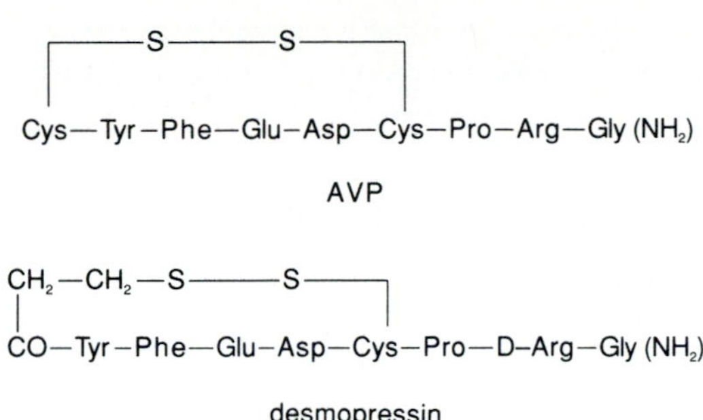

FIGURE 41-5 Amino acid sequences of arginine vasopressin *(AVP)* and an AVP analog, 1-desamino-8-D-arginine-vasopressin (desmopressin, DDAVP). See the text for further information.

Hypothalamic Hormones

GnRH Clinically, GnRH is administered by IV or SC routes. In hypogonadotropic patients, continuous SC infusions of GnRH result in steady-state concentrations that are one third less than those achieved with the IV route. Therefore SC administration of GnRH results in delayed and prolonged absorption of GnRH with consequently lower serum concentrations. In patients receiving pulsatile GnRH therapy, these absorption characteristics cause the plasma GnRH concentration peaks to be significantly damped. The lack of a pulsatile GnRH concentration waveform may diminish pituitary responsiveness and explain the lower ovulation induction success rate with SC as compared to IV administration.

GnRH is metabolized, though the pathway has not been established. GnRH is not significantly bound to plasma proteins. The primary route of excretion is renal, and renal insufficiency significantly lengthens the overall clearance rate. Moderate abnormalities of hepatic function do not affect GnRH clearance. Estimates of GnRH half-life are from 2 to 8 minutes, with metabolic clearance rates from 500 to 1600 ml/min. This wide range of estimates is probably caused by differences in the method of administration (single bolus versus continuous infusion) and the radioimmunoassay used to estimate concentrations.

GHRH In normal humans, GHRH (GHRH-40, GHRH-44), administered IV, SC, or intranasally, stimulates GH release in a dose-dependent fashion. The 29 amino acid GHRH analogs $[N1e^{27}]GHRH(1\text{-}29)\text{-}NH_2$ and $GHRH(1\text{-}29)NH_2$, have similar potency and duration of action, as GHRH 1-40 has.

After IV administration, the plasma half-life for disappearance of GHRH immunoreactivity is 63 minutes, with the maximal effect occurring 30 to 45 minutes after injection. Peptide degradation in the plasma occurs by removal of the first two amino-terminal residues with a half-life of 6.8 minutes. There is no evidence that

Table 41-1 Pharmacokinetic Parameter Values

Drugs	Administration	Absorption	$t_{1/2}$	Disposition
HYPOTHALAMIC HORMONES AND ANALOGS				
GnRH	IV, SC	—	2-8 min	R, M
GnRH agonists	SC, Intranasal	—	3 hr	—
GHRH	IV, SC Intranasal	—	63 min	M
bromocriptine	Oral	Fair (28%)	6 hr*	M (100%) B (main)
octreotide (somatostatin analog)	SC	—	80-90 min	—
PITUITARY HORMONES AND ANALOGS				
LH/FSH	IM	Good	30-60 min	M
FSH	IM	Good	Hours	—
GH	IM, SC	—	19 min	—
vasopressin	IM, SC	Good	3-15 min	M
vasopressin tannate	IM	(Erratic) Fair	—	M
desmopressin	IV, SC Intranasal	Good	75 min	M
clomiphene	Oral	Good	Long	B (main)

M, Metabolized; *R,* renal excretion as unchanged by drug; *B,* excreted in bile.
*90% bound to serum albumin.

GHRH is bound to plasma proteins or stored in peripheral tissues.

Dopamine Agonists After oral administration, approximately 28% of bromocriptine is absorbed. Ninety percent of bromocriptine circulates bound to serum albumin. The half-life of bromocriptine is about 6 hours for the parent drug and 50 hours for metabolites. In some patients, suppression of prolactin by bromocriptine lasts only 12 to 40 hours, an indication that the metabolites may be pharmacologically inactive. Although the details of bromocriptine degradation are not known, it appears that the peptide aminocyclol portion of the molecule is metabolized with subsequent scission of the amide to yield bromolysergic acid derivatives together with peptide fragments. Ninety-eight percent of the drug is excreted in the feces, with only trace amounts found in urine.

Somatostatin and Analogs IV administration of native somatostatin (somatostatin 14) results in a prompt decline in serum GH concentrations. The peptide is not absorbed orally and must be administered parenterally. The half-life is approximately 3 to 4 minutes, rendering it unsuitable for therapeutic use.

The 8 amino acid somatostatin analog octreotide has a circulating half-life of 80 to 90 minutes, but the biological effect persists for 6 to 8 hours. This analog must also be administered parenterally and is given by SC injection or continuous SC infusion.

Pituitary Hormones

LH and FSH LH and FSH are effective only if given IM. The absorption characteristics and subsequent metabolism of the gonadotropins have not been elucidated, but liver appears to be the major source of glycoprotein clearance after enzymatic removal of sialic acid. The estimated half-life of LH is between 30 and 60 minutes. FSH has a higher sialic acid content and consequently a longer half-life because of decreased hepatic uptake. The clearance of LH is about 30 ml/min in women and 50 ml/min in men; that of FSH is approximately 15 ml/min in women and has not been determined in men.

Growth Hormone IM and SC administration of GH to children who have a GH deficiency results in serum concentrations that reach maximal concentrations 2 to 3 hours after injection and that decline progressively over approximately 15 hours. The serum half-life of GH administered both endogenously and exogenously ranges from 15 to 51 minutes. In recent studies involving stimulation of endogenous GH release with GHRH and suppression of further release with somatostatin, the half-life of endogenous GH in normal men is 19 minutes; exogenously administered synthetic GH is 15 minutes in normal men. GH is not stored in tissues, and small amounts are detectable in urine.

Vasopressin Vasopressin, vasopressin tannate, and desmopressin circulate unbound to plasma proteins. All undergo metabolism in liver and kidney and may be initially inactivated by cleavage of the C-terminal glycinamide. A small amount of vasopressin (approximately 5%) is excreted as intact drug in urine.

Action durations of the three preparations are different. When administered SC or IM, vasopressin is effective for only 2 to 8 hours. After IM administration, vasopressin tannate is often absorbed erratically, with a duration of action between 48 and 96 hours. Desmopressin may be given IV, SC, or intranasally. The half-life of desmopressin is consistent with the observed duration of action, in that the distribution and elimination components are 7.8 and 75.5 minutes respectively, compared to 2.5 and 14.5 minutes for vasopressin.

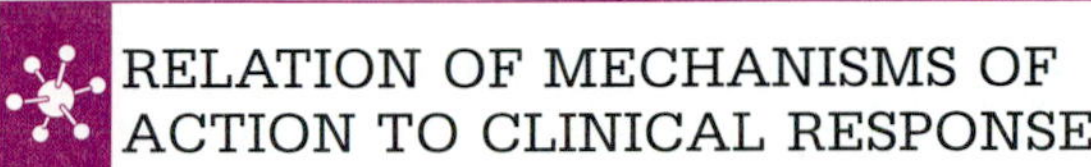

RELATION OF MECHANISMS OF ACTION TO CLINICAL RESPONSE

Hypothalamic Hormones

Gonadotropin-Releasing Hormone The approved and potential indications for therapy with GnRH and analogs can be divided into two categories: (1) replacement therapy in disorders characterized by isolated, abnormal function of the hypothalamic pulse generator and (2) continuous administration (e.g., by means of a long-acting analog) to promote pituitary desensitization and thus effect a functional orchiectomy or ovariectomy.

GnRH has recently been approved for ovulation induction in women with primary hypothalamic amenorrhea. Hypothalamic (or central) amenorrhea is characterized by abnormal function of the GnRH pulse generator. This deficiency results in inadequate gonadotropin secretion, consequent failure of ovarian follicular development, and amenorrhea. The pituitary, however, is intrinsically normal and releases LH and FSH in response to GnRH. Pulse administration of GnRH by a portable infusion pump may compensate for the underlying defect, and IV administration of the hormone frequently results in LH, FSH, estradiol, and progesterone profiles being indistinguishable from those observed in normal, spontaneous cycles. Several hundred women have been treated using IV or SC hormone delivery with results indicating successful ovulation induction in over 90% of women treated with IV GnRH. Subcutaneous administration requires larger doses and results in a pattern of LH release that does not approximate the normal cycle as closely as IV GnRH does. The success rate is lower with SC therapy, but still more than 50% of patients achieve ovulation.

Traditional treatment of central amenorrhea includes clomiphene or human menopausal gonadotropin. These methods are clearly successful in inducing ovulation but are associated with two major complications: (1) a mild form of ovarian hyperstimulation (ovarian enlargement and abdominal pain) in approximately 15% of clomiphene cycles and 25% of human menopausal gonadotropin cycles, and (2) increased incidence of multiple pregnancies with both. Because pulsatile GnRH therapy maintains the integrity of the pituitary-ovarian axis (i.e., allows for the appropriate negative and positive feedback of gonadal hormones) and more accurately reproduces the physiology of the normal menstrual cycle, the incidence of complications may be less.

Faulty GnRH secretion in men is referred to as *idiopathic hypogonadotropic hypogonadism*. The pituitary still responds to GnRH by secreting LH and FSH. Long-term pulsatile administration of GnRH was tested in a small number of men for at least 3 months. Significant increases in serum testosterone concentrations and testicular size were noted associated with clinical manifestations of the increasing androgen concentrations. Mature spermatogenesis may be achieved in 50% of patients and, in men with unfused epiphyses, linear growth may occur. Standard treatment of this disorder included testosterone injections for masculinization and other hormones for fertility. As more experience is gained with pulsatile GnRH for normalization of the pituitary-testicular axis and the induction of fertility, this approach may emerge as an acceptable alternative for the treatment of idiopathic hypogonadotropic hypogonadism.

The observation that orchiectomy causes regression of prostatic cancer (the second most frequent type of cancer for males in this country) leads to therapeutic approaches to decrease serum androgen concentrations in men with metastatic disease. Estrogens, acting through suppression of gonadotrope secretion and direct inhibition of androgen effects on the prostate, are also effective. Although the optimum hormonal regimen is controversial, current approaches to advanced cancer employ castration or estrogens. This is associated with significant side effects, including the psychological impact of orchiectomy, with thromboembolism, cardiovascular disease, and gynecomastia related to estrogen therapy. In addition, the effect on long-term survival is disappointing, with a death rate of nearly 50% at 2 years for disease with bone metastases. Partial explanations for the high failure rate may be (1) persistent production of adrenal androgen precursors, which can be converted to active androgens by the prostate, and (2) effective androgenic activity of very low (i.e., castrate) concentrations of testosterone.

Long-acting GnRH agonists can be used to down-regulate pituitary gonadotrope receptors and suppress pulsatile LH release. They have been approved for the treatment of advanced prostatic cancer (Figure 41-6).

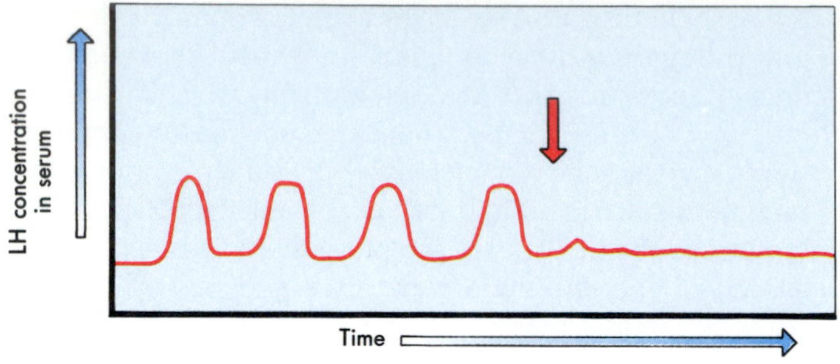

FIGURE 41-6 Schema of LH serum concentration profile in a normal subject showing initial LH pulses resulting from GnRH pulse generator. Administration of a long-acting GnRH agonist at arrow downregulates receptors and leads to decreased LH secretion.

GnRH agonist therapy initially causes a temporary rise in serum testosterone concentrations, which could cause an acute exacerbation of disease symptoms, but coadministration of the antiandrogen flutamide can prevent this. This regimen produces side effects of hypoandrogenism (hot flashes, decreased libido) without symptoms of hyperestrogenism. It therefore appears to be better tolerated than orchiectomy and estrogen therapy. When used as the initial treatment of advanced prostate cancer, the combination of a long-acting GnRH analog and flutamide produced response rates of 95% at the initiation of treatment. After 2 years of treatment, the response rate was 70% and the death rate was 11% (as compared to 10% and 50% respectively, with conventional modalities).

GnRH analog therapy has received approval recently to obtain a *medical oophorectomy* for the treatment of endometriosis. Treatment with GnRH agonists for 6 months has been shown to be as effective as danazol in reducing the size of endometrial implants and decreasing clinical symptoms including pelvic pain, dysmenorrhea, and dyspareunia.

Idiopathic precocious puberty, which results in maturation of the external genitalia, accelerated linear growth, and advanced bone age, has been treated experimentally with GnRH analogs, with very encouraging results.

GnRH analog therapy is being investigated as a means of female and male contraception. Preliminary studies in women are successful, but further trials are required to test for long-term side effects (e.g., osteoporosis secondary to low serum estrogen concentrations). Studies in males show failure to achieve azoospermia; therefore this approach holds little promise for further development.

Growth Hormone–Releasing Hormone GHRH is not approved for general use as a diagnostic or therapeutic agent in the United States. However, because the results of the experimental clinical trials are so compelling, certain potential applications are discussed.

Initial results of GHRH therapy in 55 children treated for up to 2 years for GH deficiency are promising. The majority of children with GH deficiency treated with the 40 or 44 amino acid peptide have an increase in growth velocity.

Dopamine Agonists The dopamine agonist bromocriptine is approved in the United States for the treatment of hyperprolactinemia (both physiological and pathophysiological), acromegaly, and Parkinson's disease.

In physiological hyperprolactinemia, circulating concentrations of prolactin, elevated during pregnancy, remain increased after delivery in preparation for lactation because prolactin plays a major role in milk secretion. If the mother does not breast-feed, serum prolactin concentrations decrease and are often within the normal range by 2 weeks after parturition. However, early in the postpartum period, breast engorgement and mastodynia (breast pain) may occur, thus prompting efforts to suppress lactation. Treatment with bromocriptine is a highly effective approach in that it suppresses secretion of prolactin—the primary stimulus to the breast. Used in this manner, bromocriptine is as effective as estrogen in preventing engorgement. Similarly, bromocriptine is more effective than estrogen/androgen combinations in inhibiting breast engorgement and lactation. In contrast to estrogen, bromocriptine does not increase the risk of thromboembolic disease, offering a significant advantage over estrogenic preparations.

A prolactin-secreting adenoma is the common cause of pathological hyperprolactinemia. The goals of treatment of these prolactinomas, as for all pituitary tumors, include reduction of tumor mass with concurrent restoration of visual fields and cranial nerve function, preservation of other anterior pituitary function, suppression of the secretion of tumor product, and prevention of recurrence or progression of the disease.

Bromocriptine lowers serum prolactin concentrations in patients with microadenomas and also lowers circulating prolactin concentrations and reduces tumor mass. Bromocriptine inhibits prolactin secretion by adenomatous cells by stimulating dopamine receptors present on these cells. Because dopamine receptor–second messenger systems seem intact in prolactinomas, a relative dopamine deficiency likely exists in patients with such tumors.

If hyperprolactinemia represents a dopamine deficiency, one would predict that withdrawal of the dopamine agonist bromocriptine would allow a return of elevated prolactin concentrations, and such is the case. Even more dramatic is the effect of bromocriptine withdrawal on tumor size. Bromocriptine shrinks prolactin-secreting macroadenomas in the majority of cases, apparently by effecting a return of the secretory machinery from a hypersecretory to a quiescent state. However, withdrawal of the agent results in a prompt reexpansion of tumor with a concurrent increase in serum prolactin concentrations. Thus the use of bromocriptine for the treatment of prolactinomas may be considered as replacement therapy because bromocriptine corrects the relative dopamine deficiency if it is administered repeatedly.

The clinical effects attributed to therapy of prolactinomas with bromocriptine are impressive. With decreasing prolactin concentrations, galactorrhea is abolished or greatly reduced in virtually all patients. Gonadal function, frequently compromised in hyperprolactinemic subjects, is restored in the majority, though in women, normal ovulatory menstrual cycles may not return for a year. Previously infertile women achieve pregnancy rates indistinguishable from those of normal women. Signs and symptoms of intracranial tumor expansion (headache, visual field defects) show extraordinary improvement within a few days, and remain stable as long as the drug is continued. No adverse effects of chronic treatment with bromocriptine are demonstrated. Bromocriptine therapy of prolactin-secreting microadenomas and macroadenomas is a reality. Although bromocriptine does not offer a cure, it is a feasable alternative to surgery.

Bromocriptine reduces (albeit rarely to normal) circulating concentrations of GH in at least 70% of patients with acromegaly, presumably by a direct effect on the adenomatous somatotropes.

For the effect of bromocriptine in Parkinson's disease see Chapter 27.

Somatostatin and Analogs Somatostatin's role in pathogenesis of disease is relatively small. The rare somatostatin-secreting tumor (usually pancreatic) is associated with mild diabetes mellitus, suppressed GH release, cholelithiasis, and gastrointestinal malabsorption.

Several therapeutic uses for somatostatin are proposed, but this peptide is not available for general use in the United States. Additionally, the short half-life (3 to 4 minutes) and the requirement for continuous parenteral administration limit its therapeutic usefulness. Proposed uses for this agent (or its analogs) include treatment of poorly controlled type 1 diabetes mellitus, acromegaly, gastrointestinal hemorrhage, hemorrhagic pancreatitis, prophylaxis for pancreatitis in patients undergoing pancreatic surgery, and suppression of hormone secretion from a variety of hyperfunctioning endocrine tumors. These include GH-secreting adenomas, insulinomas, carcinoids, glucagonomas, gastrinomas, and VIPomas.

Because the major therapeutic limitation is its short half-life, numerous analogs have been synthesized with longer durations of activity and more specific suppressive effects. The analog in current clinical use is the 8 amino acid cyclic peptide octreotide, approved for treatment of patients with carcinoid tumors and VIP-secreting tumors. Clinical trials for treatment of acromegaly and other hypersecretory endocrine tumors and various GI disorders are in progress.

Pituitary Hormones

Luteinizing Hormone and Follicle-Stimulating Hormone Human menopausal gonadotropin is a purified preparation of LH and FSH extracted from urine of postmenopausal women used to treat infertility in women and men. Human menopausal gonadotropin induces follicular growth and, because of its similarity to LH and its ability to stimulate the LH receptor, is administered to induce ovulation. It successfully induces ovulation in approximately 90% of women, with subsequent pregnancy resulting in 20% to 30% who achieve ovulation. Human menopausal gonadotropin therapy directly stimulates the ovaries and bypasses the normal feedback controls of the hypothalamic-pituitary-ovarian axis. Consequently, more than one follicle may develop and ovulate with multiple pregnancies, mostly twins, occurring in about 20% of women who become pregnant in this way. A mild hyperstimulation syndrome characterized by ovarian enlargement and abdominal pain or distention occurs in 20% of patients. A more severe form with ascites is infrequent.

Quite recently a highly purified FSH preparation has become available. Urofollitropin is extracted from the urine of postmenopausal women, as is menotropin, but is subsequently purified such that less than 1 IU of LH remains per 75 IU of FSH. Urofollitropin has been approved for ovulation induction in women with the polycystic ovary syndrome who have failed to respond to clomiphene citrate.

Clomiphene (Figure 41-7), with or without human chorionic gonadotropin, is commonly administered before human menopausal gonadotropin or urofollitropin. Compared to human menopausal gonadotropin, clomiphene administration has a decreased incidence of multiple births and ovarian hyperstimulation syndrome. Human menopausal gonadotropin and urofollitropin are reserved for women in whom clomiphene therapy has failed.

Human menopausal gonadotropin therapy is indicated for inducing fertility in men with hypogonadotropic hypogonadism. Adequate sperm counts are obtained in about 75% of cases, and pregnancy results in approximately 75% of patients' wives. Occasionally, men can achieve complete spermatogenesis with hu-

clomiphene

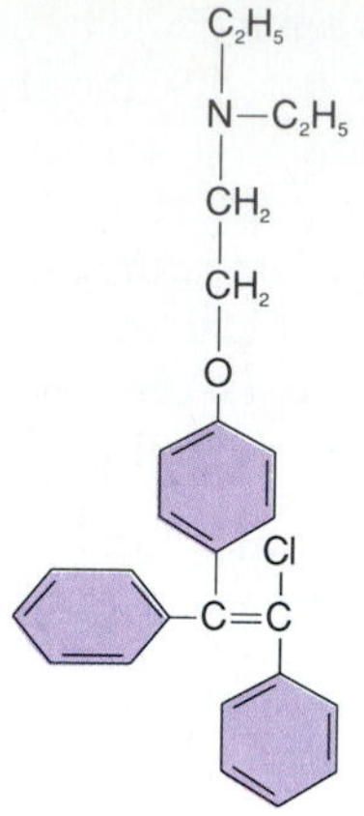

FIGURE 41-7 Clomiphene, a nonsteroidal stimulator of pituitary release of human gonadotropin. See the text for further information.

man chorionic gonadotropin therapy alone.

Growth Hormone GH promotes linear growth by generation of IGF-1 and influences all aspects of metabolism. This hormone is described as *anabolic, lipolytic,* and *diabetogenic.* Replacement of GH in children with GH deficiency stimulates amino acid incorporation into muscle protein, as indicated by decreased serum amino acid concentrations and decreased urinary nitrogen excretion. Treatment of GH deficiency with GH does not promote glucose intolerance or diabetes mellitus; the excessive GH in acromegaly is associated with glucose intolerance and diabetes mellitus. The evidence that GH is lipolytic resides primarily in in vitro studies of isolated adipose tissue. Its role in the regulation of lipid metabolism in humans is unclear.

Excessive GH secretion results in gigantism or acromegaly. Gigantism occurs if GH hypersecretion is present before epiphyseal closure during puberty, and acromegaly occurs with hypersecretion after puberty. Excessive GH secretion may cause thickening of the skin and soft tissues and result in skeletal changes such as mandibular, frontal, zygomatic bone, and acral enlargement with osseous overgrowth. These skeletal changes result in degenerative arthritis of the hips, knees, shoulders, and elbows.

Growth hormone is used therapeutically to treat children with GH deficiency. With the development of human GH using recombinant DNA technology, the supply problem for GH is resolved. Growth hormone treatment of children with GH deficiency is associated with a significant increase in linear growth rate.

Vasopressin Three forms of vasopressin are approved for clinical use: native arginine vasopressin, vasopressin tannate, and 1-desamino-8-D-arginine-vasopressin (desmopressin). Each may be employed for the treatment of diabetes insipidus.

Neurogenic diabetes insipidus is a disorder characterized by polyuria and polydipsia that results from inadequate secretion of AVP (see Chapter 39). Over 80% of the hypothalamic neuronal system responsible for synthesizing and secreting AVP must be dysfunctional before symptoms develop.

Vasopressin increases circulating concentrations of factor VIII (antihemophilic factor) (see Chapter 21), perhaps by stimulating its release from cells in the vascular endothelium. Vasopressin is used to treat mild hemophilia A and mild-to-moderate von Willebrand's disease. However, desmopressin, because of its relative lack of untoward side effects compared to AVP, is more often used. In patients with factor VIII concentrations greater than 5%, hemostasis may be maintained during and after surgical procedures if patients are treated 30 minutes before the procedure. In addition, desmopressin may be used in certain situations in which bleeding is a complication of trauma.

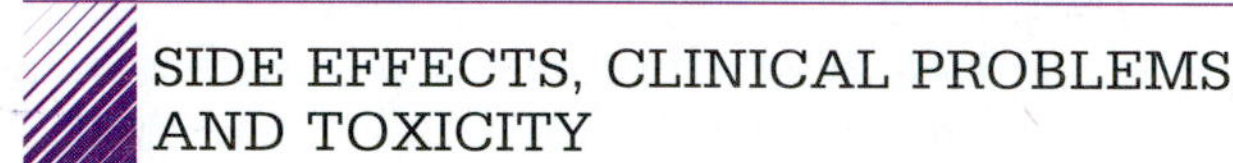

SIDE EFFECTS, CLINICAL PROBLEMS, AND TOXICITY

Clinical problems are summarized in the box. p. 559.

Hypothalamic Hormones

GnRH GnRH is generally well tolerated with the frequency of adverse reactions quite low, but occasionally nausea, light-headedness, headache, and abdominal discomfort result from relatively large doses. Subcutaneous administration is associated with antibody formation in a small number of patients.

Side effects from SC and IV administration of GnRH through portable infusion pumps include inflammation, infection, phlebitis, and hematoma at the catheter site. Frequency of these reactions can be significantly decreased by thorough patient education regarding aseptic technique and management of the infusion pump.

GHRH Side effects of GHRH include facial flushing with higher doses given IV. Repetitive, prolonged administration may result in development of circulating antibodies, but their clinical significance is not known, because the children treated demonstrate continued acceleration of linear growth. Antibodies either disappear or decrease in titer when GHRH is discontinued. No interactions with other drugs have been described.

Dopamine Agonists Adverse effects of bromocriptine may be grouped into three categories: (1) effects occurring during initiation of therapy and occasionally during chronic treatment of hyperprolactinemia and ac-

CLINICAL PROBLEMS

HYPOTHALAMIC HORMONES AND ANALOGS	
GnRH	Adverse reactions infrequent Occasional nausea, headache, abdominal discomfort Anaphylaxis (rare) with IV use Localized problems at injection site
GHRH	Facial flushing Antibodies with repeated use
bromocriptine	Nausea, orthostatic hypotension initially Confusion, hallucinations in Parkinson's disease Erythromelalgia, dyskinesia worsening Discontinue during pregnancy
somatostatin analogs	Hyperglycemia, loose stools, gallstones
PITUITARY HORMONES AND ANALOGS	
LH and FSH	Multiple pregnancy Gynecomastia in men Occasional febrile reactions
GH	Antibodies Misuse in athletes, constitutional delay of growth
AVP	Nausea, vertigo, headache Anaphylaxis Angina, myocardial infarction Water intoxication
DRUG INTERACTIONS	
bromocriptine	phenothiazine or butyrophenones, prevents dopamine agonist action
Vasopressin analogs	carbamazepine, chlorpropamide, clofibrate, urea, fludrocortisone, tricyclic antidepressants, potentiate action demeclocycline, norepinephrine, lithium, heparin, alcohol, inhibit action

romegaly, (2) effects occurring during treatment of Parkinson's disease, and (3) problems of teratogenicity and treatment of tumor expansion during pregnancy.

When bromocriptine is first administered, patients experience nausea with or without vomiting, dizziness, or orthostatic hypotension. These effects can be minimized if therapy is begun with low doses given with food and at bedtime and with a gradual increase in the frequency to a full-dose regimen. Most patients quickly develop a tolerance. A few patients complain of headache, fatigue, abdominal cramping, nasal congestion, drowsiness, or diarrhea, either at the onset of treatment or with chronic administration. An occasional patient will be intolerant of bromocriptine.

The treatment of Parkinson's disease with bromocriptine may result in special problems. In addition to the nausea and orthostatic hypotension commonly encountered, confusion and visual or auditory hallucinations or erythromelalgia (limb pain) may occur. Moreover, in some patients their dyskinetic symptoms may worsen. These effects may represent interactions of bromocriptine with a disordered CNS. Fortunately, a substantial number of patients who manifest symptoms become tolerant of the drug, allowing treatment to continue.

The fact that infertility associated with hyperprolactinemia may be successfully treated with bromocriptine raises concerns that the drug may be teratogenic. Therefore what role to assign to bromocriptine in treating tumor expansions if it occurs during pregnancy is raised. Thus far, well over 1400 bromocriptine-associated pregnancies have been described with no increased risk to the fetus. Specifically, no differences are detected in the rates of spontaneous abortion, the incidences of multiple births, or the presence of minor or severe congenital abnormalities when compared with control women not treated with bromocriptine. Although there is no evidence for teratogenicity, it is recommended that fetal exposure to bromocriptine be minimized. Fortunately, the majority of women with tumor-associated hyperprolactinemia have microadenomas and appear to have a very low rate of complications (<1%) during pregnancy. The percentage of women with macroadenomas who develop headaches and visual field defects during pregnancy is significantly higher, perhaps approaching 25%. Based so far on extremely small numbers, no untoward effects on fetal development are noted when bromocriptine is administered during pregnancy.

Because bromocriptine is a dopamine receptor agonist, the concurrent administration of dopamine receptor blocking agents may negate or diminish its clinical effects. The phenothiazines (e.g., chlorpromazine) and butyrophenones (e.g., haloperidol) may modify the dopamine agonist activity of bromocriptine if used simultaneously.

Somatostatin and Analogs The adverse effects of native somatostatin are limited to suppression of insulin release. Prolonged administration results in mild hyperglycemia. Administration of the analog octreotide is similarly associated with mild hyperglycemia, particularly postprandially. This can be minimized by administration of the drug 2 to 3 hours after meals. Gallstone or sludge formation in the gallbladder may occur with octreotide therapy. Prospective studies indicate that the incidence of stone/sludge formation may be approximately 18%. Symptomatic cholelithiasis was uncommon. Patients usually develop acholic loose stools during the first 1 to 2 weeks of therapy, but clinically significant malabsorption is not reported. No adverse effects on the cardiovascular system have been noted.

Pituitary Hormones

LH and FSH Human menopausal gonadotropin is generally well tolerated; common adverse reactions are multiple pregnancies and ovarian hyperstimulation. Gynecomastia occasionally occurs in men, and thromboembolism is a serious but very rare complication.

Growth Hormone Administration of human GH may promote development of anti-GH antibodies; however, only a small minority of children who received GH have impairment of growth. Pituitary derived GH is no longer available for use in the United States because several young adults developed Creutzfeldt-Jakob disease after being treated with pituitary-derived GH. The currently approved human GH preparation is that produced by recombinant DNA methodology. Preliminary studies with this human GH indicate that formation of anti-GH antibodies occurs less frequently, by 10% to 20%.

A potential problem with GH resides with its misuse, particularly in the field of competitive athletics. GH use by athletes is related to its suggested anabolic properties on muscle development. Excessive, unsupervised GH administration may result in medical problems associated with acromegaly, including hyperhidrosis, arthropathy, extremity enlargement, and visceromegaly. Growth hormone administration to short children with normal endogenous GH production is another area of concern. It is not established that such treatment alters ultimate height and may result in side effects of excessive GH.

Vasopressin Nonspecific adverse reactions that may occur with AVP desmopressin include nausea, vertigo, headache, and anaphylaxis. Other signs and symptoms may relate directly to specific pressor and antidiuretic effects. With regard to the former, vasoconstriction may occur and cause relatively mild problems such as skin blanching or abdominal cramping, or more serious effects such as angina or myocardial infarction. Although all preparations should be used with caution in patients with known coronary artery disease, desmopressin has lower pressor effects and may be the drug of choice. All vasopressins may cause water intoxication. Signs and symptoms of this disorder include drowsiness, listlessness, weakness, headaches, seizures, and coma. Care must be taken to closely watch for such signs and symptoms and titrate the dose appropriately.

Several drugs, if administered simultaneously, potentiate or inhibit the effects of vasopressin. Potentiators include carbamazepine, chlorpropamide, clofibrate, urea, fludrocortisone, and tricyclic antidepressants. On the other hand, inhibitors include demeclocycline, norepinephrine, lithium carbonate, heparin, and alcohol.

NEW DIRECTIONS

GnRH and certain GnRH agonists have just recently been approved for primary hypothalamic amenorrhea, advanced prostate cancer, and endometriosis. Clinical trials are continuing to assess the utility of such agonists for the treatment of precocious puberty, and approval is expected within the next year. The search for a true GnRH antagonist is continuing at a rapid pace. Such an agent should inhibit gonadotropin secretion as

TRADE NAMES

In addition to generic and fixed-combination preparations, the following trade-named materials are available in the United States.

HYPOTHALAMIC HORMONES AND ANALOGS

Lupron, leuprolide acetate, GnRH analog
Parlodel, bromocriptine mesylate
Sandostatin, octreotide, somatostatin analog

PITUITARY HORMONES AND ANALOGS

APL, Profasi, Pregnyl, human chorionic gonadotropin
DDAVP, desmopressin acetate
Pergonal, luteinizing hormone/follicle stimulating hormone
Pitressin, arginine vasopressin
Pitressin Tannate in Oil, arginine vasopressin tannate
Protropin, human growth hormone
Serophene, clomiphene citrate

do the GnRH agonists, but be devoid of the initial stimulatory effect on gonadotropins commonly encountered with he GnRH agonists. Today, allergic responses to the various candidate antagonists have hampered the development of a pharmacological agent suitable for widespread use in humans.

GHRH remains experimental for treatment of children with GH deficiency. It is used for diagnostic purposes to assess GH responsiveness and residual GH function in patients who have undergone pituitary surgery or pituitary radiation. It may also be used to diagnose GH deficiency in children. However, this is not the standard test and may produce variable results. It is anticipated that there will be developed in the future a depot GHRH preparation or long-acting GHRH analog that may be useful to treat GH deficiency or restore diminished GH secretion in elderly adults with a potentially normal pituitary gland.

The only available somatostatin analog is octreotide. Other analogs are under development. It is anticipated that an oral form of octreotide may be developed, thus eliminating the need for subcutaneous injection. Up to now, octreotide is approved for treatment of carcinoid and VIP-secreting tumors. Approval for treatment of acromegaly is anticipated in the near future.

For many years the primary source of the gonadotropins LH and FSH has been the urine of postmenopausal women. Although the recovery and purification of the gonadotropins from urine has been satisfactory in many ways, recombinant DNA technology provides an attractive alternative. Several laboratories are using this technology to produce both LH and FSH, and clinical trials should be underway in the very near future.

Growth hormone therapy in prepubertal girls with Turner's syndrome appears to increase final adult height. It is too early to know if final adult height will be altered in non–GH deficient short children, but preliminary studies indicate that it will not. Growth hormone is currently under investigation as replacement in GH deficient adults and in older adults with diminished GH production.

New dopamine agonists undergoing clinical evaluation include a nonergot derivative, CV 205-502, and a long-acting ergot derivative, cabergoline. Both drugs effectively suppress serum prolactin and produce reduction in tumor size in patients with prolactinoma.

REFERENCES

Baylis PH: Vasopressin and its neurophysin. In DeGroot L, editor: *Endocrinology,* vol 1, Philadelphia, 1989, Saunders.

Conn PM: The molecular basis of gonadotropin-releasing hormone action, *Endocr Rev* 7:3, 1986.

Evans WS, Kolp LA, Sollenberger MJ: Ovulation induction with gonadotropin-releasing hormone. In Loriaux DL, editor: The *Endocrinologist* 1:187-193, 1991.

Labrie F. Dupont A, Belanger A, et al: Treatment of prostate cancer with gonadotropin-releasing hormone agonists, *Endocr Rev* 7(1):67, 1986.

Marshall JC, Dalkin AC, Haisenleder DJ, et al: Gonadotropin-releasing hormone pulses: regulators of gonadotropin synthesis and ovulatory cycles, *Recent Prog Horm Res* 47:155-189, 1991.

Moller DE, Moses AC, Jones K, et al: Octreotide suppresses growth hormone and growth hormone releasing hormone in acromegaly secondary to ectopic GHRH secretion, *J Clin Endocrinol Metab* 68:499, 1989.

Reichlin S: Somatostatin, *N Engl J Med* 309:1495, 1983.

Robinson AG: DDAVP in the treatment of central diabetes insipidus, *N Engl J Med* 294:507, 1976.

Vance ML, Thorner MO: Prolactin: hyperprolactinemic syndromes and management, *Endocrinology* 1:408-418, 1989.

Vance ML, Evans WS, Thorner MO: Bromocriptine, *Ann Intern Med* 100:78, 1984.

Veldhuis JD, Fraioli F, Rogol AD, et al: Metabolic clearance of biologically active luteinizing hormone in man, *J Clin Invest* 77:1122, 1986.

SELF-ASSESSMENT QUESTIONS

1. Hypothalamic hormones and their analogs known to stimulate or inhibit hormone release by the anterior pituitary gland and that have been used clinically as pharmacologic agents include all of the following *except:*
   a. gonadotropin releasing hormone.
   b. growth hormone–releasing hormone.
   c. prolactin releasing factor.
   d. dopamine.
   e. somatostatin.
2. Hypothalamic-pituitary hormones and their analogs that have been used to promote ovulation in anovulatory women include each of the following *except:*
   a. gonadotropin releasing hormone.
   b. gonadotropin releasing hormone agonists.
   c. human menopausal gonadotropin.
   d. urofollitropin.
   e. dopamine agonists.
3. Of the vasopressin/vasopressin analog family available for clinical use, the agent (or agents) having excellent antidiuretic effects but minimal pressor effects is (are):
   a. arginine vasopressin.
   b. arginine vasopressin tannate.
   c. desmopressin acetate.
   d. a and b.
   e. none of the above.

4. Patients treated with the somatostatin analog octreotide are at risk for:
   a. peptic ulcer disease.
   b. gallstone formation.
   c. rash.
   d. hyperglycemia.
   e. b and d.

5. Growth hormone is currently approved for treatment of:
   a. short children.
   b. GH-deficient children.
   c. the elderly.
   d. athletes.
   e. all of the above.

CHAPTER 42

Calcium-Regulating Hormones and Other Agents Affecting Bone

PAULA H. STERN

MAJOR DRUGS

vitamin D and metabolites
parathyroid hormone
calcitonin

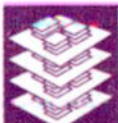

THERAPEUTIC OVERVIEW

The calcium concentration in the blood is normally maintained within narrow limits, approximately 8.8 to 10.4 mg/dl. When the calcium concentrations exceed this normal range, the functions of many tissues are affected. Hypocalcemia can lead to increased neuromuscular excitability and tetany. Hypercalcemia can result in life-threatening cardiac arrhythmias, renal damage, soft-tissue calcification, and CNS abnormalities. Various disorders can cause perturbations in calcium homeostasis. These, as well as disorders that may not necessarily affect serum calcium, can lead to changes in the skeleton that interfere with its normal function of support and protection. This chapter focuses on organs that regulate calcium concentrations in plasma and extracellular fluid (i.e., bone, kidney, and intestines).

The treatment of disorders of bone and calcium metabolism involves the use not only of calcium-regulating hormones and other agents with specific effects on mineral metabolism, but also of drugs from other pharmacological categories, including gonadal and adrenal hormones, antiinflammatory drugs, diuretics, and cancer chemotherapeutic agents. The sites at which the different agents act to produce their effects on calcium metabolism include the gastrointestinal tract, the kidney, and bone (Figure 42-1). Approximately 10% to 20% of the dietary calcium is normally absorbed. Absorption is impaired in the absence of vitamin D and augmented by excess vitamin D. Renal tubular reabsorption normally recovers 99% of the 10 to 20 g of calcium filtered per day. Bone is the major storehouse for calcium, containing approximately 1 kg per 70 kg human. Of this, more than 99% is in a stable pool, with a daily turnover of 0.3 to 0.5 g. Changes depend on cellular activity. An exchangeable pool of 4 to 5 g turns over at the rate of approximately 20 g/day. Turnover of the exchangeable pool is a passive physicochemical process.

Diseases associated with hypocalcemia and rickets (inadequate bone mineralization during development) or osteomalacia (inadequate bone mineralization in the adult) are listed in Table 42-1. These disorders, which are treated with vitamin D and calcium, result from inadequate vitamin D or resistance to its action. Disorders that lead to hypercalcemia are more diverse in nature and cause. The therapy is determined partly by the cause of the disease, but also by severity of the hypercalcemia and the need for rapid correction. Various pharmacological approaches, including inorganic ions, diuretics, antiinflammatory agents, diuretics and anticancer agents, are employed to treat hypercalcemia. Table 42-1 also lists disorders of bone turnover not usually associated with abnormal serum calcium and phosphate, which are amenable to therapy. Paget's disease of bone is characterized by both excessive formation and resorption occurring in an irregular manner in one or more bones. In osteoporosis, there is excessive loss of bone, leading to fractures.

The therapeutic overview is summarized in the box.

ABBREVIATIONS

EDTA	ethylenediaminetetracetic acid
PTH	parathyroid hormone

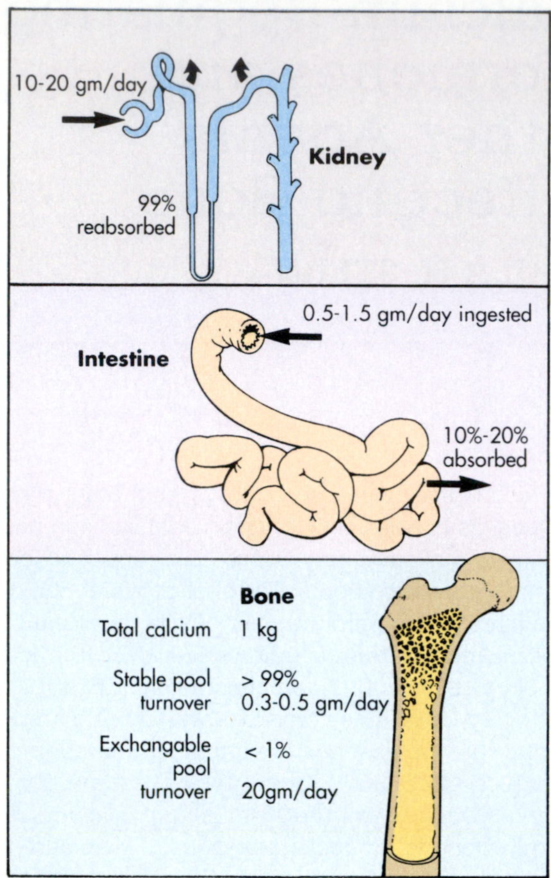

FIGURE 42-1 Sites of calcium regulation. Ten percent to 20% of dietary calcium is absorbed in the gastrointestinal tract, and the renal tubules recover 99% of filtered calcium. Bone is the primary storage site, containing approximately 1 kg of calcium.

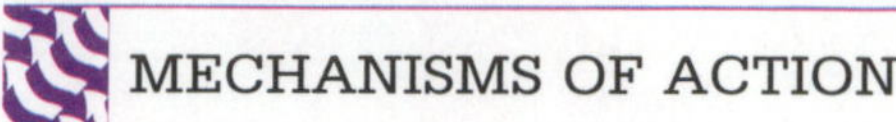

MECHANISMS OF ACTION

Vitamin D and Metabolites

Vitamin D is a secosteroid, a steroid derivative in which the B ring has been cleaved and has undergone a rearrangement. Figure 42-2 shows the structures of vi-

THERAPEUTIC OVERVIEW

VITAMIN D AND ITS METABOLITES
Rickets
Osteomalacia
Hypocalcemia
Hypoparathyroidism (10 × larger doses)
Vitamin D–resistant rickets

PARATHYROID HORMONE
Diagnostic agent for pseudohypoparathyroidism

CALCITONIN
Paget's disease of bone
Osteoporosis
Hypercalcemia of malignancy

EDTA, FUROSEMIDE, ETHACRYNIC ACID, AND MANY OTHER AGENTS (see text)
Hypercalcemia

CALCIUM, ESTROGEN, CALCITONIN
Osteoporosis

Table 42-1 Disorders of Bone and Calcium Metabolism

Type of Disorder	Treatment	Examples
Disorders leading to hypocalcemia	Usually treated with vitamin D compounds and calcium	Inadequate dietary calcium or vitamin D, or both Malabsorption caused by defective activation of vitamin D Malabsorption caused by end-organ resistance to vitamin D Hypoparathyroidism, pseudohypoparathyroidism Renal failure
Disorders leading to hypercalcemia	Treatments include fluids, low calcium diet, sulfate, loop-acting diuretics, glucocorticoids, calcitonin, plicamycin, diphosphonates	Hyperparathyroidism Hypervitaminosis D Sarcoidosis Neoplasia Hyperthyroidism Immobilization
Disorders of bone remodeling	Treated with diphosphonates, calcitonin, and plicamycin	Paget's disease of bone
	Treated with estrogen (female), calcium, and calcitonin	Osteoporosis

tamin D_2, ergocalciferol, which is synthesized from ergosterol by yeast, and vitamin D_3, cholecalciferol, synthesized from cholesterol by animals and higher plants. Vitamin D is not biologically active and first must be activated by two metabolic steps (Figure 42-3). The first step, a hydroxylation in the carbon 25 position, occurs in the liver, predominantly in the endoplasmic reticulum. The product, 25-hydroxyvitamin D, is more potent and acts more rapidly than vitamin D. 25-Hydroxyvitamin D is further activated in the kidney to 1,25-dihydroxyvitamin D by a cytochrome P-450 enzyme-dependent hydroxylation. The 1-hydroxylation step is feedback regulated and is stimulated by parathyroid hormone and by low plasma phosphate concentrations. 1,25-Dihydroxyvitamin D is the most potent and most rapidly acting vitamin D metabolite.

The active vitamin D metabolites bind to receptors in the nucleus of the cell that interact with sites in the promoter region of genes and initiate the synthesis of specific proteins. Among these protein products are two high-affinity calcium-binding proteins, calbindins, which may play a role in the stimulation of calcium transport by vitamin D, and osteocalcin or bone gla protein, a lower-affinity calcium-binding protein found extracellularly in normally and abnormally mineralized tissues. The active vitamin D metabolites have two major effects that lead to an increase in serum calcium (Figure 42-4). The first is to increase the absorption of dietary calcium and phosphate by stimulating their uptake across the GI mucosa. Rapid membrane effects to stimulate ion fluxes, as well as genomic actions, may contribute to this response. The effect of vitamin D on

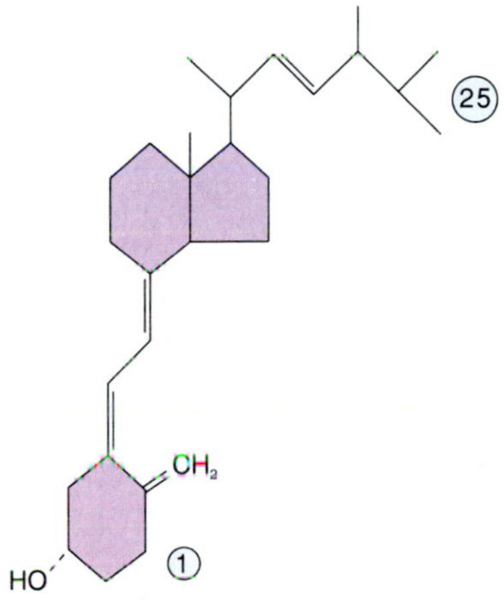

Vitamin D_2, ergocalciferol

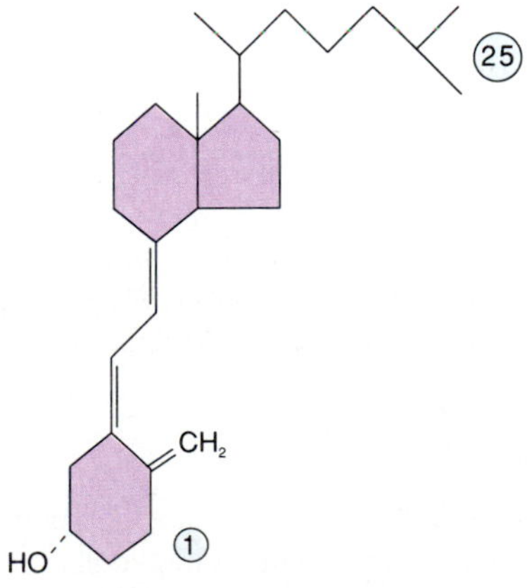

Vitamin D_3, cholecalciferol

FIGURE 42-2 Structures of vitamin D_2 and vitamin D_3 with carbon positions 1 and 25 indicated. Notice difference in side chains.

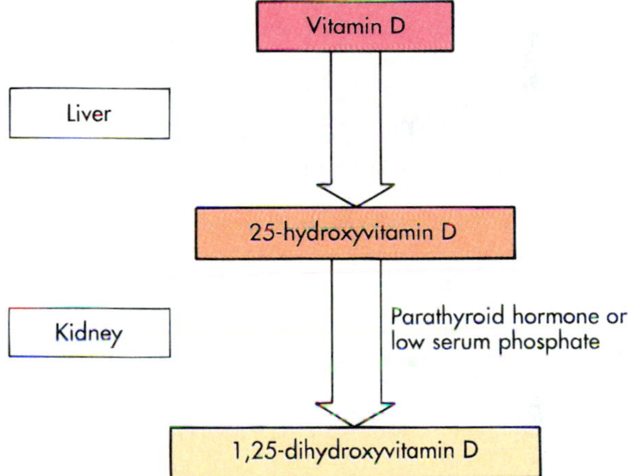

FIGURE 42-3 Vitamin D activation pathway. The first step in dihydroxylation occurs in the liver, with further activation in the kidney by cytochrome P-450 enzyme-dependent hydroxylation to 1,25-dihydroxyvitamin D.

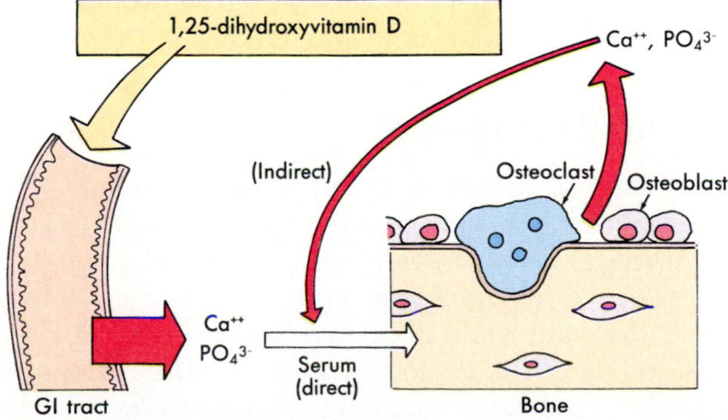

FIGURE 42-4 Major sites and effects of calcium regulation by 1,25-dihydroxyvitamin D: direct and indirect effects. Increased absorption from gastrointestinal tract into serum (direct) and stimulated release from bone into serum (indirect) are shown.

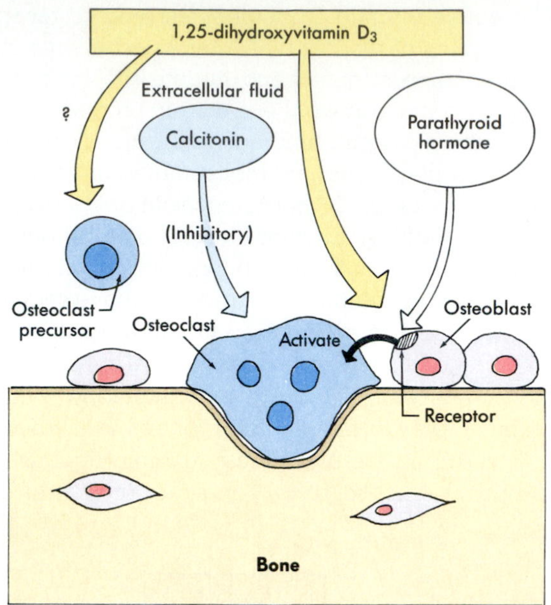

FIGURE 42-5 Cellular sites of action of calcemic hormones on bone. Hormone-osteoblast complex activates osteoclast. Receptors on osteoblasts stimulate the activity of osteoclasts, releasing Ca^{++} from bone. Calcitonin inhibits the activity of osteoclasts.

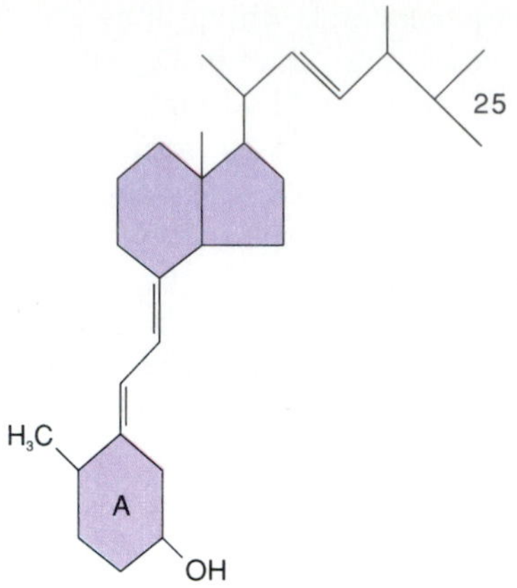

FIGURE 42-6 Structure of dihydrotachysterol. Notice position of groups in A ring. See the text for further information.

bone mineralization, the antirachitic effect, is an indirect result of the increased calcium and phosphate absorption. The elevated $(Ca^{++}) \times (PO_4^{3-})$ product results in the deposition of more mineral in the bone. The second action is to stimulate the release of calcium from bone. This action requires cellular activity, and the current concept (Figure 42-5) is that receptors are present on osteoblastic cells, which subsequently stimulate the activity of osteoclasts, releasing calcium from the bone. Effects of vitamin D metabolites on the differentiation of osteoclast precursors may also play a role. Dihydrotachysterol (Figure 42-6) is a synthetic analog of vitamin D_2. It is maximally activated by 25-hydroxylation and acts more rapidly than vitamin D.

Parathyroid Hormone

Parathyroid hormone (PTH) is an 84 amino acid polypeptide. It is processed from a 115 amino acid polypeptide precursor, preproparathyroid hormone (Figure 42-7), which is cleaved in the endoplasmic reticulum of the parathyroid gland to a 90 amino acid polypeptide, proparathyroid hormone. The latter is further cleaved in the Golgi apparatus and secretory vesicles to an 84 amino acid polypeptide. Parathyroid hormone binds to membrane receptors in target cells and acts to stimulate protein phosphorylation. Cyclic adenosine monophosphate and intracellular calcium, both of which are increased by parathyroid hormone action in target tissues, are involved as second messengers. PTH has two major direct and one indirect site of action for mediating its effects on serum calcium and phosphate (Figure 42-8). PTH acts directly on the kidney to decrease renal tubular reabsorption of phosphate and to increase renal tubular reabsorption of calcium. These effects lead to an increase in serum calcium and a decrease in serum phosphate concentrations. Acting on bone, PTH stimulates resorption and thereby increases serum calcium concentration through an effect on osteoblasts (Figure 42-5). PTH indirectly enhances calcium absorption by stimulating the formation of 1,25-dihydroxyvitamin D (Figures 42-3 and 42-8). Low concentrations of PTH also have an anabolic effect on bone and increase bone formation. Analogs of PTH that act as antagonists at the receptor have been synthesized but are not yet in current therapeutic use. A recently discovered protein, the PTH-related protein, has significant amino acid sequence homology to parathyroid hormone at the N-terminal of the molecule. It is produced by several types of tumors and is likely to play a role in some malignancy-related hypercalcemias. It may also be involved in normal calcium metabolism in tissues such as the mammary gland and the placenta.

Calcitonin

Calcitonin is a 32 amino acid polypeptide (Figure 42-9) secreted by the parafollicular cells of the thyroid. It decreases postprandial absorption of calcium; increases the excretion of calcium, sodium, magnesium, chloride, and phosphate; and inhibits the activity of osteoclasts (Figure 42-5). This latter action on bone is probably its most effective means of lowering serum cal-

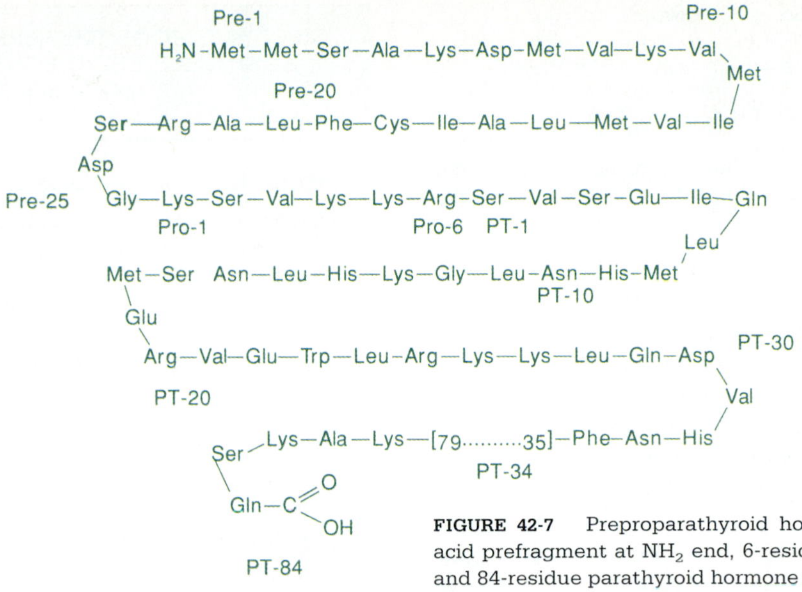

Pre-1
Pre-10
H₂N-Met-Met-Ser-Ala-Lys-Asp-Met-Val-Lys-Val
Met
Pre-20
Ser-Arg-Ala-Leu-Phe-Cys-Ile-Ala-Leu-Met-Val-Ile
Asp
Pre-25
Gly-Lys-Ser-Val-Lys-Lys-Arg-Ser-Val-Ser-Glu-Ile-Gln
Pro-1
Pro-6
PT-1
Leu
Met-Ser Asn-Leu-His-Lys-Gly-Leu-Asn-His-Met
PT-10
Glu
Arg-Val-Glu-Trp-Leu-Arg-Lys-Lys-Leu-Gln-Asp
PT-30
PT-20
Val
Ser-Lys-Ala-Lys-[79..........35]-Phe-Asn-His
PT-34
Gln-C=O OH
PT-84

FIGURE 42-7 Preproparathyroid hormone showing 25 amino acid prefragment at NH_2 end, 6-residue profragment in center, and 84-residue parathyroid hormone (PT) portion at COOH end; PT activity mainly in residues PT-1 through PT-34.

Parathyroid hormone
Ca⁺⁺
Osteoclast
Osteoblast
Ca⁺⁺
25-hydroxyvitamin D
1,25-dihydroxyvitamin D
Bone
Kidney
PO₄³⁻
Ca⁺⁺
Intestine

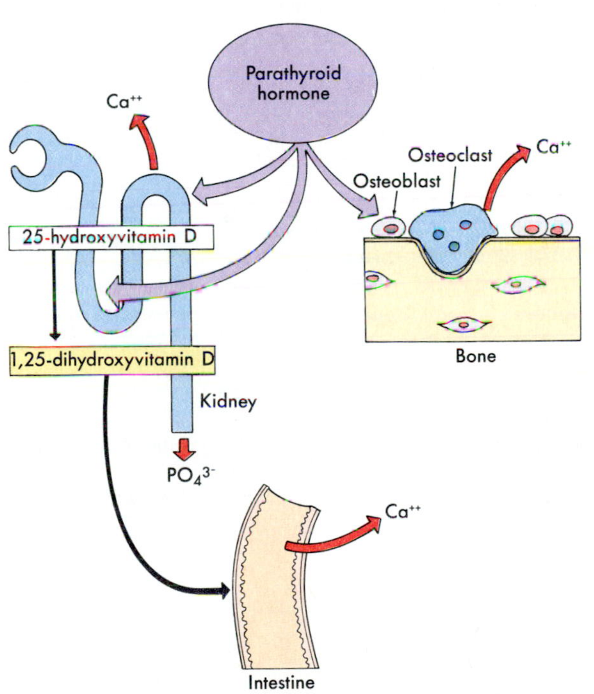

FIGURE 42-8 Direct and indirect effects of parathyroid hormone on calcium metabolism. Renal tubular reabsorption of PO_4 decreases and that of calcium increases; hormone stimulated osteoblast activates osteoclast to release calcium into extracellular fluid.

cium concentration. The effects of calcitonin on bone exhibit a phenomenon termed *escape,* a loss of effectiveness with continued use. This is unrelated to the formation of antibodies to the hormone and is related to a cellular event within bone itself.

H₂N-Cys-Gly-Asn-Leu-Ser-Thr-Cys-Met-Leu-Gly-Thr-Tyr
S-S
Thr
Gln
Asp
Phe
Asn
Lys
H₂N O
C
Pro
Ala
Gly-Val-Gly-Ile-Ala-Thr-Gln-Pro-Phe-Thr-His-Phe

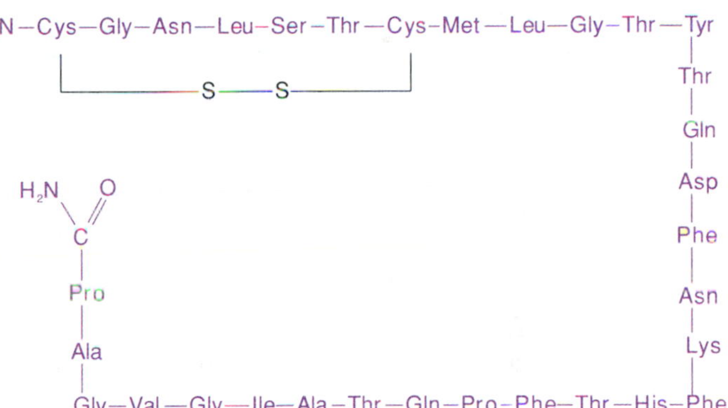

FIGURE 42-9 Calcitonin structure. See the text for further information.

Other Agents Affecting Bone and Calcium Metabolism

Phosphate salts can increase calcium deposition in bone by a physicochemical action and can rapidly lower serum calcium concentration. Sodium sulfate and ethylenediaminetetracetic acid (EDTA) form poorly dissociable calcium salts and will increase calcium excretion. Certain diuretics (specifically the loop-action diuretics ethacrynic acid and furosemide) increase both calcium and sodium excretion. This action is not shared by the benzothiadiazides, which decrease calcium excretion. Bone resorption is inhibited by estrogens, diphosphonates, plicamycin, and glucocorticoids. Estrogen inhibits bone resorption. The use of estrogens as hormone replacement therapy after menopause for the prevention of osteoporosis is discussed in Chapter 36. These are the main effects of estrogens in bone. Bisphosphonates,

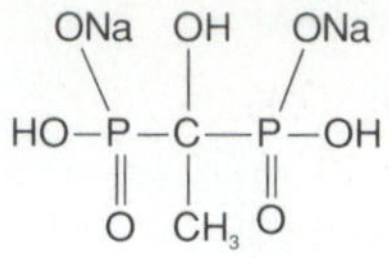

FIGURE 42-10 Etidronate disodium, showing P—C—P basic bisphosphonate structure. See the text for further information.

such as etidronate disodium (Figure 42-10), inhibit the formation, growth, and dissolution of hydroxyapatite crystals. Their effects on crystal dissolution are likely to play a role in inhibiting resorption. Some bisphosphonates can also inhibit mineralization. Plicamycin, formerly called mithramycin, which inhibits bone resorption, is an antitumor agent that inhibits RNA synthesis. It has a selective effect on bone, inhibiting bone resorption at one tenth of the antineoplastic dose. Glucocorticoids can decrease the hypercalcemia elicited by vitamin D metabolites and by other factors. This effect of glucocorticoids results from decreased calcium absorption and decreased bone resorption. Glucocorticoids also decrease the synthesis of collagen and the formation of bone by decreasing protein synthesis in osteoblasts. The decreased calcium absorption, increased PTH secretion, and antianabolic activity probably play a role in the effect of glucocorticoids to elicit osteoporosis. Nonsteroidal antiinflammatory agents are somewhat effective in inhibiting resorption but only that caused by increased prostaglandin synthesis. Fluoride can stimulate osteoclast activity and increase formation of bone. It is also incorporated into bone matrix, forming fluoroapatite in lieu of hydroxyapatite, making it resistant to resorption. However, in a recent clinical study, fluoride increased fractures at the dose tested. The box summarizes many of the effects just described.

MECHANISMS OF THERAPEUTIC ACTIONS OF AGENTS ALTERING BONE AND CALCIUM METABOLISM

MECHANISM	AGENTS
Increase intestinal calcium absorption	Vitamin D metabolites Parathyroid hormone (indirect)
Increase renal calcium excretion	Sodium sulfate, EDTA Loop-acting diuretics Calcitonin
Increase bone resorption	PTH Vitamin D metabolites
Increase bone formation	Fluoride PTH (low concentrations)
Decrease intestinal calcium absorption	Glucocorticoids Calcitonin (postprandial)
Decrease renal calcium excretion	PTH Benzothiadiazide diuretics
Decrease bone resorption	Sodium phosphate Bisphosphonates Glucocorticoids Plicamycin Calcitonin Estrogen Fluoride

Table 42-2 Pharmacokinetic Parameters

Agent	Route	$t_{1/2}$	Disappearance
vitamin D	Oral*	14 days	Bile†
1,25-Dihydroxy-vitamin D	Oral*	1-3 days	
parathyroid hormone	SC, IV	2-5 min	Metabolized, renal
calcitonin	SC, IM	20 min	Metabolized, renal
bisphosphonate	Oral	—	Renal
fluoride	Oral or topical	—	Renal, sweat, milk, GI tract

*Bile salts needed.
†Binds to a special protein.

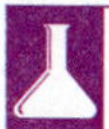

PHARMACOKINETICS

Vitamin D

Vitamin D, 25-hydroxyvitamin D, and 1,25-dihydroxyvitamin D are rapidly absorbed after oral administration (Table 42-2). Bile salts are required and absorption is impaired in biliary cirrhosis. Absorption is also decreased by steatorrhea. The vitamin D compounds circulate bound to a specific vitamin D–binding protein (DBP), a slightly acidic monomeric glycoprotein of 55,000 daltons that is synthesized in liver. Metabolic fates of these compounds include conversion to the inactive glucuronide metabolites and side-chain metabolism. It has been proposed that 24,25-dihydroxyvitamin D may have unique mineralization properties, though this possibility is not well established. Clearly, 1,24,25-trihydroxyvitamin D is a less active calcemic agent than its precursor, 1,25-dihydroxyvitamin D. 1,25-Dihydroxyvitamin D has a half-life of 1 to 3 days, dihydrotachysterol has a half-life of 7 to 25 days, and vitamin D_2 has a half-life of 2 weeks. Vitamin D is stored in body tissues, including liver, fat, and muscle for long periods of time.

Parathyroid Hormone

PTH is rapidly metabolized in the liver and kidney to both active and inactive products. The half-life of the intact hormone in plasma is 2 to 5 minutes. The N-terminal fragment, with a molecular weight of 4000 daltons, is active, whereas the C-terminal 6000-dalton fragment is inactive. The N-terminal fragment is more rapidly eliminated. Parathyroid hormone is administered by injection for diagnostic purposes only.

Calcitonin

Calcitonin is administered intramuscularly or subcutaneously. In Europe, it is also administered intranasally, and this route is being studied in the United States. It is weakly bound to plasma proteins. The intact molecule has a plasma half-life of 20 minutes and is rapidly metabolized to smaller fragments in the liver and kidney.

Bisphosphonates

The diphosphonates are poorly absorbed (1% to 6%) after oral administration; they are not metabolized. Approximately 50% of the absorbed drug is excreted by the kidneys in 24 hours. The remainder is bound to hydroxyapatite in bone and is retained in the body for years.

Fluoride

Fluoride is well absorbed after oral administration. Calcium and nonabsorbable antacids can interfere with its absorption. Fluoride is concentrated in skeletal tissues. Excretion is largely renal.

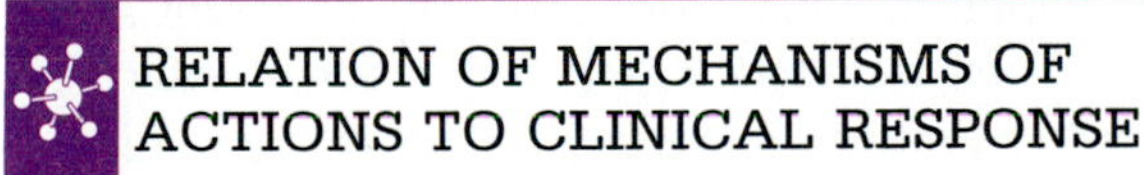

RELATION OF MECHANISMS OF ACTIONS TO CLINICAL RESPONSE

Vitamin D and Metabolites

Vitamin D and its active metabolites are primarily used in the treatment of rickets, osteomalacia, and hypocalcemia. The actions of the vitamin D compounds to increase calcium absorption are the basis of their antirachitic activity. Effects on calcium release from bone probably contribute to the hypercalcemic effect. The use of the metabolites 25-hydroxyvitamin D and 1,25-dihydroxyvitamin D rather than vitamin D per se is logical when this disorder results from a defect in their formation. Alternatively, larger doses of the precursor can result in the production of sufficient active metabolite to bring about an adequate increase in serum calcium. Therefore doses of vitamin D more than 10 times greater than those used for simple replacement therapy are used to treat hypoparathyroidism or vitamin D-resistant rickets.

Parathyroid Hormone

PTH is used diagnostically. The hormone increases urinary cyclic adenosine monophosphate subsequent to binding to renal receptors. This response is impaired in pseudohypoparathyroidism, a disorder in which there is resistance to the action of parathyroid hormone. In some cases, this disorder has been associated with a defective G protein in the adenylate cyclase system. Either the complete 84 amino acid polypeptide or the active N-terminal 1-34 fragment is administered intravenously in this test.

Calcitonin

Calcitonin has been used in the treatment of Paget's disease of bone to prevent abnormal bone turnover. It is also used to treat osteoporosis because it inhibits the loss of bone. Although used in the treatment of hypercalcemia of malignancy, its effects are somewhat delayed and less dramatic than those of other agents.

Hypercalcemia is also treated with sulfate, EDTA, furosemide, ethacrynic acid, glucocorticoids, diphosphonates, and plicamycin. All these agents decrease serum calcium concentration by the effects previously described. The use of phosphate is not recommended. Recently the use of phosphate has been reported to cause death because of metastatic calcification, in many or-

CLINICAL PROBLEMS

VITAMIN D AND METABOLITES

Hypercalcemia
Benzothiadiazides can increase hazards of hypercalcemia

PARATHYROID HORMONE

Hypercalcemia (unlikely with diagnostic use)

CALCITONIN

Local hypersensitivity
"Escape" loss of effectiveness

BISPHOSPHONATES

Osteomalacia
Bone pain

FLUORIDE

GI side effects, including nausea
Musculoskeletal pain
Joint swelling
Mottled teeth enamel
Dose related bone fracture possibility

gans, particularly in the lung. Pharmacological treatment of hypercalcemia is carried out in conjunction with a low calcium diet and administration of oral and parenteral fluids. Paget's disease of bone is treated with bisphosphonates and plicamycin as well as by calcitonin. All of these agents decrease the abnormal bone turnover. Osteoporosis therapy currently is an attempt to prevent fractures or to limit the number of fractures by using agents that decrease bone resorption, including estrogen, and more recently, calcitonin. Estrogen, started at the time of menopause, prevents bone loss and decreases fractures. The National Institutes of Health Consensus Conference on Osteoporosis recommended a calcium intake of 1500 mg/day for women starting about the time of menopause. Calcium per se appears to be less effective than estrogen in preventing bone loss. Calcium may act by inhibiting the secretion of parathyroid hormone.

TRADE NAMES

In addition to generic and fixed-combination preparations, the following trade-named materials are available in the United States.

Calciferol, ergocalciferol, vitamin D_2
Calcimar, calcitonin
Calderol, calcifidiol, 25-hydroxyvitamin D_3
DHT, dihydrotachysterol
Didronel, etidronate disodium (a bisphosphonate)
Fosamax, alendronate
Mithracin, plicamycin (formerly called mithramycin)
Parathyroid hormone, commercial status is not clear (not listing diagnostic materials)
Rocaltrol, calcitriol, 1,25-dihydroxyvitamin D_3
Vitamin D is also present in a larger number of nutritional supplements

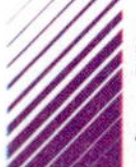

SIDE EFFECTS, CLINICAL PROBLEMS, AND TOXICITY

The problems are summarized in the box.

Vitamin D

Excess vitamin D and its metabolites can lead to hypercalcemia, a potentially fatal side effect. The immediate risk of this is greatest with 1,25-dihydroxyvitamin D, since the metabolic step that is feedback regulated, the renal 1-hydroxylase is bypassed. However, since 1,25-dihydroxyvitamin D has the shortest biological half-life, the hypercalcemia and the possibility of cumulative effects are potentially less than with the other metabolites. There is an increased risk of toxicity in patients with impaired renal function. Serum calcium concentrations are monitored in patients on vitamin D therapy, and the drug is discontinued if hypercalcemia occurs. Benzothiadiazide diuretics can increase the hazard of hypercalcemia. Drug interactions can occur with phenobarbital, phenytoin, and glucocorticoids, all of which can interfere with vitamin D activation, as well as with the action of vitamin D metabolites on target tissues.

Parathyroid Hormone

Hypercalcemia is also a potential side effect of PTH administration. However, it is unlikely to occur when the hormone is used diagnostically.

Calcitonin

Local hypersensitivity reactions, including skin rashes, other allergic reactions, and nausea, have been noted with calcitonin. Although calcitonin could potentially elicit hypocalcemia, this is not a common side effect. The major problem with calcitonin is the loss of effectiveness because of *escape*. Another limiting factor in the usefulness of calcitonin is its ineffectiveness when administered orally.

Other Agents

The bisphosphonate etidronate decreases bone mineralization, and osteomalacia and bone pain have occurred with their use. Gastrointestinal irritation is also a problem with this drug. Fluoride has GI side effects including nausea. Musculoskeletal pain and joint swelling have been reported. The possible dose-related risk of increased fractures has recently been recognized. The side effects of other agents are discussed in other chapters of this text.

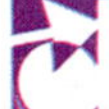

NEW DIRECTIONS

Among the drugs likely to become available for the treatment of osteoporosis within the next few years are newer bisphosphonates, which are more selective, inhibiting bone resorption while producing less inhibition of mineralization. Vitamin D analogs with greater selectivity for intestinal calcium absorption relative to bone resorption should become available. These, administered together with low intermittent PTH, could promote bone formation and mineralization. Vitamin D analogs with more selective effects on differentiation and immunosuppression should be available for treatment of malignancy, transplantation, and other applications for which effects on systemic calcium metabolism can be limiting factors. There may be clinical application of thiazide diuretics to diminish bone loss. Antiestrogens have estrogenic actions on bone, while lacking some of the undesirable effects of estrogens on other target tissues. They are being developed for the treatment of osteoporosis. A new frontier is the potential use of growth factors that stimulate osteoblast proliferation, such as insulin-like growth factors I and II and transforming growth factor β, to promote bone formation. The challenge is to develop means to target these growth factors to bone.

REFERENCES

Ettinger B, Genant HK, Cann CE: Long-term estrogen replacement therapy prevents bone loss and fractures, *Ann Intern Med* 102:319-324, 1985.

Martin TJ, Mosely JM, Gillespie MT: Parathyroid hormone–related protein: biochemistry and molecular biology, *Crit Rev Biochem Molec Biol* 26:377-395, 1991.

Marx SJ, Lieberman UA, Eil C: Calciferols: actions and deficiencies in action, *Vitamins and Hormones* 40:235, 1983.

Ozono K, Sone T, Pike J: The genomic mechanism of action of 1,25-dihydroxyvitamin D_3, *J Bone Miner Res* 6:1021-1027, 1991.

Primer on the metabolic bone diseases and disorders of mineral metabolism, ed. 1, American Society for Bone and Mineral Research, 1990.

Riggs BL, Hodgson SF, O'Fallon WM: Effect of fluoride treatment on the fracture rate in postmenopausal women with osteoporosis, *N Engl J Med* 322:802-809, 1990.

Riggs BL, Melton LJ: The prevention and treatment of osteoporosis, *N Engl J Med* 327:620-627, 1992.

Storm T, Thamsborg G, Steiniche T, et al: Effect of intermittent cyclical etidronate therapy on bone mass and fracture rate in women with postmenopausal osteoporosis, *N Engl J Med* 322:1265-1271, 1990.

Vernava AM, O'Neal LW, Palermo V: Lethal hyperparathyroid crisis: hazards of phosphate administration, *Surgery* 102:941, 1987.

SELF-ASSESSMENT QUESTIONS

1. All of the following are true of renal calcium and phosphate metabolism *except* that:
   a. approximately 10 g of calcium is filtered per day and 99% of that is reabsorbed.
   b. furosemide and ethacrynic acid inhibit Na-linked calcium reabsorption.
   c. thiazide diuretics can prevent nephrolithiasis (renal stones) by decreasing calcium excretion.
   d. parathyroid hormone decreases renal phosphate reabsorption.
   e. a high level of phosphate stimulates the renal [25-hydroxyvitamin D] 1-α-hydroxylase.
2. All of the following are therapeutically useful inhibitors of bone resorption *except:*
   a. prostaglandin E_1.
   b. calcitonin.
   c. bisphosphonates.
   d. mithramycin.
   e. estrogen.
3. All of the following are true of parathyroid hormone (PTH) *except* that:
   a. PTH acts through a G-protein coupled receptor.
   b. PTH stimulates 25-hydroxylation of vitamin D.
   c. PTH has direct effects on bone to stimulate bone resorption.
   d. low concentrations of PTH have anabolic effects on bone.
   e. PTH increases intestinal calcium absorption through an indirect (vitamin D–mediated) action.
4. All of the following are true of vitamin D *except* that:
   a. a calcium-binding protein is one of the gene products resulting from vitamin D action.
   b. the most potent and rapid-acting vitamin D metabolite is formed mainly in the liver.
   c. actions of vitamin D on intestine and bone can be antagonized by glucocorticoids.
   d. vitamin D increases both mineralization and resorption of bone.
   e. activation of the vitamin D precursor in the skin by sunlight exposure is attributable to cleavage of the B ring.
5. Vitamin D therapy can normalize calcium metabolism in all of the following *except:*
   a. hypoparathyroidism.
   b. sarcoidosis.
   c. X-linked (hypophosphatemic) rickets.
   d. renal osteodystrophy.
   e. renal [25-hydroxyvitamin D] 1-α-hydroxylase deficiency.

NEOPLASTIC CELLS: DRUGS AFFECTING CELL GROWTH AND VIABILITY

PART VI

Neoplastic mammalian cells and tissues are characterized by abnormal genetic content, altered chromosome structures, and uncontrolled growth, usually accompanied by loss of cellular differentiation (anaplasia). Abnormal genetic content includes mutations, deletions, and translocations, which can result in structural changes in the karyological appearance of cancer cell chromosomes. These chromosomal changes lead to modified cellular regulation and abnormal structures of affected enzymes. The diseased cells and cell aggregates are described as tumors, neoplasms, or cancers and occur in benign (nonvirulent) or malignant (virulent) states. Malignant neoplastic cells typically invade surrounding tissues, violating the basement membrane of the tissue of origin, eventually undergoing metastasis, with malignant cells released from the primary neoplasm and disseminating to other tissues and organs. Over 100 types of malignant neoplasms affect humans, with classification based primarily on anatomical (organ) location and type of cell from which the neoplasm develops. The advent of molecular diagnostic methods seems certain to increase this number.

In the United States, malignant neoplasms are responsible for about 500,000 deaths per year (20% to 25% of total mortality), with about 1,000,000 new cases developing each year. Lung, large intestine, breast, and prostate neoplasms account for about 55% of both new cases and cancer deaths in the United States. Solid tumors arising from epithelial cells are termed *carcinomas,* whereas those originating from connective tissue and often of a fibrous nature are termed *sarcomas*. Malignancies that arise from the hematopoietic system include the *leukemias* and *lymphomas*.

The mechanisms by which malignant neoplasms originate in humans are still not clear. Carcinogenesis (i.e., the creation of malignant neoplastic cells) appears to be caused by activation of specific dominant growth genes, called **oncogenes,** or loss of functional negative effectors, called **tumor suppressor genes.** In the best-studied tumors, both kinds of genetic changes are now believed to be essential for the development of a full malignant phenotype, and so multiple lesions may exist when a tumor is detected. Proto-oncogenes, when activated, form oncogenes, which encode modified proteins that cause cellular differentiation and proliferation characteristics of the neoplastic state. Activation of proto-oncogenes can occur by several pathways that often involve exposure of cells to chemicals, radiation, or viruses. Activation can result from a single-point mutation. The most common oncogenes found thus far in human tumors belong to the *ras* gene family, which codes for guanosine triphosphate (GTP)-binding proto-oncogenes. When the *ras* proto-oncogene is converted to the activated form, it does not readily dephosphorylate GTP, and it transforms cells to the neoplastic state. Over 100 proto-oncogenes are known to exist. Clearly, most if not all products of these variously dominantly acting oncogene are components of cellular signaling pathways. Other genes known as tumor-suppressing genes also are present in human cells and function to suppress excessive cellular growth. Retinoblastoma (tumor of the eye) is a prototype of a malignancy caused by genetic loss of the tumor-suppressor gene Rb. A second common tumor suppressor gene is p53. Mutations in p53 are now believed to be the single most prevalent lesions in human cancer. Inactivation of these tumor-suppressing genes appears to be another route that leads to the formation of neoplastic cells.

Neoplastic cells traditionally are characterized by the inability to undergo differentiation yet still capable of cell division. This definition may be too simplistic, since some tumor cells are capable of differentiation. Since most oncogenes and tumor-suppressor genes seem to alter cell signaling pathways, many investigators now believe that neoplasia is a "disease of faulty cell signaling." This includes both growth factors and cell-death signals. For example, it is now known that tumor growth represents a balance between cell division and cell death. One important form of cell death in tumors is apoptosis, and oncogenes such as bcl-2 block apoptosis. Oncogenes such as p53 may also permit the genetic instability associated with neoplasia.

From the clinical standpoint, the primary difficulty in the successful control and treatment of malignant neoplasms is that by the time malignant cells are detected, the neoplasm is relative large ($>10^9$ cells) and often has metastasized, presenting a much more difficult therapeutic problem. With a disseminated disorder, one no longer uses only local treatments such as surgery or radiation. Antineoplastic agents can be used alone, after surgery (adjuvant chemotherapy), or before surgery (neoadjuvant chemotherapy).

The overall approach in the therapy of neoplastic diseases (as shown in Figure VI-1) remains the removal or destruction of the neoplastic cells, while minimizing toxic effects on nonneoplastic cells. It has been a long-standing question whether drugs effective against one type of neoplasm should be effective against all types. Clinical experience, however, has shown a wide range of drug activities among different types (sarcoma, carcinoma, leukemia, lymphoma) and anatomical locations (breast, colon, lung) of tumors. Therefore interest has focused on treating each of the over 100 clinically important forms of cancer as separate disease states with development of suitable drug therapies. Some of the therapeutic approaches listed in Figure VI-1 are not available for clinical use but represent research approaches that are under study. For example, drugs that function specifically to return neoplastic cells to normal differentiating cells capable of surviving after differentiation, or drugs that prevent metastases in general are not available or are highly experimental. Drugs that stimulate the immune system to destroy those neoplastic cells not killed by antineoplastic drugs are of clinical importance and are discussed in Chapters 44 and 45.

The three chapters in this section present the mechanisms of action and the problems associated with the clinical use of antineoplastic drugs in humans. Individual drugs are discussed in Chapter 43 and their clinical uses, usually in multiple drug protocols, are discussed in Chapter 44.

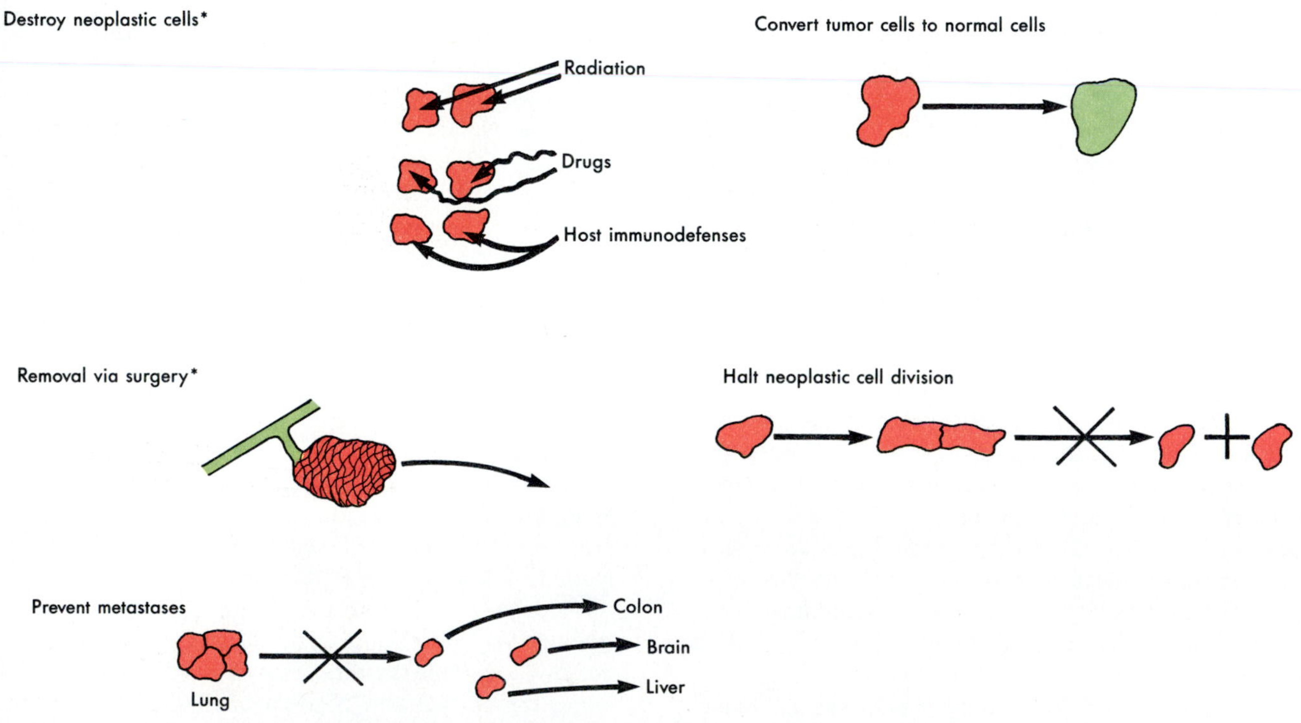

FIGURE VI-I Major approaches to therapy of cancers. Tumor cells are shown in red and non-tumor cells in green.* In clinical use. Others are experimental.

CHAPTER 43 Individual Antineoplastic Drugs

JOHN S. LAZO
JAMES M. LARNER

MAJOR DRUGS

alkylating agents (e.g., melphalan, cyclophosphamide)
antimetabolites (e.g., methotrexate, thioguanine)
antibiotics (e.g., doxorubicin, bleomycin)
hormonal agents (e.g., prednisone, flutamide)
plant alkaloids (e.g., etoposide, vinblastine)
Others (e.g., hydroxyurea)

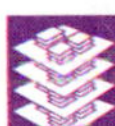

THERAPEUTIC OVERVIEW

Antineoplastic agents are used to treat most of the more than 100 types of neoplastic diseases, with the goal of destroying malignant cells. Additional drugs (discussed in Chapter 45) are used to enhance host natural defense mechanisms to eradicate those neoplastic cells not killed by the antineoplastic drugs. Although in clinical practice nearly all neoplastic diseases are treated using multiple drugs, in this chapter the mechanisms of action, pharmacokinetics, and side effects of the individual antineoplastic drugs are presented. These form the rationales for multiple drug protocols, which are described in the following chapter.

The effectiveness of antineoplastic drugs varies greatly with the type of cancer, the general biological and physiological condition of the patient (i.e., patient performance status), and the degree to which the tumor has grown or spread (i.e., tumor stage or grade). Moreover, the endpoint used to evaluate the effectiveness (e.g., tumor response, patient survival) is also important. The effectiveness of most antineoplastic agents is greater on cells that are progressing through the cell cycle (Figure 43-1), compared to cells that are resting

ABBREVIATIONS

Ara-C	cytarabine
ATPase	adenosine triphosphatase
FH_4	tetrahydrofolate
5-FU	5-fluorouracil
MESNA	sodium 2-mercaptcethane sulfonate
6-MP	6-mercaptopurine
MTX	methotrexate
6-TG	6-thioguanine

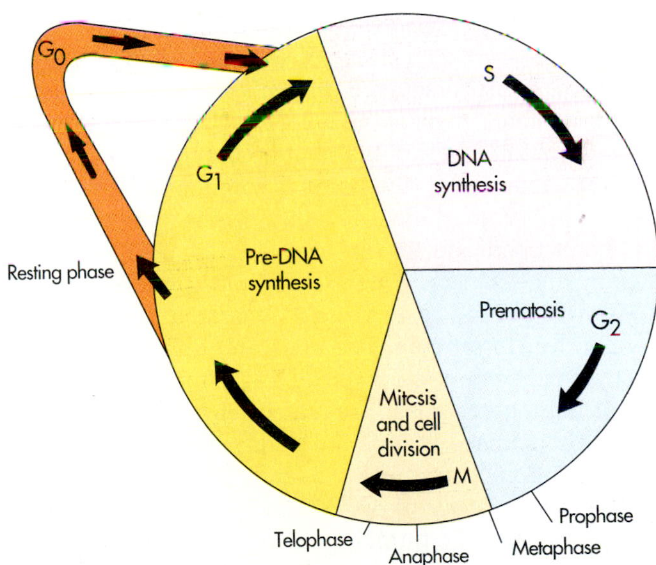

FIGURE 43-1 Growth cycle for mammalian cells. In the G_0 (resting) phase, the cells are dormant. A variety of stimulants, often of unknown origin in clinical situations, cause cycling of cells to begin by entry into the G_1 phase (pre-DNA synthesis). Here, precursors for DNA are formed. In the S, or synthetic, phase, DNA synthesis occurs. This is followed by premitotic synthesis and structural developments in the G_2 phase. Mitosis occurs in the M phase to produce two cells, each of which can continue to cycle, by entry again into G_1, or can enter the resting phase, G_0. Growth fraction is defined as the total cells in the growth cycle (G_1, S, G_2, M) divided by the total cells (G_1, S, G_2, M, G_0).

in the G_0 phase. The "growth fraction," defined in Figure 43-1, is the fraction of cells progressing through the cycle. In addition to tumor cells that may be proliferating, certain nonneoplastic cells also are undergoing cell division. In particular, the nonneoplastic cells of hair follicles, bone marrow, and intestinal epithelium are the most rapidly dividing and are especially sensitive to inhibition by antineoplastic drugs. Inhibition of these nontumor cells accounts for many of the undesirable side effects found with the use of antineoplastic drugs.

The number of cultured neoplastic cells that survive exposure to each antineoplastic drug typically shows a first-order relationship to the concentration of drug (Figure 43-2). This means that the same fraction of cells are killed with each dose of drug (log cell kill), and a series of several doses does not kill 100% of the neoplastic cells. The log cell kill hypothesis is compatible with clinical observations that a functional host immune system is needed to obtain complete kill of all neoplastic cells and thereby obtain a cure of neoplastic disease. For cytotoxic anticancer drugs, endogenous cellular defenses, such as thiols or DNA repair enzymes, can produce a "shoulder," or drug threshold, in the survival curves (Figure 43-2).

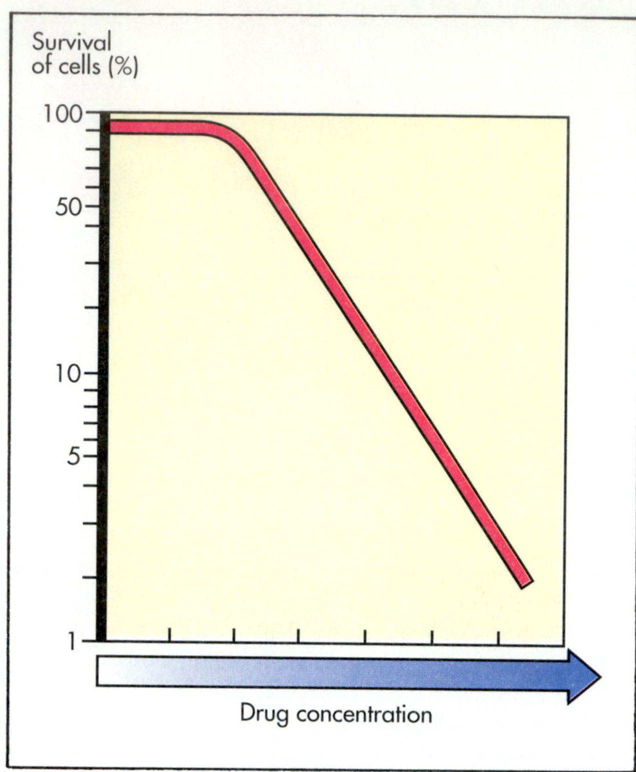

FIGURE 43-2 Decline in viable cells is first order with respect to drug concentration. Many antineoplastic agents and cultured tumor cells follow this relationship, thus establishing the principles of a fixed percentage of viable cells killed per concentration of drug. This same relationship appears to apply in vivo, although the actual situation may be more complex. A threshold concentration of drug is often required to cause a noticeable decrease in cell survival. This phenomenon, called *survival shoulder,* may reflect an endogenous repair process.

Of the four major types of tumors, the faster growing hematological (nonsolid) types (leukemias and lymphomas) are more responsive to treatment with drugs than the slower growing solid types (carcinomas and sarcomas) are. Primary factors in this difference are the more rapid doubling times of the hematological malignancies and the greater ease of distribution of drug to leukemia or lymphoma cells as compared to carcinoma or sarcoma cells. The outer or more recently synthesized portions of many solid tumors are well vascularized and are readily accessible to drugs. This is attributable in part to growth of new blood vessels generated in a process termed **angiogenesis.** The inner and older portions of many solid tumors are hypoxic and often necrotic because angiogenesis is inadequate. Consequently the inner cells of these tumors are poorly accessible to the drugs. The necrotic inner cells may be dead or merely in the resting phase of the cell cycle and therefore may still be capable of returning to the cycling state. The delivery of drugs to the inner portions of solid tumors is a major unsolved problem.

Antineoplastic drugs must enter the cell to produce their desired cytotoxic effects. Some drugs can pass through the cell membrane by passive diffusion, with the concentration gradient of drug between the outside and inside of the cell driving drug uptake. Other drugs require binding to carrier proteins, which then transport drug through the cell membrane and release the drug on the cytoplasmic side; this is especially common with antimetabolites. Carrier-mediated transport of antineoplastic drugs is an active process that is not concentration driven, and the rate of transport often is limited by a fixed number of carrier molecules per cell.

Once the antineoplastic drug enters the cell and diffuses into the nucleus or other subcellular sites, the drug can react with target molecules to disrupt key processes that are necessary for cell viability. The target molecules and their reactions with antineoplastic drugs are described in the next section.

The main therapeutic considerations are summarized in the box.

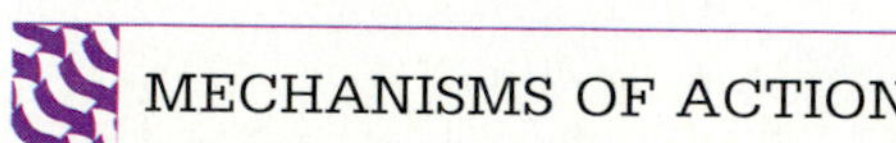

MECHANISMS OF ACTION

Basic Approaches

A generalized summary of the basic mechanisms by which antineoplastic drugs are used for killing tumor cells is given in Figure 43-3. Only those compounds that

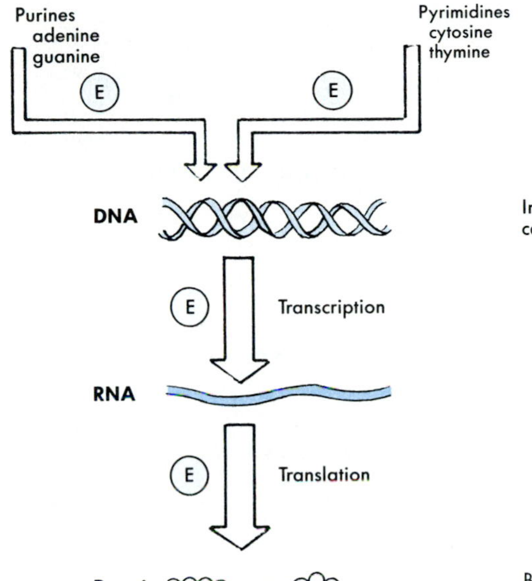

FIGURE 43-3 Basic approaches in which antineoplastic drugs are used for the selective killing of tumor cells. *E* stands for enzymes, some of which are inhibited by these drugs. Inhibition of DNA or RNA synthesis or replication, production of miscoded nucleic acids, and formation of modified proteins are key mechanisms of action for many of these drugs.

show some selectivity for neoplastic cells are used clinically. In general, antimetabolites inhibit, or make less effective, DNA synthesis. Alkylating agents, intercalators and antibiotics damage or disrupt DNA, interfere with topoisomerases, or alter RNA structure. Other agents, including steroids, interfere with transcription, whereas several plant alkaloids disrupt mitosis. Agents such as asparaginase destroy essential amino acids needed for translation.

A significant number of clinically used antineoplastic drugs must undergo either chemical or enzymatic modification to generate the active cytotoxic species. The pertinent modes of activation are described later in this section.

The principal types of antineoplastic drugs are listed in the box, on p. 578. Discussion of these drugs follows.

Alkylating Agents

Alkylation refers to the covalent attachment of alkyl groups to other molecules. This approach to cancer therapy came about as a result of observations on the effects of the mustard war gases on cell growth. Although the sulfur mustard war gases were too toxic for clinical use as antineoplastic agents, the related nitrogen mustard alkylating agents produced the first effective antineoplastic agents, including mechlorethamine, which is still in use today.

The process of alkylation takes place through chemical formation of a positively charged carbonium ion (also

THERAPEUTIC OVERVIEW

GOAL

Kill tumor cells selectively with no side effects

USES

Treatment of systemic disease (curative and palliative)
Decrease tumor burden
Treatment of carcinomas, sarcomas, leukemias, lymphomas

EFFECTS

Some but not all tumors respond

CONSIDERATIONS

Drug-delivery problems to individual cells
Cycling versus noncycling cells
Log-cell kill (same fraction of cells killed per dose)
Need for active immune system (host defenses) to eradicate remaining neoplastic cells
Problem of central hypoxic zone of tumors
Drug resistance

called *carbocation*). This positively charged group subsequently reacts with an electron-rich site, particularly on DNA or RNA, to form modified nucleic acids. Most of the clinically used alkylating drugs have two alkylating groups, thus promoting the formation of covalent cross-links between adjacent strands of nucleic acids, which are more difficult to repair than monofunctional adducts. The cross-links prevent subsequent separation of the dual strands of DNA during cell cycling. For maximal kill, it is important to administer the maximum tolerated dose. The alkylation sequence is shown schematically in Figure 43-4 for mechlorethamine (nitrogen mustard) reacting with the N-7 position of deoxyguanylate. With free DNA or RNA, alkylation occurs predominately at the N-7 position of the guanine base, with only minor alkylation at O-6 or N-3 of guanine, at N-1, N-3, or N-7 of adenine, or at N-3 of cytosine. With cultured human tumor cells, alkylation selectivity for guanine N-7 has been shown to be 70 times that for the other unpaired ring oxygen or nitrogen atoms in the bases. Although many other nucleophilic constituents, including RNA, proteins, and membrane components, become alkylated within cells, it is generally believed the primary cytotoxic events occur through alkylation of DNA, especially by coupling to the N-7 position of the deoxyguanylates of either single- or double-strand DNA.

The structures of several clinically used alkylating agents are shown in Figure 43-5. Cyclophosphamide undergoes a combination of enzymatic and chemical activation to form the active phosphoramide mustard alkylating agent (Figure 43-6). Exposure of cells to cyclophosphamide and other alkylating agents can lead to carcinogenesis (i.e., the formation of neoplastic cells). For example, leukemia is a well-described long-term complication in patients treated with a regimen that includes the nitrogen mustard mechlorethamine for Hodgkin's disease.

Another group of antineoplastic alkylating agents in clinical use is the nitrosoureas. The structures and mechanism of activation for these compounds are

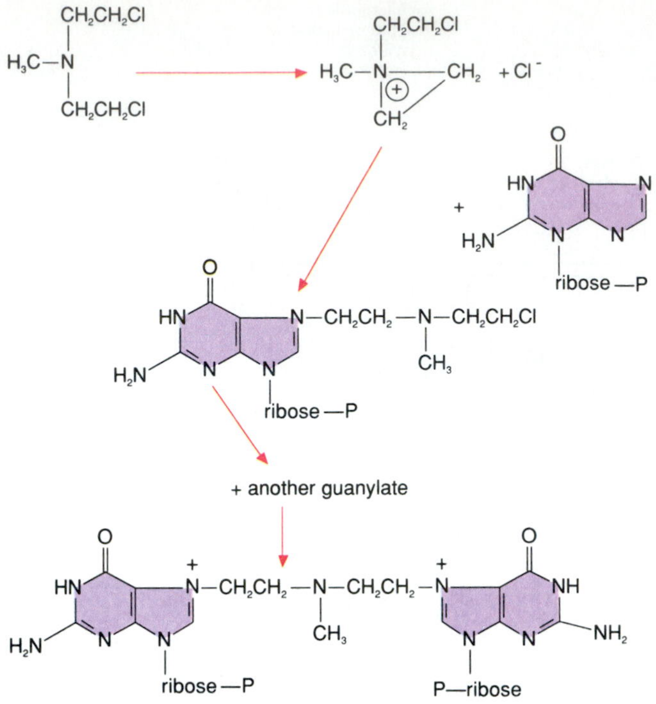

FIGURE 43-4 Alkylation by mechlorethamine, showing positively charged intermediate ion and its covalent attachment to the N-7 position of two deoxyguanylate nucleotides of DNA.

ANTINEOPLASTIC DRUGS

ALKYLATING AGENTS

nitrogen mustards
- mechlorethamine HCl (nitrogen mustard, HN_2, HCl)
- melphalan L-phenylalanine, L-PAM)
  - chlorambucil
- cyclophosphamide
- ifosfamide

nitrosoureas
- carmustine (BCNU)
- lomustine (CCNU)

other
- cisplatin (*cis*-diamminedichloroplatinum)
- carboplatin (Paraplatin)
- busulfan
- dacarbazine (DTIC)
- procarbazine
- triethylenethiophosphoramide (thio-TEPA)

ANTIMETABOLITES

methotrexate (MTX)
mercaptopurine (6-MP)
thioguanine (6-TG)
fluorouracil (5-FU)

ANTIMETABOLITES—CONT'D

cytarabine (cytosine arabinoside, ara-C)
trimetrexate
pentostatin (2-deoxycoformycin)

ANTIBIOTICS

daunorubicin (daunomycin)
doxorubicin (Adriamycin)
idarubicin
bleomycin
dactinomycin (actinomycin D)
mitomycin C
plicamycin (mithramycin)

HORMONAL AGENTS

prednisone
tamoxifen
flutamide
leuprolide
goserelin

OTHERS

asparaginase
hydroxyurea

PLANT ALKALOIDS

vincristine
vinblastine
etoposide (VP-16)
teniposide (VM-26)
Taxol (paclitaxel)

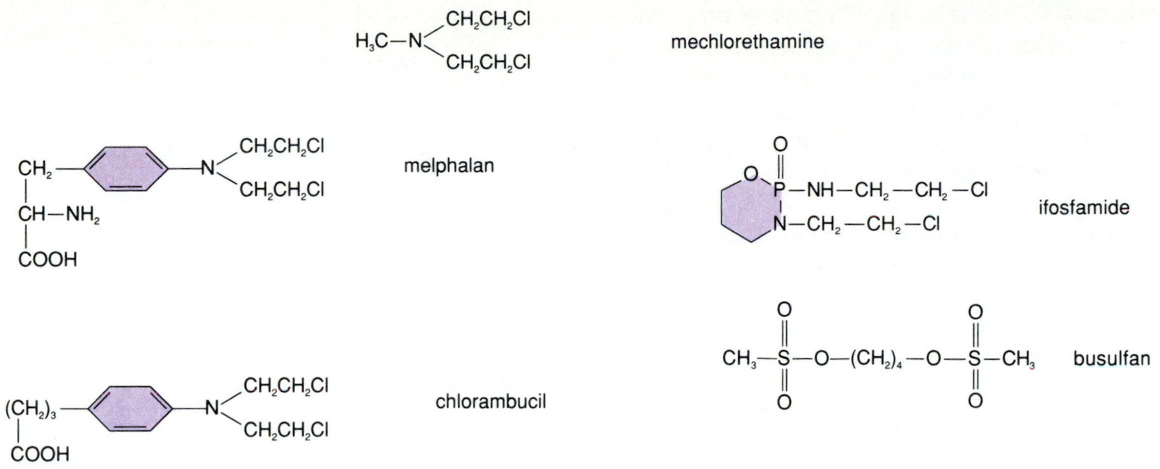

mechlorethamine

melphalan

ifosfamide

chlorambucil

busulfan

FIGURE 43-5 Structures of nitrogen mustards. See the text for further information.

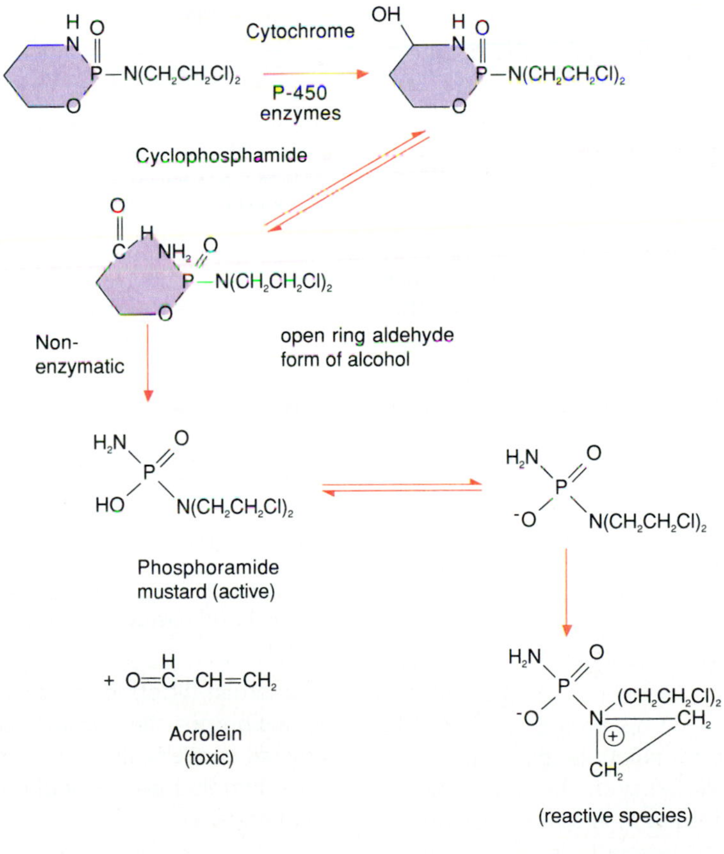

Cytochrome P-450 enzymes

Cyclophosphamide

open ring aldehyde form of alcohol

Non-enzymatic

Phosphoramide mustard (active)

Acrolein (toxic)

(reactive species)

FIGURE 43-6 Mechanism of enzymatic and chemical activation of cyclophosphamide to form active phosphoramide mustard. Acrolein has some antitumor activity but much less than that of the phosphoramide mustard.

shown in Figure 43-7. Although alternative pathways are available by which nitrosoureas can form active alkylating species, the principal route is shown in Figure 43-7. Carbamoylation of proteins also occurs with nitrosoureas (Figure 43-7); the carbamoylated proteins may play a role in producing cytotoxicity. The alkylation route however is considered to be the major cause of cytotoxicity during antineoplastic therapy. Nitrosoureas are lipophilic and are able to cross the blood-brain barrier. They are therefore frequently used to treat brain tumors.

Other clinical compounds that form covalent bonds with DNA are cisplatin and the newer platinum analog, carboplatin. Structures of cisplatin and carboplatin are shown in Figure 43-8. Cisplatin, $Pt(NH_3)_2(Cl)_2$, is a square planar complex of platinum with two ammonia molecules and two chloride ions at the corners of the plane. The detailed reaction sequence of the pharmacologically active species is complex and not completely known. Hydroxyl replacement of a chloride must occur before the formation of the platinum-nitrogen bond with DNA. Subsequently, the second chloride is aquated and reacts with DNA. The stereochemistry of the complex enables the *cis* but not the *trans* isomer to form two covalent platinum-nitrogen bonds, primarily at the N-7 positions of two adjacent deoxyguanylates of DNA. This intrastrand cross-link prevents replication of the DNA and is cytotoxic. Similar DNA cross-links are formed at the dicarboxylate sites on carboplatin.

Several other clinically useful alkylating agents include busulfan, dacarbazine, procarbazine, ifosfamide, and melphalan. The busulfan type of compounds alkylate nucleic acid bases, primarily at the N-7 of guanine, and also alkylate SH groups of glutathione and protein thiols.

The specific reaction sequences by which dacarbazine or procarbazine alkylate DNA are not well understood. For dacarbazine, hydrolysis to form a reactive aryldiazonium ion, a corresponding arylcabonium ion, or an alternative methylcarbonium ion are possibilities. In the case of procarbazine, hydrolysis to form a methyl free radical has been proposed for the alkylation mechanism, but this is not certain. Melphalan is a phenylalanine derivative and is actively transported into the cell by the same carriers that transport leucine and glutamine. Melphalan is associated with the induction of secondary leukemias. Chlorambucil is structurally similar to melphalan and is used primarily in chronic lymphocytic leukemia. Ifosfamide, like its structural analog cyclophosphamide, is activated by hepatic microsomes. Early studies with ifosfamide showed a significant incidence of hemorrhagic cystitis. Ifosfamide is now given with a systemic thiol MESNA (sodium 2-mercaptoethane sulfonate). MESNA becomes a free thiol after glomerular filtration and combines with the products responsible for the cystitis. Ifosfamide is active against several cancers, including small cell lung cancer, sarcomas, lymphomas, testicular carcinoma, and gynecological cancers.

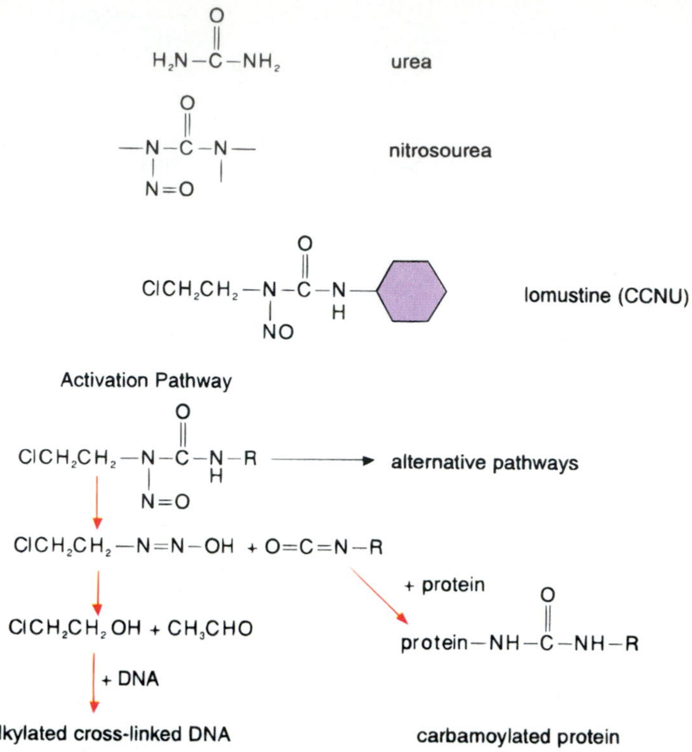

FIGURE 43-7 Structures and activation pathways for nitrosourea alkylating agents. Carbamoylation of proteins also occurs but is believed to be a lesser cause of cell cytotoxicity than the alkylation of DNA is.

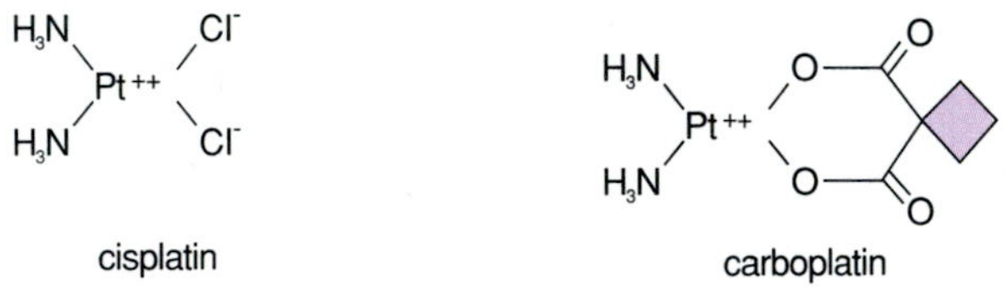

FIGURE 43-8 Square planar complex of *cis*-diamminedichloroplatinum (II), cisplatin, and a new platinum derivative, carboplatin.

Antimetabolites

The antimetabolites are compounds that mimic the structures of normal metabolic constituents, including folic acid, pyrimidines, or purines, well enough to inhibit enzymes necessary for folic acid regeneration or for pyri-

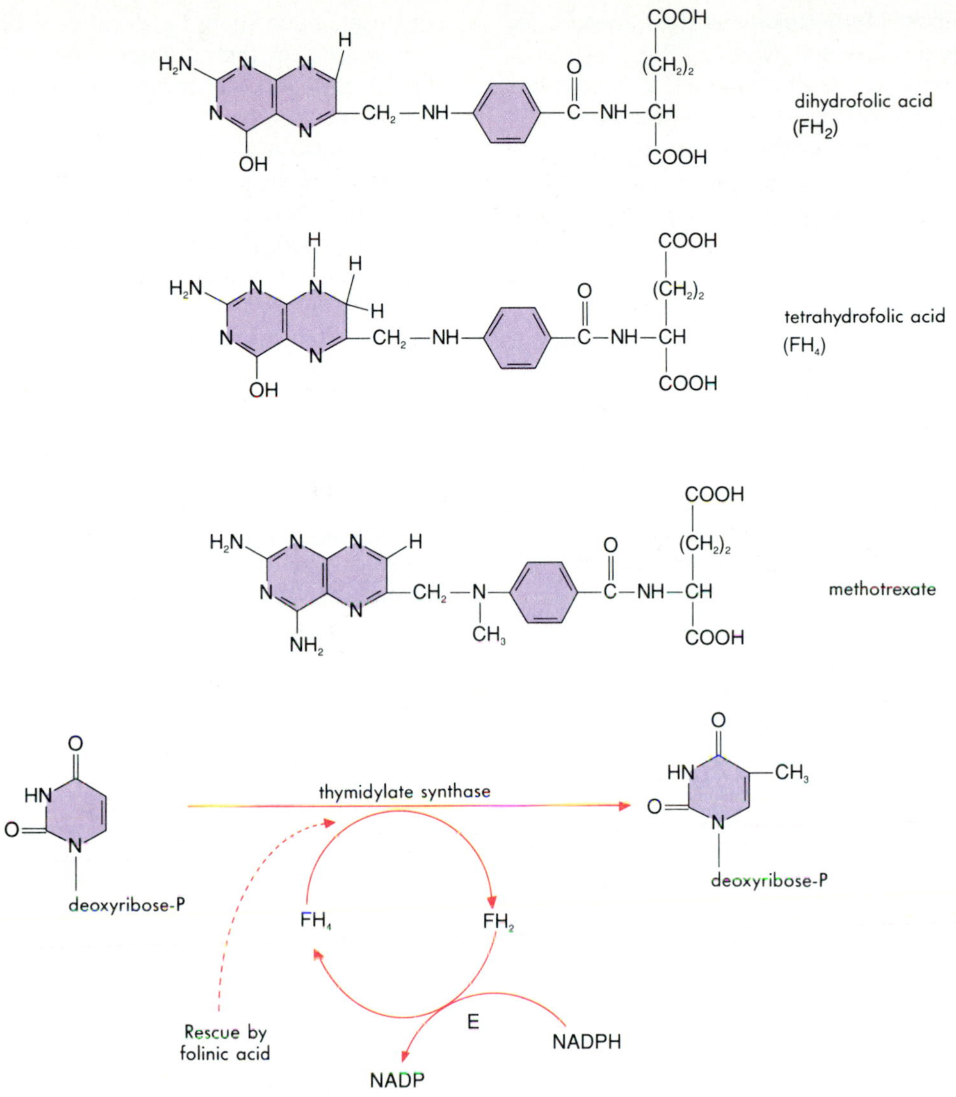

FIGURE 43-9 Structures of tetrahydrofolic acid (FH_4) and methotrexate. The reaction shown is a pyrimidine synthesis (thymidine monophosphate from deoxyuridylic acid) catalyzed by thymidylate synthase and requiring FH_4 as cofactor. *E* is dihydrofolate reductase, which is reversibly inhibited by methotrexate, thus preventing regeneration of FH_4 from dihydrofolate (FH_2). The rescue path is discussed in the text. The pyrimidines are needed for DNA formation.

midine or purine activation for DNA or RNA synthesis in neoplastic cells. Antimetabolites frequently kill cells in s-phase (Figure 43-1). Methotrexate (MTX), 5-fluorouracil (5-FU), cytarabine (ara-C), 6-mercaptopurine (6-MP), and 6-thioguanine (6-TG) are the primary clinical antimetabolites. The antimetabolite methotrexate shows enhanced selectivity for neoplastic cells because methotrexate is selectively polyglutamated by tumor cells. The tetrahydrofolates act more efficiently as enzyme cofactors when present as polymers with glutamate than as monomers. Methotrexate is transported in the blood as a monomer but undergoes enzyme-catalyzed polymerization within cells and becomes trapped intracellularly as a polymer. Tumor cells have higher polymerizing enzyme activity than nonmalignant cells have. Thus a higher concentration of polymerized (more active) methotrexate is trapped within the tumor cells to act as an antimetabolite.

Folic acid is essential for enzyme-catalyzed reactions that transfer methyl groups and related groups during purine and pyrimidine synthesis. Methotrexate competitively inhibits the enzyme dihydrofolate reductase, which catalyzes the reduction of dihydrofolate to tetrahydrofolate (FH_4) (Figure 43-9). This blocks the regeneration of FH_4 and thereby prevents the synthesis of purine and pyrimidines. Methotrexate is thus specific for cells in the S phase of the cell cycle.

Cellular transport of methotrexate is a carrier-mediated process. To overcome the limitations of carrier uptake and to enhance entry of drug into the cells by passive diffusion some investigators have infused high-dose methotrexate IV (≤16 g/day) over several hours. When high-dose methotrexate is used, it is mandatory that the methotrexate infusion be followed by a "rescue process" of leucovorin (citrovorum factor or N^5-formyl-FH_4). This is a substitute for FH_4, which is believed to enter nonmalignant cells by a carrier-mediated process enabling purine and pyrimidine synthesis to proceed. The clinical efficacy of this high-dose methotrexate-leucovorin rescue approach, however, is still being debated.

Another antimetabolite, 5-FU (Figure 43-10) acts primarily by inhibiting pyrimidine synthesis and thus DNA formation. Its structure is shown in Figure 43-10. Fluorouracil is metabolized to the 5-fluoro analog of deoxyuridylic acid, which in turn inhibits thymidylate synthase by covalent coupling to the enzyme. Modulation of the activity of 5-FU with folinic acid, α-interferon, or the anthelminthic levamasole has been an interesting area of clinical investigation. Response rates of colorectal cancer are significantly increased when folinic acid or α-interferon is given with 5-FU. Folinic acid enhances the activity of 5-FU by stabilizing the ternary complex of thymidylate synthase. Therefore, less thymidylate synthase is available to convert deoxyuridine monophosphate to deoxythymidine monophosphate, and DNA synthesis is reduced. The mechanism by which α-interferon enhances activity of 5-FU is unknown. Recent trials have shown a significant benefit in an adjuvant setting for the combined use of 5-FU and levamisole for patients with colorectal cancer with lymph node involvement.

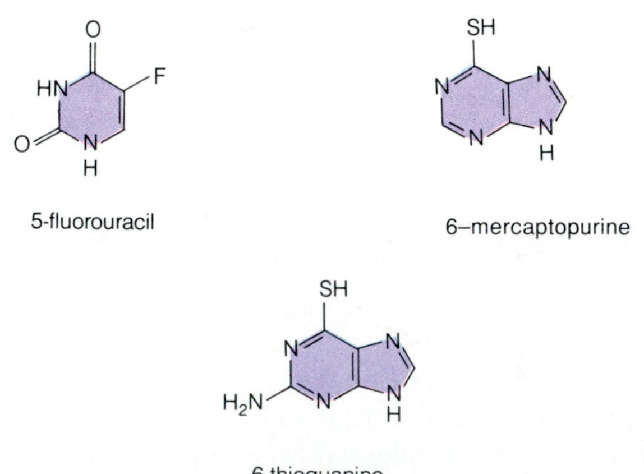

FIGURE 43-10 Structures of prototype purine and pyrimidine antimetabolites. See the text for further information.

Ara-C also acts to inhibit pyrimidine synthesis but through a more complex pathway (Figure 43-11). The drug must undergo enzymatic conversion to the cytosine triphosphate derivative, which is the active form, and which is incorporated into DNA. At high doses ara-C also binds and inhibits DNA polymerase competitively. In some patients cytidine deaminase activity is high and deoxycytidine kinase activity is low. This results in considerable inactivation of drug before its conversion to its active form.

The purine analogs 6-MP and 6-TG (Figure 43-10) also must undergo activation to form nucleotides, which then act as competitive inhibitors of several enzymes in purine synthesis pathways. The adenosine deaminase inhibitor pentostatin (2-deoxycoformycin) is highly active against hairy cell leukemia.

Antibiotics

Several antibiotics of microbial origin are very effective in the treatment of certain tumors. These antibiotics include doxorubicin, daunorubicin, bleomycin, actinomycin D, and mitomycin C. The anthracycline structures of daunorubicin and doxorubicin are shown in Figure 43-12.

Bleomycin is a mixture of several basic glycopeptides with one called A_2 predominating. Bleomycin forms a tertiary complex with oxygen and Fe (II) competent to cause nucleotide–sequence-specific single and double DNA strand scission. Plicamycin (mithramycin) intercalates into DNA with preferance for guanine-cytosine base pairs. The drug may have a direct action on osteoclasts, and it lowers serum Ca^{++}. Plicamycin is active against testicular carcinoma. The double strand DNA cleavage that results is thought to be lethal.

Doxorubicin and daunorubicin are anthracyclines that act (1) through intercalation between the bases in double-stranded DNA, (2) by inhibition of topoisomerase II, (3) by generation of free radicals, and (4) possibly by an action on the cell membrane. It is generally believed that the major antitumor action is through inhibition of DNA topoisomerase II (Figure. 43-13). DNA topoisomerase II is essential for DNA replication and catalyzes the uncoiling and breakage of both strands of double-stranded DNA to modify the number and the types of linkage twists. The enzyme is inhibited by doxorubicin and daunorubicin by stabilizing a covalent complex of an enzyme-DNA intermediate, preventing the DNA breaks from rejoining, thereby leading to cell death. Inhibition of topoisomerase II occurs also with

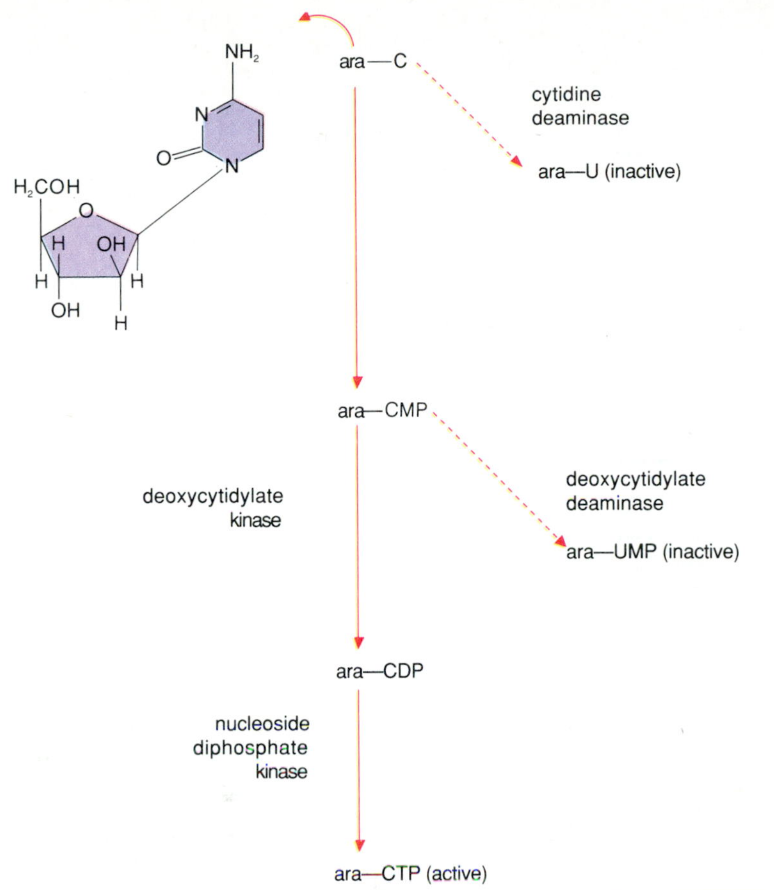

FIGURE 43-11 Competing activation and deactivation pathways for conversion of ara-C (cycosine arabinoside) to the active form that inhibits DNA polymerase.

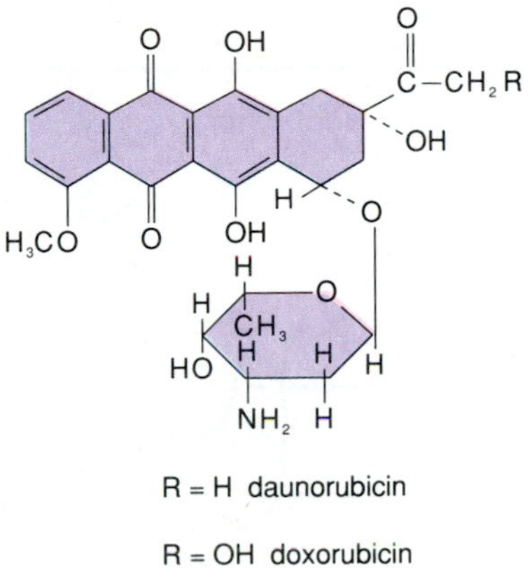

R = H daunorubicin

R = OH doxorubicin

FIGURE 43-12 Structures of daunorubicin and doxorubicin. See the text for further information.

etoposide (VP-16), and teniposide (VM-26). Doxorubicin is the single most active agent against breast cancer, whereas daunorubicin and idarubicin are frequently used to treat leukemias.

Actinomycin D intercalates into DNA at the same site as plicamycin. Thus transcription is blocked and this appears to be a major cause of antitumor activity. In addition, actinomycin causes single-strand DNA breaks possibly through free radical production and it prevents the synthesis of RNA. Mitomycin C first undergoes chemical activation within cells resulting in the formation of a derivative that acts by cross-linking DNA by alkylation.

Plant Alkaloids

The primary compounds in this group, vincristine and vinblastine, bind avidly to tubulin, block microtubule polymerization, and thereby disrupt mitotic spindle formation during mitosis at the metaphase phase of the cell cycle (Figures 43-1 and 43-14). Cell death results from an inability to segregate chromosomes properly. Taxol, which acts as a mitotic inhibitor, binds specifically and reversibly to tubulin, but unlike other antitubule drugs it stabilizes microtubules in the polymerized form. Taxol appears to be active against solid tumors including ovarian carcinomas. Etoposide is a semisynthetic derivative of podophyllotoxin that is prepared from the mandrake plant (mayapple). This inhibitor of hopoisomerase II has significant activity against small cell cancer of the lung and testicular carcinoma and is used in most first-line regimens for these diseases. Teniposide is a close analog of etoposide and is active against acute leukemias in children.

Hormonal Agents

Steroids act by passing through the cell membrane and binding to cytoplasmic receptors, which then enter the nucleus and interact with specific hormone-responsive chromatin to induce the synthesis of special mRNAs. Translation of these mRNA species leads to

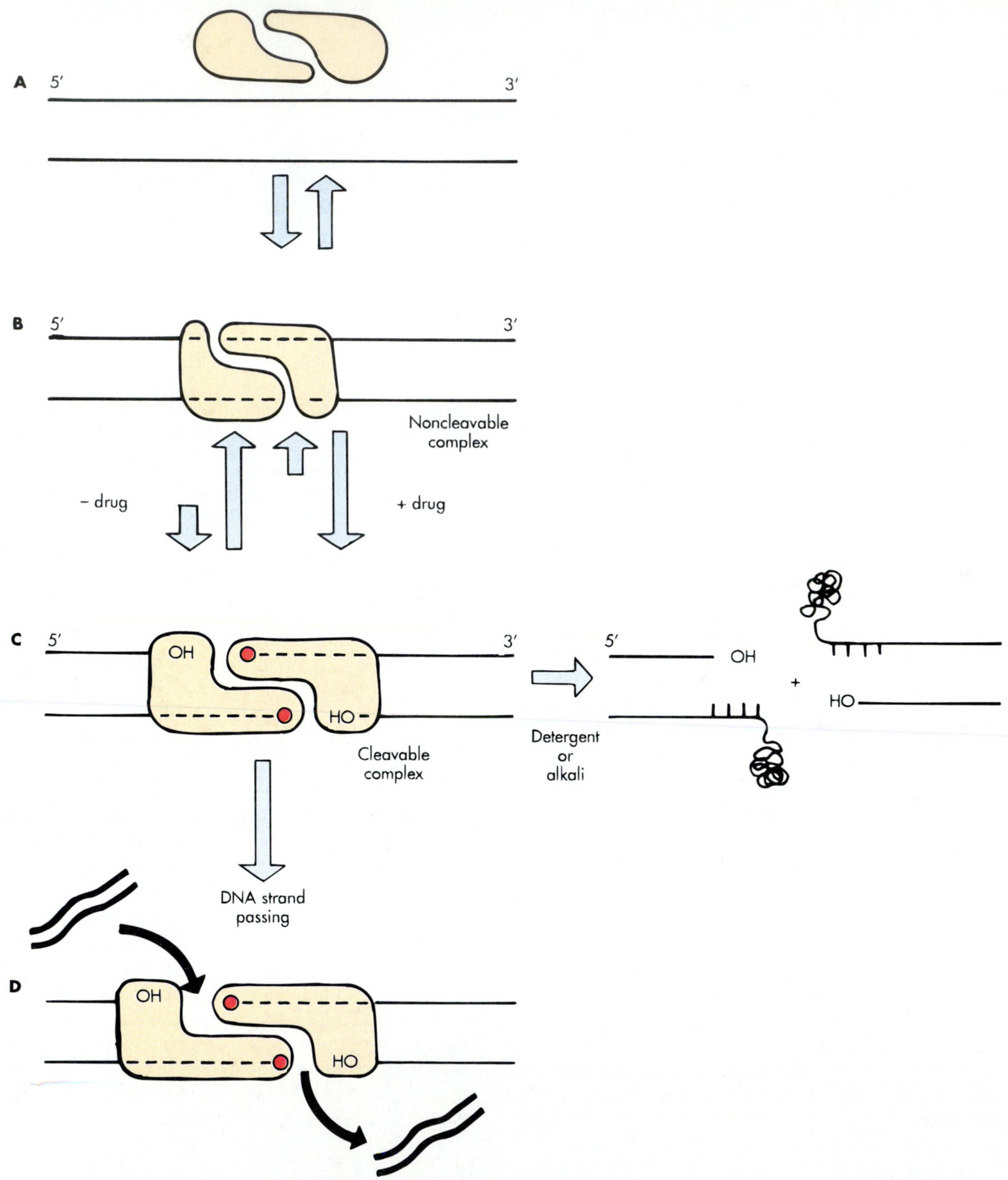

FIGURE 43-13 A scheme of mammalian DNA topoisomerase II mechanism and anticancer drug action. Mammalian DNA topoisomerase II forms two different types of protein-DNA complex that are in rapid equilibrium: the noncleavable complex *(B)* and the cleavable complex *(C)*. These complexes can be identified in vitro by the ability of detergent or alkali to separate DNA strands. The cleavable complex is transient but is stabilized by doxorubicin, daunorubicin, etoposide, and actinomycin D. In the absence of drug, DNA strand passage occurs, whereas drugs block DNA strand passage and DNA replication.

new proteins that alter physiological or biochemical reactions in a beneficial way. Most of the new proteins, however, have not yet been identified and characterized.

Hormonal drug treatment strategies for breast cancer have included (1) attempts to eliminate estrogen production by the adrenals and (2) blockade of estrogen receptors using antiestrogen drugs. In postmenopausal subjects, complete elimination of adrenal-produced estrogens is not always possible because the adrenals secrete androstenedione, which undergoes peripheral conversion to an estrogen (estrone) or to testosterone. Estrone in turn undergoes conversion to estradiol.

About 70% of all postmenopausal patients whose breast tumors show the presence of estrogen receptors respond favorably to antiestrogen therapy, whereas only about 10% of those that show a negative receptor assay respond to antiestrogen therapy. Tamoxifen is the main antiestrogen used clinically and acts by binding to the estrogen receptors and blocking estrogen-dependent transcription in cells in the G_1 phase. By blocking the binding of estrogens, tamoxifen (see Chapter 36 for structures) may decrease estrogen stimulation of the production of transforming growth factor α and secretion of associated proteins.

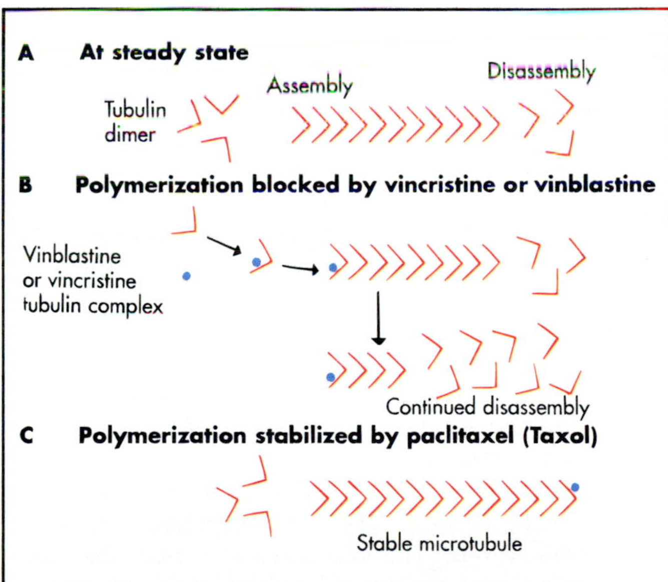

FIGURE 43-14 Scheme of microtubule dynamics in the presence of vincristine, vinblastine, or paclitaxel (Taxol). A dynamic steady state exists, with microtubules assembly occurring at one end and disassembly at the other **(A)**. Vincristine and vinblastine **(B)** bind to tubulin dimers and block polymerization, allowing disassembly to predominate. In contrast, Taxol **(C)** blocks disassembly, causing stable microtubules to form even in the absence of normally essential cofactors. Cells treated with any of these agents are blocked in mitosis.

In metastatic prostate cancer, like breast cancer, objective responses are seen, with hormonal manipulations. For prostate cancer this involves either orchiectomy or pharmacological castration. Testosterone concentrations can be reduced by the estrogen diethylstilbestrol or by suppression of the pituitary gonadotropic axis. Leuprolide and goserelin are analogs of gonadotropic-releasing hormones that inhibit release of gonadotropins and result in castrate testosterone concentrations. Both agents are available in depot form and can be given monthly. Both are agonists as well as antagonists of luteinizing hormone–releasing hormone. They produce an initial rise in gonadotropin concentrations, followed by a decline in 2 to 3 weeks.

Flutamide is an antiandrogen that inhibits androgen binding to receptors in the nucleus. Unlike other agents discussed, it leads to increased concentrations of testosterone. The testosterone is ineffective because flutamide blocks the action of testosterone. There has been recent interest in achieving total androgen blockage (both testis and adrenal) with the concurrent use of flutamide and luteinizing hormone–releasing hormone analogs.

Others

L-Asparaginase is administered to hydrolyze asparagine, required for growth in tumor cells in higher amounts than in normal cells. This depletes asparagine concentrations to well below 10 μM, thereby shutting off protein and eventually nucleic acid synthesis. This approach is selective for those neoplastic cells devoid of asparagine synthetase and thus unable to synthesize the essential asparagine.

Hydroxyurea acts to inhibit ribonucleotide reductase, which reduces ribonucleoside diphosphates to deoxyribonucleotides required for DNA synthesis. It presumably complexes with non-heme Fe required by the enzyme for activity. It is therefore an S phase-specific agent.

Targeting the Antitumor Drugs (see also Chapter 6)

Extensive side effects produced by the actions of antitumor drugs on nonneoplastic cells have resulted in efforts to develop procedures for targeting these drugs to tumor cells. The idea is to maximize the exposure of tumor cells to the drugs while minimizing the exposure of nonneoplastic cells. Regional infusions through intraarterial catheters are used where the circulatory system of the tumor can be localized, and intracavitary infusions (e.g., into the peritoneal cavity) are employed as well. Monoclonal antibody-drug conjugates are being investigated for targeting drugs to the tumor cell surface, but the heterogeneity of tumor cell surface antigens makes this approach difficult. Encapsulation of drugs in liposomes also is an investigational technique.

Mechanisms of Resistance

Some patients initially respond favorably to antitumor drugs, but later the tumor may return and the same drugs may be ineffective. In other patients a drug protocol may show few positive results, even though the same protocol has proved beneficial with other patients. These situations all are typical of resistance either present initially or developing after exposure of the patient to one or more antitumor drugs.

In resistant subjects, the reduced effectiveness can be attributed to a decreased intracellular concentration of drug, to repair of drug-induced damage, or to modified drug targets. Several mechanisms account for these differences, as indicated in the box.

Decreased drug uptake by cells is one mechanism of resistance, especially for drugs, such as methotrexate, that require carrier proteins for transmembrane transport. Actinomycin D resistance is also based on decreased cellular uptake. Cyclophosphamide requires metabolic activation and, in the absence of this metabolic pathway, tumor cells can be resistant. Enhanced conversion of the active agent to an inactive metabolite is a third mechanism. Increased activity of aldehyde dehydrogenase leads to enhanced metabolism of cyclophosphamide and drug resistance.

Enhanced cellular efflux of drug is a fourth mechanism. Mammalian cells possess a 170,000-dalton phosphoglycoprotein called *P*-glycoprotein that acts like an adenosine triphosphate–driven membrane-associated transport protein. This *P*-glycoprotein functions to transport complex ring system containing, hydrophobic, positively charged antitumor drugs, as well as other compounds, out of the cell. Doxorubicin, daunorubicin, actinomycin D, etoposide, teniposide, vincristine, and vinblastine are all antitumor drugs that show resistance in cells possessing elevated concentrations of the multidrug-resistance *P*-glycoprotein. Intracellular drug concentrations are decreased because of energy-dependent removal of drugs by the *P*-glycoprotein. Efforts are underway to develop compounds that will block the drug efflux action of the *P*-glycoprotein pumps and thus develop drugs that circumvent multidrug resistance. Verapamil and other calcium-channel blockers block the *P*-glycoprotein pump, but unacceptably high concentrations are required. Analogs of cyclosporin that lack immunosuppressive properties of cyclosporin may be more promising.

Bleomycin resistance exemplifies the fifth mechanism in which cells rapidly repair the DNA breaks caused by this drug. DNA repair mechanisms may be a source of resistance for other DNA-directed antitumor drugs as well. An example could be the repair of covalent cross-links between DNA strands.

Intracellular targets are a sixth mechanism of resistance, for which MTX serves as an example. In one mechanism, cells have increased intracellular concentrations of the target enzyme dihydrofolate reductase, resulting from gene amplification.

In another, seventh, mechanism, an altered enzyme is present, still enzymatically active, but with a lower binding affinity for methotrexate. In yet another example, methotrexate is not conjugated with polyglutamates and is therefore not retained within the tumor cell. The more active MTX-polyglutamate conjugate is less lipid soluble and therefore less likely to traverse the cell membrane. A higher unconjugated MTX concentration is required to inhibit dihydrofolate reductase. Thus, in these examples, the enzyme is no longer inhibited to the same degree by the usual concentration of intracellular methotrexate. This also illustrates how cells can have multiple mechanisms of resistance to a single aspect.

Sulfhydryl compounds, including glutathione and metallothioneins, act as cellular protective groups, particularly against alkylating agents. Increased concentrations of such protective compounds scavenge highly reactive compounds and represent the eighth mechanism. Cells in a ninth mechanism can also decrease the available target to produce a resistant phenotype. For

POSSIBLE MECHANISMS FOR THE DEVELOPMENT OF RESISTANCE TO ANTINEOPLASTIC AGENTS

ANTINEOPLASTIC AGENT

Decreased uptake of active agent into cancer cell
Failure of agent to be metabolized to a chemical species capable of producing a cytotoxic effect
Enhanced conversion of agent to inactive metabolite
Increase in transport of agent from the cancer cell

CANCER CELL (DNA, TARGET ENZYME, OR OTHER MACROMOLECULE)

Repair of drug-induced DNA damage
Gene amplification or increased gene transcription leading to greater amount of target enzyme within the cancer cell
Reduced ability of target enzyme to bind agent
Increase in concentration of sulfhydryl scavengers
Altered concentrations of target protein

Table 43-1 Pharmacokinetic Parameters

Drug	Administration	Disposition	Notes
nitrogen mustard	IV	M	
melphalan	Oral	M	
cyclophosphamide	IV, oral	M	
nitrosoureas	IV, oral	M	Lipid soluble, crosses blood-brain barrier
cisplatin	IV	R	90% protein bound
carboplatin	IV	R	3-6 hr half-life
busulfan	Oral	M	Few-minute half-life
methotrexate	IV, oral	R	50% to 60% plasma protein bound
5-fluorouracil	IV	M	
cytarabine (ara-C)	IV	M	Few-minute half-life
6-MP and 6-TG	Oral	M*	Large first-pass effect
doxorubicin	IV	M	(10-minute half-life)
daunorubicin	IV	M	
bleomycin	IV	R (50%), M	
asparaginase	IV, IM	—	
vincristine	IV	M, B	Minimal entry into CSF
vinblastine	IV	B	
etoposide (VP-16)	IV, oral	R (main), M, B	97% plasma protein bound
tamoxifen	Oral	M (main)	Enterohepatic cycling

M, Metabolized; *R*, renal excretion; *B*, biliary excretion.
*See text for drug interaction.

example, a decrease in topoisomerase II leads to resistance to etoposide and teniposide.

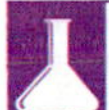

PHARMACOKINETICS

Numerous measurements have been made to determine the plasma concentration decay curves for antitumor drugs. A standard compartment model is used to explain the plasma concentration versus time decay curves. It is a sum of one to three exponentials. It is useful in providing pharmacokinetic guidance to dosing schemes that maximize drug tumor contact while minimizing drug tissue contact. A more complex type of pharmacokinetic model, called a flow model, provides more help but is much more difficult to construct and is usually unsuccessful in obtaining parameter values for individual patients. For those antitumor agents where the drug disappears rapidly from the plasma, continuous IV infusion rather than bolus injection often is needed to obtain a high enough drug concentration to obtain a suitable therapeutic effect. The modes of administration and disposition of several antineoplastic agents are listed in Table 43-1.

6-Mercaptopurine undergoes enzyme-catalyzed metabolism with xanthine oxidase as the principal enzyme. Allopurinol, a drug used in the treatment of gout, also is metabolized by the same enzyme. A drug interaction occurs if the two compounds are given orally concurrently. A major reduction in 6-MP dosage must be instituted in patients receiving allopurinol. Coadministration of these drugs leads to slower disappearance of both. Allopurinol also lengthens cyclophosphamide half-life and increases myelotoxicity, possibly because of decreased renal elimination of cyclophosphamide metabolites. MTX and weak organic acids such as nonsteroidal antiinflammatory agents compete for plasma binding and for renal tubular excretion. Significant increases in MTX concentrations have also been noted when both agents are administered.

The other drugs that undergo metabolism also may show interactions during multiple-drug antitumor dosing, resulting in prolonged plasma concentrations of the involved drugs.

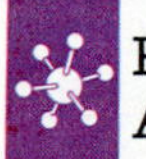

RELATION OF MECHANISMS OF ACTION TO CLINICAL RESPONSE

Most antineoplastic drugs are used in multiple agent protocols where the cytolytic effects of the different agents interact in a complex manner. The clinical use of combination chemotherapy is discussed in a separate chapter (Chapter 44).

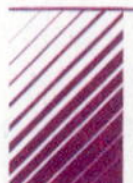

SIDE EFFECTS, CLINICAL PROBLEMS, AND TOXICITY

Typical undesirable side effects experienced with many antitumor drugs are listed in Table 43-2. Many of these side effects reflect effects of the drug on populations of rapidly proliferating normal cells. Nausea and vomiting are quite common and can be attributable to effects on both cycling, and noncycling cells. Strategies for ameliorating these effects are available (see Chapter 44).

Combinations of different drugs are generally designed based on nonoverlapping, dose-limiting toxicities, such as those listed in the box below. These toxicities are unrelated to rapidly proliferating populations of normal cells.

Nephrotoxicity, peripheral neuropathy, and ototoxicity remain the major side effects with cisplatin, though the severity of the renal toxicity can be reduced through hydration of the patient and administration of mannitol. The renal damage arises from toxicity of cisplatin to renal tubules, resulting in decreased glomerular filtration rates and increased reabsorption. Nephrotoxicity does not develop until a week or two after treatment is begun and may be worsened by coadministration of an aminoglycoside for treatment of an infection. Cisplatin-induced neuropathy occurs mainly in large sensory fibers and results in numbness and tingling followed by loss of a sense of joint position and a disabling sensory ataxia. The toxicity is reversible after discontinuation of drug but may require a year or longer to resolve. Nephrotoxicity is more common when patients receive a bolus injection of cisplatin while fractionating the dose over several days has reduced the intensity of this toxicity. Cisplatin neuropathy is a more recently observed cumulative dose-limiting side effect. Carboplatin has less neurotoxicity and nephrotoxicity but more pronounced myelosuppression than cisplatin.

Bleomycin and busulfan both result in drug-induced pulmonary fibrosis, with this side effect dose limiting.

CELL PROLIFERATION–INDEPENDENT SIDE EFFECTS

bleomycin: pulmonary fibrosis ("bleomycin lung")
busulfan: pulmonary fibrosis ("busulfan lung")
doxorubicin: cardiotoxicity
cisplatin: nephrotoxicity and peripheral neuropathy
cyclophosphamide: hemorrhagic cystitis
vincristine: neurotoxicity
cytarabine: cerebral damage

Table 43-2 Typical Undesirable Side Effects with Antineoplastic Drugs in Humans*

Tissue	Undesirable Effects
Bone marrow	Leukopenia and resulting infections
	Immunosuppression
	Thrombocytopenia
	Anemia
GI tract	Oral or intestinal ulceration
	Diarrhea
Hair follicles	Alopecia
Gonads	Menstrual irregularities, including premature menarche; impaired spermatogenesis
Wounds	Impaired healing
Fetus	Teratogenesis (especially during first trimester)

*Many of these effects are caused by drug action on nontumor cells that usually are growing (i.e., cycling).

Bleomycin is excreted in the urine 50% or more as unchanged drug. The dose should be reduced when creatinine clearance drops below 30 ml/min (from 120 ml/min standard). Bleomycin accumulates in the lungs and skin where bleomycin hydrolase (which in other tissues actively metabolizes the drug) is present at very low activity. The continued presence of elevated concentrations of bleomycin leads to recruitment of lymphocytes and polymorphonuclear leukocytes in bronchoalveolar fluids. It is not known how this leads to fibrosis. Hypersensitivity pneumonitis also is observed with bleomycin therapy but is less frequent with methotrexate, mitomycin C, nitrosoureas, and alkylating agents.

The major side effects with cytarabine are myelosuppression and dose-limiting cerebral damage. Ocular toxicity also has occasionally been associated with higher doses. Nausea and vomiting are seen in almost all patients receiving higher doses of cytarabine administered to overcome drug transport resistance.

Doxorubicin, daunorubicin, and idorubicin are associated with the long-term, dose-limiting side effect of myocardial failure. Doxorubicin usually is discontinued when the cumulative dose reaches 500 mg/m^2 of body surface area of when cardiac ventricular ejection fraction shows a significant decrease. The acute cardiac effects of hypotension, tachycardia, and arrhythmias are usually not clinically significant, but long-term effects leading to congestive heart failure can be life threatening and necessitate discontinuance of drug therapy. The chronic effects appear after weeks to months of therapy and have been reported up to several years after discontinuing treatment especially in pediatric cancer patients. At a cumulative dose of $>$600 mg/m^2, 35% of patients experience congestive heart failure, which is refractory to medical management. The detailed mechanism is complex not well understood, but appears to involve Ca^{++}-activated adenosine triphosphatase (Ca^{++}ATPase), cyclic adenosine monophosphate, and lipid peroxidation. The principal metabolite of doxorubicin, doxorubicinol (carbonyl side chain converted to an alcohol), is a potent inhibitor of Na^{+}, K^{+}-ATPase, Mg^{++}-ATPase, and Ca^{++}-ATPase. This may contribute to this serious side effect of an otherwise highly efficacious antitumor drug. Bone marrow and gastrointestinal toxicity vary with the plasma concentrations of doxorubicin.

Cyclophosphamide, which undergoes metabolism to form an active compound and other reactive metabolites (Figure 43-6), occasionally produces hemorrhagic cystitis. This can be largely eliminated with vigorous hydration of patients during cyclophosphamide administration. As little as a single IV dose of cyclophosphamide can produce the cystitis. For very high doses of IV cyclophosphamide, MESNA is used as a protectant. The cause appears to be acrolein, which is produced as a toxic by-product of the metabolism of cyclophosphamide. This side effect is not age or sex related and leads to a 9 to 45 times greater risk of developing bladder cancer. The likelihood of developing bladder cancer is not so severe for orally as compared to intravenously administered cyclophosphamide.

With MTX, vinblastine, etoposide, and 5-fluorouracil the main side effect is bone marrow suppression. Vinca alkaloids such as vincristine can cause peripheral neuropathy, but this is less frequent with etoposide (or vinblastine).

Nearly all antineoplastic drugs have side effects that are considered by the patient as very objectionable.

TRADE NAMES

In addition to generic and fixed-combination preparations, the following trade-named materials are available in the United States.

Adriamycin, doxorubicin HCl
Alkeran, melphalan
BiCNU, carmustine (BCNU)
Blenoxane, bleomycin sulfate
CeeNU, lumustine (CCNU)
Cerubidine, daunorubicin HCl
Cosmegen, dactinomycin, actinomycin D
Cutoxan, Neosar, cyclophosphamide
Cytosar-U, cytarabine
DTIC-Dome, dacarbazine
Efudex, Adrucil, 5-fluorouracil
Elspar, asparaginase
FUDR, floxuridine
Hydrea, hydroxyurea
Intron A, interferon alfa-2b, recombinant
Leukeran, chlorambucil
Matulane, procarbazine HCl
Mexate, methotrexate sodium
Mustargen, mechlorethamine HCl
Mutamycin, mitomycin
Myleran, busulfan
Nolvadex, tamoxifen citrate
Novantrone, mitoxantrone
Oncovin, Vincasar, vincristine sulfate
Paraplatin, carboplatin
Platinol, cisplatin
Purinethol, 6-mercaptopurine
Roferon-A, interferon alfa-2a, recombinant
Thioguan tabloid, thioguanine
Velban, Velsar, vinblastine sulfate
VePesiol, etoposide
Vumor, teniposide
Zanosar, streptozocin

SELF-ASSESSMENT QUESTIONS

1. All of the following antineoplastic agents are antimetabolites EXCEPT:
   a. Cisplatin
   b. Methotrexate
   c. Cytarabine
   d. Thioguanine
2. A 28 year old male is being treated for testicular carcinoma and develops severe and irreversible pulmonary fibrosis. Which of the following drugs are most likely responsible for this adverse effect?
   a. Vinblastine
   b. Cisplatin
   c. Doxorubicin
   d. Bleomycin
3. Most antineoplastic agents kill malignant cells by:
   a. zero order kinetics
   b. first order kinetics
   c. hypoxic sensitization
   d. enzyme inhibition
   e. oncogene suppression
4. All of the following anticancer drugs are thought to function by blocking topoisomerase II EXCEPT:
   a. Etoposide
   b. Doxorubicin
   c. Daunoribicin
   d. Mitomycin C
5. Of the following drugs, which functions to block ribonucleotide reductase?
   a. Bleomycin
   b. Hydroxyurea
   c. L-Asparaginase
   d. Chloroambucil

6. Antimetabolites frequently act to kill cells in which phase of the cell cycle?
   a. M phase (mitotic phase)
   b. G_1 phase
   c. S phase (DNA synthetic phase)
   d. G_2 phase
   e. Phase nonspecific

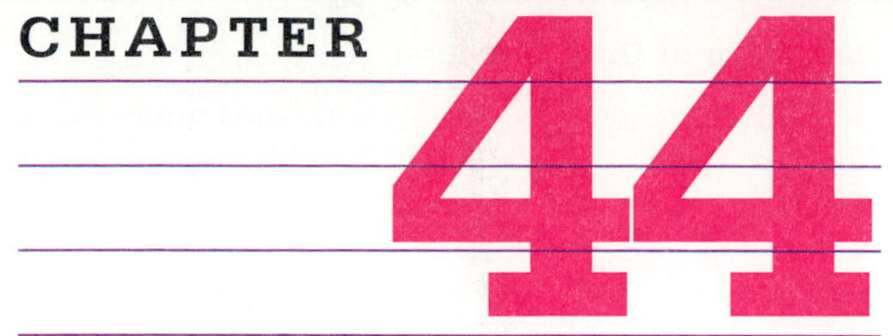

Clinical Effects with Antineoplastic Drugs

JAMES M. LARNER
JOHN S. LAZO

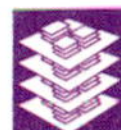

THERAPEUTIC OVERVIEW

A growing number of tumor types now respond to treatment with antineoplastic drugs. The types of clinical response to chemotherapy of advanced stage tumors in patients of various ages are listed in the box.

For children, 5-year survival data for 1993 show about 90% success for Hodgkin's disease, about 70% for acute lymphocytic leukemia, and 90% for Wilms' tumor. Acute lymphocytic leukemia is the most common of the childhood neoplastic diseases, and expectations in the 1990s are that about 95% should attain remission, with at least one half of those being probable cures.

It is of interest to compare the list of tumor types (in the box on p. 592), in which therapy has been aided greatly by antineoplastic drugs with the leading causes of cancer mortality to see if chemotherapy is effective on any of the most common forms of neoplastic diseases. Figure 44-1 summarizes the anatomical sites associated with the highest rates of cancer mortality for different patient ages. Overall, carcinoma of the lung accounts for the greatest number of deaths from cancer in men and women. Some of the leukemias, lymphomas, breast tumors, and small cell lung tumors appear in the box and Figure 44-1, an indication that these high-mortality tumors are ones in which chemotherapy has proved beneficial. The small cell lung tumors represent only about 20% of lung neoplasms, with squamous cell carcinoma, adenocarcinoma, and large cell carcinoma making up another estimated 60% of lung neoplasms. Thus, despite progress, there is still a great need for more effective chemotherapy for the major neoplastic diseases.

DRUG SELECTION AND PROBLEMS

The Nature of the Problem

One of the difficulties in treating neoplastic diseases is that the tumor burden often is excessive by the time the diagnosis is made. This is shown schematically in Figure 44-2, where the number of cells in a typical solid tumor is shown versus time. With 10^9 cells roughly equivalent to a volume of 1 cubic centimeter and representing the minimum size for usual detection, the large number of cells already established at detection becomes readily evident. An upper limit of 10^{12} to 10^{13} tumor cells leads to the death of the patient. Thus, by the time a tumor is detected, it has undergone many doublings. For acute lymphocytic leukemia, the cell doubling time during log phase (first-order) growth is 3 to 4 days, whereas for lung squamous cell carcinoma it is estimated to be about 90 days. Thus in roughly 100 days, two lymphocytic leukemia cells in theory could keep doubling and reach 10^9 cells. Such a cell burden is extremely large to treat only with drugs and is cited here to emphasize the difficulty of the therapeutic task under a typical diagnostic timetable.

Primary versus Adjuvant Therapy

In carrying out chemotherapy against a specific tumor type in an individual patient, the objective may be (1) curative, to obtain complete remission and cure the patient (e.g., Hodgkin's disease); (2) palliative, to improve symptoms but with little expectation of complete remission or cure (e.g., carcinoma of the esophagus with

RESPONSES OF CANCERS TO CHEMOTHERAPY

CANCERS IN WHICH COMPLETE REMISSIONS TO CHEMOTHERAPY ARE COMMON AND CURES ARE SEEN EVEN IN ADVANCED DISEASE*

Acute lymphocytic leukemia (adults and children)
Hodgkin's disease (lymphoma)
Non-Hodgkin's lymphoma
Choriocarcinoma
Testicular cancer
Acute myelogenous leukemia
Burkitt's lymphoma
Ewing's sarcoma
Wilms' tumor
Small cell lung cancer
Ovarian cancer
Hairy cell leukemia

CANCERS IN WHICH OBJECTIVE RESPONSES ARE SEEN BUT CHEMOTHERAPY DOES NOT HAVE CURATIVE POTENTIAL IN ADVANCED DISEASE

Multiple myeloma
Breast cancer
Head and neck cancer
Colorectal carcinomas
Chronic lymphocytic leukemia
Chronic myelogenous leukemia
Transitional cell carcinoma of bladder
Gastric adenocarcinomas
Cervical carcinomas
Medulloblastoma
Soft-tissue sarcoma
Neuroblastoma
Endometrial carcinomas
Insulinoma
Osteogenic sarcoma

CANCERS IN WHICH ONLY OCCASIONAL OBJECTIVE RESPONSES TO CHEMOTHERAPY ARE SEEN

Non–small cell lung cancer
Melanoma
Renal tumor
Pancreatic carcinomas
Hepatocellular carcinoma
Prostate carcinomas (hormone nonresponsive)

*Depending on tumor type, complete remission may result in cure of tumor.

chemotherapy used to improve dysphagia); or (3) adjuvant, to improve chances for cure or to increase the period of disease-free survival when no detectable cancer is present, but subclinical numbers of neoplastic cells are suspected (e.g., chemotherapy for breast cancer after surgical resection of all known tumor).

Selection of Drug Regimen

Although choriocarcinoma (gestational trophoblastic disease) and hairy cell leukemia are treated using single drugs, nearly all other neoplasms are treated with drug combinations.

The choice of drugs and dosing schedule for multiple drug therapy has been and remains largely empirical. There are continuing efforts to try to understand why some combinations are more effective than others for certain tumor types. Despite the empirical approach, several guidelines still need to be appreciated in selecting a combination of drugs. These guidelines are as follows:

1. Use drugs that show activity against the tumor type being treated. The rationale is that only rarely will a compound that shows no activity alone have an effect when used in combination.
2. Use drugs that have minimal or no overlapping toxicities. This requirement may broaden the range of the undesirable side effects of the drug combination. However, the goal of this guideline is to reduce the possibility of encountering life-threatening side effects that act in concert. For that reason, the side effects of the drugs selected should be diverse and not centered on the same organ system.
3. The dosing schedule for each drug should be optimal, and the doses should be given at consistent times. In establishing how often to repeat a dosing sequence, it is usual to allow sufficient time between the sequences to allow the most sensitive tissues (often bone marrow) to recover.
4. Evaluate the degree of success of the combination chemotherapy on the basis of clinical effectiveness.

Many sophisticated approaches have been used to select the drugs and dosing schedules for combination chemotherapy, but the results have been disappointing. Some approaches include drugs that have different mechanisms of action in hopes that one mechanism would succeed where the others fail. Another goal of the multiple mechanism approach has been the hope of finding synergistic combinations. Several combinations are synergistic when tested against cultured tumor cells in vitro, including sequential methotrexate–5-fluorouracil; doxorubicin-cyclophosphamide; and cisplatin-etoposide. A major problem of this approach is that the observed in vivo clinical results often do not correlate with the in vitro data.

The relative sequence of drugs and the timing of drug administration may play a significant role. Most of these drugs are more effective against tumor cells that are cycling than cells resting in the G_0 phase, but, in vivo, cells may be present in any part of the cycle. The effective-

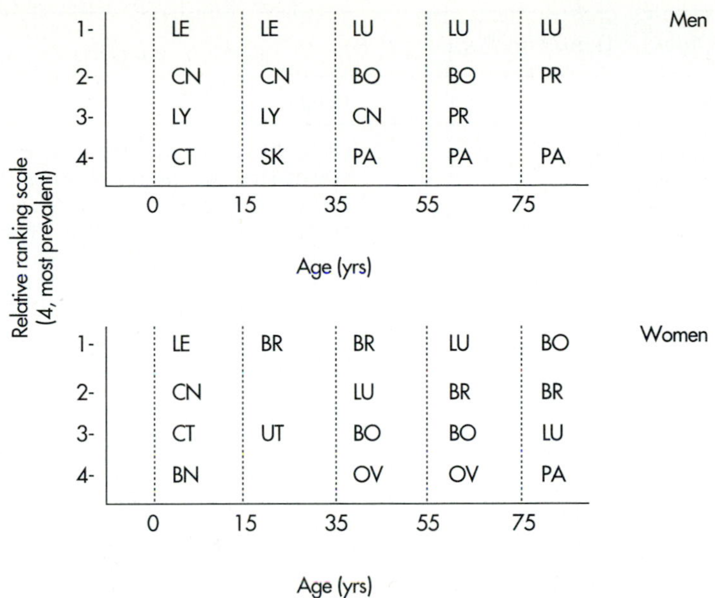

FIGURE 44-1 Leading sites of cancer mortality in 1986. *BN,* Bone; *BO,* colon/rectum; *BR,* breast; *CN,* central nervous; *CT,* connective tissue; *KY,* kidney; *LE,* Leukemia; *LU,* lung; *LY,* lymphoma; *OV,* ovary; *PA,* pancreas; *PR,* prostate; *SK,* skin; *UT,* uterine.

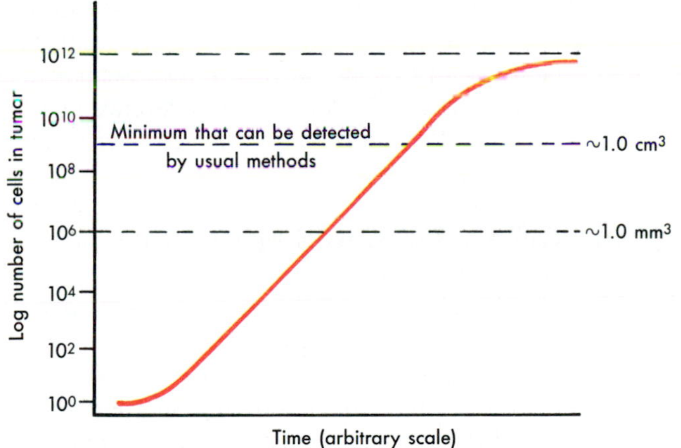

FIGURE 44-2 Typical tumor growth curve indicating roughly 10^9 cells needed for usual diagnosis.

ness of some drug combinations may be in part attributable to activation of cells from G_0 to start cycling or to cycle more rapidly. Thus are placed a greater number of cells in those portions of the cell cycle where the antineoplastic drugs can exert their cytotoxic actions. Because of this possibility, it is important that multidrug dosing schedules be followed accurately. Although existing antitumor drugs may affect the cycling of cells, the timing and sequence of drug combination administration and cellular results remains largely empirical.

Antineoplastic drugs are used as the primary mode of therapy when the tumor is known to be sensitive or when the feasibility for surgical removal or radiation destruction of the main tumor mass is poor. A more difficult situation is presented when the patient fails to respond to first-line regimen of chemotherapy. Such patients are difficult to treat because the tumor volume may be large, the cells may be resistant to one or more of the usual drugs, and the general health of the patient is likely to be poor. An easier situation is the patient in which drugs can be used as an adjuvant after surgical or radiation removal of the primary tumor, as in breast cancer.

Some examples of popular combination drug regimens are given in Table 44-1.

A trend exists toward the use of high-dose protocols with other drugs besides methotrexate to try to push higher concentrations of drug into the tumor site and into the tumor cells. This trend is also being used with those drugs that undergo rapid degradation in plasma (e.g., cytarabine). In most cases the detailed studies needed to substantiate the efficacy of the higher dose protocols are missing or the conclusions are controversial. The emergence of granulocyte colony stimulating factor and granulocyte macrophage–colony stimulating factor as clinical agents to reduce chemotherapy-induced neutropenia and infections will certainly increase this high dose trend.

Table 44-1 Current Combination Drug Regimens

Terminology	Cancer	Drugs
MOPP	Hodgkin's	mechlorethamine, vincristine, procarbazine, prednisone
ABVD	Hodgkin's	doxorubicin, bleomycin, vinblastine, dacarbazine
CMF	Breast	cyclophosphamide, methotrexate, 5-fluorouracil
CAF	Breast	cyclophosphamide, doxorubicin, 5-fluorouracil
—	Acute lymphocytic leukemia	vincristine, prednisone, asparaginase, daunorubicin
—	Acute myelogenous leukemia	cytarabine, plus mitoxantrone or idarubicin or daunorubicin
—	Chronic myelogenous leukemia	hydroxyurea, interferon
—	Wilm's	actinomycin D, vincristine, doxorubicin
—	Small cell (lung)	etoposide-cisplatin or cyclophosphamide, doxorubicin, vincristine
VBP	Germ cell cancers	etoposide, bleomycin, cisplatin
BIP	Cervical cancer	bleomycin, ifosfamide, cisplatin
—	Ovary	cyclophosphamide, carboplatinum
CHOP	Lymphoma	cyclophosphamide, doxorubicin, vincristine, prednisone
—	Head and neck	5-fluorouracil, cisplatinum
—	Colon/rectum	5-fluorouracil, leucovorin

Special Clinical Problems

Two problems are particularly troublesome: (1) the risk of the patient developing leukemia (or other neoplastic condition) as a result of chemotherapy and (2) the frequent nausea and vomiting side effects with many of these drugs.

Several retrospective studies have been carried out to try to define the specific variables that increase the risk of leukemia developing in patients treated initially for Hodgkin's disease and others for ovarian tumors. From the roughly 30,000 patients with Hodgkin's disease, 163 developed leukemia between 1 and 10 years after being diagnosed with Hodgkin's disease. Many of them received mechlorethamine, vincristine, procarbazine, and prednisone (MOPP) (Table 44-1) for chemotherapy of the Hodgkin's disease. Because this rate of leukemia formation is much higher than expected, the conclusion is reached that chemotherapy for Hodgkin's disease greatly increases the risk of leukemia, and the data indicate that it occurs in a dose-dependent manner. Recent evidence indicates that the use of ABVD (doxorubicin, bleomycin, vinblastine, dacarbazine) for the treatment of Hodgkin's disease may be associated with a significantly lower risk of leukemias.

Similarly, from 99,000 patients with ovarian tumor, 114 developed leukemia in about 1 to 10 years after being diagnosed with ovarian cancer. Chemotherapy (not radiotherapy or surgery) was associated with the higher incidence of leukemia, with the risk greatest with chlorambucil and melphalan and less with cyclophosphamide and thioTEPA. The increased leukemia risk was also enhanced with higher doses of these drugs. It should be noted that not all chemotherapeutic drugs are associated with an increased risk of leukemia. The increased risk is mainly with the use of alkylating agents.

Nausea and vomiting can be expected in a high fraction of patients receiving antineoplastic drugs. Some of the drugs that are most and least likely to trigger the emesis are listed in the box on p. 595. Although clinical management of nausea and vomiting can become a serious problem, antagonists as antiemetics appear likely to greatly decrease this. In addition, 5-HT$_3$ antagonists, oral phenothiazine, dexamethasone, butyrophenone, metoclopramide, and diphenydramine are useful as antiemetics, and sedation with benzodiazepines is also possible.

BIOLOGICAL-RESPONSE MODIFIERS

Biological-response modifiers are a class of agents that stimulate the human immune system to destroy tumor cells. The α and β human interferons are efficacious in hairy cell leukemia and in certain skin cancers and may become aids for treating chronic myelogenous leukemia and non-Hodgkin's lymphoma. Interleukin-2 is another endogenous compound that has possibilities for applications in treating lung, renal, colorectal, and several other tumor types. Still other compounds include tumor necrosis factor, human growth factors, and monoclonal antibodies. These compounds are discussed in detail in Chapter 45 on immunopharmacology.

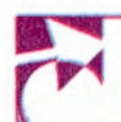

NEW DIRECTIONS

Although significant advances have been made in the treatment of the hematological neoplastic diseases over the past several decades, only minimal progress

TENDENCY OF ANTINEOPLASTIC DRUGS TO INDUCE NAUSEA OR VOMITING

STRONG TENDENCY

cisplatin, dacarbazine, mechlorethamine, cyclophosphamide, doxorubicin, lomustine, carmustine

MODERATE TENDENCY

daunorubicin, actinomycin D, catarabine, procarbazine, methotrexate, mitomycin C, etoposide

LOW TENDENCY

chlorambucil, vincristine, tamoxifen, vinblastine, bleomycin, hydroxyurea, fluorouracil

has been made in the treatment of most solid tumors. During this same time period, there has been an explosion in our understanding of the basic science of cancer. For example, the last few decades have witnessed the description of RNA and DNA tumor viruses, oncogenes, and antioncogenes *(tumor suppressor genes)* as well as dramatic advances in the understanding of cell-cycle regulation. Thus far, these advances have led to only a minimal number of new treatment strategies. However, over the next several years many cancer treatments are certain to be devised based on our understanding of cancer. For example, now underway are gene therapy trials for glioblastoma multiforme in which a retrovirus is used to introduce a thymidine kinase gene into the tumor cells in order to sensitize them to the antiviral agent ganciclovir. Also underway are trials in which antisense oligonucleotides are used to inactivate oncogenes as an attempt to eliminate the growth advantage of these cells. In general, the chasm between the molecular biology of cancer and clinical oncology is likely to be narrowed as more molecular-based treatment methods are adapted.

REFERENCES

Chabner BA, Collins JM, editors: *Cancer chemotherapy: principles and practice,* Philadelphia, 1990, Lippincott.

Foon KA: Biological response modifiers: the new immunotherapy, *Cancer Res* 49:1621, 1989.

Itesketh PJ, Giandara DR: Serotonin antagonists: a new class of antiemetic agents, *J Natl Cancer Inst* 83:613-620, 1991.

Skeel RT, editor: *Handbook of cancer chemotherapy,* ed 3, Boston, 1991, Little, Brown & Co.

Williams C: *Cancer biology and management: an introduction*, Chichester, 1990, John Wiley & Sons.

SELF-ASSESSMENT QUESTIONS

1. Which of the following diseases is potentially curable with combination chemotherapy even when both the liver and lung are involved by metastatic disease?
   a. breast cancer
   b. Hodgkin's disease
   c. colon cancer
   d. non–small cell carcinoma of the lung
   e. stomach cancer
2. Which of the following regimens is both effective for Hodgkin's disease and not associated with a significant risk of secondary leukemia?
   a. CMF (cyclophosphamide, methotrexate, fluorouracil)
   b. MOPP (methotrexate, vincristine, procarbazine, prednisone)
   c. ABVD (Adriamycin, bleomycin, vinblastine, decarbazine)
   d. CAF (cyclophosphamide, Adriamycin, fluorouracil)
   e. BIP (bleomycin, ifosfamide, cisplatin)
3. Which of the following antineoplastic agents is associated with the greatest likelihood of nausea and vomiting?
   a. vincristine
   b. tamoxifen
   c. methotrexate
   d. cisplatin
   e. fluorouracil
4. Which of the following cancers is associated with only a minimal <20% objective response rate to chemotherapy?
   a. acute myelogenous leukemia
   b. large cell lymphoma
   c. renal cell carcinoma
   d. small cell carcinoma of the lung
   e. seminoma
5. When patients fail to respond to first-line chemotherapy the likelihood of a response to a second-line regimen may be diminished because of:
   a. tumor cell resistance caused by multidrug resistance gene
   b. tumor cell resistance caused by selection of resistant clones
   c. decreased performance status of patient
   d. increased tumor burden
   e. all of the above

CHAPTER 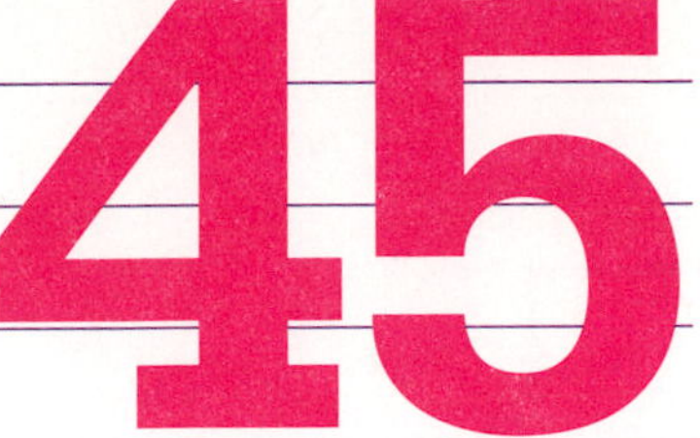

Immunopharmacology

THOMAS T. KAWABATA
ALBERT E. MUNSON

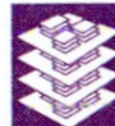

THERAPEUTIC OVERVIEW

The immune system defends the body against invading organisms, foreign antigens, and host cells that have become neoplastic. In addition, the immune system is an active participant in autoimmune diseases, hypersensitivity reactions, and transplant tissue rejections.

The ability of the immune system to discriminate between foreign molecules and antigenic sites of foreign cells and normal endogenous molecules and cells of the host results in elimination of most diseases before an overt pathological condition is established. Moreover, after an infection or neoplasm becomes established and chemotherapy initiated, drugs kill only a fraction of the invading organisms (Chapter 46) or neoplastic cells (Chapter 43), and a functional immune system is needed to eradicate the remaining organisms or cells. This ability to recognize foreign antigens allows destruction and removal of invading organisms by various effector mechanisms of the immune system. However, in autoimmune diseases, inappropriate immune responses against host cells (self-antigens) may occur. In addition, an overt response to an antigen may result in tissue-damage reactions known as *hypersensitivity responses.*

Pharmacological modulation of the immune system can stimulate or suppress the response, as summarized in the box on p. 598.

ABBREVIATIONS	
CSF	cerebrospinal fluid
CTL	cytolytic T lymphocytes
G-CSF	granulocyte–colony stimulating factor
GM-CSF	granulocyte macrophage–colony stimulating factor
IFN	interferon
IG	immunoglobulin
IL	interleukin
LAK	lymphokine-activated killer cell
M-CSF	macrophage–colony stimulating factor
MHC	major histocompatibility complex
TNF	tumor necrosis factor

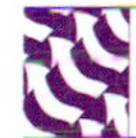

MECHANISMS OF ACTION

Immune System Components

Cell Types The cells of the immune system are formed from pluripotent stem cells produced in bone marrow. These stem cells undergo a sequence of cellular differentiations, outlined in part in Figure 45-1, to form B lymphocytes, T lymphocytes, erythrocytes, polymorphonuclear leukocytes, monocytes, macrophages, and mast cells.

Lymphocytes are one of the primary cell types involved in the immune response. There are two general types of lymphocytes, B and T. Both are derived from bone marrow lymphoid stem cells, but T cells go through an additional maturation process in the thymus. Although the morphology of T cells and B cells is similar, the functions of these two types are distinct. After antigen exposure, B cells develop into antibody-producing plasma cells, whereas T cells are divided into functional subtypes that possess distinct cell surface antigens.

The other major participant in the immune response is the bone-marrow–derived macrophage (see Figure 45-1). When unactivated and circulating, it is referred to as a *monocyte;* however, when it migrates into the extravascular spaces, it is known as a *macrophage.* In comparison to unactivated lymphocytes, macrophages are larger and possess a greater cytoplasmic to nuclear

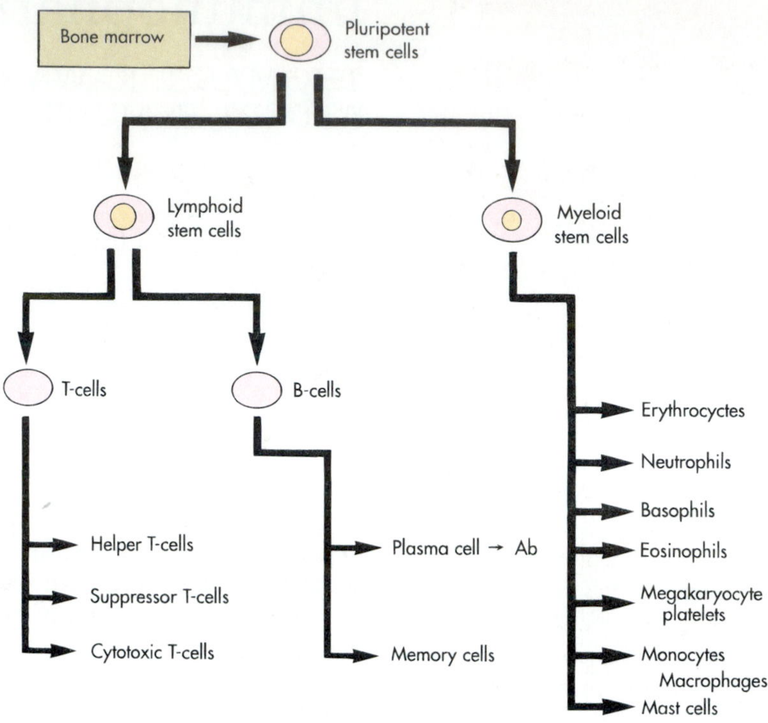

FIGURE 45-1 Terminology, sources, and interrelationships of components of the immune system. Terms in () with T-cells represent names of markers. *Ab,* Antibody.

PHARMACOLOGICAL MODULATION OF THE IMMUNE SYSTEM

SUPPRESSION

Overcomes organ/tissue transplantation rejection
Reduces effects of autoimmune diseases

STIMULATION

Enhances activity of immune system against viruses, microorganisms, or other invading organisms
Enhances immune system activity against neoplastic cells of the host.

ratio. The macrophage contains lysosomes filled with various catabolic enzymes. The macrophage membrane possesses digestive enzymes and receptors for binding complement components and the constant or Fc region (Figure 45-2) of antibodies (immunoglobulins). The size and cytoplasmic contents are determined by the activation state. The primary functions of macrophages are phagocytosis, antigen presentation, and cytokine production. Phagocytic macrophages are distributed throughout many tissues (Table 45-1) and collectively are called the *reticuloendothelial system.* The genera-

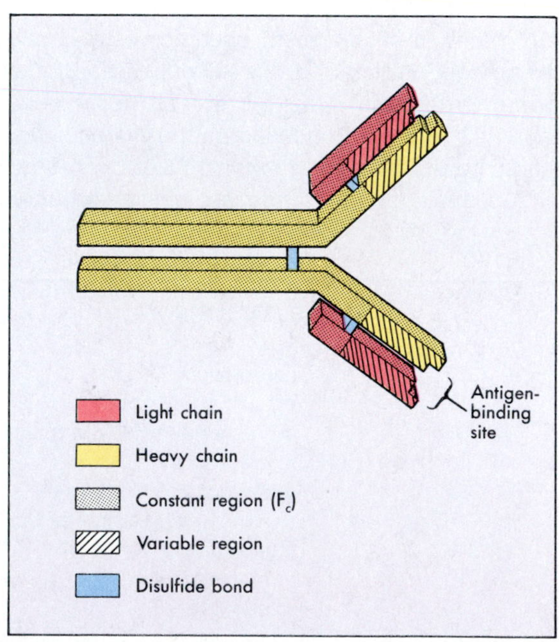

FIGURE 45-2 Antibody structure, showing light and heavy chains, variable regions, constant regions, and disulfide bonds.

Table 45-1 Cells That Constitute the Reticuloendothelial System

Tissue	Cell Type
Liver	Kupffer cells
Brain	Microglial cells
Spleen	Macrophages
Lymph node	Macrophages
Lung	Aveolar macrophages

tion of superoxide free radicals and digestive enzymes allows the macrophage to destroy other phagocytized organisms or molecules. This phagocytic process is also important in altering and cleaving large antigen molecules before presentation to T lymphocytes (antigen processing).

Polymorphonuclear granulocytes and mast cells also participate in immune system processes. Three types of polymorphonuclear granulocytes (neutrophils, eosinophils, and basophils) originate from bone marrow and are located primarily in the vascular system. These cells constitute 50% to 60% of the total circulating leukocytes, with most being neutrophils (90%) and eosinophils (3% to 5%). Granulocytes can move out of the vascular system between endothelial cells and into tissue. Neutrophils have an important role in host resistance to microorganisms. Opsonized organisms bind neutrophils via complement and Fc receptors and are phagocytized. Although eosinophils are morphologically similar to neutrophils, they are believed to be mainly involved with reactions against parasitic infections. Basophils and mast cells are important effector cells in IgE-mediated allergic reactions. The binding of IgE to these cells stimulates the release of vasoactive amines (e.g., histamines, see Chapter 58). IgE binds to these cells via the Fc portion. The binding and cross-linking of antigen to cell-bound IgE results in the release of histamine, prostaglandins, leukotrienes, and cytokines. These factors cause the clinical symptoms of an immediate (Type I) hypersensitivity response causing vasodilatation and loss of vascular fluids into tissue. Basophils and mast cells are functionally very similar but differ in that basophils may circulate in the blood and may migrate into inflamed tissue and have a polymorphonuclear nucleus. Mast cells are residents of connective tissue and have nuclei with a more oval mononuclear shape. Although similar in function, these cells arise from different cell lineages.

Organs and Tissues Immune system cells migrate from the bone marrow via the circulatory system to secondary lymphoid organs, lymph nodes, spleen, and mucosal tissue (gastrointestinal, respiratory, urogenital). The centralization of immunocompetent cells in secondary lymphoid tissue, rather than dispersal throughout the circulatory system, provides a location where antigen may be retained and presented to lymphocytes. Moreover, activated lymphocytes may interact more readily with neighboring lymphocytes in the lymphoid tissue. These cells may then migrate out of the secondary lymphoid organs and function at distant sites in the body. Lymph nodes are distributed throughout the body and are interconnected by lymphatic vessels and the circulatory system. This allows lymphocytes to circulate between different organs and to contact foreign antigens more readily. The lymphatic circulatory system drains into the thoracic duct and then back into the vascular system. Secondary lymphoid organs are organized as reticular structures to allow cells to migrate into the lymphoid tissue where they may contact antigen and then migrate out into the periphery as mature, antigen-specific lymphocytes. Different types of immunocompetent cells are distributed in distinct regions in the tissues.

Antibodies One of the primary effector components of the immune response is antibodies. Antibodies are immunoglobulins secreted from B cells that have been stimulated with antigen. Antibodies produced in response to a specific antigen bind only that specific antigen. Immunoglobulins are composed of two heavy and two light chains, as shown schematically in Figure 45-2. Antigen binds to a portion of the variable region (V) and affords specificity to the immunoglobulin. The other region is named the *constant region* (Fc). There are five classes of immunoglobulins: IgA, IgD, IgG, IgE, and IgM. The IgA and IgM immunoglobulins contain multiple immunoglobulin units joined by disulfide bonds (Figure 45-3).

Antigens, which stimulate the formation of antibodies, may be molecules of various types (e.g., proteins, carbohydrates, lipids, nucleic acids). However, many low molecular weight compounds such as drugs and environmental contaminants are not capable of inducing antibody production. If these small molecules are bound to high molecular weight molecules (carriers), these compounds (called *haptens*) can become antigenic. Antibodies are produced against either haptens or hapten-carrier conjugates.

Immune defenses against infectious organisms and neoplastic cells are commonly classified as innate or acquired (also known as adaptive). Responses that are antigen-independent are considered innate, whereas acquired immunity involves antigen recognition and is characterized by an antigen-dependent action. In many host defense responses, both innate and acquired immunity occur.

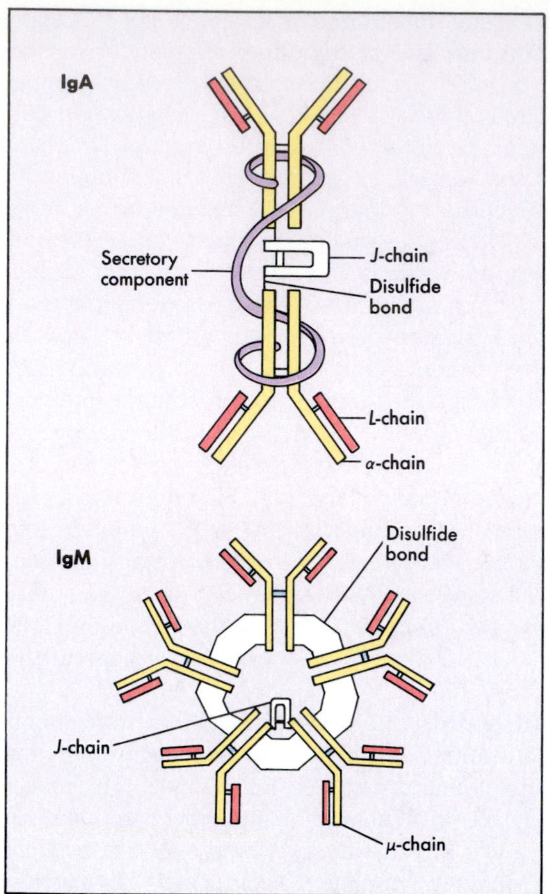

FIGURE 45-3 IgA and IgM structure. The secretory IgA is composed of two immunoglobulins connected by a J-chain and secretory component. IgM is composed of five immunoglobulin molecules joined with a J-chain. *L-chain,* Light chain; *μ-chain,* heavy chain.

Immune Response

Innate Immunity Commonly referred to as the first line of defense, innate immunity encompasses a wide variety of cell types and mechanisms of action. Microorganisms and tumor cells are phagocytized by macrophages and neutrophils after activation by cellular components of the invading organism (e.g., endotoxin) or cytokines (e.g., macrophage activating factor). Tumor cells may be lysed in an antigen nonspecific manner by natural killer cells or lymphokine-activated killer cells (LAKs). Another important component of the innate response is the complement cascade, in which certain components act as substrates for other enzyme components. The substrates are then activated to form enzymes that convert other components of the cascade to active enzymes. The activated complement components form complexes that are capable of lysing the invading organisms. These complexes may be activated by cellular constituents or bacteria (alternate pathway) and thus do not require antigen recognition.

Acquired Immunity Antigen stimulation of lymphocytes may result in the development of humoral or cell-mediated immune responses. Humoral responses involve the participation of antibody. Macrophages and T-helper cells are required in addition to B cells in most humoral immune responses (Figure 45-4). This collaborative effort involves the production of cytokines (e.g., interleukin-1, IL-1) and antigen presentation to T cells by antigen presenting cells (macrophages, dendritic cells, and antigen-activated B cells). The CD4-containing T-helper cells will recognize antigen only when associated with major histocompatibility (MHC) class II antigens (Figure 6-5). The combination of antigen activation and cytokine costimulation of T cells results in the production of IL-2 and other cytokines. Antigens bind to specific immunoglobulin receptors on B cells. Lymphokines produced by T cells stimulate the antigen-activated B cells to proliferate and differentiate into antibody-producing plasma cells. Concurrent with the generation of activated T cells and B cells, antigen also induces the generation of suppressor T cells. These cells are believed to down-modulate the immune response by the secretion of suppressive factors. However, since several laboratories have been unable to characterize the factors, the area of suppressor cells remains controversial.

Cell-mediated responses also require antigen-presenting cells to present antigen to T cells and produce various cytokines (Figure 45-5). These steps may lead to the generation of cytolytic T cells or activation of macrophages. In the generation of cytolytic T cells, antigen is presented to the cells, and production of interleukin-2 by the activated T-helper cells stimulates the proliferation and differentiation of cytolytic T cells to mature cytolytic T cells. Cytolytic T lymphocytes may be produced against graft cells, tumor cells (Figure 45-6), or virus-infected cells. Antigen recognition and binding of cytolytic T cells to antigen of cells results in the lysis of target. In delayed-type hypersensitivity reactions, antigen-stimulated T-helper cells secrete lymphokines, which recruit and activate macrophages. These macrophages are then capable of phagocytizing the foreign organisms or host cells in an antigen-nonspecific manner. This can occur in reactions against tuberculosis and with chemicals such as urushiol from poison ivy (contact hypersensitivity).

Modulation of Response by Hormones and CNS The interplay between hormones and neurotransmitters and the immune response is very important in presenting a multiorgan response to stimuli. Glucocorticoids secreted by the adrenal cortex during stress can lead to suppressed immune responses and movement of lym-

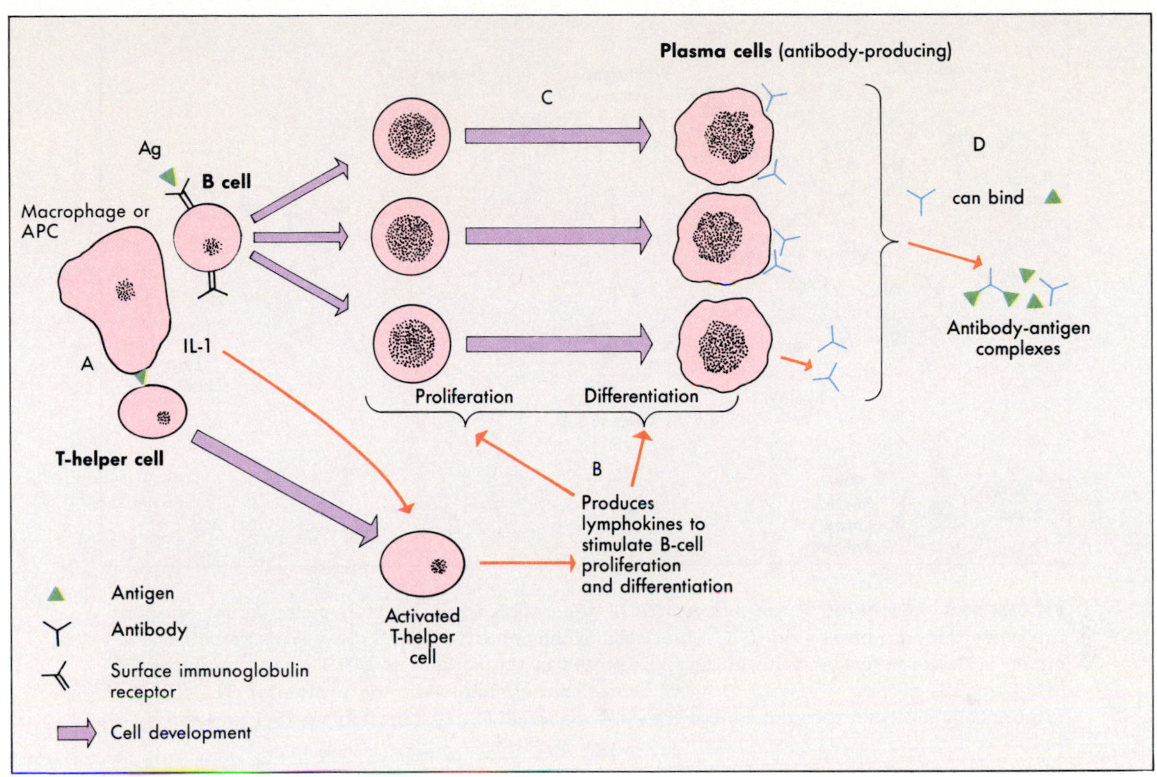

FIGURE 45-4 Generation of a humoral immune response. There are several cell types required in the generation of the antibody-producing plasma cells. Antigen *(Ag)* is processed and presented to T-helper cells with class II MHC antigens *(A)* (see Figure 45-5). This results in the synthesis and secretion of lymphokines, which act on B cells, macrophages, and T-helper cells *B)*. Antigen-activated B cells proliferate and differentiate to plasma cells *C)*. Antibodies are produced that bind antigen *(D)*. *(IL,* Interleukin; *APC,* antigen-presenting cells such as macrophages B cells and dendritic cells.)

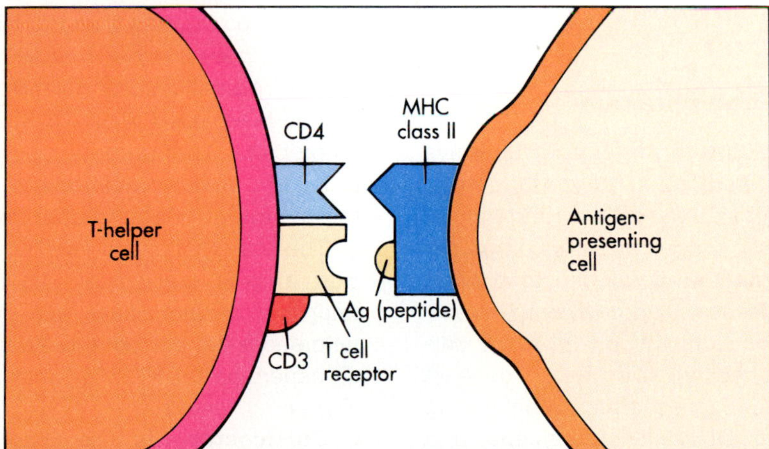

FIGURE 45-5 Molecular interaction between a macrophage and a T-helper cell. The CD4 molecules on T-helper cells act as receptors for major histocompatibility *(MHC)* class II antigens. CD8 molecules on cytotoxic T lymphocytes recognize MHC class I *(not shown)*. Close association of the T-cell receptor and CD4 allows for the presentation of antigen-class II antigen complex. This binding results in the transduction of a signal via the CD3 molecule. MHC class II antigens are found on macrophages, B cells, and other specialized antigen-presenting cells (APCs). MHC class I antigens are present on all somatic cells.

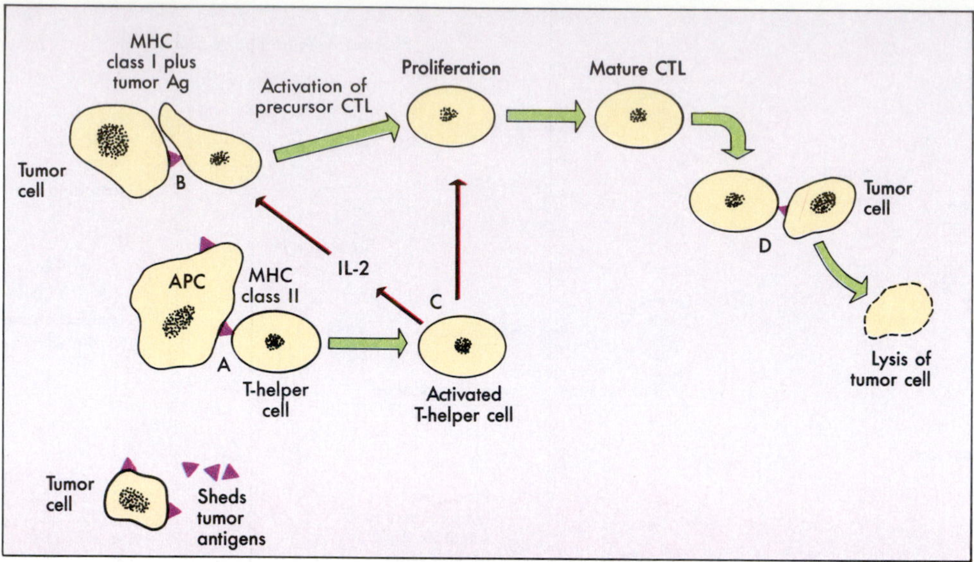

FIGURE 45-6 Cytolytic T lymphocyte *(CTL)* generation against tumor cells. Tumor antigens are processed and presented to T-helper cells in the context of MHC class II antigens *(A)*. Precursor CTL are activated with antigen presented in the context of MHC class I antigens *(B)*. T-helper cells secrete a variety of lymphokines that stimulate the maturation of CTL *(C)*. The tumors cells are then recognized and lysed by mature CTL *(D)*. (See Figure 45-4 for key.)

phocytes out of the vascular space. Prolactin is believed to enhance the immune response by binding to prolactin receptors on lymphocytes. CNS control of the immune response is suggested by decreased immune responses in patients bereaved by death of a spouse. Neuroanatomical studies demonstrate the presence of neurons in lymph nodes and spleen in close contact with lymphocytes. Receptors for neurotransmitters are present on lymphocytes.

Pharmacological Immunosuppression

Pharmacological approaches for immunosuppressive therapy stress selective eradication of certain cells, similar to selective killing of tumor cells during cancer chemotherapy (Chapter 43). Target immunocompetent cells must be selectively altered or deleted to prevent adverse effects on other tissues. Approaches to obtaining immunosuppression can be divided into four categories according to their relative selectivity. The least selective (category 1) approaches affect proliferating cells and include irradiation, DNA alkylating agents, and antimetabolites. Nontarget tissues with high proliferative rates such as bone marrow and gastrointestinal tract epithelium also are adversely affected. Depletion of immunocompetent cells (category 2) may be accomplished by physical removal of cells (e.g., splenectomy, thoracic duct drainage) or by use of antilymphocyte serum. A more selective method (category 3) affects only certain subpopulations of lymphocytes, as is obtained with cyclosporin or monoclonal antibodies specifically against cell surface antigens. A still more ideal method (category 4) is selective alteration of only those antigen-specific cell populations that mediate the response. In this manner, immune responses against pathogenic organisms and tumors are not altered. Suppression of the immune response by drugs is obtained currently by means of categories 1 and 3. Different immunosuppressive therapies involve the use of more than one drug to obtain optimal results. Currently, numerous treatment regimens are used, many of which have been developed empirically. The primary uses of immunosuppressive drugs are in the prevention of transplant rejection and the treatment of autoimmune diseases.

The principal drugs used to obtain immunosuppression include corticosteroids, cyclophosphamide, azathioprine, methotrexate, and cyclosporine. Experimental monoclonal antibody to lymphocyte subsets, as well as experimental FK-506, a cyclosporine-like drug, are also being tested.

Corticosteroids The actions of the corticosteroids are discussed in Chapter 35.

Glucocorticoids secreted by the adrenal cortex affect a wide range of normal physiological functions; the immune system is a major target. The effectiveness of glucocorticoids in treating autoimmune diseases and preventing graft rejection is mediated by its immunosuppressive and anti-inflammatory effects. The administration of glucocorticoids to patients results in decreased numbers of circulating lymphocytes, basophils, and eosinophils over a 24-hour period, whereas the number of neutrophils increases. In addition, changes in corticosteroid concentrations during the normal diurnal cycle and in stressful situations correlate with decreases in the number of circulating lymphocytes. The lymphopenia observed in humans is attributed to the migration of cells into extravascular spaces, with a greater T-cell migration than B-cell or monocyte migration. A majority of the cells migrate to bone marrow. Some studies suggest that changes in membrane proteins produce the altered migratory behavior. High dose glucocorticoid therapy is also known to reduce the size of lymphoid organs.

Although corticosteroid-induced lymphopenia is well documented, the importance of this effect on immunosuppression is not clear. It is apparent, however, that corticosteroids alter the immune response by directly changing immune cell function. The macrophage is the primary target responsible for the decreased immune response. Exposure of macrophages to corticosteroids results in decreased IL-1 production, decreased expression of MHC class II antigens, and decreased phagocytosis of virus-infected cells, tumor cells, bacteria, and fungi. T and B cells are also directly affected, with T cell mediated responses being affected to a greater extent.

Cyclophosphamide The structure, activation to phosphoramide mustard and acrolein, and antitumor mechanism of action of cyclophosphamide are discussed in Chapter 43.

The roles of the active phosphoramide mustard and acrolein in mediating the actions of cyclophosphamide on the immune response are unclear. The mustard is believed to alkylate DNA and mediate the antiproliferative and immunosuppressive effects. This is consistent with the hypothesis that the selective cytotoxic effects on B cells are attributable to a greater proliferative rate. However, the highly reactive, sulfhydryl-binding acrolein may also play an important but unclear role in the drug action.

Azathioprine The structure of azathioprine is shown in Figure 45-7. This drug undergoes metabolism to the antiproliferative drug 6-mercaptopurine (see Chapter 43), which is further metabolized to the active antitumor and immunosuppressive thioinosinic acid. This inhibits hypoxanthine-guanine phosphoribosyltransferase, which mediates conversion of purines to the corresponding phosphoribosyl-5′ phosphates and conversion of hypoxanthine to inosinic acid. This leads to inhibition of cellular proliferation. The mechanism of immunosuppression is mediated by azothraprine's antiproliferative actions. However, as with cyclophosphamide, immunosuppression by azathioprine may be mediated in part by other mechanisms. Thus inosine reverses the 6-mercaptopurine–induced suppression of an in vitro immune response but does not reverse the suppression of azathioprine.

Methotrexate Methotrexate is discussed in Chapter 43. The immunological and antitumor mechanisms are similar.

Cyclosporine Cyclosporine is a cyclic endecapeptide purified from two strains of fungi imperfecti, *Tolypocladium inflatum* Gams and *Cylindrocapon lucidum* Booth (see Figure 45-7).

Cyclosporin primarily affects T cell–mediated responses, whereas most humoral immune responses not requiring T cells are spared. The effectiveness of cyclosporin is based on selective inhibition of T-helper cell activation and slight enhancement of T-suppressor cell activity. The major effect on T-helper cells is by inhibition of interleukin-2 production. Messenger RNA concentrations for interleukin-2 and γ-interferon are decreased. The decreased interleukin-2 production in turn leads to decreased numbers of interleukin-2 receptors and functional unresponsiveness of CTL precursor cells. Because there is positive feedback through interleukin-2 production and interleukin-2 receptors, the decreased interleukin-2 production of T-helper cells also leads to decreased interleukin-2 receptors on T-helper cells. Cyclosporin does not, however, affect the proliferative response of activated cytolytic T lymphocytes (CTL) to interleukin-2 or the lytic activity of CTL. Consistent with this is the observation that cyclosporin is effective only during the very early stages of antigen activation of T-helper cells. There is also evidence for inhibition of macrophage antigen presentation and interleukin-1 production by macrophages.

The exact molecular mechanism of action has not been determined. Recent evidence indicates that cyclosporin inhibits T-cell activation by binding to a cytoplasmic receptor called *immunophilin*. This receptor is a propyl *cis-trans* isomerase, an enzyme involved in the folding of proteins. Cyclosporin binding is known to inhibit isomerase activity. How this binding can selectively alter T-helper function is not clear. It has been proposed that the cyclosporine-immunophilin drug complex binds and inhibits calcineurin, a Ca^{++}- and calmodulin-dependent phosphoprotein phosphatase. This results in the inhibition of the translocation of an IL-2 transcription factor from the cytosol to the nucleus. This transcription factor is required for expression of the IL-2 gene.

FK-506 FK-506 is an immunosuppressive macrolide undergoing human trials in renal, heart, and liver transplant patients with early success. The mechanism of action may be similar to cyclosporine. The structure is shown in Figure 45-7. It inhibits the synthesis of inter-azathioprine

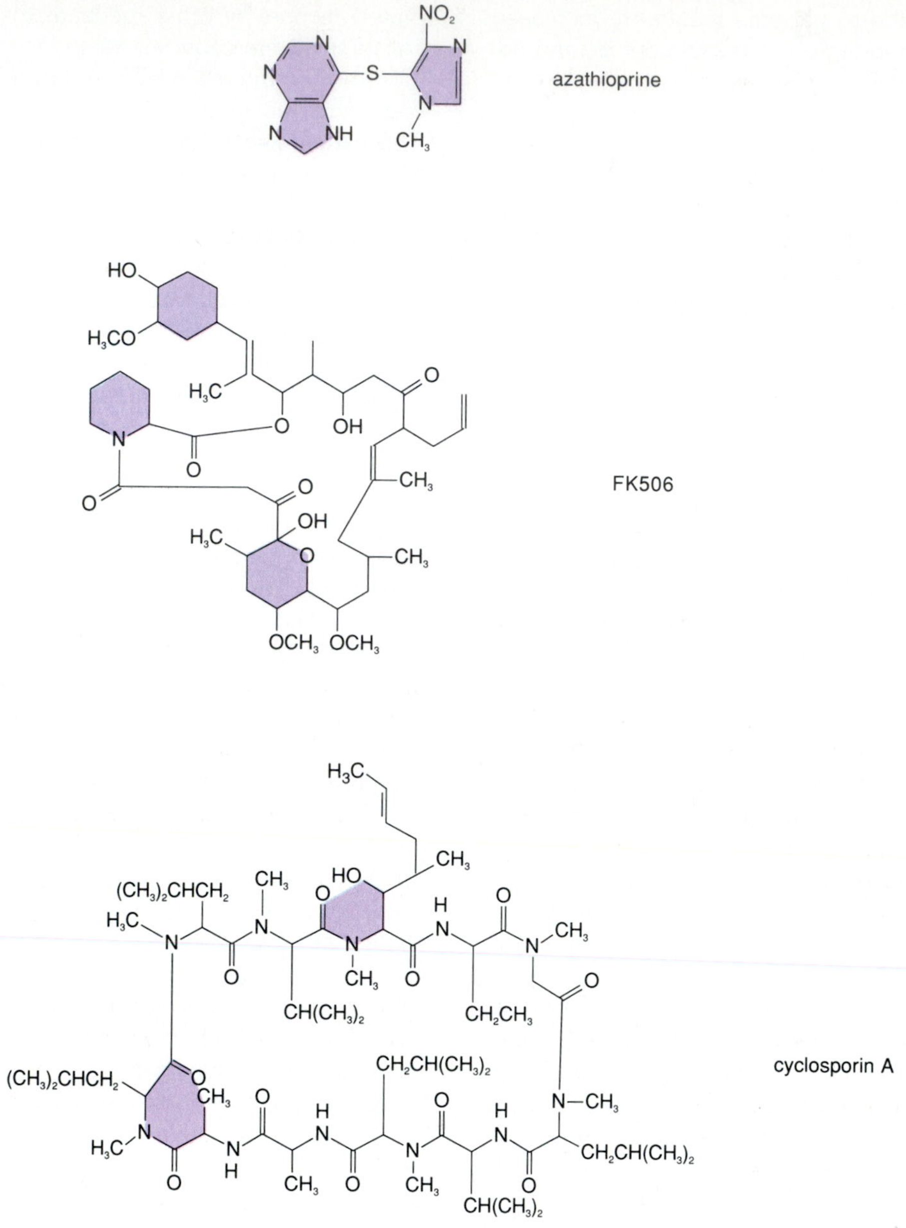

FK506

cyclosporin A

FIGURE 45-7 Structures of several immunosuppressants, including the 11–amino acid cyclosporin A. See the text for further information.

leukins 2, 3, and 4, granulocyte macrophage–colony stimulating factor (GM-CSF), tumor necrosis factor-α, and γ-interferon. FK-506 also binds to a protein with peptidylprolyl *cis-trans* isomerase activity that is distinct from immunophilin. This binding protein–FK-506 complex also binds and inhibits calcineurin. A summary of the major effects produced by these immunosuppressive effects is shown in Figure 45-8.

Monoclonal Antibodies Antibodies have been used recently as pharmacological agents to obtain greater therapeutic specificity. A purified monoclonal antibody represents a reagent that can be approximately 100% reactive against a single antigenic epitope. The generation of antibodies by injection of antigen into different animal species results in generation of numerous B-cell clones, each producing antibodies against different antigenic sites of a large molecule. However, the amount of antiserum obtained is limited, significant amounts of antigen must be purified, the quality of antibody varies between batches, and the antiserum may contain antibodies against certain unwanted determinants. The development of monoclonal antibodies al

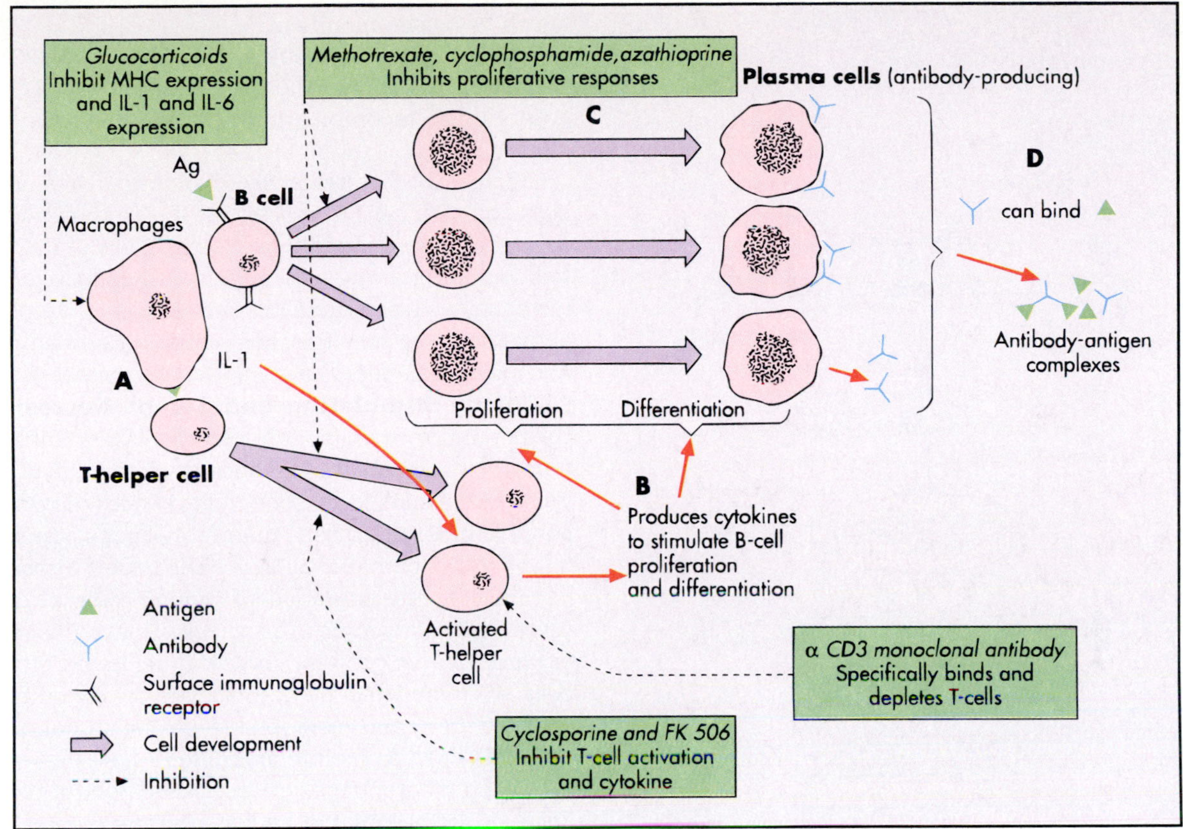

FIGURE 45-8 Primary mechanisms of immunosuppressive drugs. The antibody response shown in Figure 45-4 is used as an example to demonstrate the primary targets and mechanisms of action of immunosuppressive drugs.

lows circumvention of these problems. Fusion ofantibody-producing plasma cells with neoplastic myeloma cells yields a cell population called a *hybridoma*, capable of secreting a specific antibody and continually proliferating (Figure 45-9). Isolation, characterization, and cultivation of single clones of hybridomas can result in the generation of one type of antibody against a specific antigen in almost unlimited supply.

The use of antibodies with drugs can be divided into (a) targeting drug-antibody conjugates to cell surface tumor antigens and (b) using antibodies as drugs against specific cell surface components important for the immune response, such as antigen binding sites or lymphokine receptors. The latter is employed in immunosuppressive treatment for specific inhibition of lymphocyte function or depletion of certain cell populations. Polyclonal antilymphocyte and antithymocyte sera are successfully used in the prevention of graft rejection. Such sera are produced by the injection of human thymocytes or lymphocytes into sheep, horses, or goats. Monoclonal antibodies to lymphocyte antigens may replace the use of polyclonal sera. Monoclonal antibodies against the CD3-receptor complex on T cells and the interleukin-2 receptor are the most widely studied. The use of anti-CD3 antibodies in the treatment of acute rejection of renal transplants has now been approved.

The anti-CD3 preparation evolved out of attempts to find monoclonal antibodies to alter T cell responses clinically. In testing of antibodies of a clone that appeared to bind only T cells, it was found that the clone specifically bound to the CD3 or T3 structure on T cells. The CD3 unit is associated with the T cell antigen receptor complex involved in signal transduction to the T cell after binding of antigen to the receptor complex (Figure 45-5). Intravenous administration of anti-CD3 leads to a dramatic decrease in T3-positive cells. Although the mechanism of T cell depletion is unknown, T cells are believed to be opsonized with anti-CD3 and removed by the reticuloendothelial system.

Pharmacological Immunostimulation

The availability of drugs that stimulate the immune response against infections and tumors is desirable, but many drugs are limited as a result of low efficacy and life-threatening toxicity. Compounds that act as general

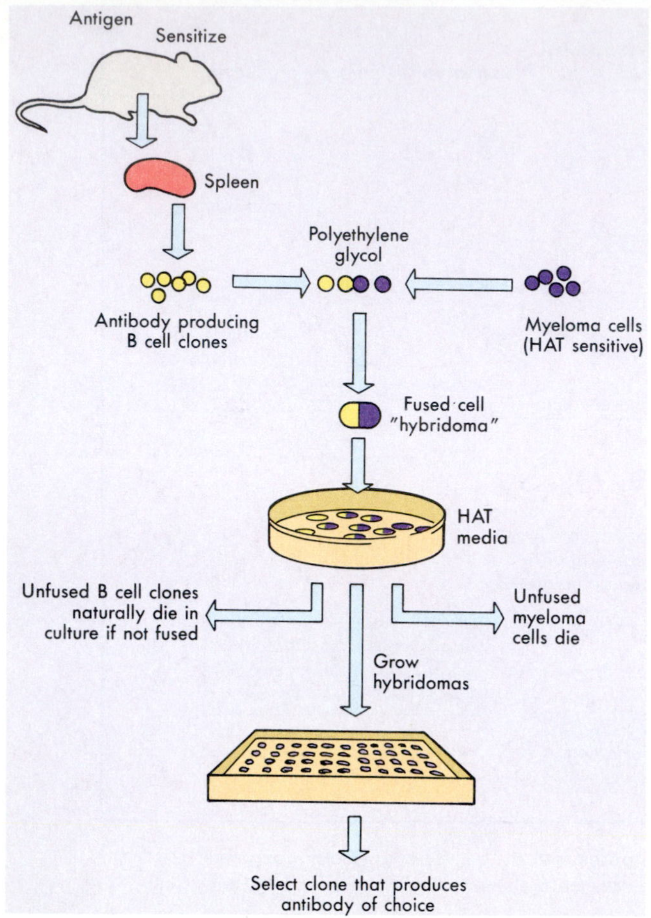

FIGURE 45-9 Preparation of monoclonal antibodies. Antibody-producing cells obtained from a mouse treated with antigen are fused with myeloma tumor cells in the presence of polyethylene glycol. The fused cells are called *hybridomas.* Each hybridoma secretes antibody against one specific antigenic site and continues to proliferate. To separate the unfused lymphocytes and myeloma cells from the hybridomas, the cells are incubated in cell culture medium containing hypoxanthine, aminopterin, and thymidine *(HAT).* Aminopterin inhibits the conversion of tetrahydrofolate to dihydrofolate (major pathway of purine synthesis). In the presence of aminopterin, normal cells survive by using xanthine and thymidine (salvage pathway). The myeloma cells lack the enzyme hypoxanthine phosphoribosyltransferase (HPRT), an enzyme required for the salvage pathway. Thus in the presence of HAT, the myeloma cells die in culture unless fused with normal B cells, which provide HPRT. These cells are grown, and the antibody secreted is tested.

stimulators of the immune response (e.g., BCG and dextran polymer) were extensively studied from the 1950s to the mid-1980s but produced only marginal effects and are seldom used today.

Cytokines such as interleukins, colony stimulating and tumor necrosis factors, and interferons are new leads that may generate more potent and safe compounds for possible use in stimulation of the immune response. These drugs are commonly referred to as "biological response modifiers."

Interleukins Interleukin 2 (IL-2) is a 15,420-dalton peptide of 133 amino acids that is produced by T-helper cells. Human recombinant interleukin-2 is commercially available.

As discussed previously, IL-2 stimulates T-helper cells and CTL cells to proliferate. IL-2 stimulation of cell proliferation is dependent on expression of IL-2 receptors with prior antigen stimulation. IL-2 incubation with lymphocytes also stimulates production of lymphokine-activated killer cells that lyse tumor cells in an antigen nonspecific manner but do not affect normal cells.

Colony-Stimulating and Tumor Necrosis Factors Four colony-stimulating factors (CSF) (Table 45-2), named for their ability to induce the formation of certain types of colonies from bone marrow cells grown in soft agar cultures, affect bone marrow cell populations at different stages of maturity. Multi-CSF (called *interleukin-3*) stimulates the primitive progenitor cells of granulocytes, megakaryocytes, mast cells, macrophages, and erythrocytes. In contrast, more differentiated progenitor cells are stimulated by granulocyte–colony stimulating factor (G-CSF) and macrophage–colony stimulating factor (M-CSF) to proliferate and differentiate into granulocytes and macrophages, respectively. Both of these cell lineages are stimulated by GM-CSF. As cells of certain lineages mature from progenitors to more committed states, they became refractory to certain CSFs and sensitive to other subtypes. The production of CFSs by various cell types and development of drugs that stimulate or inhibit their secretion by the immune system is under intense research. After exposure to a pathogen (e.g., bacteria, virus-infected cells) T cells activate and produce IL-3 and GM-CSF, whereas activated macrophages produce M-CSF, G-CSF, and GM-CSF. Activated macrophages also produce interleukin-1 and tumor necrosis factor (TNF), which stimulate the production of GM-CSF, G-CSF, and M-CSF by endothelial cells and mesenchymal cells. In this manner, the host produces more granulocytes and macrophages to combat the invading organism. CSFs also act on mature neutrophils to increase their ability to destroy the invading organism.

The discovery of TNF was based on the observation that bacterial infections in patients with tumors were correlated with the regression of the tumors. It was later found that bacterial cell wall components stimulated the secretion of TNF by macrophages. TNF is named for its ability to produce hemorrhagic necrosis of tumors by an unknown mechanism and acts on the inflammatory process and immune response.

TNF (called *TNF*-α) is a 157–amino acid protein functionally similar to another cytokine, lymphotoxin (called *TNF*-β). Recombinant TNF is produced by several companies.

Table 45-2 Classification of Colony Stimulating Factors

Colony Stimulating Factor Subtype	Cell Origin	Cell Types Produced with Stimulation
CSF-multi (interleukin-3)	T cell	Granulocytes, macrophages, megakaryocytes, mast cells, erythrocytes
GM-CSF	T cell, macrophage, endothelial cell, mesenchymal cell	Granulocytes, macrophages
G-CSF	Macrophage, endothelial cell, mesenchymal cell	Granulocytes
M-CSF	Macrophage, endothelial cell, mesenchymal cell	Macrophages

After injury or bacterial infection, a sequence of events that involves TNF occurs (Figure 45-10). In bacterial infections, granulocytes such as neutrophils migrate into the infected area and attack the microbes. These effects are potentiated by the actions of interleukin-1 and TNF on endothelial cells and neutrophils. Macrophages are also recruited, activated, and secrete interleukin-1 and TNF. Both cytokines stimulate T cells, which results in production of IL-2 and interferon. Further production of TNF by macrophages is stimulated by interferon.

Interferons The interferons (IFN) are named after their ability to interfere with viral RNA and protein synthesis. There are three types of interferons, α, β, and γ, which are synthesized by different cell types. With viral stimulation, the α form is primarily synthesized in macrophages, and the β form in macrophages and fibroblasts. The γ form is primarily produced in T lymphocytes after stimulation with antigen or mitogens.

Recombinant IFN is commercially available and is undergoing clinical trials. The structure of α-IFN and β-IFN are similar (30% homology), whereas there is no sequence homology between γ and the α-β types. α-IFN and β-IFN can bind to the same receptor. The human α, β, and γ forms each have molecular weights of 20 to 25 kilodaltons, and all three differ as to antigenicity.

Although all interferons show antiviral actions, α and β are more potent than γ. However, γ-IFN affects the immune system more than α-IFN or β-IFN. The major action of γ-IFN on the immune system is the induction of MHC expression on macrophages and B cells. This results in increased ability to present antigen. γ-IFN is a potent activator of macrophages that leads to increased cytocidal action as a result of increased secretion of hydrogen peroxide, phagocytosis, and expression of Fc receptors. These effects on macrophages are greater than those obtainable with α-IFNs or β-IFNs. γ-IFN also activates natural killer cells of the innate immune response to destroy viral infected and neoplastic cells.

The inhibition of viral replication by IFN may result from the induction of an enzyme that inhibits viral replication by catalyzing breakdown of viral RNA. The antitumor actions of IFN appear to be a result of reduced oncogene expression.

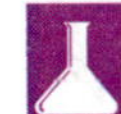

PHARMACOKINETICS

Immunosuppressive Drugs

Numerous synthetic derivatives of glucocorticoids are used as immunosuppressive agents. These preparations may be administered by oral, parenteral, and topical routes. The pharmacokinetic parameters of glucocorticoids are described in Chapter 35.

The pharmacokinetics of cyclophosphamide and methotrexate are discussed in Chapter 43.

Azathioprine is usually given intravenously as a loading dose on the day of transplantation with subsequent orally administered maintenance doses. It is rapidly absorbed from the gastrointestinal tract, even to a greater extent than 6-mercaptopurine, thus providing an advantage over 6-mercaptopurine. Azathioprine is metabolized in the liver to 6-mercaptopurine. However, other minor metabolites may account for the differences in the action of azathioprine and 6-mercaptopurine. Most of the metabolites are excreted in urine. The half-life of azathioprine is 5 to 6 hours.

Cyclosporine, a highly nonpolar compound, is administered orally in alcohol/olive oil or in a galenic formulation or intravenously in an alcohol/cremophor vehicle. When cyclosporine is given orally, absorption occurs slowly and is highly variable between individuals, with a mean oral bioavailability of only 30%. Because of variability, concentrations of cyclosporine must be monitored to maintain effectiveness and prevent toxicity, especially in patients with renal allografts. The nonpolar characteristics of cyclosporine result in a large volume of distribution. In the blood, 40% to 60% of cyclosporine is bound to lipoproteins. The disposition is biphasic with a half-life of 19 hours. Metabolism of cyclosporine

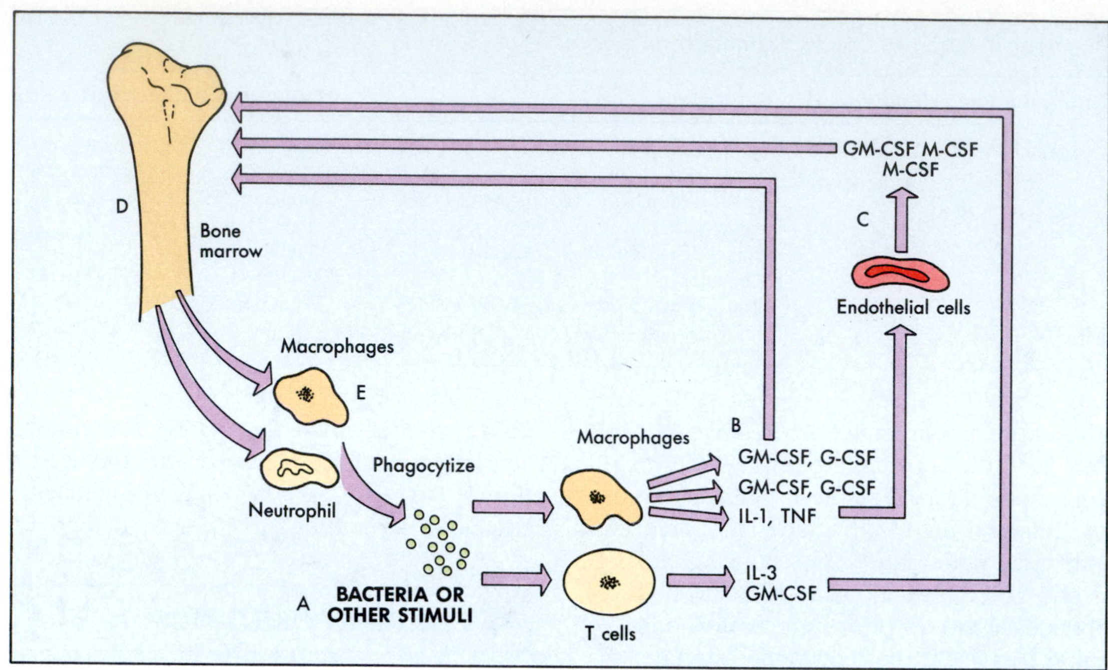

FIGURE 45-10 Secretion of colony-stimulating factors *(CSFs)* in response to immune stimulation. Bacteria or other stimuli *(A)* activate macrophages and T cells to produce a variety of CSFs *(B)*, which also stimulate endothelial cells to produce CSFs *(C)*. CSFs stimulate production of macrophages and neutrophils from bone marrow *(D)*. These cells are then able to phagocytose the bacteria *(E)*. *IL-1*, interleukin-1; *IL-3*, interleukin-3; *G-CSF*, granulocyte–colony stimulating factor; *M-CSF*, macrophage–colony stimulating factor; *GM-CSF*, granulocyte macrophage–colony stimulating factor.)

occurs in the liver, mediated by the cytochrome P-450 system. Some of the metabolites are immunosuppressive but are less potent than the parent compound. Metabolites are predominantly excreted through the biliary system, with only 10% excreted in the urine.

Monoclonal anti-CD3 antibody is administered intravenously. Blood concentrations decline to 10% of peak values after 24 hours, but the mechanism of clearance is not known.

Immunostimulant Drugs

The cytokines are proteins and are thus rapidly eliminated by serum proteases. This requires the use of various routes of administration to maintain blood concentrations adequately without reaching toxic concentrations.

IL-2 can be administered intravenously by bolus or continuous infusion; the latter results in less toxicity. Elimination of IL-2 from serum follows a first phase half-life of 6 to 7 minutes, in which most of the IL-2 is cleared, and a second phase half-life of 70 minutes.

After IV or IM injection, serum TNF concentrations decrease rapidly within 30 minutes and then continue to slowly decrease. TNF concentrates in the liver, kidneys, spleen, and gastrointestinal tract.

With interferons, the route of administration depends on the target tissue or disease, with topical, IV, IM, SC, and intranasal widely used. Because the interferons are proteins, the oral route is not effective. Most of the pharmacokinetic information on interferons is available for α-IFN. The vascular half-life is 6 to 8 hours after IM injection, but the fate of α-IFN is not known. Concentrations in the cerebrospinal fluid are about 0.08 times that in serum. Penetration into the lung and fluid compartments of the eye are poor, and little drug crosses the placenta. Virtually no interferon is recovered in urine, and blood concentrations are not altered in renal deficiency. Neutralizing anti–α-IFN antibodies are produced in some patients and may present a problem. Development of methods to monitor the generation of this antibody are under study.

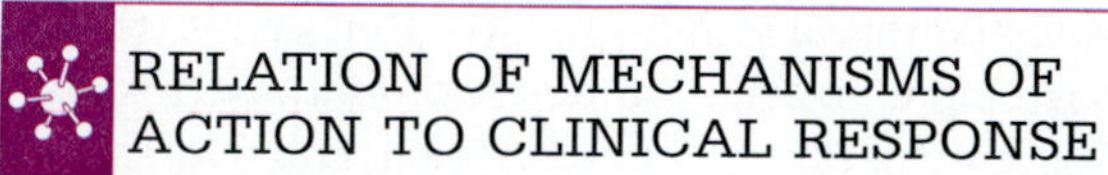

RELATION OF MECHANISMS OF ACTION TO CLINICAL RESPONSE

Immunosuppression

Graft Rejections Genetically coded antigens are the determining factor in the rejection of a graft by a host.

Most human studies of transplant rejection involve renal allografts. The types of rejection processes can be classified according to how quickly the rejection occurs. Hyperacute rejection can occur within minutes and is mediated by cytotoxic antibodies already circulating in the host as a result of prior exposure to graft antigens. Cytotoxic antibodies to type ABO blood group antigens may mediate rejection in a mismatch. Accelerated rejection occurs in 2 to 5 days, with the mechanism being an accelerated form of the acute process, again mediated by prior exposure to graft antigens (secondary immune response). Acute rejection occurs over 7 to 21 days and is mediated by a primary response requiring a longer time for generation of effector cells. Chronic rejection is observed after about 3 months. The immune process of graft rejection is divided into afferent and efferent stages.

Afferent Stage Initiation of the response is mediated by graft cells possessing MHC class II antigens that are incompatible with the host (bone marrow–derived dendritic cells, Langerhans cells, certain endothelial cells of human tissue). These cells, termed *passenger cells,* drain into the lymphatics and directly stimulate T cells in lymph nodes. Contact between circulating T cells and special antigens may also occur in the graft. It is known that tissues containing a greater burden of passenger cells are more likely to be rejected (e.g., skin and bone marrow). In addition, removal of passenger cells before transplantation dramatically increases the chances of acceptance.

Efferent Stage Activation of macrophages and T cells during different stages leads to various effector mechanisms by which the host may destroy the graft: antibody, CTL, and delayed-type hypersensitivity. The involvement of CTL and antibody in transplant rejection are more clearly documented than the role of delayed-type hypersensitivity. Common to all three responses is the role of T-helper cells. Special antigens on the graft can activate T-helper cells and production of lymphokines, which stimulate the activation, proliferation, and growth of T lymphocytes, B lymphocytes, and macrophages. In delayed-type hypersensitivity response, T-helper cell–produced lymphokines activate and recruit monocytes to the graft. These activated macrophages nonspecifically destroy surrounding tissue.

Autoimmune Diseases The basic mechanism by which the immune system selectively destroys infectious microbes and tumor cells is through its ability to discriminate between self- and non–self-antigens. A dysfunction in this ability may lead to an immune response against one's own tissue, an autoimmune disease. Although the manifestations of autoimmune diseases are well described, only within the last few years several diseases have been classified as autoimmune responses (e.g., type 1 diabetes). The discovery of an autoimmune origin has led to investigation of immunosuppressive therapy for treatment. Several contributing factors may trigger or predispose individuals to an autoimmune disease. Each type of autoimmune disease may have a different cause. There is a genetic predisposition associated with the expression of certain MHC (histocompatability leukocyte) antigens. A greater occurrence in the elderly has also been found. Mechanisms proposed include the following:

1. Possible induction of cells that possess self-antigens to express MHC class II antigens and activate autoreactive T cells
2. Dysfunction of the suppressor T-cell system removing down-regulatory actions on autoreactive T and B cells
3. Immune response against foreign agents with similar structure to self-antigens
4. Exposure of sequestered cellular antigens not normally exposed to the immune system
5. General stimulation of the immune response by viruses and bacteria, which leads to lymphokine production and nonspecific stimulation of autoreactive B-cell clones

Autoimmune diseases are categorized as organ-specific and organ-nonspecific. In organ-specific diseases, immune responses are mounted against antigens specific for a certain organ, with manifestations of the diseases being dysfunction of the specific organ. In contrast, with organ-nonspecific diseases, immune responses are against tissue components in most cell types (DNA, cytoskeletal proteins). Examples include organ-specific (Hashimoto's thyroiditis, myasthenia gravis, Graves' disease, type 1 diabetes) and organ-nonspecific (systemic lupus erythematosus). In these five examples, the antibodies that are produced are anti–thyroid hormone, anti–acetylcholine receptor, anti–thyroid stimulating hormone, anti–insulin, or antibodies to intracellular components, respectively.

Immunosuppressive Drugs

Glucocorticoids Numerous synthetic derivatives of glucocorticoids are in use as immunosuppressive agents. Only the minimal effective dose should be given if corticosteroids are to be administered over a long period (months to years) to minimize toxicity. Glucocorticoids are usually administered with other immunosuppressive agents to treat graft rejection and autoimmune diseases. Doses of glucocorticoids may be decreased when used with other immunosuppressive drugs to decrease toxicity. Because of their antiinflammatory actions, glucocorticoids are effective in treatment of immunological problems that are exacerbated by inflammatory reactions. This is especially evident with their topical use for dermatological problems such as contact hypersensitivity to poison ivy and atopic dermatitis.

Cyclophosphamide Cyclophosphamide is used to treat autoimmune diseases and to prevent rejection of grafts. However, its use has dramatically decreased since the discovery of cyclosporin. As with other immunosuppressive drugs, cyclophosphamide is given often in combination with corticosteroids. Because of the life-threatening toxicities that may occur with cyclophosphamide, extreme care should be taken to administer the minimal dose necessary.

Humoral immune responses are more sensitive to the effects of cyclophosphamide than cell-mediated responses. However, both arms of the immune response are affected at high doses. Low doses of cyclophosphamide enhance various immune responses. These findings are attributed to the selective inhibition of suppressor T-cell generation or a selective effect on suppressor T cells.

Azathioprine In contrast to cyclophosphamide, the primary targets of azathioprine are cellular-mediated immune responses. Inhibition of in vitro immune responses is maximum during initiation of the response. This time-dependent action is consistent with the clinical findings that azathioprine is ineffective against ongoing rejection of grafts. Additional in vitro investigations indicate that azathioprine primarily effects antigen-stimulated lymphocytes, whereas unstimulated spleen cells are unaffected. Primary immune responses are suppressed with azathioprine treatment, whereas secondary responses are unaffected. Azathioprine is used in combination with glucocorticoid therapy when cyclosporine therapy of graft rejection is discontinued because of signs of nephrotoxicity.

Methotrexate Although methotrexate is a potent immunosuppressive agent, its numerous adverse effects and the development of cyclosporine has limited its use in the treatment of immune-associated diseases. However, low-dose methotrexate is now used to treat rheumatoid arthritis refractory to conventional drugs. Because rheumatoid arthritis is an autoimmune disease, the immunosuppressive actions of methotrexate could account for its effectiveness. However, the low doses used may not affect the immune system and the anti-inflammatory effects may be the major contributing factors that inhibit neutrophil and macrophage function. The sudden onset of action and flare-ups after discontinuation are also suggestive of nonimmunosuppressive effects.

Cyclosporine The objective of immunosuppressive therapy is to specifically inhibit the immune response against the graft or autoantigen. However, drugs that also affect proliferating cell populations such as cyclophosphamide, azathioprine, and methotrexate produce life-threatening bone marrow suppression. Until the early 1980s, the use of these drugs in combination with corticosteroids was the preferred immunosuppressive therapy. Their use has largely been supplanted by cyclosporine, which usually is effective in preventing the onset of acute graft rejection (during the first 3 weeks). The absence of bone marrow toxicity makes it very beneficial in bone marrow transplants. Cyclosporine therapy may be replaced with azathioprine and prednisolone, or steroid therapy alone at a later date.

FK-506 FK-506 is effective in prolonging liver and other organ transplants and appears to act similarly to cyclosporin. FK-506 is used in combination with glucocorticoids. The optimal protocol for the use of FK-506 is being investigated.

Monoclonal Antibodies A commercial anti-CD3 monoclonal preparation is used to reverse acute graft rejection of patients being administered other immunosuppressive drugs and to prevent acute graft rejections. Patients are then continued on other immunosuppressive drugs. Because the anti-CD3 antibody is a murine monoclonal antibody (different constant and variable regions), patients usually develop neutralizing antibodies after 10 days of treatment. The development of antibody against the anti-CD3 antibody, however, does not result in allergic or anaphylactic reactions. When the anti-CD3 antibody is given with prednisolone and azathioprine, development of neutralizing antibodies is attenuated.

Immunostimulant Drugs

Interleukins IL-2 is administered to patients with metastatic carcinomas with marginal results, and large doses of IL-2 produce severe fluid retention. Consequently, adoptive transfer of IL-2–induced LAK-cells was conducted. In this time-consuming and costly procedure, patients are first administered low doses of IL-2. Then peripheral lymphocytes are isolated and cultured with IL-2 to stimulate LAK cell production. Finally, LAK cells are infused with IL-2. This approach is successful in the treatment of metastatic renal cell carcinoma, melanoma, colorectal cancer, and non-Hodgkins lymphoma and has been approved for use in treatment of renal cell carcinomas and melanomas. Although small amounts of IL-2 are used in this approach, severe fluid retention is still a problem. A recent modification involves removing tumor cells, isolating tumor-infiltrating lymphocytes, incubating them with IL-2 to activate and stimulate proliferation, injecting the patient with the added lymphocytes, and low concentrations of IL-2. The tumor-specific infiltrating lymphocytes are more effective than the LAK cells in killing tumor cells, but more importantly, much lower quantities of IL-2 are needed.

Colony-Stimulating and Tumor Necrosis Factors CSFs appear to have a major potential for use as pharmacological agents without major toxicities. Patients with depressed bone marrow function undergoing cancer chemotherapy or immunosuppressive therapy, receiving bone marrow transplants, or with aplastic anemia would benefit greatly. The induction of differentiation by CSFs may be possible in the treatment of certain tumors.

The results of GM-CSF from clinical trials are favorable. Patients with certain bone marrow dysfunctions from disease or cancer chemotherapy were administered GM-CSF intravenously over 2 weeks, with dramatic increases in neutrophils, eosinophils, and monocytes and minimal side effects.

Results of initial clinical trials to determine tolerated dose and adverse effects of TNF for use in tumor treatment indicate good tolerance. The antitumor effects of TNF have been demonstrated in animal models and are now being examined in clinical trials.

In the near future, multiple lymphokines may be administered to obtain greater therapeutic effects. Studies in experimental animals demonstrate that combined treatment with IL-2 and TNF results in synergistic enhancement of antitumor effects.

Interferons α-IFN is effective in the treatment of hematological cancers, especially hairy cell leukemia, chronic myelogenous leukemia, and T-cell lymphomas related to mycosis fungoides. Because γ-IFN stimulates various cell types involved in immune destruction of tumors, there is interest in the use of γ-IFN. Initial clinical studies show that administration of γ-IFN to humans results in immunoenhancement. Whether this will lead to antitumor actions is not determined from present clinical trials.

In the treatment of viral infections, α-IFN is effective against chronic hepatitis B. Intranasal administration of α-IFN is useful in the treatment of rhinoviral infections, an especially valuable procedure in immunocompromised patients.

The activity of the IFNs is quantified by their ability to inhibit viral growth in cultured cells. Because of this, care must be used when comparing preparations for immune response or antiproliferative effects.

Additional agents that induce synthesis of IFN in the body are under study. These inducers may be grouped into viral and polyanionic polymers.

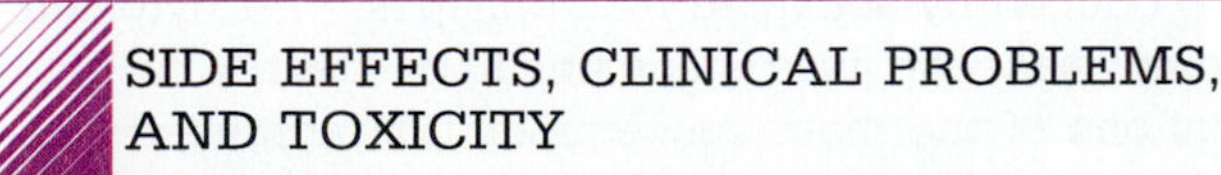

SIDE EFFECTS, CLINICAL PROBLEMS, AND TOXICITY

Clinical problems are summarized in the box.

CLINICAL PROBLEMS

- Corticosteroids
  - electrolyte imbalance
  - Cushing's syndrome
  - osteoporosis
  - peptic ulcer
  - poor wound healing
- Cyclophosphamide
  - myelosuppression
  - hemorrhagic cystitis
- Methotrexate
  - bone marrow suppression
  - gastrointestinal upsets
- Azathioprine
  - bone marrow suppression
- Cyclosporine
  - nephrotoxicity (reduced glomerolar filtration)
  - hepatotoxicity (cholestasis)
  - neurotoxicity
  - hypersensitivity to vehicle
- Interleukin (IL-2)
  - fluid retention
  - fever, chills
- Interferons (IFN)
  - fever, myalgia, fatigue
- CSF and TNF
  - fever, chills, fatigue
  - possible endotoxin shock with TNF

Immunosuppressive Drugs

One of the primary problems with prolonged immunosuppressive therapy is enhanced susceptibility to infections and cancer. Prophylactic therapy with antibacterial and antifungal drugs is commonly needed.

The side effects of the corticosteroids are discussed in Chapter 35 and those for cyclophosphamide and methotrexate in Chapter 43.

The major limiting toxicity of azathioprine is suppression of bone marrow. Leukopenia or thrombocytopenia occurs after a delay and is reversible after the drug is discontinued. The severe or prolonged suppression of bone marrow may predispose the patient to opportunistic infections. Liver toxicity is a common side effect. Since allopurinol inhibits azathioprine metabolism, its concurrent use is contraindicated.

One of the major advantages of cyclosporine is its relatively selective effect on T-helper cells and the absence of myelotoxicity in comparison to cyclophosphamide, azathioprine, and methotrexate. However, its use is limited by other toxicities. Similar toxicities are produced with FK-506. Nephrotoxicity with reduced glomerular filtration is a common and dose-limiting side ef-

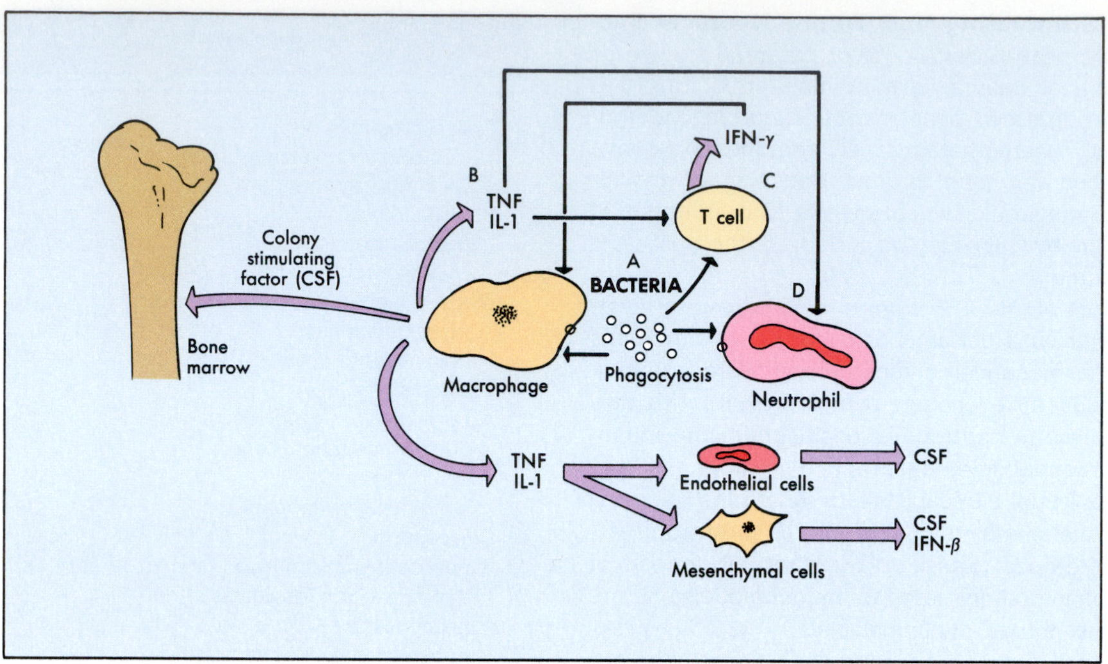

FIGURE 45-11 Role of tumor necrosis factor *(TNF)* in bacterial infections. Macrophage activation by bacteria *(A)* results in the production of TNF along with CSFs and IL-1 *(B)*. TNF and IL-1 stimulate T cells to produce IFN-γ *(C)*, which further activates macrophages. TNF and IL-1 also stimulate neutrophils and enhance phagocytosis of bacteria *(D)*. Macrophage-derived CSF also stimulates bone marrow, whereas macrophage-derived TNF and IL-1 stimulate endothelial and mesenchymal cells to produce CSF and IFN-β. *IL-1,* interleukin-1; *CSF,* colony-stimulating factor; *IFN-γ*, interferon γ; *IFN-β*, interferon β.

fect, with the mechanism unknown. The incidence of hepatotoxicity with cholestasis and hyperbilirubinemia nearly doubles in patients on cyclosporine. Neurotoxicity, including tremors, is observed in about 20% of patients, and elevated concentrations of several plasma enzymes may be seen. Moderate hypertension may also occur in 50% of patients. Hypersensitivity to the drug vehicle also occurs.

The administration of anti-CD3 intravenously may produce flu-like symptoms with fluid retention and possible pulmonary edema. The flu-like symptoms can be effectively treated by administration of acetaminophen.

Immunostimulant Drugs

Intravenous administration of IL-2 and other lymphokines results in fever and chills. Lethargy and malaise also are observed. The major limiting toxicity of IL-2 is the dramatic increase in fluid retention caused by vascular leakage. This can lead to life-threatening pulmonary edema and ascites. The mechanism of this toxicity may be related to IL-2 activation of endothelial cells, as observed in other cell-mediated immune responses.

The common adverse effect of CSFs is bone pain, which is correlated with white blood cell counts and occurs independently of dose. Some common effects observed with intravenous administration of proteins (e.g., monoclonal antibodies and IL-2) are also observed: fever, chills, myalgia, fatigue, headaches, reduced appetite, and nausea.

With TNF, the induction of endotoxic shock and wasting (cachexia) observed in patients with infections or tumors was mediated in part by IL-1 and another factor produced by activated macrophages. This cytokine, termed *cachectin,* was later found to be identical to TNF. Thus one of the main concerns of TNF administration is the possible induction of endotoxic shock. Clinical studies reveal a similar non–life threatening syndrome

TRADE NAMES

In addition to generic and fixed-combination preparations, the following trade-named materials are available in the United States.

Sandimmune, cyclosporine, azathioprine, anti-CD3 receptor
Imuran, azathioprine
Muromonab, CD3, anti-CD3

of effects observed with intravenous administration of IFN and CSF, namely, fever, chills, and malaise.

The adverse effects of IFN are dependent on source and preparation. In several human studies with partially purified recombinant α-IFN, the major side effects were fever, myalgia, headache, fatigue, and numbness of extremities. α-IFN also reportedly produces bone marrow depression.

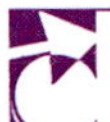

NEW DIRECTIONS

The primary research direction of many pharmaceutical companies is in the development of drugs that are more selective for specific components of the immune system. Recombinant cytokines and monoclonal antibodies to lymphocyte surface structures and cytokines are a major part of this research effort. Research to solve problems associated with delivery, metabolism, and toxicity by these proteins will greatly enhance the potential usefulness of this therapeutic approach. Another avenue being pursued is the development of traditional small-molecule drugs that may act as agonists and antagonists of cytokine receptors. In addition, the discovery of the mechanism of action of cyclosporin has fueled the search for other compounds that may act by similar mechanisms while having a minimized associated toxicity. A more selective approach to immunomodulation in the future will involve altering antigen-specific interactions. In this manner, immune responses to other antigens (e.g., bacteria) will not be compromised. For example, oral administration of autoantigens or foreign-graft antigens has been shown to produce a state of immunological tolerance to those antigens and a decrease in autoimmune and graft-rejection responses. In the treatment of cancer, tumor-antigen vaccines are being developed as a potential method to stimulate an immune response against tumor cells. These approaches will be more difficult to develop but may yield more efficacious therapy. Basic research and early clinical trials have shown some promise.

REFERENCES

Barry, JM: Immunosuppressive drugs in renal transplantation. A review of the regimens, *Drugs* 44:554, 1992.

Blick M, Sherwin SA, Rosenblum M, et al: Phase I study of recombinant tumor necrosis factor in cancer patients, *Cancer Res* 47:2986, 1987.

Bonnem EM, Oldham RK: Gamma-interferon: physiology and speculation on its role in medicine, *J Biol Respir Modif* 6:275, 1987.

Clipstone NA, Crabtree, GR: Identification of calcineurin as a key signalling enzyme in T-lymphocyte activation, *Nature* 357:695, 1992.

Handschumacher RE, Harding MW, Rice J, et al.: Cyclophilin: a specific cytosolic binding protein for cyclosporin A, *Science* 226:544, 1984.

Kaplan BD: cyclosporine, *N Engl J Med* 321:1725, 1989.

Paul WP: *Fundamental immunology,* ed 2, New York, 1989, Raven Press.

Roit IM, Brostoff J, Male DK: *Immunology,* St Louis, 1985, Mosby.

Rosenberg SA, Lotze MT, Muul LM, et al: A progress report on the treatment of 157 patients with advanced cancer using lymphokine-activated killer cells and interleukin-2 or high-dose interleukin-2, *N Engl J Med* 316:889, 1987.

Tocci MJ, Matkovich DA, Collier KA, et al.: The immunosuppressant FK 506 selectively inhibits expression of early T cell activation genes, *J Immunol* 143:718, 1989.

Turk JL, Parker D: The effect of cyclophosphamide on the immune response, *J Immunopharmacol* 1:127, 1979.

Table VII-1 Invading Pathological Organisms That Can Live in a Parasitic Invader Host Relationship in Humans Listed in Order of Increasing Complexity

Cellular type	Organism	Typical Size (nm)
Acellular	Viruses	20-200
Unicellular	*Chlamydia* (P)	1000
Unicellular	Mycoplasmas (P)	1000
Unicellular	*Rickettsia* (P)	1000
Unicellular	Bacteria (P)	1000
Unicellular	Fungi: yeasts (E)	3000-5000
Unicellular	Protozoa (E)	
Multicellular	Fungi: molds (E)	2000-10,000 and larger
Multicellular	Helminths (E)	

P, Prokaryotes (no nuclear membrane); *E,* eukaryotes (with a nucleus).

variety of infectious unicellular microorganisms may seem overwhelming to the embryonic clinician. However, by noting common aspects in the mechanism of action or chemical structure of different drugs and by noting further that some drugs are more efficacious in certain anatomical regions than in other regions, it is possible to organize this topic into an easier to understand and easier to master outline. Notice that the specific microbial strains of clinical relevance change with time. New strains of microorganisms appear, existing strains develop resistance to previously highly efficacious antimicrobial drugs, old strains disappear, and new problems develop with old, relatively benign strains. This further complicates the use of drugs in treatment and demands that the clinician stay informed.

The organizational scheme for drugs used to treat bacterial and related infections and some principles specific to the use of antimicrobial drugs are discussed in Chapter 46. A large group of agents act by inhibiting the synthesis of bacterial cell walls (Chapter 47). Another large group of agents act at the ribosomal level to inhibit bacterial protein synthesis (Chapter 48). Drugs that act on the bacterial tetrahydrofolate cofactor system are described in Chapter 49, and bacterial DNA replication inhibitors, along with drugs that create openings in bacterial membranes, are discussed in Chapter 50. Guidelines for the use of antibacterial drugs are summarized in Chapter 51. Chapter 52 is reserved for the special drugs used to treat mycobacterial infections, which are the cause of tuberculosis and leprosy.

The bacteria are characterized as unicellular, nonnuclear organisms. Higher orders of size and complexity are found in unicellular, nucleated fungi (which include yeast and filamentous forms) and in protozoa. The major differences are the addition of a membrane-enclosed nucleus and mitochondria within the cell. More complex fungi are found in the multicellular, nucleated molds. Still higher orders of parasitic invading organisms are the helminths (worms), estimated to infect 40% to 60% of the world population and are a medical problem in industrialized as well as developing countries. Drugs used in the treatment of infections resulting from these more complex invading organisms are discussed in separate chapters for fungi (Chapter 53), viruses (Chapter 54), protozoa (Chapter 55), and helminths (Chapter 56). Although antiseptics and disinfectants are not used as drugs, these compounds are important for cleansing the skin and preparing instruments and materials used during surgery and are described in Chapter 57.

The term *chemotherapy* was coined in the 1950s to indicate the use of complex chemicals for the treatment of microbial infections (i.e., administering chemicals that inhibited or killed the invading microorganisms). Since then the term has been used in a broader context to include the use of drugs to kill any type of cell, microbial or mammalian. Therefore the term no longer is applied only to the treatment of infections caused by invading organisms but also in the treatment of neoplastic diseases, as mentioned in Chapters 44 and 45.

CHAPTER 46

Principles of Antimicrobial Use

HAROLD C. NEU

The era of modern microbial chemotherapy stems from the work in the early 1900s of Paul Ehrlich, who suggested that antimicrobial drugs might be found that would be chemically allied to molecular sites of action on parasitic organisms. He suggested further that this approach would be most useful if these parasitic sites of action were not present in the organs and tissues of the human host. Ehrlich defined the selective drug action of chemotherapeutic agents, beginning with the use of arsenic compounds, which subsequently led to the development of the sulfonamides. These compounds illustrated that the activity of some agents could be predicted from their physical-chemical structures.

The next breakthrough was the 1929 discovery in Great Britain of penicillin by Fleming, who demonstrated the ubiquitous nature of these agents and that antimicrobial substances could be found in molds and other microorganisms that exist in the soil. Although thousands of potential antimicrobial agents have been found in nature or synthesized chemically in the past 60 years, only a very small percentage of these have proved to be effective, nontoxic agents when used therapeutically.

The term **antibiotic** traditionally refers to substances produced by microorganisms to suppress the growth of other microorganisms. The term **antimicrobial agents** is broader in meaning, since it encompasses agents synthesized in the laboratory as well as those natural antibiotics produced by microorganisms. Many agents used clinically today are produced industrially by chemical synthesis, even if originally produced by microbial fermentation. Many agents are semisynthetic, that is, the key portion of the compound is produced industrially by microbial fermentation, and various moieties are synthetically attached. Thus the distinction between the terms "antibiotics" and "antimicrobials," or "antimicrobial agents," has little meaning today.

ABBREVIATIONS	
CSF	cerebrospinal fluid
MBC	minimum bactericidal concentration
MIC	minimum inhibitory concentration

Antimicrobial agents can be **bactericidal** (i.e., the organisms are killed) or **bacteriostatic** (i.e., the organisms are prevented from growing) (Figure 46-1). Both bacteriostatic and bactericidal agents are effective as chemotherapeutic drugs, but both also rely upon host defenses to aid in eliminating the pathogens. In some clinical conditions, the lack of host defenses, such as complement or antibody, makes it mandatory that bactericidal agents be used. A given agent may show bactericidal actions under certain conditions but bacteriostatic actions under other conditions, depending on the concentration of drug and the target bacteria.

Antimicrobial agents can be classified into five major groups according to the point in the cellular biochemical pathways at which the agent exerts its primary mechanism of action (Figure 46-2). These are (1) inhibition of synthesis and damage to the peptidoglycan cell wall, (2) inhibition of synthesis or damage to the cytoplasmic membrane, (3) modification in synthesis or metabolism of nucleic acids, (4) inhibition or modification of protein synthesis, and (5) modification in energy metabolism. The agents that inhibit synthesis of cell walls include the β-lactams, such as penicillins, cephalosporins, and monobactams, and others such as bacitracin and vancomycin. Inhibitors of cytoplasmic membranes include the polymyxins. In fungi the cell wall is damaged by the polyene antifungal agents or by the imidazoles. Inhibitors of nucleic acid synthesis include the quinolones, which inhibit DNA gyrase, and the RNA polymerase inhibitor rifampin. Protein synthesis is inhibited by aminoglycosides, which are bactericidal, and by tetracyclines, chloramphenicol, erythromycin, and clindamycin, which are usually bacteriostatic, depending on the microorganism involved. Finally, folate antagonists such as sulfonamides and trimethoprim interfere with cell metabolism. The five major types of antimicrobial drugs according to their mechanisms of action are listed in Table 46-1.

SELECTION OF DRUG FOR INDIVIDUAL PATIENTS

Major factors that need to be considered in the selection of antimicrobial agents for therapy of individual patients are outlined in the box on page 619. If the desired procedure of identifying the organism and demonstrating susceptibility to a specific antimicrobial agent is followed, the expectation for successful therapy is high. Unfortunately, the practical use of antimicrobial agents is more complex because the initial antimicrobial therapy is often begun empirically without precise identification of the pathogen.

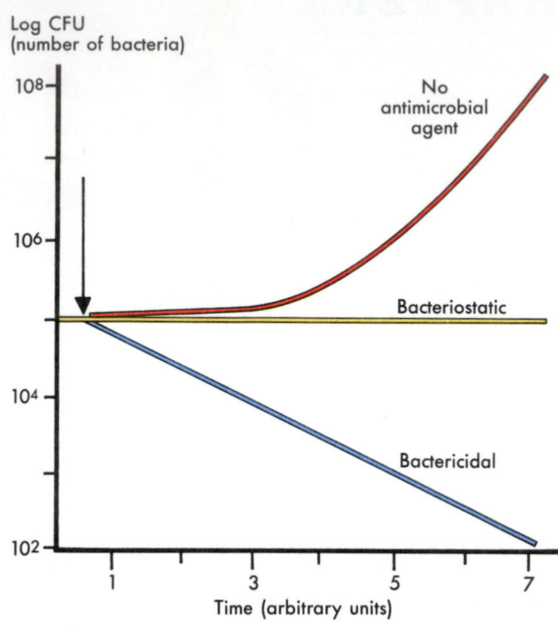

FIGURE 46-1 Bactericidal versus bacteriostatic antimicrobial agents. A typical culture is started at 10^5 colony-forming units (CFU) and incubated at 37°C for various times (time in arbitrary units). With no antimicrobial agent, there is cell growth. With a bacteriostatic agent added, no growth occurs, but neither are the existing cells killed. If the added agent is bactericidal, 99.9% of the cells will be killed during the standardized test time.

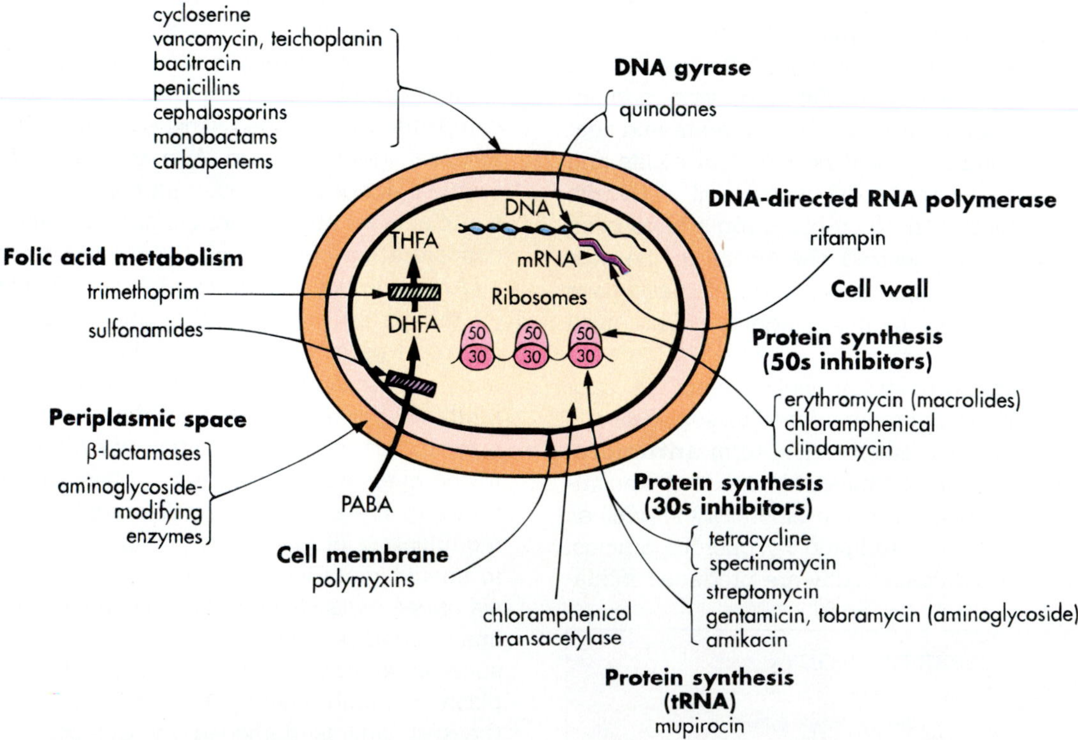

FIGURE 46-2 Antimicrobial sites of bactericidal or bacteriostatic action on microorganisms. The five general mechanisms are (1) inhibit synthesis of cell wall, (2) damage outer membrane, (3) modify nucleic acid/DNA synthesis, (4) modify protein synthesis (at ribosomes), and (5) modify energy metabolism within the cytoplasm (at folate cycle).

Table 46-1 Classification of Antimicrobial Agents by Mechanism of Action

Mechanism of Action	Agent Discussion in Chapter	
Inhibition of synthesis or damage to cell wall	penicillins	47
	cephalosporins	47
	monobactams	47
	carbapenems	47
	bacitracin	47
	vancomycin	47
	cycloserine	52
Inhibition of synthesis or damage to cytoplasmic membrane	polymyxins	50
	polyene antifungals	53
Modification of synthesis or metabolism of nucleic acids	quinolones	50
	rifampin	52
	nitrofurantoins	50
	nitroimidazoles	56
Inhibition or modification of protein synthesis	aminoglycosides	48
	tetracyclines	48
	chloramphenicol	48
	erythromycin	48
	clindamycin	48
	spectinomycin	48
	mupirocin	48
Modification to energy metabolism	sulfonamides	49
	trimethoprim	49
	dapsone	52
	isoniazid	52

Each of the factors in the box is discussed in the following pages. The goal is to provide an overall perspective of the relative importance of each of the factors before the description and discussion of individual antimicrobial agents in subsequent chapters. When reference is made to individual antimicrobial agents in the present chapter, the points are reiterated in the chapters on the individual agents. Because of the importance of microbial resistance to drugs, this topic is discussed in a separate section in the latter part of this chapter and in the chapters on the individual antibacterial drugs. Clinical guidelines for the selection of antibiotics are given in Chapter 51.

Identification of Organisms

Before initiating antimicrobial therapy, it is highly desirable to determine the possible pathogen or pathogens in the infection site. Several direct techniques are available to identify the microorganisms.

The use of Gram's stain is the fastest, simplest, and most inexpensive method to identify bacteria and fungi. Any body fluid that normally is sterile should be Gram stained. However, wound exudates, sputum, and fecal material can provide only preliminary information concerning the infecting microorganisms.

In addition to Gram's staining, agglutination, immunoelectrophoresis, and direct immunofluorescence techniques can be used for detection of some organisms. When it is not possible to obtain a specimen, knowledge of the most commonly infecting organisms can be used to direct therapy. For example, cellulitis can be caused by group A streptococci or by *Staphylococcus aureus*. Knowledge that these two species could be present, combined with knowledge of the resistance of staphylococci to certain antimicrobial drugs, should influence the choice of antimicrobial agent. Otitis media is primarily caused by *Streptococcus pneumoniae, Haemophilus influenzae,* or *Moraxella catarrhalis*. Knowledge of the incidence of β-lactamase–positive *Haemophilus* isolates in a community should influence the selection of the antimicrobial agent.

FACTORS FOR SELECTION OF ANTIMICROBIAL AGENTS FOR THERAPY IN INDIVIDUAL PATIENTS

- Identification of organism
- Antimicrobial susceptibility of organism
- Bactericidal versus bacteriostatic
- Host status
  - Allergy history
  - Age
  - Pharmacokinetic factors
  - Renal function
  - Hepatic function
  - Pregnancy status
  - Genetic factors
  - Anatomical site of infection
  - Host defenses, white cell function

Antimicrobial Agent Susceptibility of Infecting Microorganisms

The susceptibility of bacteria to specific antimicrobial agents can be determined by several methods, but the results of these tests generally are not available until 18 to 48 hours after an initial culture sample has been obtained.

One of the most common methods for determining bacterial susceptibility to antibiotics is the disk diffusion method. This is simple to perform, is inexpensive, and provides data within 18 to 24 hours; however, this method is only semiquantitative and is not useful for many slow-growing or fastidious organisms. In the disk test, the surface of an agar plate is inoculated with a swab moistened with a dilution of the unknown culture. Paper disks of standard size impregnated with an antimicrobial agent are placed on this "lawn" of bacteria and incubated for 18 to 24 hours at 37°C. The test drugs diffuse from the disk into the agar, with the concentration of antibiotic diminishing at greater distances from the disk. The amount of drug impregnated in the disk is selected to provide an inhibitory zone around the periphery of the disk for susceptible organisms. The diameter of the inhibitory zone is related linearly to the logarithm of the concentration of drug. The test procedure and typical results are shown schematically in Figure 46-3. Results from the disk test are provided as susceptible, resistant, and intermediate for the tested drugs. For example, an ampicillin disk may contain 10 μg of ampicillin. A zone of inhibition ≥14 mm indicates the organism is susceptible, whereas a zone ≤11 mm indicates the organism is resistant. A susceptible zone of inhibition correlates with the serum and urine concentrations that can be achieved by use of recommended doses of a particular agent in most patients.

Quantitative data on the antibiotic susceptibility of microorganisms can be determined by methods using broth or agar dilution. These methods detect the lowest concentration of antimicrobial agent that prevents visible growth after an 18- to 24-hour incubation. This concentration is referred to as the minimal inhibitory concentration (MIC). The agar or broth contains antibiotics in serial twofold dilutions that encompass the concentrations normally achieved in humans. The technique is described schematically in Figure 46-4. Deciding whether the results show the organisms to be susceptible or not requires an understanding of the pharmacokinetics of the antimicrobial agent. The plasma half-life of many antibiotics is short, and so for a typical dosing schedule of 3 or 4 times per day, each dose is eliminated before the next dose is administered. In general, an organism is considered susceptible to the drug when the MIC is one fourth or less of the readily obtainable peak plasma concentration. This same test procedure can be extended further to determine the minimal bactericidal concentration (MBC) or minimal concentration that kills 99.9% of the microbial cells. Samples are removed from the antibiotic-containing tubes in which there is no visible microbial growth and plated on agar that contains no additional antibiotic. The lowest concentration tube from which bacteria do not grow on the agar is the MBC (see Figure 46-4). MBC determinations are necessary in only a few clinical situations, such as endocarditis or some cases of osteomyelitis or meningitis.

Because of the large number of antimicrobial agents

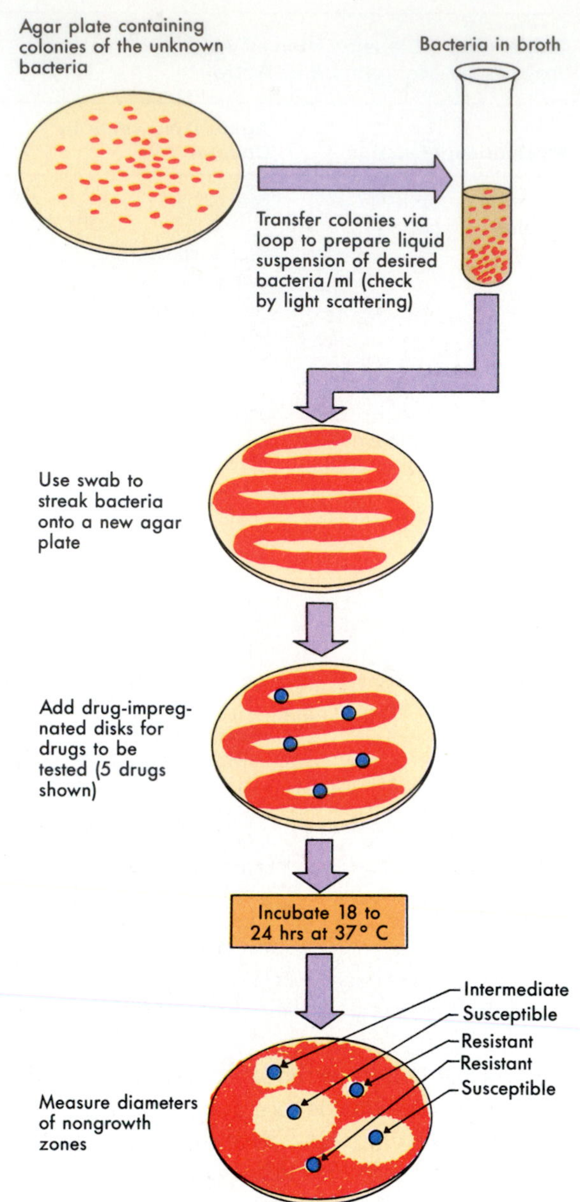

FIGURE 46-3 Disk diffusion method for testing bacteria for susceptibility to specific antimicrobial agents (see text).

available, it is difficult to test routinely all antimicrobial agents against an isolate. Laboratories often use one compound as representative of a class of compounds. For example, cefazolin is used as the prototype for all first-generation cephalosporins. However, considerable differences in pharmacokinetics and in vitro activity have prevented finding a prototype agent for second-generation cephalosporins. It is important to recognize that susceptibility tests require interpretation. Furthermore, certain organisms such as methicillin-resistant *Staphylococcus aureus* may appear susceptible to cephalosporin antibiotics, but these would not be eradicated

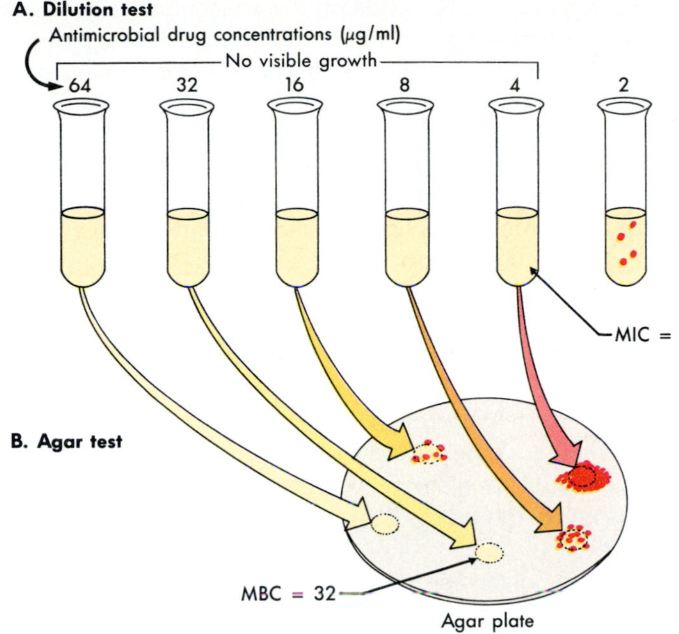

FIGURE 46-4 Dilution/agar tests for determination if MIC and MBC for a given drug and microorganism. **A,** Dilution test: each tube contains 5×10^5 colony-forming units (CFU) of bacteria, plus antibiotic at the concentration indicated. The MIC is the minimum drug concentration at which no visible growth of bacteria is observed (4 μg/ml in this example). **B,** Dilution/agar test: each tube in **A** that showed no visible growth is cultured on a section of the new agar plate (no additional antibiotic is added to the agar plate). The MBC is the lowest concentration where no growth occurred on the agar (32 μg/ml in this example).

by such drugs. Susceptibility tests are not error-proof and may also fail to identify a resistant subset population.

Bactericidal Versus Bacteriostatic Drug

One of the first decisions that must be made in antimicrobial therapy is whether a bactericidal therapy is required. In uncomplicated infections a bacteriostatic agent often is adequate, since the host defenses will contribute to the eradication of the microorganism. For example, in pneumonococcal pneumonia, tetracyclines, which are bacteriostatic agents, suppress the multiplication of the pneumococci; however, destruction of the pneumococci is achieved by the interaction of alveolar macrophages and polymorphonuclear leukocytes. For a neutropenic individual, such a bacteriostatic agent might prove ineffective and a bactericidal agent would be necessary. Thus the status of the host influences the selection of either a bactericidal or bacteriostatic agent.

In some infections, bactericidal antimicrobial agents are necessary. Effective therapy of bacterial endocarditis requires bactericidal agents. Treatment with bacteriostatic antibiotics such as tetracyclines or erythromycin has an unacceptably high failure rate in contrast to cure rates in excess of 95% with bactericidal agents such as penicillin. Meningitis is another illness where bactericidal therapy is necessary. In meningitis, concentrations of an antimicrobial agent eight- to tenfold above the MBC must be achieved within the spinal fluid to effect a cure. Thus susceptibility is not the only criterion for efficacy, but a drug must achieve concentrations four- to sixteenfold above the inhibitory concentration to be effective. Cefamandole inhibits *H. influenzae* and will cure pneumonia caused by *Haemophilus* organisms, but it will not cure most patients with *Haemophilus* meningitis, since cerebrospinal fluid concentrations of the drug are usually inadequate. Unless peak serum concentrations are eight- to sixteenfold above the MIC in neutropenic patients, there is a predictable high rate of failure.

Host Status

Allergy History A history of any previous allergic reaction is important in selecting an antimicrobial agent because a similar reaction to other members of the same drug class may occur. Allergy to penicillins is an important factor. Anaphylactic reactions to any penicillin compound preclude the subsequent use of penicillins. However, a rash after use of ampicillin in a patient with mononucleosis may not indicate true allergy to all penicillins, and in special situations penicillin could be used if the patient does not have a positive skin test. Patients allergic to one sulfonamide are allergic to all sulfonamides. Allergy to aminoglycosides is rare. However, cutaneous eruptions ranging from urticaria to exfoliative dermatitis have been reported with every class of antibiotic.

Age Factors Many antibiotics are removed from the body by renal elimination, which may undergo change with age. The pH of gastric secretions also is affected as part of the aging process and may influence selection of a drug. Certain antibiotics should not be given

Table 46-2 Antimicrobial Agents to be Avoided During Pregnancy

Agent	Potential Toxicity
ANTIBACTERIAL	
aminoglycosides	VIII nerve damage
chloramphenicol	Gray baby syndrome
erythromycin estolate	Cholestatic hepatitis
metronidazole	Possible teratogenicity
nitrofurantoin	Hemolytic anemia
sulfonamides	Hemolysis in newborn with glucose-6-phosphate dehydrogenase deficiency; increased risk of kernicterus
tetracyclines	Limb abnormalities, dental staining, inhibition of bone growth
trimethoprim	Altered folate metabolism
quinolones	Abnormalities of cartilage
vancomycin	Possible auditory toxicity
ANTIFUNGAL	
griseofulvin	Teratogenic in animals
ketoconazole	Teratogenic in animals
ANTITUBERCULAR	
isoniazid	Use with caution
rifampin	Use with caution
ANTIVIRAL	
amantadine	Teratogenic

to children. For example, tetracyclines that bind to developing teeth and bone and those that cross the placenta will affect the fetus and are to be avoided (Table 46-2). Similarly, sulfonamides should not be given to newborns because they displace bilirubin from serum albumin and can produce kernicterus (i.e., CNS disorder).

Pharmacokinetic Factors The administration of antimicrobial agents is usually by the oral, IM, or IV routes. Although absorption can occur after topical or rectal administration, these routes of drug delivery are uncommon. Most antimicrobial agents yield peak serum concentrations 1 to 2 hours after oral administration. Peak concentrations may be delayed when antimicrobial agents are ingested with food or in patients with delayed intestinal transit such as sometimes occurs with diabetics. After IM injections, peak plasma concentrations occur in 0.5 to 1 hour; after IV infusions of 20 to 30 minutes, the peak occurs at the end of the infusion.

The amount of antimicrobial agent that reaches the extravascular tissues and fluids, where the infection is usually present, depends on the concentration gradient between plasma and target tissue, the degree of drug binding to plasma and tissue proteins, molecular size, degree of ionization and lipid solubility of the drug, and rate of elimination or metabolism of the agent. Considerable variation exists in each of these factors among the many diverse types of chemical compounds that make up the list of clinically useful antimicrobial agents.

Renal Function Many antimicrobial agents are eliminated from the body by renal filtration or secretion. Since renal function changes with patient age, some antimicrobial agents can accumulate in the body and cause serious toxic reactions without a proper adjustment in dosing regimen. Toxicity may be to the kidney or to other organs. Dosage adjustments for these agents eliminated by glomerular filtration usually can be estimated on the basis of age, body size, and serum creatinine.

Aminoglycoside, vancomycin, and certain penicillin, cephalosporin, carbapenem, and quinolone dosing schedules need to be adjusted to compensate for diminished renal function. Decreased renal function promotes hypoalbuminemia caused by poor nutrition and produces substances in blood that decrease binding of drugs to albumin to give greater concentrations of free drug. Decreased renal function also leads to increased ototoxicity from aminoglycosides, some interference with platelet function by penicillins, and neurotoxicity from penicillins, imipenem, quinolones, and polymyxins.

Hepatic Function Antimicrobials that are metabolized in the liver include chloramphenicol, erythromycin, clarithromycin, rifampin, nitroimidazoles, and some of the quinolones. Reduction in dosage may be necessary to avoid toxic reactions in patients with impaired hepatic function. Chloramphenicol toxicity in newborns is related to failure to convert the drug to an inactive, nontoxic glucuronide. In combined hepatic-renal disease the half-life of some drugs, such as ticarcillin, increases significantly.

Pregnancy Pregnant patients or nursing mothers pose important problems in the use of antimicrobial agents, since most of these drugs cross the placenta to some degree. One must consider both the teratogenic and toxic potentials of these drugs on the fetus (Table 46-2). Certain agents such as metronidazole are teratogenic in lower animals and therefore may have this effect in humans. Other agents such as rifampin and trimethoprim may have teratogenic potential and should be used only when alternative agents are unavailable.

Use of tetracyclines in pregnancy should be avoided because they alter fetal dentition and bone growth. Tetracyclines have also been associated with hepatic, pancreatic, and renal damage in pregnant women. Streptomycin has been associated with auditory toxicity in children of mothers treated for tuberculosis. Sulfonamides should not be used in the third trimester of pregnancy because they may displace bilirubin from albumin binding sites and cause CNS toxicity in the fetus.

Many antibiotics are excreted in breast milk and can distort the newborn's microflora or act as a sensitizing agent to cause future allergy.

Genetic Factors Genetic abnormalities of enzyme function may affect the potential for toxicity of certain agents.

Hemolysis in glucose-6-phosphate dehydrogenase–deficient individuals can be provoked by sulfonamides, nitrofurantoin, pyrimethamine, sulfones, and chloramphenicol. Individuals who do not acetylate drugs well may not inactivate isoniazid adequately and can develop peripheral neuropathy unless treated with pyridoxine. Since 50% of the U.S. population are slow acetylators, pyridoxine usually is prescribed with isoniazid.

Anatomical Site of Infection The site of infection often determines, not only the antimicrobial agent, but also the dose, route, and duration of drug administration. The desired peak concentration of drug at the site of infection should equal at least four times the MIC. However, if host defenses are adequate, the peak concentration of antibiotic may be much lower and even be equal to the MIC and still be effective. When host defenses are absent or inoperative, peak concentrations of antibiotic eight- to sixteenfold above the MIC may be required.

Most antimicrobial agents readily enter most body tissues and compartments, except for the spinal fluid, brain, eye, and prostate gland. Concentrations adequate to treat infections of the pleural, pericardial, and joint spaces can be obtained by use of the parenteral route. Antibiotics, however, may not be active in abscesses because of the low pH and the reservoir of pus and necrotic debris.

Infected heart valves provide an example of a problem associated with the infection site. Bacteria trapped in a fibrin matrix divide at a slow rate, and many antibiotics are effective only on growing microorganisms. Antibiotics used in endocarditis therefore must be bactericidal, administered at high concentrations, and administered for prolonged periods so that diffusion of the antibiotic into the matrix is achieved and all bacteria are killed.

Meningitis is a difficult problem because many antimicrobial agents do not cross the blood-brain or blood-CSF barriers very well. Lipid-soluble agents such as chloramphenicol easily enter the CSF, as do agents like rifampin and metronidazole; however, aminoglycosides do not cross the CSF barrier even in the presence of inflammation. Penicillins, aztreonam, cephalosporins, and imipenem enter the CSF in the presence of meningitis to variable degrees depending upon the compound. Quinolones such as ciprofloxacin also enter the CSF at concentrations adequate to kill some microorganisms.

Osteomyelitis is an infection where an extended duration of therapy is required. Less than 4 weeks of drug administration usually results in high rates of failure to eradicate the infections. The concentration of antibiotic in bone is often low, and the bacteria are sequestered and thus prevented from coming into contact with the antibiotics.

Antimicrobial drug therapy frequently is ineffective in the presence of a foreign body such as an indwelling urethral catheter, an artificial joint, or a prosthetic heart valve. In the presence of the foreign body, microorganisms accumulate on the foreign surface and become covered with a glycocalyx coating. Large numbers of microorganisms growing at a slow rate in a sessile form are present on the foreign body. They are protected by the coating from attack by leukocytes and most importantly from destruction by antimicrobial agents.

Microorganisms also persist in abscesses. The impairment of circulation in an abscess reduces the delivery of antibody, complement, and leukocytes. Moreover, complement is destroyed in abscesses and cannot potentiate destruction of bacteria by leukocytes. Because of the absence of adequate oxygen and the acidic environment in an abscess, leukocytes function less effectively. Bacteria in an abscess frequently grow at a much slower rate than at other infection sites yet are not killed by antimicrobial agents, which easily kill them when they are rapidly dividing. In some situations the antimicrobial agent is destroyed by enzymes induced by the microorganisms or by enzymes released when the microorganisms are killed by the antibiotic when it penetrates into the abscess. Antibiotic therapy can rarely cure established abscesses, lesions containing foreign bodies, or infections associated with excretory duct obstruction, unless these sites are drained surgically.

Some infections are caused by microorganisms that are not destroyed when they are ingested by polymorphonuclear phagocytes or macrophages. *Mycobacterium, Legionella,* and *Salmonella* species can survive within phagocytic cells, and antimicrobial agents that do not penetrate the phagocytic cells often are not successful in eradicating infection caused by these organisms. The success of compounds such as isoniazid and rifampin in the treatment of *Mycobacterium tuberculosis* is because these agents enter mononuclear cells in which tubercule bacilli survive and the antimicrobial agents cause the death of the bacilli within the phagocytic cells.

Agents that do not readily enter phagocytic cells can still be effective in curing infections resulting from intracellular organisms such as *Listeria* if the antimicrobial agent is administered for a long enough period of time. Ampicillin can be used to cure an infection caused by *Listeria* if the antibiotic is administered for a long time. Ampicillin kills the extracellular bacteria and also alters their surface properties, increasing their destruction by macrophages. Individuals with diseases of the lymphoid system, such as chronic lymphocytic leukemia or acquired immune deficiency syndrome, can have recurrent relapses of infection such as from *Salmonella* organisms because of inadequate white cell function. Therefore there is a reduced capacity to use the modified bacterial surface properties for phagocytic destruction of the microorganisms.

Bacterial infections associated with obstructions of the urinary, biliary, or respiratory tracts tend to persist despite antibiotic therapy. Antimicrobial agent penetration into these areas is poor. Bacteria present within the obstructed regions are in a quiescent state from which they emerge when antimicrobial therapy is discontinued, since most agents do not kill resting bacteria.

Host Defenses Absence of white cells predisposes a patient to serious bacterial infection, and in such cases bacteriostatic agents are inadequate to protect these neutropenic hosts. The critical white cell count is between 500 and 1000 mature polymorphonuclear cells/mm^3. Other host defects that require use of bactericidal agents are agammaglobulinemia or asplenia. The latter predisposes to pneumococcal or *Haemophilus* infection. The absence of complement components C_7 to C_9, protect against *Neisseria* species. Knowledge of the organisms most frequently causing infections in patients with defects of white cells, complement, T-cells, or immunoglobulin production will aid in the selection of bactericidal antimicrobial agents to be used when such patients develop fever.

PROPHYLAXIS WITH ANTIMICROBIAL AGENTS

Prophylaxis should be directed at preventing a specific bacterial infection. This means that a particular species or several species have been shown to produce the infection, that an effective antimicrobial agent is available, and that the risk of the infection outweighs the hazard of using the antimicrobial agent. The antibiotic must be delivered to the site of probable infection at an appropriate time so that the agent will inhibit bacteria that would colonize the area and subsequently produce an infection. The use of the antimicrobial agent must be of limited duration to avoid toxicity and prevent selection of resistant bacterial flora by elimination of normal flora.

Prophylaxis can be considered in both medical and surgical situations. Medical conditions include the prevention of meningococcal meningitis, *Haemophilus* meningitis, recurrent rheumatic fever, postsplenectomy infections, cellulitis complicating lymphedema, recurrent lower urinary tract infections, tuberculosis, and bacterial endocarditis. A special medical problem is the prevention of infection in the neutropenic patient. Many surgical problems require prophylaxis, including upper gastrointestinal surgery, cholecystectomy, colon surgery, appendectomy, head and neck surgery, cardiac surgery, prosthetic hip and other joint surgery, hysterectomy, and cesarean section. The optimal agent for each condition has not been established.

An important prophylactic use of antibiotics is to prevent bacterial endocarditis. Individuals with valvular or structural lesions of the heart, where endocarditis is common, should receive antibiotic prophylaxis at the time of surgical, dental, or other procedures that may produce a high degree of bacteremia. Prophylaxis is administered just before the procedure. This method prevents the selection of resistant bacteria, reduces the number of organisms that could lodge on the valvular tissue, and alters the surface properties of the microorganism so they have reduced affinity for cardiac tissue. Since *viridans*-group streptococci from the mouth or intestine, enterococci from the intestine or genitourinary tract, and staphylococci from skin have the greatest propensity to cause endocarditis, prophylaxis should be directed against these organisms.

The use of oral antibiotics to reduce aerobic fecal flora of neutropenic patients is controversial. Some studies indicate that aerobic gram-negative bacterial infections in neutropenic patients are caused by passage of bacteria across the intestinal wall with resultant bacteremia. The use of agents that eliminate aerobic bacteria but do not destroy anaerobic and streptococcal flora reduces the incidence of bacteremias in the neutropenic patient.

Prophylaxis can also be effective without eradication of all bacteria. Topical application of silver sulfadiazine to a burn wound will reduce the number of bacteria in the burn eschar to less than 10^5 per gram of tissue and prevent burn wound sepsis.

For the prevention of postoperative wound infections, the antimicrobial agent must be present at the probable site of infection when the area may be exposed to the bacteria. The antibiotic must be given immediately preoperatively or during the operation and should inhibit the most common and important bacteria likely to produce infection.

Prophylaxis should also be used in procedures in which contamination is probable. The surgical procedures that require prophylaxis are those in which there is insertion of a foreign body, such as a heart valve or an orthopedic prosthesis. In these situations, if infection develops, the consequences are so drastic that the short use of antibiotics is a minor risk.

There are disadvantages to the prophylactic use of antibiotics. Toxic or hypersensitivity (allergic) reactions may occur and superinfection with a more resistant flora can develop. Infection may be temporarily masked or there may be alteration of the ecology of the hospital flora, leading to the selection of more resistant bacteria.

MONITORING ANTIMICROBIAL THERAPY

It is critical that serum or plasma drug concentrations be determined for some antimicrobial agents to ensure that therapeutic but not toxic concentrations are attained. This is particularly important in patients with diminished renal function who are receiving antibiotics that undergo renal elimination.

The measurement of serum bactericidal titers to monitor antimicrobial therapy has primarily been used in treatment of bacterial endocarditis. Although guidelines have been developed for the size of bacterial inoculum, composition of the bacterial growth medium, amount of serum added, and so forth, results of this test are subject to great variability even in the most trained hands. A peak serum bactericidal titer greater than 1:8 has been correlated with successful outcomes in osteomyelitis, septic arthritis, and empyema, and peak titers ≥ 1:64 have been correlated with bacteriological "cures" of bacterial endocarditis. However, results of this test have not been predictive of bacteriological failure in the treatment of endocarditis.

ANTIMICROBIAL COMBINATIONS

Many infections can and should be treated with a single antimicrobial agent. The combination of two or three antimicrobial agents may result in one of three responses: (1) indifferent, (2) synergistic, or (3) antagonistic.

Antimicrobial combinations are considered to elicit *indifferent* effects if the activity in combination equals the sum of separate independent activities. Synergism is present if the activity of the combined antimicrobial agents is greater than the sum of the independent activities. Synergism is frequently defined as a fourfold or greater reduction in the MIC or MBC for both agents. For example, the MBC of ampicillin against *Streptococcus faecalis* is 64 μg/ml, and the MBC of gentamicin is 64 μg/ml. In combination, the MBCs are 4 and 0.5 μg/ml respectively. Each is reduced by at least a factor of four,

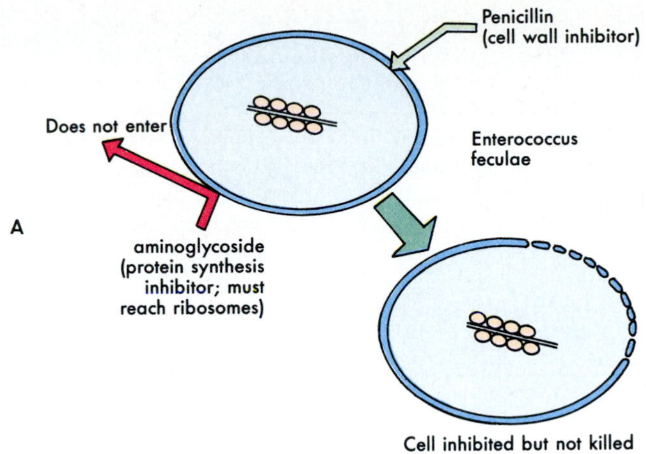

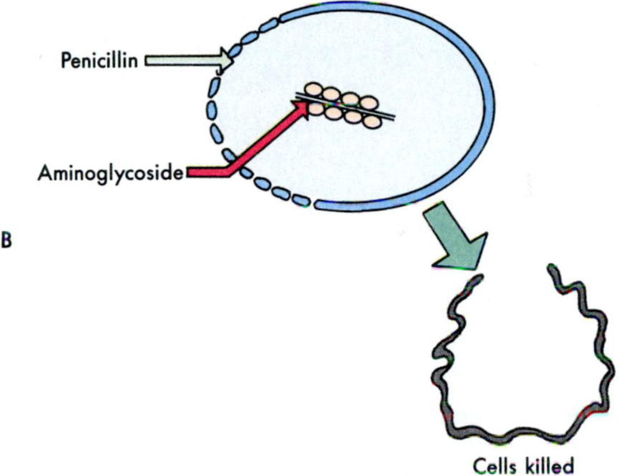

FIGURE 46-5 An example of synergy between two antibiotics. **A,** Penicillin or aminoglycoside is given, but not both; the cells are inhibited only. **B,** Penicillin and aminoglycoside are given concurrently; penicillin opens holes in the cell wall through which aminoglycosides can enter and reach the ribosomes and halt protein synthesis; therefore the cells are killed.

and thus the drugs are synergistic against this organism (Figure 46-5). Combinations of antibiotics are *antagonistic* when the activity of the combination is fourfold less than the sum of the activities of the independent agents.

The reasons to use combinations of antimicrobial agents are listed in the box on p. 626.

The evidence that combination antimicrobial therapy is of value in life-threatening infections has been shown for those infections occurring in neutropenic patients. Combination of an anti-*Pseudomonas* penicillin and an aminoglycoside have yielded better survival in *Pseudomonas* sepsis. The major disadvantages to combination therapy in serious infections are the added cost and the possibility of toxicity. However, if therapy is modified within 24 to 48 hours, the risks of toxicity are minimal.

Combination therapy for polymicrobial infections,

REASONS FOR CONCURRENT USE OF MORE THAN ONE ANTIMICROBIAL AGENT IN A PATIENT

- To treat a life-threatening infection
- Treatment of polymicrobial infection
- For synergy of the drugs (obtain enhanced antibacterial activity)
- Prevent emergence of resistant bacteria
- Permit use of a lower dose of one of the antimicrobial agents

such as those occurring at intraperitoneal and pelvic sites, has been used for years. Recently, single agents have become available that are effective in the therapy of many intraperitoneal and pelvic infections, and combination therapy is used less for such infections. Other examples of polymicrobial infections are brain abscesses often caused by a *Bacteroides* species and anaerobic and microaerophilic streptococci. Penicillin is excellent for suppressing the streptococci but may fail with the *Bacteroides* species. Metronidazole is excellent for the *Bacteroides* species but may not adequately control the streptococci. As a further example, many acute pelvic inflammatory infections are treated with two agents because one is necessary to treat the chlamydial component that may be present and the other is needed to treat aerobic or anaerobic gram-negative and gram-positive bacteria, which may also be involved.

The prevention of emergence of resistance has been well-studied in the treatment of tuberculosis. When the mycobacteria are in a cavity, the organisms are sheltered from contact with drugs, and some of the bacteria in a cavity are intrinsically resistant to the drug. Therefore the use of two drugs prevents the resistant organisms from surviving.

The use of combinations of antimicrobials to achieve a synergistic effect has been documented for three types of interactions: (1) combination of an inhibitor of cell-wall synthesis with an aminoglycoside antibiotic, (2) combination of agents acting on sequential steps in a metabolic pathway, or (3) combination of agents in which one (such as an inhibitor of β-lactamases) inhibits an enzyme that inactivates the other compound, such as clavulanate with amoxicillin.

Penicillins affect enterococci in a bacteriostatic fashion, with a large difference between the inhibitory and bactericidal concentrations. Aminoglycosides would inhibit enterococci if the drug could get inside the bacteria, but this does not occur at readily achievable concentrations. Because uptake of aminoglycosides by enterococci is enhanced by penicillins (see Figure 46-5), the use of both drugs enables the aminoglycoside to enter the bacterial cell. This synergism can be demonstrated in the treatment of endocarditis in humans.

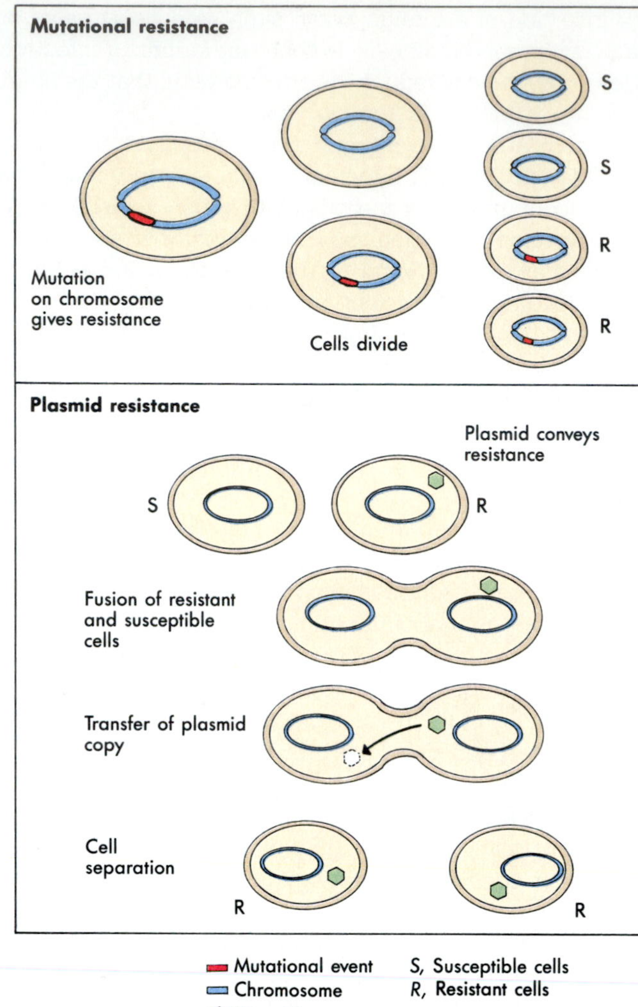

FIGURE 46-6 Propagation of resistance by chromosome versus plasmid mechanisms. See the text for further information.

BACTERIAL RESISTANCE

Bacteria have proven adept at developing resistance to new antimicrobial agents and such developments likely will continue in the future. There are several pathways by which bacterial resistance becomes apparent and several routes by which the resistance is propagated (Figure 46-6). The purpose of this section is to summarize the problem and the mechanisms, with details amplified in subsequent chapters on specific drugs.

Early studies of bacterial resistance focused on single-step mutational events, chromosomal in origin, with sulfonamide resistance an early example. With the discovery of penicillin, and even before enough penicillin G had been produced on an adequate scale to treat patients, the Oxford group reported an enzyme in *Bacillus coli* (now known as *Escherichia coli*) that inactivated penicillin G. By 1944, it was shown that some *Staphylococcus aureus* strains also were capable of inactivating penicillin G. Resistance to streptomycin soon followed.

Although resistance to the tetracyclines and chloramphenicol was noted in the 1950s, it was the Japanese who found that some strains of *Shigella dysenteriae* had become resistant not only to sulfonamides but also to tetracyclines, chloramphenicol, and streptomycin. This resistance turned out not to be caused by chromosomal change but to come from a transmissible, extrachromosomal piece of DNA now referred to as a **plasmid.**

Resistance-conferring plasmids have been identified in virtually all bacteria (Table 46-3) and are widely dispersed in nature. Resistance also is present in the form of genes on transposons and can be transferred to plasmids or become integrated into chromosomes. Chromosomal genes that code for resistance also can be transferred in the reverse direction and become attached to transposons and the resistance transferred by plasmids.

Antimicrobials are a major selective factor for the development of both chromosomal and plasmid-mediated bacterial resistance. The use of antibiotics, whether in an individual patient or in a hospital with its special environment and microorganisms, will destroy antibiotic-

Table 46-3 Resistance Mechanisms

Antibiotic(s)	Mechanisms	Genetic basis	Pathogens with Potential for Resistance Development
β-lactams Penicillins Cephalosporins Monobactams Carbapenems	Altered penicillin-binding proteins	Chromosomal	*Staphylococcus aureus* *S. epidermidis* *Streptococcus pneumoniae* *Streptococcus sanguis* *Haemophilus influenzae* *Neisseria gonorrhoeae* *N. meningitidis* *Escherichia coli* *Pseudomonas aeruginosa*
	Reduced permeability	Chromosomal	*P. aeruginosa* *Enterobacter cloacae* *Serratia marcescens* *Klebsiella pneumoniae* *K. oxytoca*
	β-lactamase	Plasmid* and chromosomal	*S. aureus* *S. epidermidis* Enterococci *P. aeruginosa* Enterobacteriaceae *N. gonorrhoeae* *N. meningitidis* *Moraxella* *Bacteroides* *Acinetobacter*
Fluoroquinolones Norfloxacin Ofloxacin Ciprofloxacin	Altered DNA gyrase	Chromosomal	*S. aureus* *S. epidermidis* Enterobacteriaceae *Pseudomonas*
Lomefloxacin	Reduced permeability	Chromosomal	Enterobacteriaceae *P. aeruginosa*
Aminoglycosides Gentamicin	Decreased ribosomal binding	Chromosomal	Streptococci

Continued.

Table 46-3 Resistance Mechanisms—cont'd

Antibiotic(s)	Mechanisms	Genetic basis	Pathogens with Potential for Resistance Development
Tobramycin Amikacin Netilmicin	Reduced uptake Modifying enzymes	Chromosomal	*Bacteroides* *Pseudomonas* Enterobacteriaceae
		Plasmid*	Staphylococci Enterococci Streptococci Enterobacteriaceae *Pseudomonas*
Macrolides lincosamides Erythromycin Clindamycin	Methylating enzymes	Plasmid and chromosomal	Streptococci S. pneumoniae Enterococci Staphylococci
Chloramphenicol	Acetyltransferase	Plasmid* and chromosomal	Staphylococci Streptococci *S. pneumoniae* Enterobacteriaceae *Neisseria*
Tetracyclines Tetracycline Minocycline Doxycycline	Efflux	Plasmid*	Staphylococci Streptococci Enterococci Enterobacteriaceae *Bacteroides*
	Ribosomal protein protected	Plasmid*	*N gonorrhoeae* *Mycoplasma* *Ureaplasma*
Rifampin	Reduced DNA polymerase binding	Chromosomal	Staphylococci Enterococci Streptococci Enterobacteriaceae Pseudomonads
Folate-inhibitors TMP/SMX	Altered targets	Plasmid and chromosomal	Staphylococci Streptococci *S. pneumoniae* Enterobacteriaceae *Neisseria*
	Reduced permeability	Chromosomal	*Pseudomonas* Campylobacter
Glycopeptides Vancomycin Teicoplanin	Altered target	Plasmid and chromosomal	Enterococci *Leuconostoc* *Leuconostoc dextranicum* *Pediococcus* *Lactobacillus* *Streptococcus pyogenes*
Mupirocin	Altered target	plasmid	*S. aureus*
Fusidic acid	Altered target	Chromosomal	*S. aureus*
Fosfomycin	Altered transport	Chromosomal Plasmid	*S. aureus* *Serratia*

From Neu HC: *Science* 257:1064, 1992.
*Also on transposons.

susceptible bacteria and permit the proliferation of bacteria intrinsically resistant or that have acquired extrachromosomal resistance. From an epidemiological point of view, plasmid resistance is most important, since resistance in this form is transmissible and may be associated with other properties that enable a microorganism to colonize and invade a susceptible host.

The basic mechanisms of microbial resistance to antimicrobial agents are (1) the development of altered receptors or enzymes that interact with the drug, (2) a decrease in the concentration of drug that reaches the receptors (by altered rates of entry or removal of drug), (3) enhanced destruction or inactivation of drug, (4) synthesis of resistant metabolic pathways, and (5) failure to metabolize the drug. These are summarized in Table 46-3. Microorganisms can possess one or all of these mechanisms simultaneously.

Resistance Based on Altered Receptors for Drug

An important example is the production of altered proteins to which β-lactams, penicillins, cephalosporins do not bind. This is a key step in the action of these antibiotics as inhibitors of bacterial cell wall synthesis. This was first encountered with *Staphylococcus aureus,* but in 1977 *Streptococcus pneumoniae,* resistant to penicillin G, was found in South Africa. These organisms had altered penicillin-binding proteins that had decreased affinity for penicillins. Resistance of *S. pneumoniae* to penicillins, because of altered penicillin binding proteins, has been increasing, and there are relatively resistant isolates in many parts of the world. This is discussed further in Chapter 47.

Erythromycin and clindamycin resistance in clinical isolates of staphylococci and streptococci is discussed in Chapter 48.

Resistance to rifampin has been found based on altered DNA-directed RNA polymerase. A change of one amino acid in the β subunit of the DNA-directed RNA polymerase alters the binding of rifampin.

The presence of an altered or new dihydropteroic synthetase that binds paraaminobenzoic acid better than the sulfonamides do is the basis for sulfonamide resistance (see Chapter 49). Resistance to quinolones is attributable to an altered DNA gyrase.

Decreased Entry of Drug

Aminoglycoside uptake by Enterobacteriaceae is a biphasic process with the initial energy independent rapid phase believed to represent binding of the drug to cell surface with passage by diffusion through the outer layers of the cell wall. The second phase of uptake is energy dependent, as aminoglycoside crosses the cytoplasmic membrane, probably with energy supplied by a gradient. Resistance to aminoglycosides occurs as a result of a drug efflux pathway and a reduced rate of influx.

Destruction or Inactivation of Drug

Many gram-positive and gram-negative bacteria, including some *H. influenzae,* are resistant to chloramphenicol because they possess the enzyme chloramphenicol transacetylase. Acetylated chloramphenicol binds poorly to the ribosome. Protein synthesis, which normally is inhibited by the nonacetylated drug, is unaffected.

The most widely recognized example of bacterial drug resistance is that of the β-lactamases. β-Lactamase enzymes catalyze the hydrolysis of penicillins, cephalosporins and other β-lactams to produce inactive products. Thus those bacteria that contain significant concentrations of these enzymes are resistant to many penicillins and cephalosporins. The β-lactamases are discussed in Chapter 47.

Synthesis by Resistant Metabolic Pathway

Some thymidine-requiring streptococci are not inhibited by trimethoprim and sulfonamides because the microorganisms fail to undergo the thymineless death that occurs normally when bacteria are exposed to these agents. The resistant bacteria produce adequate concentrations of thymidine nucleotides by an alternative pathway and as a result survive exposure to these drugs.

Failure to Metabolize Drug

Anaerobic bacteria such as the rare *Bacteroides fragilis* do not metabolize the nitroimidazole metronidazole to the active metabolite, which causes DNA damage, and so these bacteria are not killed by metronidazole. In addition, *Candida* species that fail to metabolize 5-flucytosine to 5-fluorouracil are not inhibited by this drug, since it is the 5-fluorouracil that causes the inhibition through an abnormality in RNA synthesis.

REFERENCES

Hirschman JV: Antimicrobial prophylaxis for non-surgical infections. In Gorbach SL, Bartlett JG, and Blacklow NR, editors: *Infectious diseases,* Philadelphia, 1992, Saunders, pp 403-407.

Neu HC: The crisis in antibiotic resistance, *Science* 257:1064, 1992.

Nichols RL: Prophylaxis for surgical infection. In Gorbach SL, Bartlett JG, Blacklow NR, editors: *Infectious diseases,* Philadelphia, 1992, Saunders, pp 393-402.

SELF-ASSESSMENT QUESTIONS

1. In which of the following infections is it necessary to have a drug with bactericidal activity?
   a. Bacterial exacerbation of bronchitis
   b. Pneumonia
   c. Meningitis
   d. Urinary tract infection
2. Which of the following agents should be avoided in treating an infection in a pregnant woman?
   a. Ampicillin
   b. Tetracycline
   c. Cephalexin
   d. Erythromycin
3. The combination of ampicillin and gentamicin is an example of?
   a. Indifference
   b. Synergy
   c. Antagonism
   d. Bacterial symbiosis
4. Prophylaxis of infection has been used with success in which of the following clinical situations?
   a. Prevention of bacterial infection after a viral upper respiratory infection
   b. Infection after clean surgery such as a breast biopsy
   c. Prevention of urinary infection in a patient with an indwelling urethral catheter present for a long time
   d. Endocarditis in an individual with underlying valvular heart disease
5. Plasmid-mediated resistance to antimicrobial agents has been found in all except which of the following?
   a. *Streptococcus pneumoniae*
   b. *Staphylococcus aureus*
   c. *Haemophilus influenzae*
   d. *Streptococcus faecalis*

CHAPTER 47 Bacterial Cell Wall Inhibitors

HAROLD C. NEU

MAJOR DRUGS
penicillins
cephalosporins
carbapenems
monobactams
β-lactamase inhibitors
vancomycin
bacitracin

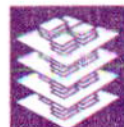

THERAPEUTIC OVERVIEW

A large group of antimicrobial agents act by inhibiting synthesis of bacterial cell walls. Included are the β-lactam antibiotics and vancomycin and bacitracin. The discovery and development of the β-lactam antibiotics is one of the milestones of medicine, since these agents encompass the widely used penicillins and cephalosporins in addition to newer structures. The discovery of penicillin in 1929 and the development of methods for its large-scale manufacture by fermentation in the early 1940s led to the demonstration that penicillin could be used for effective clinical therapy for a large number of infections. This new therapy revolutionized the treatment of infectious diseases and added years to the life-span of the population. The cephalosporins, carbapenems, and monobactams are added classes of β-lactam agents that differ chemically from the general structure of the penicillins.

Vancomycin is also a bactericidal cell wall inhibitor but not of the β-lactam family. It came into prominence as a result of (1) the occurrence of methicillin-resistant staphylococci (2) the presence of pseudomembranous colitis caused by *Clostridium difficile,* and (3) increasing numbers of infections, which are not inhibited by the present β-lactams. Bacitracin, another cell-wall active agent, is limited to topical use because of severe renal toxicity when administered parenterally.

ABBREVIATIONS	
CSF	cerebrospinal fluid
PBP	penicillin-bound protein

Since the initial clinical use of penicillin, strains that previously were inhibited by penicillin G and related agents have become "resistant" to inhibition by these drugs (see Chapter 46). The development of resistance to the β-lactams is an ongoing clinical problem. Much of the resistance to the β-lactam antibiotics is caused by β-lactamase, hydrolytic enzymes in the resistant microorganisms. "β-lactamase inhibitor" drugs are now available to limit the hydrolytic deactivation of β-lactam antibiotics.

β-lactam agents are bactericidal but may be bacteriostatic under some conditions. Many of these agents can be used effectively against gram-positive and gram-negative organisms. The clinically used β-lactam antimicrobial agents differ in (1) the organisms against which they are effective, (2) their pharmacokinetics, stability, and suitable modes of administration, and (3) the type and extent of resistance encountered with specific bacterial strains.

The inhibition of cell wall synthesis normally leads to death of the bacteria. The osmotic pressure in the cytoplasm is high, and the cytoplasmic membrane often does not remain intact when the outer rigid cell wall is damaged or when filamentous growth (which also is lethal) occurs. Because these agents act by inhibiting cell wall synthesis, drug activity is maximal in microorganisms that are growing. A therapeutic summary of the cell wall–inhibiting antibiotics is listed in the box on p. 632.

Because the β-lactams constitute a large number of drugs, they are discussed in their entirety before inclusion of the mechanism and clinical factors for vancomycin and bacitracin. The chemical structural variations of the different β-lactam drugs and the mechanisms of action and resistance are discussed later.

THERAPEUTIC OVERVIEW FOR BACTERIAL CELL WALL INHIBITORS

INHIBITOR ANTIBIOTICS

β-Lactam Agents
Bactericidal
- Inhibit many gram-positive and many gram-negative organisms

Agents differ by
- Organism inhibited
- Pharmacokinetics
- Bacterial resistance encountered

Agents include
- Penicillins
- Cephalosporins
- Carbapenems
- Monobactams
- β-Lactamase inhibitors

Vancomycin
Bactericidal
- Inhibits methicillin-resistant staphylococci

Bacitracin
Topical use only for gram-positive bacteria

β-Lactam Drugs and β-Lactamase Inhibitors

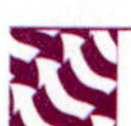

MECHANISMS OF ACTION

Mechanism of Therapeutic Effects

All β-lactam antimicrobial agents have the β-lactam ring structure (Figure 47-1). A lactam is a cyclic amide, similar to the more familiar cyclic ester (lactone). The β indicates that the amine group used to form the amide is on the second carbon from the carbonyl (C = O). Thus the β-lactam structure is a four-membered ring. Such a small ring normally is a strained structure of inherent low stability. This explains why some of the penicillins readily undergo acid or base hydrolysis and are not effective when given orally, as a result of the high acidity of the stomach.

The general structures of penicillin and cephalosporins are shown in Figure 47-2. Both classes of compounds have a second ring in addition to the β-lactam ring. Many variations are possible through addition of different R-groups. Monobactams have a single ring, and carbapenems have an unsaturated ring with the sulfur external to the ring. The sulfur of cephalosporins can be replaced by an oxygen to produce oxycephems.

The β-lactam antibiotics interfere with bacterial cell wall synthesis. The cell wall of bacteria is assembled in a series of steps, originating within the cytoplasm of the bacteria and ending outside the cytoplasmic membrane. The outer cellular coverings of gram-positive and gram-negative bacteria differ (Figure 47-3), but both classes have a rigid cell wall composed of a cross-linked peptidoglycan matrix. In aerobic and anaerobic gram-negative bacteria, an outer membrane of lipopolysaccharide is located exterior to a few layers of peptiglycan. In gram-positive bacteria the lipopolysaccharide layer is missing, and many more (15 to 30) layers of peptidoglycan are present. It is at the final cross-linking step, during the cellular synthesis of this rigid peptidoglycan matrix, that the β-lactam antibiotics exert their action.

The glycan part of the peptidoglycan matrix is composed of repeating disaccharide units of *N*-acetylglucosamine and *N*-acetylmuramate connected through β-1,4-linkages. The muramate group is composed of lactic acid, CH_3-CH(OH)-COOH, coupled to position 3 of

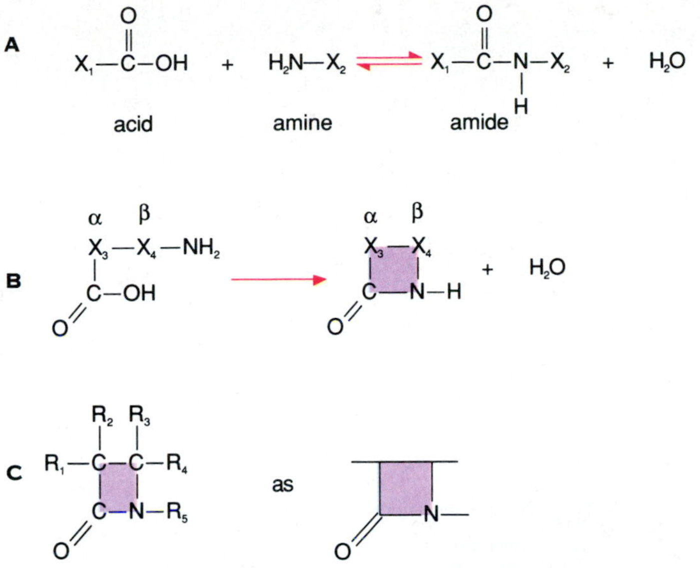

FIGURE 47-1 Description of β-lactam ring structure. **A,** Typical reaction to form an amide. In **B,** the product is a cyclic amide, called a *lactam;* X_3 and X_4 are carbons with side groups with the amine on the second, or β, carbon from the acid end. **C,** β-Lactam ring structure with the five R-groups that can be varied and in the skeletal form are R_2 and R_3 hydrogens. For many β-lactam drugs, R_1 is an acyl side chain, and R_4/R_5 are components of a second ring.

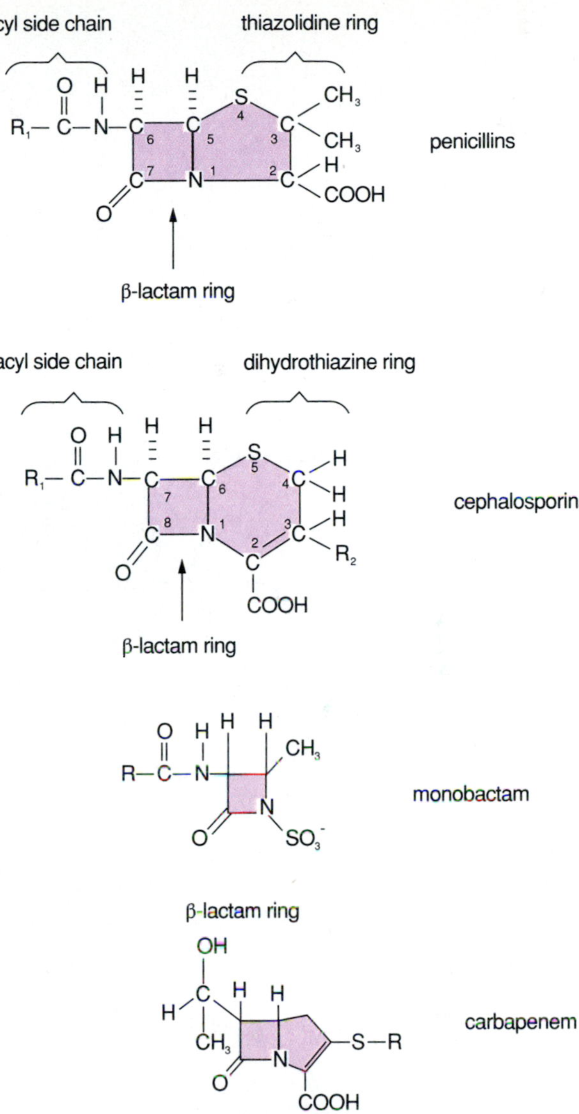

FIGURE 47-2 General structures of the two main classes of β-lactam antibiotics. Additional variations are possible at some of the non–R group positions. The arrow points to the bond that is broken during β-lactamase-catalyzed hydrolysis.

the *N*-acetylglucosamine through an ether linkage (Figure 47-4). A pentapeptide is attached to the glycan. This peptidoglycan monomer uses 20 to 25 enzymes for its synthesis.

The synthesis of the cross-linked peptidoglycan matrix is divided into four stages. In the first stage, which occurs in the cytoplasm, uridine nucleotide precursors are synthesized, using uridine triphosphate, to make UDP-*N*-acetylmuramyl-peptide-and-UDP-*N*-acetylglucosamine. The muramyl pentapeptide has D-alanine-D-alanine as a terminus. This is produced by racemization of L-alanine, followed by condensation using alanine racemase and synthetase enzymes. In the second stage, in the cytoplasmic membrane the nucleotides are displaced by a membrane carrier lipid that is a 55-carbon isoprenyl alcohol phosphate. The carrier lipid brings about the translocation of *N*-acetylmuramyl peptide and *N*-acetylglucosamine across the cytoplasmic membrane. In the third part, the saccharide units are linked in sequence to form chains of alternating disaccharides (Figure 47-4) of 10 to 50 or more repeating units. The fourth step in the formation of the rigid peptidoglycan cell wall is cross-linking between chains to form continuous two-dimensional sheets. This occurs outside of the cytoplasmic membrane but is accomplished by use of cytoplasmic membrane enzymes. During the cross-linking reaction, release of the membrane carrier lipids also occurs.

The cross-linking reaction is catalyzed by transpeptidase enzymes, and it is through inhibition of these enzymes that the β-lactam antibiotics exert their action. In this reaction (Figure 47-5), the third amino acid from the muramyl end of the pentapeptide (chain X) of a disaccharide chain is coupled between the two terminal alanines of the pentapeptide of an adjacent disaccharide chain (chain Y). In this process, the terminal alanine is released. The thickness of the peptidoglycan cell wall varies from 1 to about 50 cross-linked sheets in different bacteria. The biochemical pathways for cell wall

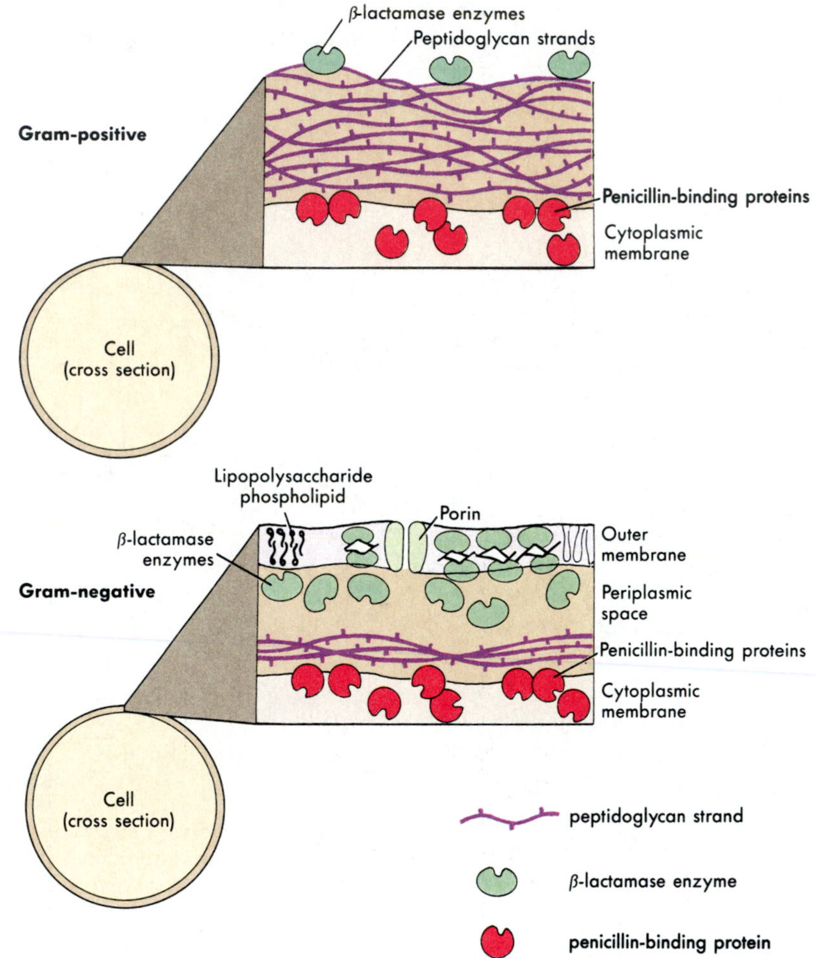

FIGURE 47-3 Outer coating of gram-positive (20 to 30 strands) and gram-negative bacteria showing thinner (3 to 5 strands) rigid peptidoglycan structure but added outer membrane for gram-negative cells. β-Lactam drugs act by inhibiting the synthesis of the rigid peptidoglycan part of the cell wall.

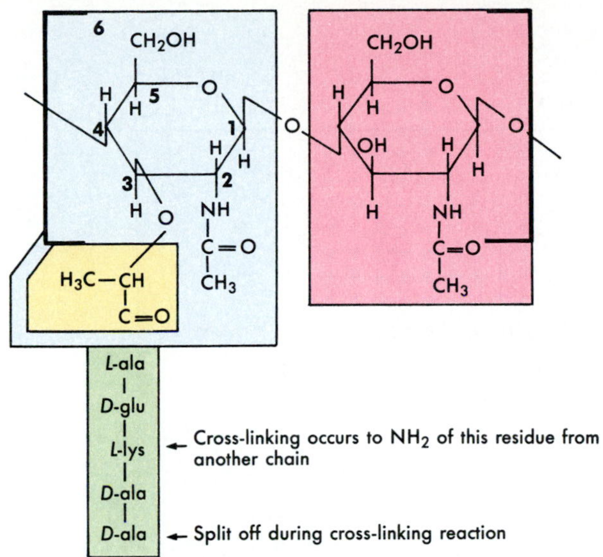

FIGURE 47-4 Repeating glycan portion of peptidoglycan matrix (shown as *n* units), consisting of the disaccharide *N*-acetylmuramate plus *N*-acetylglucosamine connected through the β-1,4-link and with the lactyl and pentapeptide attached as shown.

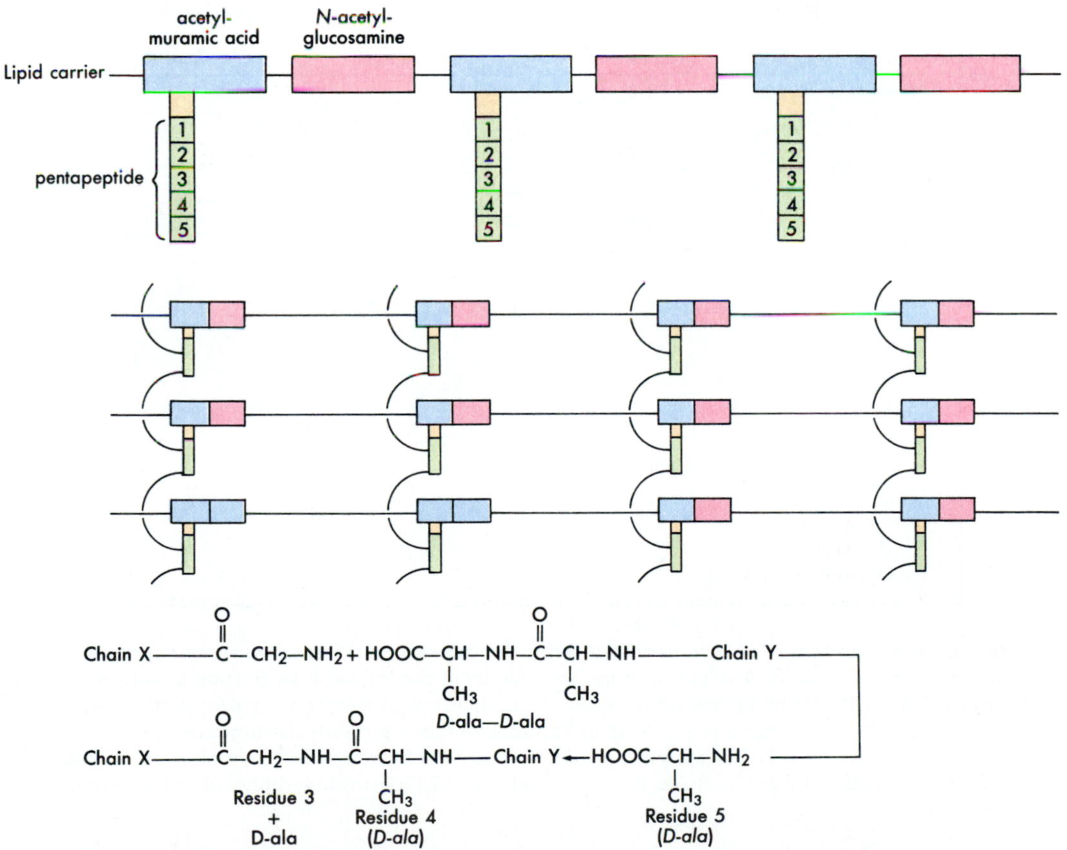

FIGURE 47-5 Cross-linking reaction to join strands and to form sheets of peptidoglycan and at the same time displace carrier.

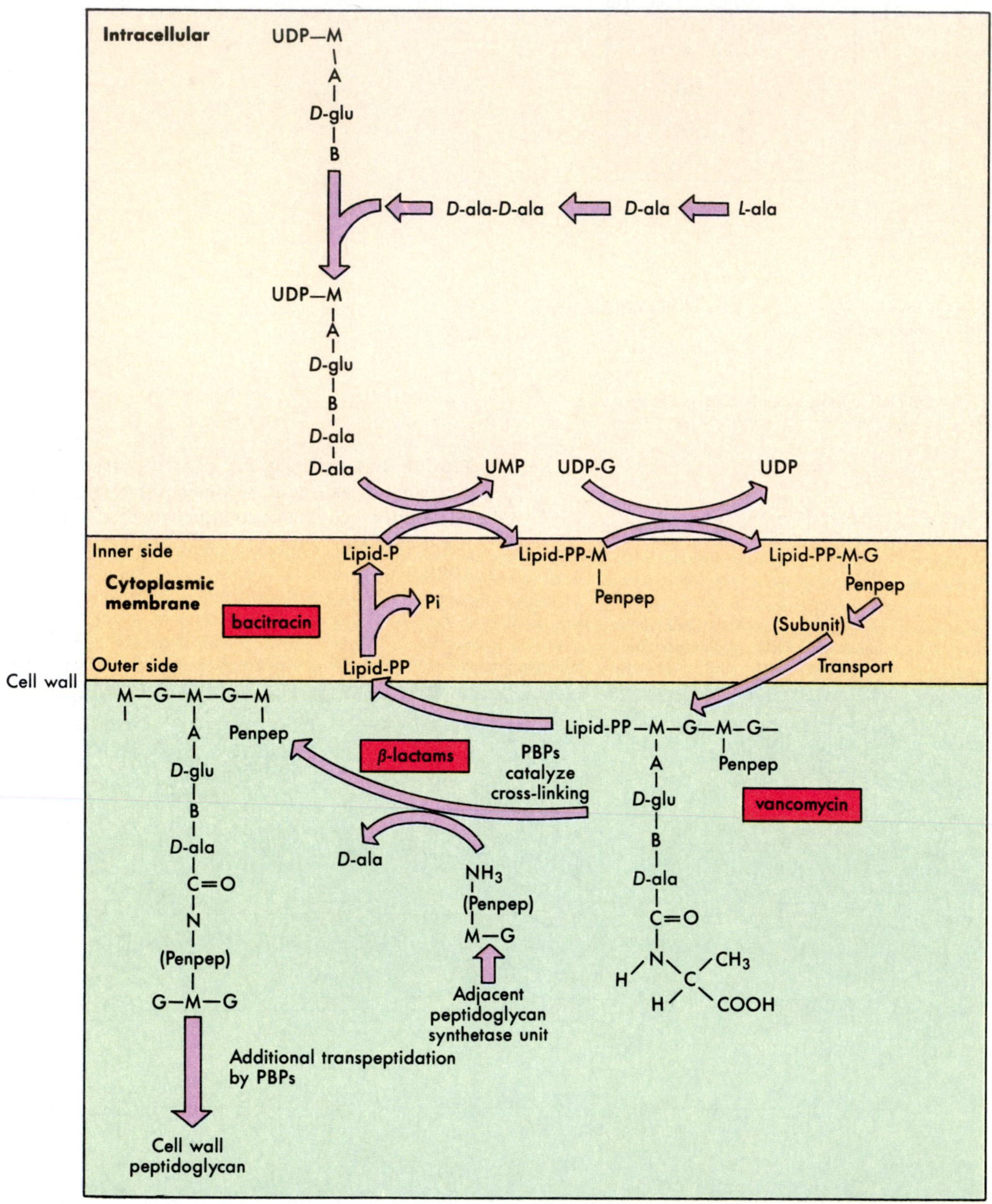

FIGURE 47-6 Summary of peptidoglycan cell wall synthesis and transport showing where in the sequence the cell wall–inhibitor drugs act. Details in the intracellular portion are shown in Figure 47-4. *UDP,* Uridine diphosphate; *M,* acetylmuramate with lactyl group; *Ala,* alanine; *D-Glu,* D-glucose; *B,* another amino acid (lysine in Figure 47-4 can vary with the organism); *UMP,* uridine monophosphate; *G, N*-acetylglucosamine; *P* and *PP,* phosphate and pyrophosphate; *penpep,* pentapeptide of A-Glu-B-Ala-Ala; *A,* L-alanine; *UDP-G,* uridine-diphospho-*N*-acetylglucosamine.

Table 47-1 Penicillin-Binding Proteins

PBP Number	Molecular Weight (daltons)	Relative Amount in Bacteria (%)	Effect if Inactivated	Function of PBP
GRAM-NEGATIVE BACTERIA				
1A	90,000	6*	None unless 1B absent	Compensates for loss of 1B
1Bs†	87,000	2*	Rapid cell lysis	Cell elongation
2	66,000	<0.5*	Oval cell formation	Maintains rod shape
3	60,000	2*	Long filaments form	Septation
4	49,000	4‡	None	May increase cross-linkage
5	42,000	65‡	None	—
6	40,000	21‡	None	Regulate cross-linkages
STAPHYLOCOCCI (GRAM-POSITIVE) BACTERIA				
1	80,000	10	Contributes to lethality	—
2§	70,000	80	Death of bacteria	—
3	60,000-70,000	80	Death of bacteria	— —
4	46,000	10	Not essential	

*Transpeptidases.
†Several proteins.
‡Carboxypeptidase.
§Production of new PBP-2, i.e., PBP-2a, results in resistance to β-lactam antibiotics.

synthesis and the points of antibiotic attack are summarized in Figure 47-6.

The multiple β-lactam–sensitive transpeptidase enzymes in bacterial cytoplasmic membranes are called penicillin-binding proteins (PBPs), since they covalently bind radiolabeled penicillin G. Some of the PBPs are cross-linking enzymes that are inhibited by the β-lactams. The PBPs in a given organism are numbered in order of decreasing molecular weight. The PBPs of gram-negative and gram-positive bacteria differ, with usually five PBPs in gram-positive and six PBPs in gram-negative organisms. However, the particular numerical designations are not the same protein in different organisms. For example, PBP-3 from one organism is not the same as PBP-3 from a different organism. Specific PBPs vary considerably in their relative abundance; all the PBPs make up about 1% of the total membrane protein in a bacterial cell. The PBPs differ between gram-negative and gram-positive bacteria, as shown in Table 47-1. In addition to transpeptidase action, some of the PBPs show carboxypeptidase or endopeptidase activity and function as β-lactam hydrolytic enzymes.

During the cross-linking reaction to connect the peptidoglycan chains, the D-Ala-D-Ala terminus of the lactyl pentapeptide reacts with a transpeptidase enzyme to displace the final D-Ala and form an acylenzyme intermediate along with the remaining free D-ala. The acylenzyme intermediate is reactive and readily couples to the free amino group of the third residue of the pentapeptide of an adjacent chain, thus completing the cross-linking and also regenerating the enzyme. Molecular modeling shows that penicillins and cephalosporins can assume a conformation that is very similar to that of the D-Ala-D-Ala peptide, with the reactive β-lactam ring in the same position in which the PBP acylation site is believed to sit (Figure 47-7). Therefore β-lactam antibiotics undergo acylation, with the β-lactam ring forming a covalent compound with a PBP. It is thought that the β-lactam ring opens and reacts with the OH group on a serine residue at the active site of the enzyme. This drug-PBP compound is not subject to further reaction, as is the D-Ala-D-Ala-PBP intermediate. Thus with the drug, the PBP enzyme is inactivated and the cross-link to the peptidoglycan chains is not carried out. The resulting morphological effects depend on the bacterial species and the PBP on which the β-lactam drug is bound. Some bacteria swell rapidly and burst. Some develop into long filamentous structures that do not divide but eventually fragment with disruption of the organism. Others show no morphological change and cease to be viable. The lysis of gram-positive bacteria treated with β-lactams may be related to murein hydrolyases, which are normally involved in the synthesis of the new wall when cells divide. Some bacteria may lack these autolysins and hence be only inhibited, not killed, by β-lactam antibiotics.

The structures of common penicillins, cephalosporins, and other β-lactam antimicrobial agents are given

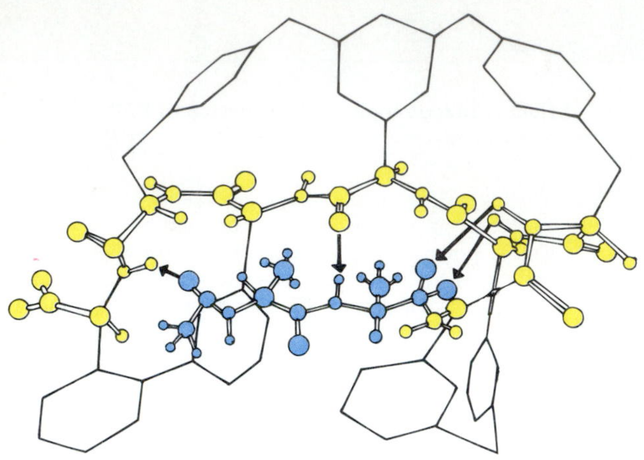

FIGURE 47-7 Schema of the interaction between a glycopeptide (structure simplified) and acyl-D-alanyl-D-alanine. The arrows indicate hydrogen bonds.

in Figure 47-8. The structure of moxalactam has a nucleus that is not naturally occurring; the sulfur at position 1 is substituted by an oxygen.

Mechanisms of Bacterial Resistance to β-Lactams

There are three major mechanisms of resistance to β-lactam antibiotics. These include (1) destruction by β-lactam enzymes, (2) failure to reach the target PBP, and (3) failure to bind to the target PBP (Figure 47-9). Another possibility, increased production of a PBP, was created in the laboratory but so far has not been detected clinically.

The major forms of resistance of gram-positive bacteria to β-lactam drugs are from β-lactamases or from altered PBPs (see Figure 47-9). Within a few years of the initial widespread use of penicillin G, most *Staphylococcus aureus* demonstrated resistance to the drug, resulting in major problems for hospitals, where this microorganism is usually present. Over 90% of staphylococci are resistant to penicillin G and to ampicillin. The resistance occurs by spread of a plasmid-mediated β-lactamase, which acylates the β-lactam ring to produce inactive drug. In gram-positive species, such as staphylococci, the β-lactamases are induced by penicillin and secreted into the environment as exoenzymes.

The presence of an altered PBP confers resistance to β-lactams, especially in gram-positive organisms, and results in failure of a particular drug to bind to a key PBP. The important clinical example is the methicillin resistance of staphylococci, with methicillin-resistant *S. aureus* posing a serious hospital problem. These staphylococci are not inhibited by any of the currently available β-lactams because of the poor affinity to PBP-2a (see Table 47-1). *Streptococcus pneumoniae* is penicillin resistant because of alteration of several PBPs. The failure to bind to PBPs is also the reason cephalosporins do not inhibit enterococci, such as *Streptococcus faecalis* and *S. faecium*. Aztreonam also does not inhibit gram-positive species, since it fails to bind to the PBPs.

In gram-negative bacteria, the common forms of resistance are the presence of β-lactamases and failure of the drug to reach the PBPs in the periplasmic space adjacent to the outer lipopolysaccharide membrane (see Figure 47-9). The synthesis of β-lactamases of gram-negative bacteria can be by chromosome-directed routes or by plasmid-directed routes. A wider variety of β-lactamases are produced by gram-negative bacteria than by gram-positive bacteria.

Gram-negative bacteria have an outer lipid membrane through which β-lactam drugs must pass to reach the PBPs located on the cytoplasmic membrane (see Figure 47-3). Channels contain outer membrane proteins referred to as porins which allow β-lactams to pass through the membrane. Changes that reduce the amount of drug reaching the PBPs via porin proteins have been observed. Some β-lactam antibiotic structures are extremely stable to β-lactamase exposure but do not readily pass through porins of gram-negative outer membranes and thus fail to inhibit these bacteria. If less drug crosses the membrane to reach the enzyme and the concentration of β-lactamase is large, resistance may occur, since small amounts of even very stable agents can be destroyed. But compounds that have poor affinity and high stability for β-lactamases can inhibit the resistance. *Pseudomonas aeruginosa* can lose its outer membrane proteins and become resistant to imipenem, which is extremely β-lactamase resistant.

Amino acid sequence data indicate that there are three classes of β-lactamases: classes A and C include serine enzymes and Class B includes metalloproteins. The molecular weights of the β-lactamases range from 12,000 to 32,000 daltons. The β-lactam inhibitors, clavulanic acid, sulbactam, and tazobactan, are strong inhibitors of class A, but not of classes B or C, β-lactamases. Coadministration of a β-lactamase inhibitor with a β-lactam antibiotic is an alternative approach to the use of β-lactam antibiotics inherently resistant to β-lactamases.

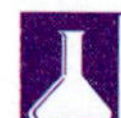

PHARMACOKINETICS

Penicillins

Penicillins differ greatly in their oral absorption, binding to serum proteins, metabolism, and renal excretion.

Text continued on page 645.

Penicillins

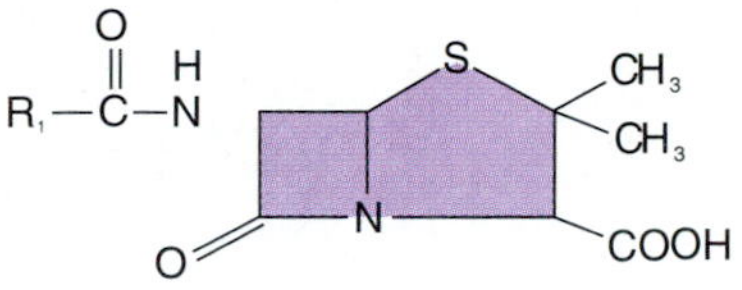

R$_1$—C(=O)—N(H)— ; S ; CH$_3$; CH$_3$; N ; O ; COOH

Name	Group R_1
penicillin G (benzylpenicillin)	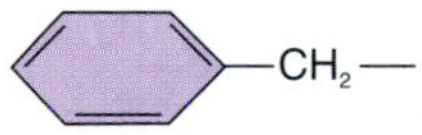 —CH_2—
penicillin V	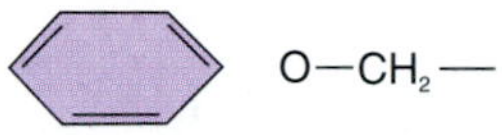 O—CH_2—
methicillin	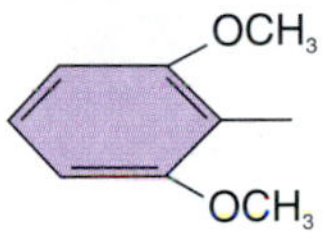 OCH_3, OCH_3
oxacillin	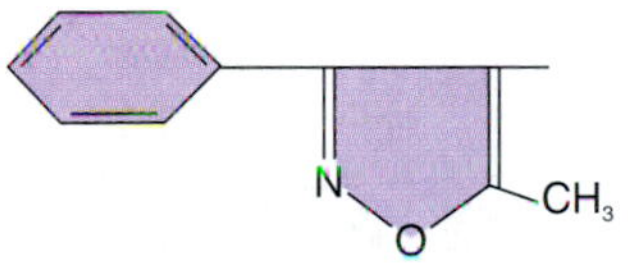 N, O, CH_3
cloxacillin	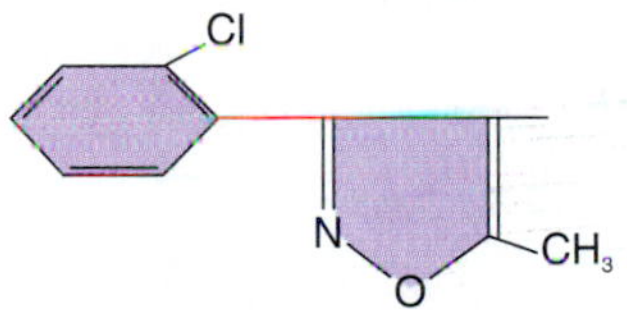 Cl, N, O, CH_3
dicloxacillin	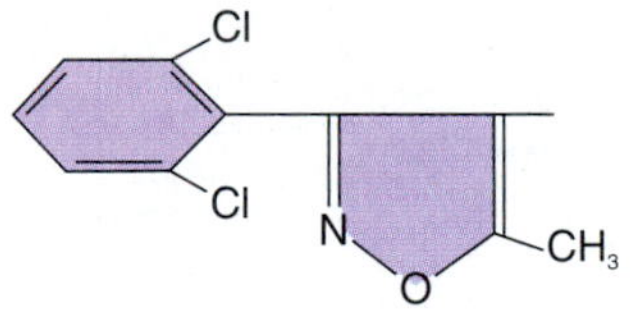 Cl, Cl, N, O, CH_3
nafcillin	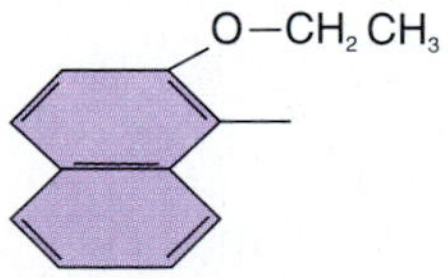 O—CH_2CH_3
ampicillin	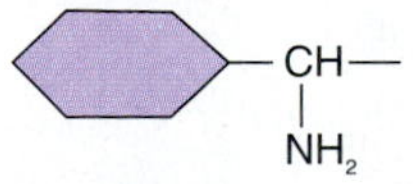 CH—, NH_2

FIGURE 47-8 Structures of β-lactam antibiotics of clinical interest, including penicillins, cephalosporins, carbapenems, monobactams, and β-lactamase inhibitors.

Continued.

amoxicillin

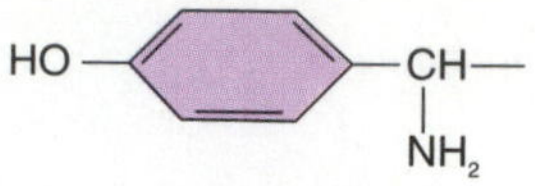

HO—C_6H_4—CH(NH$_2$)—

carbenicillin

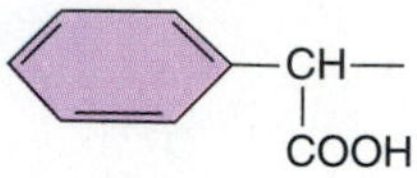

C_6H_5—CH(COOH)—

ticarcillin

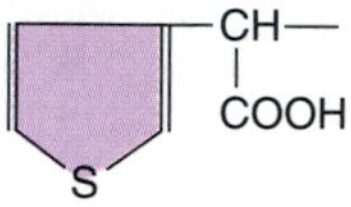

thienyl—CH(COOH)—

azlocillin

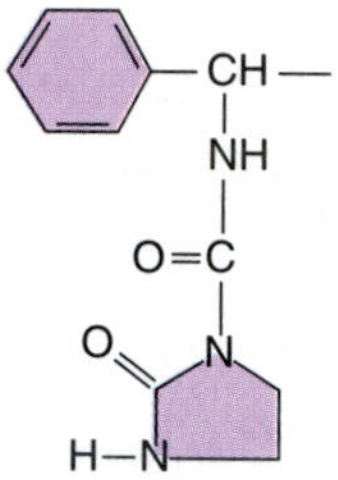

C_6H_5—CH(NH—C(=O)—N)—

mezlocillin

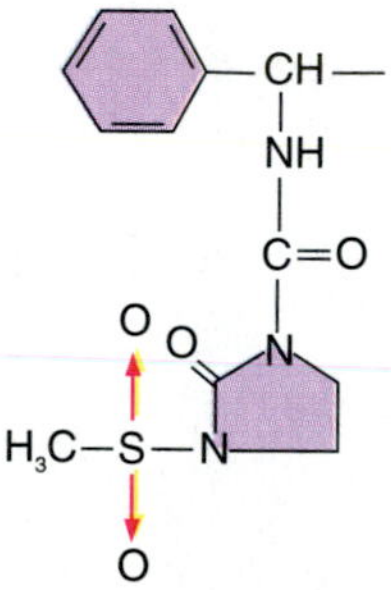

C_6H_5—CH(NH—C(=O)—N)—; H_3C—SO_2—N

piperacillin

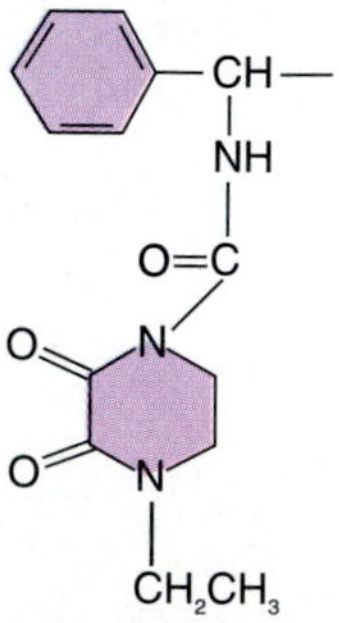

C_6H_5—CH(NH—C(=O)—N)—; N—CH_2CH_3

amdinocillin

N—CH=N—; S; CH_3; CH_3; N; O; COOH

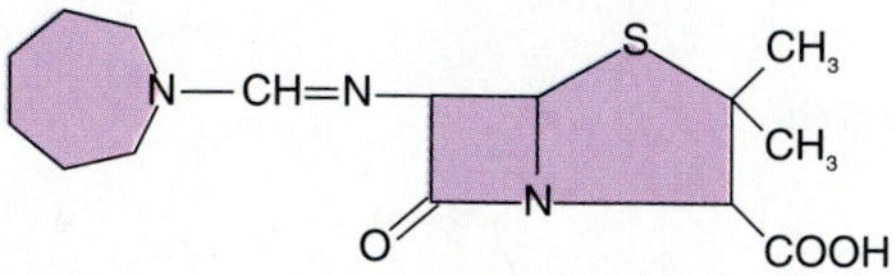

FIGURE 47-8, cont'd For legend see p. 639.

Cephalosporin

Name	R_1	R_2
First Generation		
cephalexin	–CH– NH$_2$	CH$_3$
cephalothin	S CH$_2$–	O CH$_2$ O C CH$_3$
cepazolin	N–CH$_2$– N N N	–CH$_2$–S– N N S –CH$_3$
cephradine	–CH– NH$_2$	CH$_3$
cefadroxil	HO– –CH– NH$_2$	–CH$_3$
Second Generation		
cefaclor	–CH– NH$_2$	–Cl
cefamandole	–CH– OH	–CH$_2$–S– N N N N CH$_3$
cefuroxime	O C– N–OCH$_3$	CH$_2$OCONH$_2$
Cefonicid	–CH– OH	–CH$_2$–S– N N N N N CH$_2$SO$_3$H

FIGURE 47-8, cont'd For legend see p. 639.

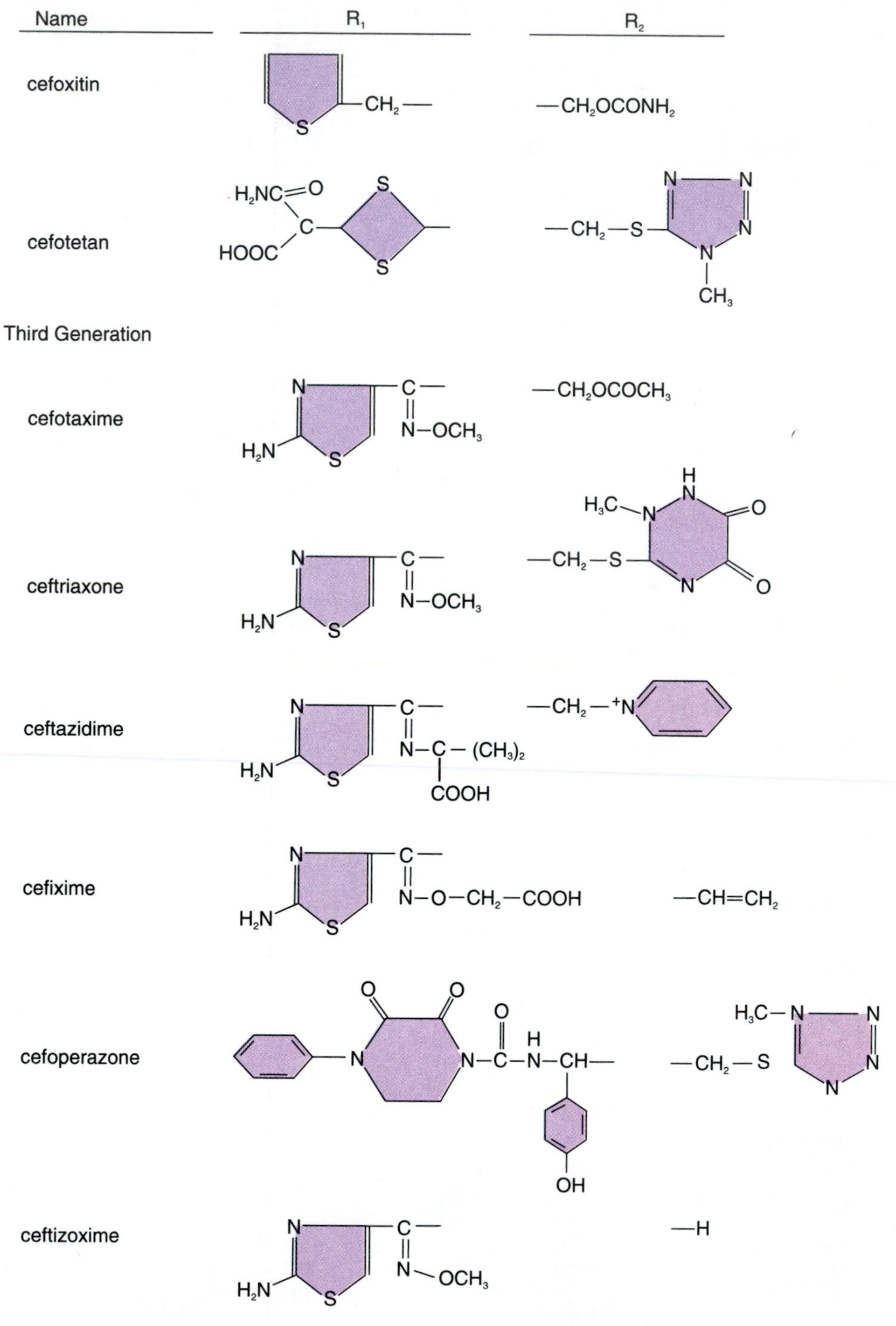

Name	R_1	R_2
cefoxitin	S, $-CH_2-$	$-CH_2OCONH_2$
cefotetan	$H_2NC{=}O$, C, HOOC, S, S	$-CH_2-S-$, N, N, N, N, CH_3
Third Generation		
cefotaxime	N, H_2N, S, $C-$, $N-OCH_3$	$-CH_2OCOCH_3$
ceftriaxone	N, H_2N, S, $C-$, $N-OCH_3$	H, H_3C-N, N, O, $-CH_2-S-$, N, O
ceftazidime	N, H_2N, S, $C-$, $N-C-(CH_3)_2$, COOH	$-CH_2-{}^{+}N$
cefixime	N, H_2N, S, $C-$, $N-O-CH_2-COOH$	$-CH{=}CH_2$
cefoperazone	N, O, O, $N-C-N-CH-$, O, H, OH	$-CH_2-S$, H_3C-N, N, N, N
ceftizoxime	N, H_2N, S, $C-$, $N-OCH_3$	$-H$

FIGURE 47-8, cont'd For legend see p. 639.

Name	R_1	R_2
moxalactam		

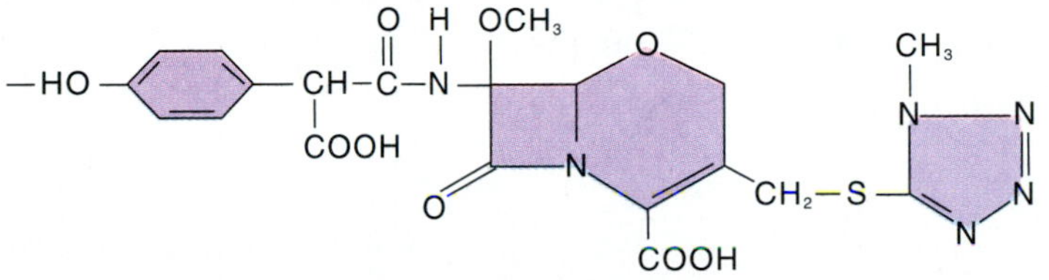

Carbapenems

imipenem

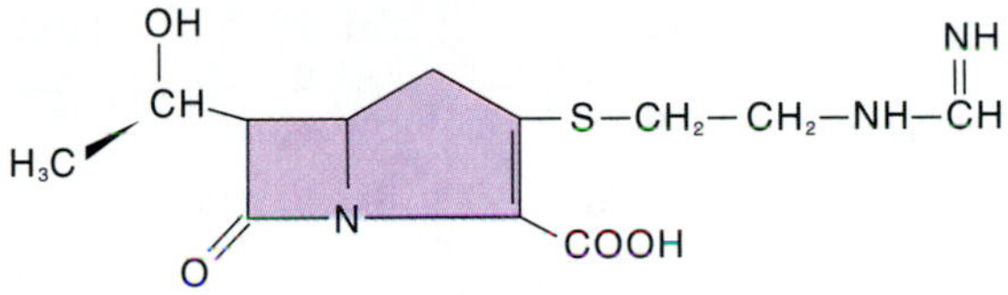

Monobactams

aztreonam

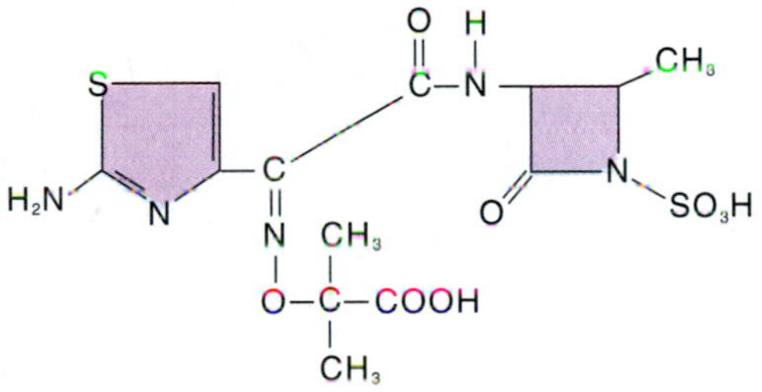

ß-Lactamase Inhibitors

clavulanate

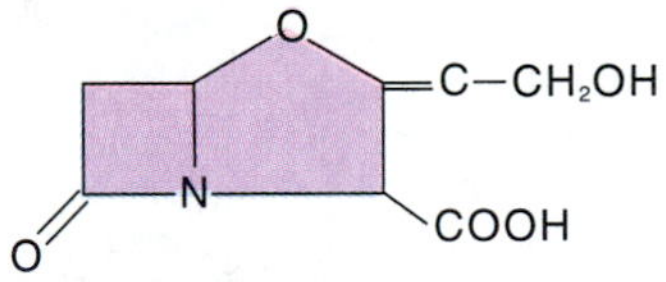

sulbactam

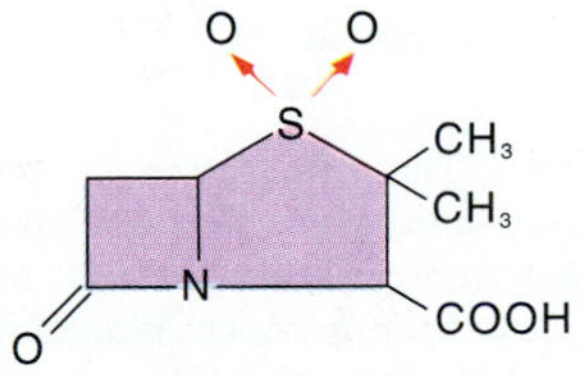

FIGURE 47-8, cont'd For legend see p. 639.

Table 47-2 Pharmacokinetic Parameters of Penicillin

Penicillin	Oral	IV	$t_{1/2}$ (hr)	Protein Bound (%)	Elimination
penicillin G	*	Yes	0.5	55	R (main), M
penicillin procaine G	No*	Yes	12 hours	55	R (main)
benzathine penicillin G	No*	Yes	14 days	55	R (main)
penicillin V	Yes	Yes	1.0	60	R (main)
methicillin	Poor	Yes	0.5	35	R (main), M
oxacillin	Yes	Yes	0.4	92	R (main), M
cloxacillin	Yes	Yes	0.4	94	R (main), M
dicloxacillin	Yes	Yes	0.6	97	R (main), M
nafcillin	Poor	Yes	0.5	90	R(some); mainly B
ampicillin	Yes	Yes	1.0	15	R(some); some B
amoxicillin	Yes	Yes	1.0	15	R (main)
carbenicillin	No*	Yes	1.2	50	R (main), M
ticarcillin	No*	Yes	1.2	50	R (main), M
azlocillin	No	Yes	0.8	30	R (main), some M
mezlocillin	No	—	1.0	50	R (main), M
piperacillin	No	—	1.3	50	R (main), M
amdinocillin	No	Yes	1.0	20	R (main), M

M, metabolism; *B*, biliary; *R*, renal.
*Poor acid stability.

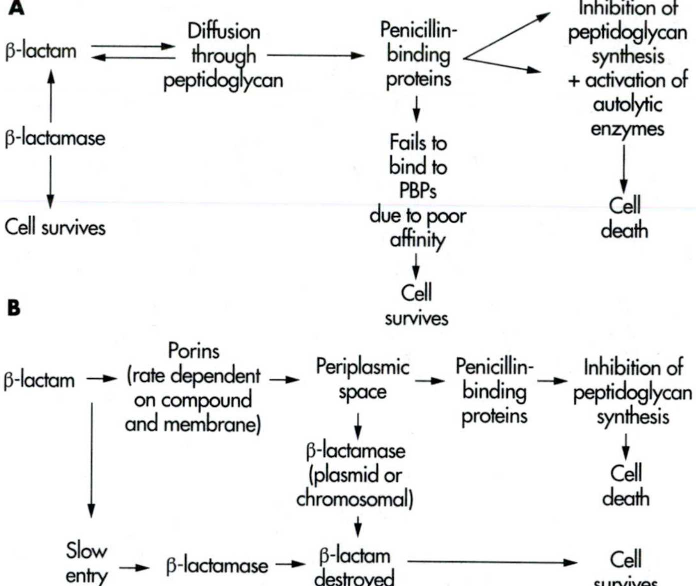

FIGURE 47-9 The interaction of β-lactam antibiotics with gram-positive and gram-negative bacteria. **A,** Gram-positive bacteria. **B,** Gram-negative bacteria. In resistant gram-positive bacteria such as Staphylococci, β-lactamases are excreted as exoenzymes and destroy the β-lactams, or the bacteria contain transpeptidases, which fail to bind the β-lactams. In gram-negative bacteria, β-lactam antibiotics enter the periplasmic space of bacteria through outer membrane proteins, porins. In the space between the outer wall and the cytoplasmic membrane, β-lactamases can destroy the β-lactams before they reach and bind to penicillin bound proteins.

Most penicillins are excreted as unchanged drug via renal tubular mechanisms, and adjustment of dosage is necessary in the presence of severely depressed renal function.

In general, penicillins are well distributed to most areas of the body, achieving therapeutic concentrations in some abscesses and in otic, pleural, peritoneal, and synovial fluids. Distribution to eye, brain, and prostatic fluid is low, whereas urinary concentrations generally are high. Concentrations of penicillins in cerebrospinal fluid are less than 1% of plasma values in uninflamed meninges and rise to 5% of plasma concentrations during inflammation. Penicillins do not enter phagocytic cells to any major extent, since the drug that enters is extruded by an anion pump.

Pharmacokinetic parameters for specific penicillins of clinical interest are summarized in Table 47-2.

Penicillins G and V and β-Lactamase-Resistant Penicillins

Penicillin G is not acid stable and is rapidly hydrolyzed in the stomach when ingested with food. Absorption is rapid, primarily in the duodenum, and is enhanced in persons with achlorhydria. Unabsorbed penicillin is destroyed by bacteria in the colon. In contrast, penicillin V is acid stable and well absorbed even if ingested with food.

After IM injection of penicillin G, a peak plasma concentration is achieved in 15 to 30 minutes but falls quickly because the drug is rapidly removed by the kidney. The half-life is 30 minutes. Repository forms of penicillin are available as procaine or benzathine salts. Procaine penicillin is an equimolar mixture of procaine and penicillin that delays the peak concentration by 1 to 3 hours. Serum and tissue concentrations of penicillin G are present for up to 12 hours after 300,000 units, and for several days after doses of 2.4 million units.

Benzathine penicillin is a combination of 1 mol of penicillin and 2 mols of the ammonium base, that is slowly absorbed and produces a detectable plasma concentration for up to 15 to 30 days.

Penicillin G is widely distributed throughout the body, with a volume of distribution equivalent to that of extracellular fluid. In the presence of inflammation, cerebrospinal fluid (CSF) concentrations reach approximately 5% of peak plasma values, and penicillin secretion from the CSF can be blocked by probenecid.

Approximately 10% of penicillin G is eliminated by glomerular filtration and 90% by tubular secretion. Renal clearance is equivalent to renal plasma flow, with a maximum rate of approximately 3 million units eliminated per hour. The excretion of penicillin can be blocked by probenecid, prolonging the plasma half-life. Renal elimination of penicillin is considerably lower in newborns because of poorly developed tubular function; the half-life of penicillin G is 3 hours in newborns compared to 30 minutes in children 1 year of age. As age increases, renal tubular excretory ability declines, with a corresponding increase in drug half-life. In the presence of anuria, the half-life is approximately 10 hours. In general, adjustments in dosage are not necessary until renal clearance decreases below 30 ml/min. Hepatic metabolism to penicilloic acid can inactivate penicillin G to some extent when renal function fails; thus with combined renal and hepatic failure, serious accumulation of drug can occur if dosing is not reduced.

Hemodialysis will remove penicillin G from the body, but peritoneal dialysis is less efficient. A small amount of penicillin is excreted in human milk and saliva, but it is not present in tears or sweat.

Considering the β-lactamase–resistant penicillins, only methicillin is not acid stable and must be administered IV, though rapid absorption occurs after IM injection. Its plasma half-life, distribution, and excretion are similar to those of penicillin G.

β-Lactamase–resistant penicillins (oxacillin, cloxacillin, and dicloxacillin) are absorbed when administered orally, but absorption is decreased by the presence of food. Oxacillin is least well absorbed, with cloxacillin absorbed twice as well and dicloxacillin four times as well as oxacillin. Peak plasma concentrations are achieved approximately 1 hour after ingestion. All these drugs are highly bound to plasma albumin (>90%). Elimination is primarily via the kidney with some biliary excretion and some liver metabolism. These drugs are minimally removed from the body by hemodialysis. Oxacillin is less effective orally; intravenously it achieves adequate plasma and cerebrospinal fluid concentrations.

Nafcillin is erratically absorbed when ingested orally, with or without food, and plasma concentrations are low after IM injection; thus the preferred route is IV. Elimination is primarily by excretion in bile and, to a much lesser extent, via kidney. It enters the CSF in concentrations adequate to treat staphylococcal meningitis or brain abscesses.

Aminopenicillins, Carboxypenicillins, and Ureidopenicillins

Ampicillin is moderately well absorbed after oral administration, but absorption is decreased and peak plasma concentrations are delayed by food. The half-life can be prolonged by coadministration of probenecid. Ampicillin is well distributed to most body compartments and achieves therapeutic concentrations in pleural, synovial, and peritoneal fluids. CSF concentrations in the presence of inflammation are adequate to treat meningitis because of susceptible *Streptococcus pneumoniae, Haemophilus influenzae,* and *Neisseria meningitidis.* Ampicillin is excreted in bile and undergoes enterohepatic recirculation. Urinary concentrations remain high until renal function is greatly reduced (creatinine clearance <15 ml/min).

Amoxicillin is better absorbed after oral ingestion than ampicillin and is not influenced by food. Distribution is similar to ampicillin.

Bacampicillin is an inactive ester of ampicillin that undergoes hydrolysis in the intestinal mucosa and plasma to yield ampicillin.

Carbenicillin and ticarcillin are not absorbed from the gastrointestinal tract and are therefore administered parenterally. They are rarely used intramuscularly, since plasma concentrations are inadequate for treatment of *Pseudomonas* species tissue infections. Both are secreted by renal tubules. Distribution is extensive except for inadequate concentrations in CSF for treating *Pseudomonas* meningitis.

Because none of the ureidopenicillins are orally absorbed, administration is limited to IV or IM. These drugs have nonlinear pharmacokinetics, with peak plasma concentrations and area under the drug versus time curves not proportional to dose.

Cephalosporins

Many of the cephalosporins can be administered only by the parenteral route. Although cephalosporins are distributed widely into body compartments, only a few enter the CSF to yield sufficient concentrations to treat meningitis. All of the cephalosporins, including those eliminated primarily by hepatic mechanisms, provide high enough urinary concentrations to treat urinary tract infections. In the absence of common duct obstruction, biliary concentrations of cephalosporins exceed the plasma concentrations for all agents. Aminothiazolyl cephalosporins penetrate the aqueous humor and are useful in the treatment of ocular infections.

Cephalosporins with an acetoxy side-chain undergo metabolism to yield a desacetyl compound. Some are inactive; the desacetyl metabolite of cefotaxime is less active than the parent compound but more active than most first- and second-generation drugs.

Cephalosporins are generally eliminated by renal mechanisms with varying degrees of tubular secretion and glomerular filtration. Accumulation of the agents depends on the status of renal clearance mechanisms. Cefoperazone and ceftriaxone are excreted to a major degree by the biliary route.

Pharmacokinetic parameters for the cephalosporins of clinical interest are listed in Table 47-3.

First-generation Cephalosporins Cephalothin is not absorbed orally and is extremely painful when administered IM; therefore it must be administered IV. Because of the short half-life, it is not used much today. Cephalothin is metabolized to a less active desacetyl derivative.

Cefazolin can be administered IM or IV and is widely distributed but does not adequately penetrate into the CSF. Clearance is by glomerular filtration and tubular secretion with no metabolism.

Cephalexin, cefadroxil, and cephradine are extremely well absorbed orally to give wide distribution in body tissues, including bone. They are not metabolized, with elimination by glomerular filtration and tubular secretion, and renal failure requires adjustment of the dosing regimen. An orally administered agent, cefaclor, undergoes metabolism to inactive fragments in addition to renal elimination by glomerular filtration and tubular secretion. Loracarbef is similar in activity to cefaclor, but replacement of the sulfur with a carbon has produced a more stable compound.

Second-generation Cephalosporins Cefamandole is not absorbed orally, is not metabolized, and is eliminated primarily by tubular secretion. Parenterally administered cefuroxime also is not metabolized, with renal elimination by glomerular filtration and tubular secretion.

Administration of cefoxitin is limited to IV or IM with good distribution in the body except for inadequate CSF concentrations. Elimination is similar to the other cephalosporins. Cefotetan is administered IV and has a long half-life ($t_{1/2}$) of 4 hours. It is renally excreted.

Third-generation Cephalosporins Third-generation cefotaxime, ceftriaxone, ceftizoxime, and moxalactam enter the CSF and can be used to treat meningitis. Cefotaxime is partially metabolized to a desacetyl derivative, which has antibacterial activity less than that of cefotaxime but greater than that for most first-generation or second-generation cephalosporins. The metabolite acts synergistically with cefotaxime against many microorganisms. Elimination is by tubular secretion and is blocked by probenecid; half-lives of the parent drug and the metabolite are increased in renal failure.

Ceftriaxone differs from other cephalosporins by its long plasma half-life of 6 to 8 hours. In addition, its plasma protein binding (90%) is concentration dependent, with a greater fraction of free drug present at higher total concentrations, and so the drug is administered once daily. Ceftriaxone is not metabolized, with 60% excreted in the bile and the remainder eliminated by the kidney. Dosage must be adjusted in the presence of combined hepatic-renal dysfunction. Cefoperazone is eliminated by both biliary (75%) and renal (25%) mechanisms. Cefixime is moderately well absorbed orally and

Table 47-3 Pharmacokinetic Parameters of Cephalosporins

cephalosporin	Oral	IV	$t_{1/2}$ (hr)	Protein Bound (%)	Renal Elimination	Metabolized†
FIRST GENERATION						
cephalothin	No	Yes	0.5	70	Yes, T	Yes
cefazolin	No	Yes	2.0	85	Yes, T	No
cephalexin	Yes	No	1.0	15	Yes, T	No
cephradine	Yes	Yes	0.5	18	Yes, T	No
cefadroxil	Yes	No	1.5	20	Yes, T	No
cefaclor	Yes	No	1.0	25	Yes, T	Yes
cefprozil	Yes	No	1	20	Yes, T	No
loracarbef	Yes	No	1	25	Yes, T	No
SECOND GENERATION						
cefamandole	No	Yes	0.7	70	Yes, T	No
cefuroxime	Yes	Yes	1.7	35	Yes, T	No
cefonicid	No	Yes	3.5-4.0	>90	Yes, T	No
cefoxitin	No	Yes	0.8	70	Yes, T	No
cefotetan	No	Yes	3.5-4.0	85	Yes, T	No
THIRD GENERATION						
cefotaxime	No	Yes	1.0 (1.6 metabolite)	50	Yes, T	Yes (active)
ceftizoxime	No	Yes	1.8	30	Yes, T	No
ceftriaxone	No	Yes	6-8	90	Yes, T	No; bile (60%)
moxalactam*	No	Yes	2.0	60	Yes, G	No
cefixime	Yes	No	3.0-4.0	75	Yes, T	No
ceftazidime	No	Yes	1.6-2.0	15	Yes, G	No
cefoperazone	No	Yes	2.0	85	Yes, T	No; bile (75%)
cefpodoxime	Yes	No	1.2	25	Yes, T	No

G, glomerular; *T*, tubular.
*Bleeding problem
†Primary route.

has a half-life of about 4 hours. Cefpodoxime is better orally absorbed but has a short half-life.

Fourth-Generation Cephalosporins Cepirome and cefepime are fourth-generation cephalosporins, which have increased activity against gram-positive bacteria, inhibit *Pseudomonas aeruginosa,* and do not bind to β-lactamases of the type 1, cephalosporinase group as in *Enterobacter.*

Other β-Lactam Drugs

Pharmacokinetic parameters of clinical interest are summarized in Table 47-4 for imipenem, aztreonam, and the β-lactamase inhibitors.

Imipenem Imipenem is not absorbed orally because of its instability at gastric pH. In the United States, it is administered primarily IV. It is widely distributed but enters CSF only in the presence of inflammation. It has a high affinity for brain tissue. Imipenem is eliminated by glomerular filtration and tubular secretion and undergoes hydrolysis by a dihydropeptidase in the renal tubules. To overcome this hydrolysis, imipenem is combined with a renal dehydropeptidase inhibitor, cilastatin (see Figure 47-8 for structure). Cilastatin has no antibacterial activity and does not affect the antibacterial activity or pharmacokinetic properties of imipenem, except to prevent its hydrolysis. In the absence of cilastatin, less than 25% of imipenem is recovered in the urine, with nephrotoxic breakdown products. With cilastatin, 70% of imipenem is recovered as parent compound and 25% as metabolites. Minimal amounts of drug are excreted in bile, though biliary concentrations are adequate for treatment of biliary tract infections.

The serum $t_{1/2}$ of imipenem increases as creatinine clearance falls, reaching 4 hours in individuals with creatinine clearances <10 ml/min. The plasma half-life of cilastatin increases in patients with renal insufficiency, reaching 19 hours in anuria.

Meropenem Meropenem is a carbapenem with a spectrum similar to imipenem. It is not hydrolyzed by renal dihydropeptidase. It enters the CSF and is excreted by the kidneys.

Aztreonam Aztreonam is not absorbed after oral ingestion but can be administered IV or IM. It is widely

Table 47-4 Pharmacokinetic Parameters of Other β-Lactams and β-Lactamase Inhibitors

	Oral	IV	$t_{1/2}$ (hr)	Protein Bound (%)	Renal Elimination	Metabolized
OTHER β-LACTAMS						
imipenem	No	Yes	1.0	20	Yes	Yes*
aztreonam	No	Yes	1.5-2.0	45-60	Yes	No
meropenem	No	Yes	1	little	Yes	Yes (minor)
β-LACTAMASE INHIBITORS						
clavulanate (with amoxicillin or ticarcillin)	Yes (amox)	Yes (ticar)	1.0	20, 65	Yes	Yes (minor)
sulbactam (with ampicillin)	Yes	Yes	1.0	15	Yes	No
tazobactam (with piperacillin)	No	Yes	1.0	20, 50	Yes	No

*Prevented by cilastatin.

distributed to all body sites and compartments, including the CSF.

Aztreonam is removed from the body by glomerular filtration and tubular secretion. In neonates of less than 2.5 kg body weight, the $t_{1/2}$ is two to four times longer (5 to 10 hours). The $t_{1/2}$ increases from 1.6 to 6 hours when the creatinine clearance falls below 10 ml.

β-Lactamase Inhibitors Clinically, clavulanate, combined with amoxicillin or with ticarcillin, is available. Clavulanate is moderately well absorbed from the gastrointestinal tract, with peak plasma concentrations occurring 1 hour after ingestion. Combining clavulanate with amoxicillin does not alter the pharmacokinetics of either agent. Food, milk, and antacids do not affect its absorption.

When clavulanate is combined with ticarcillin and administered IV, it is rapidly distributed. Accumulation occurs when creatinine clearance is <10 ml/min. Clavulanate enters most body compartments with therapeutic concentrations in middle ear fluid, tonsillar tissue, sinus secretions, bile, and the urinary tract.

Sulbactam is combined with ampicillin for parenteral use. It will also be combined with cefoperazone. Sulbactam has pharmacokinetic properties similar to those for ampicillin and is widely distributed in the body, including the CSF in the presence of meningitis. It is not metabolized, and 75% of a dose is found in the urine. The $t_{1/2}$ is increased in renal failure to 6 hours in adults and in newborns.

Tazobactam is combined with piperacillin. Its half-life is prolonged in the presence of piperacillin and is excreted primarily by the kidneys.

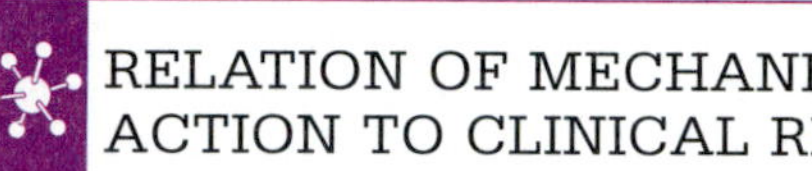

RELATION OF MECHANISMS OF ACTION TO CLINICAL RESPONSE

β-Lactam Penicillins and Cephalosporins

Antibacterial Activity of Penicillins Penicillins are classified by their main antibacterial activities, as follows:

1. Penicillin G and penicillin V are active against gram-positive and gram-negative cocci, except organisms that produce β-lactamase (penicillinase)
2. β-Lactamase (penicillinase)—resistant agents (methicillin, oxacillin, nafcillin, cloxacillin, and dicloxacillin) inhibit staphylococci and are less active than penicillin G against streptococci
3. Aminopenicillins (ampicillin and amoxicillin) are active against gram-positive and gram-negative organisms, and also inhibit β-lactamase–free strains of *Haemophilus influenzae, Neisseria gonorrhoea, Escherichia coli, Proteus mirabilis,* and *Salmonella* species
4. Carboxypenicillins (carbenicillin and ticarcillin) inhibit *Pseudomonas aeruginosa* and some *Enterobacter* and *Proteus* species but are destroyed by β-lactamases
5. Ureidopenicillins (azlocillin, mezlocillin, and piperacillin) inhibit ampicillin-susceptible organisms, *Pseudomonas,* some *Klebsiella* organisms (mezlocillin and piperacillin), and streptococci but are destroyed by some β-lactamases.

Penicillins G and V and β-Lactamase–resistant Penicillins The clinical uses of penicillins G and V are

Table 47-5 Summary of Clinical Uses of Penicillins G and V

Disorder or Organism(s)	Therapy
Streptococcus pyogenes (pharyngitis)	Penicillin V orally, procaine salt parenterally, or single benzathine injection; to reduce potential for rheumatic fever
S. pyogenes	
Less common serious types of pneumonia, arthritis, meningitis, or endocarditis	Penicillin G
Streptococcal sinusitis and otitis	Penicillin V orally
S. agalactiae, group B (meningitis or septicemia in newborns)	Penicillin G, ampicillin
Viridans streptococci as *S. mutans* or *S. mitis* (cause bacterial endocarditis)	Penicillin G; add aminoglycoside to penicillin G for some species
Pneumococcal infections (from otitis, sinusitis, and pneumonia to meningitis and other suppurative pneumococcal infections	Penicillin G; large IV doses for meningitis, endocarditis, septic arthritis, and pericarditis; lower doses for pneumonia
Anaerobic infections	
Oral area and chest	Occasionally penicillin
Intraabdominal and gynecological	Other agents preferred
Meningococcal	Penicillin G, but it will not eliminate carrier state and is not effective prophylactically
Gonococcal infections*	
Syphilis	Penicillin G main drug; for primary, secondary, or latent (<1 year) syphilis use single dose IM of benzathine penicillin; for latent syphilis (>1 year) use IV doses for central nervous system syphilis
Others	Penicillin G excellent for clostridial infections such as gas gangrene from *C. perfringens* or fusospirochetal, *Listeria* organisms, or *Pasturella* organisms from bites
Prophylaxis	Penicillins G or V will reduce recurrence of rheumatic fever in susceptible individuals. Individuals with cardiac lesions that predispose to endocarditis should receive prophylaxis during dental procedures with amoxicillin

*Increase in β-lactamase–producing *N. gonorrhoeae* has reduced effectiveness of penicillin G. Clavulanate and sulbactam add to amoxicillin, ampicillin, or ticarcillin for *Staphylococcus aureus*, coagulase-negative staphylococci, *Haemophilus influenzae, Moraxella catarrhalis, Neisseria gonorrhoeae, Escherichia coli, Klebsiella pneumoniae, Proteus vulgaris, Acinetobacter* species (sulbactam only), and *Bacteroides* species.

summarized in Table 47-5. Penicillin V is less effective than penicillin G with gram-negative species, such as *Neisseria* and *Haemophilus,* and some anaerobic species. Penicillin G inhibits most hemolytic streptococci, but most *Staphylococcus aureus* and coagulase-negative staphylococci are resistant. *Streptococcus pneumoniae* is susceptible in the United States but not in some European countries, and although *Neisseria meningitidis* remains highly susceptible, many strains of *N. gonorrhoeae* are resistant through plasmid-mediated β-lactamase production.

Many anaerobic species, except the *Bacteroides fragilis* group, are susceptible to penicillin G, but aerobic gram-negative Enterobacteriaceae and *Pseudomonas* species are resistant.

The β-lactamase–resistant penicillins include methicillin, oxacillin, nafcillin, cloxacillin, and dicloxacillin. These drugs are not destroyed by most β-lactamases of staphylococci. These penicillins are still used principally to treat staphylococcal infections, though some staphylococci contain altered penicillin-binding proteins and may show resistance to these agents. These agents are less active against oral-cavity anaerobic species than penicillin G is and show no activity against gram-negative bacilli.

The term *methicillin* resistance is used to indicate resistance of *Staphylococcus* species to all β-lactams. As discussed later, vancomycin is preferred for treating infections by such organisms.

Aminopenicillins, Carboxypenicillins, and Ureidopenicillins The aminopenicillins, ampicillin, amoxicillin, and bacampicillin (which undergoes in vivo conversion to ampicillin), are inactivated by β-lactamases of gram-positive and gram-negative bacteria. The antibacterial activity of all three compounds is similar, with two to four times more activity than penicillin G against enterococci and *Listeria monocytogenes.*

Ampicillin and amoxicillin are used to treat upper respiratory tract infections, provided that the infection is not caused by β-lactamase–producing *Haemophilus* organisms. Ampicillin and amoxicillin are also used to treat some urinary tract infections; both agents are effective against many *Salmonella typhi* strains.

The antibacterial activity of the carboxypenicillins (carbenicillin and ticarcillin) and that of three ureidopenicillins (azlocillin, mezlocillin, and piperacillin) differ in some important aspects. These agents inhibit *P. aeruginosa* but not β-lactamase–producing *S. aureus*, though they inhibit streptococcal and enterococcal species to varying degrees. All five antibiotics are inactivated by many of the β-lactamases of both gram-positive and gram-negative bacteria.

The ureidopenicillins (azlocillin, mezlocillin, and piperacillin) are ampicillin derivatives that have activities similar to ampicillin against streptococcal species. Azlocillin and piperacillin are 8 to 16 times more active than carbenicillin against *P. aeruginosa*. Mezlocillin and piperacillin have moderate activity against anaerobes and are similar to ticarcillin in activity against *Enterobacter, Serratia,* and *Providencia* species. These extended-spectrum penicillins were originally developed to treat infections of *P. aeruginosa* and, less commonly, *Proteus* and *Providencia* species but in recent years have been used to treat many other infections. These drugs are not used as single agents because of their β-lactamase susceptibility to treat serious infections but are combined with aminoglycosides or with β-lactamase inhibitors. They act synergistically with aminoglycosides to inhibit *P. aeruginosa*.

Antibacterial Activity of Cephalosporins The cephalosporins were discovered in 1945 from a fungus, *Cephalosporium acremonium,* in sea water samples obtained near a sewage outlet in Sardinia (see Figure 47-2 for structure). Compounds that possess a methoxy group at position 7 often are called *cephamycins,* but for practical purposes, these agents can be considered cephalosporins. Similarly, agents in which the sulfur at position 1 has been replaced by an oxygen are *oxycephems,* and agents in which the sulfur is replaced with a carbon are called *carbacephens,* Microbiologically and pharmacologically these agents are considered to be cephalosporins.

Cephalosporins are classified by generations based on antimicrobial activity. First-generation cephalosporins have relatively good activity against gram-positive organisms and moderate gram-negative activity, inhibiting many *E. coli, Proteus mirabilis,* and *Klebsiella pneumoniae.* Some second-generation compounds have increased activity against *Haemophilus* and inhibit more gram-negative organisms and show less activity than first-generation agents against staphylococci. Third-generation cephalosporins have less antistaphylococcal activity and more activity against streptococci, Enterobacteriaceae, *Neisseria,* and *Haemophilus* species. Some third-generation agents, ceftazidime and cefoperazone, also inhibit *P. aeruginosa.*

Like penicillins, the morphological effects of cephalosporins on bacteria depend on the penicillin-binding proteins to which the drugs bind. Resistance of bacteria to cephalosporins is caused by the same mechanisms that account for resistance to penicillins (see Figure 47-7), that is, hydrolysis by β-lactamases, failure to pass through the outer wall of gram-negative bacteria, or failure to bind to the penicillin-binding protein. Cephalosporins are more β-lactamase stable than penicillins are, in part because the cephalosporin structures are more resistant to β-lactamases.

First-generation Cephalosporins First-generation cephalosporins are cephalothin, cephradine, cefazolin, cephalexin, cefadroxil, and cefaclor. The spectra of activity are similar, with cephalothin inhibiting most gram-positive cocci (except for enterococci), many *E. coli, Klebsiella,* and *P. mirabilis.* Most other Enterobacteriaceae are resistant, and *Pseudomonas, Bacteroides,* and *Haemophilus* species are not inhibited. First-generation cephalosporins are used to treat respiratory, skin structure, and urinary tract infections and are also used as prophylaxis before surgery on the heart or before orthopedic prosthesis procedures.

Cefaclor shows greater intrinsic activity towards *H. influenzae* but less β-lactamase stability than cephalexin. It is used to treat upper respiratory tract infections in children. Cefprozil and loracarbef inhibit β-lactamase–producing *H. influenzae* and respiratory pathogens.

Several other first-generation cephalosporins (cephapirin, cephradine, and cefadroxil) are similar to cephalothin in antibacterial properties but differ in pharmacokinetic properties.

Second-generation Cephalosporins Second-generation cephalosporins include cefamandole, cefuroxime, cefonicid, cefoxitin, and cefotetan. Cefamandole and cefonicid are more active than the first-generation agents against gram-negative *Haemophilus* species, some *E. coli, Klebsiella* species, and other Enterobacteriaceae. They have adequate activity against gram-positive species but do not inhibit *Pseudomonas* or *Bacteroides.* Similarly, cefuroxime inhibits gram-positive organisms and also shows excellent activity against *Haemophilus* and *Neisseria* species and greater β-lactamase stability than cefamandole.

Cefoxitin is less active against gram-positive organisms than first-generation agents are, but its high β-lactamase stability and inhibition of many β-lactamase–producing Enterobacteriaceae (but not *Enterobacter* or *Citrobacter*) species and inhibition of 85% of anaerobic bacteria make it useful. In addition, it is not hydrolyzed by the plasmid-mediated β-lactamases that destroy cefotaxime, ceftriaxone, and ceftazidime. It is used to treat aspiration pneumonitis, intraabdominal, and pelvic infections. Cefotetan inhibits many β-lactamase–producing Enterobacteriaceae and most *Bacteroides.* It is used to treat intraabdominal and pelvic infection.

Third-generation Cephalosporins Third-generation cephalosporins include cefotaxime, ceftizoxime, ceftriaxone, moxalactam, cefixime (oral agent), cefpodoxime (oral), and two agents with activity against *Pseudomonas* species, ceftazidime and cefoperazone.

Cefotaxime has excellent activity against gram-positive streptococcal species, including *S. pneumoniae,* and gram-negative *Haemophilus* and *Neisseria* species. A metabolite acts synergistically with cefotaxime, and the two compounds have better activity against *Bacteroides* species than the parent compound. Ceftizoxime and ceftriaxone have similar activity to cefotaxime. These agents are used to treat nosocomial respiratory infections, urinary infections, skin structure infections, osteomyelitis, and meningitis. Ceftriaxone also is used to treat gonorrhea and Lyme disease.

Moxalactam, rarely used in the United States, inhibits Enterobacteriaceae, including β-lactamase–producing isolates, *Haemophilus* and *Neisseria,* most *Bacteroides* species and about 50% of *P. aeruginosa.*

Ceftazidime and cefoperazone inhibit *Pseudomonas aeruginosa.* Ceftazidime inhibits most streptococci, *Haemophilus,* and *Neisseria* and inhibits β-lactamase–producing isolates of these species and most of the Enterobacteriaceae. It does not inhibit *Bacteroides* species. Cefoperazone is less β-lactamase stable but inhibits many similar species.

Cefixime is an oral agent that inhibits streptococci, *Haemophilus* species, *Neisseria* species, *Moraxella* bacteria, and many Enterobacteriaceae. It does not inhibit staphylococci, *Pseudomonas* species, or *Bacteroides* organisms. It is used to treat respiratory infections. Cefpodoxime inhibits streptococci, *Haemophilus, Moraxella, Neisseria* and many members of the Enterobacteriaceae.

Other β-lactams

Imipenem Imipenem has structural chemical features that differentiate it from other β-lactams. It inhibits most gram-positive organisms such as the hemolytic streptococci, *S. pneumoniae,* viridans group streptococci, enterococci, and *S. aureus.* The majority of Enterobacteriaceae, *Haemophilus* species, *Moraxella, Neisseria* species, and *P. aeruginosa* also are inhibited by imipenem. Imipenem has extensive activity against anaerobic organisms, inhibiting most *Bacteroides* species. It also inhibits *Nocardia* and some mycobacteria. Imipenem has a high affinity for critical penicillin-binding proteins in a wide variety of organisms but not methicillin-resistant *Staphylococcus aureus* (MRSA) and *Enteroccus faecium.*

Imipenem shows an interesting postantibiotic effect on many gram-positive or gram-negative bacteria. After the concentration of drug falls below inhibitory concentrations, the bacteria that have not been killed do not resume growth for another 2 to 4 hours. Imipenem is not hydrolyzed by β-lactamases of gram-positive or gram-negative bacteria, with the exceptions of β-lactamases from *Xanthomonas maltophilia* and some *Bacteroides* species. Resistance to imipenem of *Pseudomonas aeruginosa* is attributable to lack of an outer-membrane porin protein (OD2).

The combination of imipenem-cilastatin is used to treat bacteremias and respiratory, intraabdominal, gynecological, bone and joint, and urinary tract infections because of resistant bacteria. It is used also in the treatment of aerobic or anaerobic bacterial infections, in which imipenem can be used as a single agent.

Monobactams

Aztreonam Aztreonam is a monocyclic β-lactam. The acyl side-chain, identical to that of ceftazidime, provides high affinity for penicillin-binding proteins of certain gram-negative bacteria.

Aztreonam inhibits only aerobic gram-negative bacteria, by binding to PBP-3 of Enterobacteriaceae and *P. aeruginosa* to produce long filamentous bacteria that ultimately lyse and die. It does not bind to the PBPs of gram-positive or anaerobic species. It is stable against attack by most β-lactamases, except from *Klebsiella oxytoca, Xanthomonas maltophilia,* or bacteria containing cefotoxime-ceftazidime hydrolyzing plasmid enzymes. Aztreonam is effective in the treatment of bacteremia, respiratory and urinary infections, osteomyelitis, and skin-structure infections. It can serve as a replacement for aminoglycosides and can be combined with clindamycin, semisynthetic penicillins, metronidazole, or vancomycin to treat mixed bacterial infections.

β-lactamase Inhibitors

Clavulanate Clavulanate is an inhibitor of β-lactamases of *S. aureus* and of many gram-negative bacteria, including plasmid-mediated common β-lactamases in *E. coli, Haemophilus, Neisseria, Salmonella,* and *Shigella* species and chromosomal β-lactamases of *Klebsiella, Moraxella,* and *Bacteroides* species.

Clavulanate has a β-lactam ring but has only minimal antibacterial activity, since it binds poorly to the penicillin-binding proteins of most species. It binds to serine at the active site of β-lactamases in an irreversible manner, resulting in inactivation of the enzyme. Thus clavulanate acts as a nonreversible or suicide inhibitor.

Clavulanate does not inhibit chromosomally mediated β-lactamases in *Pseudomonas, Enterobacter, Citrobacter,* and *Serratia* species. Combinations of clavulanate with amoxicillin or ticarcillin are used clinically.

CLINICAL PROBLEMS OF β-LACTAM AGENTS

- penicillin G
  - IgE antibody allergic reaction (anaphylaxis or early urticaria)
  - Neutropenia
- ampicillin
  - Delayed hypersensitivity and contact dermatitis
  - Idiopathic; skin rash and fever
  - Diarrhea
  - Enterocolitis
- oxacillin
  - Elevated aspartate aminotransferase (SGOT)
  - Neutropenia
- methicillin
  - Interstitial nephritis
- nafcillin
  - Elevated aspartate aminotransferase (SGOT)
- carbenicillin
  - Platelet dysfunction
  - Elevated aspartate aminotransferase
- carbenicillin—cont'd
  - Sodium overload
  - Hypokalemia
- moxalactam
  - Platelet dysfunction
  - Antabuse reaction
  - Prothrombin abnormality
- amoxicillin-clavulanate
  - Diarrhea
- cephalosporins
  - Idiopathic; skin rash and fever
  - Phlebitis; false-positive Coombs' or glucose tests
- cefixime, cefpodoxime
  - Diarrhea
- cefoxitin
  - Enterocolitis
- cefoperazone
  - Antabuse reaction
  - Prothrombin abnormality
- ceftriaxone
  - Precipitation in gallbladder
  - Diarrhea

See Table 47-6 for frequency of clinical problems.

The amoxicillin-clavulanate combination is used to treat otitis media in children and sinusitis, bacterial exacerbations of bronchitis, and lower respiratory tract infections in adults. It is also effective in skin structure infections, particularly when anaerobic as well as aerobic organisms are present. Human and animal bite wounds, gonorrhea, and lower tract urinary infections also can be treated with this combination. The ticarcillin-clavulanate combination is effective in treating hospital-acquired respiratory, intraabdominal, obstetric-gynecological, and skin structure infections, and osteomyelitis when mixed bacteria are present.

Sulbactam Sulbactam is a penicillanic acid derivative that has extremely weak antibacterial activity against gram-positive cocci and Enterobacteriaceae and inhibits several other organisms at elevated concentrations. Sulbactam acts as an irreversible inhibitor of the β-lactamases that are inhibited by clavulanate. Sulbactam is slightly less potent than clavulanate as an inhibitor of β-lactamases and enters the periplasmic space of some bacteria less effectively than clavulanate does. Sulbactam is available clinically as an ampicillin-sulbactam combination.

Tazobactam Tazobactam is a penicillanic acid derivative. It inhibits β-lactamases similar to clavulanate and sulbactam. It is combined with piperacillin.

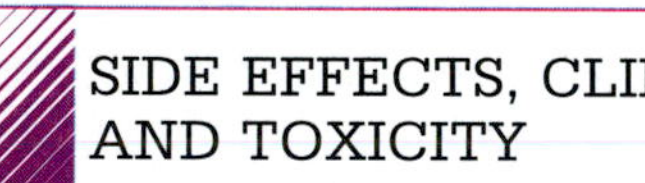

SIDE EFFECTS, CLINICAL PROBLEMS, AND TOXICITY

Problems in the clinical use of the β-lactam antibiotics are summarized in the box above.

Penicillins

Adverse reactions with penicillins fortunately are few. Hypersensitivity, which can be life threatening, is the most important. Hypersensitivity includes anaphylaxis or less severe skin eruptions. Penicillins act as haptens to produce antigens that combine with proteins to evoke IgE-mediated antibody reactions. Penicillins also can undergo partial degradation to compounds that have varying allergic potential. The major determinants of penicillin allergy are penicilloyl acid derivatives (Figure 47-10), but minor components of benzylpenicillin and benzylpenicilloate are important mediators of anaphylaxis. Anaphylactic reactions to penicillins are uncommon, occurring in 0.2% of 10,000 courses of treatment. In contrast, a morbilliform skin eruption type of allergy occurs in 3% to 5% of patients receiving penicillin.

Skin testing with benzylpenicilloyl polylysine, benzylpenicillin G, and sodium benzylpenicilloate (Figure

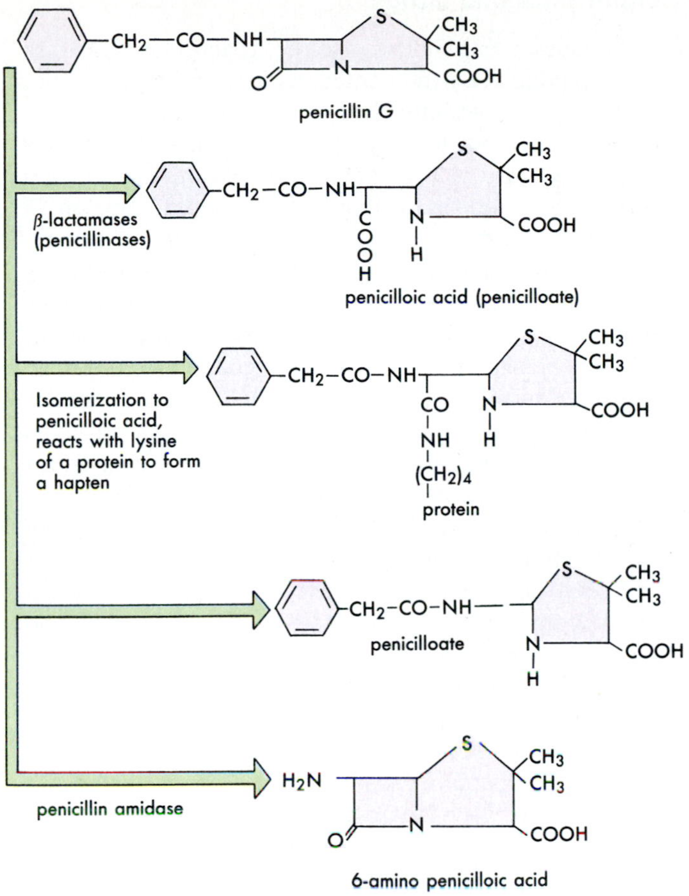

FIGURE 47-10 Some breakdown products of penicillin G in the presence of different enzymes and conditions.

47-10) has a 95% chance of identifying individuals likely to have an anaphylactic reaction if given penicillin. Failure to have a positive skin test does not exclude later development of a skin rash.

Anaphylactic reactions to penicillins should be treated with epinephrine. There is no evidence that antihistamines or corticosteroids are beneficial. Although desensitization is possible, use of a different type of antibiotic is more practical.

Although hematological toxicity to penicillins is uncommon, neutropenia may occur from suppression of granulocyte–colony stimulating factor. All penicillins, particularly high concentrations of carbenicillin and ticarcillin, alter platelet aggregation by binding to adenosine diphosphate receptors on the platelets. However, significant bleeding disorders are infrequent.

Penicillins can cause renal toxicity. Interstitial nephritis is uncommon, occurring most often with methicillin and producing fever, macular rash, eosinophilia, proteinuria, eosinophiluria, hematuria, and eventually anuria. Anatomical changes include interstitial infiltration by mononuclear and eosinophilic cells to produce tubular damage. Discontinuation of penicillin results in return of normal renal function.

Metabolic problems with penicillins occur often with the carboxypenicillins, since large doses of drug are used (18 to 30 g) causing a major load of nonresorbable anions in the distal tubule, thereby altering hydrogen-ion exchange and ultimately loss of potassium and hypokalemia. Carbenicillin, for example, contains 5 mEq Na^+ per gram and can produce congestive heart failure. Ticarcillin can be used at lower doses and has largely replaced carbenicillin in the United States.

Gastrointestinal disturbances after orally administered penicillins occur most often with ampicillin. The most serious problem is pseudomembranous enterocolitis arising from the toxin of *Clostridium difficile*. This organism is inhibited by ampicillin and amoxicillin, but these antibiotics are degraded by *Bacteroides* species in the colon, thereby allowing the *C. difficile* to survive and produce its toxin. Distortion of normal intestinal flora by penicillins can produce alteration in bowel function and colonization with resistant gram-negative bacilli or fungi such as *Candida*. The addition of clavulanate to amoxicillin and ticarcillin has not increased the adverse reactions to these compounds, though an increase in diarrhea is noted with the oral preparation compared to the use of amoxicillin alone.

Hepatic function abnormalities such as elevation of aspartate aminotransferase (SGOT) or alkaline phosphatase concentrations often follow use of high dose of antistaphylococcal penicillins or extended-spectrum antipseudomonal agents. In general, hepatic function rapidly returns to normal when agents are discontinued.

CNS-based seizures occur only in patients possessing epileptogenic foci, receiving large doses of penicillin G or other penicillins, and with impaired renal function. Penicillins do not cause vestibular or auditory toxicity. Procaine penicillin can produce cardiac and nervous system sensations if the procaine inadvertently enters directly into the bloodstream.

Cephalosporins

Allergic reactions are common adverse effects with cephalosporin use, though they occur less frequently than with penicillins. Cephalosporins can produce anaphylaxis, but the incidence is extremely low. It is estimated that less than 5% of individuals who have an anaphylactic reaction with a penicillin will have an anaphylactic reaction with a cephalosporin. However, a cephalosporin should not be administered to a patient who has had a severe immediate hypersensitivity reaction to a penicillin. Patients who have had skin reactions to penicillins in the form of a rash are at low risk to develop a similar rash to cephalosporins. However, maculopapular and morbilliform eruptions may occur with cephalosporin use.

About 1% of cefaclor-treated patients have a reaction that produces fever, joint pain, and local edema. All the cephalosporins sometimes produce fever with or without rash.

Gastrointestinal adverse effects are uncommon, though cefoperazone, because of its high intestinal secretions, and ceftriaxone may cause diarrhea. Enterocolitis from *Clostridium difficile* occurs with all the cephalosporins.

Although Coombs-positive reactions occur with the use of high doses of cephalosporins, they rarely cause hemolytic anemia. Neutropenia and granulocytopenia occur infrequently; platelet function is altered by moxalactam but not by other cephalosporins. Agents such as cefoperazone and moxalactam can cause disulfiram reactions when patients consume alcohol and can produce hypoprothrombinemia from alteration in prothrombin synthesis. Because of bleeding problems, moxalactam is rarely used in the United States.

Interstitial nephritis is uncommon but may occur with any cephalosporin. Neurological side effects also are rare. Cephalosporins are moderately irritating to the veins, and some cephalosporins produce false-positive Benedict's reactions when one is testing for glucose in the urine.

Other β-Lactam Drugs

Imipenem can cause allergic reactions similar to those produced by the penicillins and should not be administered to patients who have had anaphylactic reactions to penicillins or cephalosporins. Cutaneous eruptions can occur also. Diarrhea is infrequent, and pseudomembranous colitis is rare. Rapid infusion of imipenem-cilastatin can produce nausea and emesis, but this combination is free of hematological and renal toxicities. Imipenem alone is converted to metabolites that cause renal abnormalities in experimental animals but appear safe in humans. Imipenem binds to brain tissue with greater avidity than penicillin G does and so causes seizures, which constitute the most serious toxic reaction with imipenem. Seizures have occurred in individuals with decreased renal function and an underlying seizure focus. As a result, imipenem should not be used to treat meningitis.

Unlike other β-lactams, aztreonam does not cross-react with antibodies directed against penicillin and penicillin derivatives. It can be used in patients with known hypersensitivity to penicillins and cephalosporins, with low occurrence of skin rashes.

There are no unusual reactions noted for the ampicillin-sulbactam combination or clavulanate-amoxicillin or clavulanate-ticarcillin combinations. The incidence of rash and gastrointestinal reactions are similar to those with ampicillin used alone. The frequency of specific side reactions for β-lactam drugs is shown in Table 47-6.

Table 47-6 Frequency of Side Reactions by β-Lactams

Reaction Type	Frequency (%)	Typical Drugs	Reaction Type	Frequency (%)	Typical Drugs
IgE antibody allergy (anaphylaxis)	0.004-0.4	penicillin G	Platelet dysfunction	3	moxalactam
			Elevated hepatic aspartate aminotransferase (SGOT)	1-4	oxacillin nafcillin
Delayed hypersensitivity and contact dermatitis	4-8	ampicillin*	Interstitial nephritis	1-2	methicillin
Idiopathic, rash	4-8	ampicillin and cephalosporins	Antabuse reaction, phlebitis	Some	methicillin cefoperazine
			Hemolytic anemia, serum sickness, cytotoxic antibody, hyperkalemia, neurologic seizures, hemorrhagic cystitis	Rare	moxalactam any agent
Gastrointestinal	2-5	only oral			
Diarrhea	25	ampicillin, cefixime, ceftriaxone, cefoxitin			
Enterocolitis	1	ampicillin			
Abnormal prothrombin (vitamin K correctable)	25	moxalactam			

*Can occur with any β-lactam.

Vancomycin, Teichoplanin, and Bacitracin

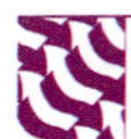

MECHANISMS OF ACTION

Vancomycin and bacitracin are two cell wall inhibitors that are structurally quite different from the β-lactam compounds and function by different mechanisms.

Vancomycin is a glycopeptide antibiotic of molecular weight 1450. It contains three substituted phenylglycines, glucose, and a unique amino sugar, vancosamine, *N*-methylleucine, and aspartic acid. Three different structures have been proposed for this compound with the definitive configuration still open to some question. Vancomycin inhibits cell wall synthesis in susceptible bacteria by binding to the free carboxyl end of the pentapeptide. This sterically interferes with elongation of the peptidoglycan backbone. The specificity of interaction of vancomycin with D-alanine–D-alanine partially explains the minimal resistance observed to this antibiotic.

Resistance to vancomycin and teichoplanin is attributable to production of a new cell wall component instead of D-Ala–D-Ala. The organism makes D-Ala–D-Lac. This prevents the bonding reaction. Resistance to vancomycin can be intrinsic or plasmid mediated (Table 47-7). Resistance to vancomycin is reported for *Enterococcus faecalis* by another pathway, that is, from a plasmid that produces a protein that interferes with the binding of vancomycin to its normal receptor. Thus far, this has occurred only in enterococci and *Streptococcus hemolyticus*.

Teichoplanin is a product of *Actinoplanus teichomyceticus*. It differs from vancomycin in that its carbohydrate moieties are D-glucosamine and D-mannose instead of D-glucose and vancosamine, and two dihydroxyphenylglycines are present instead of aspartic acid and *N*-methylleucine. The mechanism of action is inhibition of polymerization of peptidoglycan by interacting with the D-Ala–D-Ala terminal of the muramylpentapeptide which fits into a cleft inside the antibiotic molecule. Teichoplanin is far more lipophilic than vancomycin and is much higher protein bound (about 90%) than vancomycin (about 55%). The phenolic groups and terminal carboxyl and amino groups make it soluble at physiological pH, allowing absorption obtained with intramuscular injection.

Bacitracin is a polypeptide bactericidal antibiotic. It inhibits bacterial cell wall synthesis by interfering with dephosphorylation of the lipid carrier C^{55} isoprenyl pyrophosphate, which moves the early cell wall components through the membrane (see Figure 47-6).

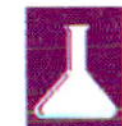

PHARMACOKINETICS

Vancomycin is not absorbed by the oral route and is irritative by the IM route. It should be administered by

Table 47-7 Resistance of Gram-Positive Bacteria to Vancomycin and Teicoplanin

Relevant Characteristics	Acquired Resistance		Intrinsic Resistance		
	High level	**Low level**	**Low level**		**High level**
MIC (μg/ml)					
Vancomycin	≥64 (R)	16 to 32 (R)	8 to 16 (R)	2 to 32 (R)	≥1000 (R)
Teicoplanin	≥16 (R)	0.5 (S)	0.5 (S)	0.5 to 1 (S)	≥250 (R)
Transferable by plasmid	Yes	No	No	No	No
Inducibility by:					
Vancomycin	Yes	Yes	No	ND	No
Teicoplanin	Some strains	No	No	ND	No
Molecular size of resistance protein (kD)	39 to 40	39.5	ND	ND	ND
Microorganisms	*Enterococcus faecium* *Enterococcus faecalis*	*Enterococcus faecium* *Enterococcus faecalis* *Staphylococcus epidermidis* *Staphylococcus hemolyticus*	*Enterococcus gallinarum*	*Enterococcus casseliflavus*	*Leuconostoc* spp. *Pediococcus* spp. *Lactobacillus* spp. *Erysipelothrix rhusiopathiae* Actinomycetes

From Neu HC: *Science* 257:7, 1992.
ND, Not determined; *R,* resistant; *S,* susceptible.

TRADE NAMES

Suprax, cefixime
Tazicef, ceftazidime
Tazidime, ceftazidime
Ultracef, cefadroxil
Velosef, cephradine
Zinacef, cefuroxime

CARBAPENEMS

Primaxin, imipenem-cilastatin

MONOBACTAMS

Azactam, aztreonam

β-LACTAM INHIBITORS

Augmentin, amoxicillin-clavulanic acid
Timentin, ticarcillin-clavulanic acid
Unasyn, ampicillin-sublactam

OTHER CELL WALL INHIBITORS

Vancocin, vancomycin
Vancoled, vancomycin
Vancor, vancomycin

histamine-release reaction and is less ototoxic and renal toxic than vancomycin is.

With bacitracin, hypersensitivity rarely occurs after topical use. If used parenterally, bacitracin can cause severe nephrotoxicity by damaging renal tubule cells.

REFERENCES

Campoli-Richards DM, Brogden RN, Foulds D: Teichoplanin: a review of antibacterial activity, pharmacokinetic properties, and therapeutic potential, *Drugs* 40:449-486, 1990.

Cooper GL, Given DB: *Vancomycin: a comprehensive review of 30 years of clinical experience,* New York, 1986, John Wiley & Sons.

Donowitz GR, Mandel GL: Beta-lactam antibiotics, *N Engl J Med* 318:419 and 490, 1988.

Frere JM et al: Mode of action: interaction with penicillin-binding proteins. In Page MI, editor: *The chemistry of β-lactams,* London, 1992, Blackie Academic, pp 129-147.

Neu HC: Structure-activity relationships: biological. In Page MI, editor: *The chemistry of β-lactams,* London, 1992, Blackie Academic, pp 102-128.

Neu HC: The penicillins. In Mandell GL, Douglas RG Jr, Bennett JE, editors: *Principles and practice of infectious diseases,* ed 3, New York, 1991, Churchill Livingstone.

Tipper DJ, editor: *Antibiotic inhibitors of bacterial cell wall biosyntheses,* Oxford, 1987, Pergamon Press.

SELF-ASSESSMENT QUESTIONS

1. Which of the following agents will not inhibit enterococci?
   a. ampicillin
   b. cephalexin
   c. vancomycin
   d. piperacillin
2. Which of the following penicillins is not destroyed by staphylococcal β-lactamase?
   a. amoxicillin
   b. ticarcillin
   c. oxacillin
   d. piperacillin
   e. penicillin V
3. Which of the following β-lactams would be an appropriate agent to treat meningitis caused by a β-lactamase–producing *Haemophilus influenzae* ?
   a. ampicillin
   b. cefazolin
   c. piperacillin
   d. cefotaxime
   e. cefoxitin
4. Which of the following cephalosporins is most effective in inhibiting *Bacteroides fragilis* strains?
   a. cefazolin
   b. cefuroxime
   c. ceftazidime
   d. cephalexin
   e. cefoxitin
5. Penicillin G is mainly:
   a. destroyed in the body.
   b. conjugated to inactive glucuronide.
   c. excreted in bile.
   d. excreted by kidney.
   e. deacylated by the liver.
6. Which of the following agents inhibits only aerobic gram-negative bacteria?
   a. clavulanate
   b. aztreonam
   c. imipenem
   d. piperacillin
7. Which of the following cephalosporins is converted to a biologically active metabolite?
   a. cephalexin
   b. cefazolin
   c. ceftazidime
   d. cefoxitin
   e. cefotaxime

8. Which of the following β-lactam agents could be used to treat an *E. coli* infection in a patient who has had an urticaria-accelerated reaction to penicillin G?
   a. piperacillin
   b. cefazolin
   c. aztreonam
   d. imipenem
   e. ticarcillin/clavulanate
9. There must be a major reduction in the dosage of which of the following penicillins when administered to patients whose creatinine clearance is <30 ml/min?
   a. penicillin G
   b. amoxicillin
   c. oxacillin
   d. ticarcillin
10. Which of the following β-lactamase–producing organisms is not inhibited by clavulanate or sulbactam?
    a. *Bacteroides fragilis*
    b. *Enterobacter cloacae*
    c. *Staphylococcus aureus*
    d. *Neisseria gonorrhoeae*
11. Which of the following agents is not removed from the body by hemodialysis?
    a. ampicillin
    b. imipenem
    c. vancomycin
    d. cefazolin
12. Which of the following agents does not inhibit *Pseudomonas aeruginosa* ?
    a. ceftazidime
    b. imipenem
    c. piperacillin
    d. ceftriaxone

CHAPTER 48

Inhibitors of Bacterial Ribosomal Actions

HAROLD C. NEU

MAJOR DRUGS
aminoglycosides
spectinomycin
tetracyclines
chloramphenicol
macrolides
clindamycin
mupirocin
fusidic acid

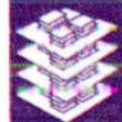

THERAPEUTIC OVERVIEW

Some antimicrobial agents act by binding to bacterial ribosomes and interfering with protein synthesis. These agents include aminoglycosides, spectinomycin, tetracyclines, chloramphenicol, macrolides, (erythromycin, azithromycin, clarithromycin), clindamycin, and mupirocin. Some of these agents exert bactericidal and others bacteriostatic actions.

The aminoglycosides are effective against gram-negative and gram-positive organisms; however, toxicity, development of bacterial resistance to these drugs and agents in the β-lactam class with similar activity make their use less common. The aminoglycosides are effective against aerobic gram-negative bacteria and are often used in combination with other classes of antibiotics but are ineffective against anaerobic organisms. Because the therapeutic index of the aminoglycosides is small and the types of toxicity can be serious, close attention must be paid to the pharmacokinetics of these drugs in individual patients. Renal function in particular must be assessed, and monitoring of the plasma concentration of these drugs is recommended.

ABBREVIATIONS	
CSF	cerebrospinal fluid
tRNA	transfer ribonucleic acid

Another ribosome-binding agent, spectinomycin, is similar to the aminoglycosides in that both are aminocyclitols, but the structures and actions are different. Whereas the aminoglycosides are bactericidal, spectinomycin is bacteriostatic.

The ribosome-binding sites for macrolides such as erythromycin, azithromycin, and clarithromycin and for clindamycin are on the same 30S subunit, but the structures of the drugs and the spectrum of activities differ considerably. Tetracyclines bind to a different 50S subunit and are effective against aerobic and anaerobic gram-positive and gram-negative organisms. Despite a wide spectrum of activity, serious side effects and development of bacterial resistance limit clinical use of the tetracyclines to selected situations. Chloramphenicol was widely used at one time, but serious side effects limit applications of this drug in the United States. Erythromycin, however, is a relatively safe antibiotic and is widely used, especially for the treatment of infections in children. Because of the success of macrolides in the treatment of pulmonary infections, these drugs continue to be used in the treatment of other respiratory infections in adults. Clindamycin displays antimicrobial activity similar to that of erythromycin, but the structures of the two compounds are different, and it is not effective for *Legionella* infections but inhibits anaerobic organisms.

Mupirocin, which interferes with transfer RNA (tRNA) synthesis, is a topical agent primarily used to treat cutaneous streptococcal and staphylococcal infection.

The therapeutic applications of these agents are summarized in the box on p. 662.

THERAPEUTIC OVERVIEW

aminoglycosides
- Small therapeutic index
- Toxicities to patient can be serious: renal, otic
- Pharmacokinetics are an important consideration
- Plasmid-mediated resistance is a problem
- Inhibit gram-negative aerobes

tetracyclines
- Broad spectrum of organisms are inhibited
- Serious toxicities to patient
- Resistance by bacteria

chloramphenicol
- Kills major meningitis pathogens
- Serious toxicity in patient

macrolides (e.g., erythromycin)
- Inhibit *Mycoplasma, Chlamydia, Legionella*
- Inhibit gram-positive organisms

clindamycin
- Inhibits gram-positive cocci and anaerobic species
- Pseudomembranous enterocolitis toxic reaction

Table 48-1 Bacterial Ribosomal Binding and Resulting Overall Effect on Bacterial Viability

Drugs	Binds to Subunit	Bactericidal	Bacteriostatic
aminoglycosides	30S, 50S, 30S/50S interface	×	—
chloramphenicol	50S	—	×*
clindamycin	50S	—	×
erythromycin	50S	—	×†
mupirocin	leu tRNA	×	—
spectinomycin	30S	—	×
tetracyclines	30S	—	×

*Bactericidal for *Streptococcus pneumoniae, Haemophilus influenzae, Neisseria meningitidis.*
†Bactericidal for *Streptococcus pneumoniae, Staphylococcus pyogenes.*

MECHANISMS OF ACTION

The bacterial ribosomal subunit to which each of these drugs binds is listed in Table 48-1, with designation of the bactericidal or bacteriostatic response of susceptible bacteria to the drug. The principal steps in bacterial ribosomal synthesis of proteins, as carried out by the 70S ribosomes and relevant RNAs, and the points at which the drugs act are summarized schematically in Figure 48-1.

Aminoglycosides

Aminoglycosides consist of aminosugars linked through glycosidic bonds to an aminocyclitol. In the aminoglycosides the aminocyclitol ring is a 1,3-diaminocyclohexitol with the amino groups in the *cis* configuration. Streptidine is the aminocyclitol in streptomycin, whereas 2-deoxystreptamine occurs in the other clinically important aminoglycosides. The structures of streptomycin and gentamicin are shown in Figure 48-2.

The structures of the other clinically important aminoglycosides are summarized schematically in Figure 48-2. The particular amino sugars and the specific locations of the amino groups on the aminoglycosides distinguish the compounds and are important for the antimicrobial effect and toxicity. The commercial form of gentamicin consists of a mixture of three species with little difference in the activities of the three components.

The aminoglycosides exert bactericidal action by entering the bacterial cell and inhibiting protein synthesis. The overall process consists of two main steps: (1) transport of aminoglycoside through the bacterial cell wall and cytoplasmic membrane and (2) binding to ribosomal sites resulting in inhibition of protein synthesis.

The aminoglycosides are more effective against gram-negative than gram-positive bacteria. These drugs can cross the more complex cell membrane structures of the gram-negative bacteria. A comparison of the cell membrane structures for gram-negative and gram-positive bacteria is shown schematically in Chapter 47 (see Figure 47-3).

The transport of aminoglycosides into bacterial cells requires several steps. Initially, there is an ionic association at the cell surface between cationic aminoglycosides and anionic surface. The aminoglycosides then penetrate the porin channel of the outer membrane of gram-negative bacteria or the water-filled areas of the peptidoglycan wall in gram-positive bacteria. In the phosphate-rich gram-negative bacteria, aminoglycosides disrupt the outer membrane and enhance their own uptake through nonporin type of channels. The aminoglycoside binds to a transport molecule that is either part of or directly linked to the electron transport chain in the cytoplasmic membrane. Movement of the drug-transporter complex across the cytoplasmic membrane occurs because of the electrical potential gradient that exists across the membrane. The transport is an energy-requiring, aerobic step that does not occur in an anaerobic environment. After crossing the cytoplasmic membrane, the aminoglycosides bind to ribosomes. This maintains a low concentration of intracellular free aminoglycoside, which helps support the con-

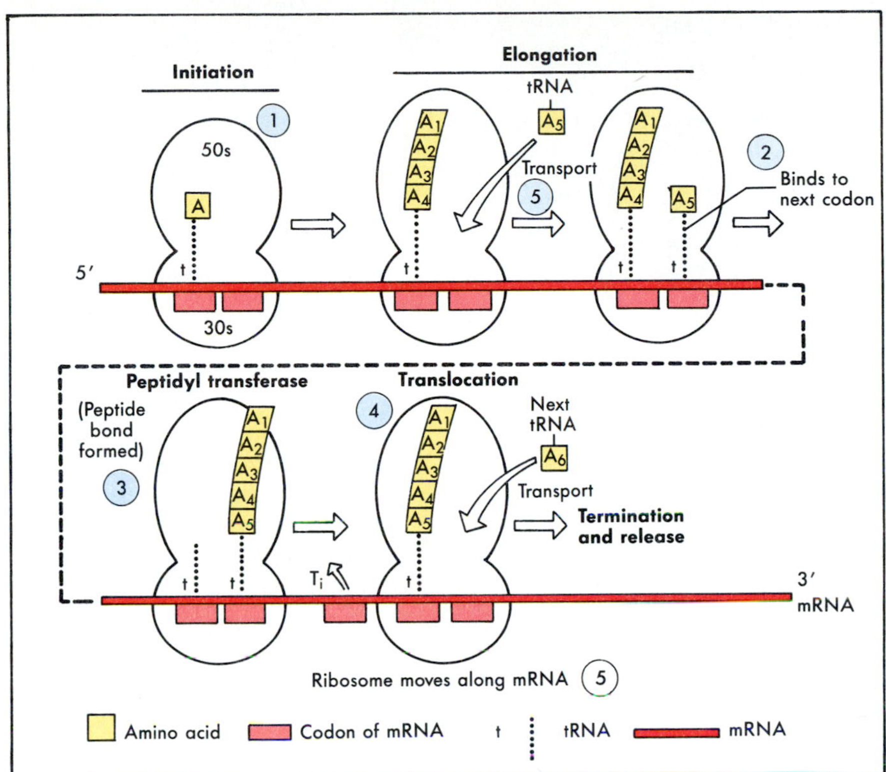

FIGURE 48-1 Bacterial protein synthesis and points where clinically used antibiotics act. The steps are as follows: (1) Streptomycin and other aminoglycosides freeze initiation; so ribosome does not progress along in mRNA and converts from polysome to monosome; (2) tetracycline and chloramphenicol prevent tRNA from binding to mRNA codon; (3) chloramphenicol and erythromycin block peptide bond formation; (4) erythromycin and clindamycin block translocation step; and (5) streptomycin and other aminoglycosides cause misreading of mRNA so that the wrong amino acid is added.

tinued transfer of drug from the cytoplasmic membrane to the ribosomes. This results in a loss of membrane integrity and eventual death of the bacteria. Calcium, magnesium, and other divalent ions inhibit the transport of aminoglycosides into the bacterial cell.

The binding to the ribosome leads to inhibition of protein synthesis. This takes place on the ribosomes where mRNA acts as the template for the addition of specific activated amino acids delivered to the synthesis site attached to tRNAs. The 70S ribosomal particles (*S* represents the sedimentation parameter) move along the mRNA template, adding the appropriate amino acid coded by the mRNA (see Figure 48-1).

Aminoglycosides bind to several ribosomal sites, usually at the interface of the 30S and 50S subunits of the 70S bacterial ribosome, but also directly to the 30S and 50S subunits. Streptomycin, the most thoroughly studied aminoglycoside, binds to the 30S subunit. Binding depends on the amino acid sequence of the adjacent S12 protein, since alteration of one amino acid in this protein can prevent binding. Binding of the aminoglycosides interferes with protein synthesis in two ways: (1) restricting polysome formation and (2) misreading mRNA. These actions prevent normal polysome function, wherein multiple ribosomes move along each strand of mRNA to synthesize multiple amino acid chains. Instead, these drugs cause polysome disaggregation to monosomes, where only one ribosome is attached to each strand of mRNA and cannot move along the mRNA to synthesize a new peptide chain. Aminoglycosides also cause misreading of mRNA. The juncture between the 30S and 50S subunits is where mRNA and aminoacyl-tRNA interact. Binding of aminoglycosides at this site causes distortion of codon recognition, resulting in misreading to produce proteins with miscoded amino acids or polypeptide chains of abnormal length. Misreading occurs more often with deoxystreptidine compounds than with streptomycin. However, the presence of miscoded proteins does not necessarily correlate with cell death.

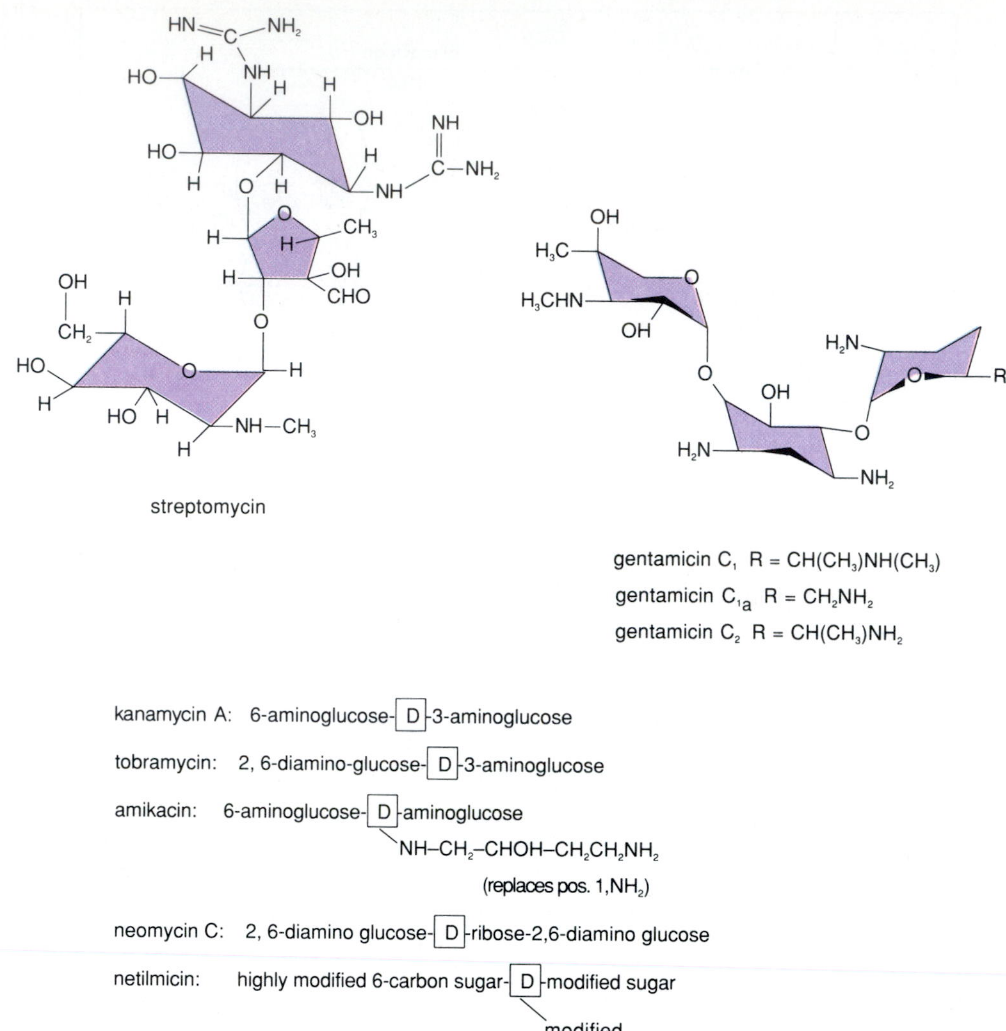

FIGURE 48-2 Structures of streptomycin and gentamicin and main components of other clinically used aminoglycosides. *D,* 2-deoxystreptamine. See the text for further information.

Bacterial resistance to aminoglycosides occurs and results from the following mechanisms: (1) altered ribosomes, (2) inadequate transport within the cell, and (3) enzymatic modification of aminoglycosides. The third mechanism is the most important clinically.

Resistance caused by altered ribosomes is relatively uncommon. Although resistance to streptomycin caused by a mutation that changes the amino acid composition of the S12 protein of the 30S ribosome has been found in enterococci, it is uncommon in gram-negative bacteria. For ribosomal resistance to other aminoglycosides to occur, there must be multiple mutational events with alteration of several binding sites.

Resistance caused by inadequate transport of drug across the cytoplasmic membrane is uncommon in aerobic or facultative species, but it is seen in strict anaerobes. Mutants with alterations in the electron transfer chain and in adenosine triphosphatase activity have been found, but they are distinctly rare. The resistance of some *Pseudomonas* species to aminoglycosides may be related to failure of the drug to distort the lipopolysaccharide of the outer membrane, thus not allowing inhibitory concentrations of drug to enter the bacterial cell.

The common form of resistance is caused by modification of the aminoglycoside, which occurs through enzyme-catalyzed phosphorylation, adenylation, or acetylation of the amino and hydroxyl groups. The genetic template for synthesis of the enzymes is located on plasmids or transposons, which means that the resistance can be spread to many different bacterial species. A large number of such enzymes have been identified. Some can inactivate only one or two compounds, whereas others can inactivate multiple aminoglycosides. For example, an enzyme that acetylates the amino group at position six of the amino hexose can inactivate kanamycin, neomycin, tobramycin, amikacin, and netilmicin but not gentamicin or streptomycin. The altered aminoglycosides do not bind as well to ribosomes, and accelerated drug uptake is not triggered by the modified compounds.

Aminoglycoside resistance varies by location and local usage patterns. One hospital may have a low resistance to gentamicin and another hospital may have a high resistance to gentamicin. Prediction of the precise resistance mechanism is not feasible at present, and there is little evidence that restricting use of an agent will prevent resistance developing to that drug, since use of other agents may select for strains possessing enzymes that inactivate the restricted drug.

Amikacin is the most resistant of the aminoglycosides to inactivation by resistant organisms, and netilmicin is the second most resistant.

Spectinomycin

Spectinomycin acts by binding to the 30S ribosome subunit and inhibiting a translocation step, perhaps by interfering with movement of mRNA along the 30S subunit. Resistance to this drug is caused by transfer of a plasmid directing the synthesis of an enzyme that acetylates the compound or changes amino acids in the S5 protein of the 30S subunit.

Tetracyclines

Tetracyclines are only slightly soluble in water, but they form soluble hydrochlorides and sodium salts (see Figure 48-3 for structures). They act by binding to 30S ribosomes, thereby preventing attachment of the aminoacyl-tRNA to the acceptor site on the mRNA-ribosomal complex. This binding prevents the addition of amino acids to the peptide chain being synthesized. Differences in the activity of the individual tetracyclines are related to their solubility in lipid membranes of the bacteria. These drugs enter the cytoplasm of gram-positive bacteria by an energy-dependent process, but for gram-negative organisms, passage through the outer membrane is by diffusion through the porins. Because minocycline and doxycycline are more lipophilic, they can enter gram-negative cells through the outer lipid membrane as well as through the porins. Once in the periplasmic space, the tetracyclines are transported across the inner cytoplasmic membrane by a protein-carrier system.

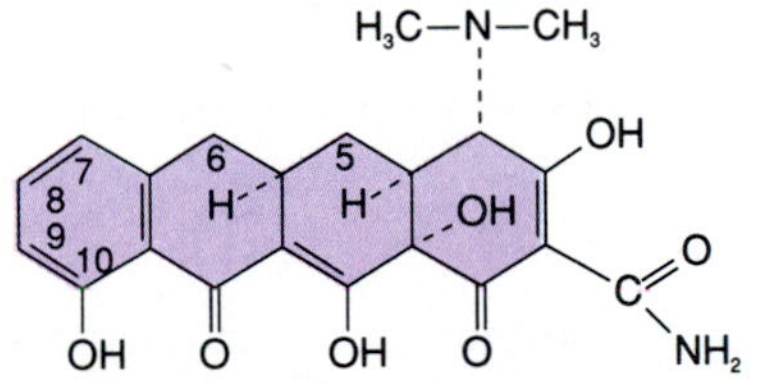

There are several mechanisms of resistance to the tetracyclines. The common mechanism, which occurs in gram-positive and gram-negative bacteria, is plasmid or transposon mediated and involves decreased intracellular accumulation and increased transport of drug out of the bacterial cell (Figure 48-4). Drug efflux occurs from the action of a new protein, probably induced by the drug. A second mechanism appears to be alteration of outer membrane proteins secondary to mutations in chromosomal genes. Another mechanism is protection of the ribosomal binding site attributable to synthesis by a plasmid-generated protein that binds to the ribosome. Resistance to one tetracycline usually implies resistance to all these compounds. However, some staphylococci and some *Bacteroides* species are resistant to tetracycline but susceptible to minocycline and doxycycline because of the lipophilicity of these latter agents. New tetracyclines that inhibit bacteria previously resistant to all the commercially available tetracyclines have recently been synthesized.

Ring position substitutions

	5	6	7
chlortetracycline	—H	—CH; —OH	—Cl
oxytetracycline	—OH	$-CH_3$; —OH	—H
tetracycline	—H	$-CH_3$; —OH	—H
demeclocycline	—H	—OH	—Cl
doxycycline	—OH	$-CH_3$	—H
minocycline	—H	—H	$-N(CH_3)_2$

FIGURE 48-3 Structures of tetracyclines. See the text for further information.

Chloramphenicol, Macrolides, and Clindamycin

Because chloramphenicol, macrolides, and clindamycin bind to the same site or sites on the ribosomal 50S subunit, they are discussed as a group. Their structures are shown in Figure 48-5. They bind to bacterial 70S ribosomes but not to the 80S ribosomes of mammalian cells.

Chloramphenicol prevents the addition of new amino acids to the growing peptide chains by interfering with binding of the amino acid–acyl–tRNA complex with the 50S subunit. This prevents association of peptidyl transferase with the amino acid and no peptide bond is formed. It is not clear whether erythromycin also inhibits the subsequent translocation step. Erythromycin inhibits binding of chloramphenicol to 70S ribosomes, but conversely chloramphenicol does not inhibit erythromy-

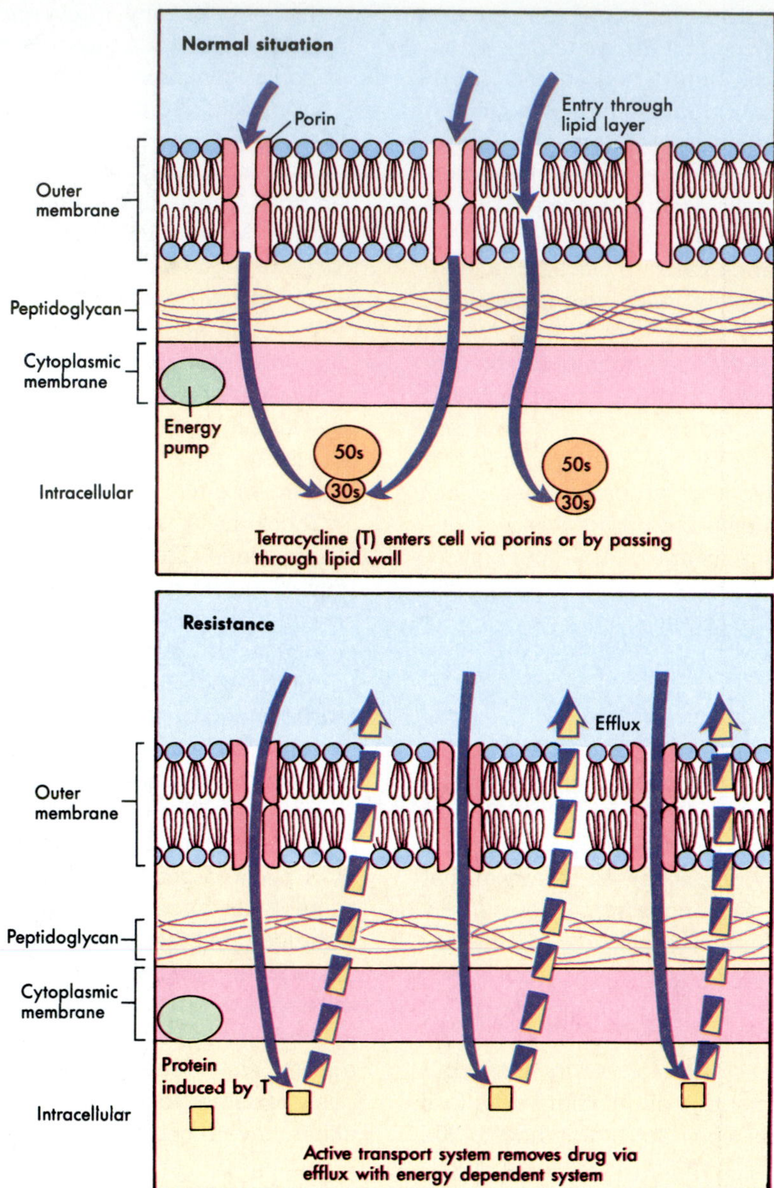

FIGURE 48-4 Mechanism for bacterial resistance to tetracycline *(T)* caused by efflux. See the text for further information.

cin binding. The new macrolides azithromycin, clarithromycin, and roxithromycin bind to the same site. The mechanism of action of clindamycin is similar to that for erythromycin. Clindamycin inhibits peptidyl transferase by interfering with binding of the amino acid–acyl–tRNA complex. The drug does not bind to polysomes containing new peptides.

Bacterial resistance is observed with all three agents. The majority of resistance to chloramphenicol is caused by chloramphenicol acetyltransferase. This enzyme catalyzes acetylation of the hydroxy groups of chloramphenicol, which eliminates its ability to bind to the 50S subunit. Less common mechanisms of resistance to chloramphenicol result from alterations in cell wall permeability or in ribosomal proteins.

One mechanism of bacterial resistance to erythromycin or clindamycin is plasmid-mediated drug induction of an enzyme that methylates 23S RNA of the 50S ribosomes. The resulting dimethyladenine 23S RNA does not bind erythromycin or clindamycin. Both drugs act as enzyme inducers, but erythromycin has greater activity. This has clinical importance because an organism resistant to erythromycin and susceptible to clindamycin can become resistant to both drugs during

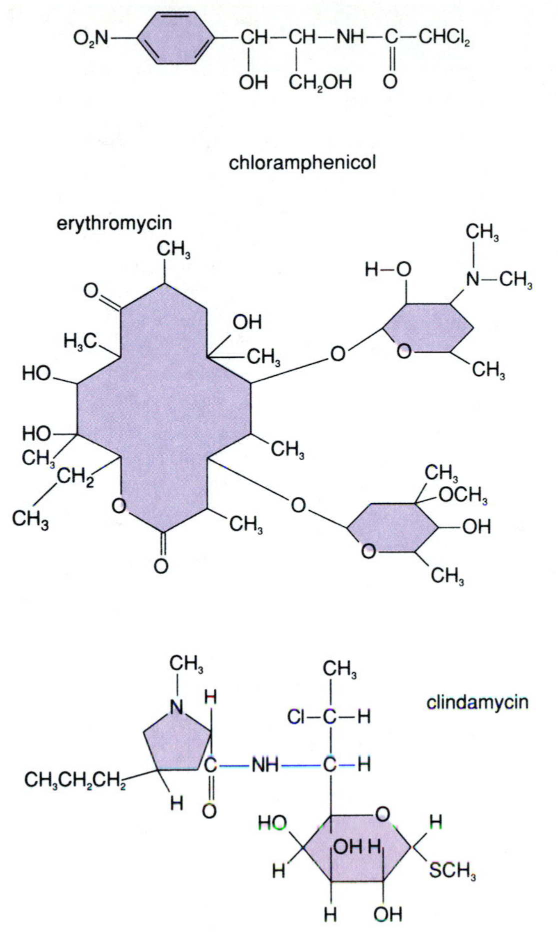

FIGURE 48-5 Structures of the additional protein synthesis inhibitors chloramphenicol, erythromycin, and clindamycin. See the text for further information.

therapy. This is applicable to treatment of infections caused by methicillin-resistant *Staphylococcus aureus,* which is often resistant to erythromycin but may appear susceptible to clindamycin. This form of resistance is present on plasmids that can pass from enterococci to streptococci and is the basis of resistance of *Streptococcus pneumoniae* and *S. pyogenes* to erythromycin and of some *Bacteroides* species and some Clostridia to clindamycin.

Although some gram-negative bacteria possess ribosomes that do not bind erythromycin or clindamycin, the common form of resistance to erythromycin is failure of the compound to pass through the outer membrane of aerobic gram-negative bacteria. For example, the amount of erythromycin that can cross the outer membrane of gram-negative *Escherichia coli* is 100 times less than that which crosses the membrane of *Staphylococcus aureus* (gram-positive). Gram-negative bacteria may possess esterases that hydrolyze erythromycin.

Fusidic Acid

Fusidic acid is a cyclopentenophenanthrene. It inhibits protein biosynthesis similarly to erythromycin by inhibiting translocation on the ribosome. It inhibits gram-positive cocci at concentrations of 0.03-0.12 mg/ml. It is bactericidal for many of the bacteria. Unfortunately resistance develops rapidly with staphylococci when used alone. It acts synergistically with other antibiotics.

Fusidic acid is well absorbed orally, but food delays absorption. Protein binding is 95%. The drug is well distributed in the body with high concentrations in bone. It is excreted in bile. It has been used to treat staphylococcal infections. It causes occasional rash and gastrointestinal upset. Jaundice has occurred when it was used intravenously.

Mupirocin

Mupirocin is a topical agent, previously known as *pseudomonic acid,* that inhibits gram-positive and some gram-negative bacteria by binding to isoleucyl-tRNA synthetase. This binding prevents isoleucine incorporation into bacterial proteins during synthesis. Mupirocin has been shown to eliminate nasal carriage of Methicillin-resistant-staphylococci.

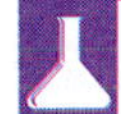

PHARMACOKINETICS

The pharmacokinetic parameters for the antibiotics that act by inhibiting bacterial protein synthesis are listed in Table 48-2.

Aminoglycosides

Aminoglycosides are not absorbed by oral or rectal administration except after oral use in newborns with necrotizing enterocolitis. If there is renal impairment, even the small amount of drug absorbed by the oral route may accumulate and cause toxicity in adults. After IM injection, peak plasma concentrations occur in 30 to 60 minutes, with plasma concentrations comparable to those achieved after a 30-minute infusion. Shock decreases absorption from the IM site of injection, and thus the IM route is rarely used to treat life-threatening infections.

Topical application of aminoglycosides results in minimal absorption, except in patients with extensive cutaneous damage such as burns or epidermolysis. Intraperitoneal and intrapleural instillation produces such rapid absorption that toxicity may develop, but irrigation (of bladder), intratracheal, and aerosol delivery do not result in significant absorption. However, new techniques of aerosolization with correct particle size can

Table 48-2 Pharmacokinetic Parameters

Drug	Administration	Absorption	Plasma $t_{1/2}$ (hr) Normal	Plasma $t_{1/2}$ (hr) Anuric	Disposition	Plasma Protein Binding (%)
aminoglycosides						
gentamicin	IV, IM	Poor	2	35-50	R (100)	<10
streptomycin	IM	Poor	2-2.5	35-50	R (100)	35
kanamycin	IV, IM	Poor	2-2.5	35-50	R (100)	<10
tobramycin	IV, IM	Poor	2	35-50	R (100)	<10
amikacin	IV, IM	Poor	2-2.5	35-50	R (100)	<10
netilmicin	IV, IM	Poor	2	35-50	R (100)	<10
tetracyclines						
tetracycline	Oral, IM, IV, topical	75%	8	>50	R, M	55
doxycycline	Oral, IV	93%	16	20-30	R, M, B	85
oxytetracycline	Oral, IM	Good	9	Long	R (20-35), M	30
minocycline	Oral, IV	95%	16	20-30	R (5%), M	75
chlortetracycline	Oral	30%	6	>50	R, M	50
other drugs						
chloramphenicol	Oral, IV	Good	3	—	M (90%), R	50
erythromycin	Oral, IV	Usually good but variable	1.5	4	M (main), R	<70
azithromycin	Oral	Good‡	10-50	Fecal	7-50	
clarithromycin	Oral	Good	4	Fecal, R		
roxithromycin	Oral	Good	12	Fecal, R	95	
clindamycin	Oral, IM, IV	90%	2.4	6	M (90%), R	90
spectinomycin	IM	Poor	2.5	—	R (100%)	<10

M, Metabolized; *R*, renal excretion as unchanged drug; *B*, biliary.
*Aminoglycosides have long $t_{1/2}$ values in tissue (25 to 500 hr).
‡Decreased by food.

produce concentrations over 100 μg/ml in the lung and 4 μg/ml in plasma.

Because of their high polarity, aminoglycosides do not enter phagocytic or other cells, the brain; or the eye. They are distributed into interstitial fluid, with a volume of distribution essentially that of the extracellular fluid. The highest concentrations of aminoglycosides occur in the renal cortex, where the drug concentrates in proximal renal tubular cells. Urine concentrations are generally 20 to 100 times greater than in the plasma and remain for 24 hours after a single dose. These drugs enter peritoneal, pleural, and synovial fluids relatively slowly but achieve concentrations only slightly less than those in plasma.

Concentrations of aminoglycosides in cerebrospinal fluid (CSF) after IM or IV administration are inadequate for treatment of gram-negative meningitis. Intrathecal administration into the lumbar space produces inadequate intraventricular concentrations, whereas intraventricular instillation yields high concentrations in both areas.

Subconjunctival injection produces high aqueous fluid concentrations but inadequate intravitreal concentrations.

Disposition of the aminoglycosides occurs almost completely by glomerular filtration with none metabolized and less than 1% excreted through the biliary tract. A small amount undergoes reabsorption into proximal renal tubular cells. Renal clearance of aminoglycosides is approximately two thirds that of creatinine. However, these drugs can become trapped in tissue compartments to give tissue half-lives of 25 to 500 hours, and aminoglycosides can be detected in urine for up to 10 days after discontinuation of a week-long dosing schedule. The elimination of aminoglycosides depends on renal function, and corrections to dosing schedules must be made for patients who have reduced renal capacity. Because clearance of aminoglycoside is linearly related to clearance of creatinine, the latter can be used to calculate an adjusted dosing schedule. For example, a patient with a creatinine clearance of 50 mg/ml should have the total daily dose of aminoglycoside reduced by about 50% compared to the dose for normal creatinine clearance.

Aminoglycosides can be removed from the body by hemodialysis but not so well by peritoneal dialysis.

Although aminoglycosides are not metabolized and do not bind to serum proteins, they can be inactivated by certain penicillins, particularly carbenicillin and ticarcillin in patients with greatly decreased renal function.

Spectinomycin

Spectinomycin is not absorbed from the gastrointestinal tract and therefore is administered IM. Elimination is primarily by glomerular filtration with 85% to 90% removed in 24 hours.

Tetracyclines

Some tetracyclines are incompletely absorbed and others are well absorbed when administered orally, but all attain adequate plasma and tissue concentrations. Minocycline and doxycycline are absorbed more completely and chlortetracycline is the least absorbed. Absorption is favored in the fasting state because tetracyclines form chelates with divalent metals, including calcium, magnesium, aluminum, and iron. Absorption is decreased when some tetracyclines are ingested with milk products, antacids, or iron preparations. However, food does not interfere with absorption of minocycline or doxycycline, and absorption is not reduced by histamine H_2-receptor blockers.

The tetracyclines are widely distributed in body compartments, with the apparent volume of distribution exceeding that for total body water. High concentrations are found in liver, kidney, bile, bronchial epithelium, and breast milk. These drugs can enter pleural, peritoneal, synovial, sputum, and sinus fluids; cross the placenta; and enter phagocytic cells. Penetration into the cerebrospinal fluid is poor and increases only minimally with meningeal inflammation; however, minocycline achieves therapeutic concentrations in brain tissue.

Tetracyclines do not bind to formed bone but are incorporated into calcifying tissue and into the dentin and enamel of unerupted teeth.

The disposition of the tetracyclines occurs by renal and biliary elimination and by metabolism. Although most of the biliary-eliminated drug is reabsorbed by active transport, some undergoes chelation and is excreted in the feces. This occurs even when the drugs are administered parenterally. Renal clearance of these drugs is by glomerular filtration. Filtration removes 20% of oral tetracycline, but this increases to 60% for IV administration. All tetracyclines, except for doxycycline, accumulate in the presence of decreased renal function. Only doxycycline should be given to patients with renal impairment.

Tetracyclines are also metabolized, an important mechanism for chlortetracycline but less important for doxycycline and minocycline. Metabolism of doxycycline is increased in patients receiving barbiturates or phenytoin because these agents induce the formation of hepatic drug–metabolizing enzymes. The $t_{1/2}$ of doxycycline decreases from 16 to 7 hours in such patients. Decreased hepatic function or common bile duct obstruction also prolongs the $t_{1/2}$ of tetracyclines because of reduction of biliary excretion.

Chloramphenicol

Chloramphenicol is extremely well absorbed from the gastrointestinal tract, with peak plasma concentrations about 2 hours after ingestion. It is also available as an inactive palmitate, most of which undergoes hydrolysis by pancreatic lipases in the duodenum with subsequent absorption of the active compound. Plasma concentrations are higher with the free compound than with the palmitate because of incomplete hydrolysis. Parenteral chloramphenicol is available as a succinate ester, which must be hydrolyzed by esterases in the liver, lungs, and kidney to the active compound. The succinate should not be given IM because the plasma concentrations are unpredictable.

Because it is highly lipid soluble, chloramphenicol is well distributed throughout the body and enters pleural, ascites, synovial, eye, abscess, and CSF fluids and lung, liver, and brain tissues. CSF concentrations are 50% to 60% of those found in plasma, and the drug crosses the placenta and also enters breast milk.

About 90% of a dose of chloramphenicol undergoes liver conjugation to an inactive and nontoxic glucuronide that is filtered by the kidney. Chloramphenicol palmitate is also excreted by the kidney in the hydrolyzed or palmitate forms. The normal plasma half-life is prolonged in patients with hepatic disease but not in patients with renal disease.

Infants deficient in forming glucuronides may accumulate high concentrations of free drug. In addition, hydrolysis of the succinate may be depressed in newborns and infants. Thus serum concentrations should be monitored if the drug is used in newborns or infants.

Erythromycin

Erythromycin in the free base form is inactivated by acid. Therefore it is administered orally with an enteric coating that dissolves in the duodenum. Even in the absence of food, which delays absorption, peak plasma concentrations are difficult to predict, and ester forms of erythromycin are available to help in overcoming this problem. Lactobionate and glucoheptate, water-soluble forms of the drug, are available for IV administration.

Erythromycin is well distributed and produces therapeutic concentrations in tonsillar tissue, middle ear fluid, and lung. It enters prostatic fluid to yield concentrations about one third those in plasma. It does not diffuse well into brain or CSF. Erythromycin crosses the placenta and is found in breast milk, with high concentrations also observed in liver and bile. It enters phagocytic cells.

The main routes for disposition of erythromycin are metabolic demethylation by liver and biliary excretion. Inactive metabolites are responsible for the gastric intolerance observed. Only a small percentage is excreted unchanged.

Azithromycin

Azithromycin is stable to acid compared to erythromycin. It is a 15-membered macrolide. About 37% of a dose is absorbed, and absorption is greatly reduced by food. Serum concentrations of azithromycin are low because of its rapid distribution in tissues. Azithromycin is highly concentrated in phagocytic cells, macrophages, and fibroblasts, from which it is slowly released. Therapeutic concentrations exist in lung, genital tissues, and liver. Presence of bacteria causes release of the drug from neutrophils.

Azithromycin is eliminated unchanged in feces and to a lesser extent in urine. Concentrations in the elderly and patients with decreased renal function are increased but are not significantly affected by hepatic disease.

Clarithromycin

Clarithromycin is a 14-membered macrolide that is about 55% absorbed by the oral route. With food, absorption is increased and serum concentrations exceed the concentrations needed to inhibit susceptible bacteria. Clarithromycin is widely distributed to lung, liver, and soft tissues. The concentrations in phagocytic cells are about ninefold greater than in serum. The drug is metabolized to a 14-hydroxy derivative, which has antibacterial activity greater than that of the parent compound. About 30% of drug is excreted in the urine and the remainder in feces. The half-lives of clarithromycin and its active metabolite are increased as renal function declines but are not appreciably affected by hepatic disease.

Other Macrolides

Roxithromycin is a well-absorbed macrolide used in Europe. It is highly protein bound and has a long $t_{1/2}$. Josamycin is a macrolide that is similar to erythromycin and has long been used in Europe. Spiramycin is a macrolide that is highly protein bound and less active than erythromycin. It has been used to treat intestinal *Cryptosporidium* infections but probably is not effective.

Clindamycin

Clindamycin is 90% absorbed from the gastrointestinal tract. Absorption is delayed but not decreased by the presence of food. Mean peak plasma concentrations occur within 1 hour. Clindamycin is available as a palmitate ester, which is rapidly hydrolyzed to the free drug, and also available as a phosphate ester, the latter for IM administration.

Distribution is widespread, with clindamycin entering most body compartments and achieving adequate concentrations in lung, liver, bone, and abscesses. It enters CSF and brain tissue, but concentrations are inadequate to treat meningitis and should not be relied on to treat brain infections except toxoplasmosis. This drug enters polymorphonuclear leukocytes and alveolar macrophages and crosses the placenta.

Clindamycin is metabolized to the bacteriologically active *N*-demethyl and sulfoxide derivatives, which are excreted in urine and bile. Only 10% of the dose is eliminated as unmetabolized drug in urine. The parent drug can be detected in feces 5 days after IV administration. The $t_{1/2}$ is prolonged by severe liver disease.

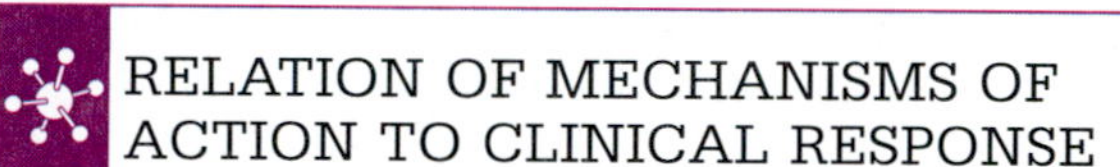

RELATION OF MECHANISMS OF ACTION TO CLINICAL RESPONSE

Aminoglycosides

The aminoglycosides are effective primarily against aerobic gram-negative bacilli such as Enterobacteriaceae or *Pseudomonas aeruginosa* and have little effect on anaerobic species. Most staphylococci are inhibited.

Aminoglycosides should be reserved for treatment of serious infections in which other agents such as penicillins or cephalosporins are not suitable. Aminoglycosides have no role as initial therapy of gram-positive infections. They are necessary in combination with penicillins to treat endocarditis resulting from enterococci or viridans streptococci. Gentamicin is the preferred agent because streptomycin resistance is common.

Treatment of suspected septic states has been initiated with an aminoglycoside such as gentamicin or tobramycin in combination with a penicillin or cephalosporin; however, newer cephalosporins and other β-lactams such as aztreonam or imipenem have lower toxicity and can replace this use of the aminoglycosides.

Aminoglycosides are particularly effective in the treatment of urinary tract infections, probably because of their elevated concentration in the kidney. However, many other agents are available for treatment of urinary tract infections, particularly the orally administered quinolones. Hospital-acquired pneumonia is treated with aminoglycosides, but the effectiveness is questionable, since the pH (6.5) of the infected lung and the large amount of cellular debris present in these lungs inhibit the activity of aminoglycosides. Nonetheless, the combination of an aminoglycoside with an anti-Pseudomonal penicillin, cephalosporin, or monobactam is usually selected when one is treating serious respiratory infections resulting from *P. aeruginosa.*

Another combination is that of an aminoglycoside with clindamycin or metronidazole, which inhibits anaerobic species to treat intraabdominal or gynecological infections. In addition, aminoglycosides can be combined with antianaerobic cephalosporin when the intraabdominal infection develops in the hospital the potential for *Pseudomonas* infection.

Although aminoglycosides have been used to treat aerobic gram-negative osteomyelitis and septic arthritis, other agents of the β-lactam or quinolone classes are preferred. Gram-negative meningitis is more appropriately treated with third-generation cephalosporins, though intraventricular instillation of aminoglycoside may be necessary for selected *Pseudomonas* or *Acinetobacter* meningitis infections. Serious endophthalmitis can be treated with intravitreal instillation of gentamicin.

THERAPEUTIC USES OF TETRACYCLINES

DRUG OF CHOICE

Rickettsial diseases: Rocky Mountain spotted fever, typhus, scrub typhus, Q fever
Mycoplasma pneumoniae
Chlamydiapneumoniae
Chlamydia trachomatis
Chlamydia psittaci
Lyme disease *(Borrelia burgdorferi)*
Relapsing fever caused by *Borrelia* organisms

ALTERNATIVE AGENT

Mycoplasma pneumoniae infection
Brucellosis
Plague
Pelvic inflammatory disease

AS TREATMENT OF SYNDROMES

Acne: low-dose oral or topical
Bacterial exacerbations of bronchitis
Sinusitis
Malabsorption syndrome resulting from bowel bacterial overgrowth

Aminoglycosides are used in combination with an anti-Pseudomonal β-lactam to treat suspected sepsis in febrile neutropenic patients. Choice of the particular agent depends on the local susceptibility patterns. In general, gentamicin is the initial agent to use, with tobramycin reserved for *Pseudomonas* infections and netilmicin or amikacin for aminoglycoside resistance. The availability of less toxic and equally effective agents allows the aminoglycosides to be restricted to situations in which their use is undeniably expected to produce a superior outcome.

Streptomycin is used primarily to treat uncommon infections, for example, those caused by *Francisella tularensis,* resistant *Brucella* species, and resistant tuberculosis strains or infections in patients allergic to the usual antituberculosis drugs (see Chapter 52).

Spectinomycin

Although spectinomycin inhibits many gram-negative bacteria, it is used to treat infections attributable only to *Neisseria gonorrhoeae,* especially penicillinase-producing *N. gonorrhoeae* of the genital tract, but not for pharyngeal or anal gonorrhea. It has been replaced by ceftriaxone or ofloxacin.

Tetracyclines

Tetracyclines are broad-spectrum agents that inhibit a wide variety of aerobic and anaerobic gram-positive and gram-negative bacteria and other microorganisms such as rickettsiae, mycoplasmas, chlamydiae, and some mycobacterial species (see Chapter 52). The tetracyclines have many clinical uses, but increasing bacterial resistance and the development of other drugs have replaced them in some of the uses. For example, some *Streptococcus pneumoniae, S. pyogenes,* and staphylococci are resistant. *Haemophilus influenzae* remains generally susceptible, but many *N. gonorrhoeae* are resistant. Among the Enterobacteriaceae, resistance has increased greatly in recent years so that many *E. coli* and *Shigella* species and virtually all *P. aeruginosa* are resistant. However, tetracyclines inhibit *Pasteurella multocida, Francisella tularensis, Yersinia pestis,* and *Brucella* organisms. Doxycycline inhibits *Bacteroides fragilis,* but most *Bacteroides* species are resistant to the other tetracyclines. Other anaerobic species such as *Fusobacterium* and *Actinomyces* are inhibited, as are *Borrelia burgdorferi* (the cause of Lyme disease) and others. *Mycobacterium fortuitum* and *M. marinum* are inhibited, and some activity is observed against *Plasmodium* species.

Tetracyclines are the preferred agents (see box on previous page) to treat rickettsial diseases such as Rocky Mountain spotted fever, typhus, scrub typhus, rickettsial pox, and Q fever. *Mycoplasma pneumoniae* respiratory infections respond to tetracyclines, which may be better tolerated by adults than erythromycin. Chlamydial infections of a sexual origin such as nongonococcal urethritis, salpingitis, or cervicitis are best treated with doxycycline. Tetracyclines are also effective for psittacosis, inclusion conjunctivitis; and trachoma caused by chlamydiae. Although tetracyclines inhibit many *N. gonorrhoeae,* they no longer are considered optimal therapy but are effective for syphilis if continued long enough.

As discussed under side effects, tetracyclines should not be given to pregnant women, children younger than 8 years of age, individuals with severe liver disease, or those with renal impairment.

Tetracyclines are no longer used in treating urinary tract infections, since so many other agents are available, nor are they useful for prophylaxis in viral illness to prevent bacterial infections. They have no role in the treatment of pharyngitis, and other agents are preferred against staphylococcal infections. In general, other agents should be used to treat osteomyelitis, endocarditis, meningitis, and life-threatening gram-negative infections. Minocycline inhibits many methicillin-resistant staphylococci and has been used to treat these infections; vancomycin remains the drug of choice.

The only prophylactic uses of tetracycline are minocycline to eradicate the carrier state of meningococci, but rifampin is the preferred agent. Doxycycline is used to prevent traveler's diarrhea, but photosensitization and resistance have decreased its value, and such use is no longer recommended.

Chloramphenicol

Chloramphenicol has an extremely broad spectrum of antimicrobial activity, inhibiting aerobic and anaerobic gram-positive and gram-negative bacteria, chlamydiae, rickettsiae, and mycoplasmas. It is particularly active against *Bacteroides fragilis.* Although chloramphenicol is bacteriostatic for Enterobacteriaceae, staphylococci, and streptococci, it is bactericidal for *H. influenzae, N. meningitidis,* and many *Streptococcus pneumoniae.*

Because of its serious diverse side effects, chloramphenicol should be used only when no other drug is suitable. The major use of chloramphenicol in the United States is centered around its entry into the CSF. It was combined with ampicillin to treat meningitis in children because of the frequency of β-lactamase–producing (and thus resistant) *Haemophilus* species. However, cefotaxime or ceftriaxone are now preferred therapy. Chloramphenicol also was used to treat brain abscesses, but metronidazole has replaced it. In other serious *Haemophilus* infections, cephalosporins or trimethoprim-sulfamethoxazole can replace chloramphenicol. The same is true for its use in intraabdominal infections in which metronidazole, clindamycin, cefoxitin, and imipenem are less toxic. In the treatment of typhoid, it can be replaced by trimethoprim-sulfamethoxazole or by norfloxacin or ciprofloxacin. The later agent appears to cure carriers, which chloramphenicol fails to do.

In rickettsial diseases, chloramphenicol is appropriate for patients who cannot be treated with a tetracycline, but it should not be used for urinary tract, respiratory, or brucellosis infections because other less toxic agents are available.

Erythromycin, Azithromycin, and Clarithromycin

The macrolides erythromycin, azithromycin, and clarithromycin are active primarily against gram-positive species such as staphylococci and streptococci but also inhibit some enterococci and gram-positive bacilli (see box below). Chlamydiae, *Mycoplasma pneumoniae, Ureaplasma, urealyticum, Legionella* and *Bordetella* species, *Campylobacter jejuni,* and most oral anaerobic species are inhibited. Most aerobic gram-negative bacilli are resistant, though azithromycin inhibits *Salmonella* species.

THERAPEUTIC USES OF ERYTHROMYCIN

DRUG OF CHOICE

Mycoplasma pneumoniae
Group A streptococcal infection (penicillin-allergic patient)
Legionella infection
Bordetella pertussis
Campbylobacter jejuni (children)
Ureaplasma urealyticum

ALTERNATIVE AGENT

Lyme disease
Chlamydia infection

AS TREATMENT OF SYNDROMES

Bacterial bronchitis
Otitis media (with sulfonamide)
Acne, topical

PROPHYLAXIS

Endocarditis, penicillin-allergic patient
Large bowel surgery
Oral surgery

Both azithromycin and clarithromycin inhibit *H. influenzae*. Azithromycin inhibits *Toxoplasma gondii* and *Mycobacterium avium*. Clarithromycin inhibits *M. avium* and other mycobacteria such as *M. chelonei* and *Helicobacter pylori* and *M. leprae*.

Erythromycin and other macrolides are used primarily as an alternative to penicillin, particularly in children, especially to treat streptococcal pharyngitis, erysipelas, scarlet fever, cutaneous streptococcal infections, and pneumococcal pneumonia. Although macrolides can cure *Staphylococcus aureus* infections, the high frequency of resistance of staphylococci does not make it an initial choice of therapy. For treating otitis media, erythromycin should be combined with a sulfonamide because of its variable activity against *Haemophilus* organisms.

Azithromycin is useful for treating sexually transmitted diseases, including ones caused by chlamydiae, and erythromycin can be used to treat chlamydial pneumonia of the newborn. Erythromycin is also useful to eradicate the carrier state of diphtheria and may shorten the course of pertussis if administered early.

As a prophylactic agent, erythromycin can be used to prevent bacterial endocarditis in penicillin-allergic patients or in patients with rheumatic fever.

Clarithromycin has been used to treat *Mycobacterium avium* infection in AIDS patients.

Clindamycin

Clindamycin inhibits most gram-positive cocci and many anaerobes but not aerobic gram-negative bacteria *Haemophilus*, *Mycoplasma*, and *Chlamydia*. Most enterococci are resistant, but *Actinomyces* species are inhibited.

The problem of serious diarrhea limits the use of clindamycin to specific indications. It is appropriate therapy for intraabdominal or gynecological infections in which *Bacteroides* organisms are likely pathogens but should not be used for brain abscesses when anaerobic species are anticipated. However, clindamycin is useful for anaerobic pleuropulmonary infections.

Clindamycin is an alternative to penicillin and may be preferable in certain situations in which β-lactamase–producing *Bacteroides* organisms are present. Clindamycin is also an alternative to penicillins in the treatment of staphylococcal infections but is usually not preferred to a cephalosporin or vancomycin and should not be used for endocarditis.

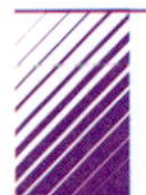

SIDE EFFECTS, CLINICAL PROBLEMS, AND TOXICITY

The major clinical problems for these drugs are summarized in the box.

Aminoglycosides

Aminoglycosides can produce serious side effects, of which vestibular, cochlear, and renal are the most important and most common.

Renal Toxicity Reversible renal impairment develops in 5% to 25% of patients receiving an aminoglycoside for more than 3 days. In a small number of patients the impairment can progress to severe renal insufficiency but is usually reversible. In the renal cortex, aminoglycosides are transported across the luminal brush border of proximal tubular cells by binding to phosphatidylinositol in the cytoplasmic membrane and undergo-

CLINICAL PROBLEMS

AMINOGLYCOSIDES
- Nephrotoxicity
- Ototoxicity
- Vestibular toxicity
- Neuromuscular blockade (infrequent)

TETRACYCLINES
- Binding to bone and teeth: can be serious in infants or children under 8 years of age and during pregnancy
- Gastrointestinal tract upsets
- Hepatic and renal dysfunction
- Vaginal candidiasis
- Vertigo with minocycline
- Photosensitivity

OTHER DRUGS
- chloramphenicol: major hematological effects can be fatal (aplastic anemia, bone marrow suppression); gray baby syndrome if glucuronidation process not well developed (for chloramphenicol elimination); drug interactions with other agents that are metabolized; optic neuritis may result
- erythromycin: relatively safe; mild gastrointestinal disturbances; infrequent hepatotoxicity; drug interaction with theophylline (metabolism); deafness with high doses
- clindamycin: pseudomembranous colitis occurs; rarely serious rash

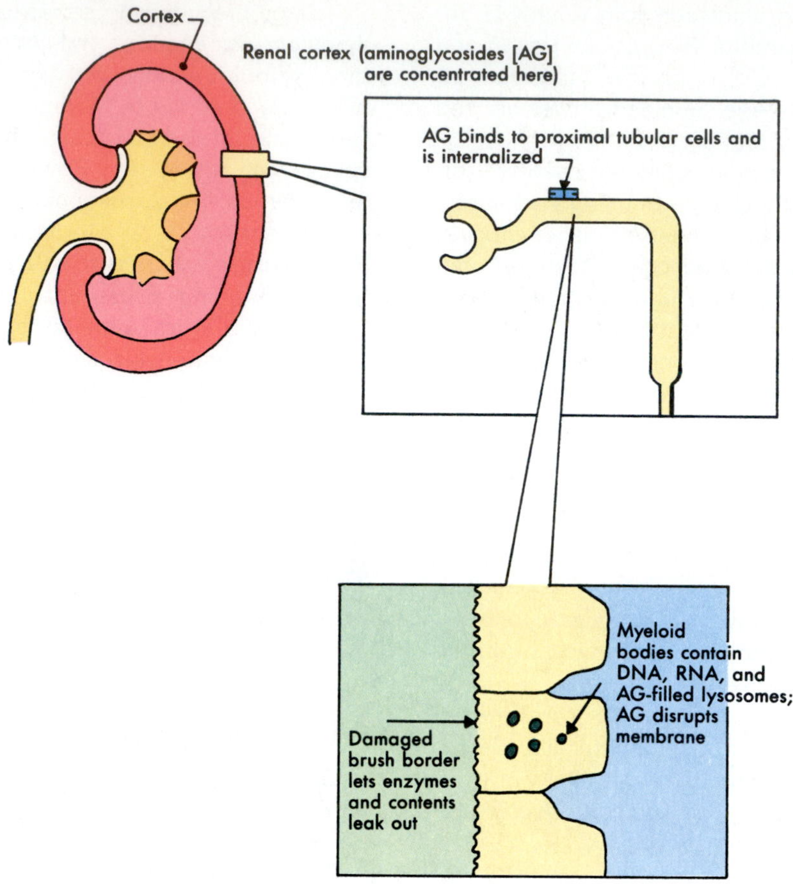

FIGURE 48-6 Schema of steps leading to nephrotoxicity caused by aminoglycosides. See the text for further information.

ing internalization by pinocytosis. Fusion with lysosomes occurs, and the aminoglycosides become trapped in the lysosomes.

Multilamellar structures, called *myeloid bodies,* also accumulate in the lysosomes (Figure 48-6), and phosphatidylinositol-specific phospholipases are inhibited. These enzymes are important in prostaglandin synthesis, and the initial decrease in glomerular filtration that occurs with aminoglycoside toxicity may result from inhibition of vasodilatory prostaglandins so that the angiotension II vasoconstrictor action is unopposed. Aminoglycosides also inhibit spingomyelinases and ATPases and alter mitochondria and ribosomes in proximal tubular cells.

The initial manifestation of aminoglycoside renal toxicity is increased excretion of brush-border enzymes such as β-D-glucosaminidase, alanine aminopeptidase, and alkaline phosphatase. However, it is not clinically useful to monitor the excretion of these enzymes, since fever and other factors also cause similar changes. Of greater clinical significance is the decrease in renal concentrating ability, proteinuria, and the appearance of casts in the urine, followed by a reduction in the glomerular filtration rate and a rise in serum creatinine.

Risk factors for development of renal toxicity are not completely understood despite extensive study. Toxicity correlates with total drug administered, but older age, female sex, concomitant liver disease, and concomitant hypotension appear to favor the development of the toxicity. Coadministration of aminoglycosides with vancomycin, cisplatin, cyclosporin, or amphotericin B is associated with increased renal toxicity, as is volume depletion and alkalosis.

Aminoglycosides themselves differ in their nephrotoxic potential. Neomycin is the most nephrotoxic, and streptomycin is the least. However, clinical trials comparing the nephrotoxicity of the other agents yield contradictory results.

Because tubules can regenerate, renal function usually returns to normal after the drug is cleared. A small number of patients require dialysis because renal function does not return to pretreatment values.

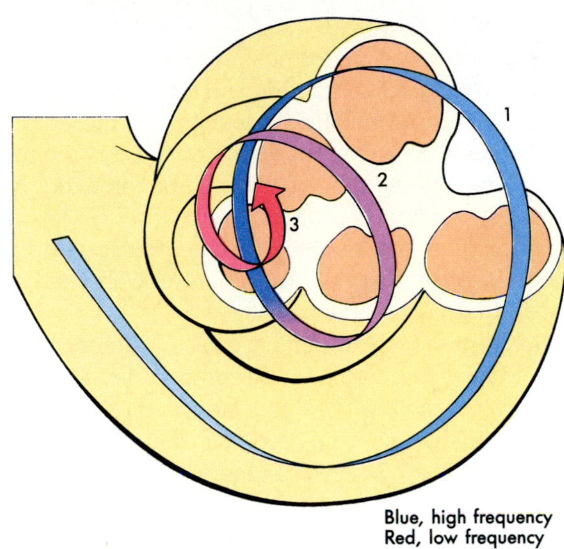

FIGURE 48-7 Cochlea, normally lined with hair cells that are destroyed by high concentrations of aminoglycosides. Aminoglycosides produce damage to the hair cells, especially in turn No. 1 and part of turn No. 2. Hairs are shed by the damaged cells to give loss of high-frequency response first (associated with turn No. 1) and low-frequency loss later (associated with turn No. 3).

Ototoxicity Aminoglycosides can damage either or both the auditory and vestibular apparatuses. The exact frequency of ototoxicity is unknown, but some damage probably occurs in 5% to 25% of patients, depending on the underlying auditory status and length of therapy. The mechanism of auditory toxicity is destruction of hair cells of the organ of Corti, particularly the outer hair cells in the basal turn (Figure 48-7). Inner hair cells and cells of the stria vascularis can also be affected. The hair cell damage is accompanied by subsequent retrograde degeneration of the auditory nerves. Aminoglycosides also damage hair cells of the ampullar cristae, leading to vestibular dysfunction and vertigo. Aminoglycosides accumulate in perilymph and endolymph and inhibit ionic transport, the cause of cochlear cell damage. Accumulation of drug occurs when the plasma concentrations are high for prolonged periods, and ototoxicity is probably enhanced by persistently elevated plasma concentrations of drug. Single daily high-dose therapy produces less ototoxicity.

The amount of auditory or vestibular function loss correlates with the amount of hair cell damage. Repeated courses of therapy continue to damage more hair cells. An unanswered question is whether loop diuretics, such as furosemide, potentiate this ototoxicity in humans as they do in animals.

Differences in toxicity exist among the agents. Streptomycin and gentamicin cause more vestibular toxicity, and kanamycin and amikacin cause more auditory damage. Whether netilmicin is less ototoxic than other aminoglycosides is not clear. Vestibular toxicity is highest for patients who receive 4 weeks of therapy, the procedure used in the treatment of enterococcal endocarditis.

Clinical signs of auditory problems such as tinnitus or a sensation of fullness in the ears are not reliable as predictors of this toxicity. The initial hearing loss is of high frequencies outside the voice range; thus, toxicity development will not be recognized unless hearing tests are performed. Eventually the loss of hearing may progress into the auditory range.

Vestibular toxicity is usually preceded by headache, nausea, emesis, vertigo, and dizziness; so patients who are ill often have difficulty in evaluating the onset of vestibular toxicity. These patients may go through a series of stages from acute to chronic symptoms that are apparent only on standing, or the patients may achieve a compensatory state in which visual cues adjust for the loss of vestibular function.

Neuromuscular Blockade Neuromuscular paralysis is rare but appears to be caused by inhibition of presynaptic release of acetylcholine and postsynaptic receptor blockade. Aminoglycoside inhibits internalization of calcium at the presynaptic nerve terminal, thus blocking the release of acetylcholine. Presynaptic blockade is more readily caused by neomycin and tobramycin than by streptomycin, whereas the opposite order is observed for postsynaptic effects.

Neuromuscular paralysis is most likely to occur during surgery when anesthesia and neuromuscular blockers such as succinylcholine are used, but it also occurs in patients with myasthenia gravis.

Other Toxicities Reversible dose-related malabsorption is observed with oral use of aminoglycosides. It is caused by direct damage to villus cells and by binding to bile salts. Absorption of fat, protein, cholesterol, iron, and digitalis is impaired.

Spectinomycin

Spectinomycin has few adverse effects.

Tetracyclines

Tetracyclines produce adverse effects ranging from minor to life threatening. Allergy precludes the use of tetracycline. Photosensitization with a rash is a toxic rather than an allergic effect and is most often seen with demeclocycline or doxycycline.

Effects on bone and teeth preclude the use of tetracycline in children less than 8 years of age because 80% of them will develop a permanent brown-yellow discoloration of teeth if treated with tetracyclines. The effect is permanent and the enamel is hypoplastic. Binding to bone may result in depression of skeletal growth, especially in premature infants.

Tetracyclines cause dose-dependent gastrointestinal disturbances including epigastric burning, nausea, and vomiting. Esophageal ulcers have been reported. Pancreatitis is rarely observed.

Hepatic toxicity is encountered most often with parenteral use but can also occur with oral administration. Pregnant women are highly susceptible to tetracycline-hepatic toxicity with development of jaundice and fatty infiltration of the liver. Tetracyclines also aggravate existing renal dysfunction.

Demeclocycline which is used to treat chronic excessive antidiuretic hormone secretion, produces nephrogenic diabetes insipidus. Other side effects include minocycline-produced vertigo, particularly in women. Superinfection caused by overgrowth of other bacteria and particularly oral and vaginal candidiasis frequently follows the use of tetracyclines.

Tetracyclines should not be used in patients receiving hyperalimentation, since they prevent new protein synthesis.

Chloramphenicol

Chloramphenicol produces serious side effects that are attributed to its action in mitochondrial membrane enzymes, cytochrome oxidases, and adenosine triphosphatases. Because of these adverse effects, chloramphenicol has only limited use, primarily when no other alternative treatment is suitable.

Hematological effects are the most important. Leukopenia, thrombocytopenia, marrow aplasia, and pancytopenia occurrence is 1:25,000 to 1:40,000, with a high death rate for those who develop an aplastic state or progress to acute leukemia. This appears to involve an idiosyncratic reaction with inhibition of stem cells and may result from a biochemical abnormality that causes formation of a toxic metabolite.

Additional hematological effects include reversible erythroid bone marrow suppression, prevention of normal response to vitamin B_{12}, and hemolysis in some patients deficient in glucose-6-phosphate dehydrogenase. The marrow suppression develops 5 to 7 days into therapy and is manifest by a decrease in hemoglobin, an increase in plasma iron, and vacuolization of erythroblasts to produce thrombocytopenia and leukopenia.

A complication known as the *gray baby syndrome* also is encountered with chloramphenicol. Neonates with excessively high plasma concentrations of drug develop pallor, cyanosis, abdominal distention, vomiting, and circulatory collapse, resulting in approximately 50% fatalities.

High concentrations of chloramphenicol are caused by inadequate glucuronidation and failure to excrete the drug by the kidneys. Children less than 1 month of age should receive only low doses of this drug, though in overdose situations, excess drug can be removed by hemoperfusion over a bed of charcoal.

Chloramphenicol also can produce optic neuritis in children, gastrointestinal overgrowth of *Candida* organisms, and hypersensitivity rashes.

Chloramphenicol inhibits hepatic microsomal enzymes of the cytochrome P-450 complex, leading to prolongation of the half-life of phenytoin, tolbutamide, chlorpropamide, and dicumarol; barbiturates in turn decrease the half-life of chloramphenicol.

Erythromycin

Erythromycin is one of the safest antibiotics, with gastrointestinal epigastric pain, abdominal cramps,

TRADE NAMES

In addition to generic and fixed-combinations of preparations that include other drugs and active compounds available as other salts, the following trade-named materials are available in the United States.

AMINOGLYCOSIDE

Amikin, amikacin sulfate
Garamycin, G-myticin, gentamicin sulfate
Kantrex, kanamycin sulfate
Nebcin, tobramycin sulfate
Netroymcin, netilmicin sulfate

TETRACYCLINE

Achromycin, Suymyin, tetracycline
Doryx, doxycycline
Minocin, minocycline HCl
Terramycin, Urobiotic, oxytetracycline or salt
Vibramycin calcium, doxycycline calcium

OTHER DRUGS

Chloromycetin, chloramphenicol salts
Cleocin, clindamycin salts
ERYC, Erycette, Ery Derm, Erygel, Ilotycin, erythromycin
Ilosone, erythromycin estolate
Pediamycin, Eryzole, Wyamycin, erythromycin ethylsuccinate (contains sulfisoxazole)
Trobicin, spectinomycin HCl
Biaxin, clarithromycin, azithromycin,
Zithromax

nausea, and emesis the primary side effects. Hepatotoxicity may occur with erythromycin sulfate, usually beginning 10 to 20 days into treatment and characterized by jaundice, fever, leukocytosis, and eosinophilia. The problem rapidly abates if drug administration is stopped. Erythromycin at high doses can cause reversible transient deafness. Erythromycin's metabolic product, spiroketal erythromycin, stimulates motulin, the gastric hormone, and causes gastric emptying. Thus erythromycin can be used in patients with gastroparesis.

Erythromycin prolongs the $t_{1/2}$ of theophylline and can lead to theophylline toxicity. It also inhibits the metabolism of carbamazepine, corticosteroids, and digoxin.

Clindamycin

The most important adverse effect of clindamycin is pseudomembranous enterocolitis, estimated to occur in 3% to 5% of patients. Diarrhea may occur in up to 20% of patients. Pseudomembranous colitis is caused by the toxin produced by *Clostridium difficile.* The illness is characterized by diarrhea, abdominal pain, and fever, with diarrhea beginning either during or after therapy with clindamycin. Orally administered vancomycin or metronidazole may be needed as therapy.

REFERENCES

Neu HC, Young LA, Zinner S, editors: *Macrolides, azalides, and streptogramins,* New York, 1993, Marcel Dekker.

Peters DH: Azithromycin, *Drugs* 44:750-799, 1992.

Peters DH, Clissold SP: Carithromycin, *Drugs* 44;117-164, 1992.

Whelton A, Neu HC, editors: *The aminoglycosides,* New York, 1982, Marcel Dekker.

SELF-ASSESSMENT QUESTIONS

1. Mupirocin inhibits which of the following organisms?
   a. *Bacteroides fragilis*
   b. *Staphylococcus aureus*
   c. *Pseudomonas aeruginosa*
   d. *Candida albicans*
2. Spectinomycin is used to treat infection caused by which of the following?
   a. *Streptococcus pyogenes*
   b. *Escherichia coli*
   c. *Klebsiella pneumoniae*
   d. *Neisseria gonorrhoeae*
3. Which of the following is used as prophylaxis of meningococcal meningitis?
   a. rifampin
   b. gentamicin
   c. erythromycin
   d. chloramphenicol
   e. clindamycin
4. Which of the following chemotherapeutic agents does not achieve adequate concentrations within phagocytic cells to kill intracellular pathogens?
   a. gentamicin
   b. rifampin
   c. clarithromycin
   d. azithromycin
5. Which of the following are toxic effects of the aminoglycoside antibiotic amikacin?
   a. hearing impairment resulting from toxic effect on hair cells of the cochlea
   b. nephrotoxicity caused by damage to proximal renal tubular cells
   c. production of neuromuscular blockade
   d. all of the above
   e. none of the above
6. Chloramphenicol is inactivated by which of the following mechanisms?
   a. oxidation to 1-oxo derivatives
   b. glucuronidation
   c. *N*-acetylation
   d. phosphorylation
   e. excretion by tubular secretion
7. Used as treatment of streptococcal pharyngitis in a penicillin-allergic patient:
   a. rifampin
   b. tetracycline
   c. erythromycin
   d. clindamycin
8. Tetracyclines should not be administered with which?
   a. furosemide
   b. potassium salts
   c. iron salts
   d. cimetidine
   e. sodium chloride
9. Which of the following is not inhibited by clindamycin?
   a. *Streptococcus pyogenes*
   b. *Enterococcus faecalis*
   c. *Bacteroides melaninogenicus*
   d. *Actinomyces israelii*
   e. *Staphylococcus aureus*

10. Aminoglycosides are removed from the body by which route?
    a. metabolism
    b. tubular secretion
    c. glomerular filtration
    d. biliary secretion
11. Which of the following aminoglycosides is most resistant to inactivation by aminoglycoside-inactivating enzymes?
    a. streptomycin
    b. neomycin
    c. gentamicin
    d. amikacin
    e. tobramycin
12. Resistance to which of the following agents can result from alteration of RNA polymerase?
    a. rifampin
    b. isoniazid
    c. gentamicin
    d. tetracycline

CHAPTER 49 Bacterial Folate Antagonists

HAROLD C. NEU

MAJOR DRUGS

sulfonamides
trimethoprim

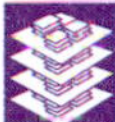

THERAPEUTIC OVERVIEW

The sulfonamides and trimethoprim are antibiotics that act through inhibition of the folate pathway in bacteria. The folate system serves in a donor-acceptor role for the transfer of one-carbon groups, such as methyl and methylene, and electrons in intracellular synthesis and degradation reactions. Most bacteria must synthesize their folic acid derivatives, whereas humans can rely on dietary sources. Thus inhibition of bacterial capability for the synthesis of folate can serve as a route for antibiotic development and is the common factor for the mechanism of action of the sulfonamides and trimethoprim, which are described in this chapter.

The introduction of the sulfonamides into clinical medicine marks the beginning of microbial chemotherapy. In the 1930s, chemists in Germany showed that the dye prontosil protected mice infected with streptococci and other bacteria and that sulfonamide was the active component. Many sulfonamide derivatives have been synthesized and tested in humans, but only a few are in clinical use. Sulfonamides formerly were preferred for the treatment of urinary tract infections. However, the development of resistant bacteria, the presence of numerous side effects, and the availability of other antibiotics have led to their discontinuation. These drugs remain of value in the treatment of nocardiosis and, topically, for burn areas. Sulfadiazine is used to treat toxoplasmosis. The trimethoprim-sulfamethoxazole combination has many therapeutic applications. The therapeutic aspects are summarized in the box.

ABBREVIATIONS

TMP/SMX	trimethoprim-sulfamethoxazole

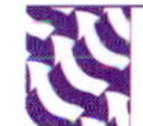

MECHANISMS OF ACTION

Folic Acid Synthesis and Regeneration

The bacterial synthesis of folic acid uses a multistep enzyme-catalyzed reaction sequence, summarized in Figure 49-1. Folic acid consists of *p*-aminobenzoic acid, pteridine, and glutamic acid linked together and can undergo reduction to dihydrofolate and further to tetrahydrofolate. The enzymes that catalyze step A, dihydropteroate synthetase, and step B, dihydrofolate reductase, are competitively inhibited by sulfonamides and trimethoprim, respectively. Thus these two drug types block the synthesis of tetrahydrofolate at different steps in the synthetic pathway. Blocking two steps also results in a feedback inhibition at the beginning of the pathway, and together the agents are bactericidal. (Figure 49-1).

Sulfonamides

The structures of many of the clinically used sulfonamides are shown in Figure 49-2. These agents are bacteriostatic. They are competitive inhibitors of *p*-aminobenzoic acid incorporation through a high affinity for dihydropteroate synthetase. Although competitive enzyme inhibition is the main mechanism of action, the sulfonamides can function as alternative substrates for the synthetase and become incorporated into a product with pteridine, thus depleting the system of pteridine.

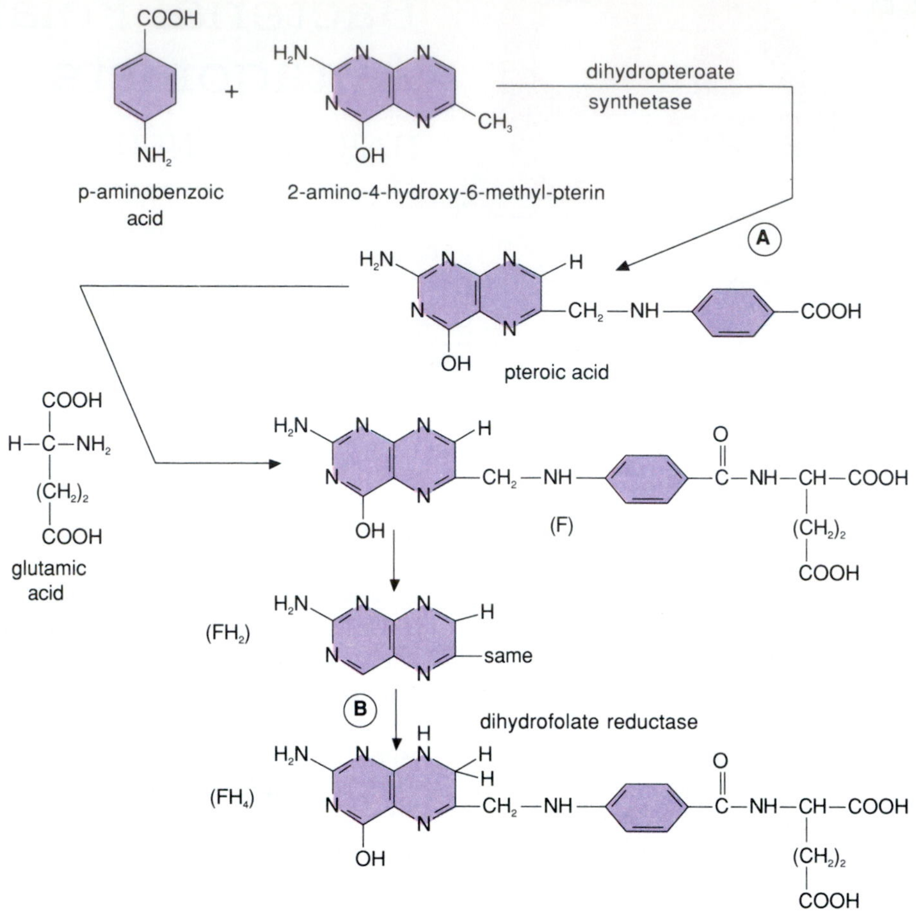

FIGURE 49-1 Bacterial synthesis of folic acid (F) and reduction to dihydrofolate (FH_2) and tetrahydrofolate (FH_2). **A** and **B** are sites of drug action.

THERAPEUTIC OVERVIEW

SULFONAMIDES

First chemotherapeutic agents
No longer urinary infection drugs of choice
- Resistant bacteria
- Significant side effects
- Other drugs available

Nocardiosis, toxoplasmosis, and burn areas: still effective

TRIMETHOPRIM-SULFAMETHOXAZOLE COMBINATION

Effective for urinary, respiratory, gastrointestinal, and gonorrhea infections with many organisms and for treatment of *Pneumocystis carinii* infections and *Isospora belli*

Microorganisms cannot use preformed pteroylglutamic acid and must synthesize their own, accounting for their sensitivity. In contrast, mammalian cells require the preformed acid. Folate metabolism is necessary for the production of thymidine, purines, and several amino acids, including methionine. Therefore, when folate synthesis is inhibited, bacterial cell growth is halted. This inhibition of cell growth can be reversed by addition of purines, thymidine, methionine, and serine.

In sulfonamides the *para*-NH_2 (or *para*-amino) group is essential for antibacterial activity and can be replaced only by groups that are converted to the free amino group in vivo. *Ortho*- and *meta*-amino substituents are inactive. The $-SO_2NH_2$ group can be substituted, but there must be a direct sulfur-carbon link to the benzene ring. Structural changes also have a pronounced effect on sulfonamide solubility. For example, sulfadiazine and sulfisoxazole are 10 and 100 times, respectively, more soluble at pH 7.5 than at pH 5.5.

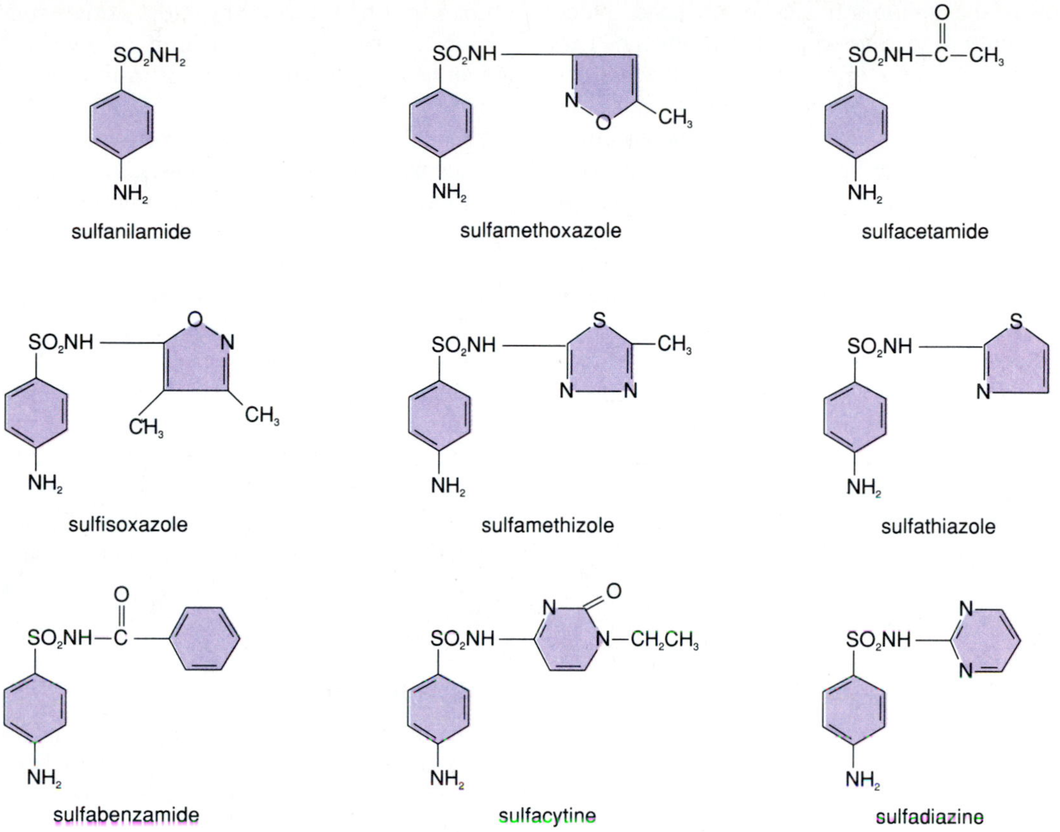

FIGURE 49-2 Structures of clinically useful sulfonamides with prototype. See the text for further information.

Bacterial resistance to sulfonamides occurs by several mechanisms. Reduced cellular uptake of drug, which can be of chromosomal or plasmid origin, is one mechanism. Another is an altered dihydropteroate synthetase, which can result from a point mutation or the presence of a plasmid that causes synthesis of a new enzyme. Replacement of a single amino acid in the enzyme alters the affinity for sulfonamides. In enteric species, plasmid-propagated resistance is the common form. A final mechanism of resistance is production of increased amounts of *p*-aminobenzoic acid, which is found with some staphylococci but is not common. Resistance stemming from an altered enzyme can develop during therapy.

Trimethoprim

Trimethoprim was initially used as an antimalarial drug but has been replaced by pyrimethamine, which acts by a similar mechanism. The antimalarial and antibacterial actions of trimethoprim (see Figure 49-3 for structure) are based on its high affinity for bacterial dihydrofolate reductase. Trimethoprim binds competitively and inhibits this enzyme in bacterial and mammalian cells. About 100,000 times higher concentrations of drug are needed to obtain 50% inhibition of the human enzyme as compared to the bacterial. This enzyme is inhibited by methotrexate, discussed in Chapter 43. Trimethoprim thus prevents the conversion of dihydrofolate to tetrahydrofolate and thereby blocks the formation of thymidine, some purines, methionine, and glycine in the bacteria, leading to rapid death of the microorganisms.

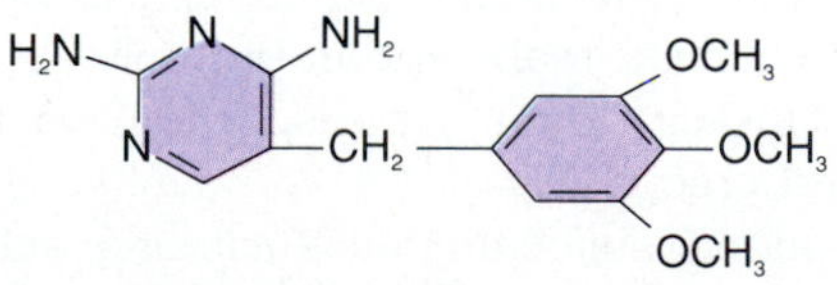

FIGURE 49-3 Chemical structure of trimethoprim. See the text for further information.

Trimethoprim and sulfamethoxazole are used effectively in combination to give synergistic effects. The two drugs block different steps in the synthesis of reduced folic acid. Moreover, sulfonamide potentiates the action of trimethoprim by reducing dihydrofolate competing with trimethoprim for binding to dihydrofolate reductase. The combination of the two drugs is bactericidal.

Resistance to trimethoprim and to the combination of trimethoprim-sulfamethoxazole (TMP/SMX) arises from permeability changes and from the presence of an altered dihydrofolate reductase. The production of this enzyme can be modified by a chromosomal mutation or by a plasmid. An increasing incidence of resistance to TMP/SMX by the plasmid mechanism is occurring. A mutation to thymine dependence has also been found, as has overproduction of dihydrofolate reductase.

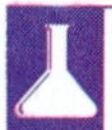

PHARMACOKINETICS

The relevant pharmacokinetic parameters are summarized in Table 49-1.

Sulfonamide

Suifonamides are generally well absorbed from the gastrointestinal tract (approximately 70% to 95%), with the majority of absorption in the small intestine. There is minimal absorption from topical application.

Sulfonamides differ in protein binding, from a low of 35% to 50% for sulfadiazine to 80% to 99% for sulfisoxazole or sulfasalazine, with less protein binding in renal failure. The drugs enter most body compartments, including ocular, pleural, peritoneal, synovial, and CSF. Highest concentrations in the CSF are achieved with sulfadiazine, reaching 30% to 80% of simultaneous plasma concentrations. Sulfonamides cross the placenta and enter the fetal circulation.

Acetylation in liver is a major mechanism of inactivation of sulfonamides. The agents vary in the degree of acetylation of the amino group, with the products being inactive and less soluble in urine. Acetylation is increased with renal disease and decreased with impaired hepatic function. Metabolism by glucuronidation also occurs with these compounds. All metabolites are excreted in the urine. Renal elimination is by filtration, with some tubular reabsorption but only slight tubular secretion. In acid urine, some sulfonamides are poorly soluble and precipitate.

Rapid-acting sulfonamides, including sulfisoxazole, sulfamethoxazole, and sulfadiazine, are rapidly absorbed and eliminated. Sulfadiazine is rapidly absorbed from the gastrointestinal tract, with peak plasma concentrations in 3 hours. It is the most active sulfonamide, but problems of crystialluria limit its use. Sulfisoxazole is acetylated, and 30% of the drug in the blood or urine is in the acetylated form. Approximately 95% is excreted in 24 hours, and urine concentrations are high. Because sulfisoxazole is highly soluble in urine, it rarely produces crystals in renal tubules. Sulfamethoxazole is similar to sulfisoxazole but is less rapidly absorbed and excreted.

Sulfadoxine is well absorbed and highly bound to plasma proteins, with an extraordinarily long half-life of 10 to 17 days. It is combined with pyrimethamine in the treatment and prophylaxis of falciparum malaria.

Sulfasalazine is poorly absorbed from the gastrointestinal tract and therefore can be used to treat gastrointestinal infections. It is metabolized by intestinal bacteria to sulfapyridine, which is absorbed from the intestine and excreted in the urine, and in turn to a second metabolite, 5-aminosalicylate, which is the active agent. Sulfasalazine can produce all the toxic reactions of the other sulfonamides.

Trimethoprim

Trimethoprim is well absorbed from the gastrointestinal tract, with peak plasma concentrations in about 2 hours. Absorption is not influenced by sulfamethoxazole.

Trimethoprim is rapidly and widely distributed to body tissues and compartments, entering pleural, peritoneal, and synovial fluids, as well as the aqueous fluid of the eye, the CSF, and brain. Because of its high lipid solubility, trimethoprim crosses biological membranes and enters bronchial secretions, prostate and vaginal fluids, and bile. Trimethoprim and sulfamethoxazole cross the placenta.

Only 10% to 20% of trimethoprim is metabolized by oxidation and conjugation to inactive oxide and hydroxyl derivatives. It is excreted in urine with 60% of the dose excreted in 24 hours with normal renal function and a linear relationship between serum creatinine and trimethoprim half-life. The half-life of 11 hours in normal adults and children is shortened to approximately 6 hours in young children. Urinary concentrations of trimethoprim are high even in the presence of decreased renal function, and a small amount of trimethoprim is excreted in bile.

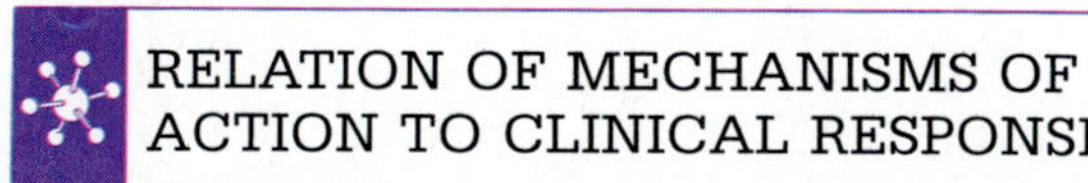

RELATION OF MECHANISMS OF ACTION TO CLINICAL RESPONSE

Sulfonamides

The antibacterial spectrum of sulfonamides varies from one community to another. Most streptococci, in-

Table 49-1 Pharmacokinetic Parameters for Main Clinical Agents

Drug	Route of Administration	$t_{1/2}$ (hr)	Disposition	Plasma Protein Bound (%)
sulfacetamide	Topical	—	—	—
sulfisoxazole	Oral	6	R, M	90
sulfamethoxazole	Oral/IV	11	R, M	70
sulfadiazine	Oral/IV	17	M, R	45
sulfadoxine	Oral	120-200	R, M	98
sulfamethizole	Oral	1, 5	R, M	90
sulfasalazine	Oral	6-10	R, M	99
trimethoprim	Oral	11	R (60%) M	70

M, Metabolized; *R*, renal excretion as unchanged drug.

cluding *Streptococcus pneumoniae, Haemophilus influenzae,* and chlamydiae, are susceptible, and *Neisseria meningitidis, N. gonorrhoeae, Brucella* organisms, and *Campylobacter* species vary from highly susceptible to resistant. Enterococci are resistant, and some strains of *Escherichia coli* that cause urinary tract infections are susceptible. However, most *E. coli* strains are resistant. *Shigella* species, most staphylococci, *Bacteroides fragilis,* and *Pseudomonas* organisms are resistant. Sulfonamides inhibit *Nocardia asteroides*.

The sulfonamides are grouped into rapidly acting, intermediate acting, long-acting, poorly absorbed, and topical agents. (See Table 49-1).

Triple sulfonamide preparations, containing sulfamerazine, sulfamethazine, and sulfadiazine in one preparation and sulfabenzamide, sulfacetamide, and sulfathiazole in another, are also rapid acting. None of these are more useful than sulfisoxazole. Sulfisoxazole is combined with erythromycin ethylsuccinate for treatment of otitis media in children.

Sulfadiazine achieves highest concentrations in CSF and brain. When sulfadiazine is used, fluid intake must be high, or alkalinization can be achieved by administration of sodium bicarbonate to reduce the risk of renal crystalluria by the drug.

The only long-acting sulfonamide used today is sulfadoxine, which is available in combination with pyrimethamine to treat malaria.

Of the poorly absorbed sulfonamides, sulfasalazine is minimally absorbed from the gastrointestinal tract and is used to treat ulcerative colitis and regional enteritis. It has no effect on intestinal flora.

Sulfacetamide, a topical agent, is used in ophthalmic preparations because it penetrates into ocular tissues and fluids. Allergic reactions are rare, though it should not be used in patients with a known sulfonamide allergy.

Silver sulfadiazine is active against a large number of bacterial species, including *Pseudomonas aeruginosa,* with the activity probably resulting from slow release of silver into the surrounding medium. This drug is used topically, particularly with burn patients, to reduce bacteria in the burn eschar to levels low enough to prevent burn wound sepsis and to hasten wound healing. Minimal silver is absorbed, but sulfadiazine can be absorbed. Adverse reactions are uncommon.

Mafenide is a sulfonamide earlier used in burn treatment. It inhibits gram-positive and gram-negative bacteria and is not inhibited by *p*-aminobenzoic acid. It is absorbed and converted to *p*-carboxybenzene sulfonamide. It has been used to prevent burn wound colonization, but adverse reactions favor the use of silver sulfadiazine. Mafenide and its breakdown products are carbonic anhydrase inhibitors, which can cause metabolic acidosis. There usually is a compensatory alkalosis caused by respiratory adjustment.

Therapeutic Uses There are few indications for use of sulfonamides because a large number of other agents are available. However, the presence of certain opportunistic infections in patients with acquired immunodeficiency syndrome has rekindled interest in these drugs.

Sulfonamides formerly were the preferred agents for treatment of urinary tract infections, but acute lower urinary tract infections now are treated with other compounds. The sulfonamides have no role in the treatment of complicated or upper urinary tract infections or in the treatment of respiratory infections, except in combination with erythromycin to treat otitis media in children. Shigellosis no longer can be treated with sulfonamides alone, and trimethoprim-sulfamethoxazole or quinolones are drugs of choice in adults.

Two additional diseases in which sulfonamides are of value are nocardiosis, which involves therapy for many months, and toxoplasmosis, using sulfadiazine or sulfisoxazole and pyrimethamine.

Although sulfonamides can be used for prophylaxis of rheumatic fever, penicillins are preferred, and in penicillin-allergic patients, erythromycin is a better alternative.

Trimethoprim

Trimethoprim inhibits many different bacteria and, with sulfamethoxazole (the TMP/SMX combination), several parasites. Trimethoprim alone inhibits most urinary pathogens, except for *P. aeruginosa*. Also, it is not highly active alone against Neisseriae.

The TMP/SMX combination inhibits most *Staphylococcus aureus;* coagulase-negative staphylococci, including *S. saprophyticus;* many methicillin-resistant *S. aureus;* hemolytic streptococci; *H. influenzae; N. meningitidis; N. gonorrhoeae; Listeria monocytogenes;* aérobic gram-negative bacteria such as *E. coli* and *Klebsiella;* and some more difficult species such as *Enterobacter, Citrobacter,* and *Serratia. Salmonella, Shigella, Aeromonas,* and *Yersinia* species are inhibited, but enterococci and *Campylobacter* species are resistant.

The TMP/SMX combination inhibits *Pneumocystis carinii* and *Isospora belli,* the parasitic organisms in immunocompromised patients that cause some pneumonias and diarrhea, respectively (see Chapter 51).

Therapeutic Uses The TMP/SMX combination is effective in the treatment of uncomplicated urinary tract infections caused by Enterobacteriaceae. Maintaining trimethoprim in vaginal secretions prophylactically is believed to contribute to reducing recurrent urinary tract infections in females. The TMP/SMX combination is also an effective therapy of prostatitis resulting from Enterobacteriaceae and in the treatment of orchitis and epididymitis attributable to susceptible bacteria and chlamydiae. Trimethoprim alone is effective therapy of uncomplicated and recurrent urinary tract infections in women and as a prophylaxis to prevent recurrences.

The TMP/SMX combination is also effective treatment of gonorrhea when continued over several days. It is efficacious for some chlamydial urethritis problems through the activity of sulfonamide. Chancroid can be treated with the combination, but not syphilis.

The TMP/SMX combination is effective treatment of acute bacterial exacerbations of bronchitis caused by *H. influenzae, Moraxella (Branhamella)* species, and *S. pneumoniae.* The combination is also effective therapy of otitis media in children resulting from the aforementioned organisms but should not be used to treat streptococcal pharyngitis. Sinusitis caused by ampicillin-resistant *Haemophilus* organisms can also be treated with the combination.

The TMP/SMX combination is effective for therapy of shigellosis and for diarrhea caused by toxigenic *E. coli.* It is also useful against *Yersinia* species, systemic *Salmonella* infections, and typhoid. *Campylobacter* diarrhea is not treated.

High-dose TMP/SMX is effective therapy of *Pneumocystis* pneumonia in immunocompromised patients, equally effective to pentamidine, but adverse effects are common.

Many other infections (brucellosis, biliary tract infections, osteomyelitis, bacteremia, and endocarditis) can be successfully treated with TMP/SMX. When administered IV, it is effective treatment of *Neisseria meningitidis* in penicillin-allergic patients.

TMP/SMX can be used successfully as prophylaxis of recurrent infection and of pneumonitis resulting from *Pneumocystis carinii.* Although reductions in other gram-negative infections may be seen in pediatric patients, the combination is less successful for such infections in adults.

TMP/SMX has proved useful as therapy of Wegener's granulomatosis (see Chapter 51).

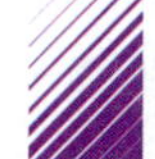

SIDE EFFECTS, CLINICAL PROBLEMS, AND TOXICITY

The major clinical problems for these drugs are summarized in the box below.

Sulfonamides

Sulfonamides unfortunately cause a large number of adverse reactions, the most important of which are hypersensitivity reactions. Allergic rashes are frequent, occurring in approximately 2% to 3% of patients receiving these drugs. Rashes may be maculopapular, urticarial, or, rarely, exfoliative, as in the Stevens-Johnson syn-

CLINICAL PROBLEMS

SULFONAMIDES

Numerous side effects
- Hypersensitivity: rashes, fever
- Stevens-Johnson syndrome (with long-acting agents)
- Renal tubule precipitation of sulfadiazine

Drug interactions
- Protein-binding displacement
- Same metabolizing enzymes as other drugs

TRIMETHOPRIM

Side effects less pronounced
Hematological reactions
Increased serum creatinine

drome. Most rashes occur after 1 week of therapy but can occur earlier in individuals previously sensitized. A serum sickness–like illness also is seen, with fever, joint pains, and rash, which can be of the erythema nodosum type. Drug fever occurs in about 3% of individuals given sulfonamides. The patients may complain of malaise, headache, chills, and pruritus. Arteritis of a periarteritis or systemic lupus erythematosus type has also been reported.

The most serious cutaneous toxicity, that of Stevens-Johnson syndrome, is distinctly uncommon with the short-acting sulfonamides but is seen with the long-acting agents. For this reason sulfadoxine is no longer used for malaria prophylaxis.

Several hematological toxicities are seen with sulfonamide use. These include agranulocytosis, megaloblastic anemia, aplastic anemia, hemolytic anemia, and thrombocytopenia. Agranulocytosis occurs in less than 0.1% patients and most recover, though the recovery can take up to a month. Neutropenia occurs occasionally but is rapidly resolved by stopping the drug. Thrombocytopenia of a mild degree is common, but severe depression of platelet counts is rare. Hemolytic anemia can occur in individuals deficient in glucose-6-phosphate dehydrogenase, in which the sulfonamide serves as an oxidant. The episode usually occurs in the first week of therapy, causing an associated reticulocytosis, bilirubinemia, urobilinuria, and pronounced decreased of hemoglobulin concentrations. Hemolysis can also occur in patients who have normal glucose-6-phosphate dehydrogenase concentrations.

Hepatotoxicity, occurring in less than 0.1% of patients receiving sulfonamides, manifests as fever, nausea, emesis, jaundice, and elevation of serum transaminases. This can rarely progress to liver failure, and the problem generally disappears with drug withdrawal. The reaction does not seem to be dose related.

TRADE NAMES

In addition to generic and fixed-combination preparations, the following trade-named materials are available in the United States.

AVC, sulfanilamide
Bactrim, trimethoprim-sulfamethoxazole, TMP/SMX
Gantanol, sulfamethoxazole
Gantrisin, sulfisoxazole
Proloprim, trimethoprim
Septra, trimethoprim-sulfamethoxazole, TMP/SMX
Sulamyd, sulfacetamide
Thiosulfil, sulfamethiazole
Trimpex, trimethoprim

Renal damage is rare with the newer sulfonamides, but sulfadiazine can precipitate in the kidneys, ureters, and bladder and lead to renal failure.

Drug interactions include potentiation of the action of sulfonylurea hypoglycemic agents, orally administered anticoagulants, phenytoin, and methotrexate. Mechanisms are displacement of albumin-bound drug and competition for drug-metabolizing enzymes.

Trimethoprim

Trimethoprim alone can cause nausea, vomiting, and diarrhea but rarely causes a rash. At the doses used for urinary tract infection, hematological toxicity is uncommon, though neutropenia and thrombocytopenia can occur. Trimethoprim can cause an increase in creatinine concentrations, since both compounds compete for the same renal clearance pathways.

The TMP/SMX combination has all the complications of both agents. Hematological toxicity in the form of megaloblastic anemia, thrombocytopenia, and leukopenia occurs more often with the combination than with the single agents and can be dose related. Other toxicities include glossitis, stomatitis, and occasional pseudomembranous enterocolitis. CNS effects include headache, depression, and hallucinations.

Patients with acquired immunodeficiency syndrome have a greater incidence of rash and neutropenia than other patients when treated with the TMP/SMX combination. The hematological toxicity can be reversed by use of folinic acid without a decrease in antimicrobial activity.

REFERENCES

Harvey RJ: Synergism in the folate pathway, *Rev Infect Dis* 4:255, 1982.

Hitchings GH, editor: *Inhibition of folate metabolism in chemotherapy,* New York, 1983, Springer-Verlag.

Kovacs JA, Masur H: *Pneumocystis carinii* pneumonia: therapy and prophylaxis, *J Infect Dis* 158:254, 1988.

National Institutes of Health Consensus Developmental Conference: Travelers' diarrhea, *JAMA* 253:2700, 1985.

Salter, AJ: Overview. Trimethoprim-sulfamethoxazole: an assessment of more than 12 years of use, *Rev Infect Dis* 4:196, 1982.

Shear NH et al: Differences in metabolism of sulfonamides, predisposing to idiosyncratic toxicity, *Ann Intern Med* 105:179, 1986.

SELF-ASSESSMENT QUESTIONS

1. What is the major mechanism of metabolism of sulfonamides?
   a. acetylation
   b. *o*-Methylation
   c. glucuronidation
   d. oxidation
2. Trimethoprim alters the excretion of:
   a. penicillins.
   b. creatinine.
   c. aminoglycosides.
   d. uric acid.
3. Which of the following organisms is routinely resistant to trimethoprim?
   a. *Staphylococcus aureus*
   b. *Haemophilus influenzae*
   c. *Pseudomonas aeruginosa*
   d. *Escherichia coli*
4. Sulfonamides lack activity against which of the following?
   a. *Escherichia coli*
   b. *Nocardia asteroides*
   c. *Toxoplasma gondii*
   d. *Neisseria meningitidis*
   e. *Candida albicans*
5. The activity of which of the following is antagonized by *para*-aminobenzoic acid (PABA)?
   a. trimethoprim
   b. sulfamethoxazole
   c. metronidazole
   d. norfloxacin
   e. polymyxin B

CHAPTER 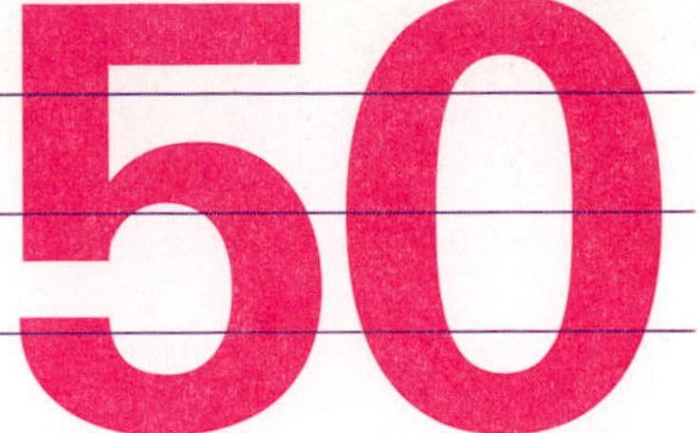

Other Antibacterial Agents

HAROLD C. NEU

MAJOR DRUGS
quinolones
nitrofurans
methenamine
polymyxins

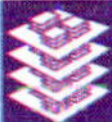

THERAPEUTIC OVERVIEW

Several types of antimicrobial agents act through inhibition or damage to bacterial DNA (quinolones and nitrofurans), through disruption of bacterial cell membranes (polymyxins), or by unknown mechanisms (methenamine). The older quinolones such as nalidixic acid, nitrofurans, and methenamine are used primarily to treat urinary tract infections; the newer quinolones are also effective against gonorrhea, diarrhea, selected respiratory infections, skin structure infections, and osteomyelitis and used as prophylaxis in neutropenic patients (see box at right). The newer quinolones will become increasingly important in the treatment of infectious diseases.

THERAPEUTIC OVERVIEW

QUINOLONES

Urinary tract infections
Gonorrhea infections
Bacterial diarrhea infections
Respiratory infections
Skin structure infections
Osteomyelitis
Prophylaxis in neutropenic patients

NITROFURANS

Urinary tract infections

METHENAMINE

Urinary tract infections

POLYMYXINS

Mainly topical uses

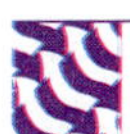

MECHANISMS OF ACTION

Quinolones

These compounds include nalidixic acid, oxolinic acid, cinoxacin, and the newer fluoro-based norfloxacin, ciprofloxacin, ofloxacin, enoxacin, and lomefloxacin (see Figure 50-1 for structures). The fluorine at position 6 provides activity against gram-positive organisms, and the piperazine ring in ciprofloxacin adjacent to the fluorine increases activity against gram-negative species, particularly *Pseudomonas aeruginosa*. The keto group at position 4 and the COOH group at position 3 facilitate entry into gram-negative bacteria by binding Ca^{++}. This neutralizes the negative charge, thus promoting hydrophobicity.

The quinolones act by inhibiting a bacterial DNA topoisomerase II known as DNA gyrase. The topoisomerases are enzymes that catalyze the direction and extent of supercoiling and other topological reactions of DNA chains (see Chapter 46). Bacterial DNA gyrase is the main target for the quinolones. DNA gyrases catalyze the introduction of negative spherohelical twists into closed circular DNA and the reversible joining of DNA circles. DNA gyrase consists of α and β subunits; quinolones affect the α subunit. The increased antibacterial activity of fluoroquinolones such as norfloxacin and ciprofloxacin correlates with increased inhibition of supercoiling, but the precise mechanism has not been established (Figure 50-2).

Altered DNA gyrase results in increased bacterial resistance to nalidixic acid, oxolinic acid, and cinoxacin,

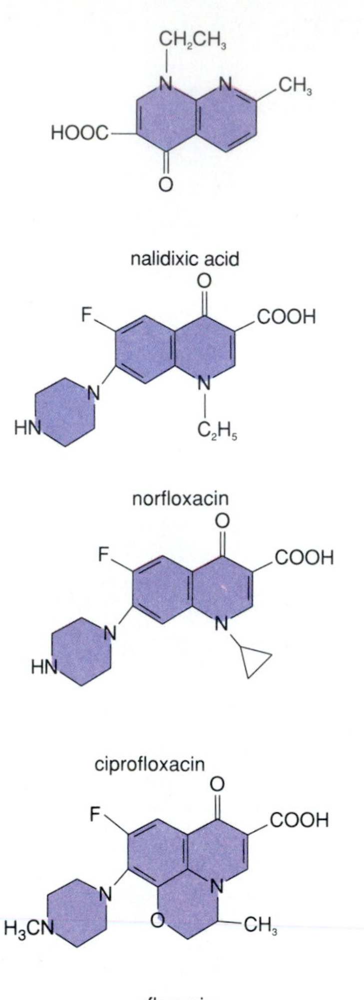

FIGURE 50-1 Structures of some quinolones in clinical use. See the text for additional information.

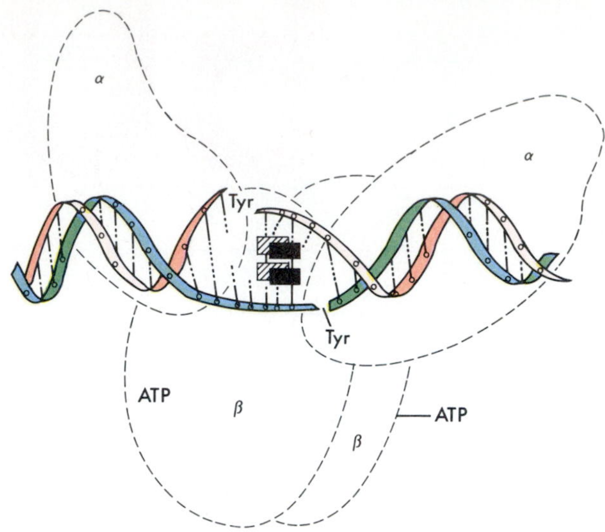

FIGURE 50-2 A model of quinolone-DNA cooperative binding in the inhibition of DNA gyrase. Illustrated are α and β subunits of the enzyme with tyrosines (Tyr). The DNA gyrase, which is inhibited by quinolones, forms normal junctions to supercoiled DNA. Although the mechanism is not established, it is known to involve the self-assembly of four molecules of quinolone shown within the opened DNA double helix in the center of the diagram. ATP binding sites on the β subunits as shown. (From Shen LE et al: *Biochemistry* 28:2886, 1989.)

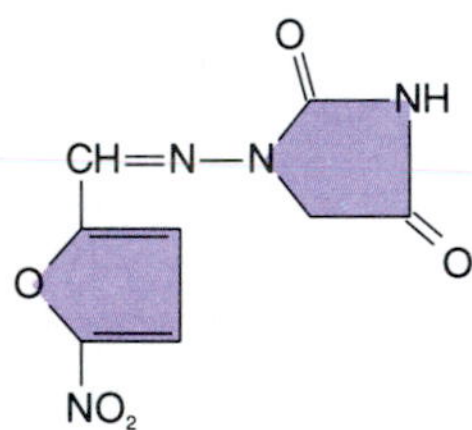

FIGURE 50-3 Structure of nitrofurantoin. See the text for further information.

but the bacteria are still susceptible to inhibition by norfloxacin or ciprofloxacin. Increases in minimum inhibitory concentration for fluoroquinolones can occur as a result of an altered DNA gyrase α subunit. Resistant bacteria have been found in patients treated for urinary tract infections and particularly in cystic fibrosis patients infected with *Pseudomonas* organisms and methicillin-resistant staphylococci. Most clinical gram-negative isolates resistant to the new quinolones appear to have lost outer-membrane porin proteins, which are important for transport of these agents into the bacteria, as well as possessing altered DNA gyrase. Plasmid resistance does not occur. Inhibition of topoisomerase II in mammalian cells requires much higher concentrations of quinolones than inhibition of the enzyme of susceptible bacteria.

Nitrofurans

Three members of the nitrofuran group are used clinically: nitrofurantoin, furazolidone, and nitrofurazone. The structure of nitrofurantoin is shown in Figure 50-3.

The precise mechanism of action of the nitrofurans is not established. They inhibit many bacterial enzyme systems, most probably through DNA damage. A nitroreductase bacterial enzyme converts the compounds to short-lived intermediates, including oxygen-free radicals, which interact with DNA to cause strand breakage and bacterial damage.

Resistance develops infrequently and is not plasmid mediated but appears to be caused by a mutation associated with loss of bacterial nitroreductase activity.

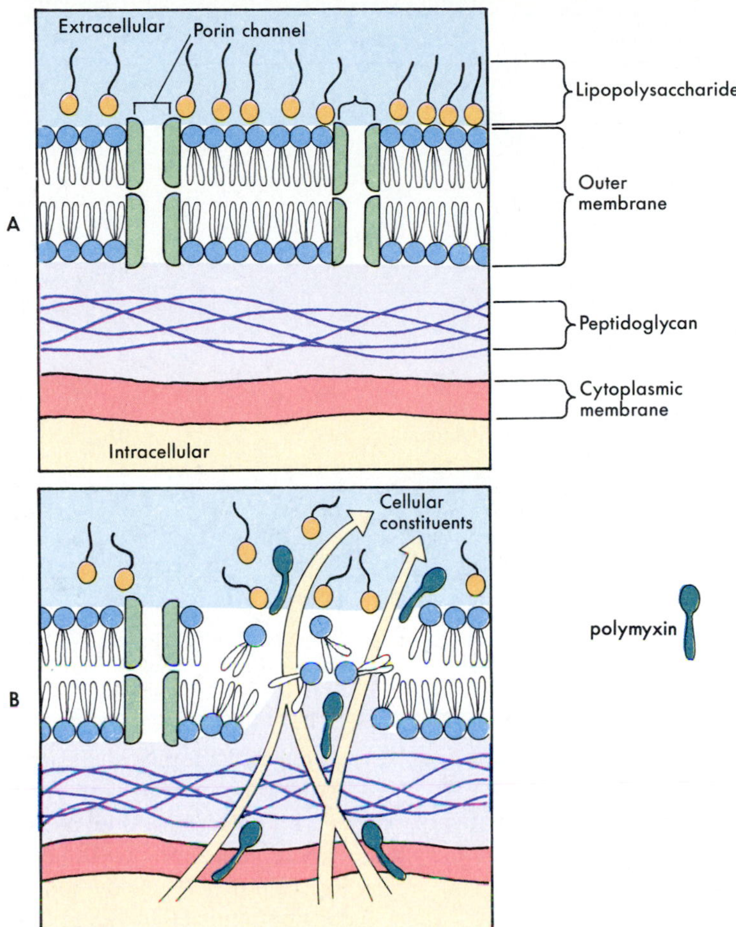

FIGURE 50-4 Mechanism of action of polymyxins. Microbial cell in, **A**, absence and, **B**, presence of polymyxin. See the text for further information.

Methenamine

Methenamine is hexamethylenetetramine, which undergoes hydrolysis at acid pH to produce formaldehyde and ammonia; formaldehyde is the antibacterial compound. At pH 5, 20% of methenamine is converted to formaldehyde, but at pH 7 only 6%; approximately 3 hours are needed for the reaction to go to completion at lower pH values.

Polymyxins

The polymyxins are branched-chain cyclic decapeptides with a molecular weight of about 1000 daltons. An analog with a similar structure to polymyxin E (colistin) is also used clinically.

They are basically bactericidal cationic detergents, with both lipophilic and lipophobic groups, that interact with phospholipids and disrupt bacterial cell membranes. The initial damage is to the cell wall with loss of periplasmic enzymes. The divalent cationic sites on the lipopolysaccharide component of the outer membrane of gram-negative organisms interact with the amino groups of the cyclic polymyxin peptide. The fatty acid tail portion of the drug molecule penetrates into the hydrophobic areas of the outer wall to generate holes in the membrane through which intracellular constituents leak out of the bacteria (Figure 50-4). Susceptibility is related to phospholipids in the bacteria cell wall interacting with the drug. The cell walls of resistant bacteria restrict the transport of polymyxin and prevent access of the drug to the cell membrane. Elevated concentrations of calcium or magnesium reduce the activity of the polymyxins.

Table 50-1 Pharmacokinetic parameters

Agent	Administration	Absorption	$t_{1/2}$ (hr)	Disposition
nalidixic acid	Oral	50%	8 (21 in anuria)	M* R
oxolinic acid	Oral	50%	—	R
cinoxacin	Oral	50%	—	R(60%)† M
ciprofloxacin	Oral	75%	4 (10 in anuria)	R (80%) M
norfloxacin	Oral	50%	4 (8 in anuria)	R M (20%)
ofloxacin	Oral, IV	98%	6	R
lomefloxacin	Oral	98%	8	R
enoxacin	Oral	80%	6	R
pefloxacin	Oral, IV	85%	11	M, R
nitrofurantoin	Oral	Adquate	0.6-1.2	R M (in tissue)
methenamine	Oral	Adequate	4	M
polymyxin B	Topical and oral IV	Not absorbed in adults; absorbed by children	6 by IV	R

M, Metabolized; *R*, renal excretion as unchanged drug.
*Metabolized to active product.
†By glomerular filtration and tubular secretion.

PHARMACOKINETICS

The pharmacokinetic parameters for these agents are summarized in Table 50-1.

Quinolones

Nalidixic acid is 95% bound to plasma proteins. It is rapidly metabolized by the liver to an active hydroxy metabolite and an inactive glucuronide. The drug is minimally distributed in the body and concentrated in the kidney, where it achieves concentrations greater than that in plasma. Nalidixic acid and the more active hydroxy metabolite are both excreted, with high concentrations occurring in urine.

Cinoxacin is metabolized to four microbiologically inactive metabolites, with 60% excreted as parent compound by glomerular filtration and tubular secretion to yield excellent urine concentrations of drug.

Ciprofloxacin is 70% to 85% absorbed orally with decreased absorption in the presence of magnesium, aluminum, calcium, zinc, and iron. Ciprofloxacin is widely distributed in the body, entering all compartments including the eye, CSF, and phagocytic cells. Concentrations in interstitial fluid equal those in plasma. High concentrations are present in salivary secretions, nasal mucosa, and bronchial epithelium, with concentrations in bile exceeding those in plasma.

Ciprofloxacin is removed primarily by glomerular filtration and tubular secretion with about 20% of a dose undergoing metabolism. There may also be some secretion by gastrointestinal cells. The $t_{1/2}$ of ciprofloxacin is 4 hours, increasing to 10 hours in anuria. Approximately 30% of a dose is recovered in the urine. The volume of distribution is 90 to 120 L. Ciprofloxacin can be removed by hemodialysis and peritoneal dialysis.

Ofloxacin and lomefloxacin are almost 100% absorbed orally. Their distribution is similar to ciprofloxacin. Both agents are cleared almost totally by the kidney with half-lives of 6 and 8 hours respectively. Half-lives are greatly increased in anuria.

Norfloxacin is 50% absorbed orally, but antacids, metals such as zinc and iron, and foods such as milk decrease absorption. Its volume of distribution is approximately 100 L, producing interstitial fluid concentrations equal to those in plasma, body tissues, and secretions. It is approximately 20% metabolized to inactive oxides and glucuronides, but renal elimination is the main excretory route.

Nitrofurans

Nitrofurantoin is 94% absorbed from the gastrointestinal tract, and the absorption is not altered by the presence of food. The drug exists in several crystalline forms; the macrocrystalline form is absorbed more slowly than the others. No drug accumulation occurs except in urine and bile. Disappearance of the drug is by excretion into bile, followed by reabsorption and elimination through glomerular filtration and tubular secretion to yield a brown urine. The half-life in normal individuals is 0.6 to 1.2 hours because of the rapid excretion and metabolism in tissues. As renal function declines, less drug enters the urine, and so treatment of urinary tract infections is ineffective in individuals with creatinine clearances less than 40 ml/min. In patients with severely depressed renal function, the drug accumulates and can cause neurotoxicity.

Methenamine

Methenamine is absorbed from the gastrointestinal tract, but 10% to 30% is hydrolyzed in the stomach. Since ammonia is produced, the drug should not be used in patients with hepatic dysfunction. Methenamine is distributed widely in body fluids, crossing most membranes to enter red blood cells, the eye, CSF, and other body fluids. Little active compound is present because at neutral pH only 7% of methenamine is converted to formaldehyde. Within 24 hours, 90% of a dose is excreted into the urine. Antibacterial activity is observed only in the bladder, since this is the only anatomical site in which the pH is acidic and the residence time is sufficient to enable the hydrolysis to formaldehyde to proceed. Even at a urine pH of 5, approximately 2 hours after the administration of methenamine is required to achieve a high enough formaldehyde concentration in urine to kill bacteria. Fluids should not be forced because this reduces the concentration of formaldehyde. An available form of the drug, methenamine mandelate, should not be given to patients in renal failure, since crystalluria can occur from the mandelic acid.

Polymyxins

Polymyxins are not well absorbed after either oral or topical administration. Polymyxin B has been given by oral, topical, endobronchial, IM, and IV routes. Colistin, an analog with a structure similar to polymyxin E, is given by the IV and oral routes. The drug may be found in urine for up to 3 days after an IV dose. Polymyxins distribute poorly to tissues and do not enter the CSF. They are excreted by glomerular filtration and accumulate to toxic concentrations in anuric patients.

Newborns can absorb toxic concentrations of polymyxin if given the drug orally. Irrigation of surfaces such as the peritoneum with solutions containing polymyxins can result in absorption of drug, leading to neurotoxicity.

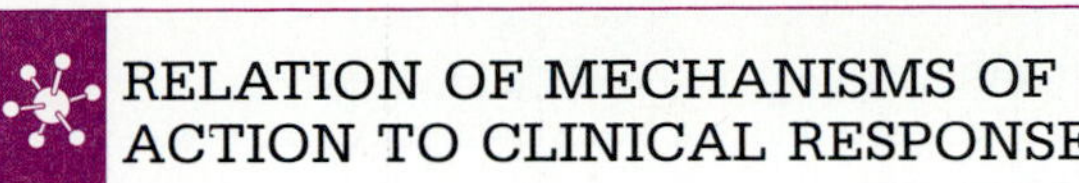

RELATION OF MECHANISMS OF ACTION TO CLINICAL RESPONSE

Quinolones

Nalidixic acid, oxolinic acid, and cinoxacin have similar activities, inhibiting most Enterobacteriaceae with concentrations of drug that can be achieved in the urinary tract. However, most *P. aeruginosa* and gram-positive organisms are resistant. These agents are used primarily for treatment of urinary tract infections, but there is little current usage because of the availability of newer fluoroquinolones.

All the new fluoroquinolones are effective for treatment of both uncomplicated and complicated urinary tract infections caused by Enterobacteriaceae and *P. aeruginosa,* with ciprofloxacin or ofloxacin also active against prostatitis resulting from *Escherichia coli.* All are used to treat gonorrhea, including infection caused by β-lactamase–producing strains. All the agents are efficacious for treating diarrhea caused by *Shigella* organisms, toxigenic *E. coli,* salmonella, and typhoid. Ciprofloxacin and ofloxacin are effective against respiratory infections resulting from *Haemophilus* species or *Streptococcus pneumoniae* in bronchitis and *Pseudomonas* infections in cystic fibrosis. Chlamydiae are inhibited, as are *Mycoplasma* and *Legionella* species, but anaerobic species generally are resistant to currently available fluoroquinolones. Ofloxacin has been used to treat nongonococcal urethritis and cervicitis caused by chlamydiae. Ciprofloxacin is effective therapy of some osteomyelitis. Ciprofloxacin and ofloxacin are effective for prophylaxis in neutropenic patients. (See Table 50-2 and Chapter 51 for uses.)

Nitrofurans

Nitrofurantoin is used to treat urinary tract infections, furazolidone for intestinal infections, and nitrofurazone only for topical applications. All three agents inhibit a variety of gram-positive and gram-negative bacteria, including most *E. coli,* staphylococci, and many *Klebsiella* species, enterococci, neisseriae, salmonellae, *Shigella* organisms, and *Proteus* bacteria.

Methenamine

Since the rate of production of the active ingredient (formaldehyde) is difficult to control, methenamine is no longer suggested as acceptable therapy.

Table 50-2 Clinical Uses of Quinolones

DISEASE ENTITY	
RESPIRATORY TRACT INFECTIONS	
Pharyngitis	Not appropriate
Otitis media	Not appropriate
Necrotizing otitis	Ciprofloxacin for *Pseudomonas aeruginosa*
Sinusitis	Ciprofloxacin, ofloxacin
Bacterial bronchitis	Ciprofloxacin or ofloxacin
Outpatient pneumonia	Rarely appropriate
Aspiration pneumonia	
outpatient	Not appropriate
hospital acquired	Ciprofloxacin or ofloxacin
Cystic fibrosis pneumonitis	Ciprofloxacin
URINARY TRACT INFECTIONS	
Cystitis, uncomplicated	All effective
Pyelonephritis	All effective
Prostatitis, hospital-acquired	Ciprofloxacin, ofloxacin, lomefloxacin
SKIN-STRUCTURE INFECTIONS	
Pyoderma	Not appropriate
Decubitus ulcers	Ciprofloxacin, ofloxacin
OSTEOMYELITIS	
Hematogenous in children	Not appropriate
Chronic infections	Ciprofloxacin, ofloxacin
DIARRHEAL DISEASES	All effective
SEXUALLY TRANSMITTED DISEASES	
Gonorrhoea	All effective
By *Chlamydia*	Ofloxacin
Chancroid	All effective
By *Mycoplasma*	Ofloxacin
Syphilis	Not appropriate

From Neu HC, *Science* 257:1054, 1992.

Polymyxins

The polymyxins are used *topically* to treat cutaneous *Pseudomonas* infections of the mucous membranes, eye, and ear. Orally administered polymyxin B or colistin can be used to prevent intestinal colonization in neutropenic patients, but adverse effects are too pronounced for systemic administration. Gram-positive and anaerobic organisms generally are resistant to the polymyxins. However, *E. coli, Klebsiella, Enterobacter, Shigella,* and several other groups of organisms are inhibited by the polymyxins. These agents can act synergistically with trimethoprim or rifampin. The mechanism appears to result form damage to the membranes, allowing increased concentrations of drug to enter the bacteria. This has not been shown to be of clinical significance.

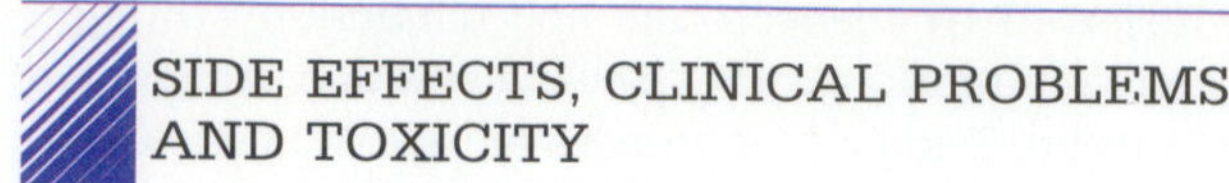

SIDE EFFECTS, CLINICAL PROBLEMS, AND TOXICITY

Quinolones

All quinolones cause gastrointestinal reactions such as nausea, vomiting, and abdominal pain, but diarrhea and pseudomembranous colitis are rare. CNS effects—dizziness, headache, restlessness, depression, and insomnia—are infrequent with occurrence of these more common in the elderly. Seizures are a rare problem. Pseudotumor cerebri, leukopenia, thrombocytopenia, hemolytic anemia, and elevated aspartate aminotransferase (SGOT) concentrations occur occasionally with nalidixic acid. Allergic reactions are uncommon, but rashes, urticaria, pruritus, and photosensitivity may occur.

Quinolones produce damage to cartilage in immature animals and therefore are not recommended for use in children, though no joint damage has been seen in children who have received nalidixic acid. Elevations of theophylline concentrations occur in patients treated with ciprofloxacin. Interstitial nephritis has occurred rarely with ciprofloxacin.

Nitrofurans

The most common adverse reactions of the nitrofurans are gastrointestinal, with anorexia, nausea, and vomiting most prevalent, though they can be reduced by administration of the drug with food. The nausea and vomiting seem to arise from CNS effects. Hypersensitivity reactions involving the skin, lungs, liver, or blood also occur and are often associated with fever and chills. Cutaneous effects include maculopapular, erythematous, urticarial, and pruritic reactions, which abate when drug administration is stopped.

Two major types of pulmonary reactions occur with nitrofuran use. An acute reaction, characterized by fever, cough, and dyspnea, begins about 10 days into the treatment. Pleural effusions and infiltrates may accompany it. This reaction appears to be immunologically mediated but resolves rapidly when the drug is stopped. A second form occurs in patients receiving long-term therapy. The onset is insidious, with cough, shortness of breath, and radiological signs of interstitial fibrosis. Patients improve when the drug is stopped, but many have residual change, which is believed to be caused by peroxidative destruction of pulmonary membrane lipids. These arise from the reactive oxygen derivatives produced by reductase action on the nitrofurans.

The nitrofurans also cause acute and chronic liver damage including cholestatic and hepatocellular disease and granulomatous hepatitis.

CLINICAL PROBLEMS

QUINOLONES

Gastrointestinal effects
CNS agitation (rarely seizures)
Damage to growing cartilage (not recommended for use in children)

NITROFURANS

Gastrointestinal effects
Hypersensitivity
Cutaneous reactions
Pulmonary reactions
Liver damage
Hematologic reactions

POLYMYXINS

Nephrotoxicity and neurotoxicity (too serious for IV use)

TRADE NAMES

In addition to generic and fixed-combination preparations, the following trade-named materials are available in the United States.

Aerosporins, polymyxin B
Cinobac Pulvules, cinoxacin
Cipro, ciprofloxacin HCl
Furacin, nitrofurazone
Furadantin, nitrofurantoin
Furoxone, furazolidone
Hiprex, Urex, methenamine hippurate
Lomefloxacin, maxiquin
Macrodantin, nitrofurantoin
Mandelamine, Thiacide, Ruoqid-Acid, methenamine mandelate
NegGram, nalidixic acid
Noroxin, norfloxacin
Ofloxacin, norfloxacin
Urised, Uro-Phosphate, methenamine

Hematologic reactions include granulocytopenia, leukopenia, and megaloblastic anemia, with acute hemolytic anemia occurring in patients deficient in glucose-6-phosphate dehydrogenase. Several neurological reactions, including headache, drowsiness, dizziness, nystagmus, and peripheral neuropathy of an ascending sensorimotor type, are also observed. Administration of drug should be stopped if the patient feels paresthesias, indicative of peripheral neuropathy.

Methenamine

Adverse effects from methenamine are uncommon and include gastrointestinal distress, painful micturition, and occasional hematuria.

Polymyxins

When used topically, the polymyxins have few adverse effects. However, when used orally, large doses cause nausea and vomiting. The IV administration of polymyxins leads to serious nephrotoxicity and neurotoxicity and thus should be avoided. The polymyxins may also damage some mammalian cell membranes and can cause neuromuscular blockade and respiratory paralysis. They can also produce persistent blockage of acetylcholine-activated endplate channels, which is not reversed by neostigmine.

The mechanism of polymyxin-induced nephrotoxicity is not established but appears to result from polymyxin binding to renal tubule cell membranes. This produces proteinuria, casts, and loss of brush-border enzymes and can progress to renal failure. Renal function usually returns when the drug is discontinued.

The clinical problems of these drug groups are summarized in the box above, left.

REFERENCES

Blumberg HM et al: Rapid development of ciprofloxacin resistance in methicillin-susceptible and methicillin resistant *Staphylococcus aureus, J Infect Dis* 163:1279, 1991.

Neu HC: Quinolone antimicrobial agents, *Ann Rev Med* 43:465-486, 1992.

Neu HC: An update on fluoroquinolones *Curr Opin Infect Dis* 5:755, 1992.

Norby SR: Side effects of quinolones *Eur. J Clin Microbiol Infect Dis* 10:378-383, 1991.

Schaad UB: Use of quinolones in pediatrics, *Eur J. Clin Microbiol Infect Dis* 10:355, 1991.

Shen LI et al: Mechanism of inhibition of DNA gyrase by quinolone antibacterials: a comparative drug-DNA binding model, *Biochemistry* 28:2886, 1989.

SELF-ASSESSMENT QUESTIONS

1. Which is the mechanism of action of nalidixic acid and norfloxacin?
   a. They interfere with peptidoglycan synthesis.
   b. They damage membranes with loss of K^+
   c. They inhibit DNA gyrase.
   d. They inhibit peptidyl transfer on ribosomes.
   e. They inhibit DNA-directed RNA polymerase.

2. Polymyxins inhibit bacteria by which of the following mechanisms?
   a. interfere with cell wall synthesis
   b. inhibit DNA gyrase β
   c. inhibit protein synthesis
   d. damage cytoplasmic membrane by interaction with phospholipids
3. Nitrofurans produce which of the following adverse reactions?
   a. pulmonary interstitial fibrosis
   b. deafness
   c. renal insufficiency
   d. seizures
4. Fluoroquinolones such as norfloxacin, ciprofloxacin, and ofloxacin do not inhibit which of the following?
   a. *Staphylococcus aureus*
   b. *Bacteroides fragilis*
   c. *Pseudomonas aeruginosa*
   d. *Neisseria gonorrhoeae*
5. Which of the following reasons explains why fluoroquinolones are not used to treat infections in children?
   a. They cause deafness in children.
   b. They cause increased intracranial pressure.
   c. They affect articular cartilage in weight-bearing joints.
   d. They cause interstitial fibrosis in the kidney.
6. Resistance to fluoroquinolones has been a major problem in the United States with which pathogens?
   a. *Klebsiella pneumoniae*
   b. *Haemophilus influenzae*
   c. *Enterobacter cloacae*
   d. methicillin-resistant *Staphylococcus aureus*

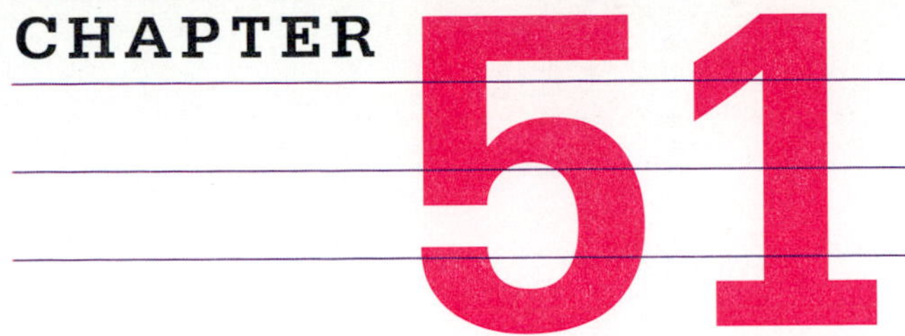

Selection of an Antibacterial Agent

HAROLD C. NEU

The basic clinical factors that need to be considered when one is selecting an antibiotic to treat a specific patient are described in Chapter 46, and some drugs are discussed further in Chapters 47 through 50. The extensive variety of pathogenic bacteria, the large number of available antibiotics, and the significant list of factors to be considered in arriving at a rational selection of antibiotic therapy can be confusing for the nonspecialist in infectious diseases. Since nearly all physicians use antibacterial agents, some additional guidelines for antibiotic selection are provided in this chapter.

These guidelines are as follows:

1. The strains of bacteria inhibited for each drug type and subtype
2. The bacteria most commonly associated with infections at different anatomical sites in the patient
3. The antibiotics that do or do not attain high enough concentrations at specific anatomical sites of infections for effective therapy
4. How special factors of the patient (allergy, disease states, pregnancy) and the bacteria (expectation of resistance developing) influence the selection of the antibiotic or antibiotics and the criteria that should be used in deciding when to switch to a different antibiotic.

ANTIBIOTIC ACTIVITY

The major classes of antibiotics discussed in Chapters 47 through 50 are listed in Table 51-1 along with the types of bacteria inhibited. The classifications are an oversimplification; for example, not all cephalosporins are active against all gram-positive or gram-negative bacteria, and several gram-negative species are not inhibited by any of the cephalosporins. More detailed listings showing the relative activities for some representative antibiotics against individual microbial species are included in Table 51-2.

Table 51-1 Activities of Antibiotics by Gram Stain of Sensitive Organisms

Antibiotics	Effective Against
penicillins	Many gram+ cocci, some gram−
cephalosporins	First generation: gram+, some gram−
	Second generation: more gram−, similar gram+
	Third generation: more gram−, less gram+; some inhibit *Pseudomonas*
	Fourth generation: better as gram+; inhibit *Pseudomonas;* don't bind to β-lactamases
imipenem	Gram+, gram−
aztreonam	Aerobic gram− only
vancomycin	Gram+ only
aminoglycosides	Aerobic gram− bacilli
tetracyclines	Aerobic and anaerobic gram+ and gram− *Mycoplasma, Chlamydia*
erythromycin, clarithromycin, azithromycin	Gram+ *Mycoplasma, Chlamydia, Legionella*
clindamycin	Most gram+ cocci, many anaerobes
sulfonamides	Some gram+ and gram−
quinolones	Some gram+ and most gram−
rifampin	Gram+

Gram+, gram-positive; *gram−*, gram-negative.

BACTERIA AND ANATOMICAL SITES

It is estimated that 75% of bacterial infections treated with antibiotics receive the initial antimicrobial therapy before the pathogenic microorganisms have been identified and that for approximately 50% of treated infections identification is never verified. It is important to

Table 51-2 Susceptability of Bacteria to Antibiotics

Organisms	Antibiotics															
	A	**B**	**C**	**D**	**E†**	**F†**	**G†**	**H**	**I**	**J**	**K**	**L**	**M**	**N**	**O**	**P**
GRAM-POSITIVE																
Streptococcus pyogenes	4	4	4	4	4	4	4	0	0	0	3	3	4	4	4	2
Streptococcus pneumoniae	4	4	4	4	4	4	4	0	0	0	4	4	4	4	4	2
Staphylococcus aureus	0	0	0	4	4	4	4	0	2	3	2	2	3	2	4	4
Enterococcus faecalis	2	4	4	3	0	0	0	0	0	0	0	1	0	0	3	3
Listeria monocytogenes	4	4	4	4	0	0	0	0	0	0	2	1	0	0	4	2
GRAM-NEGATIVE																
Escherichia coli	0	3	3	4	3	3	4	1	3	4	2	0	0	4	4	4
Klebsiella spp.	0	0	2	3	3	3	4	1	3	4	2	0	0	4	4	4
Enterobacter spp.	0	0	2	2	0	1	2	1	3	4	2	0	0	2	4	4
Neisseriae gonorrhoeae	2	2	2	4	3	4	4	1	3	2	3	0	0	4	4	4
Pseudomonas aeruginosa	0	0	3	3	0	0	1	0	3	4	0	0	0	4	4	4
Hemophilus influenzae	1	2	2	4	1	4	4	1	2	2	2	1	0	4	4	4
ANAEROBES																
Clostridium spp.	4	4	4	4	2	3	3	0	0	0	3	3	3	1	4	0
Bacteroides spp.	1	1	2	4	0	0	1	0	0	0	1	2	4	0	4	0
Actinomyces spp.	4	4	4	4	0	1	2	0	0	0	2	3	4	0	4	0

A, penicillin G; *B,* ampicillin; *C,* pipercillin; *D,* ticarcillin-clavulanate; *E,* cefazolin (first); *F,* cefuroxime (second); *G,* cefotaxime, ceftriaxone, ceftizoxime (third); *H,* streptomycin; *I,* gentamicin; *J,* amikacin; *K,* tetracycline; *L,* erythromycin; *M,* clindamycin; *N,* ceftazidime; *O,* imipenem; *P,* ciprofloxacin, ofloxacin.

*Ratings based on tissue or plasma concentration expected for normal dosing schedule; *4,* >90% inhibited; *3,* >80% inhibited; *2,* 50% to 80% inhibited; *1,* 25% to 50% inhibited; *0,* <25% inhibited.

†Generation of cephalosporin.

Table 51-3 Common Microorganisms Causing Infections

Body Site	Microorganisms	Gram Stain
Eyes	*Neisseria gonorrhoeae*	−
	Chlamydia trachomycetis	−
	Staphylococcus aureus	+
	Haemophilus spp.	−
	Streptococcus pneumoniae	+
	Pseudomonas aeruginosa	−
	Fungi	
	Herpes	
	Adenoviruses	
Oral cavity	Herpes	
	Candida	
	Actinomyces	+
	Anaerobic cocci	+
	Fusobacteria	−
Throat	*Streptococcus pyogenes*	+
	Corynebacterium diphtheriae	+
	Corynebacterium hemolyticum	+
	Neisseria gonorrhoeae	−
	Pseudomonas spp.	−
	Staphylococcus aureus	+
Lung (abscesses)	Anaerobic bacteria	
	Staphylococcus aureus	+
	Mycobacterium tuberculosis	
	Fungi	
Heart	Viridans group streptococci	+
	Staphylococcus aureus	+
	Enterococci	+
Meninges	*Streptococcus agalactiae*	+
	Escherichia coli	−
	Streptococcus pneumoniae	+
	Haemophilus influenzae	−
	Neisseria meningitidis	−
	Listeria monocytogenes	+
Brain (abscesses)	Anaerobic bacteria	−/+
	Nocardia	−
	Staphylococcus aureus	+
Sinuses	*Haemophilus influenzae*	−
	Moraxella catarrhalis	−
	Streptococcus pneumoniae	+
	Streptococcus pyogenes	+
	Anaerobic streptococci	+
	Rhinoviruses	
	Coronaviruses	
Ears	*Haemophilus influenzae*	−
	Streptococcus pneumoniae	+
	Moraxella catarrhalis	−
	Streptococcus pyogenes	+
Larynx-trachea	Respiratory viruses	
	Streptococcus pneumoniae	+
	Moraxella catarrhalis	−
Lungs	*Streptococcus pneumoniae*	+
	Mycoplasma pneumoniae	
	Legionella spp.	
	Chlamydia psittaci	
	Mycobacterium tuberculosis	
	Enterobacteriaceae	−
Bone (osteomyelitis)	*Staphylococcus aureus*	+
	Salmonella species	−
	Haemophilus influenzae	−
	Pseudomonas aeruginosa	−
	Escherichia coli	−
Urinary tract	*Staphylococcus saprophyticus*	+
	Enterobacteriaceae	−
	Pseudomonas aeruginosa	−
Peritoneum (peritonitis)	Enterobacteriaceae	−
	Bacteroides spp.	−
	Anaerobic streptococci	+
	Enterococci	+
	Clostridium species	+
	Streptococcus pyogenes	+
Skin	*Staphylococcus aureus*	+
	Herpes simplex	
	Clostridium perfringens	+
	Pseudomonas spp.	−
	Bacteroides spp.	−
	Enterobacteriaceae	−
	Fungi	
Bloodstream (septicomia)	*Staphylococcus aureus*	+
	Streptococcus pyogenes	+
	Enterobacteriaceae*	−
	Pseudomonas aeruginosa	−
	Staphylococcus epidermidis	+
	Candida albicans	−
	Haemophilus influenzae	+
	Streptococcus pneumoniae	−
	Neisseria meningitidis	

**E. coli, Klebsiella, Proteus, Enterobacter, Serratia* species.

Table 51-4 Organisms with Common Infection Sites and Drugs of Choice

Bacteria	Infection	Drugs of Choice for Treatment	
		First Choice	**Second Choice**
Staphylococcus aureus (+)	Abscess	penicillin G	l-cephalosporin
	Cellulitis, bacteremia		vancomycin
	Pneumonia endocarditis	penicillin	l-cephalosporin vancomycin
	Meningitis	nafcillin, vancomycin	TMP/SMX
Streptococcus pyogenes (+) (Group A)	Pharyngitis	penicillin V	l-cephalosporin
	Cellulitis	penicillin V	erythromycin, clindamycin
Streptococcus (Group B) (+)	Meningitis	penicillin G	cefotaxime
Enterococcus faecalis	Abscesses, cellulitis, septicemia	penicillin G	l-cephalosporin
	Urinary tract	ampicillin	quinolone
	Endocarditis	ampicillin and gentamicin	vancomycin and gentamicin
	Bacteremia	ampicillin	vancomycin
Morganella morganii	Urinary tract	quinolone	TMP/SMX
Providencia spp. (−)	Urinary tract	quinolone	TMP/SMX
	Other	3-cephalosporin, aztreonam	imipenem
Pseudomonas aeruginosa (−)	Urinary tract	quinolone	aztreonam
	Pneumonia, bacteremia	anti-*Pseudomonas*	ceftazidine, piperacillin, ceftazidime, aztreonam, imipenem
Salmonella typhi (−)	Typhoid	TMP/SMX, ciprofloxacin	amoxicillin
Salmonella enteritidis (−)	Gastroenteritis	norfloxacin, ciprofloxacin	
	Bacteremia	ampicillin	ceftriaxone
Shigella spp. (−)	Diarrhea	TMP/SMX	quinolone
Yersinia enterocolitica (−)	Diarrhea	TMP/SMX	quinolone
	Bacteremia, abscesses	3-cephalosporin	TMP/SMX
Streptococcus (viridans group) (+)	Endocarditis, bacteremia	penicillin G	cephalosporin
Streptococcus pneumoniae (+)	Pneumonia	penicillin G	l-cephalosporin
	Otitis, sinusitis	penicillin V	erythromycin
	Meningitis, endocarditis	penicillin G	cefotaxime
Listeria monocytogenes	Bacteremia, meningitis, endocarditis	ampicillin	TMP/SMX

Continued.

Table 51-4 Organisms with Common Infection Sites and Drugs of Choice—cont'd

Bacteria	Infection	Drugs of Choice for Treatment	
		First Choice	**Second Choice**
Escherichia coli (−)	Urinary tract	TMP/SMX	quinolone
	Bacteremia	3-cephalosporin	TMP/SMX
Klebsiella pneumoniae (−)	Urinary tract	quinolone	cephalosporin, TMP/SMX
	Pneumonia	3-cephalosporin	impenem
	Bacteremia	3-cephalosporin	aztreonam
Proteus mirabilis (−)	Urinary tract	ampicillin	TMP/SMX
Haemophilus influenzae (−)	Otitis	amoxicillin	amoxicillin-clavulanate
	Bronchitis	TMP/SMX	ciprofloxacin
	Epiglottitis	cefotaxime, ceftriaxone	cefuroxime
Moraxella catarrhalis (−)	Otitis, sinusitis	amoxicillin-clavulanate	TMP/SMX
Neisseria meningitidis (−)	Carrier	rifampin	ciprofloxacin
	Meningitis	penicillin G	cefotaxime
	Bacteremia	penicillin G	ceftriaxone
Neisseria gonorrhoeae (−)	Genital	ceftriaxone	quinolone
	Disseminated	ceftriaxone	spectinomycin, amoxicillin-clavulanate
Chlamydia trachomatis	Genital	doxycycline	ofloxacin, azithromycin
Bacteroides spp.	Pulmonary	penicillin G, clindamycin	cefoxitin
	Sinus, oral, brain abscess	metronidazole	clindamycin
	Abdominal infection	methronidazole/impenem	cefotetan, ampicillin-sulbactam, ticarcillin, clavulanate clindamycin
Legionella spp.	Pulmonary	erythromycin	quinolone
Clostridium perfringens (+)	Abscesses, gangrene	penicillin G	metronidazole
Clostridium difficile (+)	Diarrhea	vancomycin	metronidazole
Borrelia burgdorferi	Lyme disease	doxycycline	ceftriaxone, azithromycin
Nocardia asteroides	Pulmonary, CNS	TMP/SMX	minocycline
Mycoplasma pneumoniae	Pulmonary	erythromycin, tetracycline	ciprofloxacin
Rickettsia	Typhus	tetracycline	chloramphenicol
	Rocky Mountain spotted fever	tetracycline	chloramphenicol
Chlamydia psittaci	Pulmonary	tetracycline	erythromycin
Chlamydia pneumoniae	Pulmonary	erythromycin, tetracycline	clarithromycin
Pasteurella multocida	Bite wounds	penicillin G, amoxicillin-clavulanate	doxycycline

+, Gram positive; −, gram negative.
TMP/SMX, Trimethoprim-sulfamethoxazole.
1-cephalosporin = 1st generation cephalosporin
3-cephalosporin = 3rd generation cephalosporin

Table 51-5 Ability of Antibiotics to Enter the Cerebrospinal Fluid in Effective Concentrations

Readily Enter CSF	Enter CSF When Inflammation Present	Do Not Enter CSF Adequately to Treat Infection
chloramphenicol	penicillin G	carbenicillin
sulfonamides	ampicillin	cephalothin
trimethoprim	azlocillin	cefazolin
rifampin	mezlocillin	cefoxitin
isoniazid	piperacillin	cefotetan
metronidazole	oxacillin	erythromycin
flucytosine	cefuroxime	clindamycin
	nafcillin	tetracycline
	cefotaxime	gentamicin
	ceftriaxone	tobramycin
	ceftazidime	amikacin
	moxalactam	norfloxacin
	aztreonam	ketoconazole
	ciprofloxacin	
	vancomycin	
	ethambutol	
	pyrazinamide	
	fluconazole	

realize what bacterial strains may be present at selected anatomical sites, since this may be the only meaningful information for guidance in the selection of antibiotic therapy when the locus of infection is known. Table 51-3 lists the common organisms that lead to infections at the anatomical sites indicated, and Table 51-4 groups the organisms with the anatomical locations of the infection and the drugs often used for treatment.

Numerous infections can be treated successfully with different antibiotics, and so there may be more than one correct therapy. Proponents may argue strongly in favor of a given antibiotic for treatment of a specific type of infection, but in many cases there are few verified findings to support the argument. However, there clearly are therapies that are inappropriate for a particular organism-location combination of bacterial infection.

PHARMACOKINETIC AND DRUG CONCENTRATION CONSIDERATIONS

Although an antibiotic may show high in vitro activity against the organism present at a given infection site, the drug will not be useful clinically unless the concentration of antibiotic at this site reaches an effective value. This is especially important for antibiotics, such as carbenicillin, that are poorly absorbed and do not achieve effective plasma concentrations when administered orally. Similarly, antibiotics that do not readily cross the blood-brain barrier or enter the CSF cannot be used for effective treatment of meningeal-based infections. (See Chapter 5.) The ability of antibiotics to enter the CSF is summarized in Table 51-5.

SPECIAL FACTORS

One highly *undesirable* approach to antibiotic therapy is called "antibiotic roulette" in which the causative organism is not known and the antibiotic is changed every few days in hopes of achieving a quick cure. This action confuses the clinical situation and makes it more difficult for the follow-up physician to initiate and carry out effective therapy.

Certain agents should be avoided if possible in pregnant women. These are listed in Table 46-2.

REFERENCES

Medical Letter: Safety of antimicrobial agents in pregnancy, *Med Let* 29:61-63, 1987.

Neu HC: Side effects of antimicrobial therapy. In Gorbach SL, Bartlett JG, Blacklow NR, editors: *Infectious diseases,* Philadelphia, 1992, Saunders.

Quintiliani R: Strategies for the cost effective use of antibiotics. In Gorbach SL, Bartlett JG, Blacklow NR, editors: *Infectious diseases,* Philadelphia, 1992, Saunders.

SELF-ASSESSMENT QUESTIONS

1. Which of the following is not appropriate to treat *Legionella* pneumonia?
   a. erythromycin
   b. rifampin
   c. gentamicin
   d. ciprofloxacin
2. Which of the following is appropriate to treat meningitis caused by *Listeria monocytogenes?*
   a. cefotaxime
   b. ampicillin
   c. ceftriaxone
   d. erythromycin
3. Which of the following is appropriate to treat a lung abscess caused by *Bacteroides melaninogenicus?*
   a. clindamycin
   b. amikacin
   c. ofloxacin
   d. tetracycline
4. Tetracyclines are not used in the treatment of:
   a. Lyme disease.
   b. psittacosis.
   c. *Chlamydia* salpingitis.
   d. *Streptococcus viridans* endocarditis in a penicillin-allergic patient.
5. Which is used to treat *Clostridium difficile* colitis?
   a. rifampin
   b. amphotericin B
   c. erythromycin
   d. vancomycin
   e. clindamycin
6. Which is used to treat ampicillin-chloramphenicol–resistant typhoid fever?
   a. cefazolin
   b. trimethoprim-sulfamethoxazole
   c. vancomycin
   d. rifampin
   e. isoniazid
7. Which is used to treat methicillin-resistant *Staphylococcus aureus* infections?
   a. cefazolin
   b. trimethoprim-sulfamethoxazole
   c. vancomycin
   d. rifampin
   e. isoniazid

CHAPTER 52

Antimycobacterial Agents

HAROLD C. NEU

MAJOR DRUGS

Isoniazid
Rifampin
Theambutol
Streptomycin
Pyrazinamide
Ethionamide
Cycloserine
p-Aminosalicylic acid
Capreomycin
Kanamycin and amikacin
Fluoroquinolones

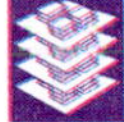 THERAPEUTIC OVERVIEW

Mycobacteria have a high waxy lipid content (approximately 40% of cell weight), with much of the lipid on the external surface of the cell. *Mycobacterium tuberculosis, M. avium, and M. leprae* are the pathogenic organisms that cause diseases of concern in humans, though other nontuberculosis mycobacteria pose occasional problems in immunocompromised patients.

Tuberculosis classically is a respiratory infection, and leprosy initially is primarily a disease of the skin but ultimately involves the peripheral nervous system. In both diseases the organism can and does spread throughout the body if not treated. Both diseases are chronic and require extended therapy over long periods of time.

Tuberculosis remains a serious and important infectious disease worldwide. Although the number of patients with tuberculosis in the past two decades has steadily declined, the number of new cases in inner cities has increased because of acquired immunodeficiency syndrome (AIDS) and the large number of homeless persons. An increase in tuberculosis has also been noted in nursing homes. Because of the nature of the disease and the microorganism, the therapy is different from that used to treat most infectious diseases. Combination therapy is required and up to four agents are used. The desired frequency of drug administration must be considered in terms of achieving compliance, since therapy may be continued for many months. Resistance is also increasingly important in determining the appropriate therapeutic program.

In the host, *M. tuberculosis* is present in three types of sites: (1) well-oxygenated extracellular cavities (abscesses) containing 10^7 to 10^9 organisms, (2) poorly oxygenated closed-caseous lesions (non-caseating granulomas) containing 10^4 to 10^5 organisms, and (3) poorly oxygenated intracellular macrophages containing 10^4 to 10^5 organisms. Drugs are effective at all three sites but especially at the extracellular cavities in which the growth of the organisms is greatest.

Leprosy is a common disease worldwide. Its epidemiology is poorly understood, but transmission appears to depend largely on the susceptibility of the individual. Children and males are most susceptible, and an incubation period of several years makes the disease difficult to detect initially. Several agents are useful in treating this chronic infection, though problems with therapy and drug resistance have occurred. The therapeutic use of drugs in the treatment of these two major mycobacterial infections is summarized in the box.

ABBREVIATION

AIDS	Acquired immunodeficiency syndrome

THERAPEUTIC OVERVIEW

TUBERCULOSIS
Mycobacterium tuberculosis is an aerobic organism.
It is a chronic disease.
Combinations of drugs are used.
Long-term treatment is needed.
Bacterial resistance is of growing importance.

LEPROSY
Mycobacterium leprae is an aerobic organism.
It is a chronic disease.
Long-term treatment is needed.
Effective drugs exist.
Bacterial resistance is developing.

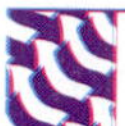

MECHANISMS OF ACTION

Tuberculosis Drugs

A number of drugs are available for the treatment of *M. tuberculosis* infections. These are listed in the box on p. 705. Chemical structures are shown in Figure 52-1 (see Chapter 48 for streptomycin, kanamycin, and amikacin.) The molecular mechanisms by which these drugs act on *M. tuberculosis* can be divided into three groups: protein synthesis inhibition, cell wall synthesis inhibition, and other mechanisms.

Protein Synthesis Inhibition Streptomycin, kanamycin, and amikacin act by inhibiting protein synthesis and are described in Chapter 48. Rifampin and capreomycin act similarly but at different points in the protein synthesis pathway.

Rifampin inhibits RNA synthesis by binding to the β subunit of DNA-directed RNA polymerase. Tight binding occurs only when the subunit is in its proper conformation and results in inhibition of initiation but not of ongoing RNA synthesis. Rifampin may subsequently inhibit DNA synthesis by preventing the binding of the initiated RNA molecule to the product-binding site on the RNA polymerase (Figure 52-2). Mammalian RNA polymerases are not as sensitive as is the mycobacterial form and thus are not affected by rifampin except at much higher drug concentrations. Microbial resistance is becoming more widespread and is caused by an altered β subunit of the RNA polymerase. However, the content of organisms with an altered RNA polymerase is much lower for *M. tuberculosis* than for bacteria, particularly Enterobacteriaceae, Neisseriae, and staphylococci. With staphylococci, resistance can develop with use of rifampin alone.

Capreomycin is a polypeptide that consists of four biologically active components. Its mechanism of action is believed to be inhibition of protein synthesis by preventing translocation of peptidyl-tRNA on ribosomes.

Cell Wall Synthesis Inhibition Cycloserine acts by inhibiting two enzymes involved in the synthesis of cell walls: D-alanyl-D-alanine synthetase and alanine racemase. (See Chapter 47 for cell wall synthesis pathways.)

Other Mechanisms Included in this category are isoniazid, ethionamide, ethambutol, pyrazinamide, and *p*-aminosalicylic acid.

The mechanism of action of isoniazid is not well established; however it has been demonstrated to be bactericidal. It inhibits the synthesis of mycolic acid, a major constituent of mycobacterial cell walls. Low concentrations also inhibit production of fatty acids that exceed 26 carbons in length and that are precursors of mycolic acid. Mycolic acids are unique to mycobacteria, and this may be the reason that only mycobacteria are inhibited. Isoniazid affects mycobacteria in several ways, which may contribute to its bactericidal effect on the growing cells. Isoniazid is taken up by mycobacterial cells through both active and passive transport and undergoes hydrolysis to isonicotinic acid, which is trapped within the cells at physiological pH. Uptake is reduced in some resistant cells. Isonicotinic acid reacts with the cofactor nicotinamide adenine dinucleotide (NAD) to form an NAD adduct, no longer active as a coenzyme for dehydrogenase reactions. These mechanisms of action are illustrated in Figure 52-3. Which mechanism is actually responsible for cell death has not been determined.

The mechanism of action of ethionamide probably involves the direct inhibition of mycolic acid synthesis, possibly with cytotoxic results similar to those for isoniazid. Little is known about the details of this mechanism.

The mechanism of action of ethambutol is also not clear. It has an effect on lipid synthesis resulting in an inhibition of mycolic acid incorporation into the cell wall. Since ethambutol forms stable chelates with metal ions, it may compete with polyamines in forming reactive complexes with transfer and ribosomal RNA, thus inhibiting protein synthesis. Ethambutol is bactericidal.

The mechanism by which pyrazinamide inhibits mycobacteria is not established.

p-Aminosalicylic acid acts as a competitive inhibitor of *p*-aminobenzoic acid in the synthesis of folate. Because aminosalicylic acid inhibits only this synthetic step in *M. tuberculosis,* the synthetase enzyme is distinct in tubercle bacilli, since sulfanomides do not generally inhibit mycobacteria.

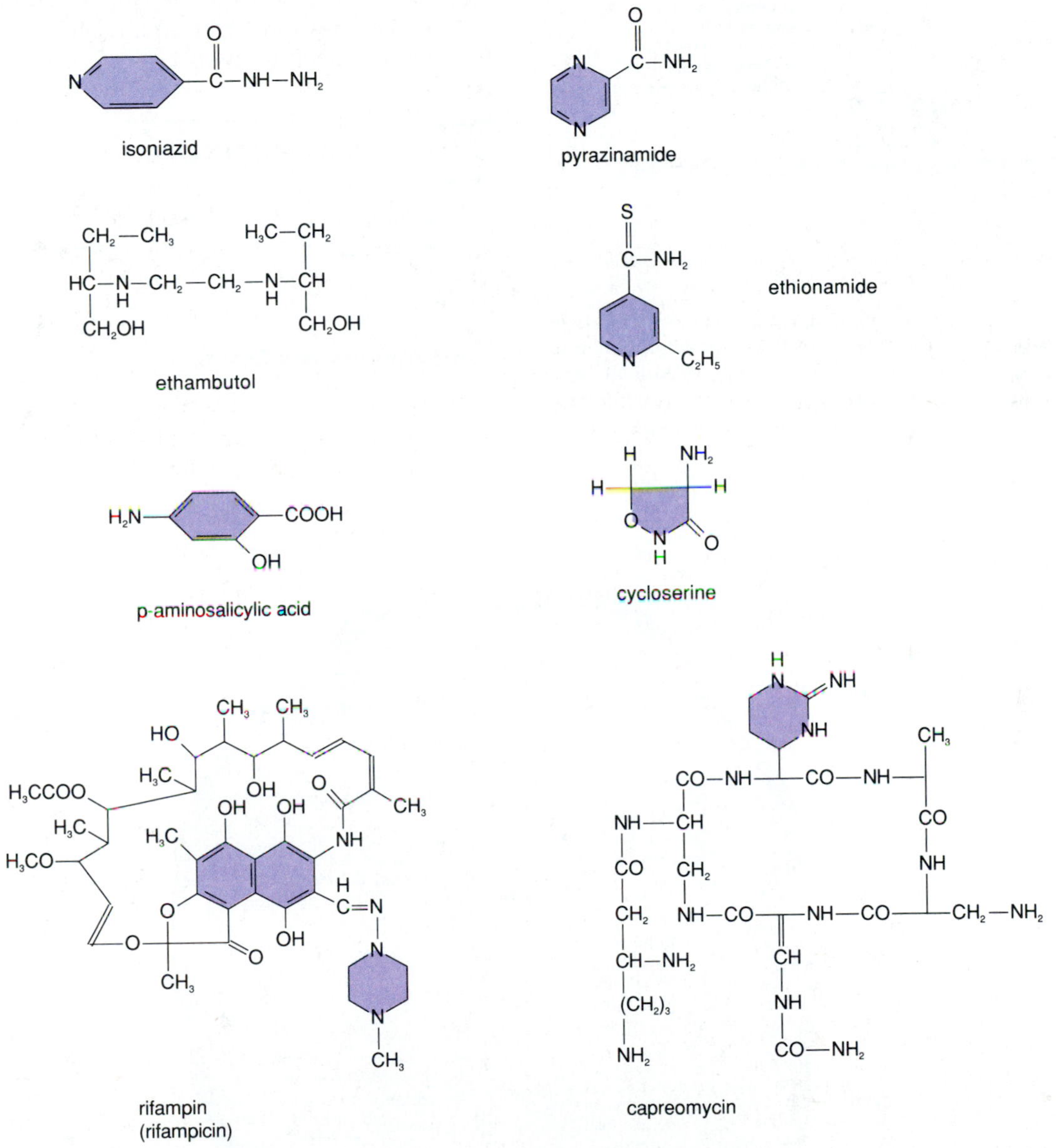

isoniazid

pyrazinamide

ethambutol

ethionamide

p-aminosalicylic acid

cycloserine

rifampin
(rifampicin)

capreomycin

FIGURE 52-1 Structures of some antituberculosis drugs. See the text for further information.

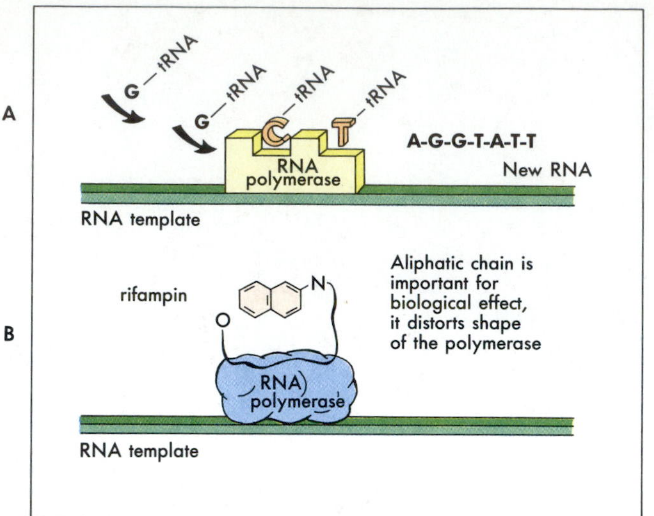

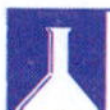

FIGURE 52-2 Mechanism of rifampin action. The drug binds to the β subunit of DNA-dependent RNA polymerase and inhibits initiation (but not ongoing) RNA synthesis. **A,** Drug is absent. **B,** Drug is bound to the polymerase and distorts the conformation of the enzyme so that it cannot initiate a new chain.

Leprosy Drugs

A major drug for inhibition of *M. leprae* is dapsone (diaminodiphenylsulfone). Similar to the sulfonamides, dapsone acts as an inhibitor of dihydropteroate synthetase in the folate pathway to produce a bacteriostatic effect. Its action is antagonized by *p*-aminobenzoic acid.

Clofazimine inhibits *M. leprae,* but its mechanism of action is unknown. Rifampin is highly active against *M. leprae,* and recently clarithromycin and minocycline have been shown to inhibit *M. leprae.*

PHARMACOKINETICS

For agents in which the information is available, the pharmacokinetic parameters are summarized in Table 52-1.

Antituberculosis Drugs

Isoniazid Isoniazid is well absorbed orally, and its absorption is decreased by aluminum antacids. Typical

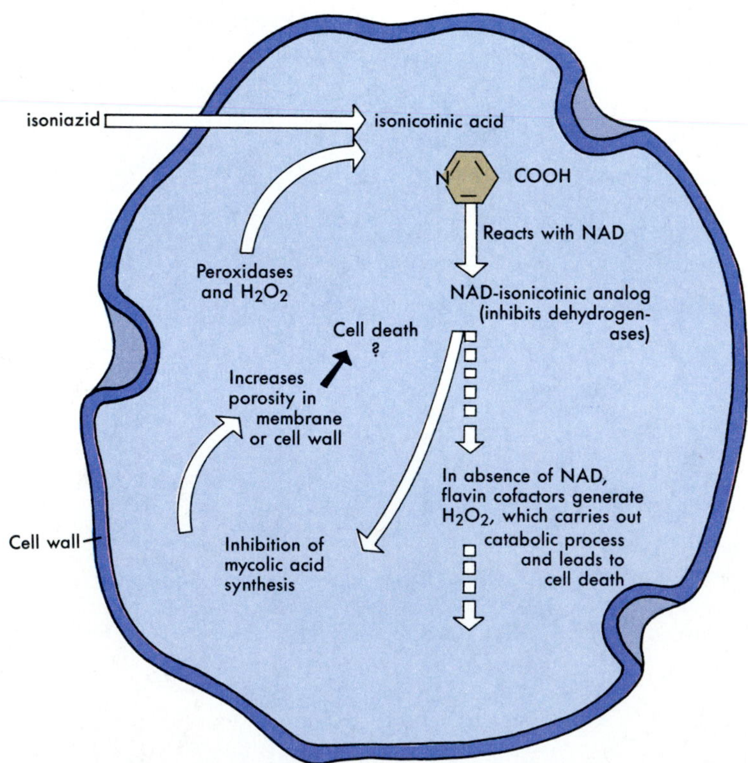

FIGURE 52-3 Postulated mechanisms of isoniazid action on *Mycobacterium tuberculosis.* See the text for further information.

peak plasma concentrations are 3 to 5 μg/ml. Isoniazid enters all body fluids and compartments, with peak concentrations achieved in the pleural, peritoneal, and synovial fluids and with CSF concentrations that are 20% to 100% of those in plasma.

Isoniazid is metabolized by a liver *N*-acetyl transferase. The rate of acetylation determines the concentration of drug in plasma and the $t_{1/2}$. Slow acetylation is inherited as an autosomal recessive trait. Approximately 50% of American whites and 15% of Orientals are slow acetylators. The mean $t_{1/2}$ in rapid acetylators is 1 hour; in slow acetylators it is 3 hours. The average plasma concentration of drug in rapid acetylators is 50% of that in slow acetylators. There is no evidence that differences in acetylation are important chemotherapeutically if the drug is administered once daily. (See also Chapter 6.)

Approximately 75% of a dose is excreted in the urine as metabolites. Toxic concentrations may accumulate in renal failure in some slow acetylators.

Rifampin Rifampin is well absorbed orally and widely distributed in the body, achieving therapeutic concentrations in lung, liver, bile, bone, and urine and entering most body fluids, including pleural, peritoneal, and synovial fluids and CSF, tears, and saliva. It enters phagocytic cells and kills intracellular bacteria.

Rifampin is approximately 75% protein bound and is metabolized in the liver to a desacetyl derivative that is biologically active. The unmetabolized drug is excreted in bile and reabsorbed from the gastrointestinal tract in the enterohepatic cycle; the deacetylated metabolite shows poor reabsorption. Approximately 30% of a dose is excreted unchanged or as metabolites (50%) in the urine.

The $t_{1/2}$ of rifampin varies during therapy from 3 to 4 hours to 2 hours after 1 or 2 weeks because of increased metabolism through induction of hepatic microsomal enzymes. No adjustment of dosage is necessary in renal failure.

Ethambutol Approximately 85% of ethambutol is orally absorbed and distributed to most body areas. CSF concentrations are 10% to 50% of plasma values. The drug crosses the placenta. Approximately 20% of ethambutol is metabolized in the liver to an aldehyde and oxidized to a dicarboxylic acid. The primary mechanism of removal involves the kidney, where the drug is both filtered and excreted. The mean $t_{1/2}$ is 4 hours, which increases to 7 hours in renal failure. Ethambutol can be

Table 52-1 Pharmacokinetic Parameters

	Administration				
	Route	**Absorbed**	**$t_{1/2}$ (hr)**	**Elimination Route**	**Plasma Protein Bound (%)**
TUBERCULOSIS					
isoniazid	Oral	Good	1* 3†	M (75%)	<50%
rifampin	Oral	Good	2-4	M (active metab.) R (15%) B	75
ethambutol	Oral	Good	4	M (20%) R (main)	30
pyrazinamide	Oral	Good	10	M (main)	—
ethionamide	Oral	Good	2	M (main)	—
cycloserine	Oral	Good	10	M (35%) R (65%)	—
capreomycin	IM	Poor	3-5	R (main)	—
p-aminosalicylic acid	Oral	Good	6-8	M, R	—
streptomycin	IM	Good	2	R	<20
kanamycin	IM	Good	2	R	<20
ofloxacin	Oral	Good	6	R	20
LEPROSY					
dapsone	Oral	Good	20-30	M (main) B	70
clofazimine	Oral	Good (70% absorbed)	7 days	M (main)	—

M, Metabolized; *R*, renal (unchanged drug); *B*, bilary.
*Rapid-acetylation patients.
†Slow-acetylation patients.

removed from the body by peritoneal or hemodialysis.

Pyrazinamide Pyrazinamide is well absorbed orally and is widely distributed in the body, readily penetrating cells and the walls of cavities. It enters the CSF if the meninges are inflamed. Pyrazinamide is metabolized by the liver to pyrazinoic acid, which is subsequently oxidized to 5-hydroxypyrazinoic acid by xanthine oxidase with the metabolite excreted by glomerular filtration. The $t_{1/2}$ of pyrazinamide is approximately 6 hours.

Ethionamide Ethionamide is well absorbed orally and is widely distributed, entering the CSF to produce concentrations equal to those in plasma. It is extensively metabolized by sulfoxidation, *N*-methylation, desulfuration, and deamination to products that are excreted in the urine. It has a $t_{1/2}$ of 2 hours.

Cycloserine Cycloserine is rapidly absorbed by the oral route and widely distributed, yielding CSF concentrations equal to plasma. About 35% of the drug is metabolized; the remainder is excreted by glomerular filtration unchanged. It accumulates in renal failure but can be removed by hemodialysis.

***p*-Aminosalicylic Acid** *p*-Aminosalicylic acid (PAS) is well absorbed orally and enters lung tissue and pleural fluid. Low CSF concentrations result from active transport out of the CSF. It is metabolized in the liver by an acetylase different from the enzyme that acts on isoniazid. PAS does prolong the isoniazid $t_{1/2}$.

Capreomycin Capreomycin is administered IM and undergoes elimination by glomerular filtration. It enters CSF poorly and accumulates in renal dysfunction states.

Aminoglycosides The aminoglycosides are discussed in Chapter 48.

Antileprosy Drugs

Dapsone is 90% absorbed from the upper gastrointestinal tract, is distributed to all body tissues, and achieves therapeutic concentrations in skin. It is approximately 70% bound to plasma proteins. Dapsone is excreted in bile and reabsorbed via enterohepatic circulation and also undergoes acetylation in the liver by the same *N*-acetyl transferase that acetylates isoniazid. The acetylation phenotype does not affect the half-life of the drug. Dapsone is excreted as glucuronide and sulfate conjugates in urine with a plasma half-life of 25 hours. The half-life is reduced in patients receiving rifampin.

Clofazimine is variably absorbed from the gastrointestinal tract and distributed in a complex pattern with high concentrations in subcutaneous fat and the reticuloendothelial system. It is unmetabolized and excreted slowly by the biliary route. The half-life is estimated to be 70 days.

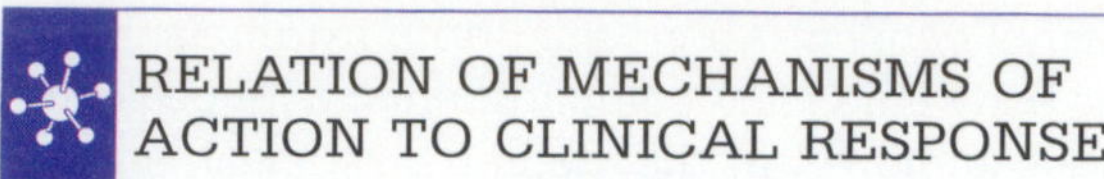

RELATION OF MECHANISMS OF ACTION TO CLINICAL RESPONSE

Antituberculosis Drugs

Isoniazid Isoniazid is the primary agent in all therapeutic and prophylactic programs for tuberculosis in which the tubercle bacilli are susceptible and the patient has no major reaction to the drug. Isoniazid is bactericidal on growing *Mycobacterium tuberculosis* and bacteriostatic on resting organisms. It inhibits *M. kansasii* but not other tubercle bacilli.

The percentage of patients infected by isoniazid-resistant *M. tuberculosis* varies depending on the geographic location. It can reach 25% in some inner-city areas but generally is approximately 5%. Resistance in Asian countries can reach 40%. Mutants are present in most organism populations at a frequency of 10^{-6}. In cavities containing 10^7 to 10^9 organisms, some *M. tuberculosis* cells will therefore be resistant and survive therapy.

Rifampin This drug inhibits most *M. tuberculosis* at concentrations of 0.005 to 0.2 μg/ml. *M. kansasii* are also inhibited, but *M. avium-intracellulare, M. fortuitum,* and *M. chelonei* are usually resistant.

Rifampin also inhibits most gram-positive bacteria such as staphylococci, streptococci, and *Steptococcus pneumoniae,* as well as many methicillin-resistant *Staphylococcus aureus.* It acts on *Listeria* organisms and enterococci, though most are inhibited but not killed, and it is extremely active against *Neisseria meningitidis* and *Haemophilus influenzae.* Rifampin inhibits many enteric species, including some *Pseudomonas* organisms, and is active against *Legionella* species, mycoplasmas, and chlamydiae. Most anaerobic species are also inhibited, including *Clostridium difficile* and *Bacteroides* organisms.

Rifampin is primarily used to treat tuberculosis, but it has several other uses. It is the drug of choice for chemoprophylaxis of meningococcal disease and for *H. influenzae* meningitis. It is also used in combination with vancomycin to treat prosthetic valve endocarditis resulting from staphylococcal infection and can be combined with antistaphylococcal penicillins or cephalosporins to treat staphylococcal osteomyelitis. Rifampin combined with cloxacillin eliminates nasal *S. aureus* in patients with recurrent furunculosis.

Ethambutol Most *M. tuberculosis* and *M. kansasii* are inhibited by this drug, but *M. avium-intracellulare* is not. Resistance can develop if the drug is used alone; when combined with other antituberculosis agents, the emergence of resistance is decreased but to a lesser degree than with rifampin or streptomycin. When used with isoniazid or rifampin, the inhibition of tubercle bacilli is additive.

Ethambutol inhibits only mycobacteria and is active against growing but not nonproliferating organisms to produce a tuberculostatic effect. It enters the mycobacteria by diffusion but encounters a lag time of several hours before inhibition of growth is observed.

Pyrazinamide Pyrazinamide is bactericidal at acid pH of 5 to 5.5 with minimal activity at neutral pH. It enters mononuclear cells, killing the bacteria present. When it is used alone, the organisms become resistant, and so it is less useful than other agents in preventing the emergence of resistance. This agent, which for years was considered a second-line drug, has recently become important as a first-line agent in multiple-drug, short-course treatment programs.

Ethionamide Ethionamide is a bacteriostatic agent that inhibits *M. tuberculosis* intracellularly and extracellularly and shows no cross-resistance with isoniazid or other agents.

Cycloserine Cycloserine inhibits *S. aureus, Escherichia coli,* Enterobacteriaceae organisms, nocardiae, and chlamydiae, as well as *M. tuberculosis* and *M. kansasii.* It shows no cross-resistance with other agents. Resistance readily develops because of reduced uptake of drug or altered enzymes involved in cell wall synthesis.

***p*-Aminosalicylic Acid** *p*-Aminosalicylic acid is bacteriostatic, inhibiting most *M. tuberculosis.* It is rarely used today.

Capreomycin Capreomycin inhibits only mycobacteria, and *M. tuberculosis* is only moderately susceptible. No cross-resistance is shown with isoniazid, rifampin, ethambutol, or streptomycin.

Aminoglycosides Streptomycin, kanamycin, and amikacin are aminoglycosides also active against *M. tuberculosis.* These drugs act by inhibiting protein synthesis and are described in Chapter 48.

Streptomycin was the first drug used to treat tuberculosis. It inhibits most *M. tuberculosis* and *M. kansasii,* but other tubercle bacilli are resistant. The primary incidence of resistance of *M. tuberculosis* to streptomycin is less than 5%, but resistant organisms appear if this drug is used alone. Streptomycin is not an ideal agent for tuberculosis because it does not enter the phagocytic cells in which the tubercle bacilli survive.

Amikacin also inhibits many of the atypical mycobacteria, but neither kanamycin nor amikacin are used as first-line therapy except for drug-resistant organisms.

Therapy of Tuberculosis The two major problems encountered in treating tuberculosis are the eradication of organisms that grow slowly or not at all in sheltered environments and the development of resistance in the large populations of organisms at the sites of infection. Because of these problems, therapy of tuberculosis includes the simultaneous use of two or more drugs, with treatment continued over prolonged periods. All earlier programs included isoniazid and a second agent to prevent the development of resistance. The problems with this approach were high cost, poor patient compliance, and risk of increased toxicity. The availability of rifampin has made it possible to use much shorter courses of therapy. Both isoniazid and rifampin are bactericidal for *M. tuberculosis* and enter phagocytic cells and cavities to eradicate persisting organisms. In combination, they prevent the development of resistance, which is normally extremely low for rifampin.

Current initial therapy uses isoniazid, rifampin, ethambutol, and pyrazinamide for 2 months and then rifampin and isoniazid given for 4 months. In areas in which drug-resistance is low, two drugs, isoniazid and rifampin, can be administered for 6 months.

More recently, longer programs have been developed that use intensive initial therapy with four drugs—isoniazid, rifampin, pyrazinamide, and streptomycin—which are administered daily for 2 months, followed by 10 months of isoniazid and rifampin therapy.

Drug resistance is probable if: (1) the acquisition of infection is in areas of the world in which resistance is high, such as Southeast Asia, the Caribbean, and in certain cities such as New York, and (2) infection of patients who received previous antituberculosis drug therapy, particularly when medication was taken irregularly because this increases the possibility for development of drug-resistant organisms. Four drugs should always be started when one is dealing with extensive pulmonary disease, miliary disease, or meningitis, and that therapy should be adjusted when the results of susceptibility testing are available.

The chemoprophylaxis of tuberculosis is directed at two different goals: prevention of infection and prevention of disease by eradication of organisms infecting the individual. Isoniazid is the most effective agent. All household contacts and close associates of a newly diagnosed patient should be treated. (This is particularly important for children younger than 7 years of age.) The second category includes individuals who have recently developed a positive skin test for tuberculosis. In these patients the risk of developing disease is highest for the first few years after the positive test results. Patients should have prophylactic therapy if (1) they have an abnormal chest radiograph and a positive tuberculin test with the length of positivity unknown; (2) they have a positive tuberculin test and a high risk of impaired cellular immunity from other agents such as prolonged therapy with glucocorticoids; (3) they are receiving immunosuppressive therapy such as azathioprine; and (4) they have a hematological malignancy, diabetes mellitus, silicosis, or a positive HIV titer. Controversy exists about whether all individuals under 30 years of age who have a positive tuberculin reaction should receive prophylaxis. Traditionally, isoniazid is administered daily for 6 months. There are no data on chemoprophylaxis for isoniazid-resistant organisms, but rifampin is a possible choice. In areas of high two-drug resistance, prophylaxis should be with ofloxacin and pyrazinamide.

Antileprosy Drugs

M. leprae can become resistant to dapsone, and resistance is increasing worldwide, varying from 2% to 40% in infected populations. Dapsone has been administered over many years for treatment of leprosy. Recently it has been used to treat and to protect against *Pneumocystis carinii* pulmonary infection in patients with AIDS.

At low concentrations, rifampin is bactericidal to *M. leprae* and rapidly reduces infectivity when used with dapsone. Clofazimine is used primarily when other treatments fail or when cases become refractory to rifampin. Clarithromycin inhibits *M. leprae.*

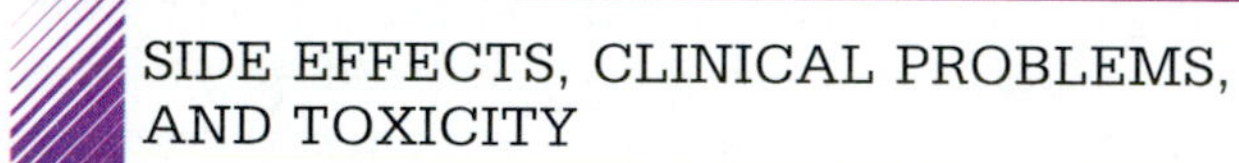

SIDE EFFECTS, CLINICAL PROBLEMS, AND TOXICITY

The main problems in the clinical use of these drugs for the treatment of tuberculosis or leprosy are summarized in Table 52-2.

Antituberculosis Drugs

Isoniazid Although adverse reactions are not common, a few are serious. About 2% of patients develop a rash, 1% fever, less than 1% jaundice, and only 0.2% peripheral neuritis. Approximately 15% of patients have elevated serum aminotransferases. Hepatic toxicity usually occurs 4 to 8 weeks after the start of treatment and is correlated with age. It is rarely seen in patients below 20 years of age but occurs in 2.3% of patients over 50 years of age. Hepatotoxicity is more common in alcoholics. Patients complain of anorexia, nausea, malaise, and fatigue. If the reaction is allowed to progress, extensive hepatocellular damage resembling viral hepatitis will develop. In many individuals, serum aminotransferase concentrations rise to 2 or 3 times normal; a further increase requires that the drug be discontinued. Some experts believe that aminotransferase concentrations should be checked monthly in elderly patients. Whether the toxicity is caused by metabolites of isoniazid or other factors remains unclear.

Peripheral neuritis occurs in patients receiving large doses, particularly individuals with nutritional deficiency attributable to vitamin lack. Pyridoxine prevents neuropathy and other CNS toxicity of isoniazid by providing the substrate for pyridoxine kinase, which is inhibited by isoniazid. Other neurological toxicities include convulsions, optic neuritis, paresthesias, ataxia, and psychoses. Mental abnormalities, such as transient memory impairment, have been reported.

Allergic reactions such as fever, rash, and a syndrome similar to lupus erythematosus occasionally occur. Arthritic symptoms have been observed, and antinuclear antibody tests may show abnormal results. Isoniazid can produce a sideroblastic anemia resulting from pyridoxine deficiency. The agent also potentiates the toxicity of phenytoin with possible production of nystagmus, altered gait, and signs of excessive sedation. Elevation of liver enzymes appears to increase further when isoniazid is administered with rifampin.

Rifampin Rifampin is generally well tolerated. It can cause gastrointestinal reactions, particularly nausea and vomiting, in 1% to 2% of individuals, but a rash is uncommon. Occasionally, patients complain of headache, dizziness, fatigue, or other CNS symptoms. Rifampin can cause hepatitis, especially in patients also receiving isoniazid or those who are alcoholics or others with previous liver disease; fulminant hepatitis is rare.

The administration of rifampin biweekly may produce a flu-like syndrome with fever, chills, muscle aches, headache, and dizziness. This occurs most often after several months of therapy and begins 1 to 2 hours after a dose. The syndrome stops with daily drug administration.

Thrombocytopenia, hemolysis, and transient leukopenia have also been reported. Interstitial nephritis occurs rarely as a renal toxicity.

Rifampin interacts with many other drugs as an inducer of microsomal P-450 enzymes. It reduces the half-lives of agents such as prednisone, digitoxin, quinidine, propanolol, metoprolol, sulfonamides, clofibrate, thyroxine, dapsone, methadone, and ketoconazole. Oral anticoagulants, oral contraceptives, and many other drugs are thus rendered less effective (see box on p. 711). Rifampin can stain soft contact lenses red. Since it causes teratogenic effects in rodents, it should be used in pregnancy only for severe tuberculosis.

Ethambutol Ethambutol has few adverse effects. The most important toxicity is a dose-related retrobulbar neuritis. There may be loss of central vision and color discrimination involving central fibers of the optic nerve. A less common problem is constriction of visual fields involving peripheral fibers of the optic nerve. In both cases no changes are seen on funduscopic examination, and the mechanism of the neuritis is unknown.

Table 52-2 Drugs Used to Treat Tuberculosis and Leprosy

Medication	Major Adverse Reactions	Recommended Regular Monitoring
Isoniazid	Hepatic enzyme elevation, peripheral neuropathy, hepatitis, increased phenytoin (Dilantin) concentrations, interaction with disulfiram (Antabuse), CNS effects	Hepatic enzymes (if base-line value abnormal)
Rifampin	Orange discoloration of secretions, urine, tears, and contact lenses. Hepatitis, fever, thrombocytopenia, flu-like syndrome Reduces concentrations of many drugs, including methadone, warfarin, birth control pills, theophylline, dapsone, and ketoconazole	Hepatic enzymes (if base-line value abnormal)
Pyrazinamide	GI upset, hepatic enzyme elevation, rash, arthralgias, hyperuricemia	Hepatic enzymes (if base-line value abnormal)
Ethambutol	Optic neuritis (decreased red-green color discrimination), decreased visual acuity, skin rash	Check color vision and visual acuity monthly
Streptomycin	Ototoxicity, nephrotoxicity, hypokalemia, hypomagnesemia	Audiometry and renal function
Ciprofloxacin	Abdominal cramps, GI upset, tremulousness, insomnia, headache, photosensitivity Drug interactions with warfarin and theophylline	
Ofloxacin	Probably similar to ciprofloxacin; possibly fewer drug interactions.	
Kanamycin, Amikacin	Auditory and renal toxicity, rare vestibular toxicity, hypokalemia, hypomagnesemia	Audiometry and renal function
Capreomycin	Auditory, vestibular, and renal toxicity, eosinophilia, hypokalemia, hypomagnesemia	Audiometry and renal function
Ethionamide	GI upset, bloating, hepatic enzyme elevation, metallic taste, hypothyroidism (esp. if patient is on para-aminosalicylic acid)	Hepatic enzymes (if base-line value abnormal)
Cycloserine	Psychosis, depression, seizures, rash, headache, increased phenytoin (Dilantin) concentrations	Assessment of mental status
Para-Aminosalicylic acid	GI upset, hepatic enzyme elevation, sodium load, decreased digoxin, increased phenytoin (Dilantin) concentrations, hypersensitivity Concentrations decreased by diphenhydramine (Benadryl)	Assessment of volume status
Clofazimine	Orange/brown skin discoloration; gastrointestinal complaints; rare visual disturbances	
Dapsone	Anemia, rash, methemagtobinemia	Check G-6-PD status

From Neu HC, *Science* 257:1054, 1992.
G-6-PD, Glucose-6-phosphate dehydrogenase.

In most patients, vision returns once administration of the drug is stopped, but recovery may take up to 6 months.

Ethambutol occasionally causes gastrointestinal upset, allergic reactions including rash, joint pains, fever, malaise, headache, and pruritus. Peripheral neuropathy develops rarely and only after many months into the treatment. This effect involves only the sensory nerves and resolves when the drug is stopped. Since ethambutol decreases the clearance of uric acid, an acute gouty attack can be precipitated, but it is rare.

Pyrazinamide Hepatotoxicity is the most serious adverse effect of pyrazinamide, and elevation of liver aminotransferase is the first sign of toxicity. The effect is dose related and is much less frequent with the lower doses currently being used. Hepatic necrosis and death may occur with higher doses. Serum aminotransferases

MEDICATIONS FOR WHICH THE HALF-LIFE IS REDUCED THROUGH INCREASED HEPATIC METABOLISM BY RIFAMPIN

Barbituates	Metoprolol
Chloramphenicol	Methadone
Cimetidine	Phenytoin
Clofibrate	Prednisone
Contraceptives, oral	Propranolol
Cyclosporin	Quinidine
Dapsone	Sulfonylureas
Digitoxin	Theophylline
Digoxin	Thyroxine
Estrogens	Verapamil
Itraconazole	Warfarin
Ketoconazole	

TRADE NAMES

In addition to generic and fixed-combination preparations, the following trade-named materials are available in the United States.

TUBERCULOSIS

Capastat, capreomycin sulfate
INH, isoniazid
Laniazid, isoniazid
Myambutol, ethambutol HCl
Rifadin, rifampin
Rimactane, rifampin
Seromycin, cycloserine
Trecator-SC, ethionamide

LEPROSY

Lamprene, clofazimine

should be determined before therapy is started and should be monitored frequently. Pyrazinamide causes hyperuricemia by inhibition of renal excretion of urate. Mild arthralgias occur in approximately 70% of patients, with occasional nausea, vomiting, malaise, and fever.

Ethionamide Ethionamide produces significant gastrointestinal reactions, and many individuals cannot tolerate elevated doses. Nausea, vomiting, abdominal pain, diarrhea, a metallic taste in the mouth, and many nervous system complaints, including depression, headache, and feelings of restlessness, are typical side effects. Seizures; peripheral neuropathy; and allergic reactions with rash, purpura, stomatitis, gynecomastia, impotence, hypoglycemia, alopecia, and hypotension rarely occur. About 5% of patients develop hepatitis, which resolves when the drug is stopped.

Cycloserine Neurotoxicity is the most important side effect, but psychotic disturbances in the form of confusion, aggression, depression, and excitement also occur. Convulsions have also been noted. Cycloserine may occasionally cause rash, fever, and cardiac arrhythmias. It should not be given to patients with a prior history of seizures or psychiatric disorders.

***p*-Aminosalicylic Acid** Gastrointestinal side effects of nausea, vomiting, abdominal pain, and diarrhea occur in up to 30% of patients, with fever, malaise, joint pains, and skin eruptions found in 5% to 10% of patients.

Capreomycin The most serious adverse effect is nephrotoxicity with loss of potassium, calcium, and magnesium in the urine. The drug may also cause tinnitus, vertigo, and deafness.

Aminoglycosides The aminoglycosides are discussed in Chapter 48.

Antileprosy Drugs

Hemolytic anemia and methemoglobinemia are the common adverse effects seen with the use of dapsone. Methemoglobinemia is caused by a dapsone *N*-oxidation product. Although bone marrow suppression is rare, agranulocytosis and aplastic anemia may occur. Anorexia, nausea, and vomiting are also found occasionally. Other problems include headache, insomnia, psychosis, paresthesia, peripheral neuropathy, nervousness, blurred vision, vertigo, tinnitus, fever, and skin rash.

Dapsone and particularly rifampin can provoke lepra reactions, which are exacerbations of the cutaneous manifestations of leprosy. Fever, erythematous nodules, malaise, and joint symptoms may occur. These reactions can be controlled by using steroids.

REFERENCES

Bartmann K, editor: *Antituberculosis drugs,* New York, 1988, Springer-Verlag New York, Inc.

Centers for Disease Control: The use of preventive therapy for tuberculosis infection in the United States, *MMWR* 39(RR8):9-12, 1990.

Hastings RC, Franzblau SG: Chemotherapy of leprosy, *Annu Rev Pharmacol Toxicol* 28:231, 1988.

Schlossberg D, editor: *Tuberculosis,* ed 2, New York, 1988, Springer-Verlag New York, Inc.

Vilarino ME et al: Management of persons exposed to multidrug resistant tuberculosis *MMWR* 41(RR-11):59-71, 1992.

SELF-ASSESSMENT QUESTIONS

1. The mechanism of action of rifampin is which of the following?
   a. interferes with bacterial cell wall synthesis
   b. inhibits DNA-dependent RNA polymerase
   c. inhibits 30S ribosome function
   d. alters membrane activity so that ions are lost from inside the bacteria
2. Which is the main elimination route of ethambutol?
   a. renal
   b. metabolized by *N*-acetylation
   c. biliary excretion
   d. oxidized
3. Which of the following mycobacterial species is inhibited by isoniazid?
   a. *Mycobacterium kansasii*
   b. *Mycobacterium avium*
   c. *Mycobacterium gordoni*
   d. *Mycobacterium chelonei*

4. Pyrazinamide interferes with excretion of which one?
   a. creatinine
   b. isoniazid
   c. uric acid
   d. ethambutol
5. Which of the following antituberculosis agents is not bactericidal?
   a. isoniazid
   b. rifampin
   c. pyrazinamide
   d. ethambutol
6. Isoniazid can produce all of the following adverse effects *except:*
   a. interstitial nephritis.
   b. hepatitis.
   c. peripheral neuritis.
   d. anemia.
7. Ethambutol produces which of the following adverse reactions?
   a. deafness
   b. blindness
   c. vestibular toxicity
   d. renal insufficiency
8. Which of the antibacterial agents are metabolized chiefly by N-acetylation?
   a. rifampin
   b. isoniazid
   c. chloramphenicol
   d. erythromycin
9. Patients who are slow inactivators of isoniazid are most likely to develop which one of the following adverse effects?
   a. renal insufficiency
   b. vestibular damage
   c. peripheral neuritis
   d. optic neuritis
   e. color blindness

CHAPTER 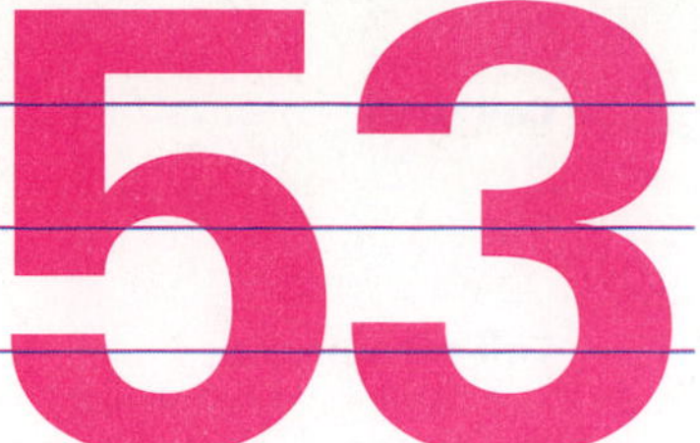

Antifungal Agents

HAROLD C. NEU

MAJOR DRUGS
polyenes flucytosine imidazoles griseofulvin

THERAPEUTIC OVERVIEW

Fungal infections (mycoses) occur less frequently than bacterial or viral infections do but may be prevalent in some geographical locations that favor the growth of specific pathogenic fungal strains. Many fungal infections are superficial and primarily annoying. Others are systemic and can be life threatening, particularly in patients with compromised host defenses, such as those receiving immunosuppressive drugs. The toxicity of many antifungal drugs limits their use, and there are unfortunately only a few agents that are useful in the treatment of systemic fungal infections.

Fungi are more complex organisms, compared to bacteria or viruses. For example, they have different ribosomes and cell wall components and possess a discrete nuclear membrane. Therefore antibacterial antibiotics are not effective against pathogenic fungi.

The major classes of fungal infections and examples of prevalent species that are often causative organisms are summarized in the box.

MECHANISMS OF ACTION

The principal antifungal drugs are polyenes, flucytosine, imidazoles, and griseofulvin. Sites of action are shown in Figure 53-1.

Polyenes

The polyene (i.e., multiple double bonds) antibiotics are macrocyclic lactones that contain a hydrophilic hydroxylated portion and a hydrophobic conjugated double bond portion. The structures of amphotericin B, the most widely used antifungal agent, and nystatin, a closely related analog, are shown in Figure 53-2.

Polyenes act by binding to sterols in the cell membrane and forming channels, allowing K^+ ions and Mg^{++} molecules to leak out of the cell. The polyenes bind to the sterol and become integrated into the membrane to form a ring with a pore in the center of about 0.8 nm diameter. K^+ leaks out of the cell through these pores, followed by Mg^{++}, and, with the loss of K^+, results in derangement of cellular metabolism (Figure 53-3). It is thought that the derangement of the membrane alters the activity of enzymes in the membrane. The principal sterol in fungal membranes, ergosterol, has a stronger affinity for polyenes than does cholesterol, the principal sterol of mammalian cell membranes. Therefore the polyenes show greater activity against fungal cells than against mammalian cells, and fungi that lack ergosterol are not susceptible to treatment by amphotericin B.

Flucytosine

Flucytosine, also called 5-fluorocytosine, is an antimetabolite that undergoes intracellular metabolism to an active form, which leads to inhibition of DNA synthesis.

Flucytosine is transported into susceptible fungi by a permease system for purines. The drug is deaminated by cytosine deaminase to 5-fluorouracil. Since cytosine deaminase is not present in mammalian cells, the drug does not undergo activation in humans. Fluorouracil, in turn, is converted by the enzyme uridine phosphate pyrophosphorylase and by other enzymes to 5-fluoro-2′-deoxyuridine 5′-monophosphate, which inhibits thymi-

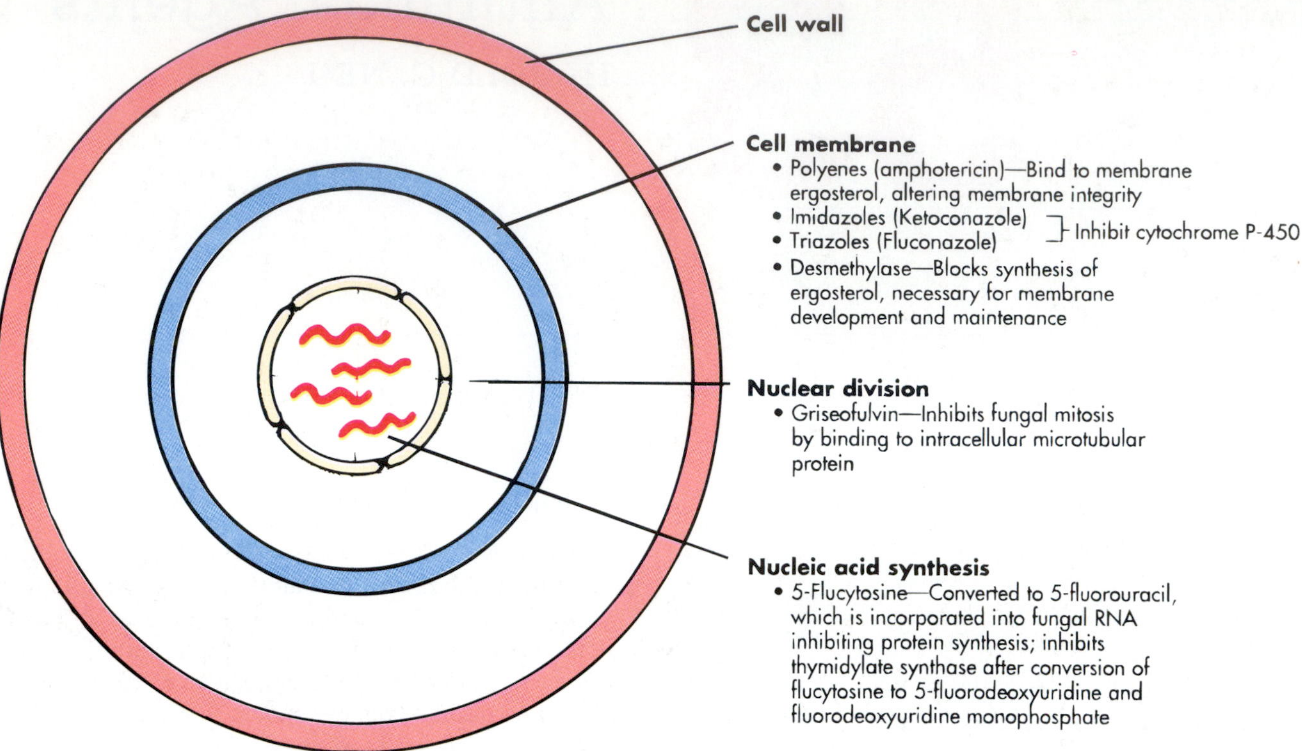

FIGURE 53-1 Mechanism of action of antifungal agents. See the text for further information.

amphotericin B

nystatin A_1

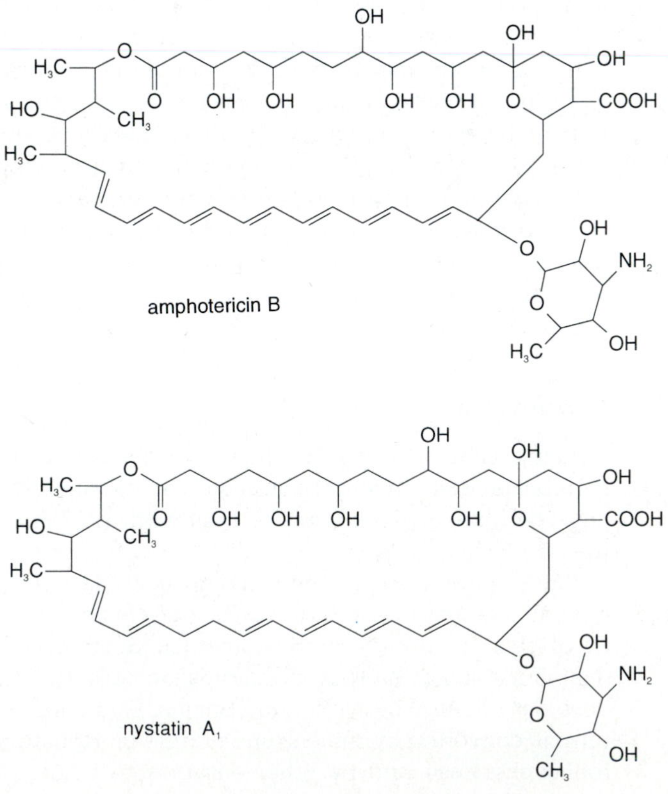

FIGURE 53-2 Structures of amphotericin B and nystatin A_1. See the text for further information.

THERAPEUTIC OVERVIEW

CUTANEOUS AND SUBCUTANEOUS MYCOSES

Epidermophyton spp.
Microsporum spp.
Sporothrix spp.
Trichophyton spp.
Treat with dermatological preparations, occasionally systemic agents

SYSTEMIC MYCOSES

Aspergillus spp.
Candida spp.
Blastomyces dermatitidis
Cryptococcus neoformans
Coccidioides immitis
Fusarium spp.
Histoplasma capsulatum
Paracoccidioides brasiliensis
Mucormycosis
Difficult to treat; available drugs often cause deleterious side effects; often need long-term therapy

dylate synthase and interferes with DNA synthesis (discussed in greater detail in Chapter 44).

Fungi can be resistant to flucytosine because they lack a permease, have a defective cytosine deaminase, or have a low concentration of the uridine monophosphate pyrophosphorylase enzyme. Whether production of faulty RNA as a result of incorporation of the fluorouracil contributes to the action of this agent is unclear.

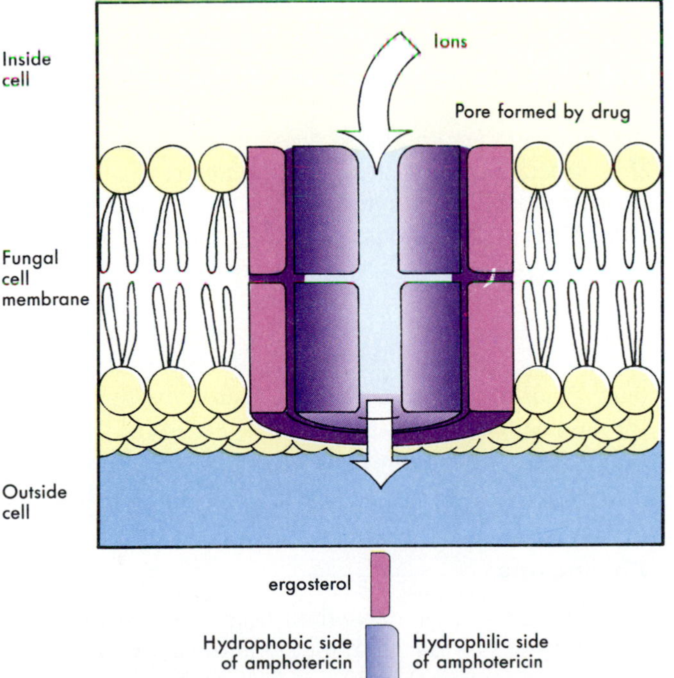

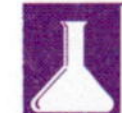

FIGURE 53-3 Action of polyene agents to form pores in the fungal cell membrane through which K^+ and Mg^{++} can leak out of the cell.

Imidazoles

The structures of the principal imidazole antifungal agents are shown in Figure 53-4. Ketoconazole, miconazole, clotrimazole, and econazole are available, as are the new agents fluconazole and itraconazole.

Depending on the concentration of drug, imidazoles can act as fungistatic or fungicidal agents. In actively growing fungi, the imidazoles inhibit synthesis of membrane sterols by inhibiting incorporation or synthesis of ergosterol. These agents interact with cytochrome P-450–dependent 14-α-demethylase, and as a result ergosterol is not produced. At high concentrations, the imidazoles cause leakage of K^+ and other components from the fungal cell. Inhibition of plasma membrane ATPase is a secondary action that may contribute to or help account for the K^+ loss. Since imidazoles inhibit fungal respiration under aerobic conditions, an alternative mechanism may be blockade of respiratory-chain electron transport.

Griseofulvin

Whether griseofulvin is fungicidal or fungistatic is not established. It enters susceptible fungi through an energy-dependent transport system and inhibits fungal mitosis. It does this by binding to the microtubules that form the mitotic spindle and blocking the polymerization of tubulin into microtubules. It also binds to a microtubule-associated protein, but the role of this protein is not known. The binding site for griseofulvin on tubulin is different from that of colchicine and the plant alkaloids (see Chapter 44). This effect on microtubule assembly probably explains the morphological changes, such as curling, that are observed in the fungi. The mechanism of resistance is unknown but may be related to decreased uptake of the drug.

The structure of griseofulvin is shown in Figure 53-4.

PHARMACOKINETICS

Pharmacokinetic parameters for the antifungal drugs are summarized in Table 53-1.

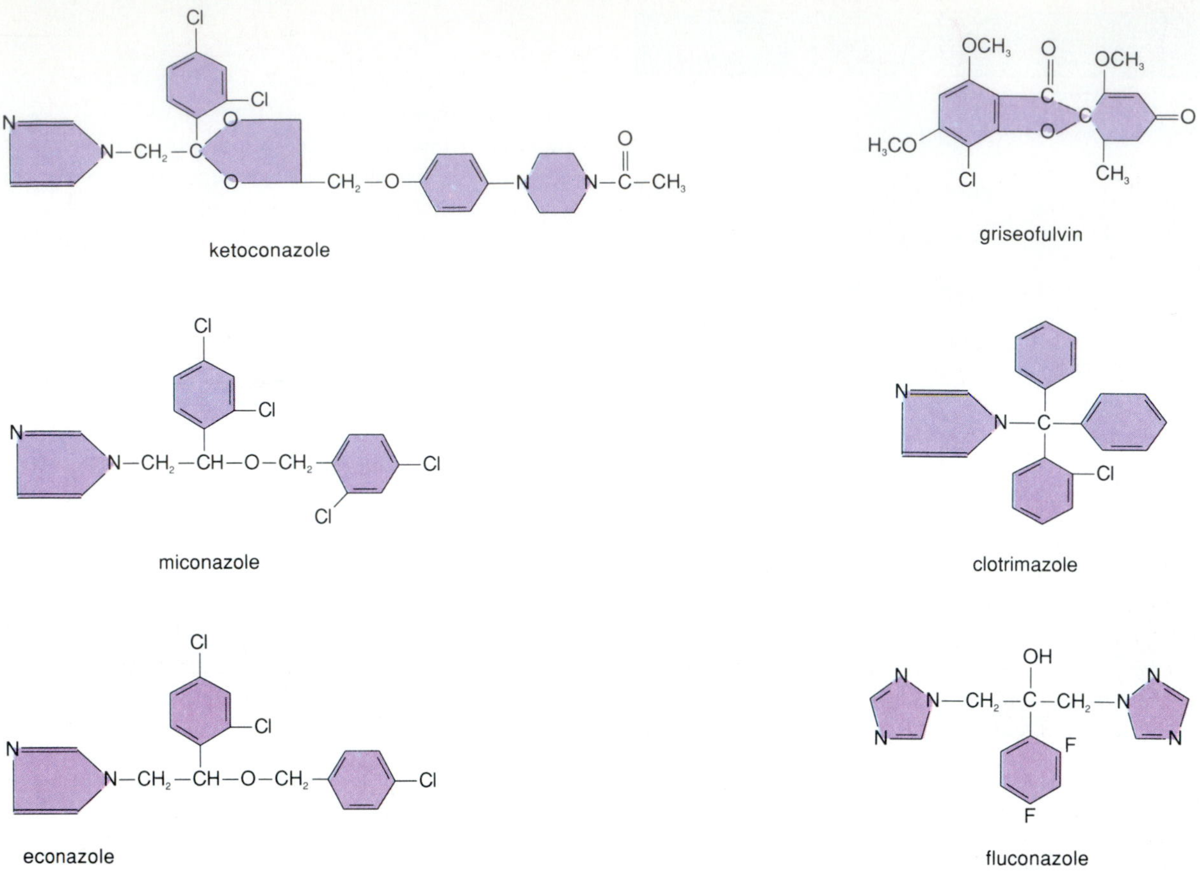

ketoconazole

griseofulvin

miconazole

clotrimazole

econazole

fluconazole

FIGURE 53-4 Structures of imidazole antifungal drugs. See the text for further information.

Polyenes

Amphotericin B is insoluble in water, has a large lipophilic domain in its structure, and is not absorbed from the gastrointestinal tract. It is administered orally only to treat fungal infections of the gastrointestinal tract, which sometimes develop as an aftermath of administration of broad-spectrum antibacterial agents because of depletion of the bacterial microflora. For parenteral use, amphotericin B is combined with the detergent deoxycholate to form a colloidal suspension.

The pharmacokinetics of amphotericin B are complex, with >90% plasma protein bound, several distribution phases, and elimination phases with half-lives of 24 to 48 hours for the initial portion and about 15 days for the terminal portions. The drug can be detected in urine and serum for up to 7 weeks after a course of therapy.

Amphotericin B enters pleural, peritoneal, and synovial fluids to achieve about 50% of serum concentrations. It crosses the placenta and is found in cord blood and amniotic fluid and also enters the aqueous but not the vitreous humor of the eye. Cerebrospinal fluid (CSF) concentrations reach one third to one half those in serum. Most of the amphotericin B in the body probably is bound to cholesterol-containing membranes in tissue sites.

The principal pathway for amphotericin B disposition is not known. Some is excreted by the biliary route, and only 3% of a dose is eliminated in urine with concentrations equivalent to those in plasma. Renal dysfunction does not affect plasma concentrations of the drug, and amphotericin B is not removed by hemodialysis.

Flucytosine

Flucytosine is well absorbed from the gastrointestinal tract and is widely distributed in the body, with CSF concentrations equal to 70% to 85% of those in plasma. It enters the peritoneum, synovial fluid, bronchial secretions, saliva, and bone.

Approximately 85% to 95% is excreted unchanged by

Table 53-1 Pharmacokinetic Parameter Values for Antifungal Drugs

Drug	Administration	Absorption	$t_{1/2}$ (hr)	Urine Concentration	Disposition	Plasma Protein Bound (%)
POLYENES						
amphotericin B	IV, topical, oral	No	24 (15 days)*	Good	B (some) ? (main)	>90
nystatin	Topical	No	—	—	—	>90
ANTIMETABOLITES						
flucytosine	Oral	Good	3-6	Good	R (85%)	<10
IMIDAZOLES						
ketoconazole	oral, topical	75%†	8	Poor	M (95%) R (3%)	99
miconazole	Topical, IV	Poor	0.5	—	M (95%)	90
econazole	Topical	<1%	—	—	M (95%)	—
clotrimazole	Topical	<1%	—	—	M (95%)	—
fluconazole	IV, oral	85%	25-30	Good	R (main), M	12
itraconazole	Oral	99% (40%‡)	17	Poor	M	99
GRISEOFULVIN						
	oral, topical	Poor§	20	—	M (main)	—

M, Metabolism; *R*, renal; *B*, biliary.
*Terminal elimination phase.
†Needs acidic pH to be absorbed.
§Particles taken up by unknown process.
‡During fasting, less well absorbed.

glomerular filtration, with a normal half-life of 3 to 6 hours increased greatly as creatinine clearance diminishes. For special conditions, the drug can be removed by hemodialysis and peritoneal dialysis. A small fraction of the dose may be converted by intestinal bacteria to 5-fluorouracil and lead to hematologic toxicity.

Imidazoles

Ketoconazole is administered orally. Since its absorption is favored at acid pH, coadministration of antacids and histamine H_2 receptor–blocking agents reduces ketoconazole absorption. Contradictory results are reported for the effect of food on absorption of this agent. For the same dose, the plasma concentration of drug varies widely between patients.

Ketoconazole is distributed into saliva, skin, bone, and pleural, peritoneal, synovial, and aqueous humor fluids. Penetration into the CSF is poor, and effective CSF concentrations are not achieved—only 5% of the plasma concentration. The plasma concentration declines in a biexponential fashion, with a distribution half-life of about 2 hours followed by an elimination half-life of 8 hours.

Ketoconazole is extensively metabolized by hydroxylation of the imidazole and by oxidative *N*-dealkylation of the piperazine rings. It does not induce its own metabolism, as clotrimazole does. However, rifampin induces microsomal enzymes that increase ketoconazole oxidation. Only 2% to 4% of a dose is excreted in urine as active drug. Renal insufficiency does not affect plasma concentration or half-life, but the half-life is prolonged in patients with hepatic insufficiency.

Miconazole is now used topically and rarely IV. It is minimally soluble in water and not adequately absorbed from the gastrointestinal tract. The half-life is only 30 minutes, and so plasma concentrations after IV doses are low. It is metabolized by *O*-dealkylation and oxidative *N*-dealkylation but does not induce its own metabolism. Only 1% is excreted in the urine as active drug. Penetration of miconazole into CSF and sputum is poor but penetration into joint fluid is good.

Fluconazole is water soluble and is rapidly absorbed after oral administration, with about 90% bioavailability, 12% protein binding, and a half-life of 25 to 30 hours. Fluconazole does not require an acid environment for absorption. It does not induce the metabolism of most other agents, but it does, however, alter metabolism of orally administered hypoglycemic agents. About 70% of the drug is eliminated unchanged through the kidneys, with small amounts of metabolites present in urine and feces. Fluconazole is widely distributed in the body, with therapeutic concentrations attained in CSF, lung, and many other areas of the body.

Griseofulvin

Griseofulvin is insoluble; however, about 50% of an oral dose passes from the gastrointestinal tract into the circulation. This uptake from the gastrointestinal tract is related to particle size and is increased when the drug is ingested with a full meal. Whether the drug diffuses through the intestinal wall or is taken up as micelles (particles of drug coated with lipid surrounded by detergent to provide a water-compatible exterior surface) is not clear. When applied topically, griseofulvin penetrates the stratum corneum, but this does not result in effective local concentrations.

Griseofulvin is widely distributed in body fluids and tissues and becomes concentrated in fat, liver, and muscle. It is deposited in the keratin layer of the skin; becomes concentrated in keratin precursor cells in the stratum corneum of the skin, nails, and hair; and is secreted in perspiration. New keratin formed during treatment with griseofulvin is resistant to fungus, but griseofulvin does not destroy fungi in previously infected outer layers of skin. Thus a dermatophyte infection can be cured only when infected skin, nails, or hair is shed and the new keratin containing the griseofulvin replaces all the old keratin. Skin and hair infections require 4 to 6 weeks of therapy, fingernails require up to 6 months, and toenails require up to a year.

Most of the absorbed griseofulvin is metabolized in the liver by dealkylation, and the inactive metabolite is excreted in the urine as a glucuronide. The half-life of the drug is about 20 hours.

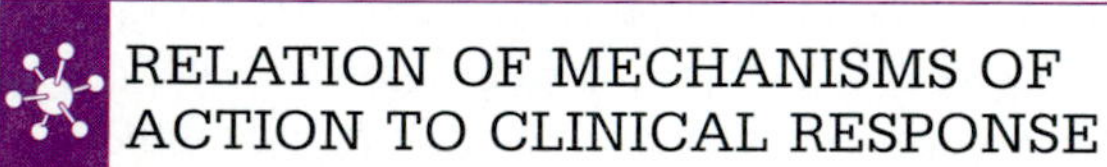

RELATION OF MECHANISMS OF ACTION TO CLINICAL RESPONSE

Polyenes

Amphotericin B inhibits all of the fungi listed in Table 53-2. *Candida* and *Aspergillus* are likely to be a cause of a systemic mycosis, as are *Mucor, Rhizopus,* and *Absidia* species, which are often present as opportunistic pathogens in debilitated patients. Amphotericin B also inhibits *Sporothrix* and *Trichosporon* species, as well as some ameboflagellates and the freshwater ameba *Acanthamoeba.* A few fungal species, such as *Allescheria boydii* and *Fusarium* species, show resistance. Amphotericin B acts synergistically with flucytosine against *Candida* organisms and cryptococci. Synergy of amphotericin B with other agents, such as rifampin and tetracyclines, can be demonstrated in vitro, but there are no clinical studies to support the use of this or other combinations of amphotericin B and antibiotics for the treatment of fungal infections.

Nystatin has a mode of action and antifungal spectrum of activity similar to those for amphotericin B. It is too toxic for parenteral administration and is only used topically.

Primaricin is a polyene used only for topical application to the eye. It has all of the activity of amphotericin B.

Flucytosine

Flucytosine inhibits *Cryptococcus neoformans,* many strains of *Candida albicans,* and *Cladosporium* and *Phialophore* species, which cause chromoblastomycosis. Resistance of *Candida* species to this drug is extremely variable. Flucytosine does not inhibit *Aspergillus* and *Sporothrix* organisms, *Blastomyces dermatitidis, Histoplasma capsulatum,* or *Coccidioides immitis.* This drug acts synergistically with amphotericin B against *Cryptococcus* organisms.

Imidazoles

The imidazoles inhibit many dermatophytes, yeasts, dimorphic fungi, and some phycomycetes. It is extremely difficult to interpret in vitro inhibition data on these drugs, since the results are method dependent and do not correlate well with in vivo responses.

Ketoconazole inhibits most of the common dermatophytes and many of the fungi that cause systemic mycoses listed in Table 53-2. However, it is not active against *Aspergillus* organisms or phycomycetes such as *Mucor* species. The membrane actions of ketoconazole also block the formation of branching hyphae, which may aid in white cell attack on the fungi.

Since ketoconazole interferes with the synthesis of ergosterol, it probably should not be used with amphotericin B because the effect of amphotericin B would be antagonized. This has been demonstrated in vitro and in an animal model of *Cryptococcus* infection.

Miconazole, econazole, and clotrimazole have a similar activity spectrum to that of ketoconazole, but miconazole inhibits *Allescheria.*

Griseofulvin

Griseofulvin inhibits dermatophytes of *Microsporum, Trichophyton,* and *Epidermophyton* species. It has no effect on filamentous fungi such as *Aspergillus,* yeasts such as *Candida* organisms, or dimorphoric species such as *Histoplasma.*

Therapeutic Usage

Amphotericin B is the drug of choice to treat most serious fungal infections (Table 53-2). Cryptococcal meningitis is treated either with amphotericin B alone

Table 53-2 Activity of Various Antifungal Agents Against Systemic Fungal Pathogens

Agent	*Aspergillus*	*Blastomyces dermatitidis*	*Candida albicans*	*Candida,* other	*Chromoblastomyces* agents	*Cryptococcus neoformans*	*Coccidioides immitis*	*Fusarium*	*Histoplasma capsulatum*	Mucormycosis agents	*Paracoccidioides brasiliensis*	*Pseudoallescheria*	*Sporothrix*
Amphotericin B	+	+	+	+	−	+	+	+/−	+	+	+	−	+
Flucytosine	+/−	−	+	+	+	+	−	−	−	−	−	−	−
Miconazole	−		+	+/−	+	+	+	−	+	−	+	+	+
Ketoconazole	−	+	+	+/−	−	+	+	−	+	−	+	−	+
Fluconazole	−	+	+	+/−	−	+	+	+/−	+	−	+	−	+
Itraconazole	+	+	+	+/−	+	+	+	+/−	+	−	+	−	+

or with a combination of amphotericin B and flucytosine. Systemic candidiasis is treated with amphotericin B, as are pulmonary, bone, joint, cardiac, and CNS infections attributable to *Candida* organisms and *Coccidioides immitis* infections of the lung or meninges. Amphotericin B is the only useful agent to treat serious *Aspergillus* species and zygomycete infections. Severe acute histoplasmosis and blastomycosis are treated with amphotericin B, though imidazoles are also useful in patients without human immunodeficiency virus infection. Other infections that respond to amphotericin B include sporotrichosis and amebic meningoencephalitis.

Amphotericin B is also used as empiric therapy in febrile neutropenic patients who have not responded to antibacterial agents. It is not effective as treatment of liver candidiasis or *Fusarium* infection.

Fluconazole is equivalent to amphotericin in treating cryptococcal infections in patients with acquired immunodeficiency syndrome. However, the initial response to therapy is slower than with amphotericin B, and fluconazole is preferred for lifetime maintenance therapy. It is also effective for therapy of *Candida* pharyngitis and esophagitis, and as a prophylactic agent against fungal infections in immunocompromised patients.

Nystatin is used to treat *Candida* infections of the skin, mucous membranes, and intestinal tract. It is effective for oral candidiasis, vaginal candidiasis, and *Candida* esophagitis. Although it is used prophylactically in neutropenic patients, it is ineffective except at very large daily doses.

Ketoconazole provides effective therapy for cutaneous mycoses and for oral and esophageal candidiasis in immunocompromised patients. The only systemic infection for which miconazole IV is appropriate is that caused by *Pseudoallescheria boydii.* Topically, it is comparable to clotrimazole for cutaneous candidiasis, ringworm, and pityriasis versicolor. Econazole is used topically because it can penetrate the stratum corneum. Itraconazole is effective therapy of histoplasmosis, paracoccidioidomycosis, blastomycosis, and coccidioidomycosis.

Clotrimazole is available only for topical use. It is not used systemically because of poor absorption and induction of microsomal enzymes, which cause its inactivation. It is used topically for *Candida* infection and superficial dermatophyte (ringworm) infections. It is also effective prophylactically for oral *Candida* colonization and infection in neutropenic patients.

Griseofulvin is used to treat only dermatophyte infections of the skin, nails, or hair, with mild forms effectively handled topically.

Tolnaftate is a topical antifungal that inhibits dermatophytes such as *Trichophyton* and *Microsporum* species but not *Candida.* Its mechanism of action is unknown. It is less effective on hyperkeratotic lesions, and scalp lesions respond poorly. It has no effect on onchomycosis. Tolnaftate has no known toxic reactions.

Haloprogin is a fungicidal agent that is effective against some *Epidermophyton, Microsporum,* and *Trichophyton* species and inhibits *Candida* organisms. Its mechanism of action is unknown. Burning sensations and peeling of the skin are the main side effects. It is used primarily to treat tinea pedis.

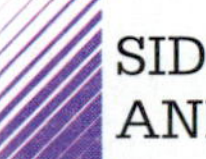

SIDE EFFECTS, CLINICAL PROBLEMS, AND TOXICITY

The clinical problems and major side effects encountered with the antifungal agents are summarized in Table 53-3.

Polyenes

Amphotericin B Unfortunately, many adverse effects are associated with the IV administration of amphotericin B. The initial reactions, usually fever to as

Table 53-3 Toxicity and Drug Interaction Profile of Antifungal Agents

Drug	Adverse Effect	Drug Interactions
POLYENES		
Amphotericin B	Nephrotoxicity; fever, chills; phlebitis; hypokalemia; anemia; GI disturbance	Azotemia with aminoglycosides; cyclosporin; pulmonary toxicity with granulocyte transfusion
FLUORINATED PYRIMIDINES		
Flucytosine	Bone marrow suppression; hepatotoxicity; GI disturbance	None, except bone marrow suppressive agents
AZOLES		
Imidazoles		
Miconazole	Headache; pruritus; thrombophlebitis; hepatotoxicity; autoinduction of hepatic degrading enzymes	
Ketoconazole	GI disturbance; hepatotoxicity	Drugs that induce hepatic microsomal enzymes, e.g., rifampicin, cyclosporin; antacids, H_2-receptor blockers
Triazoles		
Itraconazole	GI disturbance; rare hepatotoxicity	Rifampicin; phenytoin; ?cyclosporin
Fluconazole	GI disturbance; rare hepatotoxicity; rare Stevens-Johnson syndrome	Phenytoin; warfarin; ?cyclosporin

high as 40° C, chills, headache, malaise, nausea, and, occasionally, hypotension, can be controlled by antipyretics, antihistamines, antiemetics, and adrenocorticoids.

Most patients treated with amphotericin B develop some degree of renal toxicity. This is manifested by an early decrease in the glomerular filtration rate that results from vasoconstrictive action on the afferent arterioles. It may be accompanied by an effect on the distal renal tubule leading to potassium loss, hypomagnesemia caused by failure to reabsorb Mg^{++}, or tubular acidosis. Drug-induced pathological changes in the kidney include damage to the glomerular basement membrane, hypercellularity, fibrosis, and hyalinization of glomeruli with nephrocalcinosis. If the serum creatinine concentration increases above 3.5 mg/dl, drug administration should be stopped for a few days. The extent of renal damage is related to the total dose of drug, and although the majority of renal function is recovered even with continued therapy, some residual damage occurs. Hydration may reduce toxicity, but mannitol infusions have not been of benefit. Pentoxyfilline may reduce renal toxicity.

Most patients who receive a normal course of therapy develop a normochromic, normocytic anemia with hematocrits of 22% to 35%. This is the result of reduced erythropoiesis caused by inhibition of erythropoietin production. Red blood cell production returns to normal after discontinuation of therapy.

Other toxicities include rare neurotoxicity, cardiac dysrhythmias, pulmonary infiltrates, rash, and anaphylaxis. It is doubtful that amphotericin B produces liver toxicity.

Nystatin Nystatin has minimal side effects except for a bad taste when taken as an oral suspension, which in large doses can produce nausea. It is not allergenic on the skin.

Flucytosine

Occasionally patients experience nausea, vomiting, and diarrhea with flucytosine. Serious side effects are hematological: anemia, leukopenia, and thrombocytopenia. Since this drug is usually coadministered with amphotericin B, there may be reduced renal clearance of the drug. The toxicity is attributable to the metabolite 5-fluorouracil. Some cases of transient hepatotoxicity have been reported.

Imidazoles

Common side effects of ketoconazole, which occur in 3% to 20% of those treated, are nausea and vomiting, though nausea can be reduced if the drug is ingested with food. The most serious toxicity is hepatic, which is seen as transient elevations of serum aminotransferases and alkaline phosphatase in about 5% to 10% of patients. Fulminant hepatic damage is uncommon, 1 in 12,000, though a few patients develop jaundice, fever, liver failure, and even death. Thus ketoconazole use must be considered in terms of the seriousness of the infection against the risk of liver damage.

Ketoconazole can cause transient gynecomastia and breast tenderness by blocking testosterone synthesis. High doses can lead to azospermia and impotence and may block cortisol secretion and suppress adrenal response to adrenocorticotrophic hormone.

A principal drug-drug interaction with ketoconazole involves interference with the metabolism of cyclosporin, which can lead to nephrotoxicity. In contrast, warfarin metabolism is not changed.

IV infusion of miconazole produces nausea and vomiting in 25% of patients. It may also cause chills, malaise, tremors, confusion, dizziness, or seizures.

Fluconazole absorption is decreased 15% to 20% by cimetidine, and warfarin-adjusted prothrombin times are altered by fluconazole.

Griseofulvin

Many patients receiving griseofulvin initially complain of headaches, but the symptom may disappear as therapy continues. Other CNS side effects include lethargy, confusion, memory lapses, and impaired judgment in routine tasks. Nausea, vomiting, bad taste in the mouth, occasionally leukopenia or neutropenia, hepatotoxicity, skin rashes, and photosensitivity also may occur. Although renal function is not decreased, albuminuria has developed. Griseofulvin administered in very large doses is teratogenic and carcinogenic in animals, but no reports of such effects in humans are available; however, griseofulvin should not be given to pregnant women.

Griseofulvin may interact and increase the metabolism of warfarin by induction of microsomal enzymes.

TRADE NAMES

In addition to generic and fixed-combination preparations, the following trade-named materials are available in the United States.

Ancobon, flucytosine
Diflucan, fluconazole
Fulvicin, Grifulvin, Grisactin, Gris-PEG, griseofulvin
Fungizone, amphotericin B
Lotrimin, Mycelex, clotrimazole
Monistat, miconazole
Mycostatin, Nystex, Nilstat, nystatin
Nizoral, ketoconazole
Spectazole, econazole nitrate
Sporanox; itraconazole

REFERENCES

Barnett JF, Klaubert DH: Recent advances in antifungal agents, *Ann Rep Med Chem* 27:149, 1992.

Bennett JE, ed: Fluconazole: a novel advance in therapy for systemic fungal infections, *Rev Infect Dis* 12(suppl 3):5263, 1990.

Cauwenbergh G et al: Itraconazole in the treatment of human mycoses: review of three years clinical experience, *Rev Infect Dis* 9(suppl 1):146-152, 1987.

Fromtling RA: Imidazoles as important antifungal agents: an overview, *Drugs Today* 20:325, 1984.

Grant SM, Cissold SP: Fluconazole: a review of its pharmacodynamic and pharmacokinetic properties and therapeutic potential in superficial and systemic mycoses, *Drugs* 39:877-916, 1990.

Heel RC, Bragden NR, Carmine A, et al: Ketoconazole: a review of its therapeutic efficacy in superficial and systemic fungal infections, *Drugs* 23:1, 1982.

Lyman CA, Walsh TJ: Systemically administered antifungal agents, *Drugs* 44:9-35, 1992.

SELF-ASSESSMENT QUESTIONS

1. The absorption of which of the following is greatly decreased in the absence of gastric acidity?
   a. flucytosine
   b. fluconazole
   c. nystatin
   d. ketoconazole
2. Which of the following enters the CSF in adequate concentrations to treat cryptococcal meningitis in HIV-infected patients?
   a. miconazole
   b. ketoconazole
   c. fluconazole
   d. clotrimazole
3. Amphotericin B produces which of the following adverse effects?
   a. leukopenia
   b. decrease in glomerular filtration rate
   c. vestibular toxicity
   d. rash
4. Which agent is used to treat cryptococcal meningitis?
   a. bacitracin
   b. neomycin
   c. griseofulvin
   d. nystatin
   e. amphotericin B

5. Which of the following could be used to treat an *Aspergillus* infection of the lung?
   a. griseofulvin
   b. ketoconazole
   c. nystatin
   d. amphotericin B
6. Effective antifungal agent in the treatment of ringworm of skin and nails?
   a. bacitracin
   b. neomycin
   c. griseofulvin
   d. nystatin
   e. amphotericin B

CHAPTER 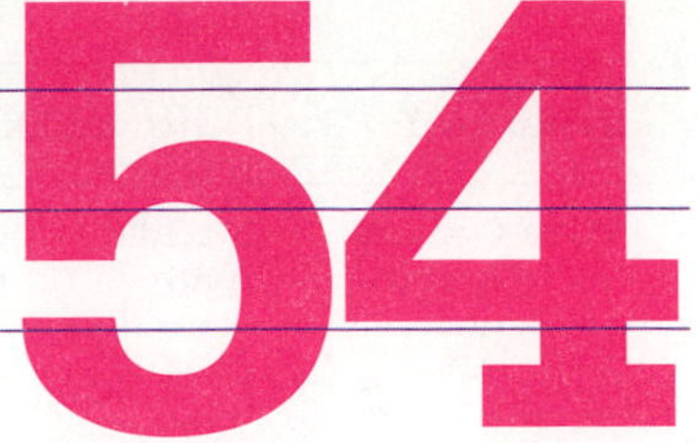

Antiviral Agents

DANIEL H. HAVLICHEK, JR.

MAJOR DRUGS

amantadine
rimantidine
vidarabine
acyclovir
ganciclovir
foscarnet
ribavirin
zidovudine
didanosine
zalcitabine
idoxuridine
trifluridine
fluorouracil
interferons
immunoglobulins

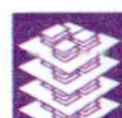 THERAPEUTIC OVERVIEW

Viruses are responsible for a large proportion of the morbidity and mortality experienced worldwide. These infectious agents consist of a core genome of nucleic acid (nucleoid) contained in a protein shell (capsid) and sometimes surrounded by a lipoprotein membrane (envelope) (Figure 54-1). Viruses cannot replicate independently. They must enter cells and use cellular energy-generating, DNA- or RNA-replicating, and protein-synthesizing pathways of the host to achieve viral replication. Some viruses can integrate a copy of their genetic material into host chromosomes, achieving *viral* latency, a condition in which clinical illness can recur without reexposure to the virus.

ABBREVIATIONS

AIDS	acquired immunodeficiency syndrome
CD	cluster of differentiation
CMV	cytomegalovirus
CSF	cerebrospinal fluid
HIV	huma-n immunodeficiency virus

Some genera of viruses known to cause human infections are listed in Table 54-1. Also listed is information about which genomic material—RNA or DNA—is present and examples of clinically important diseases attributed to each virus.

Viral biochemistry is not as well understood as bacterial biochemistry, and so antiviral drug development has been relatively slow. The way antiviral agents act is not always known. Most currently available antiviral drugs interfere with viral nucleic acid synthesis or regulation; however, some agents work by interfering with virus-cell binding, interrupting virus uncoating, or stimulating the host immune system. Because viruses generally take over host-cell nucleic acid/protein replication pathways before clinical infection is discovered, most antiviral drugs must penetrate cells already infected to produce a therapeutic antiviral response. This requirement is often the source of significant toxicity to healthy cells, thus limiting a drug's usefulness.

In vitro susceptibility testing of antiviral compounds differs significantly from that for antibacterial agents. Because viruses require cells to replicate, susceptibility systems use cell cultures. In general, a greater than 50% reduction in cell plaque formation at an achievable serum concentration classifies an agent as active against a given virus. Many antiviral compounds have in vitro activity against many different viruses but are not effective clinically. Drug distribution, timing of infection, and problems with administration can limit the usefulness of many agents. Several agents become converted in the body to active compounds (acyclovir, ganciclovir) or must be present continuously to have an antiviral effect (amantadine). The various in vitro virus sus-

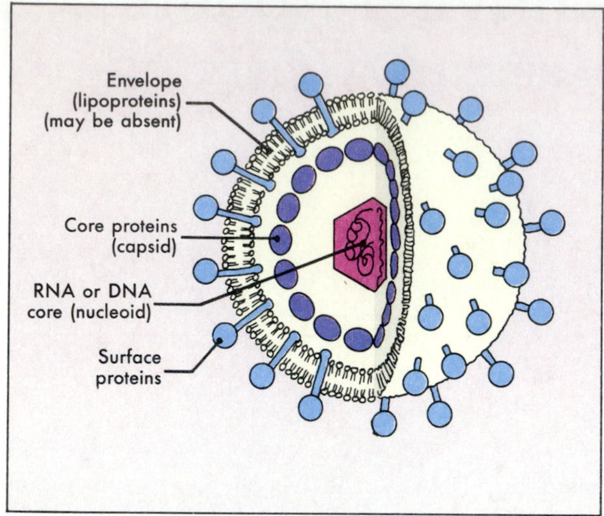

FIGURE 54-1 Basic components of virus particles. See the text for further information.

Table 54-1 Virus Groups Of Clinical Importance

Virus Genera or Groupings	Nucleic Acid	Clinical Examples of Illnesses
Adenovirus	DNA	Upper respiratory and eye infections
Hepadnaviridae	DNA	Hepatitis B, cancer (?)
Herpesvirus	DNA	Genital herpes, varicella, meningoencephalitis, mononucleosis, retinitis
Papillomavirus	DNA	Papillomas (warts), cancer (?)
Parvovirus	DNA	Erythema infectiosum
Arenavirus	RNA	Lymphocytic choriomeningitis
Bunyavirus	RNA	Encephalitis
Coronavirus	RNA	Upper respiratory infections
Influenzavirus	RNA	Influenza
Paramyxovirus	RNA	Measles, upper respiratory infections
Picornavirus	RNA	Poliomyelitis, diarrhea, upper respiratory infections
Retrovirus	RNA	Leukemia, acquired immune deficiency syndrome (AIDS)
Rhabdovirus	RNA	Rabies
Togavirus	RNA	Rubella, yellow fever

ceptibility assays cannot accurately reproduce all in vivo situations.

Many antiviral agents inhibit single steps in the viral replication cycle. They are considered virustatic and do not destroy a given virus but temporarily halt replication. Optimal antiviral effectiveness requires a competent host immune system that can eliminate or effectively halt virus replication. Patients with immunosuppressive conditions, such as leukemia, lymphoma, transplantation, and acquired immunodeficiency syndrome (AIDS), are prone to frequent and often severe viral infections that may recur when antiviral drugs are stopped. Prolonged, suppressive therapy is often necessary. Currently, no antiviral agent eliminates viral latency. Resistant strains of viruses to specific drugs can also develop.

Approaches for treatment of viral infections with drugs are summarized in the box at right.

THERAPEUTIC OVERVIEW TO APPROACHES TO TREATMENT OF VIRAL INFECTIONS

Block virus attachment to cells
Block uncoating of virus
Inhibit viral protein synthesis
Inhibit specific virus enzymes
Inhibit virus assembly
Inhibit virus release
Stimulate host immune system

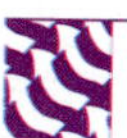

MECHANISMS OF ACTION

Viral Replication Cycle

Virions must first come into contact with an appropriate cell to initiate an infection. After contact is established, a virus penetrates the cell (Figure 54-2; step 1), disassembles (step 2), and initiates synthesis of virus components by controlling host protein and nucleic acid synthesis (step 3). Final assembly of virions (steps 4 and 5), which can then be released to enter other cells and repeat the replication cycle (step 6), occurs.

Antiviral agents that interfere with several of the steps in the virus reproductive cycle have been developed. Most are nucleic acid analogs that interfere with virus DNA/RNA production and therefore inhibit virus replication. Combination antiviral therapy with multiple agents has shown considerable promise in human immunodeficiency virus (HIV)–infected patients but not in other conditions.

Many viruses contain unique enzymes or metabolic pathways that make them more susceptible to certain agents. Herpes simplex virus encodes a thymidine kinase that monophosphorylates acyclovir significantly better than does the host cell enzyme. Since acyclovir

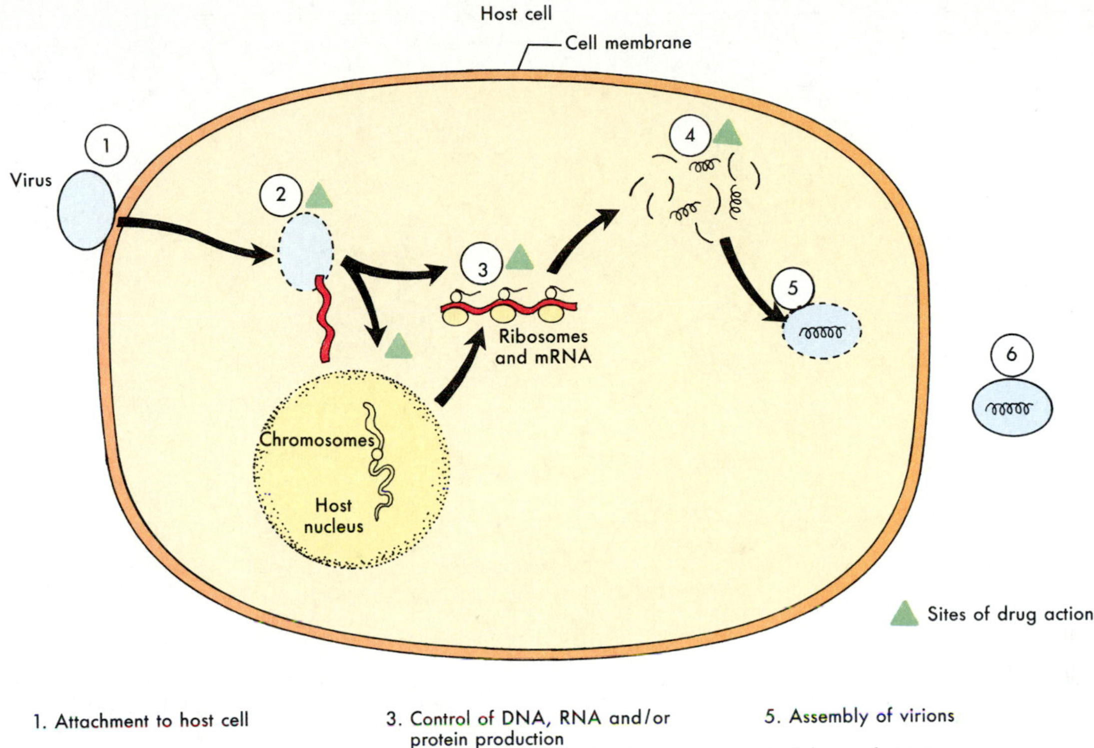

FIGURE 54-2 Schema of virus replication. Some viruses integrate into host chromosome with development of latency (see text).

monophosphate is trapped in cells, it becomes highly concentrated there, leading to greater inhibition of virus growth and few side effects on uninfected cells. Other herpes viruses (such as varicella-zoster) are less susceptible to acyclovir. Since cytomegalovirus does not encode thymidine kinase, it is inhibited only by concentrations of acyclovir not clinically tolerated. Similarly, all retroviruses use reverse transcriptase to transcribe RNA to DNA early in their replication cycle. Inhibitors of this enzyme have been developed and are useful in treatment of HIV infections.

Specific Drugs

Amantadine and Rimantidine The mechanism of action of amantadine, a symmetrical tricyclic amine (Figure 54-3), is not fully established. It does not affect influenza A virus binding, absorption or penetration, or viral RNA transcriptase. Amantadine is concentrated in lysosomes, causing increased lysosomal pH and interfering with membrane fusion. It appears to inhibit late-stage uncoating of influenza A virions. It is not effective against influenza B, which lacks the protein (M_2) to which amantadine binds in influenza A. A single amino acid change in the M_2 protein results in amantadine resistance. Resistant virus is virulent and causes disease in exposed individuals. Rimantadine is a related compound with similar antiviral action but different pharmacokinetics. Resistance develops as with amantadine.

Vidarabine Vidarabine (adenine arabinoside, also called Ara-A) is an adenosine derivative that is converted by cellular enzymes to the triphosphate that inhibits human and viral DNA polymerases resulting in decreased viral DNA synthesis (Figure 54-3). It is rapidly metabolized to produce arabinosyl hypoxanthine, which has decreased antiviral activity.

Vidarabine triphosphate formed in the cell can also act as a DNA chain terminator. Since herpes simplex DNA polymerases are approximately 20 times more susceptible to this agent than host polymerases, viral selectivity is enhanced. Vidarabine triphosphate also inhibits other enzyme systems, for example, RNA polyadenylation and red blood cell transmethylation. Changes in viral DNA polymerases can result in vidarabine resistance, but this is not a common clinical problem. Use of this agent has been significantly supplanted by acyclovir.

Acyclovir (acycloguanosine) (Figure 54-3) Acyclovir is a synthetic guanosine analog that requires phosphorylation to become active. It undergoes monophospho-

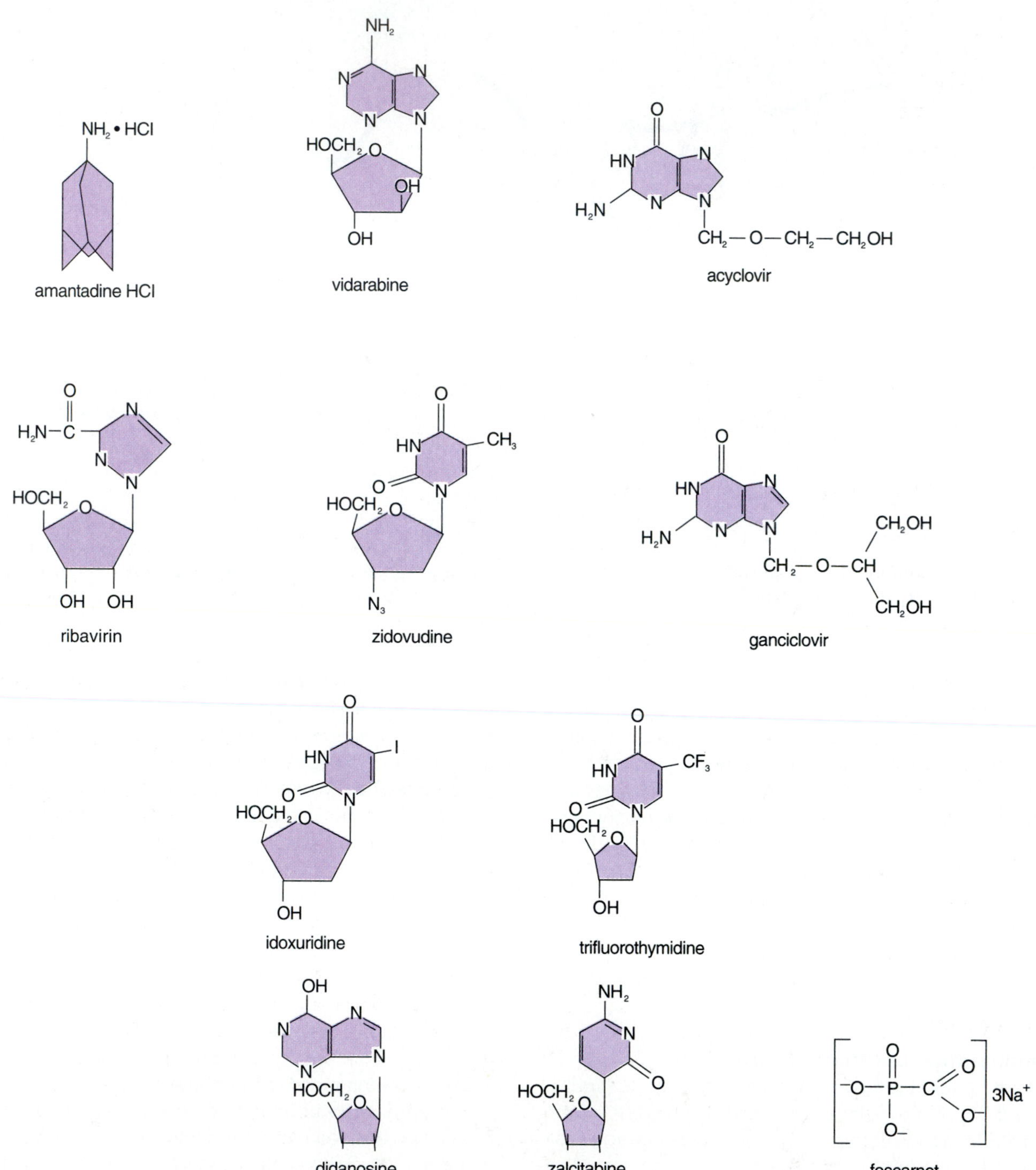

FIGURE 54-3 Chemical structures of some antiviral drugs. See the text for further information.

rylation by viral thymidine kinase. Because herpes simplex types 1 and 2 viral thymidine kinases are many times more sensitive to acyclovir than host thymidine kinase, high concentrations of acyclovir monophosphate accumulate in infected cells. Acyclovir monophosphate is then further phosphorylated to the active compound acyclovir triphosphate. The triphosphate cannot cross cell membranes and accumulates further. This increased concentration of acyclovir triphosphate is 50 to 100 times greater in infected cells than in uninfected cells.

Acyclovir triphosphate inhibits virus growth in three ways. First, it can function as a competitive inhibitor of DNA polymerases, with human DNA polymerases being significantly less susceptible to acyclovir triphosphate than viral DNA polymerases. Second, it can be a DNA chain terminator. Third, it can produce irreversible binding between viral DNA polymerase and the interrupted chain causing permanent inactivation.

The result is a several hundredfold inhibition of herpes simplex virus growth with minimal toxicity to uninfected cells. Altered thymidine kinase (acyclovir-resistant) herpes simplex viruses have developed. They occur primarily in patients receiving multiple courses of therapy or in AIDS patients. The thymidine kinase mutants are susceptible to vidarabine and foscarnet. Changes in viral DNA polymerase structures can also mediate resistance to acyclovir.

Ganciclovir The structure of ganciclovir (dihydroxypropoxymethylguanine is shown in Figure 54-3. It is a synthetic guanosine analog active against many herpes viruses, and, similar to acyclovir, it must be phosphorylated to become active. Infection-induced kinases, viral thymidine kinase, or deoxyguanosine kinase of various herpes viruses can catalyze this reaction. After monophosphorylation, cellular enzymes convert ganciclovir to the triphosphorylated form, and the triphosphate inhibits viral DNA polymerase rather than cellular DNA polymerase. Ganciclovir triphosphate competitively inhibits the incorporation of guanosine triphosphate into DNA. Because of its toxicity and the availability of acyclovir for treatment of many herpes virus infections, its use is currently restricted to treatment of cytomegalovirus (CMV) retinitis.

Foscarnet Foscarnet (phosphonoformic acid) inhibits DNA polymerases, RNA polymerases, and reverse transcriptases (Figure 54-3). In vitro it is active against herpes viruses, influenza virus, and HIV. Foscarnet is used primarily in the treatment of AIDS patients with (CMV) retinitis and acts by blocking the pyrophosphate receptor site of CMV DNA polymerase. Viral resistance is attributable to structural alterations in this enzyme. Foscarnet inhibits herpes viruses and CMV resistant to acyclovir and ganciclovir.

Ribavirin Ribavirin is a synthetic purine nucleoside analog active in vitro against many viruses, including some causing viral pneumonia, Lassa fever, and influenza (Figure 54-3). Ribavirin appears to undergo phosphorylation in host cells by host adenosine kinase. The 5′-monophosphate subsequently inhibits cellular inosine monophosphate formation, resulting in depletion of intracellular guanosine triphosphate. In some viruses, ribavirin triphosphate suppresses guanosine triphosphate–dependent capping of messenger RNA, thereby inhibiting viral protein synthesis. It also acts by suppressing viral messenger RNA initiation or elongation. Exogenous guanosine can reverse the antiviral effects of ribavirin in some viruses. Resistance to ribavirin has not been found.

Zidovudine Zidovudine (azidodeoxythymidine [AZT]) is a thymidine nucleoside analog with activity against HIV. Zidovudine becomes phosphorylated to monophosphate, diphosphate, and triphosphate forms by cellular kinases in infected and uninfected cells. It has two primary methods of action: The triphosphate acts as a competitive inhibitor of viral reverse transcriptase, and the azido group (N_3) prevents further chain elongation and acts as a DNA chain terminator. Zidovudine inhibits HIV reverse transcriptase at much lower concentrations than those needed to inhibit cellular DNA polymerases. Zidovudine is currently indicated as treatment for some stages of HIV infection.

Didanosine Didanosine (dideoxyinosine) is an adenosine derivative with activity against HIV (Figure 54-3). The exact mechanism of action of didanosine is unclear; however, after administration it must be aminated to dideoxyadenosine and phosphorylated to the triphosphate derivative ddATP. The ddATP subsequently inhibits the reverse transcriptase of HIV and can function as a DNA chain terminator. Since didanosine has little affinity for human α DNA polymerase, cellular DNA synthesis is not significantly affected. Didanosine is active against most zidovudine-resistant HIV strains. HIV resistance to didanosine occurs and is associated with changes in reverse transcriptase.

Zalcitabine Zalcitabine (dideoxycytidine) is an analog of deoxycytidine (Figure 54-3). Zalcitabine becomes triphosphorylated by cellular kinases and serves as a competitive inhibitor of HIV reverse transcriptase and as a DNA chain terminator. Resistance to zalcitabine by HIV has been reported through changes in reverse transcriptase. In combination with zidovudine, zalcitabine has shown additive or synergistic effects against HIV. It can inhibit zidovudine-resistant HIV isolates.

Idoxuridine Idoxuridine (5-iodo-2-deoxyuridine) is an iodinated thymidine nucleoside analog that is incorporated into DNA in place of thymidine and blocks further DNA chain elongation (Figure 54-3). In vitro, it inhibits many DNA viruses, and exogenous thymidine eliminates its antiviral effect. Idoxuridine affects mammalian cells, and its teratogenic, mutagenic, and immunosuppressive effects limit its use to topical preparations only, with special use in herpes simplex infections of the cornea. Herpes viruses resistant to idoxuridine occur clinically and generally have decreased thymidine kinase activity.

Trifluridine Trifluridine, or trifluorothymidine, is a pyrimidine analog that inhibits viral DNA synthesis by incorporation into viral DNA. It does not require thymidine kinase for activity and is active against thymidine kinase–deficient mutants of herpes simplex virus that are resistant to acyclovir or idoxuridine, or both. It is limited to topical use.

Fluorouracil The chemical structure of fluorouracil is shown in Chapter 44. As a fluorinated pyrimidine nucleoside analog, it blocks production of thymidylate and interrupts normal cellular DNA and RNA synthesis. Its primary action may be to cause cellular thymine deficiency and resultant cell death. The effect of fluorouracil is most pronounced on rapidly growing cells, and its use as an antiviral agent is primarily related to destruction of infected cells (warts) by topical application.

Interferons Interferons are naturally occurring glycoproteins produced by lymphocytes, macrophages, fibroblasts, and other human cells. There are three immunologically and chemically distinct classes: α, β, and γ. They act as antiviral agents by inhibiting viral protein synthesis or assembly or by stimulating the immune system. Interferons bind specific cell receptors, producing rapid changes in cellular RNA. These effects may result in inhibition of viral penetration, uncoating, synthesis or methylation of mRNA, translation of viral proteins, or assembly and release of virus. There is usually production of a 2′,5′-oligoadenylate synthetase and a protein kinase that inhibit protein synthesis in the presence of double-stranded RNA. Interferons can also protect uninfected cells from infection by mechanisms that are as yet unclear. Interferons are used for treatment of hepatitis and papillomaviruses (see also Chapter 43).

Immunoglobulins Immunoglobulins are used as antiviral agents primarily to prevent infections. Some immunoglobulin preparations have high titers against specific viruses (hepatitis B, rabies, etc.) and may be used for treatment or prophylaxis. To prevent hepatitis A infection, standard human immune globulin is used.

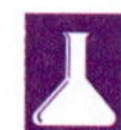

PHARMACOKINETICS

For most antiviral agents to be active they must become concentrated within cells. Many compounds are nucleoside analogs and are rapidly metabolized to inactive compounds, which are then eliminated from the body. This necessitates frequent dosing to maintain adequate drug concentrations. Some agents can be used only topically to treat certain viral infections because of severe systemic toxicity.

Because these compounds often interfere with human DNA or RNA synthesis, the use of any antiviral

Table 54-2 Pharmacokinetic Parameters

Drug	Routes of Administration	Peak Serum Concentrations (μg/ml)	$t_{1/2}$(hr)	Disposition
amantadine	Oral	0.3-0.7	12-18 (doubles in elderly)	R (90%), M (9%)
rimantidine	Oral	0.2-0.3	24-36	R (10%), M (90%)
vidarabine	IV, topical	0.3-0.6	minutes	M* (90%), R
arabinosyl hypoxanthine	(See vidarabine)	3-5	3.5	R (main)
acyclovir	Topical, oral, IV	0.6-10.0	3-4	R (80%), M (20%)
ganciclovir	IV, oral	4-6	3-4	R (90%)
foscarnet	IV	30	3	R (80%)
ribavirin	Aerosol, oral	0.8-3.5	9 (36 h final phase)	M (60%), R (30%)
zidovudine	Oral, IV (in trials)	0.05-1.5	0.8-2	M (75%), R (15%)
didanosine	Oral	1.5	0.5	R (50%), M (50%)
zalcitabine	Oral	0.01	2	R (70%)
idoxuridine	Topical	—	—	M
trifluorothymidine	Topical	—	—	—
fluorouracil	Topical	—	—	—

M, Metabolized; *R*, renal excretion as unchanged drug.
*Active metabolite.

agent in pregnancy should be done with the utmost caution and only when the potential benefits of treatment clearly outweigh the potential risks. The pharmacokinetic parameter values for the antiviral drugs are listed in Table 54-2.

Amantadine and Rimantidine

Amantadine is completely but slowly absorbed from the gastrointestinal tract, is 65% protein bound, and is distributed well throughout the body. The volume of distribution of amantadine is between 4 and 10 L/kg. Cerebrospinal fluid (CSF) and brain concentrations are approximately 50% of concurrent serum values, and concentrations in nasal mucus equal those in serum. Amantadine is excreted in breast milk.

Serum drug concentrations vary widely with the age of the patient. Peak drug concentrations occur 2 to 4 hours after ingestion. Plasma half-life for healthy, middle-aged adults is between 12 and 18 hours. In the elderly the half-life doubles, requiring dosage reduction in these patients.

Amantadine is eliminated by kidney glomerular filtration and tubular secretion, with over 90% excreted unchanged in the urine and approximately 1% excreted unchanged in stool. Amantadine is metabolized to at least eight different compounds, with *N*-acetylamantadine as the predominant metabolite. The biological activity of these metabolites is unknown.

Rimantidine is well absorbed (>90%) with peak serum concentrations between 0.2 and 0.4 μg/ml. Multiple metabolites of rimantidine are formed, and only about 10% of the drug is eliminated in the urine unchanged.

Vidarabine

Vidarabine is available for IV and topical application. After infusion, it is deaminated within minutes to the less active arabinosyl hypoxanthine. During infusion, vidarabine is detectable but not at concentrations expected to have significant antiviral activity. Arabinosyl hypoxanthine possesses only about 2.5% of the antiviral activity of vidarabine; however, the two compounds can act synergistically to produce antiviral effects. The metabolite is distributed throughout the body, and its CSF concentrations are approximately 35% of serum values in adults and 90% in children. Vidarabine is 20% to 30% protein bound.

Serum concentrations of arabinosyl hypoxanthine during continuous infusion are between 3 and 6 μg/ml, and its serum half-life is about 3.5 hours. Arabinosyl hypoxanthine has been detected in red blood cells up to 3 weeks after vidarabine administration.

Approximately 50% of the total administered drug is excreted in the urine as arabinosyl hypoxanthine and 1% to 3% as vidarabine. About 50% of arabinosyl hypoxanthine is cleared with a 6-hour course of hemodialysis. A dose should be administered after dialysis. Dosage reduction of approximately 25% is recommended for persons with renal insufficiency.

Acyclovir

Acyclovir can be used topically, orally, or IV. Oral acyclovir is only 15% to 30% bioavailable, and food does not affect absorption. For unknown reasons, bioavailability is lower in transplant patients. Acyclovir is minimally protein bound (10% to 30%), and drug interactions through binding displacement have not been reported. The drug is well distributed, with CSF and brain concentrations equaling approximately 50% of serum values. Concentrations of acyclovir in zoster vesicle fluid are equivalent to those in plasma. Aqueous humor concentrations are 35% and salivary concentrations 15% that of plasma; vaginal concentrations are equivalent to those of plasma. Breast milk concentrations exceed those of plasma. The percutaneous absorption of topical acyclovir is low and occurs primarily when large areas are treated. Plasma concentrations of about 0.3 μg/ml have been reported in patients treated topically with this drug for herpes zoster. Peak serum concentrations after oral ingestion of acyclovir average 0.6 μg/ml and occur 90 minutes after dosing, but peak serum concentrations after IV administration reach approximately 10 μg/ml.

The plasma half-life for normal adults and neonates is 3.3 and 3.8 hours respectively. In anuric patients, it increases to 20 hours. In the urine, 60% to 90% of acyclovir is excreted unchanged, by both glomerular filtration and tubular secretion. As a result, acyclovir may interfere with the renal excretion of drugs, such as methotrexate, that are eliminated through the renal tubules; probenecid significantly decreases the renal excretion of acyclovir. A major metabolite of acyclovir, 9-carboxymethoxymethylguanine, accounts for 10% to 20% of the total administered dose and is also excreted in urine. Acyclovir is effectively removed by hemodialysis (60%) but only minimally by peritoneal dialysis.

Ganciclovir

Ganciclovir is used primarily IV, since less than 5% of an oral dose is absorbed. CSF concentrations are approximately 50% of plasma with peak plasma concentrations reaching 4 to 6 μg/ml. The plasma half-life is 3 to 4 hours in persons with normal renal function, increasing to over 24 hours in patients with severe renal insufficiency. Over 90% of systemic ganciclovir is eliminated unchanged in urine, and dose modifications are necessary for persons with compromised renal function. Ganciclovir is approximately 50% removed by hemodialysis. It can be administered intravitreally with a half-life of 50 hours.

Foscarnet

Foscarnet bioavailability is approximately 20%, and foscarnet is used only IV at this time. Because foscarnet can bind with calcium and other divalent cations, it becomes deposited in bone and may be detectable for many months. Foscarnet distribution follows a three-compartment model and produces peak serum concentrations of approximately 30 μg/ml. It is eliminated by both glomerlular filtration and tubular secretion with 80% to 90% of an administered dose appearing unchanged in the urine. Dosage adjustment is required in persons with impaired renal function.

Ribavirin

Ribavirin bioavailability is about 45%, and peak concentrations after IV administration are tenfold greater than that after oral administration. It accumulates with prolonged oral use. After drug distribution the half-life is 2 hours, with a subsequent delayed half-life of 36 hours. Ribavirin is administered by aerosol in the treatment of severe respiratory syncytial virus infections. Some ribavirin is absorbed during aerosol treatments, and after 20 hours of aerosol therapy, plasma concentrations in treated infants range from 0.8 to 3.3 μg/ml. Ribavirin concentrations in respiratory secretions are approximately a thousandfold greater.

About 3% of ribavirin accumulates in red blood cells as ribavirin triphosphate to give a prolonged serum half-life of 40 days, during which the compound is slowly lost from the red cells. Concentrations in spinal fluid are about 60% those of plasma. Hepatic metabolism is the main route of elimination for ribavirin, with 30% of the drug eliminated in urine.

Zidovudine

Zidovudine is administered orally and is about 60% bioavailable with 40% metabolized by first pass. Peak concentrations occur within 30 to 90 minutes to give steady-state peak concentrations of 0.05 to 1.5 μg/ml. Zidovudine is about 40% protein bound. CSF concentrations vary widely and range from 25% to 100% of serum values. It enters brain, phagocytic cells, liver, muscle, and placenta. Plasma half-life is about 1 hour.

Zidovudine is inactivated mainly by glucuronidation (about 75% of a dose) and the 5′-glucuronide has a half-life of 1 hour. Renal elimination of unchanged drug by glomerular filtration and tubular secretion accounts for another 15% of drug elimination. Drugs that can interfere with hepatic glucuronidation (such as acetaminophen) or renal tubular transport (such as probenecid) can inhibit elimination of zidovudine and should be avoided.

Didanosine

Didanosine is extremely acid labile and is formulated with appropriate buffer to neutralize stomach acid and maximize oral absorption. Bioavailability of didanosine is approximately 40%. After administration, didanosine is taken up intracellularly and aminated by adenosine deaminase to the active compound dideoxyadenosine. The active compound then becomes concentrated intracellularly with an intracellular half-life of several hours as compared with a serum half-life of 1 1/2 hours. Peak didanosine serum concentrations are about 1.5 μg/ml. It is eliminated from the body by glomerular filtration and tubular secretion, with about 50% of an administered dose recovered unchanged in the urine.

Zalcitabine

Zalcitabine is well absorbed with average bioavailability of greater than 80%, however, drug absorption is decreased with food. Peak serum concentrations are approximately 0.01 μg/ml, and CSF penetration of zalcitabine is approximately 20%. Zalcitabine appears to be eliminated from the body primarily by renal excretion, with 70% of a dose being recovered in the urine within 24 hours. The mean elimination half-life is 2 hours. Individuals with impaired renal function have delayed elimination of zalcitabine, and dosage modification is indicated.

Idoxuridine

Idoxuridine is used only topically and systemic absorption is minimal. The small amount that is absorbed undergoes metabolism to uracil and iodouracil. In vitro resistance to idoxuridine develops easily, and resistant clinical isolates have been described, that may be a cause for treatment failure.

Trifluridine and Fluorouracil

Trifluridine is available for topical use only, especially as an ophthalmic preparation. Drug absorption is minimal, and no trifluridine has been detected in serum or aqueous humor from treated patients. Fluorouracil is also available as a topical preparation.

Interferons

Because interferons are glycoproteins, their pharmacokinetics are difficult to assess. Oral administration does not yield detectable concentrations. They are administered IM or SC. Simple detection of circulating compounds may not indicate clinical activity, since cellular binding is necessary to effect a response and biological activity may last many days despite their clearance from serum.

Interferons are effective when injected directly into condylomas or given SC or IM. Serum concentrations peak in 4 to 8 hours and decline steadily over 1 to 2 days. Biological activity of interferons begins within an hour of injection, peaks at 24 hours, and wanes over 4 to 6 days. Interferons are distributed throughout the body and are detectable in brain and CSF. Elimination of exogenous interferon is complex. Liver, lung, kidney, heart, and skeletal muscle are capable of inactivating the compounds. Negligible amounts are found in urine.

Immunoglobulins

As antiviral therapies, immunoglobulins are given SC, IM, and IV. Immunoglobulins are distributed throughout the body with only about 50% of IgG being intravascular. After IM injection, immunoglobulin serum concentrations peak in 4 to 6 days and then decline, with half-lives of 20 to 30 days. For persons with continued exposure to infectious agents such as hepatitis A, repeat immunization is often recommended every 3 to 6 months. After exposure to rabies, infiltration of the wound with high-titer immunoglobulin to neutralize virus is recommended, with administration of the remaining immunoglobulin IM. IV gamma globulin is administered every 3 to 4 weeks to agammaglobulinemic patients. It is also given to transplant patients receiving a cytomegalovirus-positive kidney or heart if the recipient is CMV antibody negative. Clearance of immune globulins is variable, with a mean half-life of 20 days.

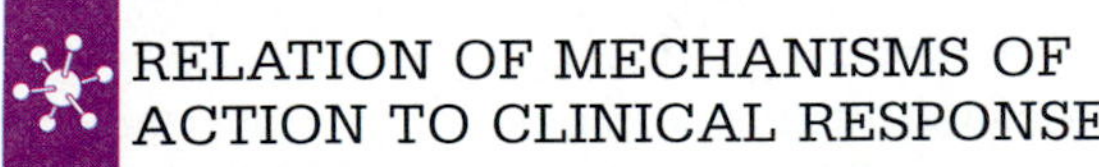

RELATION OF MECHANISMS OF ACTION TO CLINICAL RESPONSE

Human Immunodeficiency Virus and Acquired Immunodeficiency Syndrome

A retrovirus isolated in the United States and France in the early 1980s was subsequently identified and named the human immunodeficiency virus (HIV). Acute infection by HIV often leads to a typical viral illness, characterized by fever, myalgias, pharyngitis, rash, or headache, or all these signs. It generally lasts 10 to 20 days and resolves without treatment as HIV antibody develops. Some individuals acquire HIV antibody without this illness. All HIV-antibody-positive patients are considered infectious for life. The time before HIV seroconversion appears to be 6 months or less, in most instances.

After infection, most individuals experience a progressive decline in the number and function of infected cells (T-helper lymphocytes and macrophages both of which posses the CD4 receptor) leading to progressive immunodeficiency. Other cells, including those in the brain, may also be infected. Patients are therefore susceptible to opportunistic and nonopportunistic infections and tumors. When the immune system has been so severely damaged by HIV that it can no longer counteract opportunistic infections or tumors, or the person's absolute CD4 count falls below 200 cells/mm^3, the diagnosis of AIDS is established. Other AIDS-defining conditions are the wasting syndrome, dementia, recurrent pneumonia, tuberculosis, and invasive cervical cancer.

In general, patients remain relatively asymptomatic until their T-helper cell counts fall well below the normal range. This usually takes many years, and approximately 50% of antibody-positive persons will progress to AIDS in 8 years without treatment.

As patients become more severely ill, they may require suppressive or prophylactic therapy with additional antiviral, antifungal, and antiprotozoal agents. Aerosolized pentamidine, trimethoprim-sulfamethoxazole, or trimethoprim-dapsone are often used to prevent *Pneumocystis* pneumonia. Drugs used to treat HIV are considered among those below.

Specific Drugs Used to Treat Viruses

Because antiviral drugs primarily inhibit viruses after infection has occurred, they are most effective when given early in the course of the infection. Many agents are limited in their use by toxicity on noninfected cells. These compounds are primarily used as topical agents.

Some drugs (e.g., immunoglobulins and interferons) can eliminate the infecting virus from the body, but these substances are significantly less effective in immunosuppressed patients.

Amantadine and Rimantidine Amantadine is used for the treatment and prophylaxis of influenza A infections but is ineffective against influenza B. It is most effective clinically when given before exposure or within 48 hours of development of symptoms. Clinical effectiveness has been estimated at 50% protection against infection and 60% to 70% protection against illness. It also reduces fever and palliates symptoms of influenza. Amantadine does not inhibit antibody responses to influenza, and immunity develops during amantadine therapy in persons either immunized or infected. The protective effect of amantadine is lost approximately 48 hours after treatment is stopped. Groups targeted for amantadine therapy include unvaccinated persons with underlying cardiopulmonary, renal, metabolic, neuromuscular, or immunodeficiency diseases who are at increased risk for serious morbidity and mortality from influenza. Vaccination must be given, since resistant mutants may develop during therapy.

Rimantidine, the α-methyl derivative of amantidine, is approved for prevention or treatment of influenza A. Its mechanism of action is similar to amantidine. The major advantage of rimantidine is its low risk of central nervous system effects.

Vidarabine Vidarabine was used primarily in the treatment of herpes simplex encephalitis, disseminated or CNS herpes infections in the newborn, herpes keratitis (topically), and herpes zoster in immunocompromised patients. It has generally been replaced by acyclovir.

In adults with herpes encephalitis, vidarabine treatment improved survival from 30% to 70% and decreased long-term neurologic sequelae when compared with no treatment; however, only about 50% of surviving treated patients were neurologically normal 1 year after treatment. For the treatment of herpes encephalitis, vidarabine is inferior to acyclovir both in terms of survival and residual neurological sequelae.

Acyclovir Acyclovir can be used topically, orally, or IV. When used to treat herpes simplex encephalitis and most other significant herpes infections, it is more efficacious and less toxic than vidarabine.

For herpes encephalitis, acyclovir further decreases mortality to approximately 20% as compared to 50% with vidarabine. Also, about 50% of acyclovir-treated patients return to normal life as compared to about 20% with vidarabine treatment. Acyclovir should be administered as soon as possible after a diagnosis of encephalitis is made to lessen morbidity and mortality.

Systemic acyclovir is effective in reducing viral shedding, decreasing local symptoms and decreasing severity and duration of illness when treating established mucocutaneous herpes simplex infections in immunosuppressed patients. Recurrences after termination of therapy are common. Oral acyclovir is often effective in suppressing recurrences of mucocutaneous herpes simplex infections in the immunosuppressed and is often given after systemic immune suppressive therapy.

In healthy patients with recurrent oral herpes infections, oral therapy has not proved significantly beneficial and is not generally recommended. For persons with recurrent disease who are at high risk (e.g., from sun exposure), orally administered acyclovir for 1 week can decrease recurrences by approximately 75%.

Topically administered acyclovir has little advantage over a placebo when primary genital herpes simplex infections are treated. Intravenous or oral acyclovir is generally used to treat this infection. Both treatments decrease viral shedding, local and systemic symptoms, and time to resolution. Neither form of therapy decreases the rate or severity of recurrences.

Recurrent genital herpes is generally managed with orally administered acyclovir. Treatments begun within 2 days of recurrence decrease viral excretion; unfortunately, no differences in clinical symptoms are observed when compared to placebo therapy. By initiating oral acyclovir therapy at the first prodrome of clinical recurrence, improvement in clinical symptoms has been noted when compared with effects from a placebo. Patients with four to six recurrences of genital herpes infection per year are often placed on chronic suppressive therapy.

Approximately 75% of patients taking suppressive acyclovir will have no recurrences for 4 to 24 months, and total recurrences decrease by 90%. After discontinuation of acyclovir, recurrence rates generally return to pretreatment levels. Since recurrences of genital herpes tend to decrease in intensity and frequency with time, a 6- to 12-month suppressive trial with subsequent cessation of medication is generally used. If symptoms recur, another course of suppressive therapy is repeated. Herpes simplex resistance to acyclovir has been reported in persons with active lesions taking suppressive therapy. Individuals taking acyclovir are still infectious even though no lesions are visible.

Acyclovir is as effective as vidarabine in the treatment of neonatal herpes, is easier to administer, and has fewer side effects. It can also be used prophylactically with bone marrow transplant patients to prevent herpes recurrence and in renal transplant patients to decrease the incidence of cytomegalovirus infection. Therapy is most effective when begun before transplantation and continued for many weeks.

Intravenous and orally administered acyclovir at appropriate doses are capable of limiting both varicella and zoster infections in healthy and immunocompromised patients. Inhibitory concentrations of acyclovir needed for varicella zoster (3 to 7 μg/ml) are about 5 times higher than those needed for inhibition of herpes simplex virus. In zoster, acyclovir produces decreased visceral and cutaneous dissemination, shorter time to healing, and decreased duration of pain, but it needs to be given within 3 or 4 days of rash for greatest effect. Among healthy children with varicella, acyclovir decreases the total duration of illness by about 2 days.

Acyclovir is not effective in treating cytomegalovirus pneumonia or visceral disease, Epstein-Barr mononucleosis, or chronic fatigue syndrome. However, a condition in AIDS patients known as hairy leukoplakia (a proliferation of oral epithelium related to Epstein-Barr infection) is responsive to oral acyclovir.

Ganciclovir Ganciclovir is available only for IV administration and currently is approved to treat only cytomegalovirus retinitis. After 2 to 3 weeks of treatment, over 80% of AIDS patients with retinitis improve or have no further loss of vision. Clinical improvement in retinal lesions is usually observed in 10 to 14 days. After drug treatment has been completed, retinitis recurs in the majority of patients within a month if suppressive therapy is not instituted.

About 65% of AIDS patients with visceral cytomegalovirus infection have significant virological responses, but clinical improvement with ganciclovir is not as significant. Bone marrow transplant patients with cytomegalovirus pneumonia also show virological responses, but there are no differences in overall mortality with this antiviral agent.

Foscarnet Foscarnet is approved only for IV administration for treatment of cytomegalovirus retinitis. It is equally as effective as ganciclovir. In a comparative trial of foscarnet and ganciclovir in cytomegalovirus retinitis in AIDS patients, improved survival was noted in the foscarnet group with an increase in median survival times of patients of approximately 4 months. Drug-related toxicity, however, was more common with foscarnet than with ganciclovir.

Ribavirin Ribavirin is used in the United States as an aerosol for treatment of severe respiratory syncytial virus bronchopneumonia. When used for treating such infections, this drug is effective in improving oxygenation, decreasing viral shedding, and improving pneumonia symptoms. The aerosol particles must be of the proper size. Therefore, special generators are required for this treatment. Aerosol administration is given for 12 to 20 hours per day for 3 to 7 days and is most effective when started within 3 days of illness onset. Treatments may be effective in patients with underlying cardiopulmonary or immunosuppressive illnesses. Ribavirin is minimally effective for upper airway syncytial virus problems. Ribavirin orally or IV is the therapy of Lassa fever, an otherwise fatal disease. It is also useful in Korean and Argentine hemorrhagic fevers.

Zidovudine Treatment with zidovudine in asymptomatic HIV seropositive patients with less than 500 CD4 cells/mm^3 and AIDS patients produces a significant increase in absolute CD4 counts. This is associated with fewer opportunistic infections, improved physical performance, and frequently improved neurologic function.

For AIDS and AIDS-related complex patients treated with zidovudine and other therapies directed at suppression of opportunistic infections, the 2-year survival is approximately 50% and 70% respectively.

Zidovudine-resistant virus mutants have been isolated from some patients within 6 months after the initiation of therapy, but worsening of clinical status has not been uniformly noted in such patients. Resistance appears to be associated with differences in reverse transcriptase binding. When zidovudine resistance occurs, the HIV strain usually remains susceptible to didanosine and zalcitabine.

Didanosine Didanosine is approved for treatment of advanced HIV infection in individuals who are intolerant of zidovudine or are worsening while taking it. Didanosine has been shown to increase the number of circulating CD4 cells, decrease circulating HIV p24 antigen titers, and improve functional status among patients receiving it. Didanosine at 500 mg per day, but not at higher doses, was shown to be more effective than continued zidovudine in preventing opportunistic infection among HIV-seropositive patients who received zidovudine for an average of 14 months. Further studies evaluating the effectiveness of didanosine alone and in combination with zidovudine are underway.

Zalcitabine Zalcitabine is approved as a single agent or for use in combination with zidovudine. These two compounds act synergistically in vitro and when used in combination have demonstrated increased numbers of circulating CD4 cells in patients. It is approved for use in adults with progressive HIV disease who have demonstrated significant clinical or immunologic deterioration.

Idoxuridine Idoxuridine can be used to treat herpes simplex keratitis and is effective for dendritic ulcers but not for deeper stromal ulcers, which may develop. This agent is used only topically because of significant liver and bone marrow toxicity. It is not effective in genital herpes, localized zoster, or varicella.

Trifluridine Trifluridine is used topically to treat herpes simplex keratitis.

Fluorouracil Fluorouracil has been used topically to treat condylomas (warts) caused by human papillomaviruses, but this use is not well established. It acts primarily as an ablative agent, destroying infected and uninfected cells and can therefore be used only externally over relatively small areas. It also shows some success for treating intraurethral warts.

Interferons There are at least three classes of human interferons: alpha, beta, and gamma. These proteins are nonspecific immune stimulators that also have significant antiviral activity. The licensed interferons are α-2a, α-2b, and α-n3. The approved antiviral uses of interferon are in the treatment of condyloma acuminata and for the treatment of chronic hepatitis B or C. Both α-2a and α-2b-interferons are effective when injected

VIRAL INFECTIONS AMENABLE TO IMMUNOGLOBULIN TREATMENT

Cytomegalovirus	Rabies
Hepatitis A	Varicella*
Hepatitis B	Measles*

*Immunoglobulin treatment reserved for persons at high risk for complications.

directly into lesions or administered systemically. Interferons are also effective for the treatment of Kaposi's sarcoma.

Immunoglobulins Some human immunoglobulins have high titers against specific viruses such as hepatitis B and rabies and are more efficacious against these viruses than nonspecific immunoglobulin. Some viral infections amenable to immunoglobulin therapy are listed in the box. Immunoglobulins are usually given IM, as close as possible to the time of exposure to the virus. In some circumstances an immunoglobulin should also be given very close to the lesion (as in rabies) to provide high concentrations to lymphatic tissues. In most situations, IM injection provides adequate systemic immunoglobulin concentrations to prevent the development of clinical infection. Since immunoglobulins do not provide long-term immunity, they must often be given as a series of injections together with vaccine therapy.

The uses for the individual antiviral drugs are summarized in Table 54-3.

Table 54-3 Summary of Principal Uses of Antiviral Drugs

Drug	Clinical Indications
amantadine	Influenza A prophylaxis and treatment
rimantidine	Influenza A prophylaxis and treatment
vidarabine	Significant herpes simplex and herpes zoster infections
acyclovir	Herpes simplex and herpes zoster infections; suppression of recurrent herpes simplex
ganciclovir	Cytomegalovirus retinitis, possibly systemic disease
foscarnet	Cytomegalovirus retinitis
ribavirin	Severe respiratory syncytial virus pneumonia, Lassa fever
zidovudine	HIV infection, AIDS
didanosine	HIV infection, AIDS
zalcitabine	HIV infection, AIDS
idoxuridine	Herpes simplex corneal infections
trifluorothymidine	Herpes simplex corneal infections
fluorouracil	Condyloma acuminatum
interferons	Condyloma acuminatum, hepatitis B, C
immunoglobulins*	Prophylaxis against hepatitis A and B, rabies, measles, varicella

*Specific immunoglobulin preparations available for some infections.

SIDE EFFECTS, CLINICAL PROBLEMS, AND TOXICITY

Because most antiviral drugs are derivatives of nucleic acids, which must penetrate cells to be active, significant toxicities to uninfected cells often occur. Most toxicities involve bone marrow suppression with resultant loss of granulocytes, platelets, and erythrocytes. In many instances, systemic toxicities are so severe that drug administration is limited to topical use only. Several clinical problems are summarized in the box on p. 737.

Amantadine and Rimantidine

The most common side effects of amantadine therapy are gastrointestinal upsets and CNS side effects such as nervousness, insomnia, and headache. These develop within the first week of therapy and decrease with time, despite continued treatment. Side effects are reversible after discontinuation of the drug and are less if lower doses are used. Adverse events occur in 5% to 33% of persons taking amantadine for influenza prophylaxis.

Amantadine also has anticholinergic properties that can cause dry mouth, urinary retention, ventricular arrhythmias, pupillary dilatation, and psychosis with excess dosing. Therefore, amantadine should be used with caution in patients with glaucoma or urinary retention. The anticholinergic effects of amantadine are enhanced by antihistamines and anticholinergic drugs. Amantadine is embryotoxic and teratogenic in rodents at high doses. Because safety during pregnancy and breastfeeding are not established, caution should be exercised. Physostigmine given every 1 to 2 hours in adults may temporarily reverse serious neurological reactions.

Rimantidine is better tolerated than amantidine. This is likely attributable to lower serum concentrations, since, at serum concentrations comparable to those of amantidine, the rate and severity of side effects are virtually identical.

Vidarabine

Vidarabine causes mild to moderate anorexia, nausea, and vomiting in approximately 15% of patients. Bone marrow suppression, neurotoxicity with tremors, aphasia, seizures, and coma, as well as a syndrome of intense muscle cramps lasting up to several weeks af-

CLINICAL PROBLEMS	
amantidine	GI upset CNS effects (nervousness, insomnia) Anticholinergic effects
rimantidine	GI upset, CNS effects
vidaribine minor	Anorexia, nausea, vomiting Bone marrow suppression Muscle cramps, fluid balance
acyclovir	CNS effects (nervousness, headache) Decreased renal function
ganciclovir	Bone marrow suppression CNS effects Rash, fever
ribavirin	Headache, GI upset, dyspnea, teratogenic
zidovudine	Bone marrow suppression Granulocytopenia Myositis
didanosine	Pancreatitis Neuropathy
zalcitabine	Neuropathy

ter stopping vidarabine, have been reported. Theoretically, allopurinol may increase vidarabine concentrations and the subsequent toxicity resulting from blockade of vidarabine metabolism. However the clinical importance of this drug interaction is unknown. Because vidarabine is poorly soluble, large fluid volumes are administered daily and fluid and electrolytes monitored.

Topically, vidarabine can cause pain, itching, photophobia, and hypersensitivity reactions. Patients generally have fewer allergic reactions to vidarabine than to idoxuridine.

Vidarabine is teratogenic, mutagenic, and oncogenic in some animals and should not be used during pregnancy unless potential benefits outweigh potential risks.

Acyclovir

Acyclovir is well tolerated with few side effects. Because the pH of IV administered acyclovir is 9 to 11, phlebitis is the most common side effect, occurring in 15% of patients. Temporary elevations of serum creatinine concentrations and rash each occur in 5% of patients. About 1% of patients experience headache, confusion, nervousness, or other CNS side effects, and coma has been reported. Elevations of creatinine are more common with rapid infusions of less than 1 hour especially if the patient is dehydrated. Crystalline nephropathy can occur. Coadministration of probenecid reduces renal clearance of the drug and prolongs the serum half-life.

In animal experimental systems, acyclovir has not shown increased teratogenicity, but mutagenicity has been observed at extremely high doses. Its safety in pregnancy is unknown, and acyclovir should be given only when its potential benefits and risks are carefully evaluated.

Ganciclovir

Most clinical experience with ganciclovir is in the treatment of cytomegalovirus retinitis in AIDS patients in which the most common side effects are bone marrow suppression (up to 40%), CNS abnormalities (up to 15%), rash (6%), and fever (6%). Neutropenia (less than 1000 granulocytes/mm^3) and thrombocytopenia (less than 50,000 platelets/mm^3) are the most common manifestations of bone marrow suppression. These effects are most often observed in the second week of therapy but may occur after several months. Effects are usually reversible, but fatal infections during granulocytopenia can occur. Concurrent use of zidovudine increases bone marrow toxicity, with about 33% of treated patients developing CNS or bone marrow toxicities significant enough to interrupt therapy. AIDS patients who have received long-term ganciclovir therapy have significant increases in follicle-stimulating hormone, luteinizing hormone, and testosterone concentrations.

Ganciclovir is teratogenic and mutagenic in several different experimental systems.

Foscarnet

Foscarnet is a strongly anionic compound and can chelate divalent cations. This has resulted in hypocalcemia and hypomagnesemia in up to 20% of patients receiving the drug. Foscarnet also causes renal insufficiency, and dosages must be adjusted in patients with decreased creatinine clearance. Up to 30% of AIDS patients receiving foscarnet therapy for cytomegalovirus retinitis have increases in their serum creatinine, and renal function must be monitored closely. Additionally, 65% of persons receiving this medication have associated fevers. Seizures and cardiac arrythmias may occur presumably secondary to hypocalcemia. Foscarnet is less myelosuppressive than ganciclovir. In comparative trials, fewer AIDS patients were required to terminate use of zidovudine if they received foscarnet.

Ribavirin

Aerosolized ribavirin is generally well tolerated, but some bronchospasm may occur. In adults with chronic obstructive pulmonary disease and among asthmatics, significant deterioration of pulmonary function has been reported with aerosol therapy. Aerosols may also cause rash or conjunctivitis, but no significant effects on bone marrow have been reported. Ribavirin may be passively absorbed by employees working with patients treated with aerosols. The clinical importance of this is unclear, but pregnant women should not be exposed to the aerosol.

Ribavirin aerosols must be generated with a small-particle aerosol generator approved for this purpose. Care should also be taken to prevent aerosol condensation in the delivery tubing, and ribavirin should not be given with other aerosols.

In HIV-infected patients receiving chronic oral ribavirin therapy, headaches, gastrointestinal complaints, insomnia, lethargy, mood swings, and dyspnea on exertion occur. Ribavirin can cause extravascular hemolysis with resultant increases in serum bilirubin, uric acid, and iron concentrations. A dose-dependent macrocytic anemia may develop after about 2 weeks of ribavirin therapy. After administration of ribavirin has ended, a reticulocytosis is frequently observed.

Ribavirin is teratogenic or embryolethal in all species tested up to now and is contraindicated in pregnant women or women who may become pregnant during exposure to the drug.

Zidovudine

The greatest problem associated with zidovudine therapy is bone marrow suppression, which occurs in 20% to 30% of patients. These effects were significantly related to baseline host status, since granulocytopenia (less than 750 cells/mm^3) developed in 50% of zidovudine recipients when their initial absolute T-helper cell counts were below 100 cells/mm^3. But granulocytopenia developed in only 20% of recipients when initial T-helper cell counts were above 100 cells/mm^3. Similarly, transfusions were required in 40% versus 20% of persons with T-helper cell counts of less than and greater than 200 cells/mm^3, respectively.

Megaloblastic erythrocyte changes occur within 2 weeks of therapy in most recipients. By using zidovudine earlier in the course of HIV infection with lower doses (500 to 600 mg/day), there has been a decrease in the number of patients experiencing side effects.

The most common nonhematological side effects of therapy are headache, nausea, insomnia, and myalgias. Long-term studies of zidovudine therapy indicate that these symptoms usually improve despite continued therapy, but dose modification may be necessary. Severe neurotoxicity such as seizures, encephalopathy, and polymyositis can occur. Proximal muscle weakness and rhabdomyolysis can also develop. Black nail pigmentation may occur with therapy and is more common in persons of African descent.

Several drug interactions with zidovudine have been reported. Probenecid inhibits the renal excretion of zidovudine and may increase marrow toxicity. Agents, such as acetaminophen, that may interfere with drug glucuronidation should not be taken concurrently. When used with ganciclovir, zidovudine greatly increases the risk for bone marrow suppression. Concomitant dapsone use with zidovudine has been reported to cause severe anemia. Neurotoxicity has been reported with the combined use of acyclovir and zidovudine.

The teratogenicity and mutagenicity of zidovudine have not been completely evaluated. Acute overdose does not produce bone marrow toxicity but can cause coma.

Didanosine

Didanosine's major toxic side effects are pancreatitis and peripheral neuropathy. Pancreatitis has been reported in 5% to 10% of all didanosine recipients. This condition has sometimes been fatal (0.4%). Thus monitoring of pancreatic enzymes has been recommended by some authorities. Pancreatitis is more common among individuals who have a prior history of pancreatitis (30%), and this is a relative contraindication to didanosine use. Peripheral neuropathy has been reported in about 30% of patients and improves upon discontinuation of the drug. Retinal depigmentation has been reported in a few pediatric patients. Biannual retinal ex-

TRADE NAMES

In addition to generic and fixed-combination preparations, the following trade-named materials are available in the United States.

Cytovene, ganciclovir
Foscavir, foscarnet
Flumadine, rimantidine
H-BIG, Hyperhep, Hyperab, VZIG, immunoglobulins
Hivid, zalcitabine
Retrovir, zidovudine
Roferon, (Actimmune, Introna, Alferon) interferon
Stoxil, Dendrid, Herplex, idoxuridine
Symmetrel, amantadine
Vira-A, vidarabine
Virazole, ribavirin
Videx, didanosine
Viroptic, Trifluridine, trifluorothymidine
Zovirax, acyclovir

aminations are recommended for children receiving therapy.

Because didanosine is extremely acid labile, complete neutralization of stomach acid must occur for proper absorption of the compound. Didanosine is administered as two chewable tablets. The need for gastric acid neutralization requires a sufficient amount of buffer to be contained in the two tablets or a water soluble powder. Because the buffer contains divalent metal cations, it can interfere with absorption of other medications, including tetracyclines and fluoroquinolones. Further, absorption of dapsone and ketoconazole may be decreased in patients who are taking didanosine since these medications need acid for full absorption, and these medications should be taken at least 2 hours before a patient takes didanosine.

Zalcitabine

Zalcitabine is approved as monotherapy or as combination therapy with zidovudine in HIV-infected patients. The primary toxicities of zalcitabine are peripheral neuropathy, which occurs in about 30% of drug recipients, gastrointestinal upset (including esophageal ulcers), and headache.

Others

Idoxuridine is generally well tolerated; however, it can cause mild local irritation, headaches, and nausea. Idoxuridine is teratogenic and mutagenic and should be used only when the potential benefits outweigh the potential risks of therapy.

Adverse effects are uncommon with trifluorothymidine. Mild transient burning of the eyes occurs in approximately 5% of patients, and palpebral edema develops in about 3% of patients. Many topical ophthalmic agents have been used in conjunction with trifluorothymidine without interference or adverse effects. These agents include antibiotics (erythromycin, polymyxin B, gentamicin, and sulfacetamide); steroids (prednisolone, dexamethasone, and hydrocortisone); and other ophthalmic drugs (atropine, scopolamine, pilocarpine, and epinephrine). Trifluridine has teratogenic and mutagenic potential and should be used in pregnancy only when the potential benefits outweigh the potential risks.

The most common side effects of topical fluorouracil therapy are local pain, pruritis, and irritation. Contact dermatitis with scarring has also been reported.

Intralesional interferons produce pain at the injection site and leukopenia; malaise and fever also occur. In about 10% of patients the side effects are severe enough to warrant discontinuing therapy. For patients receiving systemic interferon therapy, more significant systemic side effects are reported.

Immunoglobulins are well tolerated, with pain at the injection site and brief low-grade fever the most commonly reported side effects. True allergic reactions with urticaria or angioedema rarely occur, but IV gamma globulin can activate the alternative complement pathway, producing an anaphylactoid reaction.

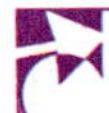

NEW DIRECTIONS

Research in antiviral therapy has been rapidly accelerated by the need for effective therapies against HIV and opportunistic viral infections. New products that are being evaluated against HIV include many nucleic acid derivatives and research continues with compounds (soluble CD4) designed to prevent attachment of viruses to healthy cells. Additionally, with computer assistance the active sites of HIV proteases and other HIV-specific enzyme inducers have been mapped and drugs have been designed as inhibitors. The utility of mismatched RNA to inhibit viral growth is also being evaluated.

Several new compounds are being evaluated for treatment of herpes simplex and varicella-zoster infections. These include acyclovir analogs including prodrugs with better oral absorption and a longer half-life for increased patient convenience. Examples include penciclovir and valacyclovir. Famciclovir was recently approved for use in zoster. Management of cytomegalovirus infections in the immunocompromised patient continues to be problematic, and agents more effective against this infection are anxiously awaited.

REFERENCES

Chrisp P, Clissold SP: Foscarnet: a review of its antiviral activity, pharmacokinetic properties and therapeutic use in immunocompromised patients with cytomegalovirus retinitis, *Drugs* 41:104-129, 1991.

Connolly KJ, Hammer SM: Antiretroviral therapy: strategies beyond single-agent reverse transcriptase therapy, *Antimicrob Agents Chemother* 36:509-520, 1992.

Faulds D, Brogden RN: Didanosine: a review of its antiviral activity, pharmacokinetic properties and therapeutic potential, *Drugs* 44:94-116, 1992.

Kahn JO, Lagakos SW, Richman DD, et al: A controlled trial comparing continued zidovudine with didanosine in human immunodeficiency virus infection, *N Engl J Med* 327:581-587, 1992.

Spector SA, editor: *Ganciclovir therapy for cytomegalovirus infection,* New York, 1991, Marcel Dekker.

Volberding PA, Lagakos SW, Koch MA, et al: Zidovudine in asymptomatic human immunodeficiency virus infection: a controlled trial in persons with fewer than 500 CD4-positive cells per cubic millimeter, *N Engl J Med* 322;941-949, 1990.

Whitley RJ, Gnann JW Jr: Acyclovir: a decade later, *N Engl J Med* 327:782-789, 1992.

SELF-ASSESSMENT QUESTIONS

1. Which of the following is not at least partly responsible for the increasing concentration of acyclovir in infected cells compared with uninfected cells?
   a. monophosphorylation of acyclovir by viral thymidine kinase
   b. triphosphorylation of acyclovir monophosphate by cellular kinases
   c. amination of acyclovir to the active compound by the enzyme adenosine deaminase
   d. alterations of acyclovir that prevent the movement of activated drug extracellularly
2. Which of the following drugs does not require modification to become active?
   a. amantadine
   b. acyclovir
   c. ganciclovir
   d. zidovudine
3. Which of the following drugs is not approved as monotherapy for HIV-infected individuals?
   a. zidovudine
   b. didanosine
   c. zalcitabine
   d. none of the above
4. Which of the following drugs is administered as an aerosol for severe respiratory syncytial virus infection?
   a. amantadine
   b. ribavirin
   c. idoxuridine
   d. foscarnet
5. Immunoglobulins have been shown to be effective in modifying the following viral diseases except:
   a. rabies
   b. hepatitis A
   c. hepatitis B
   d. condyloma acuminatum
6. Which of the following compounds can be used only topically?
   a. idoxuridine
   b. acyclovir
   c. both
   d. neither

CHAPTER 55

Drugs Effective Against Parasitic Helminthic Infections

JAMES L. BENNETT

MAJOR DRUGS

albendazole
diethylcarbamazine
ivermectin
mebendazole
metrifonate
niclosamide
oxamniquine
praziquantel
pyrantel pamoate
suramin
thiabendazole

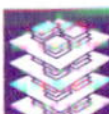

THERAPEUTIC OVERVIEW

Human infections caused by helminths (worms) produce significant medical problems, not only in developing countries in tropical climates, but also in highly industrialized countries in more temperate climates. About 300 million people are infected with blood-dwelling flukes (*Schistosoma* spp.), and hookworms and ascariasis are among the 20 infections that cause the highest morbidities in much of Africa, Asia, and South America. Although their prevalence is higher in certain regions of the world, helminths have no geographical boundaries and are carried by their hosts (parasitized humans) throughout the world.

The life cycle of the helminths is often complex and plays a critical role in the spread of the organism and its infection of humans. The life cycle for schistosomes is summarized in Figure 55-1. Some organisms live in the bloodstream (portal blood) of the intestinal tract; lay approximately 300 eggs per day; and through the action of elastases, break through the intestinal wall and leave the host via the feces. The eggs hatch in water, forming parasites that use snails as carriers (intermediate host). The parasite undergoes asexual multiplication to produce thousands of infective parasitic cercariae, and humans are infected through skin contact with the cercariae in infested water. In Africa, only one snail in 5000 harbors the parasite, but 65% to 95% of the people in nearby villages are infected when exposed to infected water. Some parasites evade the immune system of the host by coating themselves with host antigens or simply avoiding damage to their surface by shedding and repairing areas that have been damaged by the host immune system.

ABBREVIATIONS

ATP	adenosine triphosphate
GABA	γ-aminobutyric acid

The helminths are divided into three groups: nematodes (roundworms), trematodes (flatworms, flukes), and cestodes (flatworms, tapeworms). These three groups, the important species within each group, and the drugs available for the treatment of the different groups are summarized in Table 55-1. Some of the helminths are potentially dangerous, such as certain tissue-dwelling larval tapeworms. The life cycle of human-infecting hookworms (nematodes) is shown in Figure 55-2.

MECHANISMS OF ACTION

The strategy for the use of drugs to treat helminthic infections differs greatly from that employed in the treatment of bacterial or fungal infections. Most anthelmintic drugs are targeted at the nonproliferating adult stage of the organism, whereas with bacterial and fungi the targets are young, growing cells. The helminthic life cycle (see Figures 55-1 and 55-2) is strongly dependent on the following factors: (1) neuromuscular coordination for worm feeding movements and for maintaining a favor-

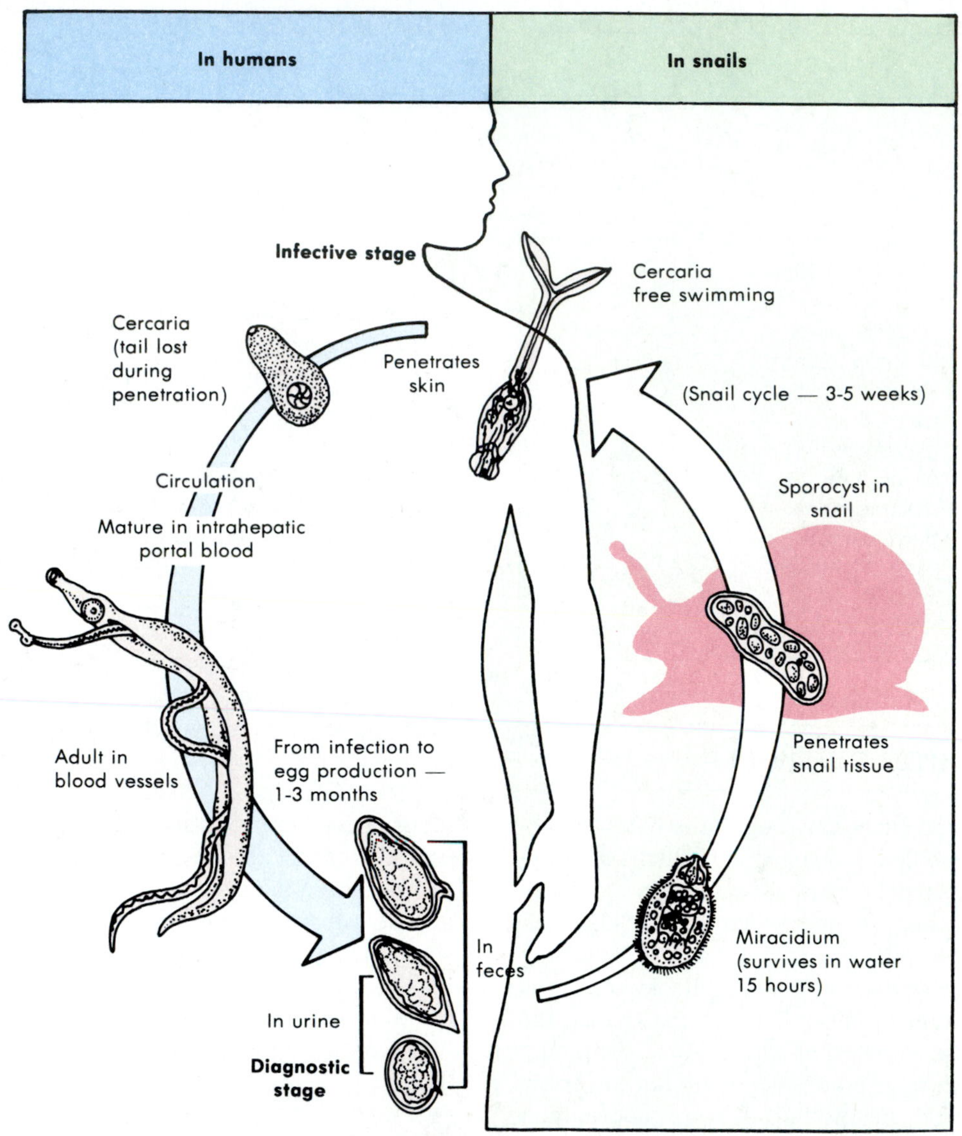

FIGURE 55-1 Life cycle of schistosomes (see text). (From Murray PR, Kobayashi GS, Pfaller MA, Rosenthal KS: *Medical microbiology,* ed 2, St Louis, 1994, Mosby.)

Table 55-1 Therapeutic Overview

Helminth Infection	Drug of Choice	Alternate Drug
INTESTINAL NEMATODES (ROUNDWORMS)		
Capillaria philippinensis	mebendazole	pyrantel pamoate
Ascaris lumbricoides	mebendazole	pyrantel pamoate
Enterobius vermicularis (pinworms)	mebendazole	pyrantel pamoate
Necator americanus	mebendazole	pyrantel pamoate
Ancylostoma duodenale	mebendazole	pyrantel pamoate
Strongyloides stercoralis	thiabendazole	mebendazole
Trichinella spiralis	mebendazole	thiabendazole
Trichuris trichiura (hookworm)	mebendazole	pyrantel pamoate
EXTRAINTESTINAL NEMATODES (ROUNDWORMS)		
Dracunculus medinensis	thiabendazole, metonidazole	niridazole
Onchocerca volvulus (adult)	suramin†	
Onchocerca volvulus (microfilariae)	ivermectin	diethylcarbamazine
Wuchereria bancrofti (adult)	diethylcarbamazine§	ivermectin‡
Wuchereria bancrofti (microfilariae)	diethylcarbamazine§	ivermectin‡
Brugia spp. (adult)	diethylcarbamazine§	ivermectin‡
Brugia spp. (microfilariae)	diethylcarbamazine	ivermectin‡
Loa loa	diethylcarbamazine	ivermectin‡
LARVAL NEMATODES (ROUNDWORMS)		
Strongyloides stercoralis	thiabendazole*	mebendazole
Cutaneous larva migrans	thiabendazole	
Visceral larva migrans	thiabendazole	
Trichinella spiralis	thiabendazole, mebendazole	
INTESTINAL CESTODES (TAPEWORMS)		
Taenia saginata (beef tapeworm)	praziquantel	niclosamide
Taenia solium (pork tapeworm)	praziquantel	niclosamide
Diphyllobothrium latum	praziquantel	niclosamide
Hymenolepis nana	praziquantel	niclosamide
LARVAL CESTODES (TAPEWORMS)		
Taenia solium	praziquantel	niclosamide
Echinococcus granulosus	albendazole	
Echinococcus multilocularis	albendazole	
BLOOD-DWELLING TREMATODES (FLUKES)		
Schistosoma mansoni	praziquantel	oxamniquine
Schistosoma haematobium	praziquantel	metrifonate
Schistosoma japonicum	praziquantel	niridazole
INTESTINAL TREMATODES (FLUKES)		
Heterophyes heterophyes	praziquantel	
Metagonimus yokogawai	praziquantel	
LIVER TREMATODES (FLUKES)		
Clonorchis sinensis	praziquantel	
Opisthorchis spp.	praziquantel	
Fasciola hepatica	praziquantel	bithinol
LUNG TREMATODES (FLUKES)		
Paragonimus spp.	praziquantel	bithinol

*Some success reported for ivermectin, but this drug is for investigational use only in the United States.
†The microfilaricidal drug ivermectin is given first, followed 2 to 3 weeks later by suramin.
‡This drug is for investigational use only in the United States.
§Effectiveness of diethylcarbamazine against these adult filariae is questionable.

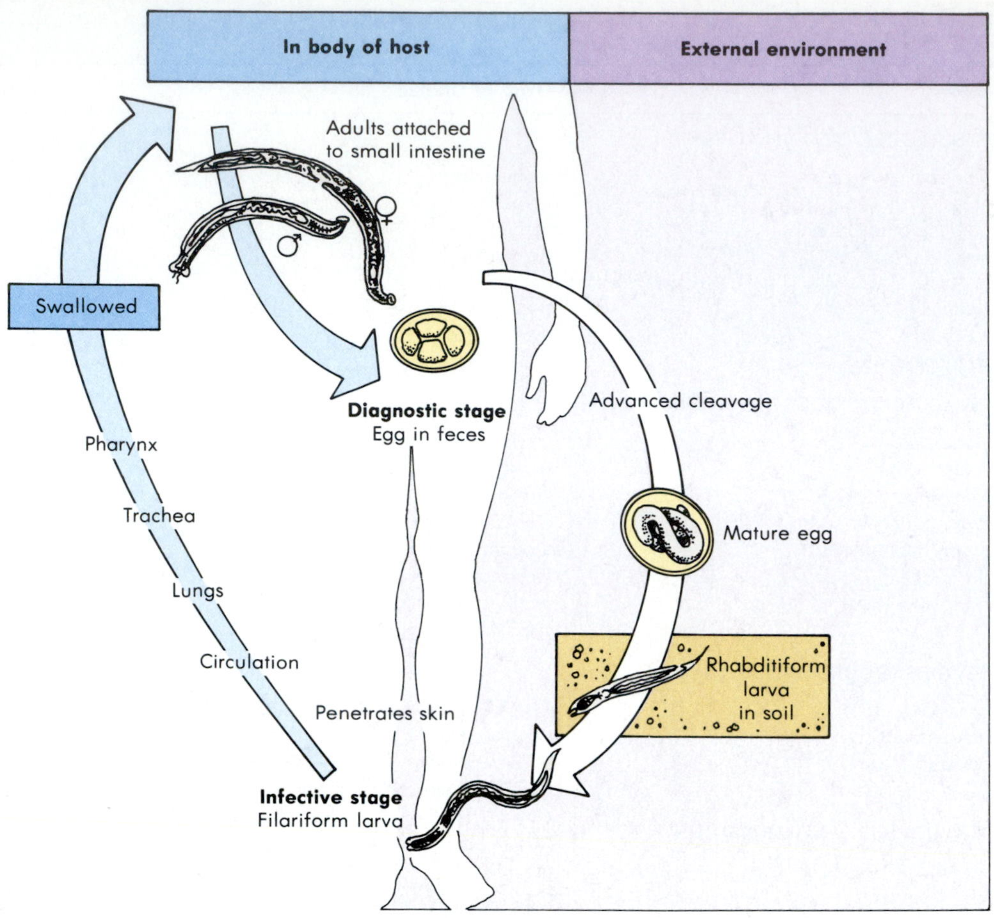

FIGURE 55-2 Life cycle of hookworms (see text). (From Murray PR, Kobayashi GS, Pfaller MA, Rosenthal KS: *Medical microbiology,* ed 2, St Louis, 1994, Mosby.)

able location of the worm within the host; (2) carbohydrate metabolism as the source of energy, with glucose the primary substrate; and (3) microtubular integrity, since egg laying and hatching, larval development, glucose transport, and enzyme activity and secretion are hindered when the microtubules are modified. Most anthelmintic agents are targeted at one of these three biochemical functions in the adult organism.

The structures of the primary anthelmintic agents are shown in Figure 55-3. The sites of action and the physiological effects of each of the agents is listed in Table 55-2.

Mebendazole and Thiabendazole

Mebendazole, thiabendazole, and albendazole (not available in the United States) are embryotoxic to mammals and extremely embryotoxic to helminth larval nematode development in utero *(Onchocerca volvulus)* or within the egg. In adult nematodes these compounds suppress production of secretory products such as acetylcholinesterase and result in disappearance of cytoplasmic microtubules from nematode tegumental and intestinal cells. Mebendazole and thiabendazole block the assembly of tubulin dimers into tubulin polymers (Figure 55-4) in a process mimicked by colchicine, a powerful antimitotic and embryotoxic drug.

Pyrantel Pamoate

The nervous system of helminths appears to be the target for pyrantel pamoate, ivermectin, and metrifonate, since all three produce a rapid change in motor activity of the helminth. Pyrantel pamoate produces a powerful cholinomimetic effect on the nematode muscle cells by binding to cholinergic receptors, which results

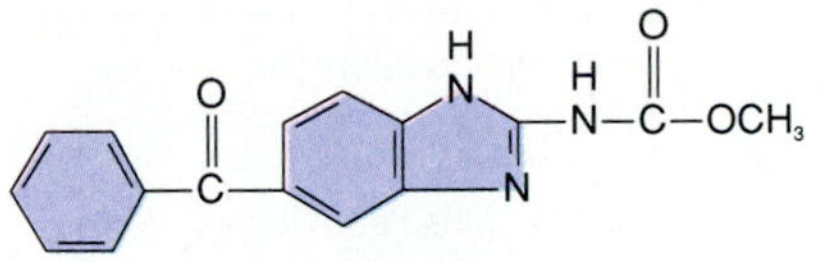

mebendazole

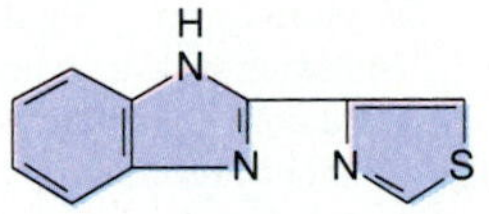

thiabendazole

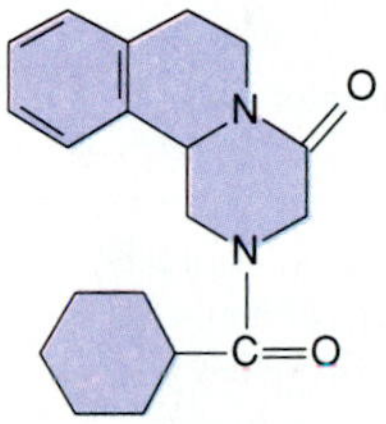

praziquantel

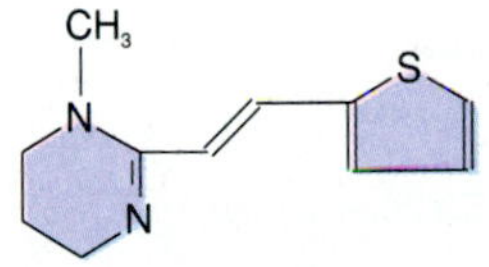

pyrantel

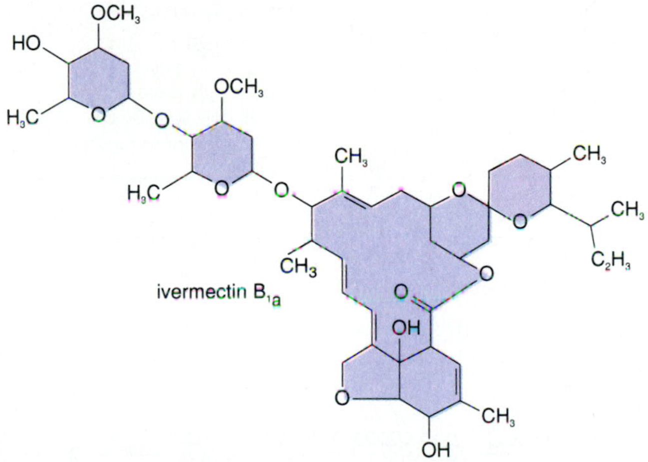

ivermectin B_{1a}

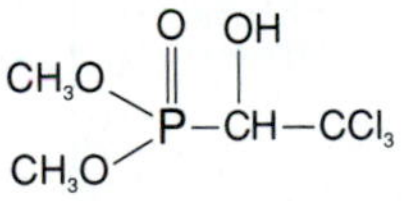

metrifonate

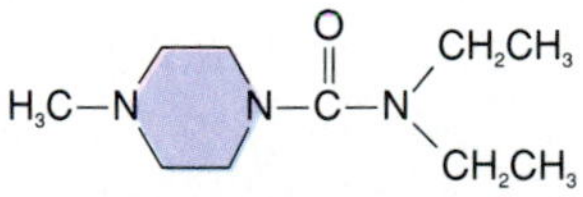

diethylcarbamazine

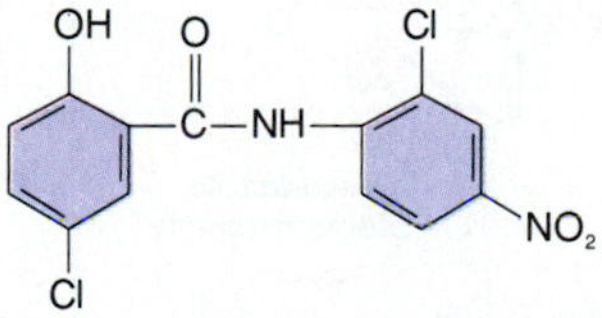

niclosamide

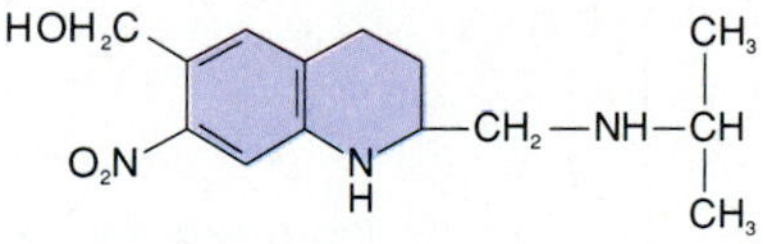

oxamniquine

FIGURE 55-3 Structures of primary anthelmintic agents. See the text for further information.

Table 55-2 Sites and Mechanisms for the Major Anthelmintics

Drug	Site of Action	Physiological Effect	Molecular Mechanism
mebendazole thiabendazole	Cytoplasmic microtubules in tegumental and intestinal cells of nematodes	Inhibit protein secretion and glucose transport	Binds to colchicine receptor on tubulin dimers
praziquantel	Tegument and muscle	Contracts muscle; disrupts tegument that attracts antibody and phagocytes	Change in membrane permeability; synergy with host immune system
pyrantel pamoate	Cholinergic synapse on muscle cells of nematodes	Contraction of muscle cells	Binds to cholinergic receptor
ivermectin	Uterus of female *Onchocerca volvulus*	Blocks release of microfilariae	Not known
diethylcarbamazine	Surface of microfilariae	Exposes antigens on surface that bind antibody and attract phagocytes	Not known
metrifonate	Cholinergic synapse	Causes flaccid paralysis of muscles	Inhibits acetylcholinesterase
niclosamide	Mitochondria	Gradual paralysis of muscles	Uncouples anaerobic phosphorylation
suramin	Appears to alter cells lining intestinal tract	May block absorption from intestinal tract	Inhibits many enzymes, including dehydrogenases, dihydrofolate reductase, protein kinases
oxamniquine	No particular site	Reduction in protein synthesis followed by degeneration of tegument	Alkylates parasite DNA

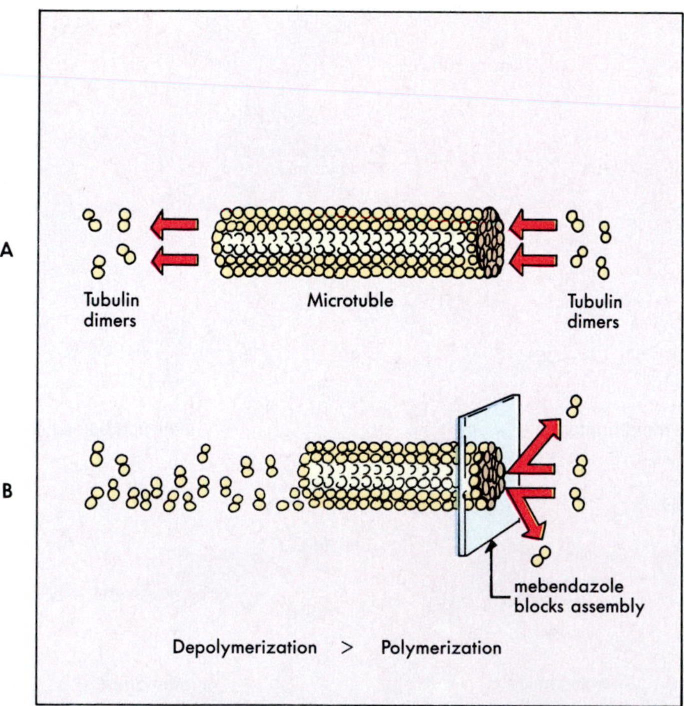

FIGURE 55-4 **A,** Under normal conditions, tubulin dimers are continually being polymerized and depolymerized from the ends of the microtubule. **B,** Mebendazole or colchicine can bind a high affinity site on the tubulin dimer and prevent polymerization or assembly, leading to depolymerization or complete breakdown of the microtubule.

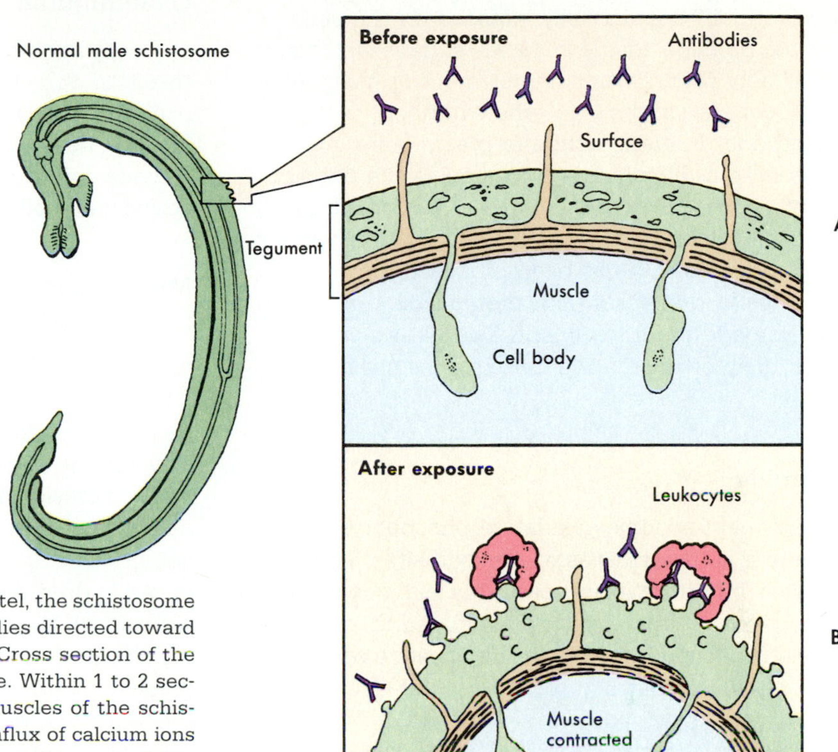

FIGURE 55-5 Before exposure to praziquantel, the schistosome is capable of avoiding the numerous antibodies directed toward surface and internally located antigens. **A,** Cross section of the dorsal surface of a normal male schistosome. Within 1 to 2 seconds after exposure to praziquantel, the muscles of the schistosome contract because of drug-induced influx of calcium ions into the schistosome tegument. **B,** The change in permeability of the schistosome surface toward external ions initiates the appearance of small holes and balloon-like structures, making the parasite vulnerable to antibody-mediated adherence of host leukocytes, which kill the helminth.

in cell depolarization and muscle contraction. This paralytic action on gut-dwelling nematodes leads to expulsion of the helminth from the host intestinal tract into the feces.

Diethylcarbamazine

Diethylcarbamazine shows no activity in vitro but kills the microfilariae readily in vivo (Figure 55-2), possibly altering the parasite surface membrane and thus activating the host immune system. There is a decrease in muscle activity and subsequent paralysis of the worms.

Ivermectin

Ivermectin produces rapid and pronounced inhibition of nematode movement by interacting with the chloride channel on the helminth's α-aminobutyric acid receptor complex. This receptor mediates inhibitory effects on nematode muscle cells. Ivermectin is used extensively to control gut-dwelling nematode infections in domestic and farm animals, and because it concentrates in the hides of animals, it prevents insect damage. Its use in humans is limited to treating the filarial parasite *Onchocerca volvulus.* The drug has no lethal effect on the adult *O. volvulus* but dramatically acts on microfilariae produced by the female parasite. First, ivermectin alters the ability of the microfilariae to evade the host immune system, thus allowing the immune system to recognize this body as a foreign antigen. Second, ivermectin alters the reproductive system of adult female *O. volvulus* by reducing its capacity to produce microfilariae. The exact mechanism and receptor associated with this action of ivermectin on nematode reproductive function is not known.

Praziquantel

The action of praziquantel on *Schistosoma mansoni* and other schistosomes is described schematically in Figure 55-5. Synergy between the drug and the response of the humoral immune system of the host is observed (Figure 55-5, *B*). This occurs through disruption of the surface, which protects the parasite from the host immune system and thus allows antibodies to attack parasite antigens not normally exposed on the surface. Irreversible damage to the parasite surface and tegument probably occurs when complement or host leukocytes are recruited to the sites where antibody is bound. This rapid and dramatic action of praziquantel may be attributable to a drug-induced change in the helminth permeability toward divalent cations. The result is an elevation of calcium-ion concentration within various cells of the helminth. It has been proposed that this action initiates in the worm both the spastic contraction and the damage to its tegument. The nature of the receptor or receptors mediating these events has not been identified.

Niclosamide

Niclosamide uncouples oxidative phosphorylation in mitochondria in mammals as well as parasites. The drug is absorbed by gut-dwelling cestodes but not by gut-dwelling nematodes. Cestode mitochondria generate adenosine triphosphate (ATP) in the absence of oxygen through pathways that use other terminal electron acceptors. These novel pathways generate a hydrogen gradient across the parasite mitochondrial membrane susceptible to the action of niclosamide. Thus cestodes exposed to niclosamide cannot generate ATP. Loss of helminth ATP ultimately immobilizes the parasite within the intestine so that it is expelled with the feces.

Oxamniquine

Oxamniquine inhibits DNA, RNA, and protein synthesis in *Schistosoma mansoni*. Compounds similar to oxamniquine are highly mutagenic, although oxamniquine itself is not. The parasite may have a unique enzyme capable of esterifying oxamniquine to form a reactive metabolite whose action alkylates helminth DNA.

Metrifonate

The paralytic action of metrifonate, an organophosphate, on the motor activity of *Schistosoma mansoni* and *S. haematobium* is directly related to inhibition of parasite acetylcholinesterase. Inhibition of this enzyme elevates the concentration of the inhibitory neurotransmitter acetylcholine within the helminth. The drug is active against *S. haematobium* but not extremely active against *S. mansoni*. This may be attributable to differences in drug accessibility, in that adult *S. mansoni* reside within the mesenteric veins, whereas *S. haematobium* live within the veins surrounding the bladder. The paralytic action of the drug dislodges the parasites from the veins. On rare occasions when *S. mansoni* infestations are located in the urinary bladder, this organism is just as susceptible to the drug as *S. haematobium*.

Suramin

Suramin inhibits numerous enzymes of filarial helminths, most notably lactate dehydrogenase, malate de-

Table 55-3 Pharmacokinetic Parameters

Agent	Administration	Absorption	$t_{1/2}$ (hr)	Disposition
diethylcarbamazine	Oral	Rapid	9-13	R (50%), pH dependent M (50%)
ivermectin	Oral	Rapid	28	M (main)
niclosamide	Oral	Poor	—	—
mebendazole	Oral	Poor* (5%-10%)	0.9-1.1†	M (main) first pass
albendazole	Oral	Good	—	M (active metabolites)
praziquantel	Oral	Rapid (80%)	4	M (90%) first pass
thiabendazole	Oral	Poor	—	M (main), R
oxamniquine‡	Oral	Rapid	1-2	M (main)
metrifonate	Oral	Rapid	1.5-3	M (active metabolite)
suramin	IV	Poor	36-49	R (main), B
pyrantel pamoate	Oral	Poor	—	R (10%-20%), F

M, Metabolized; *R*, eliminated unchanged by renal mechanisms; *B*, bile; *F*, feces.
*Increased by food, bioavailability only 22% (first pass).
†2-5 hr in other studies.
‡50% bioavailability (vs IM).

hydrogenase, dihydrofolate reductase, and various protein kinases. It is a large polyanion that complexes proteins readily.

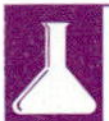

PHARMACOKINETICS

The pharmacokinetic parameter values are summarized for the anthelmintic agents in Table 55-3.

For treatment of intestinal helminthic infections, the drugs should not be absorbed but remain in the gastrointestinal tract where the organisms are usually located. However, with the more difficult to treat extraintestinal or systemic helminthic infections, it is necessary that the drugs be absorbed and enter the systemic circulation.

Mebendazole is poorly absorbed from the intestinal tract and shows a large first-pass effect. Bioavailability is increased by food. Thiabendazole is well absorbed but rapidly metabolized to 5-hydroxythiabendazole and the latter conjugated with glucuronic acid or sulfate and excreted in the urine.

Albendazole is moderately well absorbed, and its metabolites inhibit *Echinococcus* in extraintestinal sites such as the liver and the chest.

Niclosamide is also poorly absorbed but reaches the systemic circulation because it binds tightly to albumin.

Pyrantel pamoate is poorly absorbed and thus acts effectively in the gastrointestinal tract. The bulk of the drug is present in the feces, with only 10% to 20% excreted in urine. Unlike drugs used almost exclusively against gut-dwelling nematodes, diethylcarbamazine is completely absorbed within 1 to 2 hours and undergoes rapid metabolism, with most of the metabolites being excreted in the urine.

Similar to diethylcarbamazine, *praziquantel* is rapidly and almost completely absorbed, with peak plasma concentrations appearing 1 to 2 hours after administration. This drug is rapidly metabolized to a 4-hydroxycyclohexyl derivative, which is then conjugated and excreted in the urine. High concentrations of the drug are found in liver, bile, and muscle. Both parent and metabolite are present in the brain and CSF. Approximately 80% is bound to plasma protein. Recent studies of ivermectin in humans show a prolonged-disposition half-life, probably because of drug deposition in fatty tissue from which it slowly diffuses.

Oxamniquine and *metrifonate* are rapidly absorbed from the intestine, with peak plasma concentrations appearing 1.5 to 3 hours after administration. Food delays the absorption of oxamniquine and limits the concentration achieved in the plasma. The major metabolite of oxamniquine is formed in the intestine before absorption, and its concentration in the plasma can be 8 to 10 times greater than that of oxamniquine. This metabolite is devoid of any anthelmintic activity and is excreted in the urine within 12 hours after administration of oxamniquine.

Metrifonate undergoes extensive metabolism, including spontaneous rearrangement at neutral pH to form active dichlorvos. *Dichlorvos* is the metabolite responsible for the antischistosomal activity associated with metrifonate. *Suramin,* the only anthelmintic to be given parenterally, has an unusually long half-life because it binds so strongly to plasma proteins. Metabolism of suramin appears to be negligible.

Ivermectin is administered orally or intravenously. It is widely distributed in the body with concentration in liver and fatty tissue. Most is excreted in feces, with minimal amounts found in the urine. A single dose can be detected in tissues for up to 28 days.

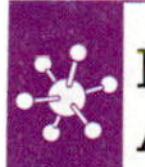

RELATION OF MECHANISMS OF ACTION TO CLINICAL RESPONSE

Anthelmintics for Intestinal Nematode Infections

Many nematodes reside as adults within the intestinal tract. Examples are *Ascaris lumbricoides* (large roundworm), *Enterobius vermicularis* (pinworm), *Necator americanus* with *Ancylostoma duodenale* (the hookworms), *Strongyloides stercoralis, Trichinella spiralis,* and *Trichuris trichiura* (whipworm). The anthelmintic used to treat these intestinal roundworms is mebendazole, with the exception of *Strongyloides* infections, for which thiabendazole is recommended, though mebendazole may be adequate. The drug acts slowly on these helminths, and so organism elimination from the intestinal tract may take 3 days following a course of therapy.

Pyrantel pamoate is also extremely effective against the major gut-dwelling nematodes and is not readily absorbed from the intestine. The drug is well tolerated with no reported toxic side effects and no contraindications. An analog, *oxantel,* is used in combination with pyrantel to provide effective therapy for the three major soil-transmitted nematodes: *Ascaris* roundworms, the hookworms, and *Trichuris* whipworms.

Anthelmintics for Extraintestinal Nematode Infections

Adult nematodes of clinical significance also reside outside the gastrointestinal tract. Infections by adult nematodes in tissues are termed *filariasis,* and the larvae that are released are called *microfilariae.* Special note should be taken concerning the lack of effective drugs against the extraintestinal nematodes, a group of helminths that inflict a considerable amount of human suffering worldwide. *Dracunculus medinensis* (guinea worm) and adult *O. volvulus* along with their microfilariae live within subcutaneous tissues and are devastating parasites. Unfortunately, no effective drugs for either adult parasites exist, though treatment of *D. medinensis* with thiabendazole or niridazole (not available in the United States) allows the worm to be mechanically withdrawn from the ulcer more easily by virtue of an antiinflammatory effect of these agents. The microfilariae released by female *O. volvulus* can be destroyed by diethylcarbamazine, but the destruction increases a pathological condition in the skin (Mazzoti reaction) and eye.

A new microfilaricidal drug, ivermectin, has fewer side effects than diethylcarbamazine, and a single dose can eliminate microfilariae for up to 6 months. Ivermectin has a dramatic effect on the tissue-dwelling microfilariae of *O. volvulus.* These microfilariae are responsible for widespread blindness in rural West and East Africa.

Wuchereria bancrofti and *Brugia* species are filarial nematodes that dwell within lymph glands, causing lymphedema of the extremities (elephantiasis). Multiple doses of diethylcarbamazine eliminate some of the adult parasites and most of the circulating microfilariae. Recent clinical trials with ivermectin indicate that this drug may be superior to diethylcarbamazine in the treatment of these filarial infections. Another less pathogenic filarial parasite that resides in subcutaneous tissues, *Loa loa,* can be effectively controlled with diethylcarbamazine.

In addition to adult nematodes, many larval forms are pathogenic. For example, larvae released by adult *Strongyloides stercoralis* can cause serious damage to the lining of the gut, and in patients with a depressed cell-mediated immune system the larvae can invade many organ systems and cause death. *Trichinella spiralis* larvae migrate from the gut-dwelling adult to the skeletal muscles predominantly but also to the heart, lungs, and nervous system, where the larvae cause myositis and trichinosis.

Thiabendazole should be used for trichinosis and visceral larva migrans, and thiabendazole and mebendazole can be considered for *S. stercoralis* or cutaneous larva migrans. These drugs may significantly suppress the immune response. This action may be more important than the drugs' effects in destroying the tissue-dwelling larvae. Antiinflammatory steroids are often coadministered in cases where the infection is intense.

Anthelmintics for Cestode Infections

Adult tapeworm infections are predominantly not symptomatic. Parasites such as *Taenia saginata* (beef tapeworm); *T. solium* (pork tapeworm); *Diphyllobothrium latum* (fish tapeworm), which can cause vitamin B_{12} deficiency; and *Hymenolepis nana* (dwarf tapeworm) live within the intestinal tract of man and can be easily eliminated with praziquantel or niclosamide.

The problem with some cestode infections arises when the larval forms take residence in an organ system. If a human ingests the eggs of *T. solium,* the hatching pork-tapeworm larvae invade various organs. The pathogenic response (referred to as *cysticercosis*) depends on the organ invaded, with the most serious ef-

CLINICAL PROBLEMS

DIETHYLCARBAMAZINE

Onchocerca volvulus infections
- Intense pruritus and papular rash
- Swelling of inguinal lymph nodes
- Chorioretinitis and optic nerve atrophy

Brugia malayi and *Wuchereria bancrofti* infections
- Nausea
- Vomiting
- Pain in joints
- Fever

Loa loa infections
- Similar to *B. malayi*
- Encephalitis caused by *Loa* organisms should not be treated until encephalitis subsides

IVERMECTIN

Onchocerca volvulus infection
- Similar to but milder than diethylcarbamazine
- No adverse ocular effects

MEBENDAZOLE

Contraindicated during pregnancy

METRIFONATE

Avoid treating patients recently exposed to insecticides

PRAZIQUANTEL

Cerebral edema, aqueductal stenosis (prevented by steroids)

SURAMIN

Toxic compound to be used with caution especially with patients having renal insufficiency

THIABENDAZOLE

Severe hepatitis with prolonged use

fect associated with larvae invading the CNS. Praziquantel effectively eliminates cysticercosis. However, worm death causes ingress of white blood cells and cerebral edema. Patients should be treated with steroids (prednisone or dexamethasone) before and during therapy. If humans consume the egg of the tapeworm *Echinococcus granulosus* or *E. multilocularis,* the resulting infection can be fatal, especially with ingestion of *E. multilocularis.* The larvae from these eggs migrate principally to the liver or lung where they form small cysts, which can increase in size. Treatment with mebendazole gives marginal results, but albendazole (not available in the United States) is effective.

Anthelmintics for Trematode Infections

Preeminent in medical and economic importance are the schistosomes, or blood-dwelling flukes, of *Schistosoma mansoni, S. japonicum,* and *S. haematobium.* They cause schistosomiasis, which is a source of morbidity in many countries of Africa and the Caribbean Islands. Although oxamniquine and metrifonate are used to control schistosomiasis, praziquantel has become the drug of choice. Liver flukes (*Opisthorchis* spp.) and lung flukes (*Paragonimus* spp.) are important parasites in Asia. Other clinically troublesome flukes are intestinal flukes *Heterophyes heterophyes* and *Metagonimus yokogawai* and the liver fluke *Fasciola hepatica.* Praziquantel is now used to treat all these trematode infections, except for *Fasciola hepatica,* in which results have been mixed.

Oxamniquine is still used in some areas to treat *S. mansoni* infections. Drug resistance has been detected in Brazil, and Egypt.

Metrifonate, an organophosphate that is converted to the active antischistosomal compound dichlorvos, is still used for *S. haematobium* infections in some countries.

SIDE EFFECTS, CLINICAL PROBLEMS, AND TOXICITY

With some notable exceptions most of the major anthelmintics present few problems when administered to infected patients (see box on facing page). Side effects associated with diethylcarbamazine are frequent but usually not severe.

Some anthelmintic agents accumulate as a result of binding to lung tissue, as in the use of diethylcarbamazine for treating patients with *Wuchereria bancrofti* or *Brugia* species (organisms that dwell mainly in lymph glands). The resulting side effects include headache, weakness, joint pains, nausea, and vomiting. In heavily infected patients, effects may include small localized reactions of pain, tenderness, and inflammation in the groin and thigh, especially in *Brugia* infections. Initiating therapy with a low dose and gradually increasing to a higher dose can attenuate these side effects. With *Loa loa,* microfilariae can migrate to the CNS and produce encephalitis, which can be greatly exacerbated by treatment with *diethylcarbamazine.* Treatment should be delayed in favor of corticosteroid therapy to suppress encephalitis, which then allows the use of diethylcarbamazine. When diethylcarbamazine is given to patients with onchocerciasis, an intense hypersensitivity reaction associated with drug action on tissue-dwelling microfilariae may occur. Itching within minutes after dosing is followed by a fine papular rash and hyperpyrexia, tachycardia, and headache. The severity of this reaction is often proportional to the number of microfilariae. The reaction can sometimes be severe, and the patient may remain prostrate for 24 hours. In addition, diethylcarbamazine can cause eye lesions including chorioretinitis and optic nerve atrophy, along with a pronounced increase in punctate keratitis and limbitis, an eye inflammation.

Problems associated with *ivermectin* treatment of onchocerciasis are fewer than with diethylcarbamazine. The pruritus is less prominent, and eye lesions are not observed. In an extremely small number of cases, a mild hypotensive response is observed.

With *niclosamide,* undesirable side effects include malaise, fever, abdominal discomfort or pain, and pruritus. There are no contraindications to the use of niclosamide, and it has been administered to debilitated patients and pregnant women.

Poor absorption of *mebendazole* is responsible for the few side effects associated with its use even in sick and debilitated patients. With high doses, alopecia and reversible neutropenia are seen. This drug is embryotoxic and teratogenic and thus should not be given to pregnant women. Thiabendazole induces anorexia, nausea, vomiting, and dizziness, and approximately 30% of patients receiving it will be incapacitated for several hours; this may increase to 50% with higher doses. Unlike mebendazole, thiabendazole is not embryotoxic or teratogenic in rats, but its safety in humans has not been evaluated. The drug can produce a severe allergic hepatitis when used for longer than 2 days, as is necessary in severe infestations of the small intestine. It may also interfere with xanthine metabolism.

The high degree of safety associated with *praziquantel* makes it possible to control human trematode and cestode infections. Three groups of side effects have been identified: abdominal discomfort, headache and dizziness, and skin manifestations. Most of these side effects appear within the first 12 to 24 hours after dosing. The third effect may result from antigens released

TRADE NAMES

In addition to generic and fixed-combination preparations, the following trade-named materials are available in the United States.

Antiminth, pyrantel pamoate
Biltricide, Distocide, praziquantel
Mintezol, thiabendazole
Niclocide, niclosamide
Vansil, oxamniquine
Vermox, mebendazole

by dying parasites that initiate an allergic reaction. Most patients tolerate the drug without serious side effects. Even patients with advanced schistosomiasis, Symmers' periportal fibrosis, or esophageal varices have been treated without complication. Treatment of CNS lesions always requires premedication with steroids.

Side effects associated with oxamniquine and metrifonate usually are minor, and both drugs are well tolerated. Some dizziness and drowsiness has been reported along with a mild fever after the administration of *oxamniquine,* and patients with a history of epilepsy may experience convulsions after exposure to this drug. Oxamniquine can be used in patients with severe hepatosplenic schistosomiasis. Side effects with metrifonate include mild vertigo, colic, lassitude, and nausea. Patients receiving this drug should avoid contact with insecticides containing anticholinesterase agents.

Suramin must be used with great care. Within hours after administration of suramin, papular eruptions, paresthesias, photophobia, lacrimation, hyperesthesias of the palms of the hand and soles of the feet, and palpebral edema are commonly observed. The drug is administered parenterally and accumulates in the kidney and can induce albuminuria. In addition, hematuria and urinary casts may appear. One should manage a persistent albuminuria by altering the treatment schedule or discontinuing use of the drug if casts appear in the urine.

NEW DIRECTIONS

Triclabendazole, a benzimidazole that is highly selective for trematodes, has been successfully employed, using a single dose, in the control of *Paragonimus* infections in South America. Single-dose application is very significant for public health programs, since the present drug of choice, praziquantel, requires dosing over several days.

REFERENCES

Campbell WC, Rew RS, editors: *Chemotherapy of parasitic diseases,* New York, 1986, Plenum Publishing.

Edwards G, Breckenridge AM: Clinical pharmacokinetics of anthelminthic drugs, *Clin Pharmacokinet* 15:67, 1988.

Vanden Bossche H, Thienpont D, Janssens PG, editors: Chemotherapy of gastrointestinal helminths. In Vanden Bossche H. Thienpont D, and Janssens PG, eds: *Handbook of experimental pharmacology,* vol 77, New York, 1985, Springer-Verlag.

SELF-ASSESSMENT QUESTIONS

1. Helminth infections are the result of:
   a. lack of effective drugs.
   b. poor public health infrastructure, e.g., lack of good sanitary facilities.
   c. poor understanding, among the infected population, of how these diseases are transmitted.
   d. resistance of many helminths to the anthelmintic drugs.
   e. rapid rate at which people become reinfected after treatment.
2. The major physiological system of the helminth that is the focus of the action of most anthelmintics is the:
   a. reproductive system
   b. nervous system
   c. cytoskeletal system
   d. tegument, or cuticle
   e. digestive system
3. This drug could be used to treat patients that are infected with cestodes and trematodes:
   a. praziquantel
   b. mebendazole
   c. levamisole
   d. ivermectin
   e. pyrantel
4. Adult filarial parasites can be eliminated with:
   a. mebendazole
   b. ivermectin
   c. diethylcarbamazine
   d. pyrantel
   e. none of the above
5. Of the following anthelmintics, which one would be considered the most toxic?
   a. ivermectin
   b. praziquantel
   c. mebendazole
   d. suramin
   e. pyrantel

CHAPTER 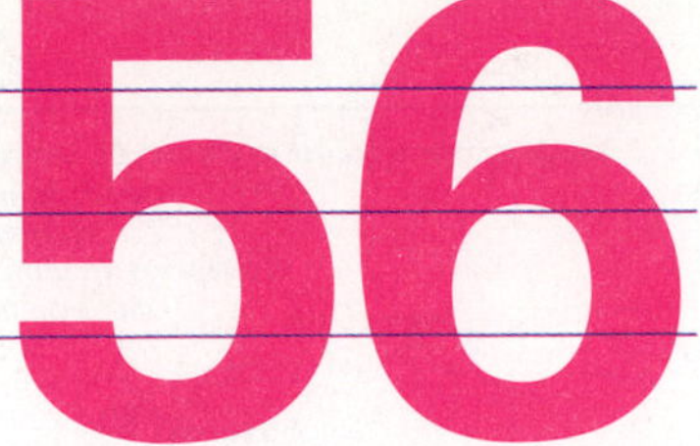

Drugs Effective Against Parasitic Protozoal Infections

ELIZABETH A. VANDEWAA

MAJOR DRUGS

antimalarial agents
antileishmaniasis agents
antitrypanosomal agents
antiamebiasis agents
antigiardiasis and antitrichomoniasis agents

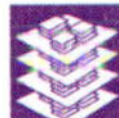

THERAPEUTIC OVERVIEW

Parasitic protozoa infect a significant percentage of the world population to produce malaria, leishmaniasis, trypanosomiasis, amebiasis, giardiasis, trichomoniasis, and other diseases. Protozoal diseases are more prevalent in tropical climates but are also found in the United States. International travel and immigration of persons from other countries to the United States provides opportunities for exposure of U.S. inhabitants to these organisms.

Protozoa invade host cells, multiply, and eventually destroy the host cells. Infections with these organisms typically have acute and primary phases that result in death or development of a chronic latent stage, interspersed with relapses.

Malaria is the most significant protozoal disease in terms of morbidity and mortality, with over 1 million infant deaths a year directly attributable to this disease in Africa. Other protozoal diseases, such as amebiasis, giardiasis, and trichomoniasis are widely distributed, whereas leishmaniasis and trypanosomiasis are found primarily in tropical areas. Some protozoal infections are becoming increasingly associated with immunocompromised individuals, including those with acquired immuno deficiency syndrome (AIDS).

The prevention and treatment of protozoal diseases follows four strategies: control the vector, improve hygiene and sanitation, provide vaccination, and administer chemotherapy. Chemotherapeutic approaches are used effectively to treat and prevent many protozoal infections, though some agents have adverse effects or are eventually met with resistance. Thus optimal treatment involves use of all four strategies.

The primary therapeutic considerations with protozoal diseases are summarized in the box on p. 755.

ABBREVIATION	
AIDS	acquired immunodeficiency syndrome

MECHANISMS OF ACTION

Antimalarial Agents

Malaria is caused by protozoa of the genus *Plasmodium* present in the human host either in the erythrocytic (blood) stage or the exoerythrocytic (tissue) stage. The life cycle of a malaria parasite is summarized in Figure 56-1. Drug treatment chiefly involves the use of aminoquinolines, such as chloroquine, its analogs, and several additional drugs, for the erythrocytic stage and chiefly primaquine for the exoerythrocytic stage. Newer compounds, such as mefloquine, *qinghaosu* (*ch'inghaosu,* green-*Artemisia* factor, or *artemisinine),* and halofantrine are also used. Several antibiotics that are also antiparasitic are often administered in combination with the antimalarial agents. Older agents that have wide use include quinine and quinidine. The structures of some of the antimalarial drugs are shown in Figure 56-2.

The mechanism of antimalarial action of chloroquine and other 4-aminoquinolines is still unclear. Several

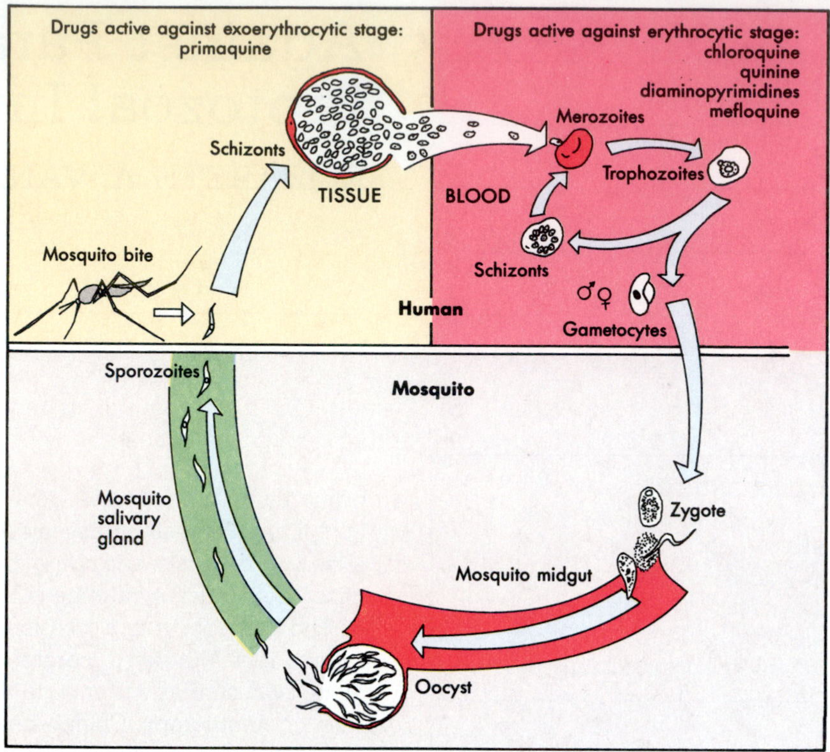

FIGURE 56-1 Life cycle of *Plasmodium* protozoa. Drugs used to treat infection are effective against either erythrocytic or exoerythrocytic stages of the parasite.

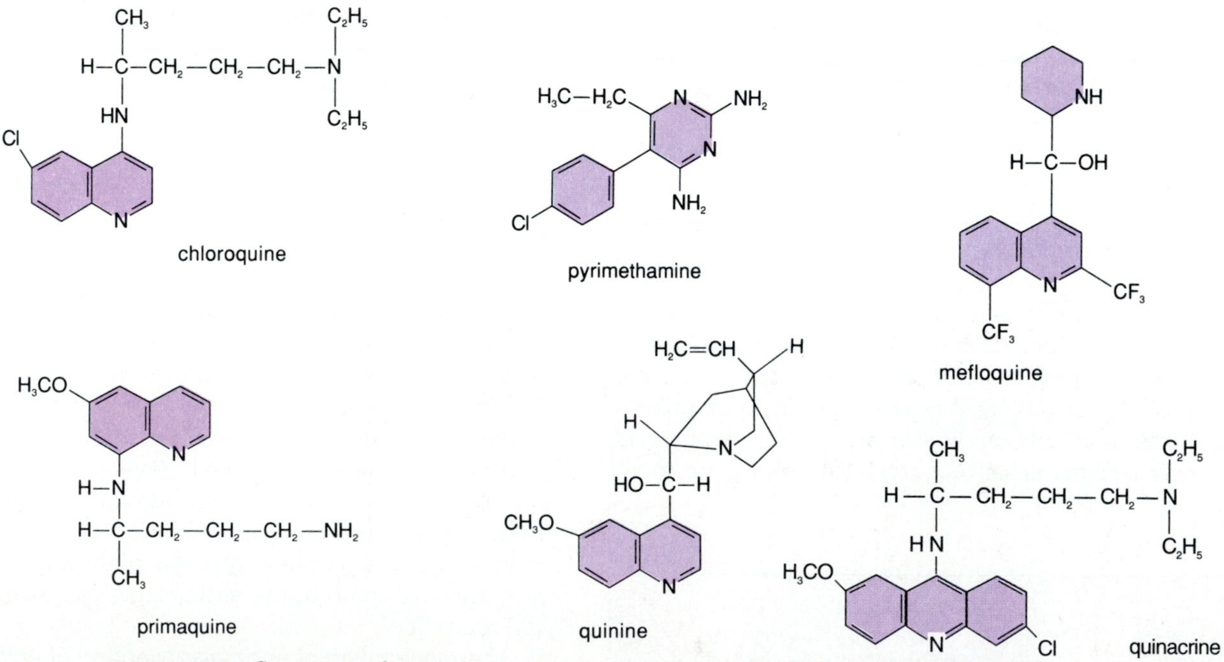

FIGURE 56-2 Structures of some drugs used in the treatment of malaria. See the text for further information.

THERAPEUTIC OVERVIEW

THERAPEUTIC STRATEGIES

Control disease vector
Improve hygiene and sanitation
Vaccination attempts
Drugs

PROTOZOAL INFECTION ENDEMIC INFECTION-VECTOR

Malaria—mosquito
Leishmaniasis—sandflies
Trypanosomiasis—tsetse fly
Amebiasis—food, water
Giardiasis—food, water
Toxoplasmosis—meats, cats

RESISTANCE DEVELOPS TO SPECIFIC DRUGS

mechanisms have been proposed. In one, binding of drug to ferriprotoporphyrin IX, released from hemoglobin in infected erythrocytes, produces a complex that is toxic for plasmodial and red blood cell membranes. In a second mechanism, uptake and concentration of drug into the parasites raises the pH of intracellular acidic vesicles. The elevated pH impairs the ability of the parasite to degrade hemoglobin and causes the characteristic morphological changes seen microscopically.

The mechanisms of action of quinine and mefloquine are believed to be similar to that of chloroquine. Quinidine (see Chapter 14) also has some antimalarial properties. Both quinidine and quinine display potentially hazardous cardiac toxicity.

The diaminopyrimidines, such as pyrimethamine and trimethoprim, inhibit dihydrofolate reductase in malarial parasites. These agents are effective at concentrations far below those needed to inhibit the mammalian enzyme (see Chapter 49), and so selectivity can be attained. Inhibition of parasite dihydrofolate reductase blocks the synthesis of tetrahydrofolate, a precursor necessary for the formation of purines, pyrimidines, and certain amino acids (see Chapter 49). Parasites exposed to these agents do not form schizonts in the red blood cells or liver. When a diaminopyrimidine is used with a sulfonamide or sulfone, a synergistic effect is achieved by blockade of two steps in the same metabolic pathway (see Chapter 49). Sulfonamide inhibits the synthesis of paraaminobenzoic acid to dihydropteroic acid while the diaminopyrimidine blocks the reduction of dihydrofolate to tetrahydrofolate.

Sulfonamides, tetracyclines, and clindamycin are often administered with antimalarial agents. The mechanism of action of sulfonamides is discussed in Chapter 49 and that for the tetracyclines and clindamycin in Chapter 48. The molecular mechanisms of the newer experimental *qinghaosu* and halofantrine are not known.

Antileishmaniasis Agents

Tissue forms of leishmania are the target for pentamidine isethionate, meglumine antimoniate, sodium stibogluconate, and amphotericin B. The structures of some of these drugs are shown in Figure 56-3. (Meglumine antimoniate is a compound similar to sodium stibogluconate.) (See Chapter 53 for the structure and mechanism of action of amphotericin B.)

Meglumine antimoniate and sodium stibogluconate are antimonials and the drugs of first choice against leishmaniasis. They inhibit the glycolytic enzyme phosphofructokinase and certain Krebs cycle enzymes in *Leishmania* organisms. The resulting decreased energy production is parasiticidal.

Pentamidine isethionate acting against *Leishmania* species may interact with DNA or with nucleotides, or it may interfere with the uptake and function of polyamines. Amphotericin B prevents the synthesis of ergosterol, an important membrane sterol in *Leishmania* and thus increases membrane permeability to cause loss of low-molecular-weight nucleotides, cations, and amino acids. Both pentamidine and amphotericin B are second-line drugs to treat leishmaniasis.

Antitrypanosomiasis Agents

African trypanosomiasis (sleeping sickness) is treated with the arsenicals tryparsamide and melarsoprol, or suramin and pentamidine. For Chagas's disease, nifurtimox and benznidazole are the agents of choice. The structures of some agents are shown in Figure 56-4.

Once the infection has reached the CNS, melarsoprol or tryparsamide is the preferred drug. These arsenical drugs act on sulfhydryl groups of enzymes, which are essential catalysts in carbohydrate metabolism. Melarsoprol inhibits parasite pyruvate kinase, causing decreased concentrations of adenosine triphosphate (ATP), *pyruvate,* and phosphoenolpyruvate. These drugs also inhibit *sn*-glycerol 3-phosphate oxidase, needed for regeneration of nicotinamide adenine dinucleotide in trypanosomes but not found in mammalian cells. Inhibition of parasite metabolism at two sites produces a trypanocidal effect.

Suramin inhibits parasite *sn*-glycerol 3-phosphate oxidase and glycerol 3-phosphate dehydrogenase (Figure 56-5), causing a net decrease in ATP synthesis. An alternative to suramin is pentamidine. In trypanosomes, pentamidine may bind to the adenine- and thymine-rich

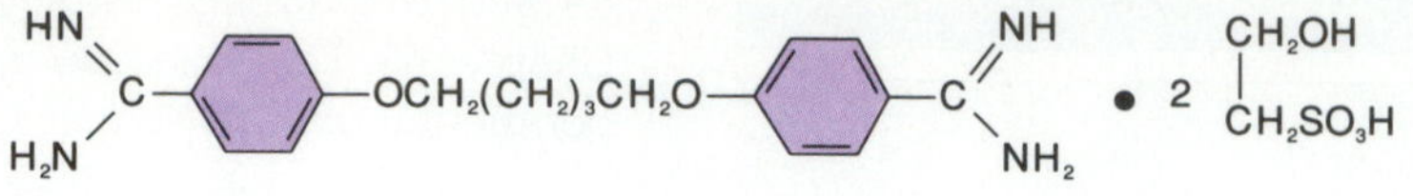

pentamidine isethionate

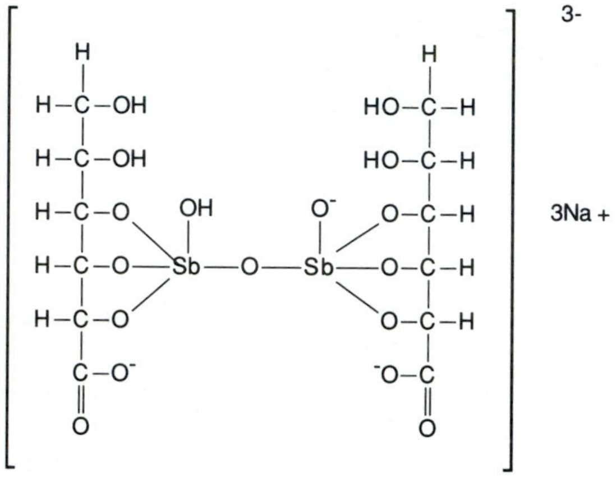

sodium stibogluconate

FIGURE 56-3 Structures of drugs used in the treatment of leishmaniasis. See the text for further information.

tryparsamide

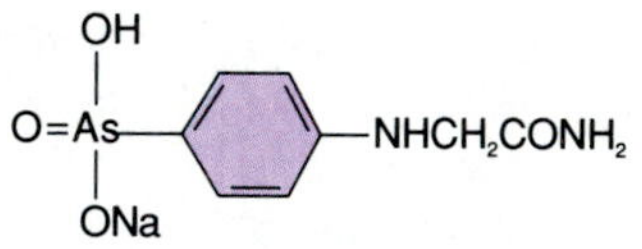

melarsoprol

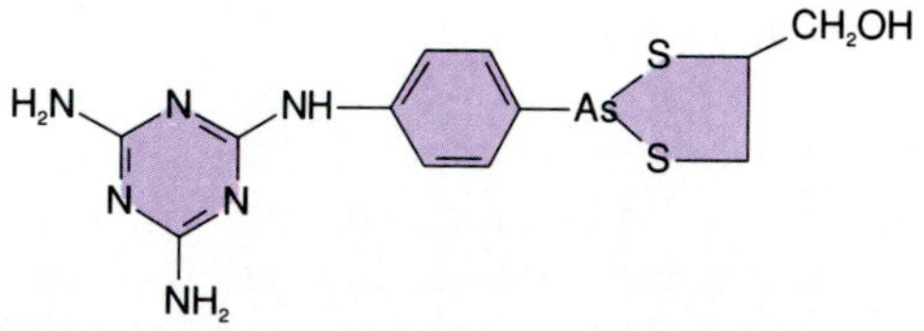

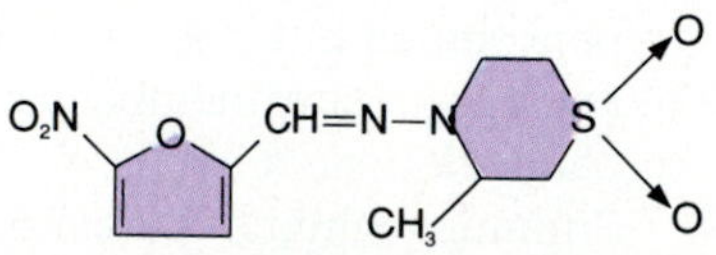

nifurtimox

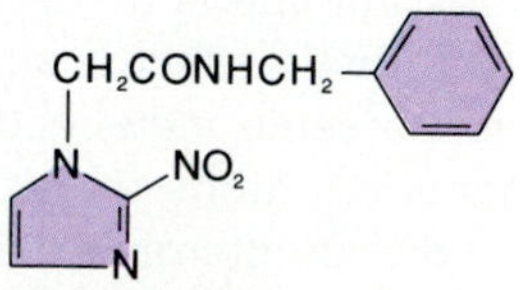

benznidazole

FIGURE 56-4 Structures of drugs used in the treatment of trypanosomiasis. See the text for further information.

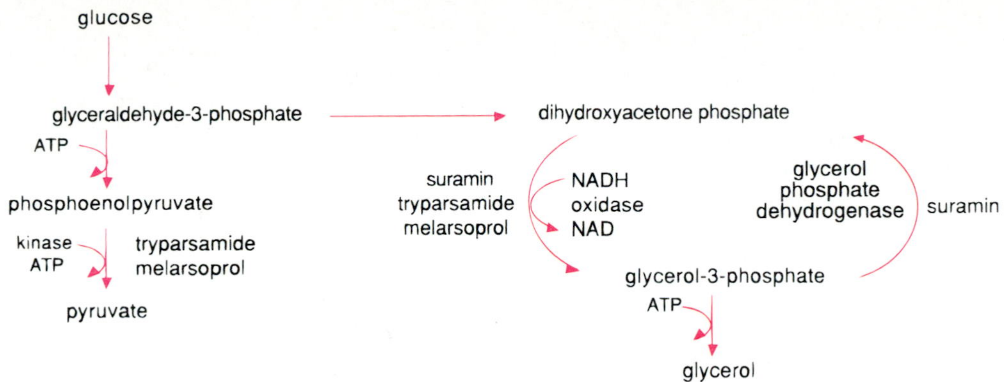

FIGURE 56-5 Glucose metabolism in African trypanosomes. Suramin inhibits *sn*-glycerol phosphate oxidase and *sn*-glycerol phosphate dehydrogenase, preventing reoxidation of NADH and decreasing ATP synthesis. The arsenicals (e.g., tryparsamide and melarsoprol) inhibit *sn*-glycerol phosphate oxidase as well as pyruvate kinase, resulting in a parasiticidal effect.

regions of DNA, inhibiting DNA replication. Like suramin, pentamidine does not penetrate into the CNS and therefore is not useful in late CNS stages of infection with *Trypanosoma brucei gambiense*. Similarly, because *T.b. rhodesiense* invades the CNS so rapidly, pentamidine is effective only in the very early stages of infection.

Eflornithine, a new agent, may prove very useful in the treatment of African trypanosomiasis. This drug is an irreversible inhibitor of the enzyme ornithine decarboxylase, which catalyzes the first step in polyamine biosynthesis. In the trypanosome, a major use for polyamines is for the synthesis of trypanothione, a nucleophile that protects the organism from reactive oxygen species. Since eflornithine is able to penetrate the CNS, it has been found to be particularly useful in arousing patients from the comatose state.

Nifurtimox, the drug of choice for treatment of Chagas's disease, exerts its trypanocidal action by forming free radicals. The free radicals react with molecular oxygen to form superoxide anion ($O_2^{\overline{\cdot}}$), hydrogen peroxide (H_2O_2), and hydroxyl-free radical ($OH^{\overline{\cdot}}$) (Figure 56-6). Trypanosomes are susceptible to these reactive intermediates, which cause peroxidation of lipids and DNA, because these organisms contain no catalase or glutathione peroxidase to inactivate the toxic products. Nifurtimox is highly toxic to human cells as well, but limited selectivity is achieved because the rates of radical formation are much decreased in human cells than in trypanosomes.

Antiamebiasis Agents

Iodoquinol, diloxanide furoate, and paromomycin are used against intestinal forms, emetine or dehydroemetine against systemic amebic forms, and metronidazole against both forms of *Entamoeba histolytica*. The structures of these agents are shown in Figure 56-7.

Iodoquinol is the drug of choice for asymptomatic individuals who pass amebic cysts; an alternative drug, diloxanide furoate, is amebicidal; and a third agent, paromomycin, is an aminoglycoside antibiotic that is amebicidal and acts by inhibition of protein synthesis (see Chapter 48). Emetine and dehydroemetine also inhibit protein synthesis, probably by blocking translocation along the mRNA of the ribosome during chain elongation.

Metronidazole interacts with amebic DNA, destroying the ability of the DNA to serve as a template for further DNA and RNA synthesis. It covalently binds to guanine and cytosine residues, causing loss of helical structure and breakage of DNA strands.

Antigiardiasis and Antitrichomoniasis Agents

Metronidazole and quinacrine are the main drugs used to treat these infections. The structure of quinacrine is shown in Figure 56-2. It presumably acts by intercalation into parasite DNA, preventing replication.

PHARMACOKINETICS

Some of the drugs discussed in this chapter may not be generally available in the United States. The Centers for Disease Control in Atlanta should be contacted to check on availability, since it maintains stocks of these agents for disbursement on special request.

Pharmacokinetic characteristics of trimethoprim and sulfonamides are discussed in Chapter 49, those of tetracyclines and clindamycin are in Chapter 48, and those of suramin are in Chapter 55. The information on the pharmacokinetic parameter values for these drugs is summarized in Table 56-1.

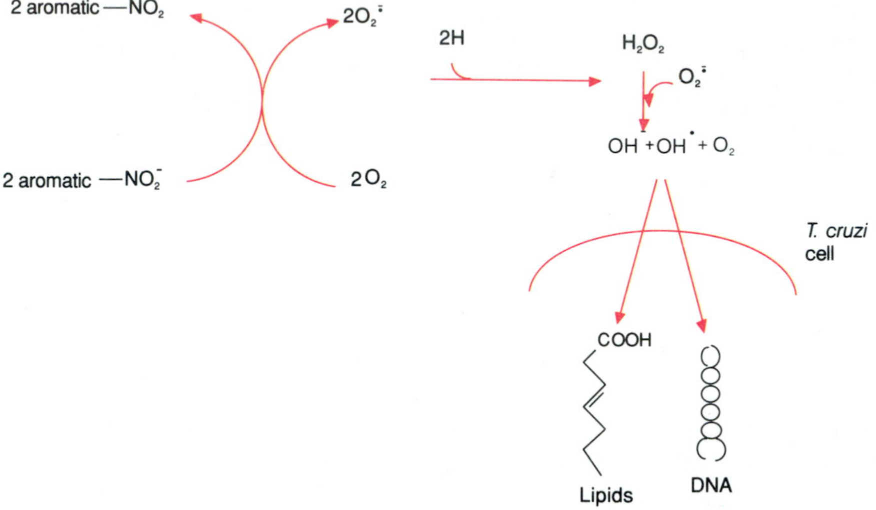

FIGURE 56-6 Generation of reactive intermediates by the aromatic nitro group of nifurtimox. The anion free radical reacts spontaneously with O_2 to form superoxide anion ($O_2^{\cdot -}$. H_2O_2, subsequently formed by superoxide dismutase, can react with $O_2^{\cdot -}$ to generate the hydroxyl radical, OH^-. Once formed, $OH^{\cdot -}$ causes peroxidation of lipids and DNA in *Trypanosoma cruzi.*

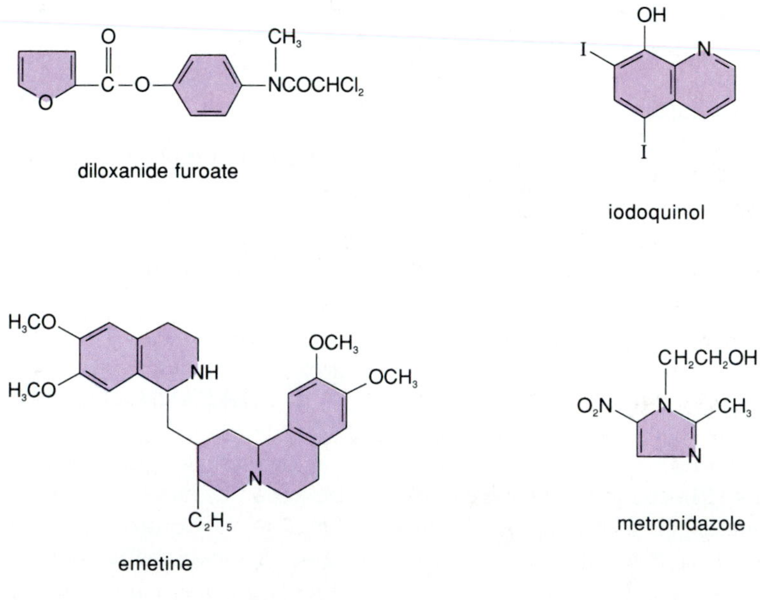

diloxanide furoate

iodoquinol

emetine

metronidazole

FIGURE 56-7 Structures of drugs used in the treatment of amebiasis. See the text for further information.

Table 56-1 Pharmacokinetic Parameter Values

Drug	Administration	Oral Absorption	$t_{1/2}$ (hr)	Disposition	Plasma Protein Binding (%)
MALARIA					
chloroquine	Oral, IM	Good	3-4 days	M, R	50
pyrimethamine	Oral	Good	110	M (90%)	Tissue bound
quinine	Oral, IM, IV	Good	10	M (95%)	70
mefloquine	Oral	Fair	14 days	M enterohepatic cycle	99
primaquine	Oral	Good	3-6	M (95%)	50%
LEISHMANIASIS					
meglumine antimoniate	IM, IV	No	2,35†	R	Tissue bound
sodium stibogluconate	IM, IV	No	2, 35†	R	Tissue bound
pentamidine isethionate*	IV, IM	No	6-8 weeks	R	Tissue bound
TRYPANOSOMIASIS					
tryparsamide	IV	No	—	R (main)	—
nifurtimox	Oral	Good	—	—	
benznidazole	Oral	Good	—	M	—
AMEBIASIS					
iodoquinol	Oral	Fair	—	M	—
diloxanide furoate	Oral	Good	—	M	—
paromomycin	Oral	Poor	—	—	<10%
emetine	IM	No	Long	R	Tissue bound
metronidazole	Oral, IV	Good	8	M, R	20
tinidazole	Oral	Good	8	M, R	20-30
ornidazole	Oral	Good	8	M, R	20-30
GIARDIASIS					
quinacrine	Oral	Good	—	R	Tissue bound
metronidazole (see above)					

M, Metabolized; *R,* eliminated unchanged by renal mechanisms.
*Aerosol available for *Pneumocystis carinii.*
†Initial and terminal.

The absorption of *chloroquine* is rapid and complete; food may increase bioavailability. Fifty percent is bound to protein and serum lipids, and thirty percent is metabolized in liver to *N*-deethyl derivatives. After a single dose, the $t_{1/2}$ is 48 hours; however, because of accumulation in liver, spleen, kidney, lung, and leukocytes, the effective $t_{1/2}$ is 3 to 4 days. Chloroquine is detected in serum and urine up to a year after treatment. It can be administered IM but not IV.

Primaquine interferes with metabolism of chloroquine and should be administered after treatment for *Plasmodium vivax* but with a period of overlap. It is well absorbed orally and is eliminated in 24 hours. It is widely distributed, with retention in tissues, and is converted to carboxyprimaquine. Less than 5% appears in urine.

Mefloquine is slowly absorbed from the gastrointestinal tract, and peak concentrations are not reached until 36 hours. It has a $t_{1/2}$ of 14 days, is 99% protein bound, and undergoes extensive enterohepatic recirculation.

Pyrimethamine is completely absorbed after oral ingestion. It is slowly eliminated and has a $t_{1/2}$ of 4 days, with suppressive concentrations present in plasma for almost 2 weeks. It undergoes minor metabolism.

Pentamidine is not absorbed from the gastrointestinal tract. It is administered IV or IM and is slowly eliminated from the body because of accumulation in tissues, but it is rapidly cleared from the blood. Fifteen percent is excreted in urine in 24 hours, but detectable amounts are found up to 8 weeks after a 2-week course of therapy.

Aerosol *pentamidine* produces sustained lung concentrations without clearance for 48 hours. Apical segments of the lungs are less well supplied than the lower lobes are.

Melarsoprol, a trivalent arsenical compound, is administered IV. Plasma concentrations decrease rapidly after administration, and no drug is detectable after a few days. It is excreted by the kidney.

Nifurtimox is rapidly absorbed and metabolized with

little drug detected in plasma after 24 hours. Metabolites are excreted in the urine.

Benznidazole is rapidly absorbed orally, widely distributed throughout the body, and metabolized with metabolites excreted in the urine.

Tryparsamide is administered IV. CSF concentrations are achieved within 20 hours. It is excreted unchanged in the urine.

Suramin is administered IV. It is extensively bound to serum proteins, and elimination is slow. It is distributed widely, and significant concentrations can be found in tissues up to 3 months after therapy. The drug is not appreciably metabolized, and the free drug is excreted in urine.

Sodium stibogluconate and *meglumine antimoniate* are administered IM or IV. Pharmacokinetics are quite complex with an initial $t_{1/2}$ of 2 hours and a terminal $t_{1/2}$ of 30 to 35 hours after IV and over 700 hours after IM administration. Conversion of pentavalent antimony to trivalent antimony probably occurs, which may explain the toxicity. Antimonials are concentrated in reticuloendothelial cells.

Diloxanide furoate is rapidly and almost completely absorbed from the gastrointestinal tract, with ester hydrolysis occurring in the intestine. It has a $t_{1/2}$ of 6 hours and is excreted in urine as the glucuronide.

Eflornithine (DL-α-difluormethylornithine) is administered IV in 4 daily doses for 2 weeks. Large doses of 20 g/day are necessary. It crosses the blood-brain barrier into the CSF. It is also present in lung tissue. The CSF to serum ratio is from 0.09 to 0.45.

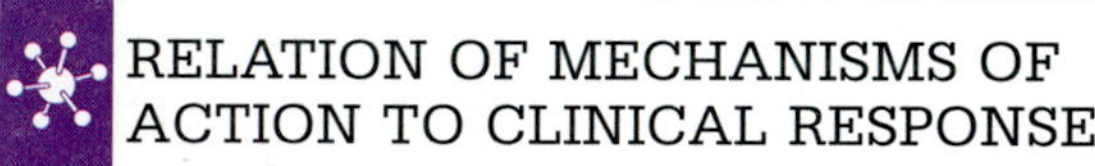

RELATION OF MECHANISMS OF ACTION TO CLINICAL RESPONSE

Antimalarial Agents

Human malaria is caused by four species of obligate intracellular protozoa of the genus *Plasmodium*. *P. vivax* is the most common, *P. falciparum* the most severe, and *P. ovale* and *P. malariae* are less common and of intermediate severity. These parasites reproduce asexually in humans and sexually in mosquitoes of the genus *Anopheles*. In the asexual stages, the malaria parasites invade erythrocytes where they multiply and ultimately burst the cells to release a new invasive population of parasites. The pathological condition and symptoms of malaria are caused strictly by the asexual blood forms of malarial parasites, and many drugs that selectively target these stages have been developed. Figure 56-1 depicts the malaria life stages within the human host. Sexually differentiated forms (gametocytes), which are infective to the mosquito, are also found in the circulation and offer another site of action of certain antimalarials.

When an individual is infected from the bite of a mosquito, some parasites leave the mosquito and enter the circulation and localize in hepatic parenchymal tissue. Here the parasites multiply and form exoerythrocytic schizonts; this is an asymptomatic stage of the disease and represents another target for drug treatment. After a period of 5 to 16 days, the exoerythrocytic schizonts rupture, releasing thousands of merozoites, the infective blood stage of the parasite, into the circulation. The rupture and reinvasion of red blood cells by the merozoite form of the parasite are responsible for the fever and clinical manifestations of the disease.

Chloroquine and related compounds remain the drugs of first choice (Table 56-2) for the treatment of susceptible malaria strains. Chloroquine has no effect against the exoerythrocyte stages of plasmodia and thus does not prevent recrudescence of infection. It is highly toxic to the asexual blood stages of most *Plasmodium* species but not *P. falciparum*. During an acute febrile attack, chloroquine lowers fever within 24 to 48 hours, and parasites are no longer visible in the blood 48 to 72 hours after treatment. The drug completely cures chloroquine-susceptible *P. falciparum*, the most lethal of the malaria species in humans. Chloroquine is well tolerated, inexpensive, and effective orally. Unfortunately, resistance of *P. falciparum* to chloroquine is widespread in Asia, Africa, and South and Central America, greatly limiting the use of this agent.

Quinine is used orally to treat mild attacks and intravenously to treat acute attacks of multidrug-resistant *P. falciparum*, which causes cerebral malaria. Quinine is never used alone but is often combined with a sulfonamide or tetracycline antibacterial agent. *Quinidine* is

Table 56-2 Drugs of Choice

Infection	Primary Drugs
Malaria	chloroquine*
	pyrimethamine
	quinine, quinidine†
Leishmaniasis	meglumine antimoniate
	sodium stibogluconate
Trypanosomiasis	melarsoprol
	suramin
	nifurtimox
Amebiasis	iodoquinol, metronidazole
Giardiasis	metronidazole, quinacrine
Trichomoniasis	metronidazole

*Mefloquine is used as prophylaxis in areas where *Plasmodium falciparum* is resistant to chloroquine.

†Quinine and quinidine are used to treat *P. falciparum* malaria of the CNS.

available in all developed countries and should be used to treat *P. falciparum* if quinine is not available.

Pyrimethamine has been used in the past in combination with antibiotics or with sulfadoxine, a sulfonamide with an extremely long plasma and tissue half-life, as prophylaxis with chloroquine to treat resistant *P. falciparum* and *P. vivax* malaria. Synergism produced with a sulfonamide-diaminopyrimidine combination is desirable because lower doses of each drug can be used to obtain the therapeutic effect. However, the combination is no longer recommended for either prophylaxis or treatment since it can cause an exfoliative dermatitis reaction (Stevens-Johnson syndrome).

Mefloquine is used for the chemoprophylaxis of falciparum malaria and is recommended for treatment of chloroquine-resistant *P. falciparum*. Resistance to mefloquine has been reported but is rare.

Primaquine is extremely effective against the tissue schizonts (exoerythrocytic phase) of *P. vivax* and *P. ovale*. Recurrent attacks of both *P. vivax* and *P. ovale* can be controlled by a combination of chloroquine and primaquine. Methemoglobinemia and potential homolysis limit primaquene's use.

Antileishmaniasis Agents

Leishmania parasites exist intracellularly in phagolysosomes of mononuclear tissue phagocytes, but infected cells are found throughout the body, including the bloodstream. The tissue forms of the parasite are called *amastigotes* and serve as the chemotherapeutic target for the treatment of the disease. Prevention or cure of leishmaniasis has been hampered significantly by both the lack of effective drugs and the toxicity associated with existing agents. Meglumine antimonate and sodium stibogluconate (antimony sodium gluconate) are first-line drugs for treatment of leishmaniasis, with pentamidine and amphotericin B being alternative drugs for treatment of various forms of the disease (Table 56-2).

Antitrypanosomiasis Agents

Trypanosomiasis, caused by *Trypanosoma brucei rhodesiense,* leads to progressive CNS involvement and almost always death. Trypanosomiasis from *T.b. gambiense* causes a chronic debilitation known as sleeping sickness with severe CNS involvement.

Once CNS involvement is apparent, melarsoprol and tryparsamide are the drugs of choice (Table 56-2). Both are effective for the treatment of the meningoencephalitic stage of African trypanosomiasis. Because melarsoprol acts more rapidly and causes fewer side effects, it is surpassing tryparsamide in use. Melarsoprol is also effective against tryparsamide-resistant trypanosomes. Eflornithine is able to penetrate the blood-brain barrier. Ornithine decarboxylase turns over in 30 minutes in humans, but in parasites it turn over is several days. Mammalian cells are rescued from drug effects by new enzyme synthesis.

Suramin is the drug of choice for African sleeping sickness (Table 56-2). When given IV, it is active against blood forms of *T.b. gambiense* and *T.b. rhodesiense,* particularly in the early stages of the disease. Once the disease has progressed to involve the CNS, suramin cannot prevent progression, since it does not penetrate the blood-brain barrier.

For the treatment of Chagas's disease caused by *T. cruzi,* nifurtimox is the drug of choice (Table 56-2), with benznidazole as an alternative that is efficacious against nifurtimox-resistant *T. cruzi.*

Antiamebiasis Agents

Amebiasis, caused by *Entamoeba histolytica,* is found throughout the world and is transmitted by the oral-fecal route after ingestion of infective cysts. The cysts change into trophozoites that reside in the colon, where they form new cysts, which are passed into the environment to complete the life cycle. These organisms may produce amebic dysentery and liver abscesses. The drugs used to treat amebiasis are specific for the location of the organism. For example, diloxanide furoate, paromomycin, and iodoquinol (Table 56-2) are effective against intestinal (noninvasive) forms of the parasite. Systemic amebicides include emetine and dehydroemetine, used for the treatment of severe amebic dysentery, and metronidazole, used against both intestinal and systemic forms of the infection. Emetine and dehydroemetine are rarely used because of their serious cardiac toxicity except in the treatment of intestinal invasive amebiasis.

Metronidazole is not effective for the treatment of individuals who are asymptomatic but continue to pass cysts, though it is extremely effective for treatment of dysentery and amebic liver abscesses. Other nitroinidazole ornidazole and tinidazole are used in Europe and South America.

Antigiardiasis and Antitrichomoniasis Agents

Giardia lamblia, a flagellated protozoan, causes the most common of the intestinal protozoal infections in developed countries. Giardiasis is transmitted by the passage of infective cysts, which become trophozoites after ingestion. The trophozoites are found in the duodenum, and the presence of these organisms may result in diarrhea but frequently results in nonspecific bloating with passage of foul-smelling stools. Giardiasis is best treated with metronidazole or quinacrine (Table 56-2).

Trichomoniasis, caused by *Trichomonas vaginalis,* is a vaginal infection. Trichomoniasis is treated successfully with metronidazole, in which cure rates exceed 90% (Table 56-2).

Other Agents

Four protozoal parasites—*Cryptosporidium, Isospora belli, Pneumocystis,* and *Toxoplasma*—are particularly important sources of infection in the immunocompromised host. Although clinical manifestations of these diseases are rare except in immunocompetent individuals infected with these organisms, predisposing factors such as leukemia, lymphoma, and AIDS can cause infection by these parasites to become fatal to these individuals.

Pneumonias caused by *Pneumocystis carinii* occur exclusively in immunocompromised individuals and contribute significantly to the mortality associated with AIDS. Recommended treatment for *P. carinii* infection is initially trimethoprim-sulfamethoxazole (see Chapter 49) with pentamidine isethionate or trimethoprim-dapsone as alternative drugs. Pentamidine can be administered as an aerosol as prophylaxis against recurrence.

Toxoplasma gondii, the causative agent of toxoplasmosis, can produce systemic infection in both immunocompetent and immunocompromised individuals. Domesticated animals, particularly cats, serve as intermediate hosts for *Toxoplasma gondii,* passing infective oocysts in their feces. Treatment of toxoplasmosis is done with sulfonamides (discussed in Chapter 49) combined with pyrimethamine. However, pyrimethamine is teratogenic and should not be used in treatment of pregnant women. Alternative agents are clindamycin in the United States or spiramycin, a macrolide, in Canada and Europe. Investigational therapy is on going with azithromycin, a macrolide.

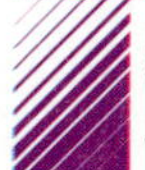

SIDE EFFECTS, CLINICAL PROBLEMS, AND TOXICITY

Although the treatment of protozoal diseases with drugs is usually successful when the treatment is begun before the disease has reached an advanced state, these drugs have serious side effects and toxicities that need to be understood. These problems are likely to become more prevalent with the growing need to increase drug concentrations in an attempt to overcome resistances to the drugs that are developing in these organisms. The clinical problems are summarized in the box.

CLINICAL PROBLEMS

ANTIMALARIAL AGENTS

Development of organism resistance to chloroquine
primaquine/cloroquine: hemolysis with use in glucose-6-phosphate dehydrogenase–deficient patients
quinine: CNS effects and cinchonism, cardiac, side effects
quinidine: cardiac side effects
pyrimethamine-sulfadoxine: may produce Stevens-Johnson syndrome

ANTILEISHMANIASIS AGENTS

pentamidine isethionate: hypotension, pancreatic β cell toxicity
amphotericin B: serious nephrotoxicity, fever

ANTITRYPANOSOMIASIS AGENTS

Nausea and vomiting with most agents
Impaired vision and even blindness with tryparsamide

ANTIAMEBIASIS AGENTS

metronidazole: disulfiramlike reaction to alcohol, seizures, peripheral neuropathy, metal taste, GI upset.
emetine: cardiac dysrhythmias.
iodoquinol: requires monitoring of thyroid function

Antimalarial Agents

Chloroquine has little toxicity unless overdosing occurs, in which case progressive retinopathy, skin lesions, ototoxicity, cardiac depression, and heart block can occur. Pruritus, vomiting, and headache can occur with normal doses, *P. falciparum* resistance to chloroquine is widespread, thus limiting the usefulness of this relatively safe agent. Chemically related mefloquin mefloquine has minimal toxicity but can cause mental confusion and seizures and is not recommended for an individual with a convulsive disorder. Primaquine has gastrointestinal side effects and, if administered to glucose-6-phosphate dehydrogenase–deficient patients, leads to hemolysis.

The side effects associated with quinine are many. This drug has a narrow therapeutic index, and toxicity occurs at concentrations only slightly above those needed for a parasiticidal effect. CNS effects, such as analgesia, antipyresis, and hypotension occur. Blood dyscrasias and *cinchonism,* which manifests as tinnitus, headache, nausea, and visual and hearing disturbances, are also associated with clinical use of quinine. An oral overdose or IV administration can result in cardiac depression.

Pyrimethamine is relatively free of problems at prophylactic doses but may produce a folic acid deficiency and severe leukopenia or thrombocytopenia, with the former reversible by administration of folinic acid. The pyrimethamine-sulfadoxine preparation may produce Stevens-Johnson syndrome, which can be lethal.

Antileishmaniasis Agents

Sodium stibogluconate is relatively safe, with muscle pains, joint stiffness, and bradycardia the principal side effects. The second-line drugs for treatment of leishmaniasis must be used much more carefully. Pentamidine isethionate produces serious hypotension when administered IV; therefore care is needed during any other parenteral form of administration of this drug. Hypoglycemia and blood dyscrasias are additional side effects that may be seen. The other second-line drug, amphotericin B, may produce serious nephrotoxicity and hypokalemia. (See Chapter 51 for further discussion of side effects.)

Antitrypanosomiasis Agents

Melarsoprol is a highly toxic agent and may cause mild myocardial damage, hypertension, colic, and vomiting but is less toxic than tryparsamide. Vomiting, nausea, impaired vision, and blindness are associated with long-term use of tryparsamide and thus limit extensive dosing with this agent. Suramin causes vomiting, pruritus, urticaria, photophobia, and peripheral neuropathy. Hypotension, hypoglycemia with pancreatic islet β cell destruction leading to diabetes, and blood dyscrasias are associated with pentamidine isethionate. Rarely it causes renal toxicity. Eflornithine causes nausea, emesis and diarrhea.

Nifurtimox and benznidazole, used in the treatment of Chagas's disease, produce gastrointestinal upsets and rashes. Nifurtimox may also cause anorexia, tremors, paresthesia, and polyneuritis. The benznidazole rash is intensified by light.

TRADE NAMES

In addition to generic and fixed-combination preparations, the following trade-named materials are available in the United States.

Aralen Hydrochloride, chloroquine HCl
Aralen Phosphate, chloroquine/primaquine phosphates
Arsobal, melarsoprol
Atabrine, quinacrine HCl
Daraprim, pyrimethamine
Fansidar, pyrimethamine-sulfadoxine
Flagyl, Protostat, metronidazole
Lampit, nifurtimox
Lariam, mefloquine HCl
Ornidyl, eflornithine
Pentam, pentamidine isethionate
Pentostam sodium, stibogluconate
Plaquenil, hydroxychloroquine sulfate
Yodoxin, iodoquinol

Antiamebiasis Agents

The side effects seen with diloxanide furoate, paromomycin, and metronidazole are mainly annoying and not substantive at normal concentrations. Diloxamide furoate may produce flatulence, nausea, or vomiting, and paromomycin may cause gastrointestinal disturbances. Metronidazole may cause nausea, headache, a disulfiramlike reaction with alcohol peripheral neuropathy, and seizures (see Chapter 19). Patients receiving iodoquinol may experience a rash, diarrhea, enlargement of the thyroid, and blindness with long-term therapy.

Considerable toxicity is associated with the use of emetine or dehydroemetine. Cardiac toxicity, especially arrhythmias, are common and can occur after the drug is no longer administered. Muscle weakness and diarrhea may also develop.

Antigiardiasis and Antitrichomoniasis Agents

Metronidazole is discussed previously; quinacrine side effects are mild but include dizziness, headache, metallic taste, gastrointestinal upset, vomiting, and occasional psychosis.

REFERENCES

Campbell WC, Rew RS, editors: *Chemotherapy of parasitic diseases,* ed 2, New York, 1995 Plenum Publishing.

Cook GC: Prevention and treatment of malaria, *Lancet* 1:32, 1988.

Miller KD, Greenberg AE, Campbell CC: Treatment of severe malaria in the United States with a continuous infusion of quinidine gluconate and exchange transfusion, *N Engl J Med* 321:65, 1989.

Monk JP, Benfield P: Inhaled pentamidine, *Drugs* 39:741, 1990.

Van Voorhis WC: Therapy and prophylaxis of systemic protozoan infections, *Drugs* 40:176, 1990.

SELF-ASSESSMENT QUESTIONS

1. Which of the following drugs or drug combinations would you select to treat a case of malaria caused by *Plasmodium vivax* ?
   a. chloroquine and primaquine
   b. quinine
   c. quinine, pyrimethamine, sulfadiazine
   d. mefloquine
   e. metronidazole
2. A 23-year-old male is seen in the ER with severe abdominal pain and protracted diarrhea. Microscopic stool examination reveals the presence of both *Entamoeba histolytica* and *Giardia lamblia*. Serology shows positive results for *E. histolytica*. Which of the following would you use to treat this individual?
   a. Administer metrifonate for both parasites.
   b. Administer diloxanide furoate for amebiasis and quinacrine for giardiasis.
   c. Administer metronidazole for both parasites.
   d. Administer mebendazole for both parasites.
   e. Administer diloxanide furoate for the amebiasis and ignore the giardiasis because it will probably be self-limiting.
3. Eflornithine, an inhibitor of ornithine decarboxylase, is useful for the treatment of which of the following?
   a. Chagas's disease
   b. leishmaniasis
   c. giardiasis
   d. African trypanosomiasis
   e. amebiasis
4. A 31-year-old woman patient presents with rapid onset of shaking chills, high fever, and profuse sweating. Her history reveals that she returned 1 week earlier from a trip to Zaïre. While there, she recalls being bitten repeatedly by mosquitoes. She assures you that she faithfully adhered to a prophylactic regimen of chloroquine phosphate. What action do you take?
   a. Draw blood samples for both thick and thin smears and wait for the results before selecting a drug based on the definitive parasitological diagnosis.
   b. Draw blood samples and order smears, but immediately begin a course of chloroquine therapy.
   c. Draw blood samples and order smears, but immediately begin a course of primaquine therapy.
   d. Draw blood samples and order smears, but immediately begin a course of quinine sulfate.
   e. Administer an antipyretic and wait 48 hours to see if the febrile episode is cyclic.
5. The drug of first choice for the treatment of tissue forms of leishmaniasis is:
   a. meglumine antimoniate
   b. metronidazole
   c. mebendazole
   d. melarsoprol
   e. ivermectin

CHAPTER 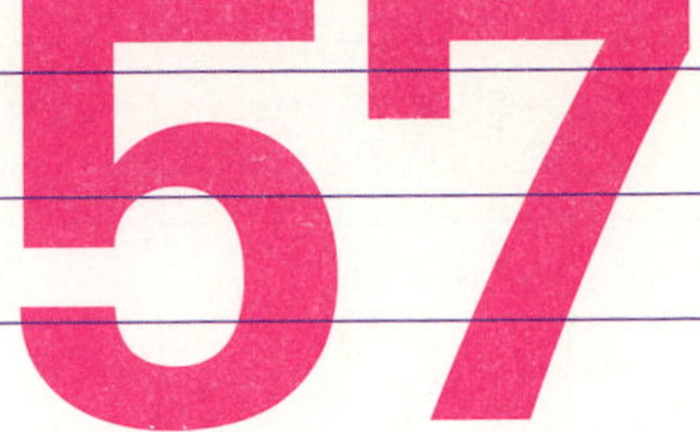

Antiseptics and Disinfectants

PAUL D. ELLNER
HAROLD C. NEU

MAJOR DRUGS

- halogens
- alcohol
- phenols
- organic mercurials
- chlorine compounds
- aldehydes
- quaternary ammonium compounds
- oxidizing agents
- gases
- alkylating agents
- chlorhexidine
- silver salts
- dyes

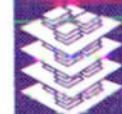

THERAPEUTIC OVERVIEW

Agents described in this chapter are not taken internally and are not used to treat disease but are employed to prevent infection by destroying or limiting the growth of microorganisms on foreign surfaces and on skin. In contrast to other antimicrobial agents, antiseptics and disinfectants lack specificity.

Sterility is the complete absence of all forms of microbial life. Substances, instruments, or devices that are introduced into normally sterile areas of the body must be free of microbes. Sterilization is best accomplished by heat—steam under pressure that provides 121°C for 15 minutes or dry heat that produces 160° to 180°C for 3 hours. Thermolabile solutions may be sterilized by passage through membrane filters that have a pore size of 0.22 μm. Optically clear solutions may also be sterilized by exposure to 254 nm ultraviolet radiation for doses of approximately 200,000 microwatt-sec/cm^2. Lensed instruments or prosthetic devices may be sterilized by high-voltage electron or gamma radiation. More often, such materials are subjected to "cold sterilization," that is, exposure to ethylene oxide gas or immersion in solutions of glutaraldehyde or alcoholic formaldehyde (20% formalin in 70% ethanol or isopropanol).

Antisepsis

Living tissue such as skin or mucous membranes cannot be sterilized, but one can minimize the risk of infection by reducing the number of microorganisms on such tissues. Antiseptics are applied to living tissues to inhibit microorganism growth. These agents are used in presurgical scrubs of the surgeon's hands and applied to the patient's skin before incisions or injections are made. The degerming action is only temporary; bacterial multiplication resumes after minutes or hours. Antiseptics may be used as solutions or incorporated into soaps, salves, ointments, dressings, mouthwashes, or douches. Commonly used antiseptics are listed in the box.

Disinfection

Sterility is not necessary in many clinical situations. Instruments used in anatomic locations normally inhabited by indigenous microorganisms, such as thermometers, specula, or proctoscopes, need not be sterile; they must be rendered free of microbial pathogens, however. It is often necessary to block the transfer of pathogens from patient to patient by fomites or other inanimate objects or surfaces. This process of destroying pathogens, termed *disinfection,* does not necessarily achieve complete sterility. Disinfectants kill pathogenic microorganisms and are used on inanimate objects or surfaces. Agents used as disinfectants include halogen-containing compounds, phenols, quaternary ammonium compounds, aldehydes, and oxidizing agents. Table 57-1 lists disinfectants currently in use.

Table 57-1 Disinfectants Commonly Used in Hospitals in the United States

Use	Agent
Cold sterilization of catheters, endoscopic instruments	Ethylene oxide Glutaraldehyde Alcoholic formaldehyde Oxidizers
For thermometers	Ethyl alcohol (ethanol)
Disinfection of floors, walls, and other surfaces	Phenolic compounds Iodophors Quaternary ammonium compounds Chlorine compounds

Table 57-2 Antiseptics and Disinfectants Listed by Mechanism of Action

Mode of Action	Agent
Oxidation	Hydrogen peroxide Ozone Peracetic acid Chlorine compounds
Alkylation	Ethylene oxide β-Propiolactone Formaldehyde Glutaraldehyde
Protein denaturation	Alcohols Phenolic compounds Iodine Heavy metals
Surface active agent	Quaternary ammonium compounds
Cation ionization	Dyes
Membrane damage	Chlorhexidine

Bacterial Inhibition versus Elimination

Antiseptics and disinfectants may be characterized as **bacteriostatic**—inhibiting the growth of bacteria, or **bactericidal**—and kill most vegetative forms of bacteria. Bactericidal agents are not necessarily effective against spores, *Mycobacterium tuberculosis,* fungi, or viruses unless specifically designated as sporicidal, tuberculocidal, fungicidal, or virucidal. Certain agents have been termed **sterilants,** since they can effectively sterilize inanimate objects or surfaces when used appropriately. Sterilants include ethylene oxide, glutaraldehyde, alcoholic formaldehyde, 20% formalin in 70% ethanol or isopropanol β-propiolactone, peracetic acid, and chlorine dioxide.

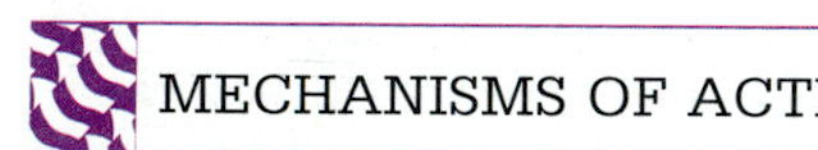

MECHANISMS OF ACTION

The mode of action of this diverse group of substances varies and, in many cases, is not well understood. Some are highly reactive oxidizing or alkylating agents and, as such, may be considered as general protoplasmic poisons. Most damage microbial cell walls or cytoplasmic membranes by denaturing proteins, lowering surface tension, or inhibiting essential enzymes. The effectiveness of these chemical agents is almost always influenced by concentration, temperature, and time of exposure. The agents are listed by their general mechanism of action in Table 57-2.

Alcohols

The commonly used alcohols are ethanol (C_2H_5OH) and isopropanol ($CH_3CH(OH)CH_3$). The bactericidal activity of aliphatic alcohols increases with increasing chain length to a maximum of 5 to 8 carbon atoms. Unbranched chains are more active than the iso configuration; tertiary alcohols are the least active. The most effective alcohol concentrations are 60% to 70%, with the activity greatly decreasing above 95% and below 60%.

Alcohols probably act as protein-denaturing agents. At low concentrations they may be used as substrates for some bacteria, but at higher concentrations dehydrogenation reactions are inhibited. Some microorganisms are lysed by alcohols.

Ethyl and isopropyl alcohols are rapidly bactericidal and are highly effective against vegetative gram-positive and gram-negative bacteria, tubercle bacilli, the pathogenic fungi, and many viruses, especially those with lipid coats. Alcohol has no effect on bacterial spores.

Alcohol is used alone or in combination with other agents as a surgical antiseptic. It evaporates rapidly and produces excessive dryness of the skin, but emollients can be added to reduce this effect.

Alcohol is also used as a disinfectant for clinical thermometers.

Halogens

Iodine and Iodophors Iodine precipitates proteins and oxidizes essential enzymes. It is rapidly bactericidal and tuberculocidal, and active against many viruses and pathogenic fungi at concentrations as low as 0.05%. Activity against spores requires prolonged exposure times.

Elemental iodine dissolves in aqueous potassium iodide, alcohol, or ether. It can also be solubilized by complexation with cationic or nonionic surfactants; such complexes are known as **iodophors.** Although iodine is effective over a wide pH range, more free iodine (the active form) is released at low pH values.

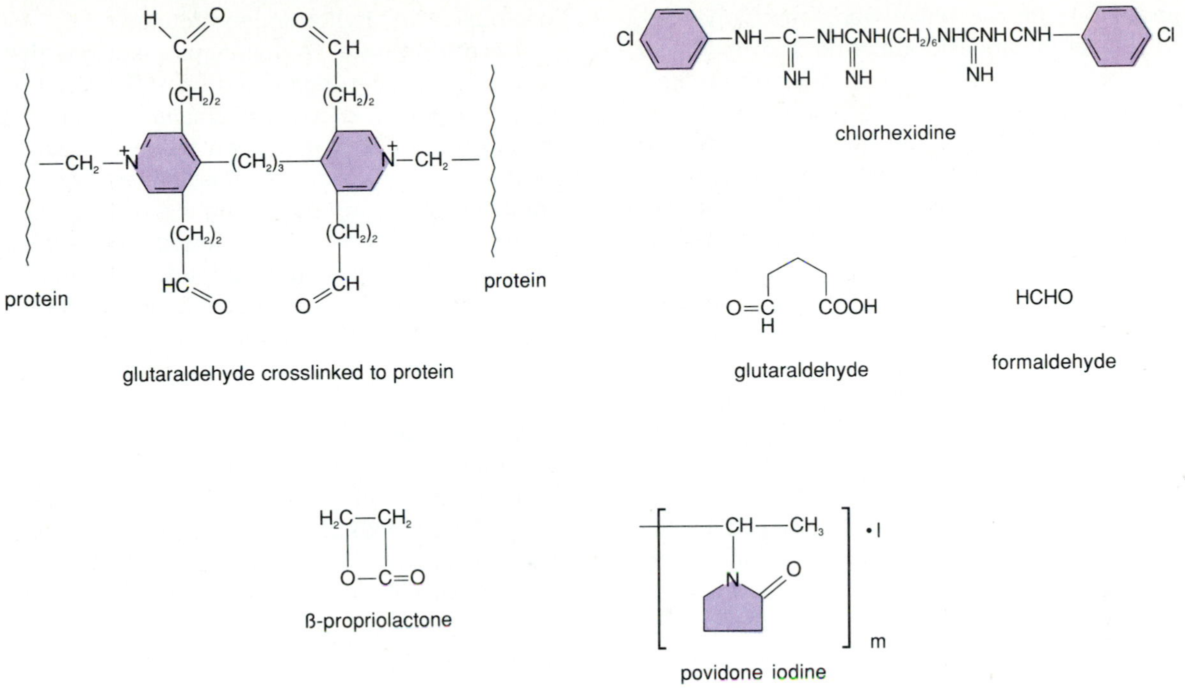

glutaraldehyde crosslinked to protein

chlorhexidine

glutaraldehyde

formaldehyde

ß-propriolactone

povidone iodine

FIGURE 57-1 Structures of antiseptics and disinfectants. See the text for further information.

Iodine acts by several mechanisms. It reacts with NH groups of nucleotide bases and some amino acids to prevent hydrogen bonding and iodinates the ring of aromatic amino acids and of histidine. The sulfhydryl group of cysteine is oxidized to a disulfide cross-link, interfering with protein synthesis and activity. Iodine also reacts with the phenolic group of tyrosine, causing steric phenolic hindrance in hydrogen bonding of the phenolic hydroxyl group. In addition, iodine interacts with the carbon-carbon double bond of unsaturated fatty acids, altering the properties of lipids and their role in membrane stabilization.

Iodine is used as an antiseptic and a disinfectant. As a skin antiseptic, Iodine Solution (2% iodine + 2.4% potassium iodide) and Iodine Tincture (2% iodine, 2.4% potassium iodine, and 44% to 50% alcohol) are used. Tincture of iodine should be dated, and discarded when outdated, because the iodine concentration increases as the alcohol-water component evaporates. Concentrations of iodine in excess of 3% may produce skin blistering. Burns can result if skin treated with tincture of iodine is covered with an occlusive dressing. Tincture of iodine should always be removed from the skin with 70% alcohol after completion of a surgical procedure.

Disadvantages of the tincture or solution of iodine are staining of skin and fabrics, skin sensitization, irritation and pain at wounds and mucocutaneous junctions, and corrosion of many metals.

Povidone-iodine iodophors (Figure 57-1), prepared by complexing iodine with polyvinylpyrrolidone, are widely used. Povidone-iodine complex is more stable than the tincture at normal ambient temperatures, much less irritating to tissues, and less corrosive to metals: fabric stains are readily removed. However, the cost is significantly higher than the tincture and the staining of some plastics is reported. Povidone-iodine is toxic to exposed fibroblasts; thus irrigation of open wounds with this substance may delay healing.

Surfactant iodine iodophors are used as disinfectants of floor areas, work surfaces, and food-handling utensils. Iodine is also used for disinfection of clinical thermometers and other instruments, and for the emergency disinfection of drinking water.

Mercurial Compounds Organic mercurial compounds have a weak bacteriostatic action and are less effective than alcohols. Serum reduces antimicrobial action, and skin sensitization can occur. Only thimerosal is available for topical use. Mercury compounds should not be applied to large areas of denuded skin. Ingestion can cause renal failure. Dimercaprol is an effective antidote.

Chlorine and Chlorine Compounds Aqueous solutions of chlorine exhibit rapid bactericidal action. Elemental chlorine reacts with water to form hypochlorous acid, but how hypochlorous acid destroys microorganisms is not clear. It may liberate nascent oxygen, which in turn oxidizes essential components of protoplasm. Or perhaps chlorine combines with cell membrane proteins to form *N*-chloro compounds that interfere with cellular metabolism. Chlorine oxidizes the sulfhydryl groups of certain enzymes, causing irreversible inactivation.

The active free chlorine and hypochlorous acid are in pH-dependent equilibrium, with rapid bactericidal, tuberculocidal, and, in many cases, virucidal actions at concentrations of 0.2 to 2.0 parts per million of available chlorine. Pathogenic fungi are more resistant and require a minimum of 100 parts per million of available chlorine. The activity of chlorine compounds increases as the concentration of available chlorine increases. In practice, concentrations of 2000 parts per million or more of available chlorine are used. With each 10°C rise in temperature, the activity of chlorine increases approximately 50%.

Chlorine is no longer used as an antiseptic because of its irritant effects and inactivation by organic matter. However, it is widely employed as a disinfectant of municipal water supplies. Its activity is quickly inhibited by dirt or extraneous material, as well as by soap or highly alkaline detergent solutions.

Widely used chlorine compounds are sodium and calcium hypochlorites, which act through nascent release of hypochlorous acid.

Chlorine dioxide is more rapidly sporicidal than hypochlorous acid, and proprietary binary systems, in which two components are mixed to produce chlorine dioxide, are useful as sterilants and disinfectants. Another compound, chlorite, is activated with an organic acid to chlorous acid, which slowly converts to chlorine dioxide, chloride, and chlorate ions.

Chloramines are produced by the reaction of hypochlorous acid on an amine, amide, imine, or imide. Organic chloramines are *N*-chloro derivatives of sulfonamides, heterocyclic nitrogen compounds, guanidine derivatives, or anilides. Various chloramine compounds have from 25% to 29% available chlorine, depending on the formulation. In general, *N*-chloro compounds are much slower in action than hypochlorites, but under acid conditions they are more effective bactericides.

Halazone, or *p*-sulfondichloramidobenzoic acid, is used for emergency water disinfection. A 4 mg halazone tablet is sufficient to render 1 liter of water safe to drink after 30 minutes. It will not inhibit *Cryptosporidium.*

Aldehydes

Aldehydes act by alkylation. Even in low concentrations, exposure of bacteria to formaldehyde (see Figure 57-1) results in accumulation of 1,3-thiazine-4-carboxylic acid, an inhibitor of methionine formation. The action of glutaraldehyde may involve reaction with bacterial sulfhydryl or amino groups.

Formaldehyde Formaldehyde is a gas that is irritating to the eyes, nose, and skin. Solutions of formaldehyde in water, known as *formalin,* contain 37% to 40% formaldehyde. At low concentrations, formaldehyde is bacteriostatic; growth of most vegetative bacteria is inhibited by 20 μg/ml. Stronger solutions, such as 8% aqueous formaldehyde (20% formalin), are bactericidal, sporicidal, tuberculocidal, and fungicidal and inactivate most viruses. The germicidal action of formaldehyde is increased by combination with alcohol; 20% formalin in 70% alcohol can be used to disinfect metal instruments.

Glutaraldehyde Glutaraldehyde (Figure 57-1) is more potent and less irritating than formaldehyde. It is more active in an alkaline environment, but when "activated" with sodium hydroxide, it has a shorter useful life. It is sporicidal and viricidal, including HIV-1. Glutaraldehyde solutions are inactivated by proteins; hence instruments must be washed before use. Glutaraldehyde must be removed from instruments by sterile water immersion; otherwise it will cause burns to skin or mucous membranes.

Phenolic Compounds

Although phenol is no longer used as a disinfectant or antiseptic, it is used as a reference compound for evaluation of other germicidal compounds. Compounds are compared in a standardized manner for antibacterial effectiveness against phenol to give values known as the **phenol coefficient.**

Halogenation of phenolic compounds potentiates their germicidal effectiveness, with *para* substitution to the hydroxyl being more effective than *ortho.* Bactericidal potency of halogenated phenols is further increased by introduction of aliphatic or aromatic groups into the nucleus. For example, *ortho*-alkyl derivatives of *p*-chlorophenol are more actively germicidal than *para*-alkyl derivatives of *o*-chlorophenols. Numerous synthetic phenols, such as *o*-phenylphenol, *p*-chlorobenzylphenol, and *p*-*tert*-amylphenol, are used as disinfectants. These substances are not inactivated by soap or organic soil and at 2% to 3% concentrations kill vegetative bacteria, tubercle bacilli, pathogenic fungi, and most lipophilic viruses, but they are not sporicidal. Spores of *Clostridium difficile* will persist on surfaces soiled with feces. Combinations of these compounds with synthetic detergents make ideal disinfectants for cleaning and disinfection of hospital floors and other hard surfaces.

Derivatives of dihydroxyphenol or resorcinol have some germicidal activity, and hexylresorcinol is employed as a topical antiseptic. Its use is limited by hepatic and myocardial toxicity and production of burns on skin and mucous membranes.

Bisphenols, two phenolic moieties linked together, possess high bacteriostatic activity. Similar to other phenolic compounds, halogenation increases the antibacterial effectiveness, particularly with gram-positive bacteria. One example, hexachlorophene, is used extensively in antiseptic soaps, with a residual film on the skin being bacteriostatic primarily for gram-positive bacteria, but such action develops only when hexachlorophene-containing soaps are used frequently and repeatedly. There is evidence that repeated use of hexachlorophene soaps causes an increase in gram-negative flora of skin. Earlier widely used 3% emulsions of hexachlorophene for preoperative scrubs, washes for neonates, and washes for burn patients have been discontinued because of absorption from the skin into the *systemic circulation,* resulting in serious central nervous system toxicity including spongiform degeneration of the brain. The use of hexachlorophene in deodorant soaps and cosmetics is banned by the Food and Drug Administration.

Phenylcarbamides, salicylanilides, and carbamilides also are used in soaps and cosmetics for skin degerming. Many of these compounds have pronounced antifungal activity but are not sporicidal. Brominated salicylanilides and trifluoromethylated salicylanilides are effective as soap germicides, particularly in low concentrations.

Chlorhexidine

Chlorhexidine (see Figure 57-1) has pronounced antimicrobial activity against gram-positive and gram-negative bacteria and many yeasts and molds. But tubercle bacilli, bacterial spores, *Aspergillus* (filamentous fungi), and viruses are not susceptible.

Chlorhexidine is absorbed on the cell surface, resulting in disorganization of the bacterial cytoplasmic membrane. Low concentrations promote leakage of cytoplasmic constituents. Chlorhexidine inhibits membrane-bound adenosine-triphosphatase, and, at the higher concentrations used for antiseptic purposes, rapidly coagulates cytoplasmic constituents.

Like hexachlorophene, chlorhexidine remains on the skin to give a cumulative and continuing antibacterial effect that persists for at least 6 hours on gloved hands.

Chlorhexidine is effective in the presence of blood and organic matter, is nonirritating, and is not absorbed from intact skin or mucous membranes into the blood. A preparation of 5% chlorhexidine and 4% isopropanol is widely used in Europe as a "frequent-use" alcohol-based hand wash.

Quaternary Ammonium Compounds

Quaternary ammonium compounds are cationic ammonium compounds with significant antibacterial activity when one of the four organic groups used in this class is between 8 and 18 carbons long. Representative compounds are benzalkonium chloride (alkylbenzyldimethylammonium chloride) and cetylpyridinium chloride (1-hexadecylpyridinium chloride).

Quaternary ammonium compounds are odorless, soluble in water and alcohol, and relatively nontoxic and nonirritating to tissues. Their mode of action is primarily through denaturation of cell membrane and cytoplasm components to produce release of nitrogen and potassium from the cells. Lipoprotein complexes throughout the cell are split, liberating autolytic enzymes. Quaternary ammonium compounds are bacteriostatic at low and bactericidal and fungicidal at higher concentrations. Certain organisms, such as *Pseudomonas aeruginosa, Mycobacterium tuberculosis, Trichophyton rubrum,* and *T. interdigitale,* are resistant to these agents. Indeed, *P. aeruginosa* and *P. cepacia* grow in solutions containing quaternary compounds. Viruses, in general, are more resistant than bacteria and fungi, and they are not effective against bacterial spores.

The quaternary ammonium compounds are neutralized by soaps and anionic detergents, and their activity is greatly decreased by organic matter and by dilution with hard water. They are selectively absorbed by fabrics, gauze, and cotton, and so a 1:1000 aqueous solution becomes a 1:2000 solution in the presence of cotton or gauze, permitting the growth of organisms such as *Pseudomonas.* The use of such contaminated solutions has resulted in many severe and fatal nosocomial infections. It is recommended that when aqueous quaternary ammonium compounds are used for antiseptics before surgical procedures they be dispensed as autoclaved solutions of 1:500 in quantities sufficient only for a single use. When used for antiseptic purposes, they are more effective as tinctures (i.e., 1:1000 diluted with 70% alcohol).

A 1% to 2% benzalkonium solution is a preferred topical agent in the treatment or prophylaxis of bite wounds from animals suspected of having rabies. However, the individual should receive rabies antiglobulin and a rabies vaccine.

A final rinse of quaternary ammonium compounds is used to impregnate the fabric of hospital gowns and bed linens to assist destruction of microorganisms in the laundry process. Control of "diaper rash" is achieved by this process by suppression of disease-producing bacteria. Quaternary ammonium compounds are also used to sanitize utensils and food-processing equipment. Care must be used by thorough rinsing of such items to avoid potential toxicity.

Oxidizing Agents

Hydrogen Peroxide The active agent of hydrogen peroxide is believed to be the hydroxyl free radical formed by the decomposition of hydrogen peroxide and possibly by the reduction of oxygen to superoxide. The hydroxyl free radical can attack membrane lipids, DNA, and other essential components of the cell. (See Chapter 56)

Hydrogen peroxide (3% to 6%) is bactericidal and virucidal; higher concentrations (10% to 25%) are sporicidal.

Hydrogen peroxide is used for disinfection of plastic implants, contact lenses, and surgical prostheses.

The presence of catalase, which inactivates peroxide, limits the usefulness of hydrogen peroxide as an antiseptic. Hydrogen peroxide is toxic to fibroblasts and may delay wound healing. Cleansing of deep wounds and lacerations with hydrogen peroxide under pressure is contraindicated because this practice has resulted in subcutaneous gas formation.

(Other oxidizing agents such as ozone and peracetic acid are discussed under sterilant gases.)

Sterilant Gases

Formaldehyde Formaldehyde is available commercially in aqueous solutions containing up to 40% of the gas (see aldehyde section). It is also available as paraformaldehyde, a solid polymer that contains 91% to 99% formaldehyde. Paraformaldehyde sublimes rapidly when heated above 150°C. The action of formaldehyde is discussed in an earlier section.

Ethylene Oxide Ethylene oxide is a colorless gas at room temperature that is soluble in water and most organic solvents and readily penetrates porous materials. Ethylene oxide is flammable and explosive; thus for practical use, it is diluted with inert gases such as carbon dioxide to 10% ethylene oxide. Ethylene oxide has a high temperature coefficient, with each 10°C increase in temperature reducing the time for sterilization by about 50%. Doubling the concentration also halves the time required to achieve sterility. The lethal effect of ethylene oxide on microorganisms depends on moisture, with maximum sporicidal activity at 28% relative humidity.

Ethylene oxide acts by alkylation, especially of terminal carboxyl, amino, sulfhydryl, and hydroxyl moieties on proteins. It also alkylates nucleic acids at the N-7 position of guanine.

Ethylene oxide is effective against all types of microorganisms, including bacterial and fungal spores, vegetative cells, rickettsiae, and viruses. It has a more rapid sporicidal action than formaldehyde. Its main advantage is that it can be used to sterilize medical and laboratory equipment that might be damaged by other sterilizing methods, especially those requiring elevated temperatures.

A disadvantage of the use of ethylene oxide is its slow action as a sterilant. The sterilizing time can be shortened somewhat if one increases the temperature, the concentration, or the pressure. The use of heat and pressure requires a special chamber. Ethylene oxide is absorbed by many materials. Thus plastics or instruments that may be in contact with patient skin or mucous membranes must be aerated for 24 hours or longer to remove all traces of the gas. Polycarbonates and various plastics will release products that can cause tissue damage. This has led to tracheal stenosis when ethylene oxide–sterilized tracheal tubes were not adequately aerated before use in intensive care units.

β-Propiolactone β-Propiolactone (see Figure 57-1) is a colorless liquid at room temperature that is effective as a vapor-phase decontaminant against vegetative cells, bacterial spores, pathogenic fungi, viruses, and rickettsiae.

β-Propiolactone is a strong alkylating agent and functions like ethylene oxide. Moisture is necessary and a relative humidity of 70% or greater is required for decontamination. It is more rapidly sporicidal than ethylene oxide, but its penetrating power is poor.

β-Propiolactone has strong lacrimator, respiratory irritant, and vesicant but weak carcinogenic properties. It has been used to disinfect hospital rooms, operating rooms, military barracks, and animal housing, but its many detrimental properties limit its use as a hospital disinfectant.

Since the decomposition products of β-propiolactone are harmless, the compound is used to sterilize blood plasma and other biologicals for medical use.

Peracetic Acid Peracetic acid is a pungent-smelling compound that is available commercially as a 40% solution. It is unstable, slowly decomposing to acetic acid, hydrogen peroxide, water, and oxygen. Its undesirable properties include those of lacrimator, respiratory irritant, vesicant, and corrosive action on metals.

Peracetic acid is highly reactive, oxidizing many organic compounds, and may be regarded as a general protoplasmic poison. It is rapidly bactericidal and sporicidal but, like other sterilant gases, requires a high relative humidity. Peracetic acid is used primarily as a solution for disinfection but is also active in the gas phase.

Ozone Ozone, highly unstable O_3, is used primarily for water purification, showing better effectiveness than chlorine for rapidly killing bacteria, viruses, and the cysts of enteric parasites. Unlike chlorine, ozone leaves no residual taste or odor and does not produce toxic chlorinated organic products in waste water.

TRADE NAMES

In addition to generic and fixed-combination preparations, the following trade-named materials are available in the United States.

Zephiran, Ionax Scrub, benzalkonium chloride
Diaparene, methylbenzethonium chloride
Betadine, Isodine, povidone-iodine
Clorpactin XCB, oxychlorosene
pHisoHex, Septisoft, hexachlorophene
Hibiclens, chlorhexidine gluconate
Cidex, glutaraldehyde

Little-Used Materials

Silver compounds, triphenylmethane dyes, and acridine dyes are used only in special situations. Free silver ions are cytotoxic to bacteria, forming silver-protein complexes that concentrate in the cytoplasmic membrane. Silver nitrate solution is still used for routine prophylactic instillation into the eyes of newborn infants to prevent gonococcal infections. Silver sulfadiazine cream (1%) is effective in the prevention of infection in severely burned individuals (see Chapter 50).

Triphenylmethane dyes such as crystal violet, brilliant green, and parafuchsin were formerly used as local antiseptics on wounds and burns. They were limited to bacteriostatic effects against gram-positive organisms, and their activity was greatly decreased by proteins. The acridine dyes acriflavine and proflavine differ from the triphenylmethane dyes in their activity against gram-negative and gram-positive bacteria and by their effectiveness in the presence of serum. The acridines bind to DNA, RNA, and other proteins to inhibit DNA synthesis, with proflavin inhibiting DNA and RNA polymerases. These dyes were formerly used to treat infected wounds and act slowly against vegetative cells but not spores. They are no longer used because of their potential carcinogenicity when activated by ultraviolet radiation.

REFERENCES

Ayliffe GAS, Babb JR, Lilly HA: Hand disinfection: a comparison of various agents in laboratory and ward studies, *J Hosp Infect* 11:226, 1988.

Block SS: *Disinfection, sterilization and preservation,* ed 4, Malvern, Penn, 1991, Lea & Febiger.

Gordon V, Parry S, Bellamy K, Osborne R: Assessment of chemical disinfectants against human immunodeficiency virus: overcoming the problem of cytotoxicity and the evaluation of selected actives, *J Virol Meths*: 45:247,1993

Hugo WB, editor: *Inhibition and destruction of the microbial cell,* New York, 1971, Academic Press. London.

Prince DL, Prince HN, Thraenhart O, Muchmore E, Bonder E, Pugh J: Methodological approaches to disinfection of human hepatitis B virus, *J Clin Microbiol*: 31:3296,1993.

Rutala WA, Cole EC, Wannamaker NS, Weber DJ: Inactivation of *Mycobacterium tuberculosis* and *Mycobacterium bovis* by 14 hospital disinfectants, *Am J Med* 91 (suppl 3B):267S,1991.

SELF-ASSESSMENT QUESTIONS

For the following questions, select the statement that is *NOT* true:

1. Agents used as disinfectants to degerm include:
   a. halogen-containing compounds.
   b. quaternary ammonium compounds.
   c. phenols.
   d. oxidizing agents.
   e. All are untrue.
2. Mechanisms of action of disinfectants include:
   a. general protoplasmic poisons.
   b. protein denaturation.
   c. lowering surface tension.
   d. inhibiting essential enzymes.
   e. All are untrue.
3. Which statement applies to iodine-containing disinfectants?
   a. They act by protein denaturation and precipitation.
   b. Iodine-containing compounds act by oxidizing essential enzymes.
   c. Iodine compounds are bactericidal and act on tubercle bacilli, viruses, and fungi as well.
   d. Active iodine is released from iodophors most effectively at high pH.
4. Which statement applies to chlorine compounds?
   a. They are effective disinfectants with bactericidal actions.
   b. Hypochlorous acid acts as an oxidizing agent to denature proteins.
   c. Chlorine is widely used as a disinfectant.
   d. Chlorine can be virucidal and fungicidal at similar concentrations.

5. Phenols are effective disinfectants in what way?
   a. Halogenated phenols are more active than phenol.
   b. Halogenated phenols are nontoxic.
   c. Halogenated phenols and the other phenols act by protein denaturation.
   d. Halogenated phenols are widely used to clean and disinfect hard surfaces and floors in hospitals.
6. For the following questions, which answer is true?
   a. At 100% concentration, alcohol is an effective disinfectant.
   b. Branched-chain alcohols are more effective than straight-chain ones.
   c. Ethyl and isopropyl alcohols are bactericidal.
   d. Alcohol is effective against bacterial spores.
1. Quaternary ammonium compounds:
   a. act as surface active agents to denature cell proteins.
   b. that are between 8 and 18 carbons long are most effective.
   c. are bacteriostatic at low and bactericidal at high concentrations.
   d. are neutralized by soaps and ammonic detergents.
   e. All statements are correct.
8. Oxidizing agents such as hydrogen peroxide:
   a. are used to sterilize plastic implants, surgical prostheses, and contact lenses.
   b. act by means of free radicals to disrupt essential cellular components.
   c. are inactivated by catalase.
   d. are toxic to fibroblasts and thus may delay wound healing.
   e. All are true.

OTHER SYSTEMS AND SPECIAL TOPICS

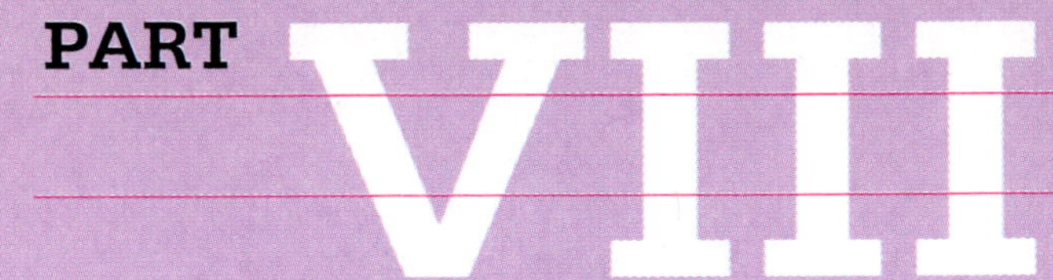

CHAPTER 58

Drugs Used in Asthma and Obstructive Lung Disease

ROBERT S. CALL
THOMAS A. E. PLATT-MILLS

MAJOR DRUGS

cromolyn sodium
inhaled steroids
oral/injectable steroids
β_2-adrenergic agonists
theophylline
ipratropium bromide

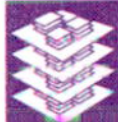

THERAPEUTIC OVERVIEW

Asthma is characterized by obstruction of the airways (predominantly in the third to seventh generation of the bronchi) that is reversible with time or in response to treatment. Even when patients have a normal air flow (which for mild asthmatics is much of the time), their lungs are hyperreactive to a variety of stimuli that occur naturally (e.g., cold air, exercise, chemical fumes) or stimuli used to test the lungs (e.g., methacholine, histamine, cold air). Bronchial hyperreactivity (BHR) correlates with inflammation of the bronchi, which includes damage to the epithelium and an eosinophil infiltration. Symptomatically, patients exhibit chest tightness, wheezing, shortness of breath, or coughing. Mild forms of the disease occur in up to 10% of the population, but asthma requiring regular treatment affects about 2% of the population. Normal bronchial smooth muscle tone is controlled by vagal innervation. In asthmatics cholinergic activity or sensitivity is often increased. However, most patients with asthma also have increased adrenergic activity, which manifests itself as increased wheezing if they are treated with β-adrenergic blocking drugs (e.g., propranolol). A variety of agents can contribute to the inflammation of asthma; however, the most common association with asthma is immediate hypersensitivity to common allergens: the major seasonal allergens outdoors (e.g., ragweed pollen, grass pollen, and the fungus *Alternaria*) or the year-round indoor allergens (dust mites, cockroaches, and domestic animals) (Figure 58-1). Although allergens release histamine and histamine can trigger bronchospasm, antihistamines are relatively ineffective in the treatment of asthma. The probable reason is that other mediators, such as leukotriene D_4, are the primary bronchoconstrictors in man. Compounds that block the synthesis of leukotrienes or block their actions at the receptor may have a major role in the treatment of asthma and are currently being tested (Chapter 18). Calcium-channel blockers (Chapter 16) would be expected to block mediator release from mast cells; however, clinically they have very little effect on asthma, probably because the calcium channels in mast cell membranes are different from those in cardiac muscle. Calcium-channel blockers are the drugs of choice for the treatment of angina or hypertension in asthmatic patients.

There are three main approaches to the treatment of asthma:

1. Avoidance of the causative factors where possible. This is the primary form of treatment in all occupational asthma and an important form of "antiinflammatory" treatment for patients sensitive to indoor allergens.

ABBREVIATIONS

BHR	bronchial hyperreactivity
cAMP	cyclic adenosine monophosphate
COPD	chronic obstructive pulmonary disease
EIA	exercise-induced asthma
FEV_1	forced expiratory volume in 1 second (liters)
MDI	metered dose inhaler

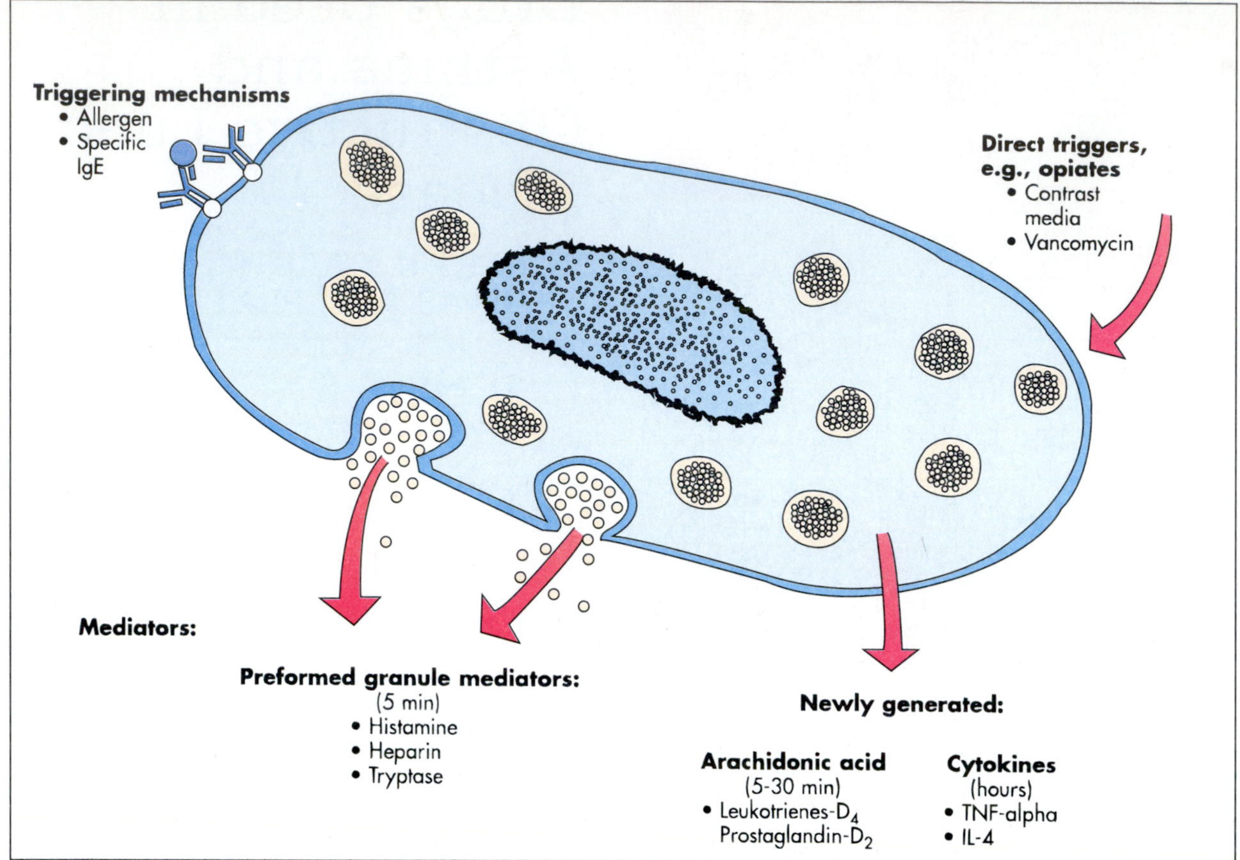

FIGURE 58-1 Mast cell mediator release. *Mediators also produced by basophils. †Tryptase can be assayed in serum or secretions as a marker of mast cell degranulation.

2. Antiinflammatory drugs, which include cromolyn sodium, nedocromil, inhaled steroids, and orally administered steroids. These drugs used regularly can reduce symptoms and bronchial hyperreactivity.
3. Drugs that can reverse bronchoconstriction or inhibit the development of it. These include epinephrine, a range of progressively more selective β_2-adrenergic agonists, xanthines, and the anticholinergic agent ipratropium bromide.

There are three special considerations with asthma treatment: (1) the inhaled route is very important and has special requirements; (2) the pharmacokinetics of drugs used in asthma are primarily based on lung-function response; blood concentrations are relevant only for the xanthines; (3) the most commonly encountered side effects of asthma medicines are short-term side effects of xanthines and cumulative side effects of orally administered steroids. However, because of the large numbers of patients using inhaled steroids or β-adrenergic receptor agonists (or β-agonists), relatively infrequent side effects of these drugs may also be important.

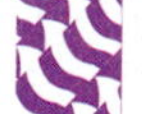

MECHANISM OF ACTION

Cromolyn Sodium

Cromolyn sodium, purified from the umbelliferous plant *Ammi visnaga,* was originally shown to inhibit release of histamine from mast cells in vitro (Figure 58-1). Subsequently it was demonstrated that inhaled cromolyn would inhibit exercise-induced asthma, could progressively decrease bronchial hyperreactivity, and inhibit seasonal rises in bronchial hyperreactivity in patients allergic to grass pollen. Whether these effects are primarily attributable to inhibition of mediator release from mast cells or basophils is not clear. Cromolyn and nedocromil are active only on the lung when given by the inhaled route and have no direct bronchodilator effect (Figure 58-2).

Corticosteroids

Corticosteroids have profound effects on multiple aspects of inflammation in asthma. In mast cells, they

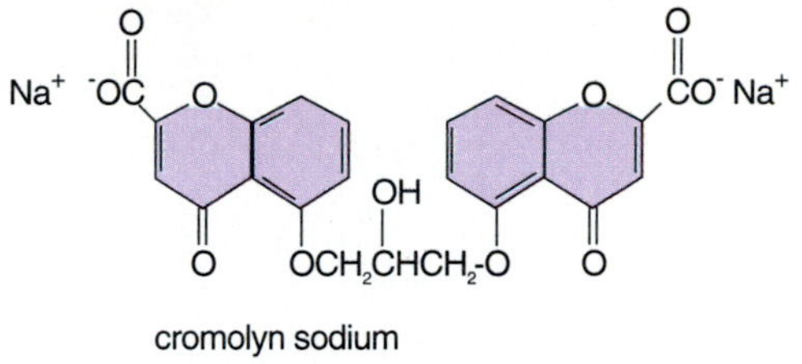

THERAPEUTIC OVERVIEW

GOALS

Reverse acute attacks
Control recurrent attacks
Reduce bronchial inflammation and the associated hyperreactivity

EFFECTS

Cromolyn for control of mediator release from mast cells and other cells; generalized membrane-stabilizing effects
Corticosteroids, local or systemic, for control of edema, mucus production, and eosinophil infiltration (also control of transcription of genes for mediators)
β_2-Agonists, for relaxing smooth muscle and causing vasoconstriction in bronchial mucosa
Theophylline (xanthines), for reduction of recurrent attacks of bronchospasm (adenosine antagonist, phosphodiesterase inhibitor?)
Ipratropium bromide, for inhibition of muscarinic effects of acetylcholine on smooth muscle

USES

β_2-Agonists and ipratropium bromide for short-term control of airway obstruction
Theophylline, steroids, and cromolyn for regular use to control attacks
Avoidance of causative factors (i.e., allergens and triggers); cromolyn sodium and inhaled steroids to control inflammation in bronchi.

have inhibitory effects on the production of arachidonic acid metabolites, such as leukotrienes, prostaglandins, and platelet-activating factor from mast cells. Steroids increase production of lipomodulin in the nucleus, which in turn inhibits the action of phospholipase A to release arachidonic acid (Figure 58-3). In mast cells or T cells, steroids also inhibit production of cytokines such as interleukin-4, interleukin 5, or tumor necrosis factor–α. These steroid effects probably result from an inhibition of nuclear gene transcription. Steroids have profound effects on eosinophils, which may be multifactorial; thus steroids cause decreased bone marrow production of eosinophils and rapid removal of eosinophils from the circulation by adherence of these cells to capillary walls (margination). Steroids also reduce local accumulation of eosinophils secondary to inhibition of the release of eosinophil chemotactic factors such as leukotriene B_4 and the cytokine tumor necrosis factor–α. Steroids have almost the opposite effect on neutrophils, by inhibiting margination and causing increases in peripheral blood counts.

cromolyn sodium

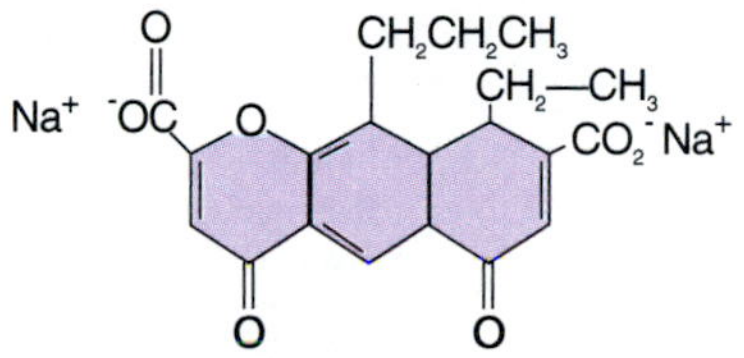

nedocromil sodium

FIGURE 58-2 Chemical structures of cromolyn sodium and nedocromil sodium.

The mechanisms of action of corticosteroids, which reduce inflammatory responses, are shown below.

β_2-Adrenergic Agonists

Epinephrine is a powerful bronchodilator but also has direct effects on the heart and on the peripheral circulation. The bronchodilator effect may be complex but is believed to be primarily attributable to a direct action on β_2-adrenergic receptors of the bronchial smooth

ANTIINFLAMMATORY EFFECTS OF STEROIDS

MECHANISMS OF ACTION OF CORTICOSTEROIDS

Control of eosinophils
- Margination of circulating eosinophils
- Decreased bone marrow production
- Reduced local recruitment

Reduced mucosal edema
- Decreased vascular permeability secondary to vasoconstriction

Increased synthesis and sensitivity of β-adrenergic receptors

CONTROL OF STEROID-RESPONSIVE GENE TRANSCRIPTION

Negative regulatory effects on cytokines, lipoxygenase, endothelin, and possible cyclooxygenase
Positive regulatory effects on lipocortin-1, and β-adrenergic receptors

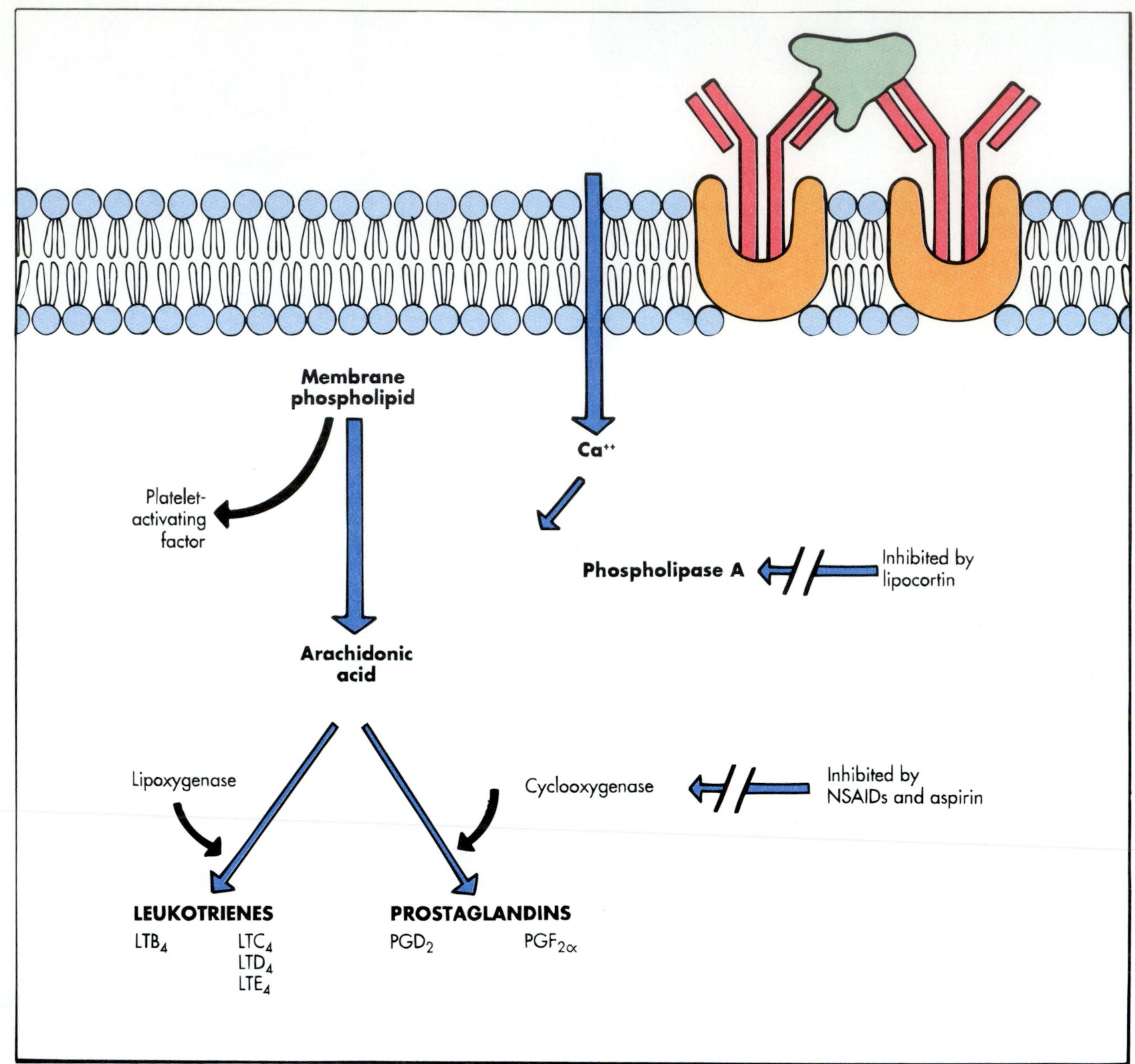

FIGURE 58-3 Newly generated lipid mast cell mediators. Nuclear transcription inhibited by steroids. Specific leukotriene D_4-receptor antagonists are effective in the treatment of asthma. *NSAIDs,* Nonsteroidal antiinflammatory drugs.

muscle. Alternative hypotheses include a vasoconstrictive effect on bronchial vessels and suppression of parasympathetic ganglia. Other β_2-adrenergic receptor agonists include albuterol, terbutaline, pirbuterol, and salmeterol.

Stimulation of β_2-adrenergic receptors raises cyclic adenosine monophosphate (cAMP) concentrations within the cell and inhibits smooth muscle contraction (see Chapter 17). There is no evidence for an antiinflammatory effect of adrenergic agents, or any beneficial effect on bronchial hyperreactivity.

Methylxanthines

Theophylline is a methylxanthine, similar to caffeine (Figure 58-4). It was generally accepted that theophylline caused bronchodilatation by acting on smooth muscle cells to inhibit cAMP phosphodiesterase. Although an increase in cAMP leads to bronchodilatation, the clinical significance of the phosphodiesterase-inhibition mechanism is questionable because concentrations required to inhibit this enzyme exceed those achieved with usual doses of theophylline.

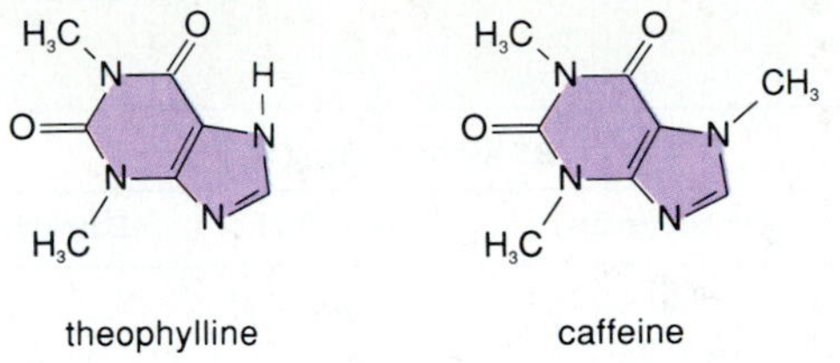

theophylline caffeine

FIGURE 58-4 Chemical structures of theophylline and caffeine.

Theophylline is also an adenosine antagonist in bronchial smooth muscle and in other tissues. Inhalation of adenosine causes bronchoconstriction in patients with asthma but does not affect nonasthmatics. It also causes contraction of isolated airway smooth muscle and an increase in histamine release from lung cells. This proposed mechanism, however, does not explain why enprophylline, another xanthine derivative without adenosine-antagonistic properties, is a more potent bronchodilator than theophylline. It has also been proposed that theophylline may act by altering intracellular calcium transport, but there is limited evidence for this mechanism. Thus the molecular mechanisms of action of theophylline remain unclear.

Anticholinergic Drugs

The main innervation of bronchial and smooth muscle is the parasympathetic nervous system, its activation causes bronchoconstriction. In the past, stramonium and other belladonna alkaloids were smoked as a treatment for asthma. Atropine (Figure 58-5) can be used as a bronchodilator in the lungs or to reduce secretions in the nose, but its use is limited by systemic toxicity. Ipratropium bromide is a quaternary nitrogen derivative of atropine that antagonizes muscarinic acetylcholine receptors in bronchial smooth muscle (see Chapter 9).

PHARMACOKINETICS

General Considerations

The pharmacokinetics of drugs used in asthma are complicated by routes of absorption as well as differences in the rate of response. Blood concentrations are irrelevant for all asthma drugs, except the xanthines, and so mean pulmonary function response times are generally used as the indicator of pharmacokinetics. Response rates are very individual, presumably reflecting differences in the detailed pathological condition of obstruction in the lung. Although bronchodilatation to inhaled β_2-adrenergic receptor agonists is fairly consistent, that is, onset within 10 to 30 minutes (see box p. 780), a response to inhaled or systemic steroids can occur within 4 hours but may take as long as 2 weeks, the time depending on the underlying lung disorder (Table 58-1 and Figure 58-6).

Cromolyn Sodium

Both cromolyn sodium and the newer agent nedocromil act on inflammatory cells and neurons in the bronchial epithelium and are only active when inhaled. Thus blood concentrations are largely irrelevant. Cromolyn sodium is very poorly absorbed from the gastrointestinal tract (i.e., <2%) and has few systemic side effects. The reason for lack of side effects is that cromolyn is excreted rapidly unmetabolized, 80% renal and 20% biliary. Although cromolyn has no direct bronchodilator activity and should not be used to treat an acute attack, it prevents exercise-induced asthma (EIA) within 10 minutes. The standard regimen to control EIA is to use inhaled β-$_2$-agonist and inhaled cromolyn sodium 10 to 20 minutes before exercise. In contrast to the rapid effect in controlling EIA, the antiinflammatory effect of cromolyn requires chronic treatment taking several days or even weeks to achieve an optimal effect.

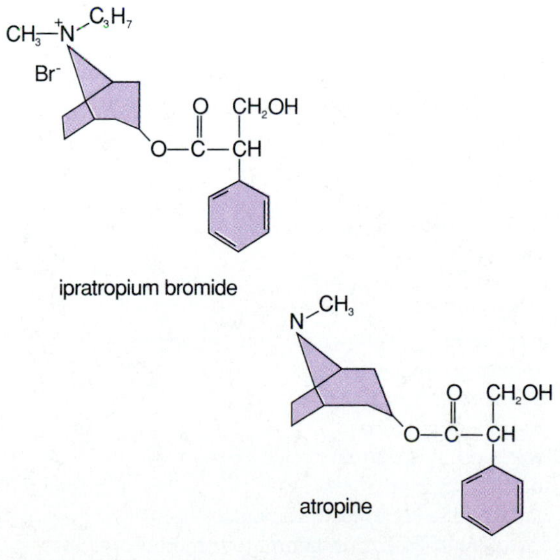

ipratropium bromide

atropine

FIGURE 58-5 Chemical structures of atropine and ipratropium bromide.

Table 58-1 Comparison of Bronchodilators

Adrenergic Agents	Selectivity*	Route	Bronchodilator Response: Onset (min)	Peak (hr)	Duration (hr)
Epinephrine	None	Inhalation	3-5	—	1-2
		Subcutaneous	6-15	0.5	<1-4
Metaproterenol	β_2+++	Inhalation	5-15	1-2	3-6
		Oral	15-30	0.5	4-8
Albuterol	β_2++++	Inhalation	5-15	1-2	3-6
		Oral	15-30	2-3	4-8
Terbutaline		Injected	15	0.5	1-2
Salmeterol	β_2++++	Inhaled	5-15	2-4	12
ANTICHOLINERGIC AGENTS					
Ipratropium	Blocks muscarinic +++ and nicotinic + (locally active)	Inhaled	15	1-2	6
Atropine	Blocks muscarinic +++	Inhaled	15	1-2	3

*Relative activity for receptor indicated by plus sign.

Corticosteroids

Pharmacokinetic values for the corticosteroids are given in Chapter 35. Responses to inhaled or oral steroids can occur within 4 hours but may take as long as 2 weeks.

β_2-Adrenergic Receptor Agonists

Most patients with asthma can detect improvement in tightness of the chest within 10 minutes after injection of epinephrine or inhaling of β_2-adrenergic receptor agonist. Optimal effect is usually within 20 minutes to 1 hour and may last for 2 to 4 hours. In most circumstances β_2-agonists are effective for approximately 6 hours. Prolonged use of β_2-agonists can cause a significant increase in bronchial hyperreactivity in a small proportion of patients. Recent development of a longer acting β_2-agonist (salmeterol), which lasts for more than 12 hours, may help resolve this problem.

SUMMARY OF MECHANISMS OF ACTION OF ANTIASTHMATIC DRUGS

- Increased cAMP
  - β-adrenergic receptor agonists
  - theophylline (?)
- Antagonize adenosine
  - theophylline
- Decrease cyclic guanosine monophosphate
  - ipratroprium bromide
- Prevent mediator release
  - cromolyn sodium
- Block mediator effects
  - antihistamines
  - leukotriene receptor antagonists
- Control synthesis of inflammatory mediators
  - corticosteroids

Methylxanthines

Theophylline clearance is influenced by food, smoking, age, a variety of disease states, and other drugs that are metabolized in the liver (see Table 58-2). Monitoring serum theophylline concentrations is necessary for any patient taking more than a minimal dose orally because of the multiple factors that influence blood concentration and because the range of safe therapeutic concentrations is narrow. The therapeutic range is 5 to 15 μg/ml and serious toxicity is increasingly likely at concentrations above 20 μg/ml.

Intravenously administered aminophylline can act rapidly on the lungs as a bronchodilator; however, this requires large bolus doses, which are now only occasionally used because of toxicity. It is easier to maintain blood concentrations by the oral route by use of delayed-release preparations.

Ipratropium Bromide

Like cromolyn sodium, ipratropium bromide is poorly absorbed and has few systemic side effects. The peak bronchodilator effect occurs 1 to 2 hours after inhalation with a duration of action of 3 to 5 hours (see Chapter 9).

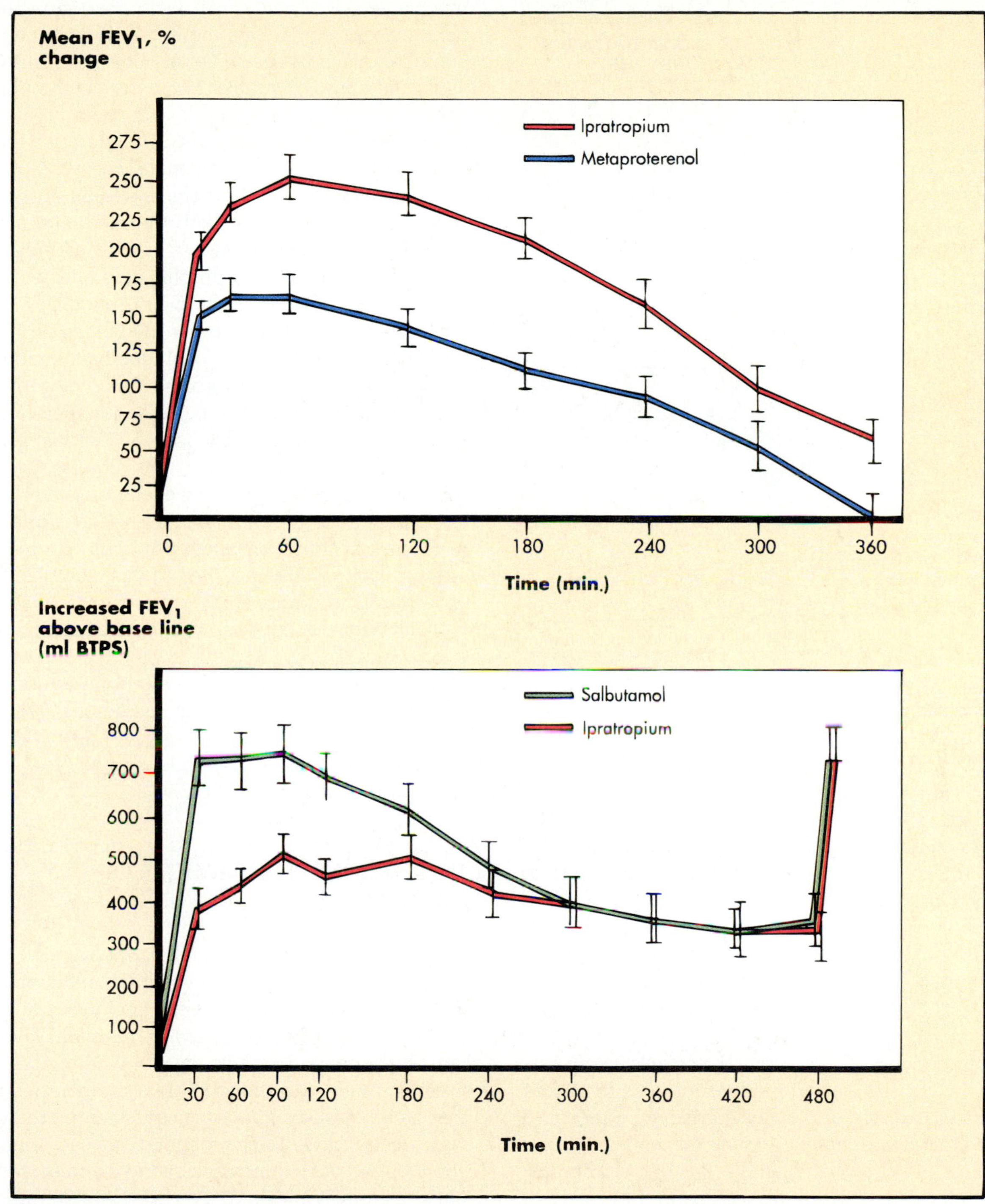

FIGURE 58-6 **A,** Response of patient with chronic obstructive pulmonary disease to ipratropium 40 μg or metaproterenol 1.5 mg. *BTPS,* At body temperature and ambient pressure and saturated with water vapor. (Modified from Tashkin DT, Ashutosh K, Bleecker ER, et al: *Am J Med* 81(suppl):81, 1986. **B,** Response of patient with asthma to ipratropium 40 μg or albuterol (salbutamol) 200 μg. (Modified from Ruffin RE, McIntyre EL, Latimer KM, et al: *J Allergy Clin Immunol* 69:60-65, 1982.)

Table 58-2 Factors Influencing Blood Concentrations of Theophylline

EFFECTS ON METABOLISM	EFFECTS ON BLOOD CONCENTRATIONS	HALF-LIFE (HR)
Cigarette smoking	Decreased	4-5
Normal adults	—	6-7
Neonates	*Elevated*	8-24
Children, 1 to 16 years	Decreased	3-7
Mature subjects >50	*Elevated*	—
DRUGS AFFECTING METABOLISM		
Erythromycin		
Cimetidine		
Ciprofloxacin	*Elevated*	Prolonged
Oral contraceptives		
Propranolol		
Phenobarbital		
Phenytoin	Decreased	Decreased
Rifampin		
DISEASE STATES		
Hepatic disease		
Congestive heart failure		
COPD (chronic obstructive pulmonary disease)	*Elevated*	Prolonged
Fever		

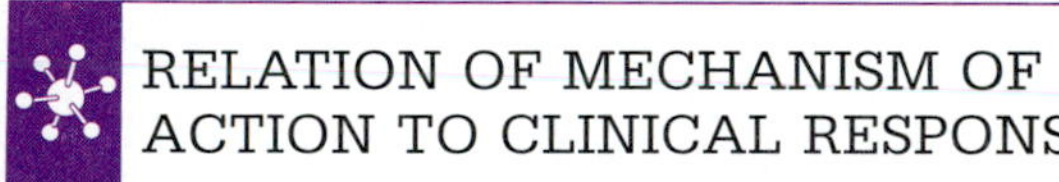

RELATION OF MECHANISM OF ACTION TO CLINICAL RESPONSE

The central problem in managing asthma is that the symptoms range from occasional tightness in the chest after exercise (which may require no treatment) to continuous airway obstruction (forced expiratory volume in 1 second, FEV_1, <60% predicted), which in some cases can be controlled only with high-dose orally administered prednisone. In all cases it is essential to establish that the symptoms correlate with changes in airway obstruction. One can achieve this by spirometry (FEV_1) or with a portable peak-flow meter. The patient should be encouraged to record peak-flow values over a 2-week period to establish a base-line value and an individual response to treatment. One can achieve this with a β_2-agonist administered by metered-dose inhaler (MDI), by nebulizer, or by tablet. For patients with more than occasional symptoms, further treatment is necessary. Reduced allergen exposure, inhaled cromolyn sodium, or inhaled corticosteroids are each recognized as antiinflammatory treatments capable of reducing bronchial hyperreactivity and improving management. Cromolyn sodium is used only prophylactically and is most effective for treating extrinsic asthma in young patients and in exercise-induced asthma. Although the mechanism or mechanisms of action of xanthines are not clear, nonetheless, regular treatment can be very effective at controlling symptoms. The action of xanthines prevents the onset of attacks of airway obstruction. Intravenous theophylline is active within minutes; orally its effect requires 1 to 2 hours. The duration of action depends on absorption and metabolism but correlates well with blood concentrations (Table 58-2).

Systemic steroids are both the most effective treatment for moderately severe or severe asthma *and* the most important cause of chronic side effects. The indication for orally received steroids is ongoing airway obstruction not relieved by other medicines within 1 to 2 days. Only a very small percentage of asthmatics (0.1%) become dependent on steroids. This may represent as many as 10 patients per 100,000 and is therefore an important cause of iatrogenic disease. Steroids have no direct bronchodilator effects and require 6 hours to achieve maximal effects. However, peripheral blood eosinophil counts fall within 2 hours, and significant effects on lung function and symptoms can be demonstrated within 4 hours of steroid use, such as IV methylprednisolone. Thus, early use of systemic steroids in management of acute asthma has become a mainstay of treatment both in outpatient practice and in the hospital. In some cases high doses of inhaled steroids can be used to abort an attack. In severe cases mucus impaction and poor ventilation of the lung prevent effective delivery of inhaled steroids, and so orally administered steroids are more effective.

OUTPATIENT TREATMENT OF ASTHMA

For a patient with occasional wheezing, one should be able to demonstrate a reversible airway obstruction and have the patient use a peak flow meter at home for 2 weeks to establish a diagnosis. Treatment involves using a β_2-agonist, two puffs by MDI when necessary. For exercise-induced asthma (EIA) it is imperative to show that breathlessness after exercise is associated with airway obstruction. Recommended are an inhaled β_2-agonist, two puffs 5 minutes before exercise and/or two puffs of cromolyn sodium by MDI, 10 to 20 minutes before exercise. Inadequate control requires identifying causes of bronchial hyperreactivity (BHR).

For frequent symptoms, including nocturnal asthma, establish that the airway obstruction is reversible and challenge the patient with methacholine, histamine, or cold air to demonstrate BHR. Skin tests may be used to identify possible sensitivity to allergens. Bronchial anti-

SPECIAL ISSUES

ASTHMA IN YOUNG CHILDREN

Among children there are special issues concerning side effects and delivery of anti-asthmatic drugs. Children can be treated with a nebulizer and face mask from age 6 months or earlier; by age 7 they can usually use an MDI with a spacer. Inhaled cromolyn is the antiinflammatory drug of choice because it has no serious side effects and is available for use in a nebulizer. In young children, total daily doses of inhaled steroids as low as 400μg have been reported to reduce growth. Chronic oral theophylline (taken as sprinklets on food) is effective and well tolerated in many children. Hyperactivity and/or learning difficulties are potential problems. Allergen avoidance should be recommended in any child who requires more than occasional treatment and has positive skin tests.

PREGNANCY

Management of asthma in pregnancy is similar to that used for all adults. Risks of uncontrolled asthma to the fetus outweigh the possible risks of drug therapy. Inhaled cromolyn, inhaled steroids, β_2-agonists, delayed release theophylline, antibiotics for sinusitis associated with asthma, and short courses of steroids are used in normal adult doses.

COPD

A reactive airway often develops in patients with chronic obstructive lung disease (COPD) as their disease progresses. While these patients are generally not allergic, drug treatment of this condition has many features in common with asthma treatment in adults. Thus, theophylline, β_2-agonists, steroids, and nebulized cromolyn are commonly used. Special issues include oxygen and monitoring of blood gases in respiratory compromised patients. Response to ipratropium bromide in patients with COPD is relatively better than that to β_2-adrenergic agonists, whereas the converse is true in asthmatics (Figure 58-4).

inflammatory treatment should include inhaled cromolyn, 2 puffs q.i.d. by MDI or inhaled steroids, 2 puffs t.i.d. by MDI. The patient should be educated on the avoidance of causative factors. For bronchospasm control use a β_2-agonist by MDI as needed, particularly when peak flow is < 70%. Oral delayed-release theophylline preparations (200-300 mg b.i.d. to t.i.d.) are also recommended. Theophylline blood concentrations after 4 days should be < 15 ug/ml.

For acute asthmatic attacks, doses of inhaled steroids should be increased to 4 puffs q.i.d. and theophylline added as needed. A short course of oral steroids (60 mg prednisone reducing to zero over 6 to 8 days), may also be necessary. In the clinic or emergency room, a nebulized β_2-agonist is the first line of treatment, which can be repeated after 20 minutes and then hourly. Patients not responding to nebulizer treatment should receive steroids (60 mg prednisone or 125 mg methylprednisolone intravenously).

Patients with unresponsive persistent symptoms may be treated with regular dose inhaled steroids (4 puffs q.i.d.); theophylline up to a maximum therapeutic range, and additional drug treatment, including cromolyn sodium and a β_2-agonist by nebulizer. Courses of oral steroids (6 days to 1 month) and other agents may also be considered. The physician should reinforce education on allergen avoidance and consider other factors such as diet, fungal infections, drug reactions, sinusitis and gastroesophageal reflux.

Antihistaminics are generally not recommended for asthma. However, many allergic patients with rhinitis and asthma use antihistaminics with no apparent harmful effects. Sedative antihistaminics should not be used in patients with acute bronchospasm. Antibiotics are commonly recommended for exacerbation of asthma because of sputum production but should be reserved for those patients with bronchial infiltrates, fever, and sinusitis.

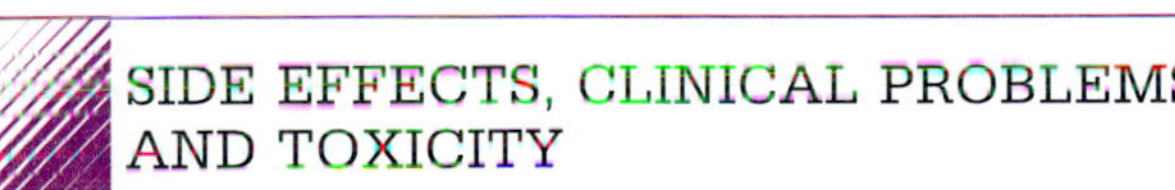

SIDE EFFECTS, CLINICAL PROBLEMS, AND TOXICITY

Cromolyn Sodium

The side effects of cromolyn sodium are restricted to irritant effects of inhaling the drug. There is very little convincing evidence for short-term or long-term drug toxicity and no recognized blood concentration that is toxic. Occasional cases of dermatitis, gastroenteritis, and myositis, apparently associated with cromolyn use, have been reported but are very unusual (see Chapter 59).

Corticosteroids

The side effects of systemic steroids are discussed in Chapter 35 and are discussed briefly here in the context of asthma. The most important issue is the difference between short-term and long-term use. Treatment with high-dose steroids can cause hypertension, diabetes, gastrointestinal bleeding, and CNS disturbances. These are uncommon. By contrast, chronic steroid use produces a wide range of severe side effects including thinning of the skin (striae, bruising); osteoporosis with

CLINICAL PROBLEMS

CROMOLYN SODIUM

Less potent than steroids
Coughing during inhalation

INHALED STEROIDS

Low dose: candidiasis
High dose: growth retardation; other systemic effects

ORAL STEROIDS

See Chapter 35 for discussion of steroid side effects

β_2-ADRENERGIC RECEPTOR AGONISTS

Tachycardia
Tremors
Increased bronchial reactivity

THEOPHYLLINE

Narrow therapeutic index
Nausea and vomiting
Seizures
Cardiac dysrhythmia

IPRATROPIUM BROMIDE

Dry mouth

rib fractures and vertebral compression; painful aseptic necrosis of the femoral head; diabetes with complications; gastrointestinal discomfort, ulceration and bleeding; and CNS disturbances including frank psychosis. Prolonged oral use of steroids causes profound suppression of adrenal function. Abrupt withdrawal after more than 1 month of usage can give rise to adrenal crisis, an uncommon problem because the dosage is reduced gradually for management of asthma. Patients must be made fully aware of the harmful effects of long-term orally administered steroids.

Inhaled Steroids

When they were initially introduced, there was great concern that inhaled steroids would produce serious side effects either locally in the lungs or systemically. In general, these fears were not borne out. The major side effect of inhaled steroids, e.g., beclomethasone dipropionate, has been oral candidiasis or occasional cases of exacerbation of symptoms triggered by the metered-dose inhaler (MDI). There are concerns that low-dose inhaled steroids can accelerate cataract formation, influence on bone formation, and delay recovery of the adrenal axis. In older patients but especially those with chronic obstructive pulmonary disease (COPD), yeast infection of the mouth is common and requires local treatment. Use of inhaled steroids in patients with COPD is not well established; there is a possibility that in patients with severe fixed obstruction (i.e., FEV_1 $\leq$40% predicted) inhaled steroids may encourage fungal colonization of the lung.

Larger doses have significant effects on adrenal axis and bone growth in children. Inhaled steroids are all locally active, and their systemic side effects depend on both absorption and drug metabolism. Some evidence indicates that budesonide and flunisolide may have fewer systemic effects because their metabolites are inactive.

β-$_2$-adrenergic Receptor Agonists

The primary side effects of adrenergic agonists are cardiac stimulatory effects, hypertension, and muscle tremor. β-$_2$-Selective agonists have fewer side effects, but tachycardia and muscle tremor still may occur with oral use. Using the inhaled route, these side effects are generally minimal. Epinephrine and isoproterenol have greater cardiotoxicity, are not widely used, and should be avoided in patients on monoamine oxidase inhibitors. With repeated β_2-agonist MDI use, the response decreases, suggestive of a receptor tolerance. These patients will respond to the same drug administered IV or by a nebulizer. Recently there have been several reports indicating that β_2-agonists are in part responsible for the increased mortality of asthma and that patients taking excessive amounts of drug should be weaned off the drug.

Methylxanthines

The side effects of theophylline can be divided into those that can occur within the normal therapeutic range and those that are very unusual with blood concentrations less than 15 μg/ml (the recommended upper limit). The most common side effects are related to the gastrointestinal tract (e.g., heartburn, abdominal pain, nausea, vomiting) relating to an increase in gastric acidity or CNS, such as headache, anxiety, tremor, or insomnia. (Similar side effects are reported with excess use of caffeine.) Side effects occur with concentrations as low as 5 μg/ml but increase greatly with blood concentrations of theophylline over 15 μg/ml. With blood concentrations over 20 μg/ml, seizures and cardiac arrhythmias are possible and become common with blood concentrations over 35 μg/ml. Seizures can result in significant mortality, and so elevated theophylline concentrations are treated as an emergency with gastric lavage, oral charcoal, and even dialysis. Considerable attention has been given to CNS symptoms in

TRADE NAMES

In addition to generic and fixed-combination preparations, the following trade-named materials are available in the United States.*

CROMONES

Intal, disodium cromoglycate
Tilade, nedocromil
INHALED STEROIDS
Aerobid and Aerobid-M, flunisolide
Azmacort, triamcinolone acetonide
Beclovent, Vanceril, beclomethasone dipropionate

B-SELECTIVE ADRENERGIC AGENTS

Alupent, Metaprel, metaproterenol
Brethine, Bricanyl, Brethaire, terbutaline sulfate
Proventil, Ventolin, albuterol
Maxaire, pirbuterol
Tornalate, bitolterol

METHYLXANTHINES

Theo-24, Slo-phyllin, Uniphyllin, Theo-dur, theophylline
Choledyl, oxitriphylline
ANTICHOLINERGIC AGENTS
Atrovent ipratropium bromide

*Trade names are capitalized; generic names are not.

children on methylxanthines, including poor attention and insomnia with resultant poor school performance.

Ipratropium Bromide (Chapter 9)

Inhaled ipratropium may give rise to drying of the mouth and upper airways. Typical side effects associated with systemic atropine are unusual.

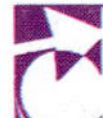

NEW DIRECTIONS

High-Dose Inhaled Steroids

High-dose inhaled steroids are widely used in Europe and are considered to be an effective method for reducing the requirement for orally administered steroids. However, inhaled steroids can have systemic side effects; for example, they can reduce growth in children. Thus, further use of high-dose inhaled steroids will need to be matched by detailed studies of the systemic side effects of these agents and their metabolites. It is likely that high-dose inhaled steroids will play an increasing role in the management of patients with moderately severe asthma.

DRUGS AFFECTING RESPIRATORY FUNCTION

DNAase has now been approved for the treatment of pulmonary symptoms in cystic fibrosis. This disease is characterized by a significant inflammatory cell burden in the lung, high cell turnover, and DNA survival. DNAase acts to hydrolyze the residual DNA, destroying the inflammatory infiltrate and alleviating some of the symptoms of the disease. Clinical trials are also underway for assessment of the effectiveness of DNAase in chronic bronchitis.

Nedocromil Sodium

Nedocromil sodium is a second-generation member of the cromolyn group. It is an active inflammatory treatment suitable for long-term use with apparently the same lack of side effects as cromolyn sodium. It has similar activity in stabilizing mast cells but has a different profile in blocking responses to a variety of medications, such as sulfur dioxide, neurokinin A, and bradykinin.

Leukotriene Antagonists and Inhibitors

Mast cells release both histamine and a range of arachidonic acid metabolites. Part of the actions of steroids are attributable to inhibition of these mediators especially leukotriene D_4 (LTD_4). Antagonists or inhibitors of production of leukotrienes have shown considerable promise in clinical trials, and it is very likely that a leukotriene inhibitor or antagonist will be introduced over the next few years.

Allergen Avoidance

Although some aspects of allergen avoidance for asthma are well established, more experience is needed, such as management of carpets and upholstered furniture. Avoidance measures are underway for dust-mite allergens and for cat and cockroach allergens, including the development of clinical treatments to control mites or cockroaches and chemicals designed to denature allergens.

Immunosuppressive Agents

In patients with severe or steroid-dependent asthma, many different treatments have been used, including gold, intravenous gamma globulin, troleandomycin, cyclosporin A, and methotrexate. The most promising results have been with methotrexate. Other immunosuppressive drugs are being evaluated including FK-506 which appears to be able to inhibit transcription of interleukin-2 and other T-cell activation genes.

Fungal Colonization in Asthma

Many patients with late-onset asthma have chronic colonization of their skin, nails, or mucosal surfaces with fungi (e.g., *Trichophyton* or *Aspergillus* species) or yeast (e.g., *Candida* or *Torulopsis* species). In some cases these patients also have immediate hypersensitivity to antigens derived from the colonizing organism. Treatment of fungi on skin or mucosal surfaces is not normally regarded as treatment for their asthma. Recent evidence has indicated that treatment with new systemic antifungals (fluconazole or itraconazole) may be helpful for the asthma in some cases.

REFERENCES

Barnes PJ, Petersen S: Efficacy and safety of inhaled corticosteroids in asthma, *Am Rev Respir Dis* 148:1-26, 1993.

Barnes PJ, Roger IW, Thomson NC, editors: *Asthma: basic mechanisms and clinical management,* ed 2, London, New York, 1992, Academic Press.

Chan-Yeung M, Lam S: Occupational asthma, *Am Rev Respir Dis* 133:686-703, 1986.

Gross NJ: Ipratropium bromide, *N Engl J Med* 319:486, 1988.

Guidelines for the Diagnosis and Management of Asthma, National Asthma Education Program, US Department of Health and Human Services, Publication No. 91:3042A, 1991.

Hendeles L, Weinberger M: Selection of a slow-release theophylline product, *J Allergy Clin Immunol* 78:743, 1986.

Platts-Mills TAE, Chapman MD: Dust mites: immunology, allergic disease, and environmental control [review], *J Allergy Clin Immunol* 80:755-775, 1987.

Schatz M, Zeiger RS, Harder KM, et al: The safety of inhaled beta-agonist bronchodilators during pregnancy, *J Allergy Clin Immunol* 82:686, 1988.

Sporik R, Holgate ST, Platts-Mills TAE, Cogswell JJ: Exposure to house-dust mite allergen (*Der p* I) and the development of asthma in childhood, *N Engl J Med* 323:502-507, 1990.

SELF ASSESSMENT QUESTIONS

1. Postulated mechanisms for theophylline's bronchodilator action include:
   a. Blockade of histamine release
   b. Phosphodiesterase inhibition
   c. Adenosine antagonism
   d. b and c
   e. a, b and c
2. Which of the following is the drug of choice for the prophylactic treatment of intrinsic asthma in young patients and in exercise-induced asthma?
   a. Cromolyn sodium
   b. Oral steroids
   c. Inhaled steroids
   d. Inhaled β-adrenergic receptor agonists
   e. Ipratropium bromide
3. Which of the following is true of theophylline?
   a. Its clearance is influenced by smoking, food and disease states
   b. Monitoring blood concentrations is necessary for all patients taking the drug on a regular basis
   c. Serious toxicity is likely at blood concentrations of 20 μg/ml or greater
   d. a and c
   e. a, b and c
4. Which of the following matching descriptions is INCORRECT?
   a. β-Adrenergic receptor agonists-Increase cAMP and relax bronchiolar smooth muscle
   b. Cromolyn sodium-Controls mediator release from mast cells
   c. Ipratropium bromide-Decreases cGMP and blocks muscarinic receptors
   d. Antihistaminics-Block mediator effects in asthma
   e. Theophylline-Inhibits phosphodiesterase and increases cAMP
5. Which of the following is NOT an effect of corticosteroids?
   a. Reduced local recruitment of eosinophils
   b. Increased sensitivity of β-adrenergic receptors
   c. Reduction of mucosal edema in asthma
   d. Reduction in mediator release
   e. Control of gene transcription for cytokines

CHAPTER 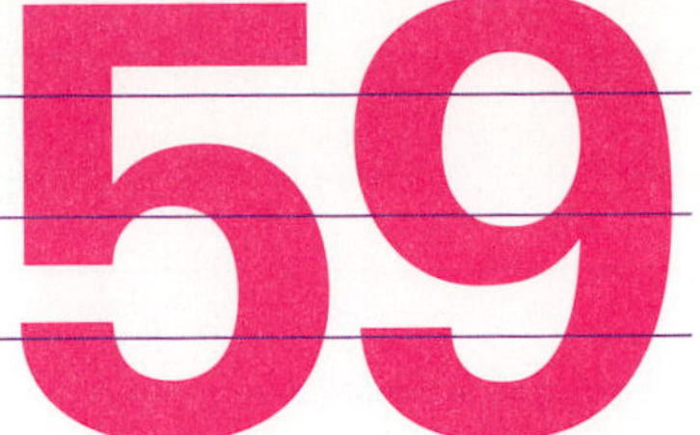

Histamine and Antihistamines

LOUIS A. BARKER

MAJOR DRUGS
histamine H_1-receptor antagonists cromolyn sodium

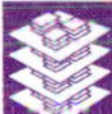

THERAPEUTIC OVERVIEW

Histamine is an endogenous compound that is synthesized, stored, and released primarily by mast cells and after release exerts profound effects on many tissues and organs. It is one of the cellular mediators of the immediate hypersensitivity reaction and the acute inflammatory response, as well as a primary stimulant of gastric acid secretion. A central neurotransmitter role for histamine has been established.

These actions of histamine preclude its use as a drug. Its importance in medicine and pharmacology lies in its pathophysiological actions, the therapeutic usefulness of drugs that prevent its release from mast cells, and drugs that block the receptors that mediate the actions of histamine.

Because the actions of histamine have considerable species variation, it is difficult to extrapolate results from studies on experimental animals to humans. Most of this discussion is based on the results of studies with human volunteers or with organs and tissues obtained from human subjects.

ABBREVIATIONS	
cAMP	cyclic adenosine monophosphate
IgE	immunoglobulin E

The experimental IV administration of histamine to human volunteers produces dose-related effects primarily in heart, vascular and extravascular smooth muscle, and secretion of the gastric mucosa. The actions of histamine are mediated by at least three distinct receptors, H_1, H_2, and H_3. Of these, the H_1- and H_2-receptors are the best characterized and mediate well-defined responses in humans. A summary of some of the actions of histamine that are mediated by H_1- and H_2-receptors is given in Table 59-1.

Responses such as bronchoconstriction are mediated by H_1-receptors and are selectively antagonized by classical antihistamines such as diphenhydramine. Responses such as facial cutaneous vasodilatation and gastric acid secretion are mediated by H_2-receptors and are selectively antagonized by agents such as cimetidine or ranitidine.

The H_3-receptor has been studied mainly in experimental animals. This receptor is found on nerve endings and mediates inhibition of neurotransmitter release. This applies to an inhibition of the release of histamine from histaminergic neurons in the CNS as well as other transmitters in the CNS and to the release of transmitters from peripheral nerves in the autonomic nervous system and the myenteric plexus.

MECHANISMS OF ACTION

Histamine

Action The structure of histamine is shown in Figure 59-1. The mechanism of signal transduction by histamine at H_1-, H_2-, and H_3-receptors differs. The direct contractile actions on smooth muscle and the neuronal actions that are mediated by H_1-receptors result from stimulation of the breakdown of inositol phospholipids. The stimulus-response mechanism for the H_1-receptor–mediated relaxation of vascular smooth muscle involves

Table 59-1 Selected Actions of Histamine in Humans

Organ/Tissue	Action	Receptor
CARDIOVASCULAR		
Vascular	Decrease in total peripheral resistance	H_1 and H_2
Facial cutaneous	Vasodilatation	H_2
Forearm	Increased blood flow	H_1, and H_2
Gastric mucosa	Increased blood flow	H_2 (?)
Carotid artery	Relaxation	H_2
Basilar artery	Constriction	H_1
Pulmonary artery	Relaxation	H_2
	Constriction	H_1
Coronary artery	Constriction	H_1
Postcapillary venules	Increased permeability	H_1
Heart	Increased sinoatrial rate	H_2
	Increased force of contraction	H_2
	Increased atrial and ventricular automaticity	H_2
RESPIRATORY		
Bronchiolar smooth muscle	Contraction	H_1
	Relaxation	H_2
GASTROINTESTINAL		
Oxyntic mucosa	Acid and pepsin secretion	H_2
Gastrointestinal smooth muscle	Relaxation and contraction	H_1
Gallbladder smooth muscle	Relaxation (?)	H_2 (?)
CUTANEOUS NERVE ENDINGS	Pain and itching	H_1 and H_2(?)
ADRENAL MEDULLA	Epinephrine release	H_1
BASOPHILS	Inhibition of IgE-dependent degranulation	H_2

These actions have been demonstrated in human volunteers or in organs or tissues obtained from human subjects. (?) means that the response was not uniformly observed or that the receptor mediating the response was not well characterized.

the synthesis and release of endothelium-derived relaxant factor, presumably nitric oxide.

The actions of histamine that are mediated by H_2-receptors may be attributable to the activation of adenylate cyclase. This occurs in H_2-receptor systems that mediate acid secretion, relaxation of vascular smooth muscle, neuronal excitation, inhibition of basophil degranulation, and increases in myocardial contractility. Such action may include H_2-receptors located at other sites.

The inhibition of transmitter release mediated by H_3-receptors is believed to involve a modulation of Ca^{++} entry into nerve endings.

Synthesis and Metabolism Histamine is synthesized in vivo by decarboxylation of the amino acid L-histidine, catalyzed by the pyridoxal phosphate–dependent enzyme L-histidine decarboxylase (Figure 59-2). Most of the histamine in tissues is stored in an inert form at the site of synthesis. Very little preformed histamine exists in a freely diffusible form. When histamine is released from its storage site, it becomes active but is rapidly converted to inactive metabolites.

Two primary pathways exist for the catabolism of histamine (Figure 59-2). The oxidative deamination path is catalyzed by diamine oxidase and leads to the formation of imidazole acetic acid. The second path involves methylation of the *tele*-nitrogen in the imidazole ring catalyzed by histamine-*N*-methyl transferase and results in the formation of *N*-methylhistamine. These primary metabolites are subject to further metabolism. In the periphery, both pathways contribute to the metabolism of histamine, but in the CNS the methylation pathway predominates.

Storage and Release The major sites of histamine storage and release are mast cells. Other sites include basophils and neurons in the CNS and cells not fully

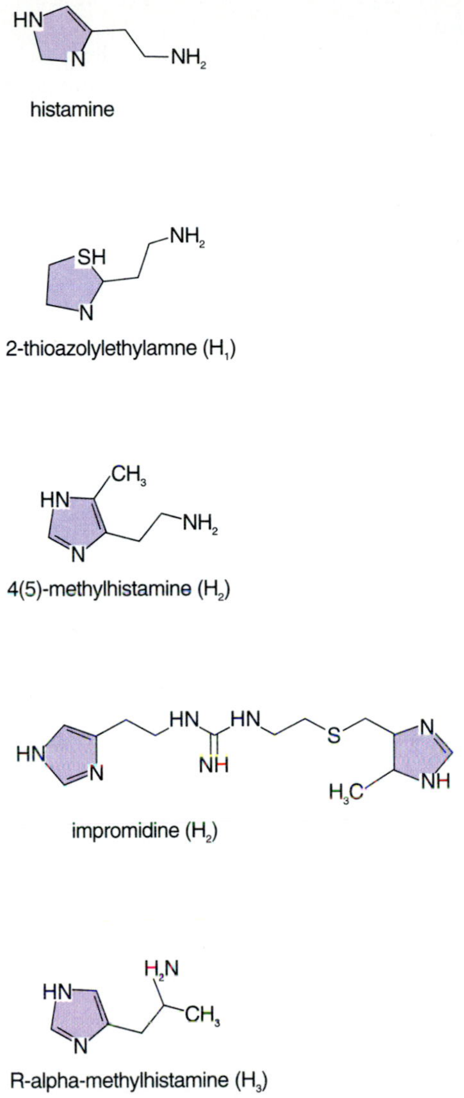

histamine

2-thioazolylethylamne (H_1)

4(5)-methylhistamine (H_2)

impromidine (H_2)

R-alpha-methylhistamine (H_3)

FIGURE 59-1 Histamine and some agonists (with specific receptor indicated).

characterized.

Histamine is distributed throughout the body, an indication that the sites of synthesis and storage also are widely distributed. However, the greatest concentrations of histamine occur in the skin, lungs, and gastrointestinal mucosa and correspond to the density of mast cells.

Basophils and mast cells are similar in that both have high-affinity immunoglobulin E (IgE) binding sites on their plasma membranes and both store histamine in secretory granules. Mast cells are heterogeneous and can be classified on the basis of staining properties, anatomical localization, or susceptibility to degranulation induced by a polyamine, compound 48/80. The anatomical classification is commonly used; the cells are denoted as mucosal or connective tissue mast cells. However, mixed populations of mast cells are in both anatomic locations, and additional heterogeneity exists within the two major classes of mast cells. Human mast cells differ with respect to the structure of the proteoglycan in storage granules, the type of proteoglycan, the types of neutral serine proteases, chymase or tryptase (or both), in the storage granules, the relative amounts of prostanoids and leukotrienes that are synthesized and released on degranulation, and the inhibition of antigen-induced degranulation by cromolyn sodium. Properties of mast cells isolated from human tissues are shown in Table 59-2.

Histamine exists in mast cell granules as an ionic complex with a proteoglycan, chiefly heparin sulfate, but also with chondroitin sulfate E. Histamine in basophils also is stored in granules as an ionic complex, predominantly with the proteoglycan chondroitin monosulfate. The release of histamine and other mediators from mast cells and basophils is common during allergic disorders but also can be induced by drugs and endogenous polypeptides to produce pseudoallergic reactions. This is shown schematically in Figure 59-3. The participation of mast cells in the immediate and delayed hypersensitivity reactions, as well as possible participation of mast cells in the pathological characteristics of nonallergic disorders, provides the therapeutic rationale for the use of agents that antagonize histamine and agents that prevent mast cell degranulation.

The release of histamine from mast cells and basophils occurs by two general processes of degranulation: noncytolytic and cytolytic. The cytolytic release of histamine from mast cells occurs when the plasma membrane is damaged. This type of release is energy independent, does not require intracellular Ca^{++}, and is accompanied by the leakage of cytoplasmic contents. Cytolytic release can be induced by a variety of substances, including phenothiazines, histamine H_1-antagonists, and some of the narcotic analgesics. The concentrations of these agents that are required to produce a cytolytic release are in considerable excess over those required for therapeutic effects.

Noncytolytic release can be induced by a variety of compounds. It is generally believed, though not unequivocally established, that noncytolytic release is evoked as a consequence of specific binding of a ligand to a receptor in the plasma membrane of the mast cell or basophil. In contrast to cytolytic release, noncytolytic release requires adenosine triphosphate for energy, depends on changes in free intracellular Ca^{++}, and is not accompanied by leakage of cytoplasmic contents. Noncytolytic release is characterized by exocytosis of the secretory granules. The classical example is the degranulation of sensitized mast cells or basophils induced by

Table 59-2 Some Properties of Isolated Human Mast Cells and Basophils

Tissue of Origin	Mast Cell Type	Histamine Release Evoked by			Inhibition of IgE-dependent Release by		IgE-dependent Release of	
		48/80	Morphine	FMLP	Cromolyn	β-Agonists	PGD_2	LTC_4
Skin	CT/TC	++++	+++	-	±	++++	+++	+
Lung								
Parenchyma	M/T	-	-		+	++++	+++	+++
BAL	M/T	-			+++	++++	+++	+++
Intestinal Mucosa	M/T	-	-	-	+	++++	++	+++
Basophils		-	-	+++	-	++++	++++	+++

BAL, Bronchoalveolar lavage–derived mast cells; *C,* chymase; *CT,* connective tissue; *FMLP, N*-formyl-methionylleucinylphenylalanine (a chemotactic tripeptide); *M,* mucosal; *TC,* tryptase and chymase. The intensity of the response is given qualitatively: (-) for no response to (++++) for a strong response. PGD_2 is a prostaglandin and LTC_4 is a leukotriene (See Chapter 18).

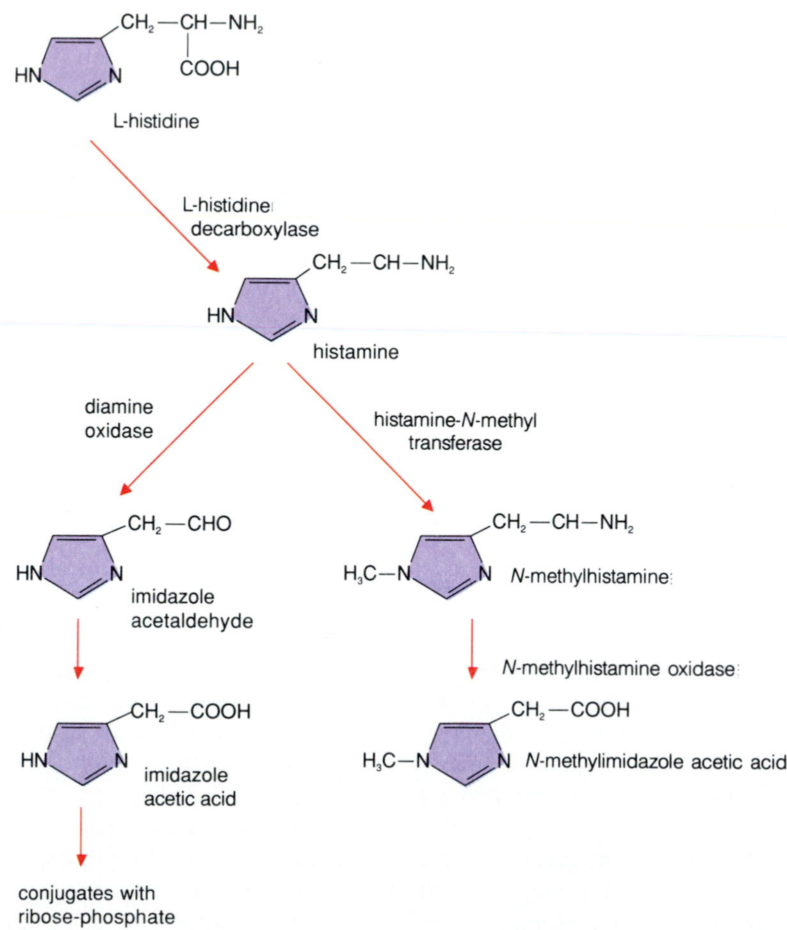

FIGURE 59-2 Synthesis and metabolism of histamine.

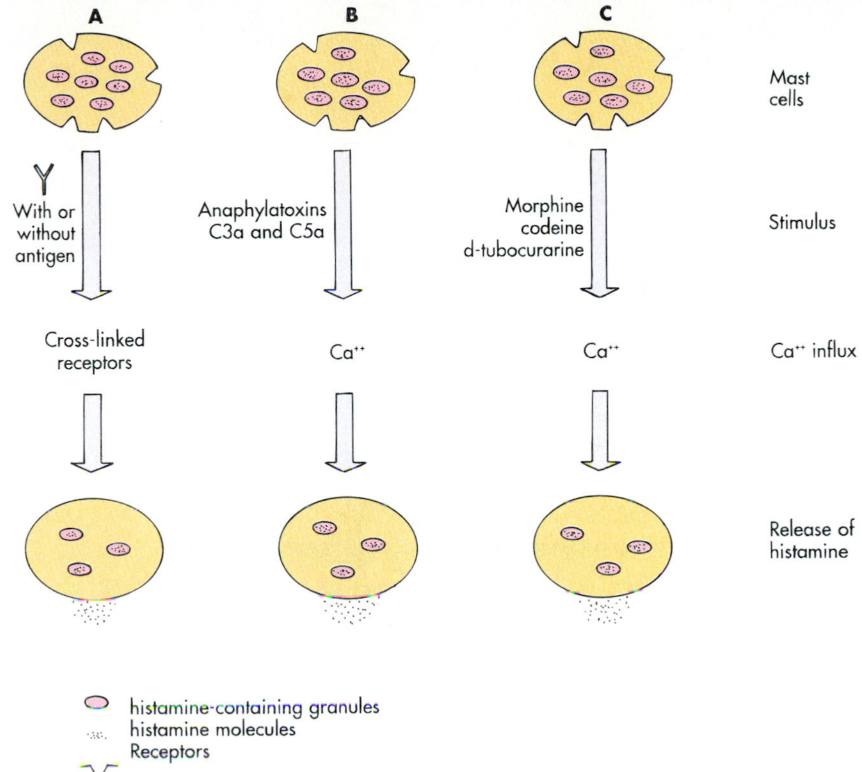

FIGURE 59-3 Summary of mast cell release of histamine. Some stimuli act indirectly through Fc receptors **(A)**, and others act directly **(B, C)** by an increase in intracellular Ca^{++} to release histamine.

cross-bridging adjacent IgE molecules bound on the membrane surface of the cell. The cascade of biochemical events that begins with the interaction of antigen and IgE molecules and culminates in the degranulation of mast cells and basophils is summarized in Figure 59-4. In addition to histamine, other constituents of the storage granules are released. These include heparin, eosinophil and neutrophil chemotactic factors, neutral proteases, and other enzymes. Also newly synthesized mediators such as prostaglandin D_2, leukotriene C_4 and D_4 (slow-reacting substance of anaphylaxis), leukotriene B_4, and platelet-activating factor are released.

Noncytolytic release also is produced by nonimmune mechanisms. A variety of agents can produce degranulation independently, without prior exposure. In general, such histamine liberators are basic in nature. Examples of polybasic substances are the polyamine 48/80 and basic polypeptides such as bradykinin, substance P, *N*-formyl-methionylleucinylphenylalanine, protamine, the anaphylatoxins ($C3_a$, $C4_a$, and $C5_a$), and the mast cell degranulating protein present in bee venom. Except for protamine, a heparin antagonist, none of these agents has any therapeutic use. Compound 48/80 is used extensively in experimental studies on mast cells. The remaining agents listed may be pathological stimuli for mast cell and basophil degranulation.

Noncytolytic degranulation can be induced by several drugs, including tubocurarine, succinylcholine, morphine and codeine, doxorubicin, and vancomycin.

Histamine release in vivo also may be produced by some plasma expanders, notably those based on cross-linked gelatin, and by radiocontrast media, especially those of high osmotic strength. The mechanism of release is not elucidated, but is believed to occur by degranulation.

The receptors mediating the noncytolytic degranulation induced by the small basic agents have not been characterized. These receptors are not the ones associated with the desired therapeutic actions of these drugs. In general, problems with histamine release by these drugs occur after IV administration of the drugs. Usually, this does not result in a serious pseudoallergic reaction; however, serious life-threatening reactions can occur.

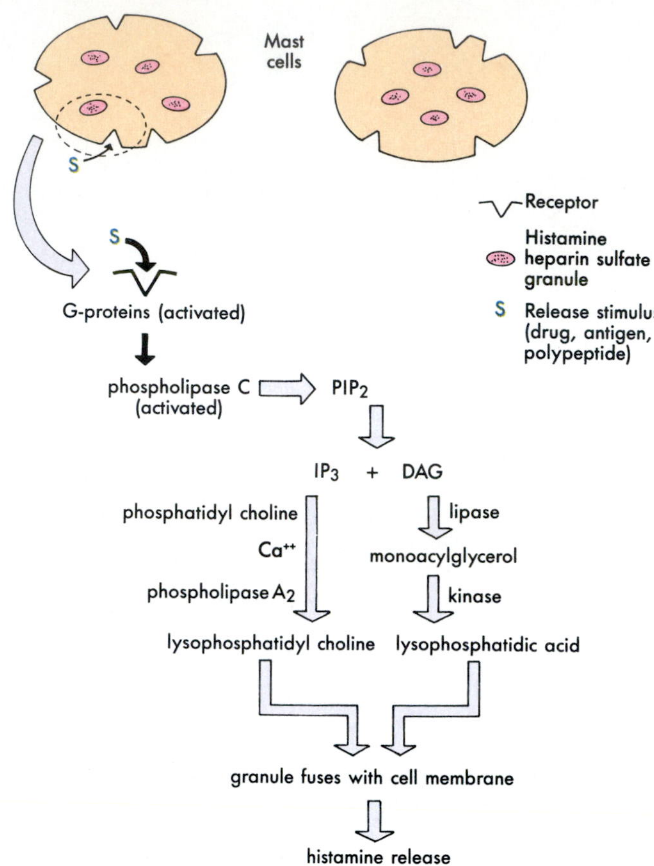

FIGURE 59-4 Release of histamine from mast cells. PIP_2 is phosphatidylinositol-4,5-bisphosphate; IP_3 is inositol 1,4,5-trisphosphate; DAG is 1,2-diacylglycerol. (See Figure 59-3 and Chapter 2 for more details.)

Inhibitors of Mast Cell and Basophil Histamine Release/Degranulation

Because many mediators are released from mast cells and basophils during noncytolytic degranulation, agents that can prevent the degranulation reaction and subsequent release of mediators are of therapeutic value.

Drugs that inhibit mast cell and basophil degranulation are used in the treatment of reversible bronchospastic disorders (see Chapter 58). Methylxanthines, such as theophylline, and β_2-selective adrenergic agonists, such as albuterol, can inhibit the degranulation of mast cells and basophils. Both classes of drugs do so by increasing intracellular concentrations of cyclic adenosine monophosphate (cAMP)—methylxanthines possibly in part by inhibition of phosphodiesterase and β_2-selective agonists by activation of adenylate cyclase. The ability to produce bronchodilation and stabilize mast cells may contribute to the actions of β_2-selective agonists. However, for the methylxanthines, bronchodilation is their major action rather than stabilization of mast cells. The concentrations of theophylline required to inhibit degranulation correspond to plasma concentrations usually associated with systemic toxicity.

Cromolyn sodium (see Chapter 58 for structure) also has been proposed to stabilize mast cells and prevent noncytolytic degranulation. Additionally, it can prevent the activation of eosinophils and neutrophils. This broad spectrum of stabilizing cells that mediate inflammatory responses account in part for its antiasthma activity. A new agent with properties similar to cromolyn, nedocromil, currently is available.

The precise mechanism or mechanisms by which cromolyn prevents noncytolytic mast cell degranulation and activation of eosinophils and neutrophils are not known. Cromolyn does not act by antagonizing any of the receptors for the known mediators of inflammation or by interfering with the interaction of IgE and antigen.

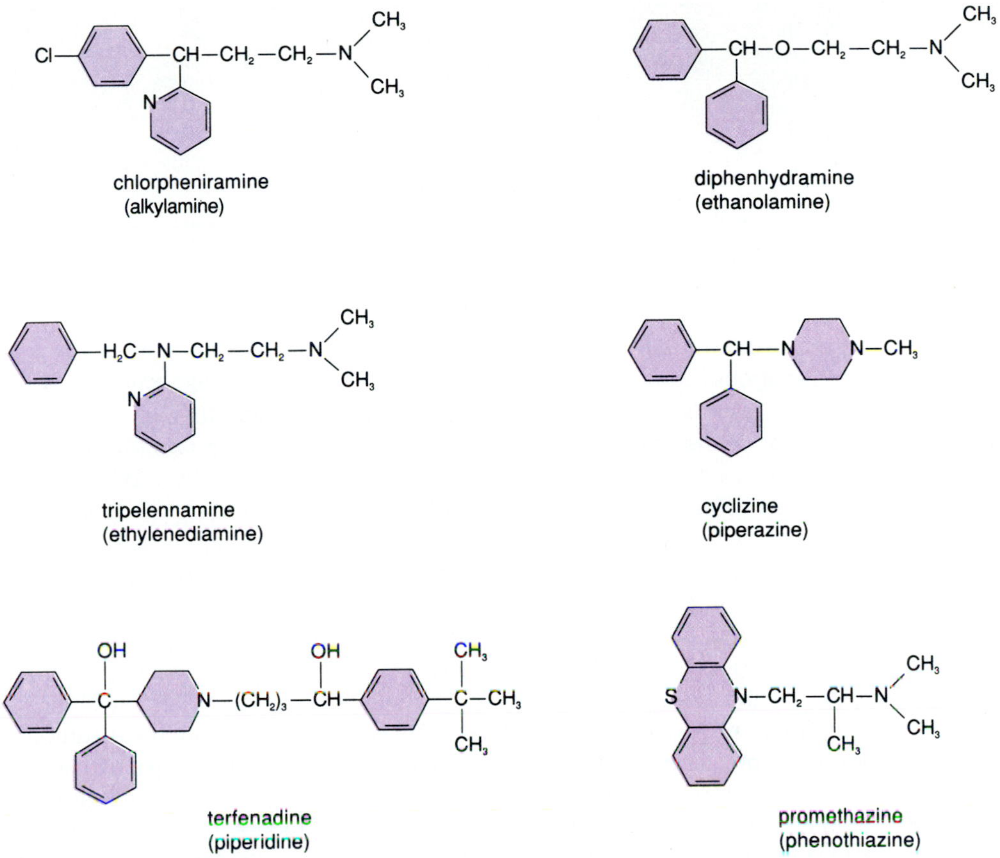

chlorpheniramine
(alkylamine)

diphenhydramine
(ethanolamine)

tripelennamine
(ethylenediamine)

cyclizine
(piperazine)

terfenadine
(piperidine)

promethazine
(phenothiazine)

FIGURE 59-5 Some H_1-receptor antagonists with chemical classification.

Cromolyn appears to act by binding with a membrane-bound receptor to promote the phosphorylation of a cytoplasmic protein. Its effectiveness is inversely related to the strength of the stimuli producing degranulation, indicating that it may produce a physiological antagonism of agents that produce degranulation. These actions occur independently of changes in the cellular content of cAMP (discussed in Chapter 58).

Histamine H_1-Receptor Antagonists

Agents referred to as *antihistaminics* are those that antagonize the actions of histamine mediated by H_1-receptors. Before the advent of selective antagonists for the H_1-receptor, histamine was believed to be the primary mediator of immediate-hypersensitivity reactions. Although the early H_1-antagonists blocked histamine-induced hypotension and bronchoconstriction, they were not very effective in true anaphylaxis. The clinical ineffectiveness of the older and the current H_1-antagonists to control anaphylaxis is attributable in part to the lipid mediators released during mast cell degranulation, that are the primary cause of hypotension and bronchoconstriction, and perhaps their lack of blockade of histamine's effects at cardiovascular H_2-receptors.

The present histamine H_1-antagonists have little structural resemblance to histamine (see Figures 59-1 and 59-5 for structures). A common structural feature is a substituted ethylamine containing a nitrogen atom in an alkyl chain or a ring. These agents are usually classified according to the chemical group containing the substituted ethylamine. The groups and representative drugs are alkylamine (chlorpheniramine), ethanolamine (diphenhydramine), ethylenediamine (tripelennamine), piperazine (cyclizine), piperidine (terfenadine), and phenothiazine (promethazine). In addition, there are other compounds that exhibit antihistamine activity.

The antihistamines act by competitive antagonism of

Table 59-3 Pharmacokinetic Parameter Values for H_1-Receptor Antagonists

Drug	Administered	Absorbed	$t_{1/2}$ (hr)	Disposition
astemizole	Oral	Good	24	M
chlorpheniramine	Oral	Good	20	M
cyclizine	Oral	Good	7-24	M
diphenhydramine	Oral	Good	4-8	M
promethazine	Oral	Good	7-15	M
terfenadine	Oral	Good	16-22	M
tripelennamine	Oral	Good	—	M

M, Metabolized.

histamine at H_1-receptors, except for terfenadine and astemizole, which act in a nonsurmountable manner. Thus the ability of most of these agents to antagonize endogenously released histamine depends on the local concentration of histamine and that of the antagonists. The latter are limited by the adverse, non–H_1-receptor effects of the antagonists, which occur more frequently above therapeutic doses. However, even at therapeutic doses, these non–H_1-receptor actions may contribute to the limited usefulness of these agents in the treatment of allergic and other disorders.

Many of the actions of these antagonists are attributable to blockade of H_1-receptors and are predictable based on the actions of histamine mediated by H_1-receptors. Differences are the result of pharmacokinetic properties that govern tissue distribution and duration of action and to actions at sites other than the H_1-receptor. In addition to blocking H_1-receptors, all these agents exhibit weak to pronounced blockade at muscarinic receptors, and some block additional receptors. For example, cyproheptadine is a fairly potent antagonist of serotonin, and promethazine exhibits weak α-adrenoceptor and moderate dopamine D_2-receptor blocking. Terfenadine and astemizole differ in that, at therapeutic doses, they exhibit very little blocking activity at sites other than the H_1-receptor.

H_2-Receptor Antagonists

The mechanism of action of the H_2-receptor antagonist drugs to inhibit gastric acid secretion is also discussed in Chapter 60. The H_2-receptor antagonists revolutionized the medical management of peptic ulcer disease. It was known for many years that the conventional H_1-receptor antagonists did not significantly inhibit histamine-induced gastric acid secretion. A deliberate effort was therefore made to develop drugs that would block parietal cell histamine receptors and provide a new approach to pharmacological regulation of acid secretion. The primary approach was systematic modification of the histamine molecule to generate H_2-receptor–selective antagonists. Whereas the H_1-receptor antagonists do not require a histamine-like nucleus, an imidazole-like nucleus is required for recognition by H_2-receptors. However, the histamine imidazole ring can exist in two tautomeric forms, only one of which is recognized by the H_2-receptor. Addition of a 4(5)-methyl (see Figure 59-1) substitution on histamine provided the appropriate tautomer for recognition, and 4(5)-methylhistamine is a moderately selective agonist at the H_2-receptor. Side-chain substitution led to the therapeutically useful antagonist cimetidine. Other H_2-receptor antagonists contain furan or thiazol rings (see structures in Chapter 60).

The H_2-receptor antagonists inhibit food-, gastrin-, and acetylcholine-induced gastric secretion of acid, as well as acid secretion induced by histamine. As expected, the H_2-receptor antagonists are especially effective in blocking the secretory effects of histamine or selective H_2-receptor agonists.

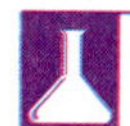

PHARMACOKINETICS

Pharmacokinetic parameter values for the H_1-receptor antagonists are given in Table 59-3. Values for cromolyn sodium are in Chapter 58 and values for H_2-receptor antagonists are in Chapter 60. For a discussion of cromolyn sodium pharmacokinetics, see Chapter 58.

H_1-Antagonists

The H_1-antagonists are well absorbed after oral administration and have onsets of action of about 30 minutes to an hour. However, astemizole must be taken for 2 days before a therapeutic effect is noted. Most have durations of action between 3 to 6 hours in adults. A notable exception is astemizole with a half-life of 24 hours and an active metabolite, desmethylastemizole, that has a half-life of 10 to 20 days. Other exceptions are meclizine with a duration of 12 to 24 hours, and terfenadine and mequitazine with durations of 12 hours.

The ability of most antihistamines to block the triple response (redness, wheal or flare) after intradermal injection of antigens or histamine can persist for 1 to 2 days after cessation of therapy.

There are two subclasses of these agents with respect to body distribution. The older, first-generation, antihistamines are distributed throughout the body and readily penetrate the CNS. The second-generation antihistamines, such as astemizole, loratidine and terfenadine, or agents currently available in Canada and Europe or currently in clinical trials in the United States, such as cetirizine, do not readily penetrate the CNS. The newer agents have a lower incidence of sedative effects than the older agents.

The antihistamines are extensively metabolized by the liver, and metabolites are eliminated by renal excretion. Some of the agents are substrates for monoamine oxidase, these agents can induce hepatic cytochrome P-450 enzymes and may facilitate their own metabolism and that of other drugs.

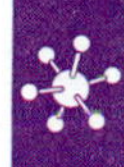

RELATION OF MECHANISMS OF ACTIONS TO CLINICAL RESPONSE

Actions of Histamine

Vascular System The effects of histamine on the systemic vasculature are complex, and different vascular beds show different responses. Most vascular beds respond with vasodilation mediated by either or both H_1- and H_2-receptors. Other beds respond with vasoconstriction mediated by H_1-receptors or vasodilation mediated by H_2-receptors.

The predominant action of histamine is dose-dependent vasodilation resulting from relaxation of arteriolar smooth muscle, precapillary sphincters, and muscular venules that is mediated by both H_1-receptors and H_2-receptors. Either receptor can mediate a maximal response; that produced by H_1-receptors occurs at lower doses and is transient. Vasodilation produced by H_2-receptors occurs at higher doses and is sustained. The complete blockade of the maximal hypotensive response requires the use of both H_1- and H_2-antagonists.

Histamine acts as H_1-receptors on endothelial cells in all postcapillary venules to produce contraction of the endothelial cells and exposure of permeable basement membrane. This results in edema from the loss of fluid and plasma protein to the surrounding tissue.

A synopsis of the actions of histamine on the vasculature is seen in the triple response that follows the intradermal injection of histamine. Initially, a small red spot is produced at the site of injection that is slowly surrounded by a flushed area. A wheal appears at the original red spot in a few minutes. The red spot and the erythema are caused by vasodilation, with the red spot resulting from the direct actions of histamine on the cutaneous vasculature and the erythema from axon reflexes that produce vasodilation. These vasodilatory responses are mediated by both H_1-receptors and H_2-receptors, with the major contribution by the H_1 component. The wheal occurs from edema formation. Histamine also stimulates nerve endings to produce pain, when injected intradermally, and itching, when administered into the epidermis. The extrapolation of the local vascular reactions of the triple response to systemic effects of large doses of histamine is one way in which cardiovascular shock can occur.

Heart Histamine exerts direct and indirect actions on the human heart. Indirectly, histamine produces an increase in heart rate and force of contraction that results from greater sympathetic tone from baroreceptor discharge in response to a decrease in blood pressure. The direct actions of histamine on the human heart are mediated primarily by H_2-receptors. The actions are a positive chronotropic response that is attributable to an increase in the rate of spontaneous depolarization of sinoatrial nodal cells, an increase in atrial and ventricular automaticity, and an increase in myocardial contractile force. Modest tachycardia, which is sensitive to blockade by cimetidine, occurs at doses of histamine that produce very little change in systemic pressure. At the lower doses of histamine, which produce a decrease in systemic pressure, its indirect actions on the heart predominate.

Other cardiac actions of histamine that may have clinical importance have been demonstrated in experimental animals. Histamine acts at H_1-receptors to decrease the rate of atrioventricular conduction and at H_1-receptors and H_2-receptors to decrease fibrillation thresholds. The actions of histamine on the electrical properties of cardiac tissue and its ability to produce coronary vasoconstriction account for the dysrhythmic actions of this compound. These actions of histamine may be clinically important in provoking cardiac shock that arises in anaphylaxis and dysrhythmias produced by drugs known to cause histamine release in vivo.

Respiratory System In most species, including humans, histamine produces contraction of airway smooth muscle. This occurs after the administration of histamine by inhalation or IV injection. Bronchoconstriction is mediated by H_1-receptors and is the major response of airway smooth muscle to histamine. In healthy humans, histamine is not especially potent; however, the airway smooth muscle of people with asthma is hyperactive to histamine, as well as to other spasmogens. Previously, aerosolized histamine was used as a provocative test for bronchial reactivity to assist in the diagnosis of asthma. Inhalational histamine is rarely used for this purpose now but is used in the clinical pharmacological evaluation of new antihistamines.

Histamine produces a modest relaxation of contracted bronchial smooth muscle by a presumed action on H_2-receptors. Because patients with asthma tolerate agents that block H_2-receptors, it is doubtful that this action of histamine has any major physiological significance.

In addition to actions on airway smooth muscle, histamine acts on H_1-receptors to increase airway fluid and electrolyte secretions. Although not demonstrated in human tissues, it is likely that histamine can produce pulmonary edema by similar processes. The actions of histamine on the respiratory system can contribute to bronchial obstruction in extrinsic asthma (see Chapter 58).

Gastrointestinal System A well-known physiological function of histamine is its role as a primary mediator in the secretion of gastric acid. This is discussed in Chapter 60.

Histamine exhibits relaxant and contractile activities on smooth muscle in the alimentary canal. This has been demonstrated in human tissues on isolated smooth-muscle preparation obtained from the large intestine and gallbladder. In the former, a biphasic effect of histamine was mediated by H_1-receptors. In the latter, the contractile response was mediated by H_1-receptors and occasional relaxant responses by H_2-receptors. The physiological significance of these actions is not established.

Other Actions In addition to the major actions discussed previously, headaches, nausea, and vomiting are also experienced by human volunteers receiving histamine. In large doses, histamine stimulates the release of catecholamines from the adrenal medulla, an effect for which individuals with pheochromocytoma are more sensitive.

Histamine in the Central Nervous System The role of histamine in the CNS is largely inferred from the result of studies on experimental animals. Postulated roles for brain histamine include thermal regulation, regulation of water balance, modulation of nociception, regulation of blood pressure, and arousal. The central effects involve H_1-, H_2-, and H_3-receptors.

Histamine Agonists

Several compounds are available that selectively bind to and activate H_1-, H_2-, or H_3-receptors (see Figure 59-1). These compounds are useful research tools and rarely are used clinically. H_1-Selective agonists have no clinical uses. The H_2-selective agonist betazole is used occasionally as a gastric secretagogue in diagnostic tests for acid secretion. Because its selectivity for H_2-receptors is moderate, it produces systemic actions as a result of activation of H_1-receptors. Pentagastrin is a preferred gastric secretagogue because it produces fewer systemic effects than betazole. Currently, H_3-selective agonists are not used clinically.

Inhibitors of Mast Cell Degranulation

Cromolyn sodium is an agent that inhibits noncytolytic degranulation of mast cells and prevents the activation of inflammatory cells. Cromolyn is effective against mucosal mast cells, particularly those in lung tissue in close contact with the alveoli. Cromolyn has little to no effect on the connective tissue mast cells or on basophils.

Cromolyn is indicated in the prophylactic management of reversible bronchospastic disorders, extrinsic asthma, and exercise-induced asthma that do not respond well to treatment with methylxanthines or sympathomimetic bronchodilators. All patients with asthma can benefit from cromolyn therapy, though young patients respond best. Cromolyn is useful in the prophylaxis of allergic rhinitis and allergic conjunctivitis. Cromolyn also can prevent bronchial pseudoallergic reactions caused by aspirin-like drugs and environmental pollutants. Clinical effectiveness of cromolyn requires at least 4 to 6 weeks of therapy. If an individual does not respond after 6 weeks, it is doubtful that cromolyn will be of any benefit. It is effective only if used before a challenge that can produce degranulation of mast cells. To maintain protective effects that can last for hours, cromolyn must be administered frequently. Unlike β_2-agonists, cromolyn is not effective in the treatment of an acute asthma attack or in the treatment of status asthmaticus (see Chapter 58).

H_1-Antagonists

All the H_1-antagonists have antiallergic properties. With varying degrees, they exhibit sedative, antiemetic, anti–motion sickness, antiparkinsonan, antitussive, and local anesthetic actions. Several antihistamines are used exclusively for one or another of these characteristics rather than for their utility in uncomplicated allergic reactions. These properties may or may not be related to the ability of these agents to block H_1-receptors.

The effectiveness of the agents in the treatment of motion sickness and extrapyramidal symptoms may be attributable to their antimuscarinic actions. Their use to promote sleep may involve the blockade of central H_1-receptors as well as muscarinic receptors. The antiemetic activity is largely confined to the phenothiazine class and probably results from blockade of dopamine

Table 59-4 Properties of Representative H_1-Antagonists and Drugs Possessing H_1-Antagonist Properties

Chemical Class/Agents	Comments
alkylamines brompheniramine chloropheniramine triprolidine	Moderately sedating in usual doses, moderate antimuscarinic activity, no antiemetic and no anti–motion sickness actions
ethanolamines clemastine dimenhydrinate diphenhydramine	Significant sedative actions, pronounced antimuscarinic and anti–motion sickness actions; diphenhydramine in many over-the-counter preparations
ethylenediamines pyrilamine tripelennamine	Low-to-moderate sedative actions, very little antimuscarinic actions, no antimuscarinic actions, no anti–motion sickness activity in usual doses
piperazines cetizine cyclizine hydroxyzine meclizine	Varying degrees of antimuscarinic, anti–motion sickness and sedative actions; cyclizine and meclizine, less sedating than hydroxyzine, used primarily in the treatment of motion sickness and vertigo; hydroxyzine, pronounced sedative and antimuscarinic actions, used as an antiemetic, sedative, and mild anxiolytic agent; cetirizine, a carboxyl metabolite of hydroxyzine, is nonsedating
piperidines astemizole cyproheptadine phenindamine terfenadine	Astemizole and terfenadine, nonsedating, little to no antimuscarinic activity; cyproheptadine, low-to-moderate sedative and antimuscarinic actions, pronounced antiserotonin activity; phenindamine, more likely to produce stimulation than other antihistamines
phenothiazines methdilazine promethiazine trimeprazine	Pronounced antimuscarinic, antiemetic, anti–motion sickness activities; α-adrenoceptor blocking activity and can cause orthostatic hypotension; sedation is common, especially with promethazine

D_2-receptors. The local anesthetic actions are attributable to blockade of sodium channels in excitable membranes. Thus the actions of antihistamines at sites other than the H_1-receptor can contribute to therapeutic uses, as well as to adverse effects. A summary of the pharmacological properties of representative H_1-antagonists is given in Table 59-4.

The release of histamine from mast cells and basophils is accompanied by the release of many other mediators of the immediate hypersensitivity response. Drugs that antagonize H_1-receptors are useful only as monotherapy in mild pseudoallergic or true allergic reactions and as adjunctive agents in the treatment of severe reactions. The treatment of severe allergic reactions requires the use of a physiological antagonist such as epinephrine that will reverse the hypotension, laryngeal edema, and bronchoconstriction produced by the mast cell mediators.

The H_1-antihistamines are used in the symptomatic treatment and prevention of allergic disorders. Their effectiveness is limited to symptoms caused mainly by the actions of histamine and not other mediators. The allergic reactions that respond best to treatment with H_1-antagonists are seasonal but also include perennial allergic rhinitis, conjunctivitis, and itching associated with acute and chronic urticaria. Antihistamines are of some value in the treatment of atopic dermatitis and contact dermatitis. The choice of a nonsedative or sedative H_1-antihistamine in treating these disorders depends on whether sedation is desirable. Tolerance may develop to the sedative properties within a few days.

The older H_1-antagonists are not beneficial in the treatment of bronchial asthma. As previously noted, this is attributable to the role of mediators other than histamine and, possibly, because local concentrations of the H_1-antagonists are too low relative to the local concentrations of histamine to produce effective blockade.

Tolerance to the antihistamines occurs. Frequently, switching to an agent in a different chemical class results in restoration of the desired therapeutic effects. It is not known if the tolerance is caused by the induction of drug-metabolizing enzymes or changes at the receptor. Experimentally, attempts to demonstrate an upregulation of H_1-receptors after chronic treatment with antagonists have been disappointing.

H_1-Antihistamines that are distributed to the CNS are used in the prophylactic treatment of motion sickness. Promethazine and diphenhydramine are the most potent but also produce a high incidence of sedation. Promethazine is effective as an antiemetic in reducing vomiting from a variety of causes. Meclazine, cyclizine, and dimenhydrinate, a salt of diphenhydramine, are used in over-the-counter preparations for prevention of motion sickness. However, none is as effective as scopolamine in preventing nausea and vomiting associated with motion. These agents also are used in the symptomatic treatment of vertigo.

H_2-Antagonists

The H_2-antagonists now used clinically are cimetidine, famotidine, nizatidine, and ranitidine. All act as competitive antagonists at histamine H_2-receptors and are used primarily in the management of peptic ulcer disease. H_2-Antagonists are also used in the management of immediate hypersensitivity reactions to block cardiac and vascular H_2-responses to histamine, which can contribute to anaphylactic shock. Their pharmacological actions are described in detail in Chapter 60.

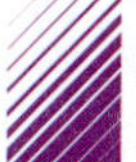

SIDE EFFECTS, CLINICAL PROBLEMS, AND TOXICITY

Clinical problems with cromolyn sodium and the H_1-antagonists are listed in the box below. Clinical problems for H_2-antagonists are given in Chapter 60.

Cromolyn Sodium

Because cromolyn sodium is not well absorbed, systemic toxicity is rare. Many patients use cromolyn for several years without adverse effects or the development of tolerance. The aerosolized powder has irritant effects that can cause coughing, wheezing, bronchospasm, and pharyngeal discomfort. The irritant properties can worsen bronchoconstriction during an acute attack. Adverse effects associated with the nasal solutions occur in about 2% of patients. Frequent adverse effects are nasal irritation, bad taste, and headache. The common adverse reaction associated with the ophthalmic solution is a transient ocular stinging or burning on instillation. The ophthalmic solution contains benzalkonium chloride and should not be used with soft contact lenses. Hypersensitivity reactions are rare.

CLINICAL PROBLEMS

CROMOLYN SODIUM

Airway irritant
Bad taste
Headache

H_1-RECEPTOR ANTAGONISTS

Antimuscarinic actions
Sedative effects
Some CNS depression (in first-generation agents)
Paradoxical excitation in children
Topical-use allergic reaction

H_1-Antagonists

The majority of H_1-antagonist adverse effects are attributable to the antimuscarinic and sedative actions of the antihistamines. With the older agents, central depressant effects are common untoward reactions and occur in about 25% to 50% of patients. Antihistamines with antimuscarinic activity may cause dryness of the mouth, blurred vision, dysuria or urinary retention, constipation, and other symptoms attributable to blockade of muscarinic receptors.

The incidences of central depression and antimuscarinic effects are less for the newer agents, such as astemizole and terfenadine. With these agents, the incidences of CNS depression and antimuscarinic effects are comparable to those produced by placebo. Additional central effects include insomnia, nervousness, tremors, and euphoria. Appetite stimulation and weight gain are reported for some agents. Paradoxical excitation can occur in children. Nausea, vomiting, diarrhea, and epigastric distress are reported.

The main signs of acute overdose are similar to those caused by classical antimuscarinic agents. In overdose, a rare but potentially hazardous quinidine-like effect is seen resulting in prolongation of the QT interval and the development of torsade de pointes, a prefibrillatory ventricular dysrhythmia. Such dysrhythmias are reported for both first- and second-generation antihistamines and in the case of terfenadine and astemizole can occur when taken with drugs that inhibit their metabolism such as erythromycin, troleandomycin, and ketoconazole.

The incidence of true allergic responses is low with systemic administration. However, allergic responses are relatively common after repeated topical use; therefore topical use is discouraged.

Teratogenic effects produced by piperazine derivatives are observed in experimental animals. Although there is no evidence that this occurs in humans, this class of antihistamines, as well as all others, is not recommended during pregnancy.

The centrally acting H_1-antagonists can potentiate the actions of other central depressant agents: hypnotic sedatives, narcotic analgesics, general anesthetics, and alcohol. Similarly, their antimuscarinic actions are additive with those produced by other agents. Monoamine oxidase inhibitors can potentiate the antimuscarinic actions of antihistamines.

TRADE NAMES

In addition to generic and fixed-combination preparations, the following trade-named materials are available in the United States.

MAST CELL STABILIZERS

Intal, Nasalcroom, Opticrom, cromolyn sodium

HISTAMINE H_1-ANTAGONISTS

Hismanal, astemizole
Atrohist, Bromarest, Bromfed, Dimetane, brompheniramine
Zyrtec, cetirizine
Chlortrimeton, Teldrin, chlorpheniramine
Tavist, clemastine
Marezine, cyclizine
Periactin, cyproheptadine
Dexchlor, Poladex, Polaramine, dexchlorpheniramine
Dimetabs, Dramamine, Marmine, dimenhydrinate
Claratin, loratidine
Anxanil, Atarax, Vistaril, hydroxyzine
Antivert, Bonine, meclizine
Tacaryl, methdilazine
Nolamine, Nolahist, phenindamine
Phenameth, Phenergan, promethazine
Seldane, terfenadine
Temaril, trimeprazine
PBZ, tripelennamine
Actidil, triprolidine

NEW DIRECTIONS

In the past two decades many advances have been made in the discovery of drugs that antagonize histamine, that is, the development of H_2-antagonists for the treatment of peptic ulcer disease and the discovery of nonsedating H_1-antagonists. Future advances may arise from agents acting at H_3-receptors. Currently they are being evaluated as potential therapeutic agents. H_3-agonists, agents that inhibit transmitter release, may find use in the treatment of asthma by virtue of their ability to inhibit neurogenic evoked bronchospasm. Similarly, such agents may provide a novel means of reducing gastric acid secretion and reducing hypermotility of the intestine. The central actions of H_3-antagonists indicate that they might be useful in increasing alertness.

The development of newer orally effective agents that exhibit antihistamine as well as cromolyn-like activity is an area for future advances. Agents in clinical trials or in preclinical testing that show such actions include azelastine, ketotifen, and epinastine.

REFERENCES

Ganellin CR, Schwartz JC, editor: *Frontiers in histamine research,* Oxford, 1985, Pergamon Press.

Garland LG: Pharmacology of prophylactic anti-asthma drugs. In Page CP, Barnes FJ, editors: *Pharmacology of asthma (Handbook of Experimental Pharmacology,* Ser. No. 98), Berlin, 1991, Springer-Verlag.

Leurs R, van der Groot H, Timmerman H: Histaminergic agonists and antagonists: recent developments. In Testa B, editor: *Advances in drug research,* vol 20, London, 1990, Pergamon Press.

Timmerman H, van der Groot H, editor: *New perspectives in histamine research (Agents and Actions Supplements* vol 33), Basel, 1991, Birkhäuser Verlag.

Uvnäs B, editor: *Histamine and histamine antagonists, (Handbook of Experimental Pharmacology,* Ser. No. 97), Berlin, 1991, Springer-Verlag.

SELF-ASSESSMENT QUESTIONS

1. First-generation antihistamines differ from second generation in that the latter have:
   a. greater affinities for H_1-receptors.
   b. partial agonist activity.
   c. greater antimuscarinic activity.
   d. less sedative effects.
   e. shorter half-lives
2. Vasodilatation produced by low doses of histamine can be antagonized by:
   a. H_1-antagonists.
   b. H_2-antagonists.
   c. H_3-antagonists.
   d. a combination of b and c.
   e. none of the above
3. Orthostatic hypotension is most likely to be produced by which of the following H_1-antagonists?
   a. astemizole
   b. promethazine
   c. diphenhydramine
   d. chlorpheniramine
   e. tripelennamine
4. Responses mediated by H_2-receptors include:
   a. bronchoconstriction.
   b. gastric acid secretion.
   c. decreased force of ventricular contraction.
   d. stimulation of basophil degranulation.
   e. inhibition of norepinephrine release.

5. Mast cells found in which location appear to be more sensitive to the 'stabilizing' actions of cromolyn sodium?
   a. skin
   b. bronchoalveolar spaces
   c. intestinal mucosa
   d. vascular wall
   e. hypothalamus
6. Which of the following is a selective agonist for H_3-receptors?
   a. betazole
   b. 4(5)-methylhistamine
   c. impromidine
   d. thiazolylethylamine
   e. *R*-α-methylhistamine

CHAPTER

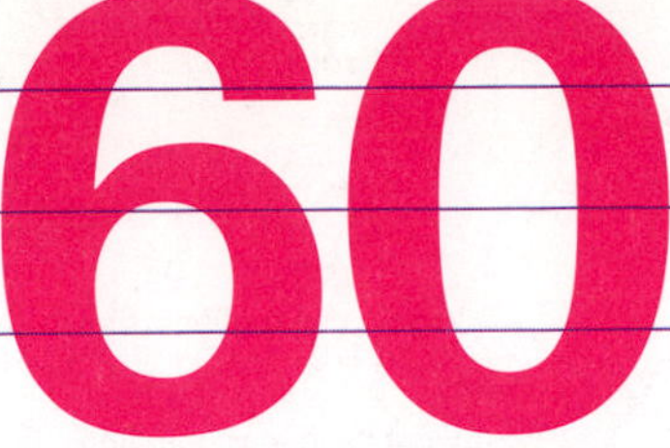

Gastrointestinal Drugs

THOMAS F. BURKS

MAJOR DRUGS

gastric antacids
antidiarrheal agents
histamine H_2-antagonists
laxatives
prokinetic agents
proton pump inhibitors
protectants

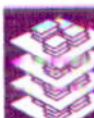

THERAPEUTIC OVERVIEW

The gastrointestinal (GI) tract stores, digests, and absorbs nutrients and eliminates wastes. Regulation of the GI organs results from control by intrinsic nerves of the enteric nervous system, neural activity in the CNS, and by an array of GI hormones. These processes are summarized in Figure 60-1.

The pharmacologically treatable impairments to normal motility, digestion, secretion, and absorption processes of the stomach and intestinal tract are reflux esophagitis, peptic ulcers, delayed gastric emptying, inadequate propulsion of chyme and solids in the small intestine, colon and rectum, diarrhea, infections, or inflammation. In each case, potential beneficial effects of drugs must be carefully considered against potential adverse effects.

Peptic ulcer is a benign lesion of gastric or duodenal mucosa occurring at a site where the mucosal epithelium is exposed to acid and pepsin. There is constant confrontation in the stomach and upper small bowel between acid-pepsin aggression and mucosal defense. Usually the mucosa can withstand the acid-pepsin attack and remain healthy; that is, a mucosal "barrier" to backdiffusion of acid is maintained. However, an excess of acid production or an intrinsic defect in the barrier functions of the mucosa can allow the defense mechanism to fail and ulcers to result. The therapeutic strategy for management of peptic ulcer disease may be directed at reduction of acid exposure of the mucosa or improvement in the integrity of the mucosal barrier.

Many patients with duodenal ulcer disease have an elevated mass of gastric parietal cells and elevated gastric acid secretion. Patients with gastrin-secreting tumors (gastrinoma, Zollinger-Ellison syndrome) secrete excess amounts of acid and almost invariably develop duodenal ulcers. In gastrinomas, excess acid production clearly overwhelms the mucosal defense. In contrast to patients with duodenal ulcers, patients with gastric ulcers often have normal or low rates of basal and stimulated acid secretion. These patients, and some with duodenal ulcers, may develop a primary defect in the mucosa that provides inadequate defense against acid-pepsin attack. The role of pepsin in peptic ulcer is not known, despite the name of the disease. Most successful therapeutic approaches to peptic ulcer are based on the adage, "no acid, no ulcer."

There is evidence that chronic colonization of the gastric and duodenal mucosae with *Helicobacter pylori* may be causally associated with peptic ulcer disease. *H. pylori* infection is known to produce inflammatory changes in the mucosa and may diminish the acid resistance (barrier function) of the mucosal defense. Eradication of the *H. pylori* infection, though difficult to achieve, may lead in some cases to long-term remission of ulcer disease (see p. 814 in New Directions).

ABBREVIATIONS

ATPase	adenosine triphosphatase
5-HT	5-hydroxytryptophan
cAMP	cyclic adenosine monophosphate

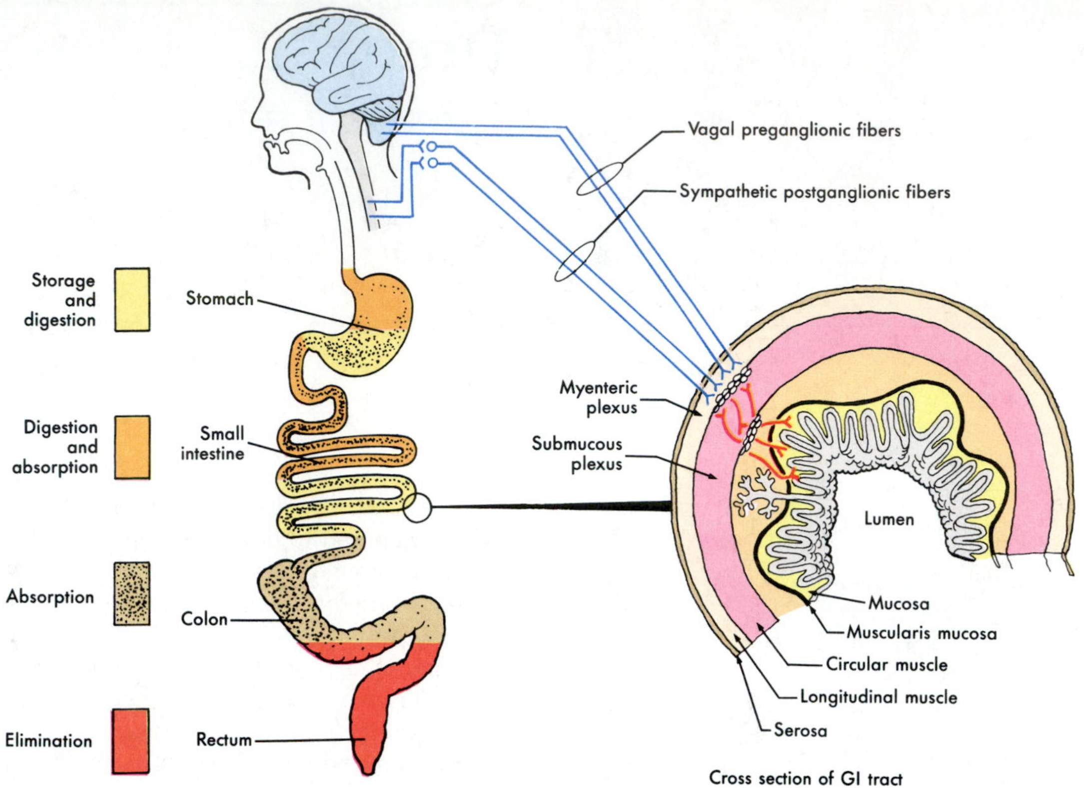

FIGURE 60-1 Overall functions of the gastrointestinal tract. Extrinsic and intrinsic autonomic efferent innervation of the wall of the intestine. The enteric nervous system of the gastrointestinal tract innervates smooth muscle and mucosa. Efferent and afferent neurons are organized in intramural plexuses; the most prominent plexuses are the myenteric plexus between the longitudinal and circular muscle coats and the submucosal plexus between the circular muscle and the muscularis mucosa.

Reflux esophagitis is most often associated with inappropriate relaxation of the lower esophageal sphincter, allowing acid gastric contents to flow into the esophagus and produce painful irritation and inflammation of the esophageal mucosa. Reflux can be reduced by drugs that increase tone of the lower esophageal sphincter, and mucosal irritation can be reduced by decreasing the concentration of acid in the stomach.

Gastroparesis is a delay in gastric emptying resulting from a complication of diabetes or other diseases that damage gastric nerves or smooth muscle. Gastric emptying can be improved by prokinetic drugs, which increase propulsive contractions of the stomach.

Frequency of defecation and the quantity and consistency of stool are subject to regulation. Dietary changes alone may be sufficient to restore normal bowel habits. However, in patients with functional intermittent or chronic constipation, treatment with a laxative may be indicated. The physician should be aware that constipation can arise from functional disorders, drug treatment, or low-residue diets. Excessive use of laxatives, especially through self-medication, can lead to adverse effects, including nutritional imbalance, abdominal cramps, fluid and electrolyte disturbance, and reliance on laxatives for bowel movements.

Diarrhea is a GI problem that can be acute, secondary to an enteric bacterial or viral infection, or chronic, secondary to inflammatory or functional bowel disease. The most effective management of diarrhea is to remove the cause. This includes eliminating the infection, removing the secretagogue-producing tumor, or curing the inflammation. The major hazard associated with diarrhea is loss of fluid and electrolytes. Serious sequelae of diarrhea can generally be avoided by replacement of fluid and electrolytes in patients with self-limiting diarrhea. However, many patients with trivial or serious acute or chronic diarrhea require antidiarrheal therapy for personal comfort and convenience.

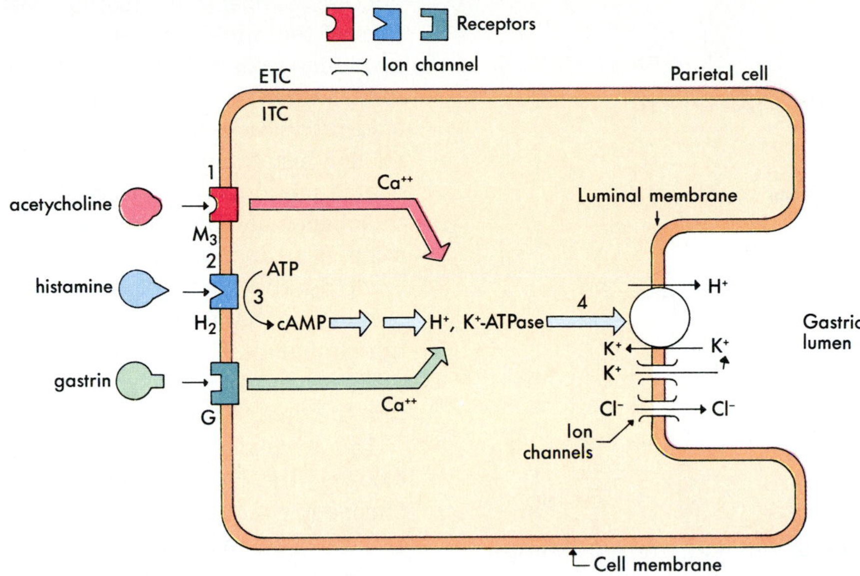

FIGURE 60-2 Diagram of the mechanisms regulating secretion of HCl by the gastric parietal cell. Receptors for acetylcholine, histamine, and gastrin interact when activated by agonists to increase availability of Ca^{++} and stimulate the H^+,K^+-ATPase of the luminal membrane. Acid secretion can be decreased pharmacologically by blockade of acetylcholine M_3-receptors (1), histamine H_2-receptors (2), intracellular adenylate cyclase (3), or the H^+,K^+-ATPase (4).

Drugs used to treat disease states or disturbances of the GI tract are summarized in the box at right.

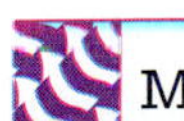

MECHANISMS OF ACTION

Drugs for Treatment of Peptic Ulcers

Secretion of acid by gastric parietal cells is regulated by histamine, acetylcholine, and gastrin (Figure 60-2). Psychic stimuli (sight and smell of food) and the presence of food in the mouth or stomach stimulates vagally mediated gastric acid secretion resulting from acetylcholine actions on parietal and paracrine cells. Acetylcholine acts at parietal cell muscarinic cholinergic receptors (M_3 in Figure 60-2) coupled to calcium channels that allow entry of extracellular calcium into the parietal cell. Gastrin is released from the antral mucosa by the presence of food that raises antral pH. The gastrin circulates through the bloodstream to act as gastrin receptors on parietal and paracrine cells. Activation of gastrin receptors is believed to mobilize intracellular calcium in the parietal cell. Histamine is released from nearby paracrine cells to act at parietal cell H_2-receptors. These receptors are positively coupled to adenylate cyclase; thus activation results in formation of intracellular cyclic adenosine monophosphate, which ultimately

THERAPEUTIC OVERVIEW

PROBLEMS	TREATMENT
Peptic ulcer	Drugs to neutralize excess acid, block acid secretion, repair mucosal barrier breakdown
Delayed gastric emptying and propulsion of contents through intestine	Prokinetic drugs
Constipation, painful elimination, elderly patients with inadequate fiber intake, impaction	Laxatives
Diarrhea	Remove source, opioid drugs

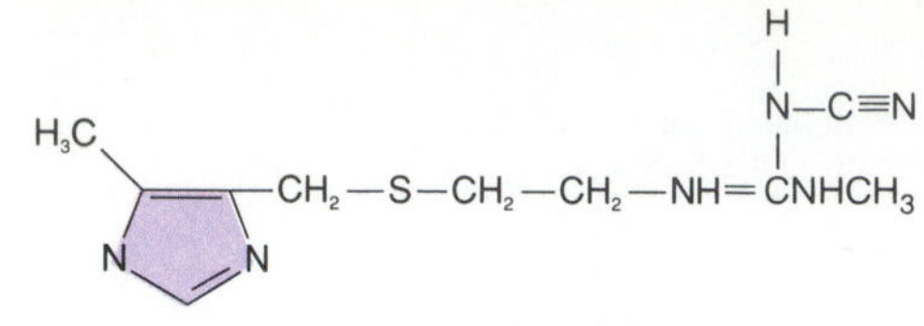

cimetidine

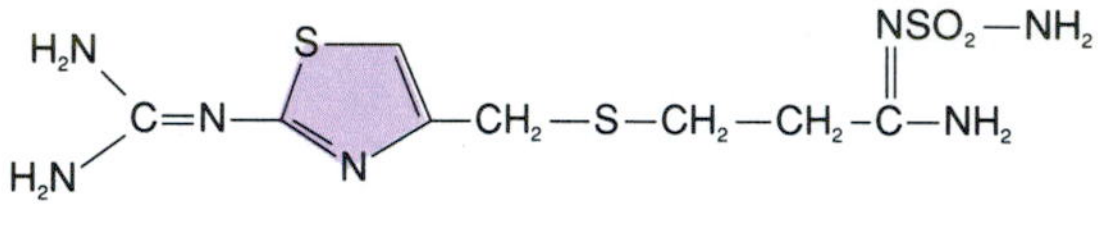

famotidine

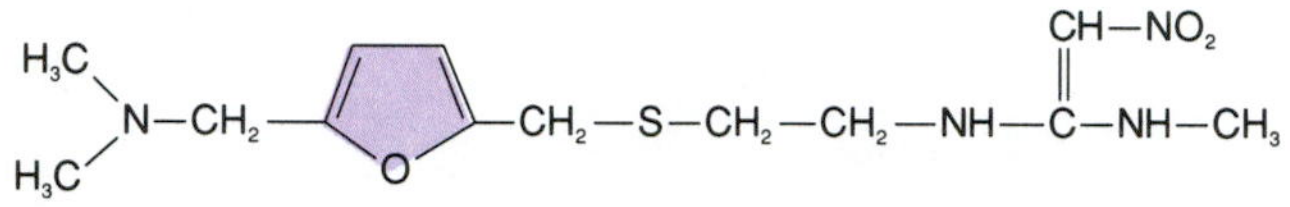

ranitidine

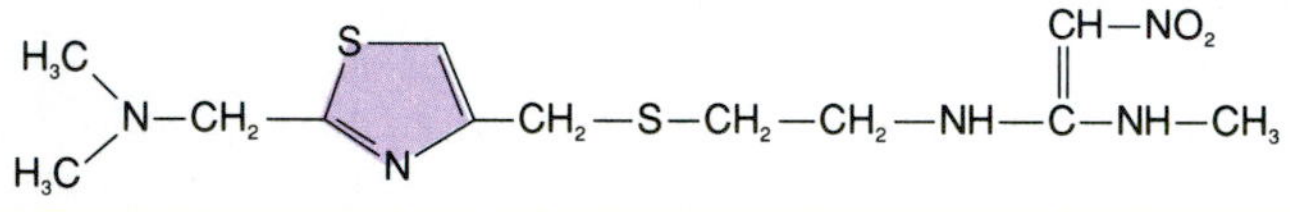

nizatidine

FIGURE 60-3 Structures of histamine H_2-receptor antagonists used in management of peptic ulcer disease.

activates a H^+,K^+-ATPase at the luminal border of the parietal cell. The H_2-receptors, muscarinic cholinergic receptors, and gastrin receptors mutually interact to augment the secretory actions of histamine, acetylcholine, and gastrin, but of these three regulatory receptors, histamine is considered to be most important and may serve as the final common pathway in regulation of gastric acid secretion.

Neurally secreted acetylcholine and circulating gastrin may exert two distinct types of stimulatory effects (one indirect and one direct) on gastric parietal cells. The indirect effect is exerted at small histamine-containing paracrine cells located near parietal cells in oxyntic glands. Acetylcholine released from secretomotor terminals of the vagus nerve act at muscarinic M_1-receptors on histamine cells to cause release of histamine, which in turn acts at parietal cell H_2-receptors to stimulate acid secretion. Acetylcholine also acts directly at parietal cell M_3-receptors to stimulate acid production. Similarly, circulating gastrin released from G cells of the antral mucosa acts at gastrin receptors on histamine cells to release histamine and also acts directly at gastrin receptors on parietal cells to stimulate acid production. Thus, both acetylcholine and gastrin release histamine as major events in their stimulation of acid production and also act directly on parietal cells to enhance and augment the secretory actions of histamine. Activation of any of the three types of parietal cell receptors appears to result in increased activity of a protein kinase that activates the H^+,K^+-ATPase located at the luminal membrane of the parietal cell. The H^+,K^+-ATPase serves as the "proton pump" that secretes H^+ into the gastric lumen.

Drugs can decrease gastric secretion (Figure 60-2) by blocking the H_2-receptors, by blocking the M_1 or M_3 cholinergic receptors, by inhibiting histamine-induced activity of adenylate cyclase, or by inhibiting activity of the H^+,K^+-ATPase of the parietal cell.

The molecular mechanism of action of histamine and antihistamines is discussed in detail in Chapter 59. A brief discussion relevant to gastric acid secretion is included here. The H_2-receptor on the parietal cell mediates the stimulatory effect of histamine on acid secretion. Activation of the H_2-receptor also augments the secretory actions of gastrin and acetylcholine on the parietal cells. The only important role of peripheral H_2-receptors in humans appears to be in regulation of acid secretion. For this reason, H_2-receptor antagonists provide remarkably specific therapy for peptic ulcer disease. In fact, the efficacy of H_2-receptor antagonists as inhibitors of acid secretion provides strong evidence for the important role of histamine as a physiological mediator of gastric acid secretion. H_2-Receptor antagonists inhibit acid secretion by histamine, as well as the secretion induced by gastrin, cholinergic agents, food, and reflex vagal stimulation.

The H_2-receptor antagonists, including cimetidine, famotidine, nizatidine, and ranitidine (see Figure 60-3 for structures), act to decrease acid and pepsin secretion by competitive antagonism at parietal cell histamine receptors (Table 60-1). H_2-Receptor antagonists do not block cholinergic receptors or gastrin receptors. The decrease in acid and pepsin secretion that results from blockade of H_2-receptors allows the mucosa, in particular the duodenal mucosa, to tolerate the diminished acid load presented and effectively promote healing of the ulcer. H_2-Receptor antagonists increase the incidence of ulcer healing, improve the rate at which healing occurs, and prevent recurrence of ulcers.

Proton-pump inhibitors, such as omeprazole, block the ability of the parietal cell H^+,K^+-ATPase to transport hydrogen ion into the lumen of the stomach (see Figure 60-2). Because all secretory stimuli ultimately in-

Table 60-1 Summary of Actions of Antiulcer Drugs

Category	Prototype	Mechanism of Action
Antacids	magnesium oxide and magnesium hydroxide	Neutralize secreted acid
Anticholinergics	propantheline	Block muscarinic receptors, decrease H^+ secretion
H_2-Antagonists	cimetidine	Block H_2-receptors, decrease H^+ secretion
Prostaglandins	misoprostol	Inhibit cAMP, decrease H^+ secretion
Protective	sucralfate	Protect mucosal barrier
Proton pump inhibitors	omeprazole	Inhibit H^+,K^+-ATPase, decrease H^+ secretion

crease acid production by increasing activity of the H^+,K^+-ATPase transporter, blockade of the enzyme provides the most effective mechanism by which acid secretion can be diminished. Proton pump–inhibitory drugs are highly efficacious in the management of peptic ulcer disease and reflux esophagitis.

Antacids act by neutralization of intragastric hydrochloric acid, and the cations (sodium, calcium, magnesium, aluminum) form soluble chloride salts (Figure 60-4). NaCl can be absorbed from the small intestine, but the divalent ions form poorly soluble bicarbonates and carbonates, which precipitate and remain in the bowel lumen to be excreted in the feces. Calcium, magnesium, and aluminum ions can also interact with fatty acids to form insoluble salts (soaps), which also are excreted in the feces.

Another type of peptic ulcer drug is typified by sucralfate, which is a basic aluminum salt of sucrose octasulfate (Figure 60-5). Unlike the other drugs presently available for management of peptic ulcer disease, sucralfate does not decrease the concentration or total amount of acid in the gastric lumen. Instead, it acts to protect the gastric and duodenal mucosa from acid-pepsin attack. Sucralfate appears to possess three relevant actions: it complexes with proteins at the ulcer site to form a protective layer, it decreases backdiffusion of hydrogen ions, and it binds to pepsin and bile salts.

Muscarinic receptor antagonists (anticholinergic drugs) historically were used in management of peptic ulcer disease; many such agents are still available for use. These antagonists block (muscarinic) M_1-receptors on histamine-containing paracrine cells in the oxyntic mucosa to inhibit acetylcholine-induced release of histamine and also block M_3-receptors on parietal cells to inhibit direct acetylcholine-induced acid secretion. Although the muscarinic antagonists are effective in reducing acid secretion and promoting healing of peptic ulcers, the spectrum of adverse side effects produced by these agents makes them less tolerable to patients. The side effects occur because the presently available muscarinic antagonists fail to discriminate among subtypes of muscarinic receptors and therefore block the muscarinic receptors responsible for gastrointestinal propulsion, regulation of heart rate, salivary secretion, ocular accommodation, and micturition. Molecular mechanisms of other drugs used in the treatment of peptic ulcers are covered in Chapter 9 (muscarinic cholinergic antagonists) and Chapter 18 (prostaglandins).

(1) $Al(OH)_3 + 3HCl \rightleftharpoons AlCl_3 + 3H_2O$

(2) $Mg(OH)_2 + 2HCl \rightleftharpoons MgCl_2 + 2H_2O$

(3) $MgCl_2 + Na_2CO_3 \rightleftharpoons MgCO_3\ (PPT) + 2NaCl$

(4) $MgCl_2 + 2R{-}COONa \rightleftharpoons Mg(R{-}COO)_2\ (PPT) + 2NaCl$

FIGURE 60-4 Intragastric and intestinal interactions of prototype antacids. (1) Interaction of aluminum hydroxide with gastric acid to form soluble aluminum chloride. (2) Interaction of magnesium hydroxide with gastric acid. (3) Soluble magnesium chloride interaction with sodium carbonate in the lumen of the intestine to form insoluble magnesium carbonate. (4) Interaction of soluble magnesium chloride with fatty acid salts in the lumen of the intestine to form an insoluble magnesium soap. *PPT,* Precipitate.

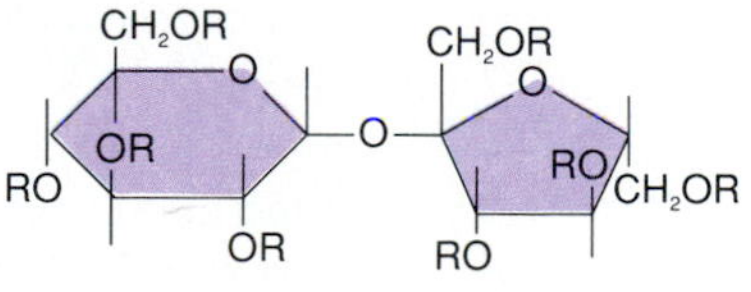

FIGURE 60-5 Structure of sucralfate.

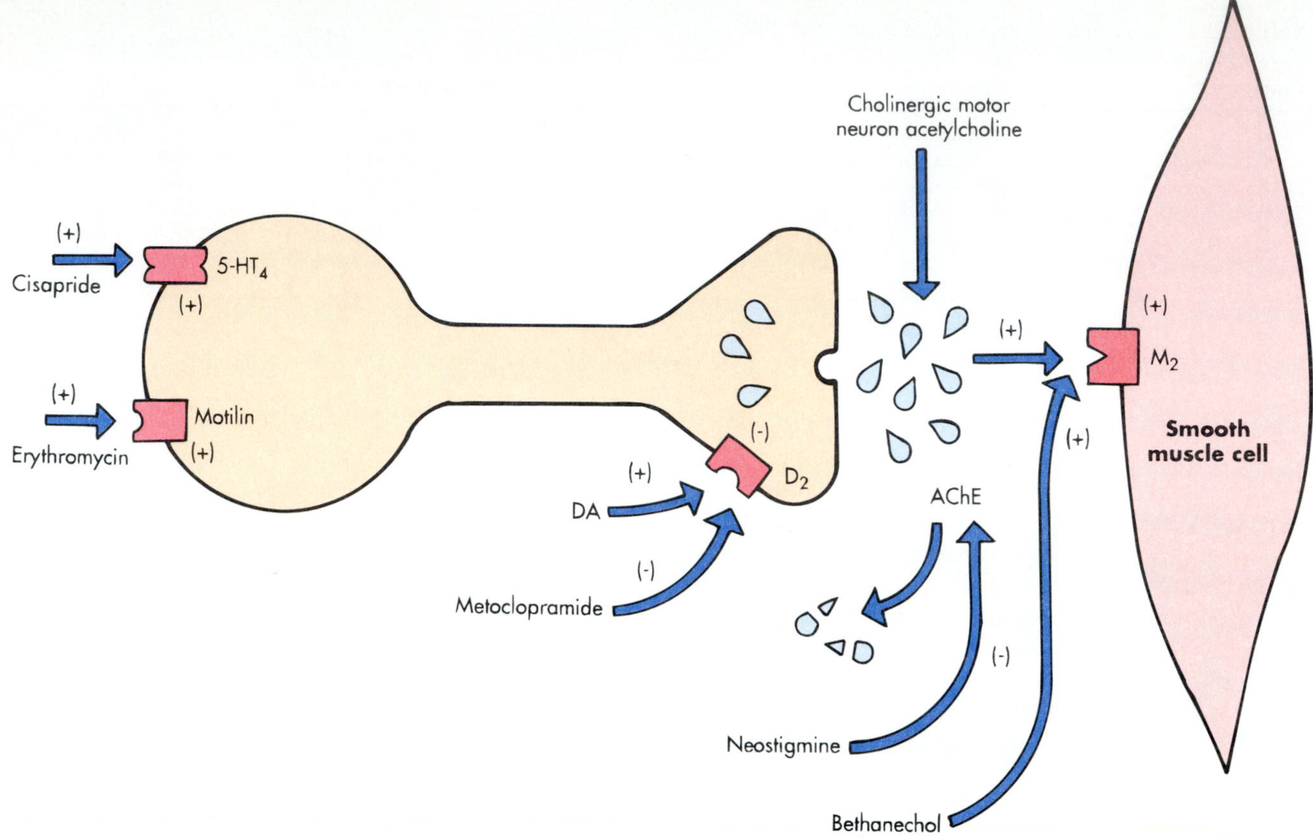

FIGURE 60-6 Mechanisms of prokinetic drugs. These agents directly or indirectly increase agonist activity at smooth muscle muscarinic M_2-receptors. Cisapride is an agonist ($^+$) at excitatory (+) neural 5-hydroxytryptamine *(5-HT₄)* receptors on enteric nervous system cholingeric motor neurons. Erythromycin is an agonist (+) at excitatory (+) motilin receptors. Metoclopramide is an antagonist (−) at dopamine *(DA)* receptors (D_2) that inhibit (−) release of acetylcholine. Neostigmine inhibits (−) hydrolysis of acetylcholine by acetylcholinesterase *(AChE)*. Bethanechol acts directly as an agonist (+) at excitatory (+) M_2 smooth muscle receptors.

Prokinetic Drugs

Prokinetic drugs increase GI contractions and propulsion by increasing cholinergic stimuli at smooth muscle cell M_2-receptors (Figure 60-6). Cholinergic stimulation can be accomplished by five different mechanisms (Table 60-2):

1. Drugs, such as bethanechol, that act directly as agonists at muscarinic receptors
2. Drugs, such as neostigmine, that block acetylcholinesterase, thereby allowing accumulation of neurally secreted acetylcholine at smooth muscle M_2-receptors
3. Drugs, such as metoclopramide, that block inhibitory presynaptic D_2-receptors of cholinergic motor neurons that innervate smooth muscle, thereby increasing release of acetylcholine from nerve terminals
4. Drugs, such as cisapride, that activate excitatory presynaptic (5-hydroxytryptamine) 5-HT_4 receptors of cholinergic motor neurons, thereby increasing release of acetylcholine from nerve terminals
5. Drugs, such as erythromycin, that activate excitatory neural and smooth muscle motilin receptors

The most useful mechanisms, in terms of therapeutic benefit/risk ratios, are those involving agonist activity at 5-HT_4 (mechanism 4) or at motilin receptors (mechanism 5). Mechanisms 1 and 2, involving cholinergic drugs, lead to significant side effects associated with excessive secretory activity. Cholinergic agonists and acetylcholinesterase inhibitors increase cholinergic stimuli at salivary, gastric, pancreatic, and intestinal secretory cells in addition to smooth muscle cells. Moreover, the cholinergic drugs fail to produce the types of closely coordinated contractions between the antrum of

Table 60-2 Summary of Action of Prokinetic Drugs

Category	Prototype	Mechanism of Action
Muscarinic agonists	bethanecol	Increase contraction of GI smooth muscle
Acetylcholinesterase inhibitors	neostigmine	Block destruction of acetylcholine
Dopamine inhibitors	metoclopramide	Block inhibitory presynaptic (dopamine) D_2-receptors
5-HT agonists	cisapride	Activate excitatory presynaptic 5-HT_4 receptors
Motilin agonists	erythromycin	Activate neural and smooth muscle motilin receptors

the stomach and the duodenum required for effective gastric emptying.

D_2-Receptor antagonists increase the tone of the lower esophageal sphincter (important in therapy of reflux esophagitis), increase the force of gastric contractions, improve coordination of gastroduodenal contractions, and enhance gastric emptying. Moreover, some drugs are highly effective as antiemetic agents, an action attributable to blockade of central dopamine receptors associated with the chemoreceptor trigger zone and other sites that control emesis. The structure of metoclopramide is shown in Figure 60-7.

The 5-HT_4 agonists, recently introduced, also increase the tone of the lower esophageal sphincter and the force of gastric contractions and improve gastroduodenal coordination. Several chemically related drugs, such as ondansetron, are antagonists at the 5-HT_3 receptor that occurs on vagal afferent nerves that activate central nervous system emetic mechanisms. The 5-HT_3 receptor antagonists are useful antiemetics.

Motilin is a gastrointestinal hormone that participates in initiation of migrating motor complexes that characterize the fasting motility pattern of the stomach and small intestine. Erythromycin and several analogs bind to nerve and muscle motilin receptors to enhance gastrointestinal contractions and increase the rate of gastric emptying. The prokinetic effect is not related to the antimicrobial activity of these agents.

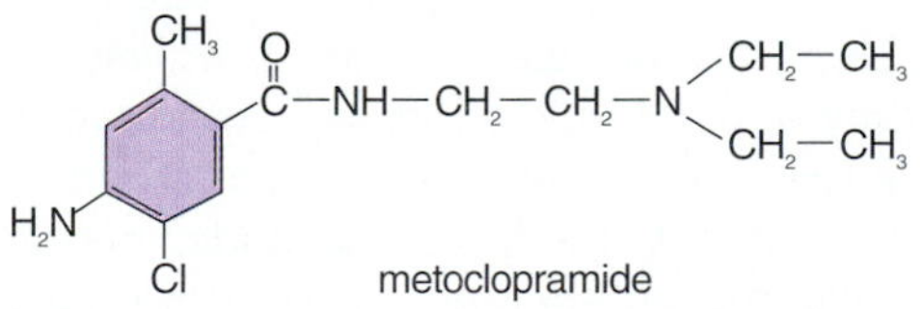

FIGURE 60-7 Structure of the dopamine antagonist prokinetic drug metoclopramide.

Laxatives

Laxatives (sometimes called *cathartics, purgatives,* or *evacuants*) can be divided into several categories depending on their mechanisms of action: secretory or stimulant, saline, emollient, and bulk forming. Certain secretory laxatives (e.g., castor oil) may act on intestinal mucosa crypt cells to open chloride channels to allow movement of chloride, sodium, and water into the intestinal lumen. Since chloride channels of enterocytes (cells lining the intestinal mucosa) are regulated primarily by cAMP, it is believed that some secretory laxatives directly or indirectly stimulate adenylate cyclase activity, thereby increasing intracellular cAMP concentrations in crypt cells. Other agents in this category act by other mechanisms. Docusate sodium is presumed to soften feces by lowering surface tension or inhibiting water absorption in the lower intestine, increasing intraluminal electrolytes and water. The precise mechanism of other secretory or stimulant laxatives has not been well established.

Saline laxatives (e.g., milk of magnesia) are salts with one or both ions poorly absorbed, thus drawing a significant amount of water into the intestine by an osmotic process. This results in increased gut propulsion and evacuation.

Emollients (e.g., mineral oil) are nonabsorbable laxatives used orally to lubricate the lower bowel in conditions of irritated anal tissues or in relieving fecal impaction.

Bulk-forming agents (e.g., psyllium) are nonabsorbable and form a large hydrophilic mass when taken with water. By increased water content and bulk, intestinal transit time is reduced.

The pharmacologic classification of laxatives is less important and less useful than a descriptive classification of their effects. Intensity, latency, and the nature of the stool produced by each agent are the major concerns.

Antidiarrheal Drugs

Diarrhea results from excessive fluid in the lumen of the intestine; this generates rapid, high-volume flow

Table 60-3 Summary of Action of Antidiarrheal Drugs

Category	Prototypes	Mechanism of Action
Opioids	loperamide, diphenoxylate	Increase resistance to flow, decrease propulsion, decrease net fluid secretion
Antisecretory agents	bismuth subsalicylate	Decrease fluid secretion
Anticholinergic drugs	dicyclomine	Reduce contractile activity
Gel-forming adsorbants	hydrated aluminum silicate, pectin, kaolin	Increase resistance to flow, increase formed stools
Ion-exchange resins	cholestyramine	Bind water and bile salts

and overwhelms the absorptive capacity of the colon. It is important to note that, in most diarrheal conditions, fluid and electrolyte absorption occurs at an essentially normal rate. However, the diarrheal stimulus increases fluid secretion into the lumen at a rate that exceeds absorptive capacity, thus leading to net accumulation of fluid in the intestinal lumen.

Diarrhea can be treated in the following ways (Table 60-3):

1. Increase resistance to flow by stimulating segmenting intestinal contractions or by increasing viscosity of luminal contents
2. Increase mucosal absorption or decrease secretion
3. Remove diarrhea-producing chemicals
4. Prevent formation of diarrhea-producing chemicals

Transport of fluid and electrolytes by the intestinal mucosa is regulated by neurons of the enteric nervous system and by the chemical composition of the luminal contents. It is believed that neurons of the submucosal plexus of the intestine terminate near mucosal epithelial cells and act to increase or decrease absorption by villus cells and secretion by crypt cells.

Natural opioids such as morphine and codeine and synthetic opioids such as loperamide and diphenoxylate are discussed with respect to side effects in Chapter 28. The opioid drugs in particular can act on intestinal neural elements to decrease secretion and promote mucosal transport from the lumen. In addition, opioids can act in the CNS to alter extrinsic neural influences on the intestine to promote net absorption of fluid and electrolytes. The specific neurotransmitters of submucosal neurons affected by opioids have not been identified. Opioids also convert propulsive patterns of motility to segmenting patterns that increase resistance to flow.

PHARMACOKINETICS

The pharmacokinetic parameters of drugs that are used systemically are summarized in Table 60-4. The present H_2-antagonists may be administered orally once or twice daily for management of acute phases of duodenal ulcer and once daily for maintenance therapy. The daily oral dose may be given at bedtime to minimize potential adverse side effects, such as somnolence or dizziness, and to control nocturnal acid secretion. Cimetidine, famotidine and ranitidine are also available for IV administration. The plasma half-lives of the H_2-antagonists are relatively short, ranging from approximately 1½ hours for nizatidine to 3 hours for famotidine and ranitidine. Cimetidine, famotidine, nizatidine, and ranitidine are excreted in the urine, primarily as intact drugs. However, there can be significant (up to 30%) formation of the corresponding sulfoxides (cimetidine and famotidine) or *N*-oxides (nizatidine and ranitidine) as well. Because renal elimination is an important terminating mechanism for all the H_2-antagonists, dosage reduction may be necessary in patients with renal insufficiency.

Sucralfate is available for oral use only. Slight absorption occurs from the intestine and most of the drug is excreted intact in the feces. The small fraction that is absorbed is excreted intact in the urine.

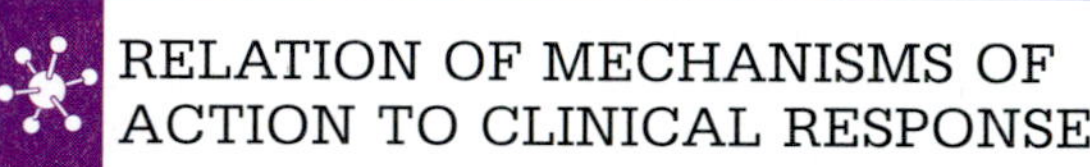

RELATION OF MECHANISMS OF ACTION TO CLINICAL RESPONSE

Drugs for Treatment of Peptic Ulcers

H_2-Antagonists Cimetidine was the first (histamine) H_2-receptor antagonist to be introduced and is widely used. It is an effective and relatively safe agent for therapy of peptic ulcer disease. Although it demonstrates a remarkable safety record, cimetidine may produce some potential side effects under certain conditions, including interference with drug metabolism. Similar to other H_2-receptor antagonists, cimetidine blocks parietal cell H_2-receptors and greatly inhibits basal acid secretion (including nocturnal secretion), as well as secretion induced by meals. By decreasing acid secretion, cimetidine decreases ulcer pain and promotes mucosal healing. A disadvantage is its relatively

Table 60-4 Pharmacokinetic Parameter Values

Drug	Administered	Absorption (%)	$t_{1/2}$ (hr)	Disposition
H_2-RECEPTOR ANTAGONISTS				
cimetidine	Oral, IV	60	2	R (main), M
nizatidine	Oral	90	1.5	R (main), M
ranitidine	Oral, IV	50	3	R (main), M
famotidine	Oral, IV	45	3.0	R (main), M
OTHERS				
sucralfate	Oral	Poor	—	Excrete in feces
propantheline	Oral	70	2	M (main), R
metoclopramide	Oral, IV, IM	80	2	R (main), M
cisapride	Oral	50	10	M
diphenoxylate	Oral	90	12	M (main), B, R
loperamide	Oral	Poor	11	B (main), R

M, Metabolized; *R,* renal excretion as unchanged drug; *B,* biliary excretion.

short duration of action requiring its administration more than one time daily during the acute phase of ulcer therapy in many patients.

Ranitidine, nizatidine, and famotidine are H_2-receptor antagonists more recently introduced for treatment of peptic ulcer. As shown in Figure 60-3, ranitidine, nizatidine, and famotidine differ chemically from cimetidine in the structures of the ring and the side chain. Ranitidine and famotidine display somewhat longer durations of action than cimetidine does, whereas nizatidine has a shorter plasma half-life. These newer drugs do not interfere significantly with drug metabolism by hepatic cytochrome P-450 enzymes.

Gastric Antacids Antacids employed for treatment of peptic ulcer disease are weak bases that neutralize gastric acid. Antacids do not decrease secretion of acid; in fact, some may increase secretion. Their ability to neutralize acid in the lumen of the stomach results in two desirable therapeutic effects: decrease in total acid load delivered to the duodenum and inhibition of pepsin activity. The activity of pepsin is significantly decreased at pH 5 and above. Antacid therapy that raises intragastric pH above 4 to 5 is adequate to achieve the desired therapeutic end point while minimizing the side effects antacids can produce.

Antacids are divided into two general categories: systemic and nonsystemic. Systemic antacids are absorbed into the bloodstream, with the potential to increase blood pH and alkalinize urine. The classic example is sodium bicarbonate. Nonsystemic antacids contain a cation (usually calcium, magnesium, or aluminum) that is poorly absorbed in the small intestine, does not alter blood pH, and does not alkalinize urine. For occasional, intermittent therapy, a systemic antacid poses no hazard. When used regularly for days or weeks, however, a systemic antacid is undesirable and a nonsystemic antacid is preferable.

Adequate treatment with antacids can provide effective management of peptic ulcers, reflected in the rate and incidence of healing. The major disadvantage of antacid therapy is the frequent dosing required and its attendant side effects. Attempts are usually made to disguise the disagreeable taste with various flavorings, but patients soon tire of antacids, and compliance is often poor. Antacids are therapeutically effective only when present in the stomach and lose their effect after gastric emptying. In addition, antacids may cause undesired or dangerous side effects. Antacids are apparently less safe than alternative forms of ulcer therapy, such as H_2-antagonists.

Sodium and potassium salts such as sodium bicarbonate or potassium bicarbonate have a rapid onset of action, providing almost immediate neutralization, and can briefly raise intragastric pH to 5 to 7 or even higher. However, the neutralizing effect is of short duration, and, as acid secretion continues, the acidity soon returns to pH 1 to 2. In contrast, most calcium salts have a relatively rapid onset of action and a neutralizing capacity in which the pH remains elevated as long as calcium is present in the stomach. However, the pH is usually raised to only 4 to 5 (still an acceptable end point). Calcium salts act directly on stimulus-secretion coupling to increase the release of gastrin and also to promote acid secretion, resulting in "acid rebound" after the calcium empties from the stomach. For these reasons, calcium salts are not recommended as antacids for the treatment of peptic ulcer. Magnesium hydroxide (milk of magnesia) has a rapid onset of neutralizing action and can raise intragastric pH to 8 to 9. By contrast, magnesium trisilicate and aluminum oxide neutralize acid slowly, and these salts have a slow onset of action. The total neutralizing capacity is adequate to maintain pH at desirable levels as long as the antacids are present in the stomach. However, magnesium (laxative) and aluminum (constipative) salts can affect consistency of the feces and frequency of defecation. Individual characteristics of antacid compounds have led to the formulation of various mixtures that combine ingredients to offer rapid onset and relatively long duration of action and balance laxative and constipating effects. Satisfactory antacid formulations are liquid dosage forms, which allow faster and more complete interaction of the antacid with H^+ and are often more effective than solid dosage forms. Different antacid products vary in sodium content. Because patients with peptic ulcers may consume large quantities of antacid, a high sodium content could constitute a health hazard, especially for patients on restricted sodium intake. Many low-sodium antacid preparations are available.

Sucralfate Controlled trials and experience with patients indicate that sucralfate can increase the incidence and rate of peptic ulcer healing with a minimum of adverse side effects. However, sucralfate is a less effective antiulcer drug than H_2-receptor antagonists or proton pump inhibitors.

Prostaglandins Several products of arachidonic acid metabolism, including prostaglandins (see Chapter 18), exert gastric antisecretory effects and cytoprotective actions on the gastric and duodenal mucosa. In most tissues, prostaglandins stimulate adenylate cyclase activity and thereby increase intracellular formation of cAMP. In parietal cells, many prostaglandins inhibit adenylate cyclase stimulation by histamine (Figure 60-2) and thereby inhibit an essential step in histamine-stimulated acid secretion.

Proton Pump Inhibitors Secretion of H^+ into the gastric lumen results from activity of parietal cell H^+,K^+-ATPase. Activity of the H^+,K^+-ATPase is evidently regulated by availability of free intracellular calcium and activity of protein kinase. Activation of the H^+ transport enzyme is brought about by activation of histamine, acetylcholine, or gastrin receptors. Blockade of these regulatory systems decreases H^+ secretion. However, direct inhibition of H^+,K^+-ATPase produces the most effective mechanism known to inhibit gastric acid secretion. Omeprazole has been introduced and other agents are undergoing clinical trials for the management of peptic ulcer disease. Initial results indicate that certain proton pump inhibitors such as omeprazole are extremely efficacious and can reduce acid secretion to almost zero. Omeprazole is essentially a prodrug that is converted to its active form in an acid environment. The secretory canaliculus of the parietal cell is the most acidic site in the body. Systemically absorbed omeprazole distributes to the parietal cell canaliculus and is converted after molecular rearrangement to an active moiety that forms a covalent bond with H^+,K^+-ATPase in the luminal portion of the cell. This reaction irreversibly inactivates the H^+ transporter. Drugs that inhibit the H^+,K^+-ATPase are useful in patients resistant to other types of pharmacological agents and in patients with gastrinomas. However, there are concerns about potential side effects of this drug.

Prokinetic Drugs

The prokinetic drugs increase gastric emptying in the treatment of diabetic gastroparesis and show promise in increasing tone of the lower esophageal sphincter in management of gastroesophageal reflux; some are used for antiemetic effects. Metoclopramide, for example, exhibits significant antiemetic activity and is often used in patients receiving antineoplastic drugs. Ondansetron may be even more effective in decreasing nausea and vomiting associated with emetogenic antineoplastic drugs. Cisapride and erythromycin have little antiemetic activity but are effective prokinetic drugs.

Laxatives

Laxatives include secretory, saline, emollient, and bulk-forming agents. Secretory laxatives (sometimes called *stimulant,* or *irritant, laxatives*) increase secretion of fluid and electrolytes into the lumen of the bowel by the intestinal mucosa, resulting in fluid accumulation and a watery luminal content that flows rapidly through the small and large intestines. The classical secretory laxative is castor oil. One of the fatty acids esterified with glycerol in castor oil is ricinoleic acid, a hydroxylated analog of oleic acid. Ricinoleic acid acts on the intestinal mucosa to allow movement of fluid into the lumen of the bowel. Other natural secretory agents—popular as lay remedies—include the anthraquinone derivatives cascara, senna, and aloe. Synthetic agents include phenolphthalein, bisacodyl, and danthron.

Saline laxatives usually contain a cation (e.g., magnesium), anion (e.g., sulfate or phosphate), or nonabsorbable sugar that carries obligatory water of hydration and is poorly absorbed from the bowel. Saline cathartics retain fluid in the lumen and promote flow through the bowel. Examples of typical saline laxatives include magnesium hydroxide, sodium phosphate, and sodium sulfate. The disadvantage of saline laxatives is that they often produce explosive, watery bowel movements. Their advantage is a rapid onset of effect, often within 3 hours of administration. Lactulose is a poorly absorbed sugar that increases accumulation of fluid in the lumen of the bowel. Emollient laxatives act as nonabsorbed lubricants to enhance flow through the bowel and to soften rectal contents.

The safest and generally preferred laxatives are the bulk-forming agents, including bran, methylcellulose, and psyllium (prepared from plantain, or *Plantago,* seeds). Bulk-forming laxatives consist of nondigestible cellulose fibers that become hydrated in the intestine, decrease viscosity of luminal contents to increase flow through the bowel, and swell to provide bulk to activate the defecation reflex. The bulk-forming agents are essentially innocuous, relatively inexpensive, and satisfy the psychological needs of nearly all patients.

Laxatives should never be prescribed for patients with undiagnosed abdominal pain or intestinal obstruction.

Antidiarrheal Drugs

Opioid Agents The most effective nonspecific antidiarrheal drugs are the natural opioids, including morphine and codeine, and synthetic opioid agents, such as loperamide and diphenoxylate. Opioids increase segmenting contractions of the small and large intestines, increasing resistance to flow through the lumen. They also decrease secretion of fluid and electrolytes into the lumen and promote mucosal absorption. These actions result in slowed transit through the GI tract, allowing time for more complete absorption of fluid. Increased segmenting activity (which increases fluid absorption) and direct inhibition of secretory processes and stimulation of absorptive processes lead to increased viscosity of luminal content and to formed stool.

Opioids, such as morphine and codeine, that effectively cross the blood-brain barrier, probably act at central sites in the brain and spinal cord to decrease transit and decrease accumulation of fluid in the lumen of the intestine. They also act locally on neural and smooth muscle elements in the intestine to increase segmenting contractions and to reduce propulsive contractions. Opioids that do not effectively cross the blood-brain barrier, such as loperamide and diphenoxylate, act primarily by local neural and smooth muscle effects to increase segmenting contractions. The natural and synthetic opioids act on neural elements in the intestine, primarily in the submucosal plexus, to inhibit secretion and promote net absorption. The increased segmenting contractions in the proximal duodenum decrease the gastroduodenal pressure gradient required for gastric emptying, causing opioids to delay gastric emptying and contributing to the overall antidiarrheal effect.

Diphenoxylate is available commercially in combination with atropine, the latter serving as a deterrent to abuse. Diphenoxylate crosses the blood-brain barrier poorly and in usual therapeutic doses does not produce CNS side effects. However, in overdose, diphenoxylate can cause respiratory depression, reversible by naloxone.

Loperamide is a more recently developed opioid antidiarrheal with the advantage of poor penetration across the blood-brain barrier and therefore with virtually no CNS effects. Loperamide is essentially devoid of opioid subjective effects when taken orally and presents a very low abuse potential.

The opioid diarrheal drugs are remarkably effective in management of acute diarrhea. Those opioids with CNS activity should be used cautiously in acute diarrheal states and generally should not be used for management of chronic diarrhea. Loperamide is effective in management of chronic diarrhea secondary to inflammatory bowel disease or irritable bowel syndrome. Opioid antidiarrheal agents should not be employed in symptomatic treatment of diarrhea induced by enteric infections with invasive organisms, especially species of *Shigella* and *Salmonella.*

Bismuth Subsalicylate Bismuth subsalicylate in several clinical trials is an effective antidiarrheal agent especially useful against enterotoxigenic strains of *Escherichia coli.* It has antibacterial activity and inhibits formation of diarrhea-producing prostaglandins.

Gel-forming Substances Substances that form a semisolid gel-like consistency within the intestinal lumen increase resistance to flow through the intestine and increase firmness of stools. Typical gel-forming substances include attapulgite, kaolin, and pectin. These substances form claylike gels when hydrated. The gel-forming substances may offer more psychological benefit than reversal of pathophysiological processes. They do not remarkably reduce the volume of fluid excreted and thus have little therapeutic benefit other than promoting formed stools.

Antifoaming Agents Small bubbles of gas, primarily air entrapped during chewing and swallowing, can lead to gastric bloating, flatulence, and uncomfortable intestinal distention. A variety of antifoaming agents, often surfactants, is used to break up gas bubbles in the stomach. The most popular agent is simethicone, used alone for this purpose or present in many commercial antacid mixtures. Although simethicone can produce a dramatic defoaming effect in the stomach, its efficacy in pathological intestinal distention has not been demonstrated.

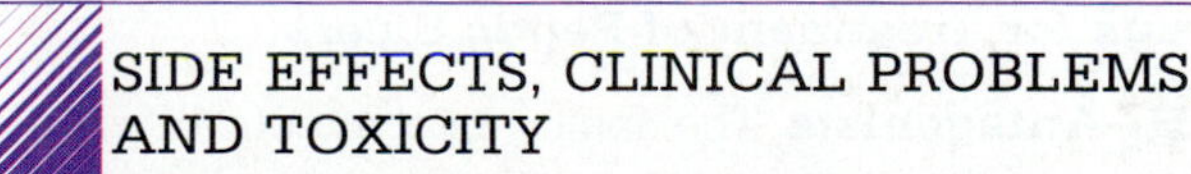

SIDE EFFECTS, CLINICAL PROBLEMS, AND TOXICITY

Clinical problems of drugs for treatment of ulcers are summarized in the box on p. 812.

CLINICAL PROBLEMS

H_2-ANTAGONISTS

cimetidine
- Interference with metabolism of many drugs (P-450 related)
- Antiandrogenic effect (binds to testosterone receptors)
- Impotence

ANTACIDS

aluminum salts
- Constipation

magnesium salts
- Diarrhea

sodium salts
- Increased plasma sodium
- Calcium salts
- "Acid rebound"

PROSTAGLANDINS

misoprostol
- Uterine stimulation

PROTON PUMP INHIBITORS

omeprazole
- Gastric mucosal hyperplasia

PROKINETIC DRUGS

bethanechol, neostigmine
- Excess GI secretions; cramps, cholinergic stimulation

metoclopramide
- Extrapyramidal effects
- Hyperprolactinemia

SECRETORY LAXATIVES

castor oil, phenolphthalein
- Electrolyte imbalance

SALINE LAXATIVES

- Magnesium absorption
- Rectal epithelium sloughing

LUBRICANTS

mineral oil
- Absorption of fat-soluble vitamins decreased
- Pulmonary aspiration

Drugs for Treatment of Peptic Ulcers

H_2-Antagonists The major side effects of cimetidine, including interference with the metabolism of certain other drugs and its antiandrogenic effects, are not directly related to blockade of H_2-receptors. Cimetidine interacts with hepatic cytochrome P-450 and slows the clearance of some drugs requiring the cytochrome P-450 enzyme system for metabolism, including hydroxycoumadin, phenytoin, propanolol, diazepam, and others. Thus cimetidine can lead to elevated plasma concentrations of and toxic responses to the other drugs.

Cimetidine can bind to testosterone receptors and thus exert antiandrogenic effects, resulting in decreased sexual libido and gynecomastia in males treated with large doses. The antiandrogenic effects have not occurred in patients treated with ordinary doses of cimetidine but have occurred in some patients with Zollinger-Ellison syndrome after treatment with very large doses. Cimetidine can induce mental confusion and disorientation in elderly and severely ill patients, particularly in those with renal or hepatic impairment. These effects disappear upon discontinuation of the drug. Some of the central actions may be a primary side effect, since cimetidine readily crosses the blood-brain barrier, and its effects might be exacerbated in the elderly or ill patient. A transient rash or diarrhea has been reported in a small number of patients.

The more recently introduced H_2-receptor antagonists famotidine, ranitidine, and nizatidine do not bind significantly to cytochrome P-450 of human liver and have not been found to alter the hepatic elimination of diazepam, metoprolol, theophylline, or hydroxycoumadin. However, ranitidine reduces hepatic renal clearance of triamterene in humans. The more recently introduced H_2-receptor antagonists do not bind significantly to testosterone receptors and have not been found to induce gynecomastia. All the H_2-antagonists produce a small incidence of mild, reversible side effects, such as dizziness, diarrhea, constipation, and headache. Collectively, the H_2-antagonists appear to be remarkably safe drugs.

Gastric Antacids Antacid therapy is complicated by the reluctance of physicians and patients to consider antacids as actual drugs, with their attendant benefits, hazards, and therapeutic ratios. Although divalent and trivalent metal ions are poorly absorbed and serve as nonsystemic antacids, small amounts are absorbed from the lumen of the intestine. Small amounts of systemically absorbed calcium, magnesium, or aluminum are normally not harmful. However, in patients with renal insufficiency, in which the cations are not adequately excreted, these cations exert systemic toxicity. Calcium salts can produce systemic hypercalcemia resulting in formation of calculi (milk alkali syndrome), and excess circulating magnesium can induce muscle weakness and fatigue. Aluminum can bind phosphate in the lumen of the gut and prevent adequate absorption of phosphate, leading to phosphate deficiency with muscle weakness and resorption of bone. The ability of aluminum to bind phosphate in the intestine is therapeutically useful in patients undergoing hemodialysis who otherwise tend to accumulate phosphate. Common problems encountered with antacids used as therapy for peptic ulcer are constipation and diarrhea. To solve this problem, an acceptable balance in stool frequency and consistency can be achieved by mixtures of magnesium and aluminum salts or by alternating doses of magnesium- or aluminum-containing antacids.

Misoprostol Many prostaglandins induce diarrhea because they promote secretion of fluid and electrolytes into the lumen of the bowel and may also inhibit intestinal segmenting contractions that retard flow of luminal contents. In contrast to their effects on parietal cell adenylate cyclase activity, prostaglandins stimulate cAMP production in enterocytes and thereby increase intestinal secretion leading to net accumulation of fluid in the lumen. Another potential problem is uterine stimulation, especially during pregnancy.

Proton Pump Inhibitors A potentially serious adverse side effect of omeprazole and possibly other proton pump inhibitors is gastric mucosal hyperplasia. This hyperplasia, demonstrated in animal studies, is believed to result from excessive secretion of gastrin from the antral mucosa as a consequence of antral alkalinization associated with profound inhibition of acid secretion. Gastrin exerts trophic effects on gastric and intestinal mucosa. If the gastric hyperplasia is caused by excessive release of gastrin, gastric hyperplasia is a theoretical side effect associated with any antisecretory drug. However, excess gastrin secretion may be associated only with extremely efficacious drugs, such as proton pump inhibitors. Up to now, significant hyperplasia has not been found in humans taking omeprazole.

Prokinetic Drugs

Cholinergic agonists, such as bethanechol, and acetylcholinesterase inhibitors, such as neostigmine, produce a variety of side effects typically associated with cholinergic stimulation: excessive salivation, sweating, urination, lacrimation, and defecation. Peptic ulcer disease, cardiac conduction disorders, and asthma can be exacerbated. Because of its activity as a dopamine-receptor antagonist, metoclopramide can induce dystonia or Parkinson's disease–like side effects. Moreover, the dopamine antagonist prokinetic drugs increase the release of prolactin and can thereby induce symptoms typical of hyperprolactinemia: gynecomastia, galactorrhea, and breast tenderness. Metoclopramide often induces sedation. More recently developed prokinetic drugs, such as cisapride, do not block dopamine receptors and do not produce extrapyramidal side effects. Some prokinetic agents without dopamine antagonist actions appear to produce antiemetic effects by antagonist actions at 5-HT_3 receptors, an indication that local gastric actions may be important in suppression of emesis. Because emesis is associated with orally progressing intestinal and gastric contractions (reverse peristalsis), some prokinetic drugs may suppress emesis by promoting aboral moving contractions.

Laxatives

The problems associated with the use of laxatives are indicated in the box on p. 812. These vary depending on the agent. Laxatives should be used only temporarily. Chronic use leads to habituation, damage to the myenteric plexus, and colonic atony. The availability of the large number of laxatives has led to their abuse.

NEW DIRECTIONS

The greatest needs in therapy of gastrointestinal disorders are drugs that can provide specific control of motility and drugs that control inflammation. No reliably effective drug is presently available, for example, for the management of irritable bowel syndrome, a condition that affects some 10% of the adult population. Among types of agents currently under investigation for treatment are improved prokinetic drugs, β-receptor adrenergic agonists, opioid agonists, and cholecystokinin antagonists. New approaches directed at bowel sensory nerve function may eventually prove fruitful. Antidiarrheal drugs without dependence liability and with nonconstipating properties need to be developed. Among candidates under investigation are δ-opioid receptor agonists, enkephalinase inhibitors, α_2-adrenergic receptor agonists, and calmodulin antagonists.

Ulcerative colitis and Crohn's disease (regional enteritis) are serious inflammatory bowel diseases not adequately managed with existing drugs. Likely approaches involve development of drugs that reduce formation of mediators of inflammation (e.g., interleukins and other cytokines) or will block their cellular receptors.

It is expected that one or more prostaglandins will soon be available for treatment of peptic ulcer disease. Misoprostol was recently introduced for prevention of mucosal damage induced by nonsteroidal antiinflammatory drugs. Administration of misoprostol to patients who are taking large doses of aspirin and related antiinflammatory drugs is expected to reduce the incidence of severe mucosal damage. The likely candidates for treatment of peptic ulcer are synthetic derivatives of prostaglandin E_1 or prostaglandin E_2 and contain substitutions at positions 15 or 16 of the side chain to protect against enzymatic attack and inactivation by prostaglandin dehydrogenase. The protected prostaglandins, such as 15,15-dimethyl and 16,16-dimethyl prostaglandin E_2, are active orally (see Chapter 18).

Many duodenal and gastric ulcers (not caused by NSAIDs) are now thought to be associated with the gram-negative bacillus *Helicobactor pylori*. If endoscopy and biopsy of the gastric antrum indicate an active infection, antibacterial treatment is indicated. Several antibacterial combinations, together with an antisecretory agent, have been evaluated. Currently the drugs of choice for patients with peptic ulcers infected with *H. pylori* appear to be amoxicillin together with either omeprazole or an H_2-receptor antagonist.

REFERENCES

Reynolds JC: Prokinetic agents: a key in the future of gastroenterology, *Gastroenterol Clin North Am* 18:437-457, 1989.

Dumuis A, Sebben M, Bockaert J: The gastrointestinal prokinetic benzamide derivatives are agonists at the non-classical 5-HT receptor (5-HT_4) positively coupled to adenylate cyclase in neurons, *Naunym-Schmiedeberg's Arch Pharmacol* 340:403-410, 1989.

Kromer W: Endogenous and exogenous opioids in the control of gastrointestinal motility and secretion, *Pharmacol Rev* 40:121-162, 1988.

Feldman M, Burton ME: Histamine H_2 antagonists, *N Engl J Med* 323:1672-1680, 1990.

Goyal RK: Muscarinic receptor subtypes, *N Engl J Med* 321:1022-1029, 1989.

Lindberg P, Brandstrom A, Wallmark B: Structure-activity relationships of omeprazole analogues and their mechanism of action, *Trends Pharmacol Sci* 8:399-402, 1987.

Schulze-Delrieu K: Metoclopramide, *N Eng J Med* 305:28-32, 1981.

TRADE NAMES

In addition to generic and fixed-combination preparations, the following trade name materials are available in the United States.

H_2-ADRENERGIC RECEPTOR ANTAGONISTS

Axid, nizatidine
Pepcid, famotidine
Tagamet, cimetidine
Zantac, ranitidine

ANTACIDS

ALternaGEL, Amphojel aluminum hydroxide
Aludrox, aluminum hydroxide/magnesium hydroxide
Gaviscon, aluminum hydroxide/magnesium carbonate
milk of magnesia, magnesium hydroxide
Mylanta, Simeco, aluminum hydroxide/magnesium hydroxide/simethicone
Mylicon, simethicone
Riopan, magaldrate

ANTICHOLINERGICS AND OTHER AGENTS USED TO TREAT PEPTIC ULCER

Bentyl, dicyclomine
Cantil, mepenzolate
Carafate, sucralfate
Cytotec, misoprostol
Prilosec, omeprazole
Pathilon, tridihexethyl
Pro-Banthine, propantheline
Robinul, glycopyrrolate
Valpin, anisotropine

PROKINETIC AGENTS

E-Mycin, erythromycin
Propulsid, cisapride
Reglan, metoclopramide
Zofran, ondansetron

LAXATIVES

Chronulac, lactulose
Colace, docusate sodium
Dulcolax, bisacodyl
Modane, danthron
Neoloid, castor oil
Prulet, phenolphthalein

ANTIDIARRHEAL DRUGS

Imodium, loperamide
Lomotil, diphenoxylate
Questran, cholestyramine
Pepto-Bismol, bismuth subsalicylate

SELF-ASSESSMENT QUESTIONS

1. Cimetidine and related antiulcer drugs act as antagonists at parietal cell:
   a. muscarinic M_3-receptors.
   b. prostaglandin receptors.
   c. histamine H_2-receptors.
   d. histamine H_1-receptors.
   e. gastrin receptors.
2. Metoclopramide produces prokinetic and antiemetic effects primarily because it acts as an:
   a. antagonist at muscarinic M_2-receptors.
   b. agonist at 5-HT_4 receptors.
   c. inhibitor of acetylcholinesterase.
   d. agonist at motilin receptors.
   e. antagonist at dopamine D_2-receptors.
3. Which one of the following is most likely to interfere with cytochrome P-450 drug metabolism?
   a. cimetidine
   b. ranitidine
   c. omeprazole
   d. sucralfate
   e. metoclopramide
4. Which of the following is most likely to induce parkinsonism-like extrapyramidal symptoms?
   a. cimetidine
   b. ranitidine
   c. omeprazole
   d. sucralfate
   e. metoclopramide
5. The major serious side effect associated with long-term use of aluminum oxide as an antacid is:
   a. diarrhea.
   b. systemic alkalosis.
   c. phosphate depletion.
   d. kidney stones.
   e. dementia.
6. Dry mouth, visual disturbance, constipation, and difficulty in urination are side effects commonly associated with use of:
   a. muscarinic antagonists.
   b. histamine H_2-antagonists.
   c. dopamine D_2-antagonists.
   d. 5-HT_3 antagonists.
   e. gastrin antagonists.
7. Which one of the following is most likely to produce constipation?
   a. neostigmine
   b. cisapride
   c. magnesium hydroxide
   d. loperamide
   e. bethanechol
8. Which one of the following drugs is most likely to improve gastric emptying in a patient with diabetic gastroparesis?
   a. loperamide
   b. cisapride
   c. magnesium hydroxide
   d. sucralfate
   e. cimetidine

CHAPTER 61

Nutritional Aspects of Pharmacology

THOMAS J. LAUTERIO
RICHARD L. ATKINSON

FOODS AS DRUGS

As interest in health and disease has increased within recent years among the general population, the use of nutrients in the prevention or cure of medical problems has also grown. It is important that medical practitioners be knowledgeable regarding the usefulness of nutrients and their possible effects in disease states, as well as their potential for abuse. It is difficult to ascertain whether consumption of a food or food product actually results in a beneficial or a detrimental effect on the body because of many confounding factors. Standard scientific methodologies used in man to examine drug efficacy must frequently be compromised. For example, it is impractical in most cases to carry out double-blind studies. Frequently, conclusions regarding beneficial actions of foods in several disease states are derived from anecdotal reports or poorly controlled studies. Although this information should not be used as a basis for therapy, it can be used as a basis for further scientific inquiry. This chapter is an attempt to describe how foods and food products affect certain conditions in man. Indications for use of certain foods and food products are shown in the box on p. 818.

ABBREVIATIONS	
BHA	butylated hydroxyanisole
BHT	butylated hydroxytoluene
cAMP	cyclic adenosine monophosphate
DEA	Drug Enforcement Administration
DES	diethylstilbestrol
FDA	Food and Drug Administration
GRAS	generally regarded as safe
HDL	high-density lipoprotein
LDL	low-density lipoprotein
LNAA	large neutral amino acid
MSG	monosodium glutamate
PPA	phenylpropanolamine
RDA	recommended daily allowance

Fiber, Oat Bran, and Starch Blockers

Dietary fiber has been promoted as useful for a variety of medical problems in recent years. Studies in Africa demonstrated that individuals consuming native diets rich in fiber and bulk had fewer gastrointestinal problems that are common to Western civilization. Dietary fiber has since been suggested to improve or cure numerous diseases or conditions including obesity, diabetes, colon cancer, diverticulitis, hemorrhoids, hiatal hernia, heart disease, varicose veins, and gallstones. However, firm data for the efficacy of fiber to improve most of these conditions is lacking. Constipation and diverticular disease are the only conditions for which fiber produces reliable benefits.

Dietary fiber has been defined as plant substances resistant to digestion by the human small intestine. Fiber is a collective term representing three types of carbohydrates: cellulose, hemicellulose A, and hemicellulose B, and one noncarbohydrate, the lignins. Although nutritional biochemists classify fiber into four groups, the food industry classifies fiber into two categories: soluble and insoluble fiber. Soluble fiber dissolves in neutral or acid detergent during extraction, whereas insoluble fiber does not (Figure 61-1). Other important properties of fiber types are the ability to hold water and cation exchange and antioxidant actions. A summary of the physiological, chemical, and clinical aspects of fiber is presented in Table 61-1.

The most familiar fiber is cellulose, a major component of plant cell walls, present in high concentration in wheat and oat bran. Cellulose is a linear polymer of glucose, but unlike the α-1,4 linkage of glycogen and maltose, the β-1,4-linkage cannot be broken down en-

THERAPEUTIC OVERVIEW

FOOD OR FOOD PRODUCT	USE
Dietary fiber	Constipation, Diverticular disease
Fatty acids	Cardiovascular disease
Vitamins	Deficiency disease
Vitamin A, Retinoids	Cystic acne Psoriasis
Niacin	Cholesterol lowering

zymatically. Hemicellulose A fiber is heteropolymeric with linkages formed between the hexoses glucose, galactose, and mannose, as well as between the pentoses xylose and arabinose. These agents are termed *gums,* or *mucilages,* since their consistency is like that of glue. They delay gastric emptying and thereby decrease the rate of small bowel absorption. Guar gum, an example of hemicellulose A, is often added to foods to bind water with other ingredients. In the plant, guar gum prevents dehydration of seeds. Hemicellulose B fiber, or pectin, also binds water as well as minerals and heavy metals in the gastrointestinal tract. Lignins, the noncarbohydrate component of fiber, exist as cross-linked polymers of oxygenated phenylpropane units. Their resistance to degradation favors their passage through the intestine, providing bulk for feces.

The use of fiber in the treatment and control of diabetes has been investigated extensively. Hemicellulose fibers (particularly the gums and pectins) reduce postprandial blood glucose and insulin concentrations. Long-term studies with high-fiber diets demonstrate improvement in glycemic control by prolonging transit time for carbohydrates, reduction in urinary glucose, and decreased ketone body losses. It is not clear whether this is an effect of the fiber or of other components of the diet. Supplements of wheat or oat bran produce only modest improvement in control of diabetes. Potential mechanisms of improvement with soluble fiber include delayed gastric emptying, increased mouth-to-cecum transit time, and delayed absorption of glucose in the small intestine.

Delay in gastric emptying caused by some soluble fibers may reduce symptoms of the "dumping syndrome," in which nutrients pass quickly down the small intestine and produce a sympathetic discharge. This syndrome is the most common effect of gastric surgery. Pectin-supplemented diets may normalize gut-endocrine responses and alter gastrointestinal motility in patients with "dumping." Diets high in insoluble fiber used to treat patients with duodenal ulcers do not speed healing but do decrease the incidence of ulcer relapse.

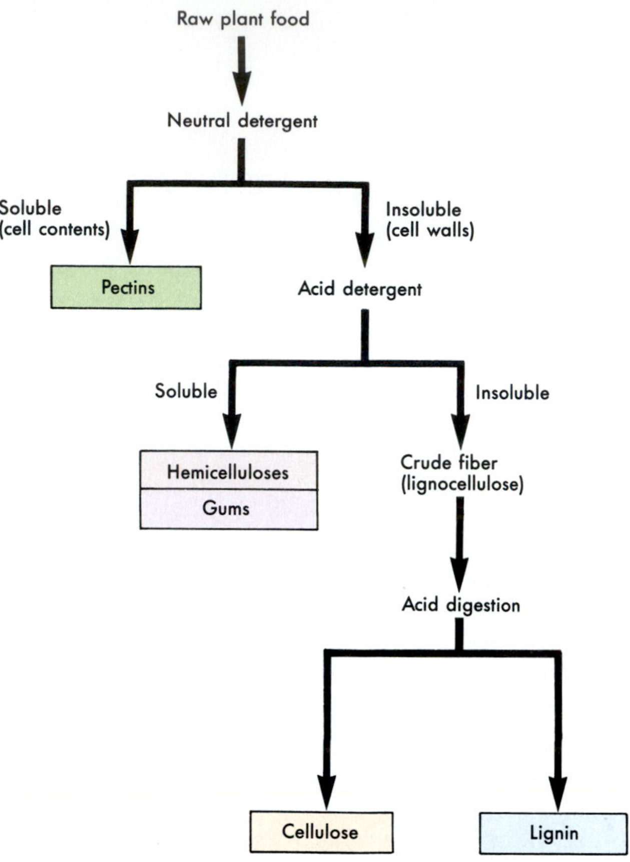

FIGURE 61-1 Classification of fiber types based on extraction procedures. Major dietary fiber groups are emphasized.

The popularity of fiber has been enhanced by advertisements promoting its ability to lower serum cholesterol. These claims are based on data from studies in which diets high in fiber and carbohydrate reduced the serum cholesterol concentrations. Again, it is not clear whether dietary fiber reduces cholesterol absorption or changes the fat and carbohydrate content of the diet. Viscous fibers were most effective in lowering blood cholesterol concentrations, whereas lignins produced variable results. Wheat bran, which is mainly insoluble fiber, does not lower serum cholesterol. Lignins decrease cholesterol and lower serum triglyceride concentrations, probably by binding bile salts, which then cannot be absorbed from the gastrointestinal tract and are lost in the feces. Gums and pectins are reported to lower low-density lipoprotein (LDL) cholesterol concentrations while maintaining high-density lipoprotein (HDL) cho-

Table 61-1 Physiological and Therapeutic Implications of Dietary Fiber

Physicochemical Property	Type of Fiber	Physiological Effect	Potential Clinical Implication
Viscosity	Gums, mucilages, pectins	↓ gastric emptying ↑ mouth to cecum transit ↓ rate of small intestinal absorption (e.g., of glucose, bile acids)	Dumping syndrome Diabetes Hypercholesterolemia
Particle formation and water-holding capacity	e.g., Wheat bran, pentosan content, polysaccharide-lignin mixtures	↑ gastric emptying ↓ mouth to cecum transit ↓ total GI transit time ↓ colonic intraluminal pressure ↑ fecal bulk	Peptic ulcer Constipation Diverticular disease Dilute potential carcinogens
Adsorption and nonspecific effects	Lignin, pectin mixed fibers	↑ fecal steroids output ↑ fecal fat and nitrogen losses (small)	Hypercholesterolemia Cholelithiasis
Cation exchange	Acidic polysaccharides (e.g., pectins)	↑ small intestinal losses of minerals (±), trace elements (±), heavy metals	Negative mineral balance, probably compensated for by colonic salvage antitoxic effect
Antioxidant	Lignin (reducing phenolic groups)	↓ free radicals in digestive tract	Anticarcinogenesis?
Degradability (colonic bacteria)	Polysaccharides (free of lignin)	↑ gas and SCFAs production ↓ cecal pH	Flatus, energy production

From Jenkins DJA. Carbohydrate. In Shils ME, Young VR, editors: *Modern nutrition in health and disease.* Philadelphia, 1988, Lea & Febiger; adapted from *Am J Clin Nutr* 32:365, 1979.
SCFAs, Short-chain fatty acids; ±, more or less.

lesterol, resulting in improvement of the LDL:HDL ratio. Lignin has a less reliable effect on the LDL:HDL ratio.

Because obesity is seldom observed among primitive cultures that consume foods high in fiber, dietary fiber has been promoted as a means for weight reduction. Fiber may promote weight loss by decreasing food intake or increasing fecal calorie loss. Fiber reduces food intake by increasing chewing time and diluting caloric density. The delay in gastric emptying produced by some soluble fibers may enhance satiety, as may changes in patterns of gut hormone secretion produced by dietary fiber. However, most controlled studies show only modest effects of dietary fiber for weight reduction.

Starch blockers, such as acarbose, have been proposed as treatment for obesity and diabetes mellitus. These agents inhibit enzymes in the gastrointestinal tract that digest carbohydrates and theoretically produce malabsorption. Clinical trials with starch blockers thus far have been disappointing, producing little weight loss or reduction of blood glucose.

Some studies suggest that dietary fiber reduces the incidence of gallstone formation, perhaps by altering the composition of the bile salt pool to increase chenodeoxycholic acid and reducing the lithogenic index of bile. Fiber also may help prevent hiatal hernia and varicose veins by increasing fecal weight and softness, thus decreasing straining with defecation. Epidemiological studies show an inverse correlation of dietary fiber and incidence of colon cancer. Several proposed mechanisms for reduction of intestinal cancers include: increased transit time of carcinogens through the large bowel, altered intestinal microflora, an altered bile salt pool, and decreased colonic pH. Further studies are necessary to confirm the beneficial effects of dietary fiber on colon cancer.

Overconsumption of fiber can produce adverse effects. Increased flatus, intestinal discomfort, and occasional diarrhea occur with increased fiber intake, especially initially. The delayed gastric emptying produced by fiber can increase esophageal reflux. Although lack of fiber can lead to constipation and irritable bowel syndrome, ingestion of large amounts of dietary fiber supplements without adequate fluid intake can also cause constipation and even intestinal obstruction, particularly in the elderly. Fiber may produce deficiencies of calcium, magnesium, iron, and zinc in people with marginal or low intakes. Again, such deficiencies occur mainly in the elderly.

Amino Acids

Therapeutic use of specific amino acids by the general population has increased with the availability of purified amino acids in health food stores. Lysine and arginine have been promoted as regulators of body composition and muscle growth by stimulating growth hormone secretion. Clinical studies have disproved these claims and indicate that this practice is ineffective and may be dangerous. Consumption of large amounts of single amino acids may produce amino acid imbalances, resulting in increased protein loss and in alteration of neurotransmitter synthesis in the central nervous system.

Tryptophan, once widely used as a sleep promoter, has been withdrawn from the market by the Food and Drug Administration because of long-term toxicity identified with high doses. Milk, long used to induce sleep, is a rich source. Tryptophan is a precursor for the neurotransmitter serotonin. Brain tryptophan concentrations can be elevated by excess dietary tryptophan, increasing serotonin turnover. This occurs because the rate-limiting enzyme for serotonin synthesis tryptophan hydroxylase is not normally saturated and is therefore regulated by substrate concentration. Generally, diets with a large amount of protein decrease brain tryptophan uptake because of competition from the large neutral amino acid (LNAA) pool that shares the same transport system. The tryptophan-to-LNAA ratio is the most important dietary index of the ability of a food to alter brain tryptophan. Increases in dietary tryptophan relative to other LNAAs (tyrosine, phenylalanine, valine, isoleucine, and methionine) or increases in dietary carbohydrate enhance the tryptophan-to-LNAA ratio and thus increase uptake into the brain.

Fish Oils, Fatty Acids, and Lipids

Fatty acids and lipids serve vital structural roles in cells and are precursors for important bioactive intermediates, including prostaglandins, thromboxanes, leukotrienes, and hydroxy fatty acids (see Chapter 18). Since the synthetic rate of these metabolites is substrate dependent, dietary manipulations can alter the level and nature of their synthesis. The essential fatty acids linolenic and linoleic acids are not synthesized by man and must be supplied in the diet. Linolenic-derived fatty acids are termed the *omega-3 (n-3) family* of compounds, and linoleic-derived fatty acids are termed the *omega-6 (n-6) family.* The double bonds are named from the methyl end rather than the carboxyl end, thus *n*-3 and *n*-6 fatty acids have a double bond inserted after the third and sixth carbons from the methyl end. There is a preference of the desaturase for the *n*-3 configuration over the *n*-6 configuration.

Oils from vegetables and legumes such as soybean, corn, peanuts, and cottonseed are rich sources of *n*-6 fatty acids. Flesh of deep-sea fish such as halibut and salmon are high in *n*-3 fatty acids. A list of representative bioactive products obtained from each of these essential fatty acids is presented in Table 61-2. Linoleic acid gives rise through intermediate desaturation and elongation to dihomo-γ-linolenic acid, which can be converted to arachidonic acid by further desaturation (Figure 61-2). Arachidonic acid (20:4, *n*-6) serves as a precursor for prostaglandin, prostacyclin, and thromboxane synthesis by the cyclooxygenase pathway (see Chapter 18) or for leukotriene and hydroxy fatty acid synthesis via the lipoxygenase pathway. By providing tissues with different precursor molecules, the final products can be altered. For example, switching from vegetable to marine oils enhances production of PGE_3 and inhibits production of PGE_2. Omega-3 fatty acids are also converted into biologically active compounds, but the major intermediates are eicosapentaenoic (20:5, *n*-3) and docosahexaenoic (22:6, *n*-3) fatty acids. Omega-3 fatty acids are preferentially incorporated in position 2 of membrane phospholipids where they function as important regulators of cell function. When cells are stimulated with phospholipase A2, there is mobilization of fatty acids from position 2 of the phospholipids, thus providing substrates for the cyclooxygenase or lipoxygenase pathways. Certain fatty acids (18:2, *n*-6; 18:3, *n*-3; and 20:3, *n*-9) are competitive inhibitors for prostaglandin and leukotriene precursors (20:3, *n*-6; 20:4, *n*-6; and 20:5, *n*-3). Not only is there a difference between *n*-6 and *n*-3 fatty acids, but there is also a great deal of variation within these groups in determining the final bioactive product. Thus the use of dietary fatty acids to alter one's physiology has potential but is extremely complex as therapy.

Increasing intake of fish or of dietary fish oil reduces plasma triglycerides. Present data do not support a role

Table 61-2 Bioactive Compounds Synthesized from the Two Essential Fatty Acids: Linoleic and Linolenic Acids

Class of Compounds	**Linoleic** (*n*-6) Fatty Acids	**Linolenic** (*n*-3) Fatty Acids
Prostaglandins	PGE_1, PGE_2	PGE_3
Thromboxans	TXA_1, TXA_2	TXA_3
Prostacyclin	PGI_3	PGI_2
Leukotrienes	8,9-LTA_3, LTA_4	LTA_5

From Myers AK: The eicosanoids: Prostaglandins, thromboxane, and leukotrienes. In DeGroot LJ, editor: *Endocrinology,* Philadelphia, 1986, Saunders.

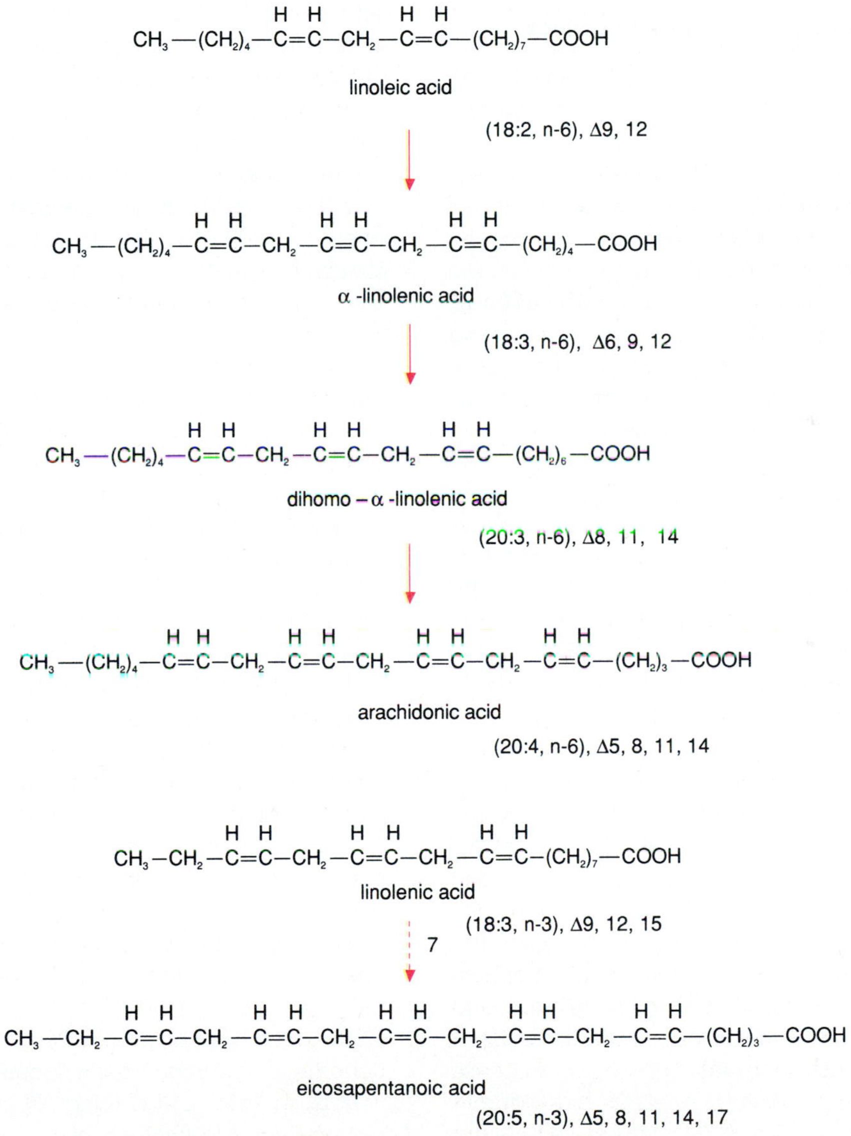

$$CH_3-(CH_2)_4-CH{=}CH-CH_2-CH{=}CH-(CH_2)_7-COOH$$

linoleic acid

(18:2, n-6), Δ9, 12

↓

$$CH_3-(CH_2)_4-CH{=}CH-CH_2-CH{=}CH-CH_2-CH{=}CH-(CH_2)_4-COOH$$

α -linolenic acid

(18:3, n-6), Δ6, 9, 12

↓

$$CH_3-(CH_2)_4-CH{=}CH-CH_2-CH{=}CH-CH_2-CH{=}CH-(CH_2)_6-COOH$$

dihomo – α -linolenic acid

(20:3, n-6), Δ8, 11, 14

↓

$$CH_3-(CH_2)_4-CH{=}CH-CH_2-CH{=}CH-CH_2-CH{=}CH-CH_2-CH{=}CH-(CH_2)_3-COOH$$

arachidonic acid

(20:4, n-6), Δ5, 8, 11, 14

$$CH_3-CH_2-CH{=}CH-CH_2-CH{=}CH-CH_2-CH{=}CH-(CH_2)_7-COOH$$

linolenic acid

(18:3, n-3), Δ9, 12, 15

⇣ 7

$$CH_3-CH_2-CH{=}CH-CH_2-CH{=}CH-CH_2-CH{=}CH-CH_2-CH{=}CH-CH_2-CH{=}CH-(CH_2)_3-COOH$$

eicosapentanoic acid

(20:5, n-3), Δ5, 8, 11, 14, 17

FIGURE 61-2 Synthesis of precursor fatty acids from linoleic (18:2, *n*-6) and linolenic (18:3, *n*-6) essential fatty acids.

for these fatty acids in lowering serum cholesterol, except when hypercholesterolemia is attributable to excess very-low-density lipoprotein as in type 5 hyperlipoproteinemia. A prudent approach to reducing serum cholesterol by dietary means is to substitute the saturated fat with a monounsaturated fat such as olive oil. Monounsaturated fats tend to lower serum cholesterol, particularly the LDL concentration.

Vitamins and Vitamin Deficiency Diseases

Dietary manipulations have long been used in the treatment of disease. The ancient Egyptians applied juice from cooked livers to their eyes to reverse night blindness. The Greeks consumed liver in addition to applying the juice topically. We now recognize the active agent present in the liver to be vitamin A.

Between 35% to 50% of the adult population in the United States supplement their diet daily with vitamins. The very young (1 to 5 years of age), the elderly, and exercising adults are the most frequent vitamin consumers. All vitamins can be used therapeutically for correction of deficiency symptoms. Claims for benefits in other diseases have not been substantiated. The Food and Drug Administration (FDA) reports that the median level of vitamin intake among users was 200% of the recommended daily allowance (RDA) and that over 4% of the users were taking potentially toxic doses of vitamin A (25,000 IU/day). Physician awareness will help in recognition and prevention of hypervitaminosis.

Vitamin A and Retinoids Vitamin A and its related natural and synthetic analogs are referred to as retinoids. Three major activities attributed to retinoids are enhancement of night vision, promotion of growth, and anticarcinogenesis. The mechanism of vitamin A action in vision is well understood. Vitamin A in its *cis*-retinal form is combined with opsin to form rhodopsin during darkness (or in the presence of specific phospholipids). When light activates rods in the retina of the eye, rhodopsin is broken down, cyclic guanosine monophosphate is hydrolyzed by a G protein that is activated, and the membrane becomes hyperpolarized. When concentrations of vitamin A fall, there is a concurrent decrease in the amount of vitamin A in the retina and pigment epithelium, and less rhodopsin is synthesized. Night blindness occurs because dark adaptation is dependent on the amount of rhodopsin in the outer rod segments. Dietary supplementation of vitamin A reverses this condition. Zinc deficiency and protein-calorie malnutrition also reduce rhodopsin content.

The link of vitamin A to cancer is conjectural but is based on the effect of retinoids on cellular growth and differentiation and also their effect on drug-metabolizing enzymes. Retinoids, for example, convert keratin-producing cells into mucus-producing cells and stimulate differentiation of certain cancer cells. Retinoids directly interact with cellular binding proteins and then enter the nucleus where they regulate gene expression by combining with receptors and interacting with chromatin. As a result, new mRNA is transcribed, and it encodes for different cellular proteins, leading to a more differentiated cell type.

Studies in animals illustrate the potential antitumor effect of retinoids. T lymphocytes from mice injected with vitamin A demonstrate increased tumor-cytotoxic activity. Retinoids produce resistance to lung, cervical, vaginal, and intestinal cancers induced by carcinogens. Vitamin A has been reported to have a protective effect in colon cancer and various chemical toxicities.

A possible alternative mechanism for the anticancer effects of the retinoids is that vitamin A affects the synthesis or activity of the drug-metabolizing enzyme systems and thereby alters the cell's ability to remove toxins.

Several therapeutic uses for vitamin A and the retinoids include treatment of cystic acne (isotretinoin) and psoriasis (etretinate). However, in the United States, excessive vitamin A intake is far more common than its deficiency. Yellowing of the skin occurs with excessive intake of vitamin A (retinol) or β-carotene. Other major symptoms of retinoid overdose are skin dryness, alopecia, hepatosplenomegaly, anorexia, headaches, and fatigue. Massive overdoses may be fatal. Excess retinoid intake during pregnancy is associated with birth defects, particularly if taken in the first trimester.

Niacin Niacin deficiency causes pellagra, which is classically characterized by the 3 *D'* s; dermatitis, dementia, and diarrhea, in addition to gastroenteritis and anemia. About 1/60 of the body's tryptophan is converted to niacin, and niacin deficiency is caused by diets deficient in both niacin and tryptophan. In large amounts (3 to 6 g/day) niacin lowers serum cholesterol in patients with hypercholesterolemia. Although vasodilation and flushing occur initially, these side effects tend to improve or disappear over time. Niacin taken in large doses over time may result in liver damage, and periodic liver function tests should be conducted to prevent this negative side effect. Nicotinamide intake does not produce the flushing observed with nicotinic acid, nor does it lower serum cholesterol (Chapter 20).

Pantothenic Acid Pantothenic acid functions as an acyl carrier in transmitochondrial fatty acid transport and activation. Reports from the late 1940s and early 1950's claimed that this vitamin was utilized in wound healing and repair of skin lesions. Although deficiency of this vitamin has not been recognized, studies investigating possible advantages of supplementation during wound healing are ongoing.

Choline and Inositol These substances serve structural and transmitter functions in cell membranes and in the nervous system. Phosphatidylcholine and phosphatidylinositol are important phospholipid components of the plasma and intracellular membranes. Phosphatidylcholine serves primarily a structural role, whereas phosphatidylinositol, together with inositol trisphosphate act as second messengers. Choline is converted to acetylcholine, and lecithin (which serves as a substrate for esterification of cholesterol by lecithin-cholesterol-acyl transferase) is also a methyl-group donor in 1-carbon metabolism in lieu of methionine and is a precursor for diacylglycerol formation. Preliminary studies indicate a possible relationship between choline and memory loss in elderly patients. Large doses of lecithin or choline may reverse memory loss in some cases, perhaps by increasing synthesis of acetylcholine. High-choline diets increase brain acetylcholine concentrations in rats.

Because tissue concentrations of acetylcholine and the phosphoinositides can be altered by diet, physiological functions ascribed to these vitamins can be modulated nutritionally. Although these substances are potentially useful, adequate studies do not as yet substantiate their effectiveness. Because overconsumption of choline and lecithin may cause depression, increased sensitivity of dopamine receptors, and excessive neurotransmitter synthesis, supplements of these substances in the diet is not recommended.

Vitamin B_6/pyridoxine Vitamin B_6/pyridoxine is an important enzyme cofactor for transamination, decarboxylation, dehydratase reactions, and side-chain cleavages. It is generally considered that improvement of diseased states obtained with B_6 supplementation occurs through stimulation of one or more of these processes. Since it is so involved in aspects of amino acid metabolism, the usual requirement of 2 mg per day increases with increased protein intake. Vitamin B_6 is used to treat sideroblastic anemia (when it is not effectively treated by folacin, iron, or vitamin B_{12}) and to improve muscle tone in patients with Parkinson's disease receiving levodopa. It is also used to treat Huntington's chorea, seizures in newborn infants, and isoniazid-induced seizures. Patients receiving isoniazid and some newborns with low concentrations of γ-aminobutyric acid find improvement with B_6 because it increases synthesis of this neurotransmitter. Pyridoxine is used to treat carpal tunnel syndrome, particularly in the elderly. Pyridoxine improves homocystinuria and primary oxalosis. Caution should be used in prescribing pyridoxine, since large doses may induce peripheral neuropathy.

Vitamin B_{12} Pernicious anemia, or combined-systems disease, is a severe disease produced by deficiency of vitamin B_{12}. It is characterized by a macrocytic anemia together with subacute degeneration of the spinal cord, cerebral white matter, and peripheral nerves. Deficiency is usually attributable to an abnormality of absorption from the gastrointestinal tract such as a lack of "intrinsic factor." Unless permanent damage has occurred, symptoms are reversible by injections of vitamin B_{12}. Vitamin B_{12} deficiency is common among alcohol abusers, as is folic acid deficiency. Treatment with folic acid alone improves the anemia, but the neurological disorder progresses. Thus care should be taken in the diagnosis of macrocytic anemia (see Chapter 65).

Vitamin C In one of the first controlled scientific experiments, Lind, a British Royal Navy physician, found that citrus fruits would control scurvy. Years later, vitamin C (ascorbic acid) was identified by Szent-Györgyi as the active agent. Vitamin C functions as a reducing agent and antioxidant in metabolic processes. Vitamin C promotes hydroxylation along with molecular oxygen, and usually with Cu^{++} or Fe^{++} as cofactors. An example of this reaction occurs during formation of collagen fiber from procollagen. Despite its obvious importance, the claim that high doses of vitamin C are beneficial in certain ailments and disease states is of questionable reliability. The use of vitamin C for prevention and treatment of the common cold was originally proposed by Nobel laureate Linus Pauling. The mild antihistaminic properties of vitamin C provide a potential mechanism for relief, but controlled studies have shown only marginal effects in reducing cold symptoms. Claims for benefits of vitamin C in lowering blood cholesterol, preventing atherosclerosis, or prolonging life in cancer patients are based on uncontrolled studies. Sudden discontinuation of large doses of vitamin C can result in the appearance of a mild vitamin C–deficiency syndrome, termed *rebound scurvy.*

Food Toxicants and Additives

Naturally Occurring Food Toxicants Contrary to popular belief, foods derived from plants contain far more toxicants than foods of animal origin. Numerous drugs have been extracted from plants and many pharmaceuticals were developed because of medicinal effects first discovered from consuming plant products.

Protease inhibitors are common in many plants with perhaps the most notable being soybean trypsin inhibitor. These substances inhibit growth in rats fed raw soybeans and are inactivated when soy is heated. Food processing will eliminate bioactivity. This is of concern mainly among health food enthusiasts who eat raw soybeans. Recent studies suggest a possible anticancer action for these compounds, but this is undocumented.

Hemagglutinins, or red blood cell agglutinators, in

NUTRITIONAL PROBLEMS

FOOD TOXINS AND ADDITIVES:

Mycotoxins
Estrogens
Antibiotics
Xanthines
Monosodium Glutamate
Preservatives
Dyes

various plants are collectively referred to as phytoagglutinins. Legumes (soybeans, kidney beans, peanuts, etc.) In particular have high concentrations of these substances; overconsumption of these foods may cause alterations in intravascular clotting. Fortunately, most of these compounds are destroyed in the digestive process and present no problem. However vegetarians may be at risk for hypercoagulability if moderation is not exercised.

Mycotoxins are fungal toxins in foods with potential toxicity for humans. Ingestion of aflatoxin, produced by a peanut fungus, has caused large-scale poisonings in India and Thailand. Susceptibility to poisoning varies with nutritional state and is increased by protein malnutrition. Aflatoxin B_1 is classified as a carcinogen by the World Health Organization, and chronic exposure to this and other mycotoxins are believed to be responsible for inducing cancer throughout Africa and Asia. In the United States, mycotoxins present in fish and shellfish products are actually of more concern than those associated with other foods. Signs of acute mycotoxin poisoning include gastrointestinal bleeding, hypertension, encephalopathy, and jaundice. Acute poisoning can be fatal.

Hormones and Growth Promoters The synthetic estrogen diethylstilbestrol (DES), when added to feed to increase the growth of livestock, was withdrawn from use when it was shown to induce ovarian and renal cancer. DES was prescribed in the 1950s to prevent premature labor. Daughters of these women later were shown to have increased ovarian cancer rates. These findings prompted the discontinuation of DES addition to cattle feedstuffs because DES was shown to have a very long half-life, which resulted in its accumulation in meat of DES-treated animals. The unfortunate experience with DES has heightened awareness of the possibility for contamination of food products by steroids. Considerable publicity has resulted from treatment of livestock with growth hormone and other growth factors, but current evidence indicates that these substances do not have adverse effects on humans consuming meat or milk from treated animals.

Antibiotics Antibiotics including tetracyclines, penicillins, and monensin have been used for about 50 years to promote health and growth of livestock and poultry. The growth-promoting ability of antibiotics apparently lies in their ability to increase intestinal absorption of nutrients by decreasing bacterial damage to the intestinal mucosa. A major concern has been their potential effect on humans consuming products from antibiotic-treated animals. Generation of antibiotic-resistant bacteria in treated animals, with subsequent transfer to humans, has been reported. Allergic reactions to antibiotics in milk or other foodstuffs (particularly to penicillins) also has been documented.

Methylxanthines and Tannins Coffee and tea are consumed by a large proportion of the population, making caffeine a widely used psychoactive drug. Other sources of caffeine include diet pills, aspirin-compound preparations, soda, and chocolate. Because of inhibitory effects on cyclic adenosine monophosphate (cAMP) phosphodiesterase activity and cAMP concentrations, as well as interactions with adenosine receptors, physicians should carefully inquire about consumption of coffee, tea, cocoa, and other caffeine-containing foods and drugs during the medical history examination. Although decaffeinated products exist, caffeine intake from caffeine-containing drinks is of major concern, particularly in children. Adverse effects including cardiac arrhythmias and CNS hyperactivity are observed with excess caffeine consumption. In children and adults, headache often occurs after withdrawal of daily caffeine consumption. A cup of coffee (5 oz) contains about 80 mg of caffeine, whereas tea has half that amount. Children who consume a soft drink receive a relatively greater dose on a weight basis than adults who ingest a cup of coffee.

Tannins exist as natural components of foods (such as those present in teas), or they may be added during processing (as in beers and wines) where they serve as clarifying agents. Tannins inhibit absorption of iron and alter the uptake of other minerals from the intestine. Consumption of normal levels of tannins has not been associated with undesirable side effects. However, heavy consumption of teas may be correlated with low blood iron concentrations, particularly among the elderly or others with marginal iron status.

Monosodium Glutamate (MSG) MSG is a flavor enhancer used in processed food and is an important ingredient in Oriental cooking. "Chinese restaurant syndrome" is caused by an inability to degrade this substance. Pyridoxine, by stimulating transamination reactions required to detoxify this compound, can help prevent or reverse the flushing and weakness that results from this syndrome. Of perhaps greater concern are the effects MSG may have on the central nervous system. In animals studies MSG causes specific brain lesions, notably in the arcuate nucleus. It is not known if MSG can adversely affect humans, but caution must be exercised in ingesting large doses, particularly in children.

Food Preservatives and Dyes The Federal Food, Drug and Cosmetic Act of 1958 describes a food additive as a compound or compounds added directly or indirectly to a food preparation. This includes radiation treatment of foodstuffs. The Delaney clause in this amendment specifically prevents use of any food additive that induces cancer at any dose in experimental animals or man. The manufacturer must demonstrate that a particular additive is safe for use in food. Exclusions from this law are made for products used before the act became effective, if no problems of usage have been demonstrated in epistemological studies, or if they are considered "safe" as a result of the judgment of a scientific panel. A list of exempted materials "generally regarded as safe" (GRAS) is published by the Food and Drug Administration.

A GRAS list exists for chemical preservatives and includes substances such as ascorbic acid, the tocopherols, and other antimicrobials and antioxidants. It also includes butylated hydroxyanisole and butylated hydroxytoluene (BHA and BHT respectively), which have been shown to cause tumors in experimental animals but not in humans. The use of the latter two preservatives is limited by quantity added, with certain acceptable concentrations. Because these substances are antioxidants and accumulate in lipids, total BHA and BHT concentrations are based on fat content. They cannot exceed 0.02% of the lipid content of the food, whereas antimicrobials are generally regulated on a percentage of total food.

Treatment of Diseases by Nutrients

Inborn Errors of Metabolism Many inborn errors of metabolism require alterations of the diet to ameliorate the symptoms or to prevent the accumulation of toxic or detrimental metabolites. Dietary therapies for the more common inborn errors of metabolism are included here, but a comprehensive review is beyond the scope of this chapter.

Glycogen Storage Disease Von Gierke's disease, one of the more common of the glycogen storage diseases, is attributable to deficiency of the enzyme glucose-6-phosphatase. This deficiency prevents the liver from breaking down stored glycogen, resulting in liver enlargement and a fasting hypoglycemia. Stimulation of glycolysis produces increased plasma lactate and pyruvate. At least seven variations of glycogen storage disease in liver, muscle, and heart are related to specific enzyme deficiencies and most can be modulated by diet. High-glucose diets should be avoided and complex carbohydrates used in place of monosaccharides and disaccharides. Although patients should avoid acute elevations of plasma glucose, the hypoglycemia in these conditions necessitates frequent meal or snack eating.

Phenylketonuria Public awareness of this inherited inborn error of metabolism has increased, since the artificial sweetener aspartame, marketed as Nutrasweet, became a popular food additive. Phenylketonurics are unable convert phenylalanine to tyrosine, which results in an accumulation of phenylalanine. Aspartame, a dipeptide of phenylalanine and aspartic acid, taken in excess amounts could result in toxic concentrations of phenylalanine. The disease is the result of a defect in or the absence of phenylalanine hydroxylase. Individuals with this disease are frequently mentally retarded, with defective myelination of nerves and hyperactive reflexes. Life expectancy is decreased dramatically, but quality and duration can be enhanced by early diagnosis and avoidance of phenylalanine.

Familial Goiter Two inborn errors of thyroid metabolism are, first, a dehalogenase deficiency, which reduces organic iodine available to the thyroid, and, second, an iodide-transport defect, which also results in low thyroid iodine. Symptoms include hypothyroidism and goiter. Dietary iodine supplementation is effective therapy for both (see Chapter 38). Endemic goiter is found in underdeveloped countries of Africa, Asia, and South America and is also treated by dietary iodine supplements.

Gout Gout is caused by deficiency in the enzymes hypoxanthine-guanine-phosphoribosyl-transferase or glucose-6-phosphatase, or by excessive activity of phosphoribosyl pyrophosphate synthetase. This heritable disorder may be exacerbated by high protein or purine diets, excessive alcohol intake, and weight loss on low carbohydrate or very low calorie diets. Symptoms of gout include hyperuricemia, tophi, and painful arthritis (see Chapter 29). Restrictions in protein, purine, and alcohol intake are indicated. Weight reduction may lower uric acid concentrations, reduce insulin resistance, and help prevent gouty episodes, but patients are at increased risk of gout during weight loss and may require drug therapy.

Wernicke-Korsakoff Syndrome The disorder Wernicke-Korsakoff syndrome, characterized by abnormal gait, impaired mental function including memory loss, and paralysis of ocular movements, is seen in individuals abusing ethanol and is caused by thiamine deficiency. Two thiamine-dependent enzymes, pyruvate dehydrogenase and α-ketoglutarate dehydrogenase, are normal in Wernicke-Korsakoff patients. However, transketolase from fibroblasts of patients with this syndrome binds thiamine pyrophosphate with only one tenth the affinity found in normal individuals. Transketolase with thiamine as cofactor transfers an aldehyde group to an aldose acceptor in the pentose phosphate pathway. Because only enzyme affinity for thiamine is affected, most symptoms of this disease may be reversed when thiamine is provided. However, in patients with advanced Korsakoff's psychosis, complete recovery of mental function is rare. Individuals with symptoms of severe alcohol abuse should routinely be treated with thiamine.

Diabetes Mellitus The initial therapy for type II (adult onset), or non–insulin dependent, diabetes is proper nutritional management. In many cases, proper nutritional guidance can obviate the need for pharmacological intervention. Some factors in diabetes treatment have been discussed previously in this chapter. In general, a low-fat, high-carbohydrate diet (50% to 60% of calories) should be followed with an emphasis on complex carbohydrate (approximately two thirds of the total). Lower carbohydrate diets with increased protein have also been advocated. In the approximately 80% of patients with non–insulin dependent diabetes who are overweight or obese, a lower calorie intake is prescribed and often leads to improvement of the disease. Artificial sweeteners can be used in moderation with no problems, and fructose may be desirable as an alternative to sucrose. There has been little evidence that supplementation of the diet with fish oils confers any advantage, but a decrease in saturated fat by substitution of monounsaturated fats may reduce the increased risk of atherogenesis in diabetes. Increased soluble fiber may be helpful in regulating carbohydrate absorption, particularly if consumed as high fiber foods. Supplements of fiber extracted from foods has limited value. Care should be taken to avoid deficiencies in minerals or vitamins when one is increasing dietary fiber. Protein should constitute about 15% of the total caloric intake leaving 20% to 30% of the calories to be supplied as fat (two thirds of this should be polyunsaturated or monounsaturated).

DRUG-NUTRIENT INTERACTIONS

Dietary Factors Affecting Drug Efficacy

There are many ways in which drug efficacy can be altered nutritionally. Foods containing pectin fiber delay food entry from stomach to duodenum. This increases the time for absorption of orally administered drugs from the intestine. The type of foods consumed and their transit times affect the amount of bile released and the pH of intestinal contents. These are important considerations if alterations in time or rate of drug absorption affect treatment efficacy. Frequent interactions of food and drugs can occur and should always be considered if a patient is not responding appropriately to a drug. Examples are the chelation of calcium with tetracycline, which decreases absorption when the drug is taken with milk or milk products, and the alteration of levodopa absorption and of theophylline metabolism with a protein meal.

Drug Effects on Nutrient Status

Antibiotics Antibiotics may interact with nutrients by causing malabsorption and maldigestion. Tetracycline reduces iron and calcium absorption by metal chelation in the intestine, forming complexes that cannot be absorbed by the gut. Neomycin, at therapeutic doses, reduces absorption of minerals, vitamin B_{12}, lipids, glucose, and nitrogen-containing compounds by affecting gastrointestinal structure as well as intestinal flora. With neomycin treatment, villi are shortened and the integrity of the crypt cells is disrupted along with infiltration of the lamina propria.

Other antibiotics that interfere with nutritional status include cephalosporins, which can cause intestinal hemorrhage (acting as vitamin K antagonists) and aminoglycosides, which cause excretion of calcium, magnesium, and potassium by inhibiting normal kidney function. Isoniazid, an antagonist of pyridoxine (vitamin B_6), can also cause niacin deficiency. Isoniazid can decrease vitamin D concentration by inhibiting kidney α-hydroxylase and liver 25-hydroxylase (Chapter 42).

Drugs that Reduce Intestinal Absorption Many orally administered drugs reduce absorption of foods from the gastrointestinal tract. Some effects such as decreased fat-soluble vitamin absorption caused by mineral oil and decreased vitamin (folate) and mineral (iron, zinc) absorption caused by binding to cholestyramine, are predictable. Presence of these two pharmacological agents shortens the contact time between nutrient and gastrointestinal mucosa and thus reduces absorption. Prevention of micelle formation (mineral oil) and cationic binding of charged particles (by cholestyramine) prevent nutrients from reaching the villi thereby decreasing gut transport. By increasing intestinal pH, any basic compound such as sodium bicarbonate, can dramatically decrease absorption of folic acid and iron by changing their oxidation state. Cimetidine inhibits the uptake of some of the water-soluble vitamins (e.g., B_{12}) by preventing secretion of hydrochloric acid in the stomach and thus increasing pH in the intestine.

Drug Effects on Vitamin and Mineral Status/Antivitamins The majority of drug effects on nutrients appear to involve vitamins or minerals. Vitamins and minerals act as enzyme cofactors, which activate specific biochemical reactions. Drugs may therefore interfere with nutrients by one or more of the following mechanisms:

1. Binding in intestine or inhibition of absorption
2. Competition with nutrients for transport
3. Direct competition at site of action
4. Destruction or deactivation of nutrient
5. Overutilization of nutrient resulting in depletion of stores
6. Alteration of metabolic half-lives of nutrients by increasing rate of removal from blood or promoting loss of nutrient from the body by increasing its excretion.

DRUGS FOR NUTRITIONAL DISORDERS

Obesity

The most common form of malnutrition in the United States is obesity, a syndrome of multiple causes. Up to 34% of the adult population may be obese. There are numerous complications, many of which can be prevented or aided by successful dietary intervention. These include diabetes mellitus, hypertension, hyperlipoproteinemia, atherosclerotic disease, myocardial infarction, cerebrovascular accidents, sleep apnea, gallbladder disease, gout, and certain cancers.

Current medical treatment of obesity, including diet, exercise, and behavioral modification, is marginally effective. Pharmacologic agents have only a minor role in treatment, mainly because of the strict state and federal regulatory agency controls. In general, treatment with obesity-controlling drugs is limited to a few weeks because of side effects and abuse potential. Table 61-3 lists drugs currently approved and those that have potential for approval for the treatment of obesity in the United States, along with their Drug Enforcement Administration schedule and mechanism of action.

Antiobesity drugs fall into two main categories: centrally active or peripherally active. Centrally active antiobesity drugs have two possible mechanisms of action: action on catecholamine neurotransmitters or an effect on central serotoninergic neurotransmitter systems. All reduce food intake, at least initially, and several agents appear to enhance energy expenditure. Some investigators believe that antiobesity drugs may lower the level at which body weight is maintained, but this concept is not established.

The first centrally acting obesity drugs developed were amphetamines, which have significant abuse potential and should not be used for obesity treatment. Except for diethylpropion, the other nonamphetamine drugs have little abuse potential based on nonhuman primate studies. Phenylpropanolamine (PPA) is the only antiobesity drug that is sold over the counter in the United States. PPA is not a Drug Enforcement Administration (DEA)–scheduled drug and has no significant abuse potential in animal studies. The effectiveness of PPA is similar to that of other antiobesity agents. *d,l*-Fenfluramine, a serotonin agonist, has central depressant rather than stimulant activity. The *d*-isomer has similar or better efficacy and fewer side effects but is not available in this country. Fluoxetine and sertraline are both approved for treatment of depression, and both cause weight loss in some individuals. These serotonin agonists should not be used with monoamine or tricyclic antidepressants because the combination may cause significant side effects.

Some peripherally active agents interfere with intestinal absorption. Acarbose is a carbohydrase inhibitor that interferes with digestion of sucrose and complex carbohydrates in the small intestine and has produced only modest weight loss in clinical trials. Tetrahydrolipostatin, a lipase inhibitor, blocks digestion of lipid in the intestine. Although it is not yet available for general use, preliminary clinical trials indicate that it may prove useful for treatment of obesity. As noted above, dietary fiber has been promoted as a treatment for obesity, but well-controlled trials with fiber supplements have shown only modest or no significant weight loss.

Antiobesity drugs have generally not been used over a long term. However, a few studies with *d*-fenfluramine alone or *d,l*-fenfluramine in combination with phentermine indicate that these drugs may promote long-term weight loss in some but not all individuals. Currently there is no way of predicting those individuals who will or will not respond to long-term treatment. More research is needed before antiobesity drugs can be recommended as safe and effective long-term treatment.

Anorexia Nervosa and Bulimia

Two types of eating disorders seen most commonly are bulimia and anorexia nervosa. Bulimia consists of episodes of binge eating, followed by self-induced vomiting, purging by laxatives or other means, and periods of limited food intake or starvation, without extreme weight loss. Anorexia nervosa is characterized by frequent incidence of food restriction or starvation, vomiting, purging, and increased activity, but without binge eating, and with an extreme weight loss.

Both humans and animals overeat after a period of starvation. Binge eating for periods as long as 2 years was observed after long-term restriction of food intake in young men in the classic studies by Ancel Keys. Although anorexia nervosa has been considered a psychi-

Table 61-3 Drugs for Obesity

Generic Name	Trade Name	Drug Enforcement Administration Schedule	Status*
CENTRALLY ACTIVE CATECHOLAMINERGIC AGENTS			
Benzphetamine	Didrex	III	A
Dextroamphetamine†	Dexidrine	II	A
Diethylpropion	Tenuate	IV	A
Mazindol	Mazanor, Sanorex	IV	A
Methamphetamine†	Desoxyn	II	A
Phendimetrazine	Bontril, Plegine, Prelu-2	III	A
Phenmetrazine	Preludin	II	A
Phentermine	Adipex, Fastin, Ionamin	IV	A
Phenylpropanolamine	Dexatrim, Acutrim	OTC	A
CENTRALLY ACTIVE SEROTONINERGIC AGENTS			
d,l-Fenfluramine	Pondimin	IV	A
d-Fenfluramine	—	—	NA
Fluoxetine‡	Prozac	None	
Sertraline‡	Zoloft	None	
PERIPHERALLY ACTIVE AGENTS			
Tetrahydrolipostatin	Orlistat	None	E
Acarbose	Glucobay	None	E

*Status: *A*, approved; *E*, experimental
NA, not available in the United States; *OTC*, over the counter.
†Amphetamine compounds not recommended for clinical use for obesity
‡Approved for other indications.

atric disorder, recent studies of activity-based anorexia in rats indicates that there may be an underlying physiological or biochemical basis.

The neuropathological mechanisms of each of these disorders is not clear, but numerous trials of various types of centrally acting pharmacologic agents have been performed, with mixed results. Both adrenergic and serotoninergic agents have been shown to have effects in some patients, an indication that the diseases can be corrected by neuropharmacological intervention. It also appears that there are multiple causes for these diseases.

Bulimia appears to respond to antidepressant medication including imipramine and desipramine. Monoamine oxidase inhibitors are effective if combined with a dietary regimen. Promising results have also been obtained with fluoxetine and other newer agents.

Anorexia nervosa responds to tricyclic antidepressants, and some studies indicate that fluoxetine and other serotonin agonists may be effective. Several open-label trials of zinc supplements have shown promising results. Controlled studies have not been performed. Drugs used to promote food intake, such as cyproheptadine, amitriptyline, clonidine, and opiate antagonists are of interest and require further evaluation. It should be emphasized that many of the recommended drugs are potent pharmacological agents and their long-term use is not without risk.

NEW DIRECTIONS

Elucidation of the pathophysiology of obesity and eating disorders may allow development of new and more effective drugs. Important future advances in nutrition and pharmacology will lead to the development of drugs to treat obesity and eating disorders. Another area of future importance is an increased awareness by clinicians of the interaction of foods and drugs. The availability of computerized pharmacy data bases will allow better information on the number of drugs, the drug doses, and the potential for identifying food-drug interactions. With major initiatives in national health care and managed health care systems, more attention will be given to the role of nutrition in disease prevention. Health maintenance organizations typically emphasize preventive medicine and development of healthy lifestyles to minimize health care costs. The role of nutritional status as it affects health should be more prominent in the decision making of clinicians and health care providers. This could lead to increased nutrition research, increased awareness of nutritional intervention in disease states, and the need for nutrition programs in medical and professional schools curricula.

REFERENCES

American Heart Association: A Joint Statement of the Nutrition Committee and Council on Atherosclerosis. Recommendations for the treatment of hyperlipidemia in adults, Dallas, 1982.

Dubick MA, Rucker RB: Dietary supplements and health aids—a critical evaluation. Part I, Vitamins and minerals, *J Nutr Educ* 15:47-53, 1983.

Grundy SM: Comparison of monounsaturated fatty acids and carbohydrates for lowering plasma cholesterol, *N Engl J Med* 314:745-748, 1986.

Linder MC, editor: *Nutritional biochemistry and metabolism,* New York, 1985, Elsevier.

Phillipson BE, Rothrock DW, Conner WE, et al: Reduction of plasma lipids, lipoproteins, and apoproteins by dietary fish oils in patients with hypertriglyceridemia, *N Engl J Med* 312:1210-1216, 1985.

Roe DA: *Diet and drug interactions,* New York, 1989, Van Nostrand Reinhold.

Shils ME, Young VR, editors: *Modern nutrition in health and disease,* Philadelphia, 1988, Lea & Febiger.

Silverstone T: Appetite suppressants: a review, *Drugs* 43:820-836, 1992.

Weintraub M: Long term weigh control study, *Clin Pharmacol Ther* 51:595-646, 1992.

SELF-ASSESSMENT QUESTIONS

1. Which of the following about drug treatment of obesity is incorrect?
   a. The two main categories of obesity drugs act on the central nervous system.
   b. Centrally acting obesity drugs are divided into noradrenergic and serotoninergic agents.
   c. Most obesity drugs have significant abuse potential.
   d. Two mechanisms of action of obesity drugs are reduction of food intake and increased energy expenditure.
   e. Current governmental regulations limit use of obesity drugs to a few weeks.
2. Which of the following statements about mechanisms by which drugs alter nutrient status is correct?
   a. Binding of nutrients in the gastrointestinal tract or inhibition of absorption
   b. Competition with nutrients for transport
   c. Direct competition with nutrients at the site of action
   d. Destruction or deactivation of the nutrient
   e. All of the above are correct
3. Which of the following statements about vitamins is correct?
   a. Pernicious anemia is treated by oral doses of vitamin B_{12}.
   b. Pernicious anemia may be treated by either vitamin B_{12} or large doses of folate.
   c. Vitamin C in large doses provides prompt relief of the common cold.
   d. Large doses of vitamin C can reverse colon cancer.
   e. Stopping large doses of vitamin C are reported to cause some symptoms of scurvy.
4. Which of the following statements about food additives and toxicants is correct?
   a. Raw soybeans contain a trypsin inhibitor.
   b. Plant foods contain more toxicants than animal sources of food.
   c. Peanuts contain aflatoxin, a potentially fatal poison and carcinogen.
   d. Antibiotics in milk and meats may induce allergy- or antibiotic-resistant bacteria in humans.
   e. All of the above.

5. Which of the following statements about dietary fiber is correct?
   a. Some types of dietary fiber cause delayed gastric emptying.
   b. Some types of dietary fiber cause delayed intestinal transit.
   c. Dietary fiber acts as a cation-exchange resin to bind bile acids.
   d. Soluble fiber delays carbohydrate absorption from the gut.
   e. All are correct.
6. Which of the following statements about vitamins is incorrect?
   a. Vitamin supplements are generally recommended for all children and elderly people.
   b. Large-dose vitamin A supplements may cause birth defects.
   c. Vitamin A deficiency produces night blindness by reducing levels of rhodopsin in the retina.
   d. Zinc deficiency simulates vitamin A deficiency in producing night blindness.
   e. Retinoids reduce cancers in animals.
7. Which of the following statements about dietary fatty acids is incorrect?
   a. Linolenic and linoleic acids are not synthesized by man.
   b. Prostaglandins, thromboxane, and leukotrienes are precursor molecules for essential fatty acids.
   c. The source of dietary fatty acids (e.g., fish versus corn oil margarine) alters the type of prostaglandin produced in the body.
   d. Increasing intake of fish or of dietary fish oil reduces plasma triglycerides.
   e. In general, fish-oil supplements are not recommended for lowering serum cholesterol.
8. Which of the following statements about vitamins is incorrect?
   a. Niacin deficiency causes dermatitis, gastroenteritis, dementia, and anemia.
   b. Large-dose niacin supplements reduce plasma cholesterol.
   c. The peripheral neuropathy caused by pyridoxine is independent of dose.
   d. Pyridoxine may reduce symptoms of the "Chinese restaurant syndrome."
   e. Requirements for pyridoxine increase with high protein diets.

CHAPTER 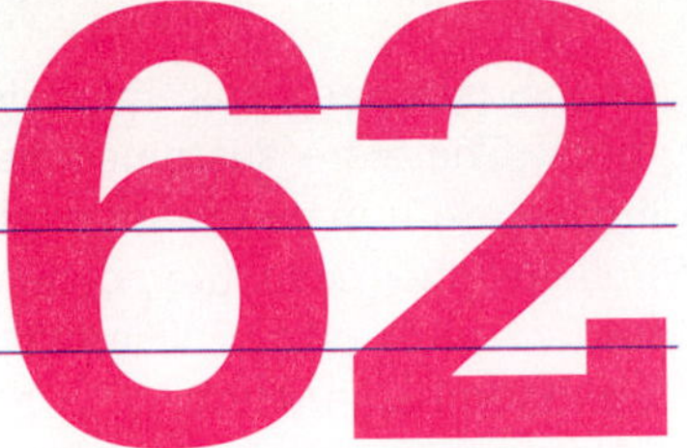

Toxicology

I. GLENN SIPES
RICHARD C. DART

WHAT IS TOXICOLOGY?

Industrial chemical and pharmaceutical development, environmental contamination, and illicit drug use present significant health hazards to the general population.

Each year in the United States it is estimated that approximately 8 million people suffer acute poisoning. About 20,000 persons die from illicit drug overdose per year. Acute toxicity from drug or poison ingestion accounts for as much as 10% to 20% of hospital admissions.

A more difficult challenge to the health care provider is the identification of health effects caused by chronic exposure to very low doses of environmental or occupational chemicals. In these cases, adverse effects may take years to develop. Physicians, nurses, and pharmacists should question their patients about the type of chemicals to which they are exposed, and they should also be alert to the potential of drug-chemical interactions.

ABBREVIATIONS	
BAL	British anti-Lewisite
CO	carbon monoxide
EDTA	ethylenediaminetetraacetic acid
FSH	follicle-stimulating hormone
IgG, IgM	immunoglobulins
LH	luteinizing hormone
TCDD	tetrachlorodibenzo-*p*-dioxin

Principles of Toxicology

Any substance injurious to humans may be classified as a poison. Substances such as sodium chloride, oxygen, and many others generally considered nontoxic can be deleterious to human health under certain conditions. The most important axiom of toxicology is that "the dose makes the poison." In other words, any chemical (NaCl, ethanol, oxygen) can be toxic if the dose or exposure becomes high enough. Similarly, the degree of injury increases as the dose increases.

The terms *poison, toxic substance, toxic chemical,* and *toxicant* are synonymous. Toxicity, or toxic response, refers to the effects manifested by an organism in response to a toxic substance.

A common test, the dose of chemical that kills 50% of animals receiving it (LD_{50}) was originally developed to quantify lethality in animals. However, LD_{50} is inappropriate in the assessment of toxicity in man. The LD_{50} is defined as the dose of a chemical that kills 50% of animals receiving it. The LD_{50} is rarely performed today, since it is more important to understand how the dose of a chemical alters biochemical and physiological processes in an organism and if these alterations produce adverse effects (i.e., toxicity).

A toxic response can occur within minutes or after a delay of hours, days, months, or years, or any interval between. These responses are often referred to as acute, subacute, subchronic, or chronic toxicities. Most acutely toxic agents rapidly interfere with critical cellular processes. For example, cyanide causes immediate injury by inhibiting cellular respiration. Acetaminophen is an example of subacute injury, since hepatic necrosis is not evident for 1 to 3 days after ingestion. Acetaminophen produces reactive intermediates that injure liver cells within a few hours. However, time is required (2 to 3 days) for this injury to become clinically manifest. Organophosphate insecticides cause an early cholinergic syndrome, which resolves before the development of peripheral neuropathy several days later.

A poison causing direct toxicity implies that direct contact and injury develops after interaction of the toxicant and the injured cell. Poisons causing indirect toxicity do so by injuring one group of cells, the injury of which precipitates injury in other cells. Similarly, interference with a normal physiological process may injure cells dependent on that process. For example, alterations of neuroendocrine function with reserpine or chlorpromazine alter sexual organ function.

Some substances such as strong acids or bases act locally. Most other toxic substances produce systemic effects or a combination of local and systemic effects. Hydrofluoric acid, a common industrial chemical, produces an extremely painful local penetrating injury at the site of skin exposure. In larger exposures, enough fluoride ions enter the blood to bind calcium and produce hypocalcemia. Most therapeutic drugs and toxicants other than strong acids or bases do not produce clinically significant local injury.

Many toxic substances are known to affect a particular target organ. The liver, nervous system, kidneys and lungs are examples in which toxicity can be related to altered physiological and biochemical functions. Because of a dual blood supply from the hepatic artery and the portal vein, the liver may be exposed to toxicants entering from the systemic circulation (as after inhalation) or from the splanchnic circulation (toxicants absorbed from the gastrointestinal [GI] tract). The leaky capillary system of the hepatic sinusoids promotes the extraction of toxicants from the blood into the liver. The liver contains a high concentration of enzymes to metabolize (biotransform) many endogenous and exogenous chemicals. In some cases, the chemical modification produced by biotransformation results in bioactivation, i.e., the production of toxic/reactive metabolites that detrimentally react within the liver. For example, acetaminophen causes hepatic necrosis. This occurs because the liver is rich in cytochrome P-450—the enzyme system that metabolizes acetaminophen to its reactive intermediates, chiefly glutathione adducts. When the rate of formation of reactive metabolites exceeds the liver's detoxification capacity, toxicity occurs. Other examples of compounds in which hepatic toxicity is caused by hepatic metabolism include solvents (carbon tetrachloride, halogenated benzenes), therapeutic agents (isoniazid), and carcinogens (aflatoxin B, aromatic amines).

The integrative role of the highly complex nervous system means that toxic injury to one part can result in adverse effects in other sites of the nervous system. Similarly, toxic injury in other organs and tissues can result in neuronal lesions. For example, chemicals that cause severe hypotension or hypoglycemia may result in neuronal cell death. Neurons have a high metabolic rate that requires a sustained delivery of oxygen and nutrients. Therefore sustained reductions in oxygen and glucose result in central nervous system (CNS) damage. Similarly, chemicals (i.e., cyanide or dinitrophenol) that interfere with oxidative metabolism can also compromise neuronal viability.

Neurons are unique among cells because the cell body must provide support for dendrites and axons. The axon is devoid of any metabolic functions (i.e., protein synthesis) and thus must rely on transport, often over long distances, of materials from the cell body to the distal axon. Acrylamide and *n*-hexane are believed to produce peripheral neuropathies by interfering with axonal transport. Diketone metabolites of *n*-hexane can derivatize and cross-link neurofilaments. As these cross-links accumulate with repeated exposure to *n*-hexane, axonal transport is retarded, ultimately causing axonal atrophy.

Another key feature of the CNS is the lack of regenerative repair mechanisms for mature neurons. Lack of repair results in the accumulation of lesions within the nervous system (Figure 62-1). Because of plasticity within the CNS, expression of these lesions as neurotoxic events is often delayed. However, the accumulation of lesions after repeated chemical exposure eventually reaches a critical concentration, and the normal neuronal reserve can no longer compensate for the chemical lesions. There is also a normal, age-related attrition of neurons. Thus chemical exposure to neurotoxicants may reduce the age at which neurological and behavioral deficits appear. If exposure to the chemical occurred in the past, a causal relationship between chemical exposure and neurotoxicity will not be apparent.

Pulmonary toxicity is primarily mediated by respiratory exposure, though blood-borne toxicants may also cause pulmonary injury. The pulmonary system is composed of the nasopharyngeal and tracheobronchial airways and the pulmonary parenchyma (alveoli). The airways are directly exposed to many gaseous or particulate toxicants. Gases may react with airway mucosal cells or penetrate to the alveoli. Chlorine gas reacts with upper airway fluids and produces hydrochloric acid, causing mucosal injury. Cyanide and chloroform penetrate to the alveoli, are well absorbed, and cause systemic, not pulmonary, toxicity. Particulates become impacted in the airway or, if small enough, reach the alveoli. If trapped in the airway, they may be cleared by the mucociliary apparatus. Substances reaching the alveoli can be eliminated only by absorption into the blood, by macrophage phagocytosis, or by biotransformation. Macrophages phagocytize toxicants in particulate form and then enzymatically degrade them or simply carry them out of the alveolus. When asbestos is involved, this function may actually produce toxicity. Macrophages engulf but cannot degrade asbestos par-

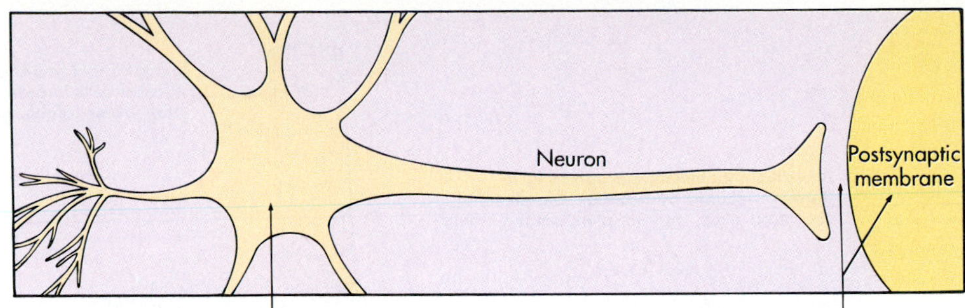

FIGURE 62-1 Summary of some toxicant actions on the central nervous system.

ticles. Ultimately, macrophages die, releasing degradative enzymes into the interstitium, which damages adjacent cells. Repetition of this process eventually leads to progressive fibrosis and restrictive respiratory dysfunction. Pulmonary biotransformation of chemicals may also lead to toxicity. The Clara cells, located in the terminal bronchioles, and the alveolar type II cells possess cytochrome P-450, which produces toxic metabolites of certain chemicals. Inhalation of benzo[*a*]pyrene and other polycyclic aromatic hydrocarbons causes lung cancer as a result of reactive intermediates produced by pulmonary cytochrome P-450.

The bloodstream is the route of exposure in the case of paraquat, a herbicide taken up by type II pneumocytes in the lung. Biotransformation of paraquat produces a reactive intermediate that undergoes redox cycling, a process that produces reactive oxygen species that injure the cell. Thus, although exposure to paraquat usually occurs after ingestion or skin contamination, death is caused by pulmonary injury. Similarly, certain pyrrolidine alkaloids are metabolized in the liver to metabolites that circulate in the blood and produce toxicity in the lung (see Figure 62-2 for summary).

The kidney is also susceptible to specific toxicants. The mechanisms of renal injury include those similar to other organs, as well as mechanisms unique to the kidney. Delivery of blood-borne toxic substances to the kidney is high because (1) the kidney receives 25% of cardiac output and (2) its functions include filtering, concentrating, and eliminating toxicants. As water is reabsorbed, the concentration of chemicals in the tubule can increase to toxic levels. In some cases, the concentration may exceed the solubility of a chemical and lead to precipitation and obstruction of the affected area (see Figure 62-3 for summary).

Although to a lesser extent than the liver, the kidney also biotransforms chemicals. Cytochrome P-450 is located in the proximal tubule. This may explain the susceptibility of this region to chemical injury. For example, carbon tetrachloride and chloroform, two halogenated hydrocarbons that injure the proximal tubule, require biotransformation by the cytochrome P-450 system to form the toxic species. In addition, many heavy metals damage the proximal tubules. Because heavy metals are not metabolized by cytochrome P-450, other mechanisms must be involved in this specificity. Heavy metals may concentrate in renal tubular cells and may also injure the blood vessels supplying the proximal tubule cells. Thus renal injury from heavy metals may result from a combination of direct and indirect toxicity.

The kidney can compensate for excessive chemical exposure. Like many organs it has a reserve mass. Thus tissue injury equal to one entire kidney must be lost before loss of function is clinically apparent. The kidney also replaces lost functional capacity by hypertrophy. In addition, the kidney has developed binding proteins to remove heavy metals. Metallothioneins, a unique protein class, avidly bind cadmium, protecting the kidney and other organs from toxicity. However, if exposure exceeds binding capacity or a large amount of the cadmium-metallothionein complex accumulates, renal toxicity will develop.

Although anatomical or functional characteristics predispose many organs to injury, designation of chemicals as specific organ toxicants (neurotoxic, cardiotoxic, etc.) is misleading for several reasons. First, toxic substances may have effects throughout the body. Although a chemical may primarily affect one organ, other organs

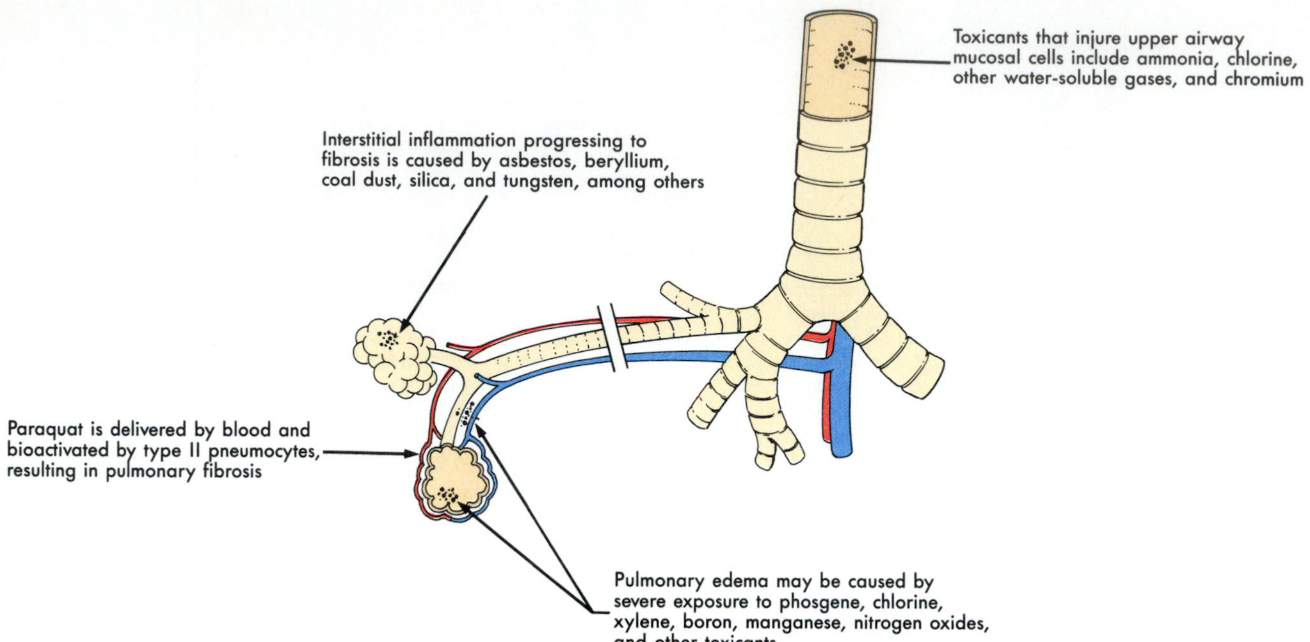

FIGURE 62-2 Summary of some toxicant actions on pulmonary tissues.

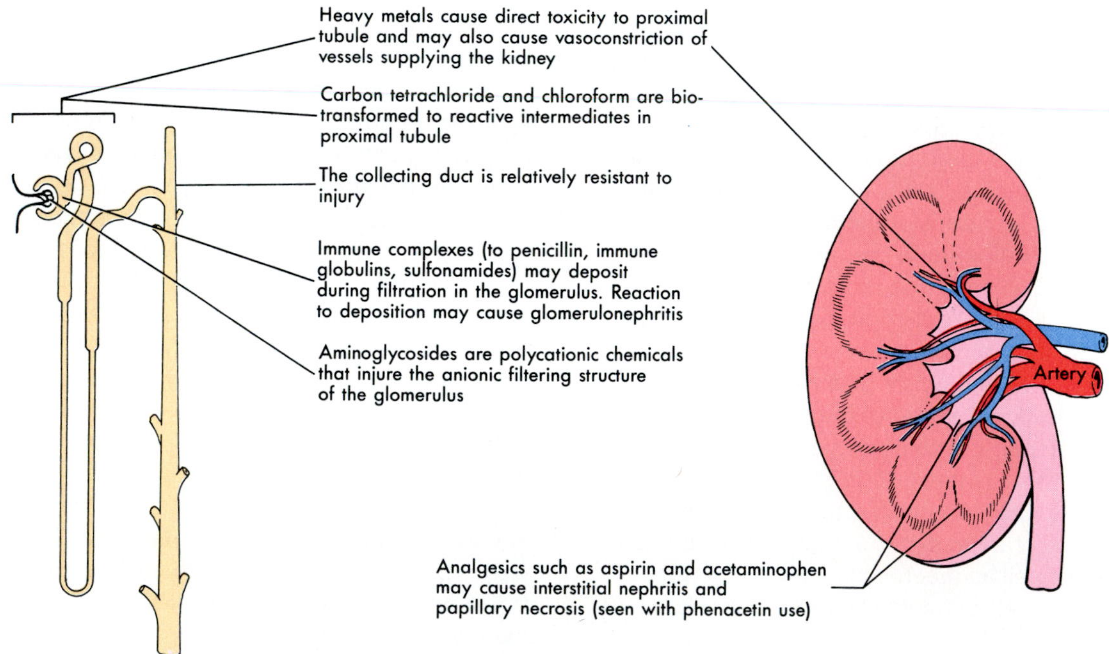

FIGURE 62-3 Summary of some toxicant actions on the kidney.

probably concurrently experience less notable degrees of injury. Second, a toxic response in one tissue will undoubtedly have serious consequences for other tissues. A toxic response represents a range influenced by the characteristics of the chemical (physical state, site of exposure, dose, and duration of exposure) and of the patient (general health, nutritional state, age, sex, enzyme induction, immune response, antioxidant concentrations). Thus a minor insult to an organ already compromised by disease may cause unexpected injury to that organ and may also affect other organs.

DETERMINANTS OF THE TOXIC RESPONSE

Generally the ability of a toxicant to reach the target organ embodies the same pharmacokinetic principles described for therapeutic agents (see Chapters 4 and 5). These pharmacokinetic principles indicate methods for reducing, reversing, or preventing the toxicity of many substances.

Poison may be absorbed by an organism by dermal, gastrointestinal (GI), or pulmonary routes. Measures to prevent absorption may reduce the concentration of toxicant at the site of the toxic action. Washing the skin, stomach lavage, and oral administration of charcoal are examples for reducing dermal or GI absorption of toxic substances. After absorption, toxic substances are distributed to the tissues through the bloodstream. In some cases it is possible to intercept the toxicant before it is absorbed or reaches its target. This can be accomplished by the following mechanisms:

1. Hemodialysis may be used to remove the toxic compound by filtration
2. Hemoperfusion may be used to remove toxicants from the blood by circulating blood through an activated charcoal filter
3. Binding of a toxicant by a chemical or antibody before it reaches the site of toxicity.

It is generally too late to prevent cell or organ damage after the toxicant reaches the target cell. However, the effects of many toxicants may still be minimized at this stage. Compounds metabolized to reactive intermediates are good examples. An antidote to prevent biotransformation of the toxicant prevents injury produced by the reactive intermediate. Competitive antagonism of methanol by ethanol is based on this principle (see Chapter 31). Similarly, drugs such as cimetidine, which inhibits certain cytochromes P-450, will reduce the biotransformation of other toxicants.

Toxic metabolites produced by biotransformation may injure the cell in which they are produced, or they may be diffused into the bloodstream and affect other areas. For a few toxic substances, this offers a final opportunity to eliminate toxic metabolites by measures (i.e., hemodialysis) that clear the bloodstream.

Another strategy for reducing cellular injury is to prevent the reactive intermediate from interacting with important cell constituents (enzymes, DNA, etc.) Treatment of acetaminophen toxicity with *N*-acetylcysteine is based on this principle (see Chapter 29).

THE IMMUNE SYSTEM

The immune system can be affected by a wide variety of toxicants. These agents often cause immunosuppression by interfering with cell growth or proliferation, resulting in a reduction of capacity. Other compounds may directly destroy immune system components. A further mechanism is the ability of toxicants to inhibit or modify cell division. Finally, some chemicals distort normal signaling mechanisms that ultimately reduce the immune response. For example, benzene causes lymphocytopenia but also affects other bone marrow elements. The functional result is a deficiency in cell-mediated immunity. Workers exposed to benzene show decreased humoral immunity, as evidenced by depressed complement and immunoglobulin concentrations.

In humans, the effect of immunosuppression may be an increased incidence of bacterial, viral, and parasitic infections. For example, polychlorinated biphenyl exposure results in an increased incidence of respiratory infections, whereas lead exposure may produce a bacterial diarrhea in children. Theoretically, immunosuppression may also interfere with the immune system's surveillance function, resulting in an increased incidence of cancer. This consequence of immunosuppression is now being investigated.

It is becoming increasingly apparent that activation and recruitment of phagocytic cells to sites of chemical-induced injury plays a major role in the progression of tissue injury. Therapeutic intervention that could minimize the effects of these activated phagocytic cells includes preventing the adhesion of phagocytic cells at the site of injury, reducing the release of cytotoxic factors from phagocytic cells, or inactivating these bioactive factors.

In addition to being a target for chemical-mediated injury, the immune system may mediate injury by producing hypersensitivity reactions (see Chapters 7, 45). Hypersensitivity reactions are adverse events caused by an immune response to foreign antigens. A type I hypersensitivity reaction (anaphylaxis) is an immediate reaction mediated by IgG bound to mast cells and basophils. Binding of antigen causes release of histamine and other mediators. Acute life-threatening responses to penicillin are an example of anaphylaxis. Type II (cytolytic) reactions involve IgG or IgM produced against a foreign compound. In some cases these immunoglobulins bind to other cells and produce destruction of that cell by stimulation of complement-mediated or other cytotoxic mechanisms. Several drugs, including penicillins, sulfonamides, and quinine can stimulate antibody formation, producing red cell hemolysis using a type II mechanism. Type III (serum-sickness) reactions involve deposition of antibody-antigen complexes in the skin and membranes. Immune reaction to these complexes can cause inflammation of the skin, joints, kidney, and other organs. Serum sickness after antivenin administration is an example of drug toxicity mediated by this mechanism. Finally, type IV (cell-mediated) hypersensitivity is caused by T lymphocytes. T lymphocytes recognize the antigen and then recruit other cells to mount an inflammatory response to the antigen. Contact dermatitis to nickel, several industrial chemicals, and poison ivy is caused by this response.

TERATOGENESIS

The term *teratogen* refers to a drug or other agent that causes abnormal fetal development. Thalidomide is a notorious example of a teratogen. However, teratogens are only one form of toxicity occurring in utero. Any known type of toxic effect caused in adults can occur in the fetus, though there are certain special considerations. An extensive treatment of teratogenesis is discussed in Chapter 63.

CARCINOGENESIS

Cancer cells are cells that escape from the fine-control mechanisms that govern growth, development, and division of normal cells (see Chapter 43). Some cancers in humans are of environmental origin, having been caused by radiation, viral infection, or chemical exposure. In 1775, scrotal cancer was associated with chimney sweeps because they were exposed to soot. Subsequent studies identified the presence of cancer-causing chemicals in the soot.

Because animals develop cancer when exposed to large doses of chemicals over their lifetime, a significant portion of the public believes that synthetic chemicals are a primary cause of cancer. These chemicals could be drugs, pesticides, or industrial chemicals that contaminate the environment. Indeed, some of these chemicals are known to cause cancer in humans after prolonged occupational exposure (vinylchloride, benzene, naphthylamine). However, it is life-style choices that result in the greatest exposure of humans to chemical carcinogens. Cigarette smoke contains many potent cancer-causing chemicals and is a causative factor of lung cancer. Similarly, chronic consumption of large amounts of ethanol is associated with an increased risk of esophageal and liver cancer. Charcoal broiling contaminates meats and fish with polycyclic aromatic hydrocarbons, which are the carcinogens in coal tars and soot. Many "natural" foods are known to contain potent carcinogens. A major percentage of cancers in humans could be prevented or delayed by reducing these "life-style" exposures to carcinogens.

Carcinogenic Process

Many steps are involved in the process by which chemicals cause cancer. Duration, dose, and frequency of exposure are important variables. Because cancer development may take 20 years or more, cause-and-effect relationships between chemical exposure and cancer incidents are difficult to establish.

Induction of cancer by chemicals is divided into three major steps: initiation, promotion, and progression. Initiation is the conversion of a normal cell into a neoplastic cell. Chemicals that cause this conversion are called *initiating agents*. The molecular target for these agents is DNA.

Within the past 20 years, significant advances in knowledge of the mechanisms of chemical carcinogenesis has led to the development of systems to test for the carcinogenic potential of a chemical. Such tests include structural comparison to known carcinogens, in vitro mutagenesis and cell transformation assays, and cancer bioassays in rodents. Some chemicals interact directly with DNA, but many require metabolic transformation to reactive species before covalent interaction with DNA can occur. If cell division occurs before enzymatic repair of the damaged DNA, a permanent mutation is encoded in the genome. Because cellular damage undoubtedly kills some cells in the target tissue, the stimulus for division of adjacent cells is high. The result is a new cell type with altered genotypic and phenotypic properties. However, additional mutational events can convert transformed cells to malignant cells.

In animal studies, some chemicals, referred to as *promoters*, increase the incidence of cancers or decrease the latency period for tumor development without interaction with DNA or production of mutations. These chemicals are effective only when administered repeatedly after an initial insult. For example, a cytosolic receptor in animals that promotes liver carcinogenesis in the presence of 2,3,7,8-tetrachlorodibenzo-*p*-dioxin has been identified. This chemical triggers a pleiotropic response that results in enhanced gene expression. Initiated cells proliferate under the influence of the promoter and undergo clonal expansion into phenotypically altered foci, nodules, or papillomas. Endogenous substances such as growth factors and hormones may also act as promoters. For example, follicle-stimulating hormone and leuteinizing hormone may promote chemical-induced ovarian cancers because of their trophic effect on the ovary. Carcinogens (i.e., initiating agents) also promote tumor development. They create the environment for selected proliferation of initiated cells or produce other cellular changes that provide a selective advantage for autonomous division and growth.

During tumor promotion, most foci and nodules regress. They do not become selective for the advantageous properties that distinguish between benign and malignant cells. The growth and division of malignant cells are not related to the growth and division of other cells within a tissue. An important property of malignant cells is metastasis (discussed in Chapter 43), but the sequence of events leading to the metastatic stage of carcinogenesis is largely unknown.

TOXIC GASES

The two most dangerous toxic gases are carbon monoxide (CO) and volatile cyanides. Both compounds are toxic because they deprive the cell of energy. Other gases, such as ozone, nitrogen oxides (NO, NO_2), and phosgene, are toxic because of their chemical reactivity. They are irritating to mucous membranes and may trigger asthmatic-like symptoms in susceptible individuals.

Carbon Monoxide

CO is the leading cause of death by poisoning. It also inflicts sublethal injuries, including myocardial infarction and cerebral atrophy.

The primary effects of CO are displacement of oxygen from hemoglobin and impairment of oxygen release from hemoglobin. CO displaces oxygen from hemoglobin because it has a >200 times higher affinity for hemoglobin than does oxygen. Even at a concentration in air of only 0.5%, CO displaces oxygen to produce 50% carboxyhemoglobin. However, CO produces more injury than simply replacing oxygen. Normally, hemoglobin binding of oxygen shows cooperativity: binding of one oxygen molecule promotes binding of subsequent oxygen molecules to a hemoglobin molecule. Similarly, hemoglobin shows cooperativity in releasing oxygen. However, carboxyhemoglobin does not release oxygen normally. CO shifts the oxyhemoglobin dissociation curve to the left and reduces oxygen release to the cell. The result of oxygen displacement and decreased release of oxygen from hemoglobin is anaerobic metabolism and cell death if not reversed.

The symptoms of CO poisoning are a reflection of oxygen deprivation to each organ. Early symptoms of nervous system dysfunction resemble the flu, including nausea, headache, malaise, lightheadedness, and dizziness. Later signs and symptoms are more ominous: depressed sensorium, loss of consciousness, seizures, and death. The histopathology of nervous system injury includes necrosis of the globus pallidus, substantia nigra, hippocampus, cerebral cortex and cerebellum, typical of all anoxic injuries.

The heart is particularly susceptible to CO poisoning. The heart has high oxygen requirements and, because it normally extracts more oxygen from the blood than other organs, compensates poorly for decreased oxygen delivery. When CO decreases oxygen delivery, severe myocardial ischemia may develop. Symptoms are similar to those of other types of myocardial ischemia, though the usual cardiac risk factors may be absent. Histopathological analysis shows patchy myocardial necrosis rather than regional necrosis found in typical myocardial infarctions.

As CO dissociates from the hemoglobin, it is expired. However, because of its high affinity for hemoglobin, this is a slow process. The half-life of carboxyhemoglobin without treatment is 3 to 4 hours, depending on the patient's ventilation. Administration of 100% oxygen by face mask shortens the time to 90 minutes. Hyperbaric oxygen reduces the half-life to 20 minutes. The patient's outcome depends on the duration and the severity of hypoxic episode.

Cyanide

The common route of exposure to cyanide is through inhalation of smoke produced by burning of plastics. Certain paints may be an additional source. Other sources are ingestion of fruit seeds (e.g., apricots and cherries) containing toxic amounts of soluble cyanide. These seeds must be crushed and then metabolized by intestinal bacteria to release the cyanide. Salts of cyanide have been used in suicide or homicide poisoning attempts.

Cyanide produces toxicity by avidly binding to ferric iron (Fe^{3+}) to prevent reduction to the ferrous (Fe^{2+}) form involved in the cytochrome oxidase electron-transport system. The transfer of electrons from cytochromes to molecular oxygen is prevented, inhibiting adenosine triphosphate (ATP) production and forcing the cell to produce energy by anaerobic metabolism. As in all cases of hypoxia, anaerobic glycolysis produces only small amounts of ATP and large quantities of lactic acid.

Thus victims of cyanide poisoning show symptoms and signs of hypoxia. Similar to CO toxicity, cyanide toxicity first affects organs that have a large oxygen use.

However, the onset of these symptoms, which depends on the route of exposure, is often faster. Inhalation may produce rapid demise, whereas ingestion delays symptoms for 30 minutes or more. CNS dysfunction causes loss of consciousness and respiratory arrest. Laboratory findings are typical of cellular hypoxia and include severe anion gap acidosis produced by lactic acid.

Treatment is based on preventing cyanide from reaching its target, cytochrome oxidase. Because cyanide has high affinity for ferric iron, ferric iron can be provided in the form of oxidized hemoglobin. This is accomplished by the administration of sodium nitrite, which converts hemoglobin to methemoglobin, the ferric form. The latter effectively competes for the cyanide with cytochrome *c* by mass action, forming cyanmethemoglobin. Cyanide is removed from the body after metabolism to thiocyanate by rhodanase and is ultimately excreted in the urine. Sodium thiosulfate is administered to facilitate thiocyanate formation. An alternative is administration of hydroxocobalamin, which reacts with cyanide to produce cyanocobalamin. Because hydroxocobalamin and cyanocobalamin have little toxicity, this is a promising treatment of cyanide poisoning.

HEAVY METALS

The widespread occurrence of metals in the environment and their numerous industrial and medical uses make them important potential toxicants.

The rate of absorption of heavy metals is dependent on their physical state. Metals may exist in their elemental state or bind to inorganic or organic ligands. The elemental and inorganic forms of metals may be well absorbed as a result of physical similarity to nutritionally essential metals. For example, lead is well absorbed by the normal transport protein for iron located in the GI mucosa. Organs containing these transport systems are predisposed to injury from these metals. Commonly injured organs include liver, kidney, and GI mucosa. Organic forms of metals are more lipid soluble than inorganic forms and may be well absorbed without specific transport systems.

Physical state also affects distribution of metals. Lipid soluble forms achieve higher concentrations in areas of high lipid content such as the CNS. For example, inorganic and elemental forms of mercury primarily injure the kidney, whereas organic forms such as methylmercury injure the brain.

The body has developed specific defense mechanisms against certain metals. The kidney has a binding protein for cadmium called *metallothionein.* The strong cadmium binding of this protein concentrates cadmium in the kidney and reduces its excretion. The binding prevents toxicity until the protein is saturated, at which time subsequent cadmium accumulation causes injury. The mechanism of heavy metal toxicity is poorly understood. Many metals function as essential cofactors of enzymes. Substitution by a similar but toxic metal may produce enzymatic dysfunction. Metals are generally very reactive and may bind to key sulfhydryl groups in active centers of enzymes, again producing dysfunction in many organ systems. Besides direct metal toxicity, metals produce hypersensitivity reactions. Nickel, chromium, gold, and others cause cell-mediated (type IV) hypersensitivity reactions (see Table 62-1 for summary).

Table 62-1 Mechanisms of Heavy Metal Toxicity

Metal	Mechanism	Target Organs
Arsenic	Reacts with sulfhydryl groups; interferes with oxidative phosphorylation	Peripheral neurons GI tract Liver Cardiovascular system
Lead	Reacts with sulfhydryl groups; interferes with heme synthesis; direct toxic effect to CNS	Hematopoietic system Central and peripheral nervous system Kidney
Mercury	Reacts with sulfhydryl groups; some forms have direct cytotoxic effect	Central and peripheral nervous system Kidney GI tract Respiratory system

Metal Chelation

Treatment for metal toxicity focuses on increasing excretion of the metal from the body. The term *chelator* drug stems from the Greek word *chēlē,* meaning 'claw.' These drugs bind the metal between two or more functional groups to form a metal-drug complex that is excreted in urine. Certain chelators work best for certain metals. The uses of chelators are summarized in Table 62-2.

Lead

Lead is one of the oldest known poisons; its toxicity was described in Roman times. Lead continues to pose a significant health problem. Industrialization, mining, and leaded gasoline dramatically increased the amount of lead in the environment and consequently in humans. (The switch to unleaded gasoline has resulted in decreases in environmental lead contamination.) Lead is also present in some ceramic glazes and paints. In older homes, paint containing lead flakes off or is present in dust and may be ingested or inhaled by children, producing chronic lead toxicity. Adults are exposed to toxic

Table 62-2 Metals Chelated by Therapeutic Agents

Chelator	Metal
dimercaptosuccinic acid (DMSA)	Lead, arsenic, mercury
deferoxamine	Iron
EDTA (ethylenediaminetetraacetic acid)	Lead
penicillamine	Copper, lead
British anti-Lewisite (BAL)	Lead, arsenic, mercury

concentrations in certain work environments.

Lead binds to sulfhydryl and other active sites in many enzyme systems, leading to enzyme inactivation. Although its effects are diffuse, certain manifestations predominate. Heme synthesis is sensitive to lead poisoning, with two enzymes in the heme biosynthetic pathway inhibited by lead, producing anemia.

Lead is particularly toxic to the nervous system, producing deleterious effects especially in children. In adults, lead exposure produces a peripheral neuropathy. Early signs and symptoms in children include anorexia, colicky abdominal pain, lethargy, and vomiting. If lead exposure continues, children are more likely than adults to develop encephalopathy manifested by irritability progressing to seizures and coma, with approximately 30% having permanent neurological sequelae.

Low-concentration lead exposure may pose special risks for children. Subtle neurological injury from low lead exposure, detected by depressed IQ scores and learning disorders, is reported. Lead may accumulate in the immature nervous system because it may cross the blood-brain barrier more easily in children, and the CNS may be less capable of removing lead than in adults. Individuals, and particularly children, with blood lead concentrations >10μg/dl are considered to be at risk.

Adults exposed to lead generally develop vague complaints of headache and light-headedness. With increased exposure, a peripheral neuropathy is manifest.

In the patient with lead-poisoning signs and symptoms, the whole-blood lead concentration is the best indicator of exposure. As concentrations rise, the danger of encephalopathy increases, though overt signs and symptoms do not usually occur until lead concentrations approach 50 μg/dl.

Lead is slowly excreted from the body. The primary treatment of lead poisoning is removal from the source. Excretion may be hastened by the use of chelators such as British anti-Lewisite.

OTHER TOXICANTS

Toxicities resulting from organophosphates or to drugs of abuse are discussed in Chapters 9 and 32, respectively.

CLINICAL MANAGEMENT OF TOXIC PATIENTS

The clinical diagnosis and management of patients subject to chemical toxicity is an extensive subject that is beyond the scope of this book. However, some overview guidelines are presented here to summarize the variety of signs and symptoms (Table 62-3), to point out the contraindications and problems associated with emesis and gastric lavage (see box below), and to provide a list of antidotes for common types of chemical toxicants (Table 62-4).

CONTRAINDICATIONS AND COMPLICATIONS OF EMESIS AND LAVAGE

CONTRAINDICATIONS	COMPLICATIONS
EMESIS	**EMESIS**
Altered mental status	Aspiration
Age less than 6 months	Prolonged vomiting
Inability to protect airway	Esophageal tearing
Ingestion of agents causing rapid deterioration of mental status	
Convulsants	
Tricyclic antidepressants	
Camphor	
Ingestion of	
Acid	
Alkali	
Hydrocarbons	
Sharp objects	
Pregnancy	
LAVAGE	**LAVAGE**
Strong acid or alkali ingestion	Aspiration
Petroleum-product ingestion	Esophageal perforation
Unconscious patients without endotracheal intubation	Intratracheal insertion

Table 62-3 Physical Findings with Exposure to Toxic Agents

Agent	Signs of Toxicity
Narcotic	Miotic pupils, CNS and respiratory depression, hypotension, may have needle-track marks
Anticholinergic	Dry, flushed appearance; mydriasis; decreased bowel motility; tachycardia; hallucinations
Cholinergic	Muscarinic—salivation, lacrimation, urination, defecation Nicotinic-muscle fasciculations, weakness, paralysis
Stimulants (cocaine, amphetamines)	Tachycardia, hypertension, hyperthermia, mydriasis, agitation, psychosis
Tricyclic antidepressants	Anticholinergic findings and electrocardiogram abnormalities (QRS widening, QT prolongation)

Table 62-4 Common Antidotes

Toxicant	Antidote	Mechanism
venoms—snake, black widow	antivenin	Immunological binding to toxicant
cholinesterase inhibitors	atropine	Blocks muscarinic receptors
cyanide	cyanide kit (Na nitrite, Na thiosulfate)	Induction of methemoglobinemia; cyanide binds preferentially to methemoglobin
digoxin	digoxin antibodies	Immunological binding to toxicant
metals	chelators	Binding of metal with subsequent urinary excretion
methanol, ethylene glycol	ethanol	Competition for alcohol dehydrogenase (enzyme-producing reactive metabolites)
acetaminophen	*N*-acetylcysteine	Provides sulfhydryl groups to detoxify reactive metabolite
opiates	naloxone	Blockade of opiate receptors
carbon monoxide	oxygen	Oxygen in high concentration displaces CO molecules from carboxyhemoglobin
isoniazid	pyridoxine HCl	Competitively reverses isoniazid effect by providing substitute for pyridoxine kinase enzyme inhibited by isoniazid
benzodiazepines	flumazenil	Blockade of benzodiazepine receptor

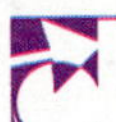

NEW DIRECTIONS

Toxicology has progressed rapidly from a descriptive discipline to a mechanistic science. Understanding of mechanisms allows physicians and paramedical personnel effectively to prevent and treat injury in individual patients. For example, elucidation of mechanistic and receptor-mediated chemical toxicity has allowed development of specific antidotes. Flumazenil, a potent benzodiazepine antagonist is approved for human use (see Chapter 25). New antidotes for toxic alcohols, cyanide, venoms, and tricyclic antidepressants are on the horizon.

Prevention will become an important part of toxicology. Using molecular biology techniques, it is becoming possible to identify individuals at risk from a given toxic substance. Individuals will soon be able to select their employment environment with the knowledge that they may be more susceptible to certain chemicals. However, the ability to predict toxicity will raise important ethical and moral dilemmas. Many individuals are presently willing to work with dangerous chemicals despite a known predisposition to chemical-induced injury. Will these persons be allowed to work under conditions known to hold a higher risk for them?

In the real world, most exposures involve multiple chemicals. Hazardous waste sites, for example, may involve pesticides, heavy metals, and a variety of industrial byproducts. Currently an area of intense research is to produce information needed to predict the toxicologic profile of such mixtures.

The increasing sensitivity of analytic methodologies will create further dilemmas. Chemicals once believed safe are increasingly being found to cause toxicity at levels already present in the environment. For example, many children are exposed to concentrations of lead predicted earlier to be safe but now known to cause injury. The near future will find governments attempting to cope with enormous costs in order to make older housing safe and to treat these children with toxic lead levels. As research progresses, other chemicals may present similar problems.

REFERENCES

Amdur MO, Doull J, Klassen CD, et al, editors: *Casarett and Doull's Toxicology: The Basic Science of Poisons,* ed 4, New York, 1991, Pergamon Press.

Goldfrank LR, editor: *Goldfrank's toxicologic emergencies,* ed 2, East Norwalk, 1982, Appleton-Century-Crofts.

Roitt I, Brostoff J, Hale D: *Immunology,* ed 2, New York, 1989, Gower Medical Publishing.

Sax NI, Lewis RJ: *Dangerous properties of industrial materials,* ed 7, New York, 1989, Van Nostrand Reinhold.

Sullivan JB, Krieger GR, editors: *Hazardous materials toxicology,* Baltimore, 1992, Williams & Wilkins.

SELF-ASSESSMENT QUESTIONS

1. Certain types of chemicals cause characteristic effects in victims poisoned with that substance. Pick the one correct answer.
   a. Narcotic syndrome consists of dry, flushed appearance with mydriatic pupils, tachycardia, and hallucinations.
   b. The anticholinergic syndrome includes miotic pupils, respiratory depression, hypotension, depression of mental activities.
   c. The cholinergic syndrome includes salivation, lacrimation, urination, and diarrhea as well as muscle weakness and fasciculation.
   d. Stimulants cause the skin to be dry and flushed and is accompanied by tachycardia, hallucinations, and mydriatic pupils.
2. Select the correct statement regarding the site of injury produced by pulmonary toxicants.
   a. Toxic substances in the form of small particulates (less than 5 micrometers) may penetrate and be deposited in the alveoli.
   b. Water-soluble chemicals are primarily absorbed in the alveoli.
   c. The route of exposure of all pulmonary toxicants is through respiration.
   d. Toxic substances in the form of large particulates (greater than 15 micrometers) are primarily deposited in the large bronchioles.

3. The kidney is a common target of toxic injury. Select the correct statement concerning renal injury by toxic substances.
   a. The most sensitive part of the kidney to toxic agents is the collecting tubule.
   b. Aminoglycoside antibiotics cause injury to the proximal tubule, which in most cases is reversible.
   c. Analgesics such as aspirin cause tubular injury.
   d. Papillary necrosis is characteristic of heavy-metal injury.
4. Lead poisoning has been a health hazard for over 2000 years. Select the correct statement concerning lead toxicity in the United States today.
   a. Low-level lead exposure has been shown to be safe for adults and children.
   b. In adults, a typical patient with lead poisoning will complain of abdominal pain, headache, and vomiting.
   c. The blood lead concentration is useful in the assessment of lead poisoning.
   d. Lead is an endogenous trace metal with important biological functions.

CHAPTER 63 Perinatal/Neonatal Pharmacology

ROBERT M. WARD
BERNARD L. MIRKIN

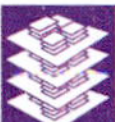

THERAPEUTIC OVERVIEW

Limited understanding of the clinical pharmacology of specific drugs in pediatric patients particularly infants, predisposes this population to problems in the course of drug treatment in younger subjects such as newborn infants. The absence of FDA requirements for pediatric studies and therefore reliance on pharmacological data derived primarily from adults to determine appropriate efficacy and dosage guidelines for therapeutic use of drugs in children is risky. The problem of establishing efficacy and dosing guidelines for use in infants is further complicated, since the pharmacokinetics of many drugs change appreciably as the subject ages from birth (sometimes prematurely) to several months after birth—the dose-response relationships of some drugs may change markedly during the first few weeks after birth.

Both pharmacokinetics and organ responsiveness change dramatically during development from the embryonic and fetal periods to adulthood. Prematurely born neonates are now surviving at gestations as short as 24 weeks in contrast to 40 weeks for a full-term gestation. This is a stage of fetal development when both structure and function are quite immature. Although these topics are mentioned briefly in Chapter 7, the dynamic changes in drug disposition and organ responsiveness during development, from fetus to adulthood, constitute the primary topic for this chapter.

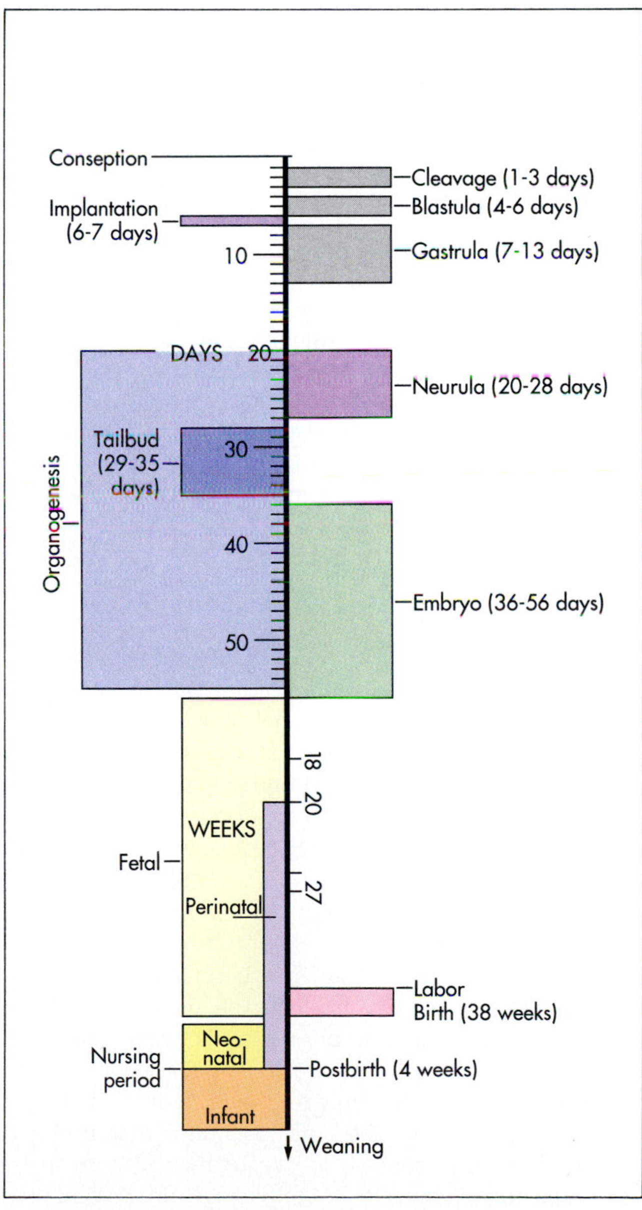

FIGURE 63-1 Sequence of normal human development timed from conception.

MATERNAL-PLACENTAL-FETAL UNIT

Maternal Pharmacokinetic Variables

Maternal physiological changes occur during pregnancy that result in differences in maternal pharmacokinetics of drugs administered during pregnancy com pared to the nonpregnant state. These modified pharmacokinetic variables ultimately determine fetal therapeutic and toxic responses to drugs, drug metabolites, or toxic compounds in the maternal circulation that are capable of crossing the placenta.

Maternal drug absorption may be enhanced or decreased from the combination of delayed gastric emptying and decreased motility. Absorption from sites other than the gastrointestinal (GI) tract also may be affected. For example, increased pulmonary absorption may result from greater minute ventilation and increased cutaneous absorption as a result of greater surface area and blood flow.

The apparent volume of distribution of many drugs increases predictably during pregnancy as maternal plasma volume expands 30 to 50% during the first trimester. Some of these are indicated in Table 63-1. Concomitant changes occur in cardiac output and glomerular filtration rates, which also increase approximately 30 to 50% during this period. The expanded apparent volume of distribution, together with an increase in renal clearance leads to lower maternal circulating concentrations of drugs, unless maternal dosage is increased. Hepatic blood flow remains constant, and so the percentage of total cardiac output distributed to the liver tends to decrease. This may diminish the metabolism of drugs that undergo "first-pass" hepatic clearance and result in unanticipated elevations in plasma drug concentrations. Cholestasis frequently develops during pregnancy and may result in decreased hepatic clearance of drugs that undergo biliary excretion.

Table 63-1 Change in Apparent Volume of Distribution of Some Drugs During Pregnancy*

Agent	Gestation (weeks)			
	10	20	30	40
ampicillin	36	45	57	68
caffeine	2	8	16	32
furosemide	1	9	20	29
meperidine	32	27	21	16

*Values represent % increase from prepregnancy values.

The Placenta

The functions of the placenta during gestation are protection of the conceptus, maintenance of pregnancy, possible prevention of maternal rejection of the pregnancy as foreign tissue, transportation of nutrients and wastes, metabolism of endogenous and xenobiotic substances, and endocrine activity. *However, any drug or environmental agent that gains access to the maternal bloodstream should be considered capable of crossing the placenta and reaching the fetus unless demonstrated otherwise.*

The chorioallantoic placenta begins to form at implantation. It gradually invades the maternal endometrial glands, stroma, and arterial walls to gain access to the maternal blood supply in a villous structure that maximizes the surface area for maternal-fetal exchange. The structure allows the high-resistance maternal arterial system to become a low-resistance system in the spiral arteries. Maternal and fetal blood circulate in proximity by the third week of gestation. Until 12 weeks of gestation, there are four tissue layers separating the maternal and fetal circulations: syncytiotrophoblast (the outer layer of the trophoblast), cytotrophoblast, villous connective tissue cores, and fetal capillary endothelium. By the third trimester, the cytotrophoblast is discontinuous, and only three layers separate the circulations.

At term, blood enters the spaces between the villi from over 100 spiral arteries; over 150 ml of blood may be contained in these spaces at a given time. The rate of blood flow increases during gestation from 50 ml/min at 10 weeks to 600 ml/min at term. Thus at term, the circulation replaces the blood volume in this space three to four times each minute.

During development, placental vessel architecture changes to facilitate the transfer of diverse substrates. The diffusion distance for these substrates between maternal and fetal circulations decreases from 50-100μm at the second month to 4-5 μm at term. This affects drug diffusion across the placenta. For example, when gentamicin is infused continuously to the mother, the maternal to fetal transfer of this aminoglycoside antibiotic appears to increase from the first half of gestation to term.

Placental Processes

The basic process by which substances cross the placenta and gain access to the fetus are similar to those that occur in adults. The Fick equation describes the transfer of substances only by simple diffusion as follows:

$$\text{rate of diffusion} = D \times \Delta c \times A/d$$

where D is the diffusion constant of the drug, Δc is the drug concentration across the placenta (maternal plasma drug concentration-fetal plasma drug concentration), A is the area across which transfer occurs, and d is the membrane thickness. For the transfer of many substances, the placenta can be viewed as a lipid membrane.

In general, lipophilic, unionized, low molecular weight drugs in their free non–protein bound state tend to cross the placenta. Some of these agents, such as bar-

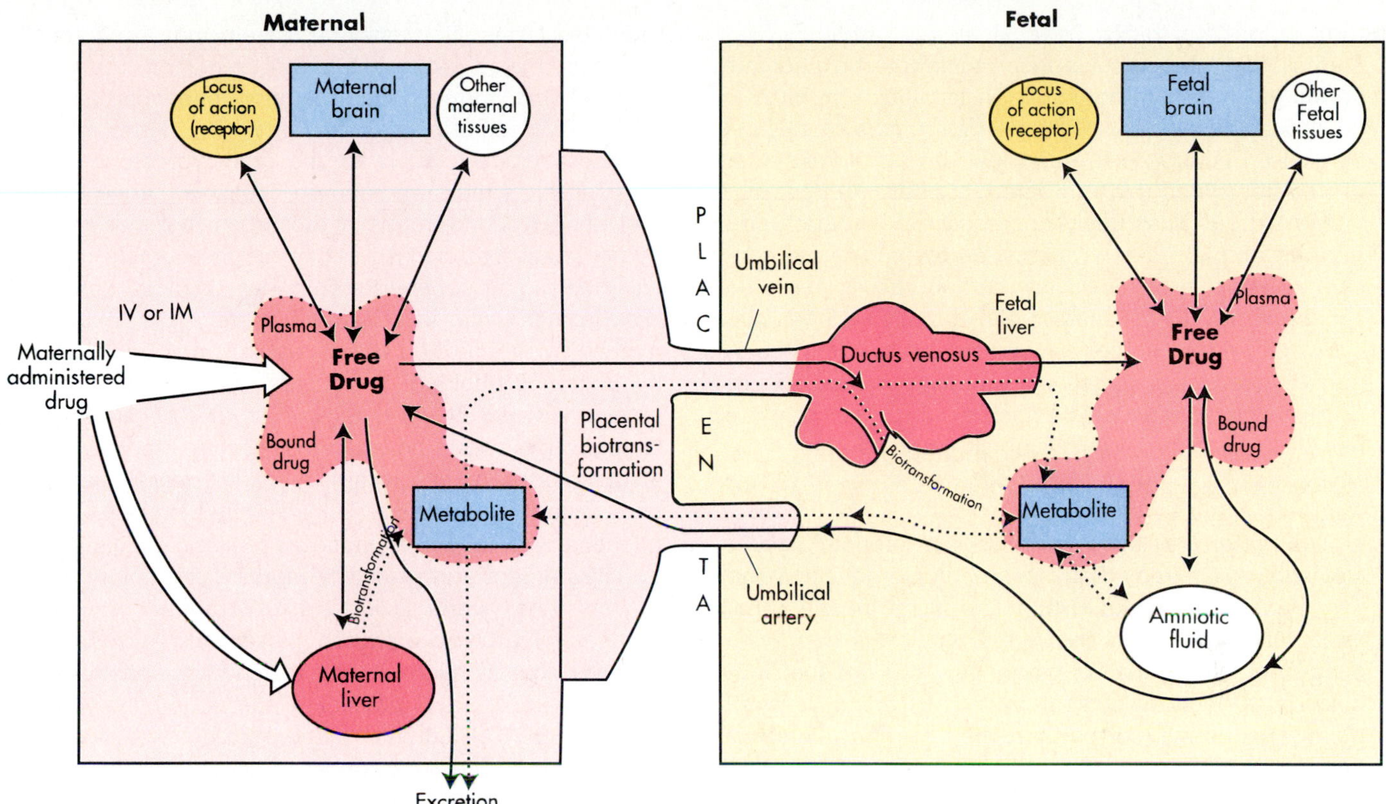

FIGURE 63-2 Schema of drug disposition in the maternal-placental-fetal unit. (Redrawn from Mirkin BL: Drug distribution in pregnancy. In Boreus L, editor: *Fetal pharmacology,* New York, 1973, Raven Press.)

biturates, narcotic analgesics, and local anesthetics, are "flow limited" in their placental transfer because a decrease in maternal blood flow to the placenta may reduce the placental passage of these agents. Normal uterine contractions during labor, oxytocic drugs, exogenously administered sympathomimetics, or β-adrenergic receptor blocking agents all affect maternal and fetal hemodynamics and therefore may modify maternal drug distribution and placental transfer. For a specific drug, maternal-fetal transfer may change during gestation.

The human placenta contains multiple enzyme systems, including those responsible for drug oxidation, reduction, hydrolysis, and conjugation. These systems are primarily involved with endogenous steroid metabolism; however, the activities of these enzymes are usually minor compared with those of maternal or fetal organs (including liver, kidney, and adrenal gland). Thus the presence of xenobiotic metabolizing systems in the placenta does not contribute greatly to overall drug clearance from the maternal-placental-fetal unit. Some of these relationships are shown in Figure 63-2. The transfer of many substances across the placenta requires energy or special carriers.

Fetal Development

Initial human development may be divided into three periods: preimplantation, embryonic, and fetal (Figure 63-1). During the preimplantation period, rapid cell division occurs, followed by embryonic differentiation and organogenesis. Because organ development includes structural formation and functional maturation, such development may continue through the perinatal period into infancy or later. For example, the lung does not mature fully until well after the end of gestation. The human brain is immature at birth and myelination of the brain and maturation of its function continues for many years. Thus the period of organogenesis bridges the late embryonic and early fetal periods and may extend into the first several years of life.

Pregnancies are timed clinically from the first day of the last menstrual period which is about 2 weeks prior to fertilization of the ovum. Full term gestation by menstrual dates averages 40 weeks compared to 38 weeks after conception. Perinatal refers to the period from the onset of labor through the first 4 weeks after birth. For comparison of neonatal mortality internationally, term gestation is defined as 38 to 42 weeks and neonatal mortality is a death occurring during the first 4 weeks after term or preterm birth. For evaluation of pharmacodynamics and pharmacokinetics, however, the neonatal period will apply to the first 4 weeks after term birth or gestational week 40 to 44 for premature neonates. Newborn also designates the first few days or weeks after birth, after which the term infant applies.

Most drugs pass freely to the postimplantation embryo. In animal model systems, embryonic tissue concentrations are generally lower than those measured concomitantly in the mother. Substances such as salicylic acid, diethylstilbestrol, and the herbicide (2,4,5-T) may be present in increasing amounts in fetal tissues as gestation advances. Even some substances that are not well-transferred to the embryo (such as phenothiazines) may be found in higher concentrations in the fetus than in the embryo.

The patterns of drug distribution in prenatal tissues also shows ontogeny. Early in embryonic development, exogenous substances accumulate in the neuroepithelium. The blood-brain barrier to diffusion is not developed until the last half of pregnancy, and the susceptibility of the central nervous system (CNS) to developmental toxins may be partly related to the preferential distribution.

Fetal Drug Disposition

Virtually every drug or its metabolite reaches the fetus through passage from the maternal compartment. The presence or absence of an effect on the fetus is dependent on the amount of drug to which the fetus is exposed and the potential for response by the fetus. The placenta is much more complex than a passive lipid bilayer. It possesses several enzyme systems, which promote the biotransformation of endogenous substrates such as glucocorticoids and other hormones. In contrast, most drugs or xenobiotics pass the placenta with minimal or no metabolic alteration (Figure 63-2).

The biotransforming enzyme systems of the fetus are first detectable at 5 to 8 weeks of gestation, and their activity increases until 12 to 14 weeks, when it reaches up to 30% of adult activity. It is not until approximately 1 year after birth that liver enzymatic activity is comparable to that of the adult. The first system expressed is the cytochrome P-450 (or microsomal mixed-function oxidase) group of enzymes. These enzymes are detectable when the smooth endoplasmic reticulum develops (40 to 60 days in human gestation). It is most active in the fetal adrenal gland and less active in the fetal liver. The fetal kidney and gut systems also have detectable activity.

The monooxygenases are composed of a number of inducible forms. This enzyme system may be divided into two major groups that are based on the substances that induce their activity, phenobarbital or polycyclic aromatic hydrocarbons. The latter group includes enzymes such as the aryl hydrocarbon hydroxylases, which metabolize benzo(*a*)pyrene, and other polycyclic aromatic hydrocarbon molecules. Aryl hydrocarbon hydroxylase activity is measurable in the blastocyst. The concentration of aryl hydrocarbon hydroxylase activity in the fetus is very low, approximately 2% to 4% of adult activity, but may be induced by maternal smoking. It appears that fetal induction of this enzyme shows ontogeny, in that a given level of maturity must be achieved before the system is inducible. There also appear to be genetic factors that govern inducibility of these hydroxylases. The phenobarbital-inducible monooxygenases appear early in development and gradually increase in activity until midgestation, when 20% to 40% of adult activity is attained. Hydrolytic enzymes, particularly epoxide hydrolases that convert stable or reactive epoxides to dihydrodiols, are also present in the fetus by 5 weeks of gestation. The activity of the epoxide hydrolases is inducible and does not appear to show interindividual variability on a genetic basis, in contrast to the mixed-function oxidases.

Alcohol dehydrogenase is expressed during the first 6 weeks of gestation. It is not certain when the reducing enzymes for subsequent detoxification of the aldehyde products are active in the fetus.

Human fetuses generally have well-developed conjugating enzyme activities, except for glucuronidation, which remains low until shortly before term. The early presence of the other conjugating systems in the human fetus may indicate a role in the modulation of activity of endogenous steroids. For endogenous compounds, conjugation may enhance activity. For example, certain steroid glucuronides and sulfates have greater potencies than the parent compound.

Considering the limited protection afforded by the placenta, the ability of the fetus to metabolize xenobiotics may appear fortuitous. However, it can sometimes be detrimental. Fetal metabolism can result in the generation of reactive intermediates that lead to fetotoxicity, indicating that the fetus and its genetic make-up may be major factors contributing to developmental toxicity. A further effect of induction of metabolism in utero is that postnatal xenobiotic metabolism may be changed after prenatal exposures. Such exposures may enhance metabolism of the same or unrelated agents; for example, the ability of the newborn infant to metabolize bilirubin by conjugation may be induced by prenatal maternal phenobarbital therapy.

TERATOLOGY

Teratology is the study of birth defects, deviations from normal development resulting from prenatal or perinatal influences. Birth defects, comprising not only congenital malformations, but also prenatal infections, chromosomal abnormalities, and genetic diseases, are the leading cause of infant mortality. Chronic illness as a result of congenital anomalies account for one half of all patient-hospital days (for patients of all ages). The medical costs of the care of children with birth defects are in excess of $13 billion annually in the United States. Currently, the overwhelming majority of birth defects are not preventable. Only a small fraction of birth defects are known to occur as a result of avoidable causes. Some toxic developmental influences include: uncontrolled maternal diseases (e.g., diabetes mellitus and phenylketonuria); infections (including rubella); and, to a lesser extent, environmental exposures (drugs, chemicals, radiation).

To be considered a teratogen, an agent must have little effect on the mother, since the presence of maternal toxicity precludes ascribing effects on the conceptus directly to the agent. The substance must cause transient or permanent, physical, or functional disorders in the fetus in the absence of toxic effects in the mother.

Not all adverse effects on prenatal development are malforming. Some agents result in death of the developing organism, whereas others produce only mild growth retardation. Death and growth retardation are not considered as teratogenic events per se. The term *developmental toxicity* is proposed as a broader categorization of outcomes. Developmental toxicity comprises four possible manifestations of abnormal development: altered growth (growth retardation), death, malformations (teras, singular; terata, plural), and functional deficits or impairments.

The concept of a behavioral teratogen is described as an agent that disrupts normal behavioral development after prenatal exposure. Because some agents clearly produce mental but not physical disturbances, it is a useful subdivision of the concept of teratogens.

Mutagens are substances that cause permanent change in germ cell lines secondary to changes in deoxyribonucleic acid (DNA). All mutagens are teratogens, but not all teratogens are mutagens.

By examining known teratogens and the factors common to their production of malformations, seven general factors on the development of teratogenesis can be described (see box on p. 848).

Vitamin A and its congeners are examples of how these principles can be applied to specific agents, as well as their shortcomings in characterizing all teratogens. Vitamin A is recognized as a teratogen in animals since 1953. Dietary vitamin A as carotene (β-carotene) is not associated with developmental toxicity in animals or humans. However, high-potency vitamin A prepared as retinol or retinyl esters is implicated as an animal teratogen. At dosages of 15 to 75 mg/kg/day and higher, it produces cranial, brain, cardiovascular, limb, or genitourinary malformations, or all five types. Human malformations are associated with daily doses of 25,000 international units of vitamin A or more, but no epidemiological studies are available to quantify the risk to humans. Isotretinoin, an agent used for the treatment of cystic acne, is an isomer of retinoic acid that may produce craniofacial, cardiac, thymic, and CNS abnormalities in humans. Etretinate, a vitamin A congener used in the treatment of psoriasis, is also a documented animal teratogen with similar potential in humans.

Direct teratogenic effects depend on the achievement of drug or active metabolite concentrations in the conceptus at a critical time period, especially during gestation weeks 3 to 12 (Figure 63-3). Thus the changes in maternal pharmacokinetic parameters and dosing requirements during pregnancy may be expected to influence the risk of malformations.

By recognizing and compensating for controllable variables, the dose-response relationships for individual anomalies or toxic effects may become clear. Because few agents appear to demonstrate a minimum teratogenic concentration for production of defects, it is a difficult task to determine the concentration at which a specific drug is safe in humans.

It should also be noted that animal models are frequently used to assess the teratogenic potential of drugs and chemicals and drug induced animal malformations sometimes do not correlate with malformations in humans.

Fetal Drug Therapy

Fetal responses to some drugs have been exploited to provide pharmacological therapy to the fetus. Potent glucocorticoid stereoisomers, betamethasone, and dexamethasone, have been intentionally administered to the mother to induce fetal enzymes needed for production and release of surfactant to prevent hyaline membrane disease after birth. Certain types of fetal arrhythmias and heart failure have been treated with drugs such as digoxin and procainamide which reached the fetus across the placenta after administration to the mother or by direct fetal injection intramuscularly or intravenously. Certain adrenal enzyme defects may cause the fetus to overproduce androgens that alter the de-

FACTORS IN DEVELOPMENT OF TERATOGENESIS

The conceptus passes through an orderly succession of developmental stages. Each stage represents a different susceptibility to teratogens (see below).

Pharmacokinetic characteristics of absorption, disposition, biotransformation, and elimination influence the ultimate amount of teratogen to reach the embryo/fetus.

The higher the dose, the more likely an adverse effect will be seen and the more severe it is likely to be. There may be a threshold dose below which defects are absent and above which defects are demonstrable.

Teratogenesis depends on the genotype of the conceptus and the manner in which it reacts with environmental factors.

The same defect may be produced by agents acting by different mechanisms. On the other hand, one agent may produce different developmental toxicities by the same initiating mechanism.

Certain agents produce developmental toxicity; other substances are associated with developmental toxicity only at doses high enough to cause signs and symptoms of toxicity in the mother.

The type of response is determined by the individual characteristics of the exposure, particularly dosage and timing, and the organism's susceptibility to it.

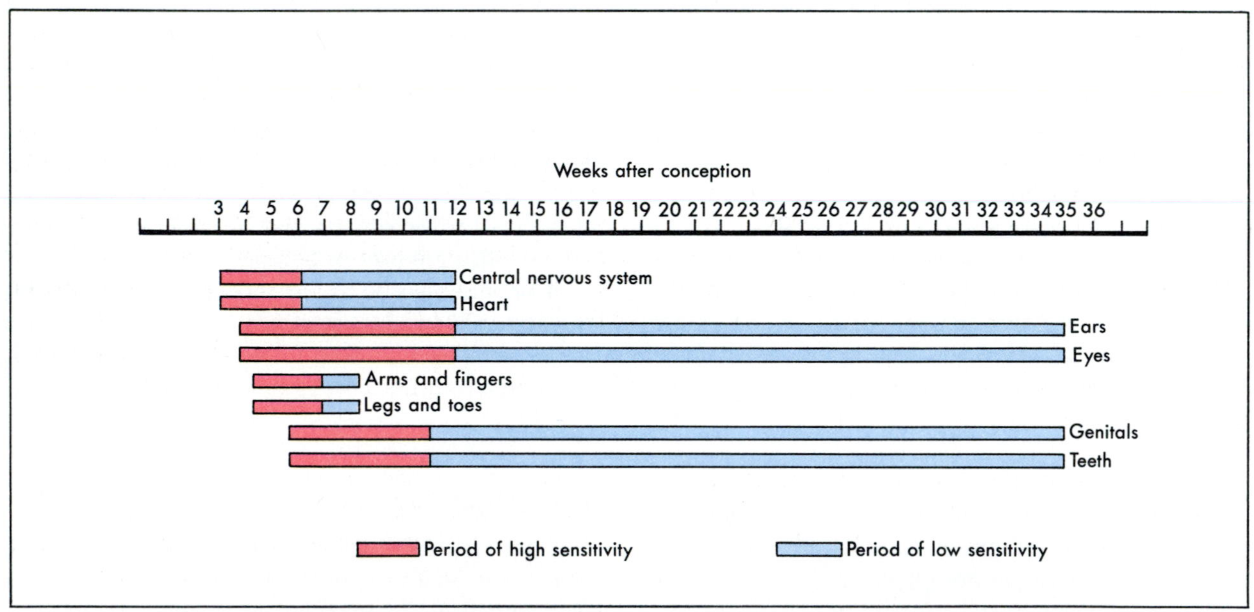

FIGURE 63-3 Most susceptible times for teratogenic actions to occur. (Adapted from Hays DP, Pagliaro LA: Human teratogens. In Pagliaro LA, Pagliaro AM, editors: *Problems in pediatric drug therapy,* Hamilton, Ill, 1987, Drug Intelligence Publications.)

DISEASE STATES THAT MAY AFFECT DRUG ABSORPTION IN THE FIRST YEAR OF LIFE

- Gastric acid secretion
  - Proximal small bowel resection
- Delayed gastric emptying and modified drug absorption
  - Pyloric stenosis
  - Congestive heart failure
  - Protein calorie malnutrition
- Intestinal transit time
  - Protein calorie malnutrition
  - Thyroid disease
  - Diarrheal disease
- Reduced bile salt excretion
  - Cholestatic liver disease
  - Extrahepatic biliary obstruction
- Decreased GI surface area for drug absorption
  - Short bowel syndrome
  - Protein calorie malnutrition

velopment of external female genitalia. These may require extensive surgical correction after birth. Female fetuses, identified by family history and enzyme analysis, may be exposed to enough glucocorticoids transplacentally to suppress the fetal adrenal gland and prevent masculinization. In the future, specific genetic treatments may be available to correct allelic disorders in the fetus. Directed pharmacologic treatment of the fetus opens up a new frontier of fetal pharmacology that revisits many old questions about placental drug passage and fetal responses.

NEONATAL PHARMACOLOGY

Basic pharmacological principles (Chapters 1 to 7) apply to neonates, as well as to children and adults. Only those processes that differ in the fetus, perinate, or neonate are discussed in this section.

Drug Absorption

At birth, gastric pH is usually between 6 and 8 but falls rapidly to 1.5 to 3.0 within several hours; however, this fall is variable and appears independent of birth weight and gestational age. In the premature infant, hydrochloric acid is decreased before 32 weeks of gestational age, and the time of acid production may be related to the initiations of enteral feedings.

The rate of gastric emptying is an important determinant of the overall rate and extent of drug absorption. The rate of gastric emptying is variable during the neonatal period and is affected by gestational maturity, postnatal age, and type of feeding. In addition, neonatal conditions of gastroesophageal reflux, respiratory distress syndrome, and congenital heart disease delay gastric emptying.

The ontogeny of bile salt formation and the colonization of bacterial flora in the gastrointestinal tract may be a determinant in the absorption of drugs and nutrients. The absorption of some drugs may be affected by disease states in neonates (see box on p ...).

Chemical agents applied to the skin of a premature infant may result in inadvertent poisoning. For example, drug toxicities in neonates are reported for percutaneous absorption of such agents as hexachlorophene, pentachlorophenol-containing laundry detergents, hydrocortisone, and aniline-containing disinfectant solutions. Extreme caution should be exercised in using topical therapy on newborn infants.

Drug Administration

Intravenous drug administration is recommended for treatment of sick newborns to ensure effective circulating drug concentrations and to avoid the unpredictability of gastrointestinal drug absorption. The small size of extremely premature neonates presents unique problems during parenteral drug delivery. Fluid infusion rates are as low as 2 ml/hr, sometimes divided between two infusion sites. Although drug is infused into the IV tubing, it may not reach the patient in the desired length of time. In small neonates, accurate infusion pumps must be used to deliver the drug as close to the circulation as possible.

Intramuscular drug administration may be used occasionally in larger infants, but it is generally not recommended. As with adults, the rate of absorption of drug from the intramuscular site is directly related to blood flow. Newborns are often hypothermic and exhibit vascular constriction, which limits circulation to muscles. With a small muscle mass, intramuscular therapy may lead to sterile abscesses, which may later require surgical intervention.

Drug Distribution

The affinity of albumin for acidic drugs and total plasma protein concentration increase from birth into early infancy. These do not reach normal adult values until 10 to 12 months of age. In addition, although plasma albumin concentrations may reach adult values shortly after birth, the concentration of albumin in blood is directly proportional to gestational age, reflecting placental transport and fetal synthesis.

Different degrees of drug-protein binding may be observed between newborns and adults. The following four mechanisms are proposed to explain the differences in the protein binding of drugs between newborns and adults:

1. Displacement of drugs from binding sites by bilirubin and free fatty acids
2. Different binding properties of cord and adult albumin
3. Different binding properties of globulins
4. Decreased binding properties of albumin as a result of interaction with globulins in newborns

Basic drugs bind to plasma α_1-acid glycoprotein. A threefold reduction in plasma α_1-acid glycoprotein concentration exists in healthy term neonates compared to maternal plasma. When the α_1-acid glycoprotein concentration in cord blood becomes increased to adult values, the protein binding of lidocaine and propranolol approaches adult values, implicating the reduced plasma concentration of α_1-acid glycoprotein as the reason for the decreased protein binding.

Bilirubin noncovalently binds to albumin, and this association is reversible. The bilirubin-binding affinity of albumin at birth is independent of gestational age and is less for the newborn compared to the adult. The binding affinity of albumin for bilirubin increases with age and reaches that of adult serum by approximately 5 months of age. The lower bilirubin-binding affinity of albumin in neonates is believed to be a contributing factor in their susceptibility to kernicterus. Other factors such as the effect of hypothermia, acidosis, hypoglycemia, hypoxia, sepsis, birth asphyxia, and hypercapnia on the permeability of the blood-brain barrier and on bilirubin-albumin binding, must also be considered.

In summary, there appears to be a reduction in binding of drugs to plasma proteins during the neonatal period.

Drug Metabolism

During fetal development, the umbilical vein carries most of the placental blood directly to the liver except for the fraction shunted through the liver via the ductus venosus. Drugs are taken up into hepatocytes by diffusion or by one of several carrier-mediated transport mechanisms. Decreased hepatic clearance of a drug may reflect either a diminution of uptake or immaturity of the intrinsic metabolic pathways. Reduced concentrations of ligandin, an intracellular binding protein identified as a glutathione S-transferase, may account for some of the reduced hepatic clearance of bilirubin as well as polycyclic hydrocarbons. In contrast, metals such as copper, iron, and zinc may accumulate in the liver of neonates and reach higher concentrations than in adults.

During fetal life, some drug-metabolizing enzymes are present at about 30% of adult activity in vitro. After correction for differences in liver weight, the specific activity in vitro for many drug-metabolizing enzymes approaches adult activities. The appearance of these enzymes correlates with the development of rough endoplasmic reticulum and indicates that these enzyme systems increase in activity when smooth endoplasmic reticulum develops. The increase in monooxygenase activity observed in the first trimester plateaus during the second trimester.

Postnatally, the hepatic cytochrome P-450 monooxygenase system appears to mature rapidly. For example, phenytoin and its metabolites appear in the urine of newborns and adults in similar proportions. Furthermore, the decline in serum drug concentration parallels the rate of urinary metabolite excretion, an indication that the rate of excretion reflects the rate of hepatic metabolism of phenytoin.

Glucuronide conjugations require the coordinated activity of uridine diphosphate–glucose dehydrogenase and UDP-glucuronyl transferase. The first enzyme is present at 25% of adult activity in fetal liver at 8 to 18 weeks of gestation, and the second enzyme is barely detectable by 20 weeks of gestation. As a result, at birth, compounds that rely on glucuronidation for elimination have greatly prolonged half-lives or are conjugated by different pathways compared to children and adults.

Conjugation with glycine appears to occur as rapidly in fetal liver as in adult liver, whereas certain methylation reactions, which do not occur in adults, appear to be functional in the fetus and newborn. Theophylline is methylated to form caffeine in fetal livers that are 12 to 20 weeks of age. Caffeine, discussed below, has therapeutic implications in the treatment of apnea of prematurity.

Renal Drug Elimination

Whether renal function is normalized to body weight or body surface area, it is reduced at birth compared to the adult. Renal blood flow increases with age as a result of increased cardiac output and reduced peripheral vascular resistance. Within the first 12 hours after birth, the kidneys receive only 4% to 6% of cardiac output, but it increases to 8% to 10% during the first week. By adult life, the kidneys recieve 25% of cardiac output. The distribution of intrarenal blood flow away from the cortex and to the medulla immediately after birth further reduces glomerular filtration. Effective renal plasma flow (ERPF) measured with para-aminohippurate (PAH) increases from 20 ml/minute/1.73 m^2 at 30 weeks' gestation to 83 ml/minute/1.73 m^2 at term. ERPF continues to increase rapidly to 300 ml/minute/1.73 m^2 by 3 months and to 650 ml/minute/1.73 m^2 by 12 to 24 months after birth. Adult levels of renal function are usually reached by 6 months of age. These developmental changes in renal tubular and glomerular function contribute to rapid changes in the elimination kinetics of drugs cleared by the kidneys.

At birth, the glomerular filtration rate (GFR) is directly proportional to gestational age. This linear relationship is not evident before 34 weeks of gestation. In contrast, GFR, as measured by creatinine or inulin clearance, remains relatively constant at low rates of 12 ml/minute/ 1.73 m^2 before 34 weeks of gestation. The reason for this is not clear but may relate to the ontogeny and functional organization of the glomerulus. The GFR for full-term infants at birth averages 20 ml/minute/1.73 m^2. In the first 2 to 3 days of postnatal life, there is a rapid increase in the GFR of full-term babies by 2-3 fold compared to increases in neonates less than 34 weeks of gestation of 1-2 fold. The increase in GFR after birth is dependent on postconceptual age and not postnatal age. Adult values for GFR are reached by 2 ½ to 5 months of age. An example of the clinical implications of the maturation of GFR is the decreasing half-life for gentamicin with increasing gestational age in infants less than 7 days of age. Gentamicin is eliminated almost entirely by glomerular filtration (Chapter 48).

Proximal convoluted tubules in the normal kidney of a full-term infant are small in relation to their corresponding glomeruli. This glomerulotubular imbalance in size is reflected by functional differences in the secretory capacity of the proximal tubular cells. A tenfold increase in *para*-aminohippuric acid secretion occurs in the first year of life, with adult values (based on body surface area) attained by 30 weeks of age. Therefore tubular drug secretion matures at a slower rate than glomerular drug filtration function.

Penicillins, which undergo renal elimination, show high variability in elimination half-life in infants, but the range generally decreases to 1 to 2 hours by 2 weeks of postnatal age. The capacity of the secretory pathways responsible for penicillin elimination appear to undergo substrate stimulation in animals, and such a process may also exist in humans. A reduction in elimination half-life for ampicillin in preterm and term infants occurs after multiple doses compared to single-dose administration.

Pharmacodynamics

The ability of the developing fetus, newborn, and child to respond to a particular concentration of drug may involve a complex sequence of events. Inadequate response to an effective concentration of a drug may result from the presence or absence of receptors, inadequate drug-receptor binding, inadequate transduction of the receptor-drug interaction to an intracellular message, or the ability of the organ or tissue to respond to that intracellular message. Each of these events progresses during development at different rates, beginning with growth to biochemical maturation, and eventually to structural maturation, at which point the organ can respond fully to the events initiated by a drug.

Receptor Maturation

The cardiovascular system exemplifies some of the developmental steps in receptor maturation. When fully matured, many cardiovascular tissues exhibit a balance between sympathetic and parasympathetic nervous system control. During development, however, these two innervations occur at different rates among different tissues and do not mature simultaneously in all tissues. This may produce imbalances in the responsiveness of postjunctional organs or tissues innervated by parasympathetic or sympathetic mediators such as acetylcholine and norepinephrine. Thus, failure of the fetal heart or that of the newborn to respond to β-adrenergic receptor stimulation may reflect incomplete innervation or a lack of receptors for that agonist or neurotransmitter.

Once receptors are present, the interactions between the agonist and receptor may differ significantly between newborn and the adult. Studies in ventricular muscle of animals have shown that the binding affinity for the β-adrenergic receptor is greater in the adult where there are more receptors. Studies of the coupling between the receptor and the adenylate cyclase system in animal models indicate that the newborn heart exhibits a greater increase in adenylate cyclase activity for a smaller number of β-adrenergic receptor interactions than does a later-aged infant.

Dose-response studies using β-adrenergic agonists comparing fetal and maternal sheep reveal similar responses, but much higher doses are required to achieve comparable responses in fetal tissues. Differences have been noted between contractile responses and chronotropic responses to β-adrenergic receptor stimulation. A complete evaluation of these developmental changes encompasses each of the steps coupling receptor interactions to organ responses.

Clinical Problems

As a result of the often compromised cardiac output and peripheral perfusion of seriously ill infants, IV drug administration is generally used to assure adequate sys-

Drugs Contraindicated During Breastfeeding

Contraindicated
- Bromocriptine
- Cocaine
- Cyclophosphamide
- Cyclosporine
- Doxorubicin
- Ergotamine
- Lithium
- Methotrexate
- Phencyclidine (PCP)
- Phenindione

Temporary Cessation of Breastfeeding Required
- Radiopharmaceuticals:
  - Gallium 67
  - Indium 111
  - Iodine 125
  - Iodine 131
  - Radioactive sodium
  - Technetium 99m

Give with Caution During Breastfeeding
- Aspirin
- Clemastine
- Phenobarbital
- Primidone
- Salicylazosulfapyridine (sulfasalazine)

Contraindicated Drugs of Abuse
- Amphetamine
- Cocaine
- Heroin
- Marijuana
- Nicotine (smoking)
- Phencyclidine

Unknown Drug Effects, But of Concern
- Antianxiety:
  - Diazepam
  - Lorazepam
  - Prazepam
  - Quazepam
- Antidepressants:
  - Amitriptyline
  - Amoxapine
  - Desipramine
  - Doxepin
  - Fluoxetine
  - Imipramine
  - Trazodone
- Antipsychotic:
  - Chlorpromazine
  - Chlorprothixene
  - Haloperidol
  - Mesoridazine
- Chloramphenicol
- Metoclopramide
- Metronidazole
- Tinidazole

Modified from American Academy of Pediatrics Committee on Drugs, (1989). The transfer of drugs and other chemicals into human milk. Pediatrics, 84, 924-936. Reprinted with permission.

temic availability. Problems can be serious and include dilution and timed administration of small dosage volumes, maintenance of fluid balance, and the effect of the specific drug administration technique on resultant serum concentrations. In addition, mistiming of peak or trough serum drug determinations can result in clinical decisions to inappropriately adjust dosing regimens that result in increased risk of drug toxicity or of ineffective concentrations.

Certain drugs pose unusual therapeutic challenges when used in neonates or during the perinatal period because of the unique character of their distribution or elimination in these patients or because of the unusual side effects they may cause. These drugs include the antibiotics, digoxin, methylxanthines, and indomethacin.

Antibiotics Antibiotics are commonly used drugs in infants and newborns. Bacterial sepsis, pneumonia, necrotizing enterocolitis, and meningitis, as primary or secondary diseases, are frequent infections in these patients and are effectively treated with β-lactams, aminoglycosides, and glycopeptides. Because these drugs are primarily eliminated from the body unchanged through the kidneys, the renal function of the patient is an important variable in establishing doses and dosage intervals.

Another type of antibiotic, chloramphenicol, is associated with the "gray baby" and "gray toddler" syndromes of drug-induced toxicities that are a direct result of excessively high and prolonged chloramphenicol serum concentrations (usually above 50 to 75 mg/L). These substantially elevated serum chloramphenicol concentrations usually arise from doses >75 mg/kg/day combined with an immature capacity for conjugation by the newborn liver.

Digoxin Digoxin is a commonly used cardiac glycoside in the treatment of myocardial disturbances in neonates, infants and children. Extensive clinical experience shows that available data describing digoxin biodisposition in neonates and infants requires cautious interpretation. The neonatal heart is also less sensitive to the cardiac glycosides than is the adult heart.

Methylxanthines The methylxanthine theophylline remains a frequently used bronchodilating drug in the United States. During the neonatal period, theophylline is used in the treatment of apnea of prematurity. However, the efficacy of theophylline in this syndrome may be related to the additive or synergistic action of caffeine, a metabolite of theophylline, which accumulates in the serum of infants receiving theophylline. The *N*-methylation of theophylline to caffeine appears to be unique to preterm and newborn infants and is clinically important because of its prolonged elimination half-life. Caffeine is rarely detectable in the serum of older infants, children, or adults receiving theophylline alone.

The pharmacokinetics of theophylline in neonates are considerably different from those for older infants, children, and adults. These differences are likely attributable to different body-water compartmentalization and decreased plasma protein binding of theophylline in neonates (averages 36% in neonates and 56% in adults). Although neonates can methylate theophylline, it is excreted largely unchanged in newborn urine as compared to only approximately 10% as unchanged drug in older children and adults.

Indomethacin The use of indomethacin in neonates to stimulate ductus arteriosus closure is associated with potentially serious drug-induced complications and thus is not without risk.

DRUGS AND BREAST MILK

Human milk represents a complex solution of proteins, carbohydrates, fat, and liquid with a composition similar to that in serum. Its composition varies during the weeks to months of lactation as well as during a single feeding. Human milk has a pH of approximately 7.0, which influences the distribution of drugs from the maternal circulation into milk. To enter human milk, a drug leaves the maternal circulation and enters the breast alveolar cell. This may occur by diffusion across cell membranes or into water-filled channels or through binding to carrier proteins. For most drugs, the milk concentration is similar to that in the maternal circulation. The usual percentage of the maternal dose transferred to the infant ranges from 0.05% to 2%. Practical measures can be used to minimize the passage of drug into milk, e.g., breastfeeding just before the administration of medication so that significant amount of drug can be eliminated before the next feeding. Few drugs are considered to be contraindicated during breastfeeding and should be avoided (see Table on p 852).

REFERENCES

American Academy of Pediatrics Committee on Drugs: The transfer of drugs and other chemicals into human milk, *Pediatrics* 84:924-936, 1989.

Dothey CI, Tserng K-Y, Kaw S, King KC: Maturational changes of theophylline pharmacokinetics in preterm infants, *Clin Pharmacol Ther* 45:461-468, 1989.

Green TP, O'Dea RF, Mirkin BL: Determinants of drug disposition and effect in the fetus, *Annu Rev Pharmacol Toxicol* 19:285-322, 1979.

Kauffman RE: Drug therapeutics in the infant and child. In Yaffe SJ, Aranda JV, editors: *Pediatric pharmacology therapeutic principles in practice,* ed 2, Philadelphia, 1992, W.B. Saunders.

Koren G: *Maternal-fetal toxicology: a clinician's guide,* New York, 1990, Marcel Dekker.

Mirkin BL: *Perinatal pharmacology and therapeutics*, New York, 1976, Academic Press.

Mirkin BL, editor: *Clinical pharmacology and therapeutics: a pediatric perspective,* St Louis, 1978, Mosby.

Polin RA, Fox WM (editors): *Fetal and neonatal physiology,* Philadelphia, 1992, W. B. Saunders.

Ward RM: Maternal-placental-fetal-unit: unique problems of pharmacologic study, *Pediatr Clin North Am* 36:1075-1088, 1989.

Ward RM: The use of therapeutic drugs. In Avery GB, Fletcher MA, MacDonald MG, editors: *Neonatology: pathophysiology and management of the newborn,* ed 4, Philadelphia, 1994, Lippincott.

Ward RM, Green TP: Developmental pharmacology and toxicology: principles of study design and problems of methodology, *Pharmacol Ther* 36:309-334, 1988.

SELF ASSESSMENT QUESTIONS

1. Which of the following statements on fetal drug disposition is NOT correct?:
   a. Alcohol dehydrogenase is poorly expressed in the fetus and is only minimally developed at birth.
   b. Most conjugating systems are reasonably well-developed except glucuronidation.
   c. Monooxygenases in the fetus are inducible by barbiturates or smoking.
   d. Enhanced fetal drug metabolism can lead to reactive intermediates with potential toxicity.
   e. Biotransformation systems in the fetus are detectable at 5-8 weeks of gestation.
2. Which statement on the development of teratogenesis is NOT correct?:
   a. Potential for teratogenesis is not dose or concentration related.
   b. The most critical period for teratogenic effects is gestation week 3-12.
   c. It is difficult to determine a minimal teratogenic dose for any agent.
   d. Pharmacokinetic characteristics of a drug or chemical influence the teratogenic potential.
   e. Widely disparate chemical species can produce the same spectrum of teratogenic effects.
3. Which of the following is NOT true of protein binding in the newborn?
   a. α_1-acid glycoprotein is low in neonates and thus may be responsible for a reduced binding of acidic drugs.
   b. Bilirubin binding at birth is low and does not achieve adult values until about 5 months after birth.
   c. The reduced binding of bilirubin to albumin contributes to neonate susceptibility to kernicterus.
   d. Binding of acidic drugs to albumin does not achieve adult capacity until 10-12 months after birth.
   e. Plasma albumin concentrations in the adult and concentrations in the infant are similar, therefore the albumin concentrations per se are not responsible for differences in drug binding.

4. Digoxin is frequently used in the treatment of myocardial problems in neonates, infants, and children. Which of the following statements about digoxin use is correct?
   a. Digoxin is less efficacious in neonates than in adults.
   b. Digoxin is more potent in the neonate or infant than it is in the adult.
   c. Digoxin is less potent in the infant because the heart is less sensitive to digoxin than is the adult heart.
   d. Differences between neonate and adult in the dose required for a positive inotropic effect are the result of differences in biotransformation.
   e. b and d are correct.

CHAPTER 64

Gerontological Pharmacology

JOHN E THORNBURG

The rational use of drugs by the elderly is challenging to patient and physician. Decline in physiological functions as part of the normal aging process can lead to altered drug disposition and sensitivity to drug effects (see box at right). Increased chronic illness, multiple diseases, hospitalization, and long-term institutionalization contribute to increase drug usage and, in turn, more adverse reactions in the elderly than in younger people. In addition, inadequate nutrition, decreased financial resources, or poor compliance for various reasons may contribute to inadequate drug therapy.

Decisions about drug selection and dosage in the elderly are largely based on trial and error, anecdotal data, and clinical impression. Sound information on drug disposition and tissue or cellular responses to drugs in the elderly has been obtained only recently.

The objectives of this chapter are (1) to relate the normal physiological changes of aging to alterations in drug pharmacokinetics and to tissue or cellular responses and (2) to describe the geriatric pharmacology of some commonly used drugs.

PHYSIOLOGICAL CHANGES AND AGING

Several physiological functions in the human body tend to decline linearly, beginning between 30 and 45 years of age, and have important influences on pharmacokinetic processes (see box, p. 856). An important caveat, however, is that rates of declines in physiological functions with aging are highly individualized and some elderly people show little changes compared to population means. For example, cardiac output decreases about 1% a year beginning at 30 years of age. In the elderly, this is associated with redistribution of blood flow favoring brain, heart, and kidney and a reduction in hepatic blood flow. The percentage of lean body mass declines with age, such that body fat increases from 18% to 35% in men and from 33% to 48% in women between 18 and 55 years of age. Total body water decreases by 10% to 15% between 20 and 80 years of age.

Plasma albumin concentrations are lower in the elderly, particularly in the chronically ill or poorly nourished. The concentrations of α_1-acid glycoprotein increase, but they do so more sharply in response to acute illness than simply to aging. Glomerular filtration rate and effective renal plasma flow decline steadily with advancing age. Note that serum creatinine does not increase as a function of aging in spite of a smaller lean body mass (see p.857). Tubular secretory capacity declines in parallel with glomerular filtration rate.

FACTORS CONTRIBUTING TO ALTERED DRUG EFFECTS

- Altered drug disposition and pharmacokinetics
  - Decreased lean body mass
  - Increased percentage body fat
  - Decreased liver mass and blood flow
  - Reduced renal function
- Altered response to drug
  - Altered receptor and/or postreceptor properties
  - Impaired sensitivity of homeostatic mechanisms
  - Common diseases: glaucoma, diabetes, arthritis, hypertension, coronary artery disease, cancer
- Social and economic factors
  - Inadequate nutrition
  - Multiple drug therapy
  - Noncompliance

PHARMACOKINETIC CHANGES ASSOCIATED WITH AGING

Drug Absorption

Several physiological alterations in gastrointestinal (GI) function occur with aging: (1) decreased gastric pa-

PHYSIOLOGICAL CHANGES WITH AGING THAT AFFECT DRUG ABSORPTION, DISTRIBUTION, AND METABOLISM

DRUG ABSORPTION

Physiological Changes	Effect on Drug Absorption
Increased gastric pH	can be ↑ or ↓
Slowed gastric emptying rate	usually ↓
Reduced splanchnic flow	↓
Slowed GI motility	can be ↑ or ↓
Thinning and reductions of absorptive surface	↓

DRUG DISTRIBUTION AND METABOLISM

Decline in body weight with advanced age
Decrease in lean body mass
Increase in body fat
Decrease in total body water
Reduction in plasma albumin
Slight and variable increase in α_1-acid glycoprotein
Redistribution of regional blood flow from liver and kidney
Reduction in hepatic microsomal enzyme activity

rietal cell function with (2) a corresponding rise in gastric pH, (3) a slowed rate of gastric emptying, and (4) decreased active transport of glucose, vitamin B_{12}, and other nutrients. The rate and extent of absorption of most drugs are determined by passive diffusion in the proximal small bowel. This likely accounts for the general lack of clinically significant alterations in drug absorption in the elderly. One exception is a threefold increase in the bioavailability of levodopa as a result of reduced activity of dopa decarboxylase activity in the stomach wall.

Drug Distribution

Reduced lean body mass, reduced total body water, increased fat, and decreased plasma albumin in the elderly can contribute to alterations in drug distribution. The effect of body composition on drug distribution depends largely on the physiochemical properties of individual drugs. Lipid-soluble drugs such as diazepam and lidocaine have a larger volume of distribution in the elderly; water-soluble drugs such as acetaminophen or ethanol have a smaller volume of distribution. Digoxin has a lower volume of distribution in the elderly, and therefore doses of digoxin must be reduced.

There is a slight trend to lower plasma albumin concentrations in the healthy elderly patient, whereas the hospitalized or poorly nourished elderly may have 10% to 20% decreased plasma albumin concentrations. This can result in increased unbound or free concentration of drug, the consequences of which can be complex. There are no guidelines available based on objective data for dosage modification to compensate for decreased protein binding.

Much of the pharmacokinetic data available for elderly patients reports only elimination half-life. Without corresponding measures of volume of distribution (V_d) and clearance, interpretation of half-life changes is not possible, as is clear from the equation (see also Chapter 4):

$$t_{1/2} = \frac{0.693 \times V_d}{\text{Clearance}} \qquad \textbf{(1)}$$

Drug Metabolism

The decline in the ability of the elderly to metabolize most drugs is relatively small and difficult to predict. In general, hydroxylation and *N*-dealkylation reactions catalyzed by hepatic microsomal mixed-function oxidase enzymes decrease slightly with aging. Conjugation reactions such as glucuronidation are not greatly affected by aging. Effects of change in cigarette smoking, diet, or alcohol consumption may be more important than physiological hepatic changes. For example, decreased dietary protein intake or reduction in cigarette consumption may lead to decreased liver microsomal enzyme activity. Studies in aging animals are not predictive in humans because of pronounced sex and species differences.

In the elderly, first-pass metabolism may be of clinical importance requiring decreased dosages. Total liver blood flow declines 40% to 45% with aging, partly as a result of reduced cardiac output. Diseases such as congestive heart failure may further compromise hepatic blood flow. Thus, as hepatic blood flow declines, clearance of flow-dependent drugs will usually decrease and blood concentrations will rise.

The ability of hepatic mixed-function oxidases to respond to inducers is retained, though there are exceptions. Cigarette smoking and phenytoin induce hepatic theophylline metabolism to a similar degree in young and old. In contrast, the clearance of antipyrine is not increased by cigarette smoking in elderly subjects. The ability of cimetidine to inhibit microsomal drug metabolism is the same in young and old.

In summary, the rate of hepatic metabolism of a drug is not a predictable consequence of well understood alterations in hepatic function. Normal values of liver function tests do not predict normal drug metabolism.

Nearly all the available data are obtained in healthy, not sick, elderly subjects.

Drug Elimination

Consistent with the physiological decline of renal function with normal aging, the rate of elimination of those drugs dependent on the kidney is reduced in the elderly. Such drugs include the aminoglycosides, lithium carbonate, chlorpropamide, and digoxin. To avoid drug toxicity, renal function must be estimated and downward adjustments in dosage made accordingly.

As discussed in Chapter 5, drug clearance is often directly proportional to creatinine clearance whether elimination is by tubular secretion or glomerular filtration. Because of difficulties in obtaining accurate 24-hour urine collections to measure creatinine clearance directly (see Chapter 5, equation 10), it is usually estimated using nomograms or equation 2, which accounts for differences in age and body weight.

$$(CL)_{Cr} = \frac{(140 - \text{age})\,(\text{weight})}{72\,[S_{Cr}]} \qquad \textbf{(2)}$$

where $(CL)_{Cr}$ is creatinine clearance in ml/min, age is in years, weight in kg, and S_{Cr} is serum creatinine in mg/dl. The formula is multiplied by 85% for females. Interpretation of serum creatinine concentration in the elderly requires caution. Because creatinine is a product of muscle metabolism, less is produced as lean body mass declines. Thus an 80-year-old man with a serum creatinine concentration of 1 mg/dl may have a creatinine clearance of 60 ml/min, only one half that of a 40-year-old man with the same serum creatinine.

There are no absolute guidelines, but two general principles apply. First, most elderly patients do not have "normal" renal function when serum creatinine appears "normal." Second, most elderly patients require dosage adjustments for drugs that are eliminated primarily by the kidneys.

The decreased rate of elimination of inhalation anesthetics resulting from declining pulmonary function with aging is an important consideration regarding general anesthesia in the elderly.

DRUG RESPONSE CHANGES ASSOCIATED WITH AGING

Changes in drug responses in the elderly have received less study than have pharmacokinetic changes (see box, p. 856). This is attributable to the relative difficulty of direct assessment of target organ responses. Nevertheless, drug responses are clearly altered with aging. In general, an enhanced response can be expected (Table 64-1). However, reduced responses to some drugs, such as the β-adrenergic receptor agonist isoproterenol, do occur, and a reduced dosage schedule is recommended to prevent serious side effects (Table 64-2).

Factors that affect the sensitivity or intensity of responses at target organs include the following:

1. Age-related changes in receptors and postreceptor molecular mechanisms
2. Age-related changes in homeostatic control
3. Disease-induced changes
4. Drug-drug and drug-nutrient interactions

Table 64-1 Altered Drug Responses in the Elderly

Drugs	Direction of Change
barbiturates	Increased
benzodiazepines	Increased
chlordiazepoxide	
diazepam	
flurazepam	
morphine	Increased
pentazocine	Increased
anticoagulants	Increased
warfarin	
heparin	
isoproterenol	Decreased
tolbutamide	Decreased

Table 64-2 Drugs Given in Reduced Dosage in the Elderly

Drug	Possible Effects of Usual Dosage
aminoglycosides	Nephrotoxicity and ototoxicity
carbamazepine	Drowsiness, ataxia
cimetidine	Confusion
digoxin	Toxicity more likely
levodopa	Hypotension
meperidine	Respiratory depression
metaclopramide	Confusion
thioridazine	Confusion
thyroxine	Myocardial infarction
vitamin D	Renal toxicity

Modified from the Report of the WHO Technical Group on the Use of Medicaments in the Elderly, World Health Organization, 1981.

Age-related Changes in Receptors and Postreceptor Mechanisms

Age-related changes may occur at receptor and postreceptor levels. In general, there is little evidence for specific alterations causing altered sensitivity or intensity in responses. Possible mechanisms include the following:

1. Changes in receptor density or affinity
2. Altered second messenger (cyclic adenosine monophosphate or cyclic guanosine monophosphate) activity
3. Alteration in a biochemical response such as glycogenolysis
4. A mechanical effect such as vascular relaxation

The β-adrenergic system of the heart has been extensively studied. The sensitivity of the heart is decreased with aging in elderly subjects. For example, a higher dose of isoproterenol is required in the elderly to cause a 25-beat-per-minute increase in heart rate. This reduced sensitivity to isoproterenol is not caused by alterations in β-receptors but to changes in the cyclic adenosine monophosphate system or in other postreceptor events proximal to calcium-troponin interaction.

The magnitude of the increased responses to benzodiazepines, diazepam, flurazepam, and nitrazepam in the elderly cannot be totally explained by pharmacokinetic differences. The occurrence of flurazepam-induced adverse effects increases dramatically with aging.

Impaired Homeostatic Mechanisms

With advancing age, several critical physiological control mechanisms become increasingly inefficient. These include decreased activity of aortic and carotid body chemoreceptors, reduced baroreceptor reflexes, impaired thermoregulation, inappropriate response of blood glucose and insulin to an orally administered glucose load, and altered neurological control of bowel and bladder. Drug toxicity may therefore result.

Decreased baroreflex sensitivity may lead to increased risk of orthostatic (postural) hypotension. In the elderly, this is a common problem with some phenothiazines and antidepressants (those with significant α_1-adrenergic antagonist properties), nitrates, and antihypertensives such as prazosin and α-methyldopa.

The normal homeostatic response of the aortic and carotid body chemoreceptors to morphine-induced respiratory depression is to increase respiratory stimulation. Impaired chemoreceptor activity may lead to greater than expected respiratory depressant effects of morphine.

Multiple mechanisms are implicated in the impaired patient. Thermoregulation may be seen in a significant number of elderly individuals and includes absence of shivering, failure of metabolic rate to rise, poor vasoconstriction, and insensitivity to a low body temperature. Chlorpromazine and many other psychoactive drugs may cause hypothermia. Alcohol tends to augment this effect.

Disease-Induced Changes

Multiple chronic diseases are common in the elderly. One third have three or more chronic diseases such as diabetes, glaucoma, hypertension, coronary artery disease, and arthritis. Multiple diseases may lead to multiple medications, an increased frequency of drug-drug interactions, and adverse drug reactions. Moreover, a disease may increase the risk of adverse drug reactions or preclude the use of the otherwise most effective or safest drug for another problem. For example, anticholinergic drugs (see box) may cause urinary retention in men with enlarged prostate glands or precipitate glaucoma, and drug-induced hypotension may cause ischemic events in persons with vascular disease.

Drug-Drug and Drug-Nutrient Interactions

Multiple drug therapies may lead to confusion, medication errors, and further drug-drug interactions. An often overlooked factor is the common use among the elderly of over-the-counter antacids, laxatives, analgesics, antihistamines, sleeping pills, and vitamins. Inadequate dietary potassium increases the likelihood of diuretic-induced hypokalemia, whereas excessive sodium chloride ingestion may attenuate the effect of an antihypertensive drug. Most drug-nutrient problems, however, are pharmacokinetic in nature.

EXAMPLES OF DRUG PROBLEMS AND PRESCRIBING IN THE ELDERLY

Many drugs require dosage modifications for use in the elderly. Two examples of problematic drug use in the elderly are described.

Anticholinergic Drug Toxicity

Anticholinergic drug toxicity illustrates some of the inherent problems of drug treatment in the elderly. Some of the large number of drugs with atropine-like activity are listed in the box. For some of those drugs, the anticholinergic response is the desired useful pharmacological effect, but for others this may be an unwanted side effect. It is common for elderly patients to concurrently receive several of these atropine-like drugs. Re-

DRUGS WITH ANTICHOLINERGIC PROPERTIES

Antipsychotics, thioridazine
Antidepressants; amitryptiline, doxepin
Antidysrhythmics; disopyramide, quinidine
Anti-parkinsonian drugs; benztropine, trihexyphenidyl
Antispasmodics; belladonna alkaloids, atropine, propantheline, clidinium
Antihistamines; diphenhydramine, chlorpheniramine
Ophthalmic preparations; tropicamide, cyclopentolate
Proprietary hypnotics, cold preparations

cently, a so-called anticholinergic syndrome (see box, below) has been recognized, particularly in the elderly, in whom the additive effects of these drugs lead to toxicity. Some elderly patients will be more susceptible than others to anticholinergic toxicity because of impaired autonomic bowel or bladder innervation, glaucoma, benign prostatic hypertrophy, or impaired cognitive capacity. Some elderly patients are especially sensitive to cognitive disruption caused by anticholinergic drugs. Thus, in the elderly, great care must be taken to avoid excessive antimuscarinic effects and to be observant for potential toxicity.

Benzodiazepine-based Depression

Benzodiazepines are more likely to cause greater central nervous system depression in elderly than in younger patients. Altered pharmacokinetics and increased tissue sensitivities are involved. Benzodiazepines, such as diazepam, which undergo oxidative hepatic metabolism, show a decline in metabolic clearance, a disproportionately longer plasma half-life, and an increase in volume of distribution. This is attributed to the relative increase in body fat and a small decline in plasma albumin with aging. Oxazepam, lorazepam, and temazepam, which are all metabolized by conjugation, exhibit little alteration in metabolism and clearance with aging. Yet these latter drugs are associated with an increased sensitivity in response. The best evidence for altered tissue sensitivity is that at equal plasma concentrations of diazepam or nitrazepam, greater CNS depression occurs in the elderly. The molecular basis for this altered sensitivity remains unknown, but in the elderly, smaller doses should be employed and drugs with extremely long half-lives should be avoided if possible.

SIGNS AND SYMPTOMS OF ANTICHOLINERGIC SYNDROME

Systemic
- Tachycardia
- Warm, dry, flushed skin
- Decreased secretions
- Decreased bowel motility
- Urinary retention
- Mydriasis, loss of accommodation
- Hyperpyrexia
- Cardiac conduction problems

Neuropsychiatric
- Anxiety
- Agitation
- Confusion
- Delirium
- Increased forgetfulness
- Hallucinations
- Seizures

GUIDELINES FOR DRUG PRESCRIBING IN THE ELDERLY

Drug prescribing in the elderly can be safe and effective by adherence to the following principles:

1. Know all of the patient's medical problems
2. Ascertain all drugs being taken, including over-the-counter preparations
3. Know the pharmacology of the drugs
4. Start with small doses and titrate the drug based on response
5. Keep dosage regimens simple
6. Be sure that visual, motor, or cognitive impairments will not result in errors or noncompliance
7. Review treatment plan and response regularly
8. Regularly consider that new symptoms or problems may be drug induced

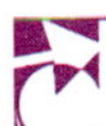

NEW DIRECTIONS

Particularly important for geriatric pharmacology is the need for greater systematic study of effects of commonly used drugs in the elderly. Despite recent efforts, there remain large and serious voids in our basic understanding of effects of specific drugs in the aging population.

Compounds such as selegiline and vitamin E have awakened a major effort to develop and use antioxidants or free-radical scavengers in a preventive fashion in the hope of slowing various degenerative diseases.

Tacrine, a centrally active acetylcholine esterase inhibitor, has been approved for treatment of dementia of Alzheimer's disease. At least twelve other compounds are being studied in Alzheimer's patients.

REFERENCES

Dawling S, Crome P: Clinical pharmacokinetic considerations in the elderly, *Clin Pharmacokinet* 17:236-263, 1989.

Tumer N, Scarpace PJ, Lowenthal DT: Geriatric pharmacology: basic and clinical considerations, *Annu Rev Pharmacol Toxicol* 32:271-302, 1992.

Vestal RE, Montamat SC, Nielson CD: (1992). Drugs in special patient groups: the elderly. In Melmon KL, Morrelli HF, Hoffman BB, Nierenberg, DW, editors: *Clinical Pharmacology*, ed 3, New York, 1992, McGraw-Hill.

SELF-ASSESSMENT QUESTIONS

1. Altered pharmacokinetics of a drug in the elderly may be attributable to:
   a. decreased total body fat.
   b. increased total body water.
   c. increased gastric acid secretion.
   d. decreased portal circulation.
   e. increased plasma albumin concentrations.
2. The hepatic drug metabolism reaction most likely not to be decreased in the elderly is:
   a. *N*-demethylation.
   b. hydroxylation.
   c. sulfoxidation.
   d. glucuronidation.
   e. deesterification.
3. Drugs requiring dosage modification in the elderly because of reduced renal function include all of the following *except:*
   a. lithium carbonate.
   b. warfarin.
   c. gentamicin.
   d. digoxin.
   e. cimetidine.
4. Evidence of anticholinergic toxicity might include:
   a. bronchospasm.
   b. diarrhea.
   c. miosis.
   d. diaphoresis.
   e. tachycardia.

CHAPTER 65

Drugs to Treat Anemia

BRENDA J. GROSSMAN
THEODORE M. BRODY

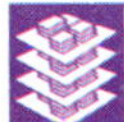

THERAPEUTIC OVERVIEW

Agents discussed in this chapter include iron, vitamin B_{12}, folate, and erythropoietin. All are used therapeutically to treat certain types of anemias.

Anemia is defined as a decrease in the number of circulating red blood cells (RBCs). A decrease in RBC production caused by cytoplasmic or nuclear maturation defects, or by an increase in destruction from intrinsic RBC abnormalities or extrinsic mechanisms, results in anemia. Regardless of cause, clinical signs and symptoms are similar and occur because of reduced oxygen-carrying capacity. Anemias are usually classified according to the appearance of the RBC on microscopic examination.

Anemias associated with cytoplasmic maturation defects exhibit peripheral blood smears that are usually hypochromic and microcytic. This category includes iron deficiency, sideroblastic anemias, thalassemia, and anemia of chronic disease. All are attributable to abnormal hemoglobin synthesis. Adequate iron, globin, and porphyrin are essential for hemoglobin synthesis. Iron deficiency, which may be caused by inadequate iron ingestion, absorption, or transport, or by excessive blood loss, leads to abnormal heme synthesis. Sideroblastic anemia (characterized by cells having a perinuclear ring of iron granules) has multiple causes but primarily results from a defect in incorporation of iron into the porphyrin ring. Abnormal globin synthesis occurs in the genetic disease thalassemia. Anemia of chronic disease is caused by an inability to transport iron from the body's storage sites to the RBC.

Anemias associated with RBC nuclear maturation defects have peripheral blood smears that appear normochromic and macrocytic. This category includes megaloblastic anemias caused by vitamin B_{12} (commonly called *pernicious anemia*) or folate deficiency. Both vitamins are essential for DNA synthesis, and a lack of either results in a decrease in DNA as well as protein synthesis.

Anemias from increased destruction (hemolysis) result from RBC abnormalities evolving from genetic defects such as sickle cell anemia, hereditary spherocytosis, and glucose 6-phosphate dehydrogenase deficiency. Other causes of increased destruction occur from external factors such as drug-induced antibodies. Diseases such as septic shock may result in RBC destruction associated with disseminated intravascular coagulation, where the RBC membrane is directly damaged by mechanical forces. The peripheral blood smear in these anemias exhibits spherocytes and fragmented RBCs.

Therapy of anemia must be tailored to the specific cause of the anemia. For example, iron is reserved solely for iron deficiency states and vitamin B_{12} for megaloblastic anemias related to B_{12} deficiency. Recently developed, human recombinant erythropoietin has been useful in diseases where inadequate erythropoietin is present because of renal disease.

Before one treats an anemic patient, it is essential that a specific diagnosis be established and that the implications of that diagnosis be considered. In general, iron therapy should not be instituted empirically, but only if studies (serum iron and ferritin) confirm the iron deficiency. The importance of initiating iron therapy is

ABBREVIATIONS

BFU-E	burst erythroid colony forming unit
CFU-E	erythroid colony forming unit
MCB	methylcobalamin
GM-CSF	granulocyte macrophage–colony stimulating factor
MTHF	methyltetrahydrofolate
PMN	polymorphonuclear neutrophil
RBC	red blood cell, erythrocyte

THERAPEUTIC OVERVIEW

IRON AND IRON SALTS

Used to treat hypochromic, microcytic anemias associated with iron deficiency

VITAMIN B_{12} AND FOLATE

Used to treat megaloblastic anemia

ERYTHROPOIETIN

Used to treat anemia of end-stage renal disease

Other anemias

overshadowed by that of pursuing a thorough gastrointestinal evaluation. Frequently men and postmenopausal women with iron deficiencies are found to have a bleeding gastrointestinal lesion. Empiric therapy, without pursuing the cause, is never appropriate in these populations.

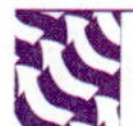

MECHANISMS OF ACTION

Iron

Anemia caused by red-cell iron deficiency is treated by iron replacement therapy until hemoglobin concentrations are normal and iron stores have been repleted. Absorption, distribution, elimination, and regulation of body concentrations of iron and management of iron-deficiency anemia are discussed in the following sections.

Vitamin B_{12} and Folic Acid

Vitamin B_{12} and folic acid are both required for normal DNA and protein synthesis. Deficiency of one or the other results in defective nuclear maturation of rapidly and continuously replicating cells in bone marrow, with development of megaloblastic, anemia. The roles of B_{12} and folic acid in the normal economy of the cell is illustrated in Figure 65-1. Vitamin B_{12} (cyanocobalamin) exists as two coenzymes, methylcobalamin (MCB, methyl B_{12}) and deoxyadenosylcobalamin (deoxyadenosyl B_{12}). While both coenzymes are important in lipid and carbohydrate metabolism, MCB promotes methionine synthesis by transmethylation from homocysteine, important for normal folate metabolism. Methyl groups contributed by methyltetrahydrofolate (MTHF) form MCB, the latter acting as the methyl donor for the homocysteine-methionine conversion. Methionine is converted to *S*-adenosylmethionine, important in transmethylation and protein biosynthesis. With either a folic acid or B_{12} deficiency, the cell increases its MTHF pool and maintains methylation reactions at the expense of nucleic acid biosynthesis. A B_{12} deficiency prevents formation of tetrahydrofolate from MTHF, blocking folate metabolism. The cyanocobalamin-folate system thus plays a key role in synthesis of purines and pyrimidines, necessary constituents of DNA, leading to hematological dysfunction (i.e., the development of megaloblastic anemia). Management of this type of anemia is achieved by the appropriate use of several preparations of vitamin B_{12} and folic acid.

Erythropoietin

Growth factors that stimulate proliferation, differentiation, and maturation of the bone-marrow pluripotent stem cell to both lymphopoietic and hematopoietic cell lines have been identified. (Lymphopoiesis is discussed extensively in Chapter 45). Several humoral and cellular factors are involved in erythropoiesis, the major one being erythropoietin. Others that may act synergistically with erythropoietin are granulocyte– and granulocyte macrophage–colony simulating factors (G-CSF and GM–CSF) and interleukin-3 (IL-3).

Erythropoietin is a heavily glycosylated 36,000-dalton glycoprotein comprising 166 amino acids. The amino acid sequence of human erythropoietin has been determined, and the gene has been cloned. Four cysteines are present, two joined by a disulfide bond. The polypeptide chain can be digested by trypsin and chymotrypsin to inactive products, and enzymatically deglycosylated erythropoietin is not active in vivo. The carbohydrate moiety of erythropoietin protects it from clearance by the liver. Antibody studies have indicated that the functional activity of erythropoietin may reside in the 111 to 129 amino acid region of the molecule.

About 90% of erythropoietin is synthesized in renal cortical cells and the remainder in extrarenal sites, primarily liver. Hypoxia is the stimulus for initiating production/secretion of erythropoietin by kidney and extrarenal tissues. Thus any condition that results in hypoxia (anemia, hypobaria, or ischemia, with a subsequent decrease in renal blood flow) will promote production of erythropoietin.

The most recent model for the production of erythropoietin, developed by Fisher (1994), involves the role of hypoxia and the ability of the kidney to respond to the oxygen deficit by increasing erythropoietin messenger RNA. A two-cell system is visualized; with one cell, per-

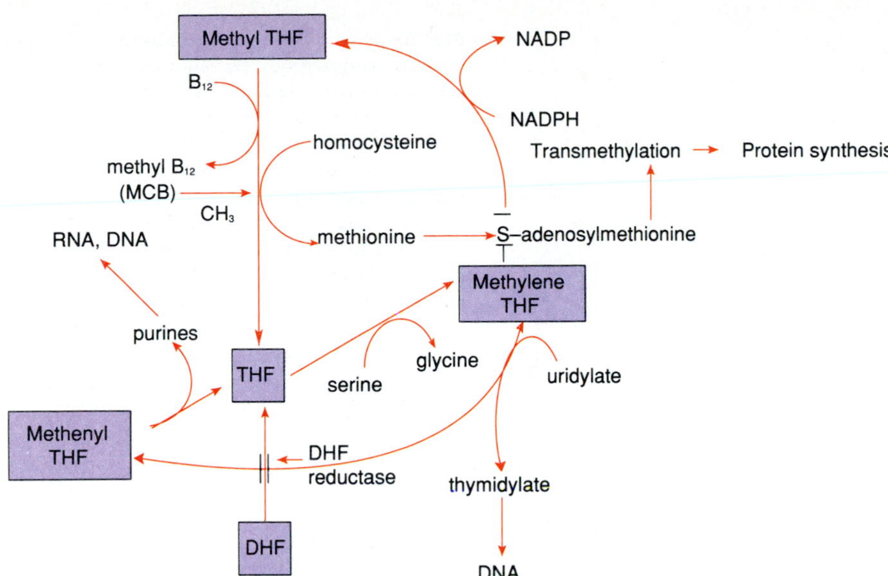

FIGURE 65-1 Folate metabolism: role of B_{12}. *DHF,* Dihydrofolate; *THF,* tetrahydrofolate.

haps the endothelial cell lining the vascular wall, sensing the oxygen concentration, and a second cell, an interstitial epithelial cell, producing erythropoietin mRNA. A current hypothesis is that adenosine triphosphate is elevated extracellularly during hypoxia, stimulating membrane receptors, which in turn activate nitric oxide synthase, generating nitric oxide in the sensing cell. Nitric oxide is released and enters the erythropoietin-producing cell and activates guanylate cyclase to increase cyclic guanosine monophosphate. The latter increases transcriptional proteins to produce erythropoietin mRNA (Figure 65-2). Although interstitial cells of the peritubular capillary bed have been implicated, the precise renal cell type actually responsible for the production of erythropoietin has not been established. In response to hypoxia, other messengers, such as adenosine, eicosanoids, and β_2-adrenergic receptor agonists coupled to G proteins and increasing cyclic adenosine monophosphate, apparently modulate the effects of erythropoietin mRNA at the posttranscriptional level and alone will not increase erythropoietin production.

In end-stage renal disease, there is no physiological mechanism for erythropoietin production, since the kidney cells are largely destroyed. Erythropoietin must therefore be provided exogenously. Targets for exogenous erythropoietin in marrow are the early erythroid colony forming unit cell (CFU-E), and the late burst erythroid colony forming unit (BFU-E). Erythropoietin expands the BFU-E compartment and stimulates CFU-E proliferation. This promotes a series of proliferation, differentiation, and maturation events from primitive stem cell to reticulocyte (Figure 65-3). Other regulatory glycoprotein factors act synergistically with erythropoietin, including interleukin-3, G-CSF, and GM-CSF. Epo apparently binds to saturable high-affinity sites on the erythroid cell to bring about its effects. Maturity of the progenitor cell determines the degree of differentiation and proliferation produced by erythropoietin.

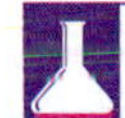

PHARMACOKINETICS

The pharmacokinetic characteristics of drugs used are shown in Table 65-1.

Iron and Iron Salts

The rate of absorption of iron reflects the total body burden of iron. Two forms of iron are available for absorption: heme and nonheme iron. Heme iron, a minor constituent of the normal diet, is readily absorbed from the gastrointestinal (GI) tract; its absorption is relatively independent of other dietary components. In contrast, nonheme iron accounts for the largest fraction of iron presented to the GI tract but is poorly absorbed and highly dependent on other components in the diet. Ascorbate, for example, facilitates nonheme iron absorption by reducing iron from ferric to the ferrous form. Meat promotes nonheme iron absorption by stimulating production of gastric acid.

Iron in the body exists in two compartments: a functional one as part of hemoglobin and myoglobin and other essential protein structures, and the nonfunctional storage form of ferritin. Ferritin is present either as a

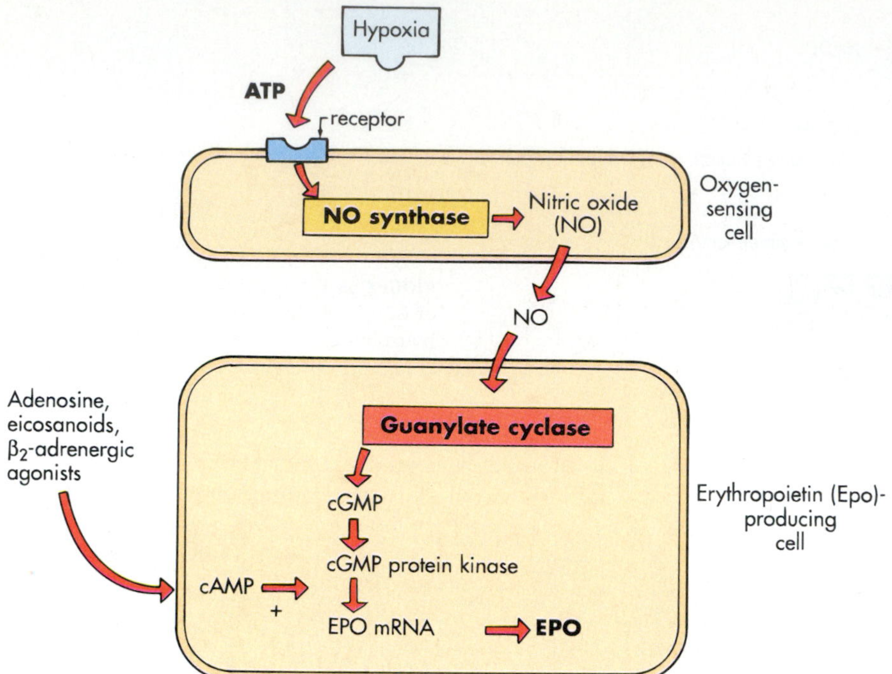

FIGURE 65-2 Model for stimulation of erythropoietin production by hypoxia: extracellular adenosine triphosphate *(ATP)* is increased, activating a membrane receptor to stimulate nitric oxide *(NO)* synthase and producing NO in the oxygen-sensing cell. NO diffuses into the erythropoietin *(EPO)*-producing cell stimulating guanylate cyclase and increasing cyclic guanosine monophosphate *(cGMP)*. cGMP promotes generation of transcriptional proteins, increasing expression of erythropoietin mRNA and erythropoietin production. Some agents, released during hypoxia, and others that increase cyclic adenosine monophosphate *(cAMP)* concentrations act as modulators of erythropoietin mRNA. In the absence of the nitric oxide synthase activation, they fail to stimulate erythropoietin production. (Modified from Fisher JA. In Massry SG, Glassock RJ, editors: *Textbook of nephrology,* ed 3, Baltimore, 1994, Williams & Wilkins.

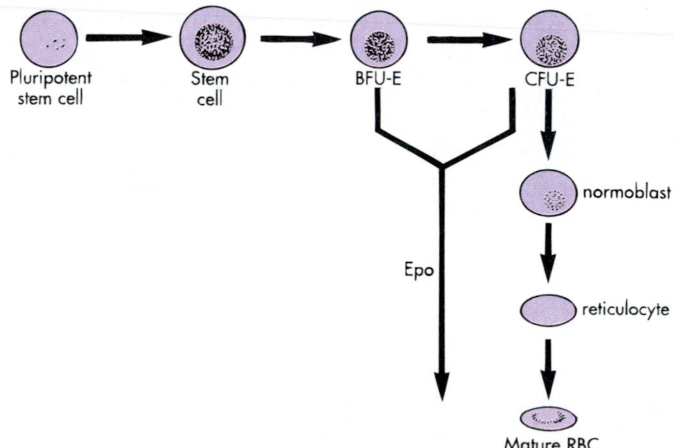

FIGURE 65-3 Erythropoietin acts on BFU-E and CFU-E and the nucleated erythroid series to produce mature erythrocytes.

Table 65-1 Pharmacokinetic Parameters

Drug	Routes of Administration	Remarks
recombinant human erythropoietin (rHuEpo)	IV, SC	SC may be as effective as IV; $t_{1/2}$ is 8 hours
iron	Oral, IM, IV	Oral absorption of ferrous good; ferric poor but enhanced by ascorbate; enteric-coated preparations unreliable
vitamin B_{12}	Oral, SC, IM	Oral route ineffective in malabsorption disease; enterohepatic cycling
folic acid	Oral, IM, IV	Oral absorption good; enterohepatic cycling

monomer termed *apoferritin* or as aggregates referred to as *hemosiderin*. Apoferritin has a molecular weight of 450,000 daltons and is made up of 24 polypeptide subunits. Distribution of iron between functional and storage compartments is accomplished by the plasma protein transferrin, a glycoprotein of molecular weight of 76,000 daltons, which binds ferric iron and controls iron movement to various transferrin binding sites located on cell plasma membranes. The iron-transferrin complex is taken up into the cell by endocytosis. The complexed iron is released intracellularly, and transferrin is extruded and returned to the extracellular compartment. The number of transferrin binding sites and the intracellular ferritin concentration are determined by the total body burden of iron. With adequate iron, fewer transferrin binding sites are synthesized and ferritin increases to promote iron storage. When the iron content is low, more transferrin binding sites are expressed by the cell and ferritin concentrations are reduced to minimize storage and maximize iron absorption. Remarkably, there is very little physiological iron loss; most iron is conserved. In men, loss is about 10% of total iron per year. Menstruating females may lose up to 20%. In pregnancy, higher iron intake is required, as in conditions associated with significant blood loss. Thus iron absorption is the most important factor determining total iron content.

Vitamin B_{12}

Deficiency of this vitamin is generally not dietary in origin. Vitamin B_{12} is available in animal products and in legumes and is readily absorbed from the GI tract with the aid of the intrinsic factor. In pernicious anemia, there is a loss of gastric parietal cell function, resulting in failure to produce the intrinsic factor, a glycoprotein with a molecular weight of 59,000 daltons that complexes vitamin B_{12} under acid conditions in the stomach and is important for its absorption. The complex of intrinsic factor–vitamin B_{12} reaches the ileum where it interacts with an ileal binding site, is absorbed, and enters the circulation. In the circulation, vitamin B_{12} binds to a plasma β-globulin (transcobalamin II) and is transported to tissues including liver, where it is stored as active coenzyme. About 90% of the body's stores of this vitamin are in hepatic parenchymal cells. Cobalamin is also secreted into bile and reabsorbed from the intestine. Thus enterohepatic cycling plays a key role in maintenance of vitamin B_{12} concentrations. Tissue availability is related to the amount stored and also to the amount bound to transcobalamin II.

Folic Acid

Folates in the diet present as polyglutamates, are hydrolyzed by a carboxypeptidase, reduced by dihydrofolate reductase in the small intestine, and methylated to MTHF during GI transport. Once absorbed, MTHF is transported to body tissues. As with vitamin B_{12}, enterohepatic cycling plays an important role in maintaining folate concentrations. Liver reduces and methylates folates and transports the methylated product (MTHF) to the bile, where it is reabsorbed from the intestine.

Erythropoietin

Recombinant human erythropoietin is administered either by the IV (during hemodialysis) or the SC route. The plasma half-life of IV erythropoietin is approximately 8 hours (range from 2 to 12 hours) in normal subjects, hemodialysis patients, or those undergoing continuous ambulatory peritoneal dialysis. After SC injection of recombinant human erythropoietin, peak serum concentrations are observed within 8 to 12 hours and maintained for an additional 12 to 16 hours. Recombinant human erythropoietin is distributed in a single body compartment after IV injection, with a mean apparent volume of distribution varying from 2 to 7 liters in a 70 kg individual, depending on plasma volume. Erythropoietin is metabolized primarily by the liver.

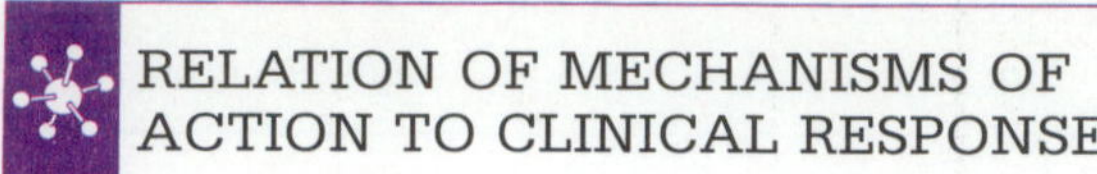

RELATION OF MECHANISMS OF ACTION TO CLINICAL RESPONSE

Iron Deficiency

Iron deficiency is the most common cause of anemia and results from a negative iron balance in which iron loss exceeds iron intake. Iron requirements depend on the amount of iron lost and the amount needed for growth. In the United States the most common cause of iron deficiency in men and postmenopausal women is GI blood loss. This may be attributable to the effects of alcohol or aspirin or to GI tract malignancies. GI bleeding is often intermittent and may be difficult to detect. In postmenopausal women, uterine bleeding is an additional common cause. Infants and pregnant women require an increase in iron intake for development; however, routine iron supplementation in these latter groups has lessened this cause of iron deficiency. In underdeveloped countries, decreased nutritional intake is an important cause. There has been a significant decline in iron deficiency anemia in developed countries, and pathological blood loss should be pursued in evaluation of most clinical cases.

Specific signs and symptoms of iron deficiency are few and are generally those associated with any chronic anemia, including pallor, fatigue, light-headedness, and in severe cases, palpitations, dyspnea, and angina pectoris. An interesting specific symptom of iron deficiency anemia is pica, a craving for nonfood substances including ice, clay, and laundry starch.

The most common laboratory manifestation of iron deficiency is a hypochromic and microcytic anemia. Microcytosis is measured by a decrease in mean corpuscular volume and hypochromia by a reduction in mean corpuscular hemoglobin concentration.

Various tests are useful in measuring body iron stores. The most sensitive and specific method is by detection of iron on bone marrow examination. Apart from this invasive procedure, serum ferritin best reflects body iron stores and is the preferred method for determining iron depletion. Patients with chronic inflammatory and liver disease may have disproportionately elevated serum ferritin concentrations. Measurements of total serum iron, total iron-binding capacity and transferrin are additional laboratory procedures for detecting iron deficiency but are diagnostic only after total body iron stores are fully depleted.

Iron deficiency occurs in multiple stages. Initially, storage iron is depleted while serum iron concentration and hemoglobin remain normal. As iron deficiency progresses, there is a decrease in the serum concentration without anemia. With further progression to the most advanced stage, iron deficiency with anemia occurs.

Iron replacement therapy is generally administered orally as ferrous sulfate. In adults, 100 to 150 mg of elemental iron should be provided daily to treat anemia. In infants, 10 to 20 mg of elemental iron may be given prophylactically to prevent iron deficiency. Iron is best absorbed in the fasting state. It should be taken 1 hour before meals and at bedtime to maximize absorption. Adverse GI effects (nausea, heartburn, abdominal cramping, vomiting, diarrhea, and constipation, resulting from effects of unbound iron acting on the stomach and intestine) may require that it be ingested with food. These conditions can reduce iron absorption by 50%. The use of ferrous gluconate, liquid iron, or enteric forms does not always significantly reduce GI effects but should be tried. Because preparations vary in content of elemental iron, dosage adjustments must be made when changing preparations.

After initiation of iron therapy, immature RBCs (reticulocytes) should increase within 7 days. Hemoglobin and ferritin concentrations should begin to increase within the first month of therapy. Iron should be continued for 6 months after correction of anemia to ensure that total body iron stores are repleted.

Parenteral iron should be used with caution and reserved for those patients with well-documented iron deficiency anemia, unable to absorb iron because of a pathological disorder of the small intestine, or unable to tolerate oral iron.

Megaloblastic Anemias

Both folate deficiency and vitamin B_{12} deficiency cause megaloblastic anemia. This anemia, which results in abnormal nuclear maturation of immature stem cells, is also observed with drugs such as dihydrofolate reductase inhibitors, antimetabolites, inhibitors of deoxynucleotide synthesis, anticonvulsants, and oral contraceptives.

Folate deficiency may be caused by inadequate nutritional intake, malabsorption, or an increase in folate requirement. Dietary sources of folate are critical because folate storage is limited in the body. Inadequate nutritional intake, which is often associated with alcoholism, is the most common cause of this deficiency. Alcohol may also affect the enterohepatic cycling of the vitamin, leading to a decrease in absorption. Increased requirements for folate occur during pregnancy and in patients with acute or chronic hemolysis. Patients with sickle cell anemia and thalassemia have rapid RBC turnover and require folate supplementation to their normal diet. Occasionally, folate deficiency may occur from malabsorption associated with diseases of the small intestine, including nontropical and tropical sprue. Deficiency also may occur concurrent with vitamin B_{12} deficiency.

Many clinical features that occur in folate deficiency are also found with vitamin B_{12} deficiency. These include the nonspecific signs and symptoms of anemia. In addition, patients with folate deficiency may have diarrhea, anorexia, and sore tongue and may exhibit irritability and forgetfulness. Physical findings associated with severe deficiency include jaundice from ineffective hematopoiesis, petechiae from thrombocytopenia, glossitis, fever, splenomegaly, weight loss, and impaired mentation.

The most common laboratory manifestation of folate deficiency is megaloblastic anemia. The peripheral blood smear shows macrocytic RBCs and hypersegmented polymorphonuclear neutrophils (PMNs). The blood cell count will reveal an increased mean corpuscular volume. Additionally, thrombocytopenia and neutropenia may be present. If a bone marrow examination is performed, a hypercellular marrow is seen with abnormal nuclear maturation occurring in all cell lines. Low serum folate concentration is an early indicator of folate deficiency; however, serum folate concentrations reflect recent folate intake and may be low because of recent inadequate intake. Similarly, the concentration may appear normal when recent intake has improved, but tissue folate concentrations remain depressed. A better indicator of tissue folate status is the RBC folate concentration, which remains constant during the lifespan of the RBC and reflects folate turnover during the preceding 2 to 3 months. Decreased RBC folate concentrations may also be observed in vitamin B_{12} deficiency. Other findings that may be abnormal include elevated serum lactic dehydrogenase, serum bilirubin, and urine formiminoglutamate concentrations.

Before folate deficiency can be treated, it is important to exclude vitamin B_{12} deficiency, since folate therapy will correct the hematological abnormalities associated with vitamin B_{12} deficiency without correcting the vitamin B_{12}–related neurological abnormalities. Folate may be given orally or IV. For mild cases of folate deficiency or prophylaxis, the oral route is preferred. In more severe cases, as in problems of malabsorption, intravenous folate should be given. The folate preparation is given until the deficiency is corrected and blood counts are normal. A rapid increase in reticulocytes normally occurs during the first week. The hematocrit should return to normal in 1 to 2 months.

Vitamin B_{12} Deficiency

Vitamin B_{12} (cobalamin) deficiency most commonly results from intestinal malabsorption. This is unlike folate deficiency, which results from poor nutritional intake and rarely from intestinal problems. Other causes of vitamin B_{12} deficiency include gastrectomy, which removes the source of intrinsic factor, and Zollinger-Ellison syndrome, a gastrin-producing tumor that increases gastric and duodenal acid and prevents transfer of cobalamin to intrinsic factor. Intestinal disorders such as extensive resection of the ileum, regional ileitis, and sprue lead to malabsorption of intrinsic factor–vitamin B_{12} complex. Other causes include malabsorption because of pancreatic disease; fish tapeworm infestation in which the worm competes with the host for ingested cobalamin; and blind loop syndrome resulting from intestinal stasis, which leads to bacterial overgrowth and bacterial utilization of cobalamin before it can be absorbed in the intestine.

Many clinical features of vitamin B_{12} deficiency are similar to those found with folate, including nonspecific symptoms such as constipation, anorexia, and fainting. Unlike folate deficiency, vitamin B_{12} deficiency results in neurological disease. Signs and symptoms include paresthesias in distal extremities, disturbances in vibratory and position sense, and memory loss. If vitamin B_{12} deficiency progresses, a spastic ataxia, called *subacute combined system disease,* may occur. This disorder is caused by degenerative changes in dorsolateral columns of the spinal cord, manifested by nerve fiber demyelination.

The findings in the peripheral smear and bone marrow examination in vitamin B_{12} deficiency are indistinguishable from those in folate deficiency. Serum B_{12} concentrations are usually low but may be normal in 10% to 20% of deficient patients. The presence of increases in urinary methylmalonic acid is the most reliable evidence for vitamin B_{12} deficiency. Schilling's test (a radiolabeled cobalt isotope test) can be performed to determine the cause of vitamin B_{12} deficiency.

In mild cases of megaloblastic anemia the underlying vitamin B_{12} deficiency should be demonstrated before instituting therapy. Since the cause of deficiency is usually malabsorption, the preferred route of administration of vitamin B_{12} is IM. In the majority of cases, maintenance therapy with monthly injections of vitamin B_{12} must be given for life.

Shortly after therapy is begun, the changes in bone marrow revert to normal morphology. Reticulocytosis begins within the first week of instituting therapy and peaks around day 7. Hypersegmented PMNs will also disappear from the circulation in the first week of therapy.

Erythropoietin

Erythropoietin is the most important growth factor responsible for the proliferation and further differentiation of the early erythroid colony forming units, and it is also instrumental in the release of reticulocytes from the bone marrow. Recently, the human erythropoietin gene has been cloned. Because of recombinant techniques, large amounts of human erythropoietin have been made available for therapeutic use. Clinical trials with recombinant human erythropoietin in patients with end-stage renal disease anemia have shown an excellent response. Over 2000 patients have been treated since the clinical trials began in 1985, and all have shown increases in their hematocrits to a target range of 33% to 38%. Some patients have been treated for 3 years without any decrease in response or generation of an antibody to erythropoietin. Recombinant human erythropoietin has been recommended for patients with end-stage renal disease and a hematocrit less than 30%. The recommended starting dose is 150 U/kg IV given 3 times a week until the hematocrit reaches 30% without blood transfusions. The dose may then be reduced and adjusted to maintain the hematocrit in the target range. Increasing the hematocrit too rapidly in these patients, who have adjusted their blood volume to the chronic anemia, may result in hypertension. Patients with end-stage renal disease are especially vulnerable because they cannot regulate blood volume. Decreasing the dose may eliminate this side effect.

Other uses for recombinant human erythropoietin have been studied. It has been approved for anemia in patients with HIV infection and associated bone marrow depression production by azidothymidine. Although not presently licensed, it has been recommended for anemias associated with rheumatoid arthritis, after chemotherapy or radiation therapy, and for patient's undergoing preoperative autologous blood collection.

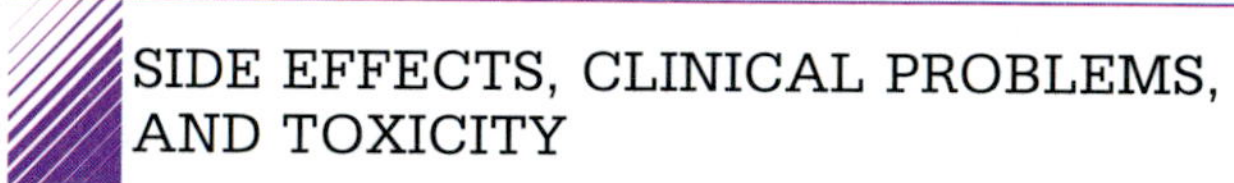

SIDE EFFECTS, CLINICAL PROBLEMS, AND TOXICITY

Iron and Iron Salts

Iron overdose most often occurs in children ingesting iron-containing products. There are four distinct phases that classically occur after the ingestion of greater than 20 mg per kg of elemental iron. Initially, vomiting and hemorrhagic gastritis are seen. Hypotension and lethargy develop early in severe intoxication. There follows a quiescent period of up to 12 hours, during which deceptive improvement occurs. Life-threatening signs, including coma, seizures, cardiovascular collapse, pulmonary edema, hypoglycemia, and metabolic acidosis, predominate 12 to 24 hours after ingestion. Gastric scarring and pyloric stenosis appear in the late phase, at 1 month. The ingestation of 200 to 300 mg per kg is lethal.

Patients with serum iron concentrations greater than the total iron binding capacity are at highest risk for serious toxicity. Treatment includes gastric lavage with sodium bicarbonate to treat the acidosis and chelation therapy parenterally with deferoxamine. Intravenous iron administration has been associated with life-threatening anaphylaxis and hypersensitivity reactions, which may occur in up to 10% of patients and should be used only under unusual circumstances.

CLINICAL PROBLEMS

IRON AND IRON SALTS

GI irritation, vomiting; overdose in children can be life threatening; parenteral administration hazardous

VITAMIN B_{12}

Transient hypokalemia

ERYTHROPOIETIN

Hypertension; clotting; very expensive

Vitamin B_{12}

Adverse effects of vitamin B_{12} therapy are rare. Transient hypokalemia from a massive increase in its use for cell production may occur when correcting severe deficiencies.

Folic Acid

Folate therapy should be restricted to replacement and prophylaxis of deficient states. Adverse effects of folate are uncommon. A rare reaction to parenteral preparation has been noted. In large doses, folate has been reported to interfere with anticonvulsant therapy.

Erythropoietin

Patients with end-stage renal disease receiving recombinant human erythropoietin should be monitored closely. Weekly hematocrits should be obtained until the target hematocrit is reached. Because iron deficiency is a common cause of anemia in patients with end stage renal disease and is a common adverse effect of therapy with recombinant human erythropoietin, serum iron, total iron binding capacity, and serum ferritin concentrations should be measured monthly for assessment of iron stores, and iron therapy should be instituted as needed. Approximately 50% of patients treated with recombinant human erythropoietin will require supplemental iron therapy. Blood pressures and serum chemistries should be monitored monthly. If blood pressure cannot be controlled by medication or dialysis ultrafiltration, the recombinant human erythropoietin may need to be discontinued until the blood pressure is within reasonable limits. In a European clinical trial, an increase in blood clotting in hollow-fiber dialyzers was also noted in some patients treated with recombinant human erythropoietin. This may be secondary to an increased blood viscosity occurring with an increase in red blood cell mass or because of an increase in platelet count occurring with therapy. Minor adjustments in the heparin dose used during dialysis easily correct the problem.

TRADE NAMES

In addition to generic and fixed-combination preparations, the following trade-named materials are available in the United States.

ERYTHROPOIETIN

Epogen, Eprex; rHuEpo, epoetin alfa

ORAL IRON AND IRON SALTS

Feosol, ferrous sulfate
Fergon, ferrous gluconate

PARENTERAL IRON

Imferon, iron dextran injection

VITAMIN B_{12}

Many oral preparations, combined with other vitamins
Redisol, cyanocobalamin injection

FOLIC ACID

Folvite, oral or parenteral use

IRON ANTIDOTE

Desferal, deferoxamine

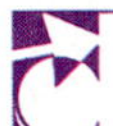

NEW DIRECTIONS

A new use for folate has been recently reported in the treatment of neural tube defects. Spina bifida and anencephaly are common serious birth defects. Annually, in the United States, about 2500 infants are born with these defects. An unknown number of fetuses with such defects are aborted. A recent British Medical Research Council multicenter randomized control study has indicated that high folic acid supplements used by women who had a prior pregnancy affected by a neural tube defect reduced the risk of a subsequent similar problem by 70%. Other intervention studies with folate have also shown a lower risk for neural tube defects. The U.S. Public Health Service has therefore recommended that all women of childbearing age who are capable of becoming pregnant should consume 0.4 mg of folic acid per day for the purpose of lowering their risk of having a pregnancy affected with spina bifida or other neural tube defects. The mechanism by which protection is afforded is presently unknown.

REFERENCES

Babior BW: The megaloblastic anemias. In Williams WJ, Beutler E, Erslev AJ, et al: *Hematology,* ed 4, New York, 1990, McGraw-Hill.

Erickson N, Quesenberry PJ: Regulation of erythropoiesis, *Anemia* 76:745-755, 1992.

Finch CA and Heubers H: Perspectives in iron metabolism, *N Eng J Med* 30b:1520, 1982.

Fisher JW, Bommer J, Eschbach J, et al: Statement on the clinical use of recombinant erythropoietin in anemia of end-stage renal disease, *Am J Kidney Dis* 14:163, 1989.

Fisher JW: Erythropoietin. In *Textbook of nephrology,* ed 3, Massry SG, Glassock RJ, editors: Baltimore, 1994, Williams & Wilkins.

Jelkmann W: Erythropoietin: structure, control of production and function, *Physiol Rev* 72:449-489, 1992.

SELF-ASSESSMENT QUESTIONS

1. The most common cause of failing to respond to oral iron therapy is:
   a. failure of bone marrow to produce adequate reticulocytes.
   b. failure to take an adequate dose.
   c. excessive amount of transferrin.
   d. small intestinal malabsorption.
2. Erythropoietin is required for:
   a. heme synthesis.
   b. proliferation of CFU-E.
   c. globin synthesis.
   d. iron absorption.
3. Which of the following agents that are used for the treatment of anemia may cause life-threatening toxicity:
   a. folate
   b. vitamin B_{12}
   c. ferrous sulfate
   d. iodine
4. Increase folate requirements occur in all of the following *except:*
   a. pregnancy.
   b. sickle cell anemia.
   c. chronic alcoholism.
   d. anemia of chronic disease.
5. Vitamin B_{12} deficiency can be caused by all of the following *except:*
   a. Zollinger-Ellison syndrome.
   b. fish tapeworm.
   c. blind loop syndrome.
   d. liver disease.
6. The major side effect from oral iron therapy is:
   a. hypokalemia.
   b. hypertension.
   c. GI irritation.
   d. headaches.
7. Before beginning folate therapy for megaloblastic anemia, one should consider which of the following to prevent neurologic disease?
   a. vitamin B_{12} deficiency
   b. zinc deficiency
   c. iron deficiency
   d. vitamin B_6 deficiency
8. All of the following are factors that may increase erythropoietin production *except:*
   a. thyroxin.
   b. estrogen.
   c. oxygen free radicals.
   d. β-$_2$ adrenergic receptor agonist.

CHAPTER 66

Regulated Drug Development and Usage

GARY E. STEIN

OVERVIEW

Discovery, development, and clinical introduction of new drugs is a process involving close cooperation between researchers, medical practitioners, the pharmaceutical industry, and the U.S. government Food and Drug Administration (FDA). The drug development process begins with the synthesis or isolation of a new compound with biological activity and potential therapeutic use. This entity must then pass through preclinical, clinical, and regulatory review stages before becoming available as a therapeutically safe and effective drug. About 20 to 30 new chemical compounds and numerous new formulations are approved for use each year in the United States.

The FDA authority over drug review and approval began with the Federal Pure Food and Drug Act of 1906. This first drug law established standards for drug strength and purity. This legislation was followed by the Federal Food, Drug and Cosmetic Act of 1938, which prohibited marketing of new drugs unless adequately tested to demonstrate safety under conditions indicated on their labels. The 1938 act was amended by Congress in 1962 to state that pharmaceutical manufacturers must provide scientific proof that new products are efficacious and safe before marketing. The amendment also required that the FDA be notified before testing of drugs in humans. More recent legislation includes controls on the manufacture and prescribing of habit-forming drugs (Comprehensive Drug Abuse Prevention and Control Act, 1970), drug development for treating rare diseases (Orphan Drug Act, 1983), and new drug applications for generic drug products (Drug Price Competition and Patent Restoration Act, 1984).

In 1990, regulations relevant to drug use aimed at reducing health care costs from unnecessary, inappropriate and unmonitored prescription drug use were passed. The act required all states receiving Medicaid dollars to submit a plan to carry out prospective and retrospective drug utilization reviews and to counsel Medicaid patients on drug use to the Health Care Finance Administration for approval. (Federal Omnibus Budget Reconciliation Act of 1990, activated in 1993).

ABBREVIATIONS	
ANDA	Abbreviated New Drug Application
FDA	Food and Drug Administration
IND	Investigational New Drug Application
IRB	Institutional Review Board
NDA	New Drug Application
PDR	*Physician's Desk Reference*
PMS	Postmarketing Surveillance

CLINICAL TESTING AND INTRODUCTION OF NEW DRUGS

Potential new drugs or biological products must first be tested in animals for their acute and chronic toxicity, influence on reproductive performance, carcinogenic and mutagenic potential, and safe dosing range. Preclinical testing often requires 2 to 5 years at a cost of millions of dollars. Chronic safety testing in animals continues during subsequent trials in humans.

After successful preclinical pharmacological and toxicological studies, the sponsor files an Investigational New Drug (IND) Application with the FDA. In addition to animal data, the IND contains protocols for clinical testing in humans. Approximately 2000 INDs are received each year by the FDA. If the IND passes FDA review, clinical trials in humans are initiated. These studies are generally conducted in three phases:

Phase 1: Conducted on a small number of normal vol unteers to determine safe dosage range and pharmacokinetic parameters

Phase 2: Conducted on several hundred patients to determine short-term safety and effectiveness of the drug in patients with specific diseases

Phase 3: Conducted on several thousand patients with specific diseases to determine overall risk-benefit relationships in specific populations of patients

These studies provide the basis for drug labeling. The completion of these clinical studies may take 3 to 10 years and often costs up to 100 million dollars.

Before initiating study of an investigational drug in humans, an investigator must also obtain approval from the local Institutional Review Board (IRB) of the hospital, university, or other institution where the planned study will be conducted. The IRB is responsible for ensuring the ethical acceptability of the proposed research and approves, requires modification, or disapproves the research protocol. To approve a clinical research study, the IRB must determine that the research design and procedures are sound and that the risk to subjects is minimized. In addition, the IRB must also approve the informed consent document that must be signed by each prospective subject or the subject's legally authorized representative. IRB approval is usually valid for 1 year (Figure 66-1).

The basic elements of informed consent include the following:

1. Explanation of the purposes and procedures of the research
2. Description of foreseeable risks
3. Description of expected benefits
4. Statement of available alternative procedures or courses of treatment
5. Statement on confidentiality of records
6. Explanation of compensation or available medical treatments if injury occurs
7. Description of whom to contact about the research and the subject's rights and the procedure to follow in the event of injury to the subject
8. Statement that participation is voluntary and refusal to participate does not involve penalty to the subject

If suitable preclinical and clinical findings demonstrate efficacy with minimal toxicity, the sponsors can submit a New Drug Application (NDA) to the FDA (see Figure 66-1). In approving an NDA, the FDA ensures the drug's safety and effectiveness for each use. Usually the sponsor and the FDA review the data and negotiate on the detailed information to accompany the drug for its use. This includes contraindications, precautions, side effects, dosages, routes of administration, and frequency of administration. The NDA approval process usually takes 2 to 3 years, with drugs having the greatest potential benefit given priority. Drug applications are now identified and placed into specific categories under a new FDA classification system (Table 66-1). Post-approval research may be requested by the FDA as a condition of new drug approval. Such research may be used to speed drug approval, uncover unexpected adverse drug reactions, and define the incidence of known drug reactions under actual clinical use.

After NDA approval, the manufacturer promotes the new drug for approved uses described on the label. Post–NDA approval or marketing period (phase 4) requires monitoring of new drug safety during clinical use. The label information does not include all conditions in which a released drug is safe and effective. It should be noted that the FDA does not restrict use of approved drugs to those conditions described on the label; the physician is allowed to determine its most appropriate use. From both the ethical and liability points of view, there should be compelling scientific evidence before a drug is used for an unapproved indication. Examples are β-blockers, which often are used interchangeably for various indications, though not all have identical FDA-approved indications (Table 66-2).

Early clinical testing of new drugs does not provide absolute assurance of safety, as evidenced by later discoveries of adverse effects after drugs are used clinically. In some instances, released drugs are withdrawn from the market after toxic or fatal adverse effects are discovered during large-scale clinical use. There are instances in which lack of efficacy of a new drug is not discovered until the drug is in large-scale clinical use with selected patient populations. The goal of postmarketing surveillance (PMS) is also important to define the true side-effect profile of a new drug.

New safety information obtained during large-scale clinical testing is used to update the current NDA and provide changes in the drug label. Side-effect profiles in patients with multiple diseases are often incomplete during early studies, and such information is vitally important for improving subsequent use. Reporting of rare and unexpected side effects not listed on the drug label is an important responsibility for prescribers; information is supplied to the FDA on the Drug Experi-

Table 66-1 FDA Drug Classification System

Designation	Meaning
AA	Drugs for AIDS or complications related to AIDS
P	Priority
S	Standard
O	Orphan

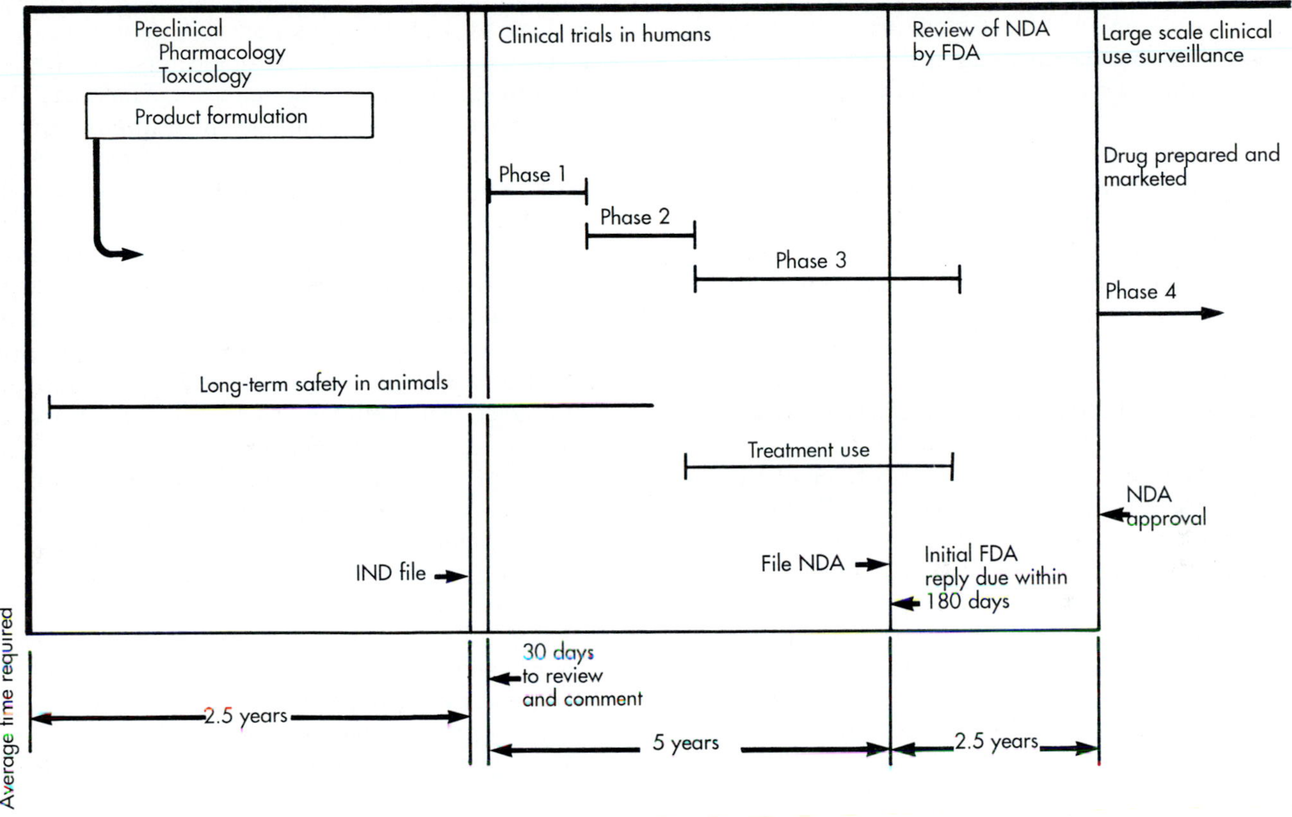

FIGURE 66-1 Stages of new drug development.

Table 66-2 Varied Uses of Several β-Adrenergic Receptor Blocking Agents

	acebutolol	atenolol	labetolol	metoprolol	nadolol	propranolol
LABEL INDICATIONS						
Hypertension	X	X	X	X	X	X
Angina	—	X	—	X	X	X
Dysrhythmia	X	—	—	—	—	X
Postmyocardial infarction	—	X	—	X	—	X
Pheochromocytoma	—	—	—	—	—	X
Hypertrophic subaortic stenosis	—	—	—	—	—	X
Essential tremor	—	—	—	—	—	X
Migraine prophylaxis	—	—	—	—	—	X

ence Form (FDA form 1639). Med Watch is a recent FDA-inetiated voluntary reporting program to encourage and facilitate monitoring by pharmacists and other health professionals of adverse events and problems with medications, medical devices and other products regulated by the Food and Drug Administration. Any adverse events or suspect problems may be reported on FDA form 3500.

Several sources of information are available to physicians concerning the safety of new drugs. These include the *Medical Letter on Drugs and Therapeutics, Facts and Comparisons, AMA Drug Evaluation,* and the *Physician's Desk Reference (PDR),* a compilation of FDA-approved drug package inserts.

ORPHAN DRUGS AND TREATMENT IND

New drugs that may benefit only a small number of patients with rare diseases, defined in the United States as fewer than 200,000 individuals, provide little economic incentive to pharmaceutical manufacturers for development and filing of an IND or NDA. The Orphan Drug Act of 1983 provides special incentives such as tax advantages and marketing exclusiveness to compensate companies for developmental costs of such agents. The National Institutes of Health also participates in development of orphan drugs, and more than 300 drugs have been given orphan status. These include human growth hormone, erythropoietin, and α_1-antitrypsin.

The FDA established guidelines to make promising investigational drugs available for treatment of patients with immediate life-threatening diseases, such as AIDS. These drugs receive highest priority at all stages of the drug-review process. The Treatment IND application enables patients not qualified for participation in ongoing studies to be treated with investigational drugs outside controlled clinical trials. The FDA generally considers Treatment INDs for drugs in later stages of clinical testing. The initial criteria include the following:

1. The drug is intended to treat a serious life-threatening disease
2. There is no comparable or satisfactory alternative to treat the disease
3. The drug is under investigation in a controlled clinical trial under an IND
4. The sponsor is actively pursuing marketing approval of the investigational drug

When no Treatment IND is in effect for an investigational drug, a physician may obtain the drug for "compassionate use." In such cases, the physician submits a Treatment IND to the FDA requesting authorization of an investigational drug for such use.

PRESCRIPTION WRITING

Prescriptions are written by the prescriber to instruct the pharmacist to dispense a specific medication for a specific patient. These include precompounded medications (prepared by the pharmaceutical manufacturer) and extemporaneously prepared medications. It is vitally important that a prescription communicate clearly to the pharmacist the exact medication needed and how this medication is to be used by the patient. Patient compliance is often related to the clarity of the directions on the prescription, and terms such as "take as directed" should be avoided. Equally important is the necessity for clarity when using proprietary drug names because of their similarities. In these instances the physician should designate the generic name, as well as the brand name, to avoid confusion.

Prescriptions contain the following elements to facilitate interpretation by the pharmacist:

1. Physician's name, address, and telephone number
2. Date
3. Patient's name and address
4. Superscription (Rx how drug is to be taken)
5. Inscription (name and dosage of drug)
6. Subscription (directions to the pharmacist)
7. Signature or transcription (directions to the patient)
8. Refill and safety cap information
9. Prescriber's (physician's) signature
10. DEA number of physician (for controlled substances)

A typical prescription blank is shown in Figure 66-2. Because both apothecary and metric systems are in use, it is important that prescribers become familiar with conversion units. Commonly used weights and measures are listed below:

2.2 pounds (lb) = 1 kilogram (kg)
1 grain (gr) = 65 milligrams (mg)
1 fluid ounce (oz) = 30 milliliters (ml)
1 tablespoonful (tbsp) = 15 ml
1 teaspoonful (tsp) = 5 ml
20 drops (gtt) = 1 ml

Patient instructions ("signature") on a prescription are sometimes written with Latin abbreviations as shorthand for prescribers giving concise directions to the pharmacist on how and when a patient takes the medication. Although instructions written in English are preferred, some common Latin abbreviations are as follows:

po: by mouth
ac: before meals
pc: after meals

Prescriber's Name, Address, and Telephone Number
Date ____________ Patient ________________
Address ________________________________

Rx
Drug name and strength
Quantity to be dispensed
Patient Instructions

Refill____ times Dr. Signature____________
No safety cap ☐ DEA No. ______________

FIGURE 66-2 Typical prescription form.

qd: every day
bid: twice daily
tid: three times a day
qid: four times a day
hs: at bedtime
prn: as needed
c̄: with
s̄: without
ss: one-half

Additional instructions may be added to the prescription to instruct the pharmacist to place an additional label on the prescription container (e.g., Take With Food). When a prescriber intends to use a drug for an unauthorized indication or when two drugs have been prescribed that may cause a clinically significant drug interaction, the prescriber should communicate to the patient and pharmacist that this is indeed the intended therapy.

In the United States a large number of drugs require a prescription from a licensed practitioner (e.g., physician, dentist, veterinarian, podiatrist) before being dispensed by a pharmacist. In addition, use of specific drugs, called **schedule drugs,** with high abuse potential are further restricted by the FDA, and special requirements are met when these drugs are prescribed. These controlled drugs (Table 66-3) are classified according to potential for abuse and include opioids, stimulants, and depressants. Schedule I drugs have no currently accepted medical use in the United States and may not be prescribed. Schedule II drugs have a high potential for abuse and cannot be refilled. In addition, Schedule II drugs may not be prescribed by telephone, and several states (e.g., Texas, Michigan, New York) require a special triplicate prescription blank. Other schedule drugs (III and V) can be refilled, but there is a 5-refill maximum and the prescription is invalid 6 months from date of issue. An exception to these regulations involves drugs in schedule V, which may be dispensed without a prescription if the patient is 18 years old, distribution is by a pharmacist, and only a limited quantity of a drug is purchased (refer to the Controlled Substance Act of 1970).

Table 66-3 Controlled Substances

Schedule	Symbol	Abuse Potential	Example
I	C-I	No accepted medical use in the United States	heroin
II	C-II	High abuse potential	morphine
III	C-III	Moderate potential for dependence	glutethimide
IV	C-IV	Low potential for dependence	diazepam
V	C-V	Lowest abuse potential	diphenoxylate

Many prescribed proprietary (brand name) drugs are available from multiple pharmaceutical manufacturers under a brand name, or trade name, or as less costly nonproprietary (generic name) preparations. Pharmacists receiving prescriptions for brand-name products may dispense an equivalent generic drug (except as noted below), without prescriber approval and pass on savings to the patient. Some states have mandatory substitution laws, and the brand-name product is dispensed only when "Dispense as Written" (D.A.W.) is stated on the prescription. Although generic products are considered to be pharmaceutically equivalent to brand-name counterparts, some may not be therapeutically equivalent.

Generic products tested by the FDA and determined to be therapeutic equivalents are listed by the FDA in *Approved Drug Products with Therapeutic Equivalence Evaluations* (Orange Book). These products contain the same active ingredients as their brand-name counterparts and also meet bioequivalence standards (see Chapter 4). The FDA recommends substitution only among products listed as therapeutically equivalent. Not all generic drugs listed in the Orange Book are therapeutic equivalents of the brand-name products. Brand-name products such as Lanoxin (digoxin), Dilantin (phenytoin), Premarin (conjugated estrogens), and Theo-Dur (slow-release theophylline) contain either unique chemicals (Premarin) or exhibit different bioavailability characteristics compared to generic products. Therefore these should not be substituted without physician approval.

NEW DIRECTIONS

Recently, four initiatives for streamlining the drug approval process have been suggested by the FDA. These changes include the use of outside expert reviewers to reduce the backlog of new applications awaiting approval, elimination of duplicate animal testing, institution of a parallel-track policy to increase patient access to treatment for those who cannot participate in controlled studies, and introduction of the use of surrogate markers (e.g., CD4* cell count for new drugs to treat HIV infection) for evaluation of efficacy of new drugs.

The FDA has also instituted a program called Med Watch to encourage and facilitate the reporting of serious adverse events and product problems.

REFERENCES

Bosso JA: The role of the institutional review board in research involving human subjects, *Drug Intell Clin Pharm* 17:828, 1983.

Cohen MR, Davis NM: Complete prescription orders reduce medication errors, *Am Pharm* 32:24, 1992.

Edlavitch SA: Postmarketing surveillance methodologies, *Drug Intell Clin Pharm* 22:68, 1988.

Kessler DA: The regulation of investigational drugs, *N Engl J Med* 320:281, 1989.

Myers AM, Moore SR: The drug approval process and the information it provides, *Drug Intell Clin Pharm* 21:821, 1987.

Steinbrook RS, Lo B: Informing physicians about promising new treatments for severe illnesses, *JAMA* 263:2078, 1990.

Strom BL: Generic drug substitution revisited, *N Engl J Med* 316:1456, 1987.

Strom BL, Melmon KL, Miettinen OS: Post-marketing studies of drug efficacy: Why? *Am J Med* 78:475, 1985.

Young FE, Norris JA, Levitt JA, et al: The FDA's new procedures for the use of investigational drugs in treatment, *JAMA* 259:2267, 1988.

SELF-ASSESSMENT QUESTIONS

1. A proprietary (brand name) drug cannot be prescribed if:
   a. the FDA has not approved it for the use that you are prescribing it.
   b. a generic form of the drug is available.
   c. the drug has a very high abuse potential.
   d. none of the above restricts prescribing a brand-name drug.
2. Phase I studies are important to:
   a. describe the adverse and toxic effects of a new drug in people.
   b. determine the efficacy of a new drug in a specific disease.
   c. determine a safe dosage range of a new drug in man.
   d. indicate the effectiveness of a new drug in animal models of disease.
3. Which of the following controlled drug schedules contain drugs that have no accepted medical use in the U.S.A.?
   a. Schedule I
   b. Schedule II
   c. Schedule III
   d. Schedule IV
   e. Schedule V
4. The Latin abbreviation, q.i.d., on a prescription, means that the drug is to be taken:
   a. twice a day.
   b. four times a day.
   c. whenever needed.
   d. every day.
   e. every other day.
5. How many milligrams (mg) are contained in 5 grains of aspirin?
   a. 30 mg
   b. 80 mg
   c. 130 mg
   d. 325 mg
   e. 500 mg

*CD is cluster of differentiation; with over 100 now known.

Answers to Self-Assessment Questions

Chapter 1

1. c
2. e
3. d
4. e

Chapter 2

1. e
2. b
3. e
4. a
5. e
6. b

Chapter 3

1. e
2. a
3. d
4. b

Chapter 4

1. d
2. d
3. e
4. c
5. c
6. d

Chapter 5

1. d
2. b
3. a
4. c
5. e
6. d
7. e

Chapter 6

1. d
2. e
3. e
4. e

Chapter 7

1. e
2. c
3. a
4. d
5. c
6. b
7. e

Chapter 8

1. c
2. a
3. e
4. d
5. e
6. c

Chapter 9

1. b
2. e
3. a
4. b
5. d
6. b

Chapter 10

1. b
2. c
3. e
4. b
5. d
6. c
7. a
8. a
9. c
10. d
11. b
12. c

Chapter 11

1. d
2. e
3. a
4. a
5. e

Chapter 12

1. d
2. b
3. e
4. a
5. d

Chapter 13

1. a
2. b
3. e
4. c
5. d

Chapter 14

1. b
2. b
3. c
4. c
5. c
6. e
7. e
8. c

Chapter 15

1. b
2. a
3. b
4. e
5. a

Chapter 16

1. d
2. e

3. e
4. a
5. b
6. c
7. a
8. e

Chapter 17

1. d
2. e
3. d
4. a
5. c

Chapter 18

1. b
2. d
3. b
4. c
5. d
6. b

Chapter 19

1. a
2. d
3. e
4. a

Chapter 20

1. d
2. b
3. c
4. d

Chapter 21

1. c
2. d
3. d
4. b
5. b
6. a
7. e

Chapter 22

1. e
2. d
3. c
4. a
5. e
6. a
7. a

Chapter 23

1. b
2. c
3. e

Chapter 24

1. a
2. b
3. e
4. a

Chapter 25

1. d
2. c
3. a
4. b
5. e
6. e
7. c
8. d
9. d
10. a

Chapter 26

1. b
2. e
3. c
4. a
5. b
6. a
7. d
8. c

Chapter 27

1. c
2. d
3. a
4. c
5. d

Chapter 28

1. d
2. c
3. a
4. a
5. d
6. b
7. d
8. a
9. b
10. d
11. b
12. a
13. b

Chapter 29

1. d
2. b
3. e
4. e
5. b
6. d
7. d

Chapter 30

1. b
2. e
3. c
4. d
5. e
6. a
7. b
8. e
9. e
10. e
11. e

Chapter 31

1. e
2. a
3. b
4. d
5. d
6. e

Chapter 32

1. c
2. b
3. b
4. a
5. e
6. c
7. e
8. b
9. b
10. a
11. d
12. a
13. c
14. b
15. d

Chapter 33

1. c
2. d
3. a
4. c
5. d

Chapter 34

1. e
2. e
3. e
4. a
5. e
6. b
7. b

Chapter 35

1. c
2. e
3. b
4. c
5. c

Chapter 36

1. c
2. c
3. a

4. c
5. d

Chapter 37

1. c
2. a
3. d
4. c
5. b
6. e
7. b
8. d
9. a

Chapter 38

1. b
2. c
3. b
4. e
5. c

Chapter 39

1. e
2. c
3. d
4. a
5. c
6. b

Chapter 40

1. c
2. d
3. d
4. c
5. a
6. b

Chapter 41

1. c
2. b
3. c
4. e
5. b

Chapter 42

1. e
2. a
3. b
4. b
5. b

Chapter 43

1. a
2. d
3. b
4. d
5. b
6. c

Chapter 44

1. b
2. c
3. d
4. c
5. e

Chapter 45

1. e
2. d
3. b
4. b

Chapter 46

1. c
2. b
3. b
4. d
5. a

Chapter 47

1. b
2. c
3. d
4. e
5. d
6. b
7. c
8. c
9. d
10. b
11. c
12. d

Chapter 48

1. b
2. d
3. a
4. a
5. d
6. b
7. c
8. c
9. b
10. c
11. d
12. a

Chapter 49

1. a
2. b
3. c
4. e
5. b

Chapter 50

1. c
2. d
3. a
4. b
5. c
6. d

Chapter 51

1. c
2. b
3. a
4. d
5. d
6. b
7. c

Chapter 52

1. b
2. a
3. a
4. c
5. d
6. a
7. b
8. b
9. c

Chapter 53

1. d
2. c
3. b
4. e
5. d
6. c

Chapter 54

1. c
2. a
3. d
4. b
5. d
6. a

Chapter 55

1. b, c, e
2. b
3. a
4. c
5. d

Chapter 56

1. a
2. c
3. d
4. d
5. a

Chapter 57

1. e
2. e
3. a, b, c
4. a, c, d
5. a, c, d
6. c
7. e
8. e

Chapter 58

1. d
2. a
3. e
4. d
5. d

Chapter 59

1. d
2. a
3. b
4. b
5. b
6. e

Chapter 60

1. c
2. e
3. a
4. e
5. c
6. a
7. d
8. b

Chapter 61

1. c
2. e
3. e
4. e
5. e
6. a
7. b
8. c

Chapter 62

1. c
2. a
3. b
4. c

Chapter 63

1. a
2. a
3. a
4. c

Chapter 64

1. d
2. d
3. b
4. e

Chapter 65

1. b
2. b
3. c
4. d
5. d
6. c
7. a
8. b

Chapter 66

1. d
2. c
3. a
4. b
5. d

APPENDIX

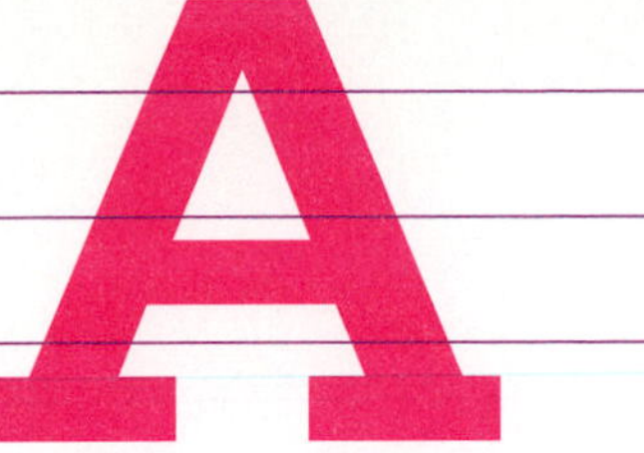

International System of Units (SI)

SI Derived Units with Special Names

Formula	Symbol	Special Name	Physical Quantity
1 kg · m/s^2	= 1 N	1 newton	force
1 N/m^2	= 1 Pa	1 pascal	pressure or stress
1 N · m	= 1 J	1 joule	work, energy, or quantity of heat
1 J/s	= 1 W	1 watt	power or radiant energy flux
1 W/A	= 1 V	1 volt	electric potential, potential difference, or electromotive force
1 A/V	= 1 S	1 siemens	electric conductance
1 V/A	= 1 Ω	1 ohm	electric resistance
1 A · s	= 1 C	1 coulomb	quantity of electricity or electric charge
1 C/V	= 1 F	1 farad	electric capacitance
1 V · s	= 1 Wb	1 weber	magnetic flux
1 Wb/A	= 1 H	1 henry	inductance
1 Wb/m^2	= 1 T	1 tesla	magnetic flux density or magnetic induction
1 cd · sr	= 1 lm	1 lumen	luminous flux
1 lm/m^2	= 1 lx	1 lux	illuminance
1 J/kg	= 1 Gy	1 gray	absorbed dose (of ionizing radiation)
1 (disintegration)/s	= 1 Bq	1 becquerel	activity (of a radionuclide)
1 (cycle)/s	= 1 Hz	1 hertz	frequency (of a periodic phenomenon)

SI Prefixes

Factor	Prefix	Symbol	Factor	Prefix	Symbol
10^{-18}	atto	a	10	deca	da
10^{-15}	femto	f	10^2	hecto	h
10^{-12}	pico	p	10^3	kilo	k
10^{-9}	nano	n	10^6	mega	M
10^{-6}	micro	μ	10^9	giga	G
10^{-3}	milli	m	10^{12}	tera	T
10^{-2}	centi	c	10^{15}	peta	P
10^{-1}	deci	d	10^{18}	exa	E

General Index

A

B

J

K

M

O

P

Q

R

T

U